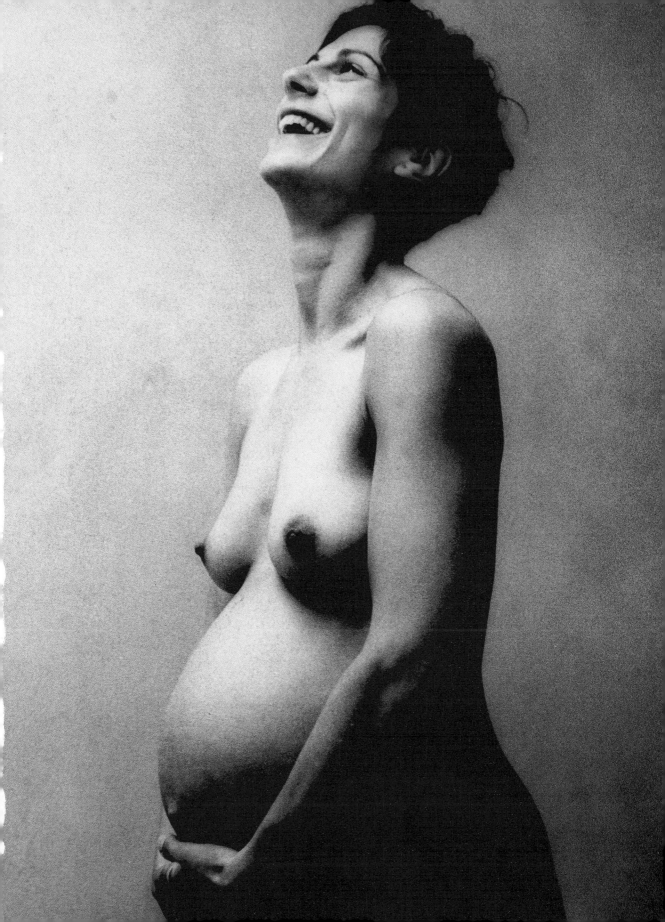

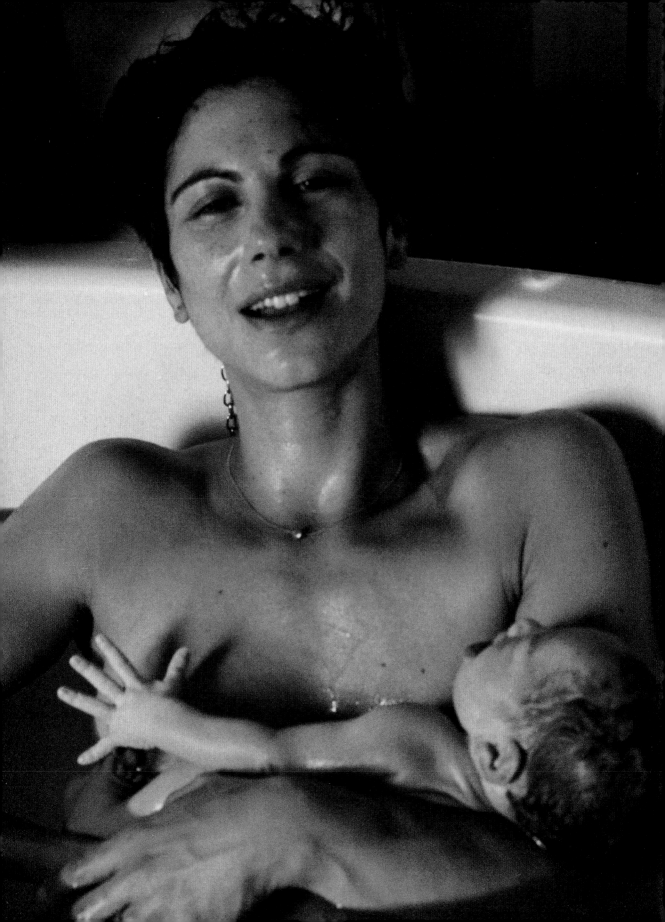

Birth

Dr Yehudi Gordon

and beyond...

Pregnancy, birth, your baby and family – the definitive guide

Vermilion
LONDON

Contents

This book is
dedicated to our
children and
grandchildren

Foreword

You're on an exciting roller coaster taking you through the changes of pregnancy and into the adventure of parenthood. This is a time of growth and revelations, trials and joys, sharing and wonder – the beginning of a new life and the birth of your new family with you and your baby at its heart. So hold tight – the adventure that begins at conception and lasts through the primal period until your baby is 9 months old may be one of the most fascinating journeys of your life.

Your pregnancy, your family

Every person experiences pregnancy, birth and parenting in a unique way. However you anticipate your life unfolding, you will probably find that you meet the unexpected in your own emotions, your partner's and family's reactions, and your child's own unique character. We hope this book will empower you and help you enjoy parenthood as you integrate changes, welcome your baby, understand medical care, listen to your emotions, watch your relationships change and cope with the practicalities of family life.

The primal period

When sperm meets egg, your baby starts the miraculous journey into life and you embark on the primal period, 18 months of growing and intense learning that end when your baby is 9 months old. During the primal period, your baby will learn more than in any other decade of her life. In the womb she hears noises and senses emotions, she dreams and experiments with movement and touch. From the moment she takes her first breath she looks to you for guidance, love, support and protection. You are her safe haven. She will learn to smile from watching the smile on your face and as she wonders at the colourful and busy world around her you are her teacher. By the end of her ninth month, she will have realised that she is a separate individual, not an extension of her mother, and will be ready for independent motion as a bold crawler.

But your baby won't do all the learning: she will communicate powerfully and be a great teacher and in the parent–baby dance you will be overwhelmed by her amazing body, her beautiful, alert eyes and her emerging personality. In the primal period, you, as parents, go through momentous change. For a mother and father this time is full of new experiences and learning opportunities, and a host of changeable and new feelings: there will be physical, emotional, spiritual and psychic ups and downs.

This book aims to be realistic and support you as you ride the rough and the smooth on the road to parenthood

so that you, your baby and your family may have the chance to build a solid foundation for the years ahead and enjoy the many rewards of family life. It is both theoretical and practical, to dip into whenever you choose. Above all, it encourages an integrated healthcare approach where the safety net of modern obstetrics and paediatrics is used in conjunction with a variety of complementary therapies, and invites you to take an active part in what is one of life's greatest transitions. This book guides you through these crucial months and gives invaluable advice on caring for yourself, your relationships and your family.

The making of this book

Birth and Beyond is the result of a powerful and wonderful collaboration of an amazing team of people who have generously given their time, energy and love. The contributors span the world of conventional medical and complementary care. Yehudi Gordon conceived, directed and nurtured the book to completion. Yehudi is an obstetrician who has practised active and water birth since 1978 and he is one of the pioneers of integrated health care for families. The major contributors are Harriet Sharkey, writer and editor, Andy Raffles, paediatrician, Genna Naccache, photographer, and homeopath Felicity Fine.

Others who have been indispensable are Mira and Tansen Elliott-Stannard, who founded the Birth and Beyond movement, and the Birth Unit midwives from St John and Elizabeth Hospital, particularly Ann Herreboudt, as well as nutritionist Marilyn Glenville, exercise consultant Shirel Stemmons, yoga and active birth teacher Jill Benjoya Miller, obstetrician and visualisations guide Dr Gowri Motha, and many other people who gave their expertise on lifestyle and Integrated health.

Our spouses – Wendy Gordon, Dee Sharkey, Jo Raffles and Barry Fine – gave their unconditional support and love. The families who were photographed and the hundreds of others on whom the book is based have our deep gratitude. It is they, above all else, who make this book what it is.

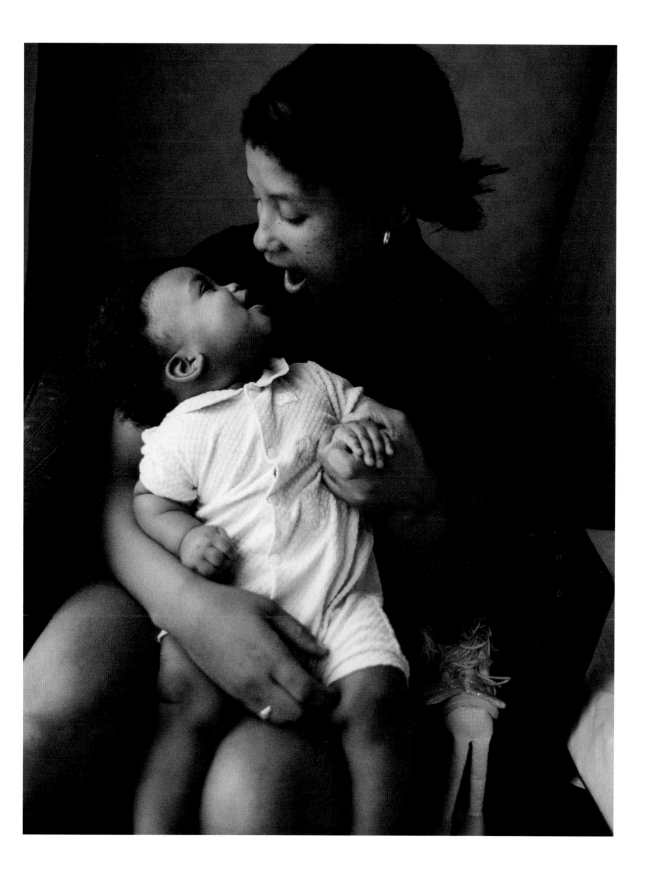

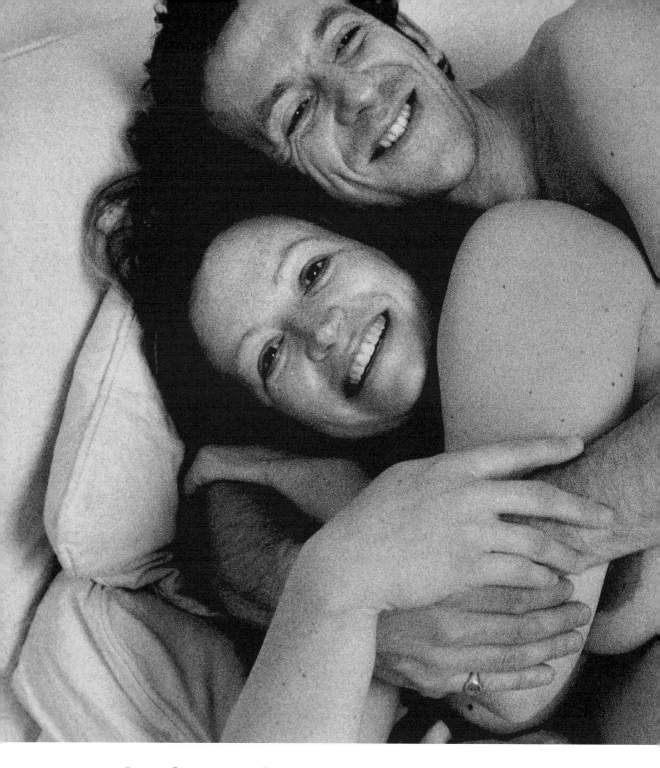

part i minus nine to plus nine

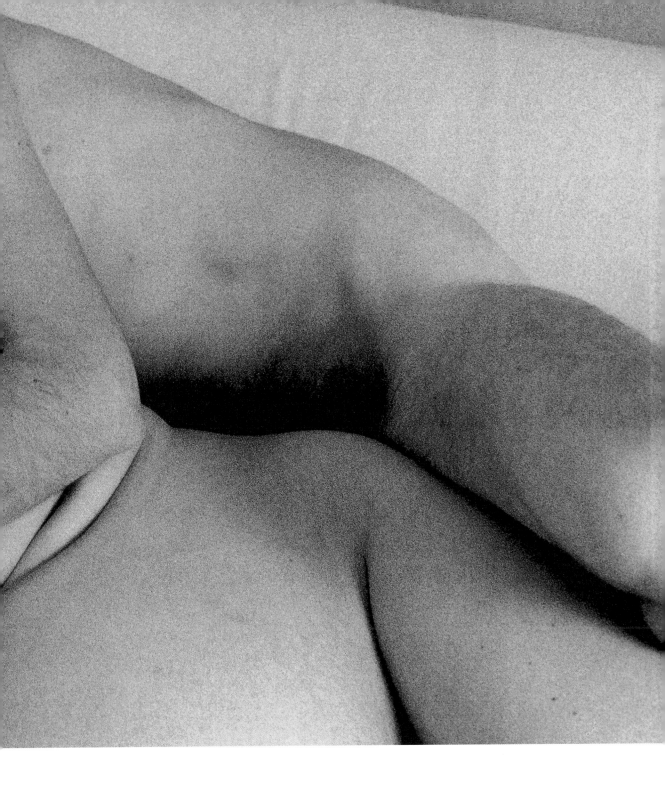

Amazing conception

When your baby's life begins, deep inside your womb, you may be doing the washing up, chairing a meeting, taking a walk or sleeping peacefully. Two cells meet and begin an amazing process of division and growth. Imprinted in these tiny cells are all the ingredients for your child that contain echoes of past generations and seeds for the future. One single moment, shorter than a breath and occurring against steep odds, heralds this new life. During every moment in your womb your baby is dependent upon you for survival. At the same time, he sends chemical messages to your body instructing it to provide the right environment and nutrition. A powerful biological and instinctual force links the two of you and this connection is also psychological and psychic.

The science of conception

Why did only one sperm out of the two hundred million ejaculated complete the journey to your waiting egg? Why was that one successful? And why did you conceive during this cycle and not the previous one? Though they can explain a lot, even scientific answers cannot hide the miracle of creation. Across the world men and women have expressed this magic with stories and songs. In some cultures babies are thought to come from the spirit world, their arrival reliant on good harvest rains, cycles of the moon or ritual. Some women believe conception only happens when the time is right, others believe the child growing in their womb has been waiting patiently to join his pre-destined parents. When sperm and egg meet, a single cell forms. For this to happen, conditions must be perfect: the egg must be in the right place, sperm must be present and your womb ready. If these factors coincide there is a high chance that, between 3 and 36 hours after sexual intercourse, one sperm will meet with one egg and the two will unite. Following this, conditions need to remain optimal if this conception is to develop into a baby.

Menses: the monthly cycle

The menstrual cycle is named after the phases of the moon. The cyclic renewal within your body allows the release of an egg and brings about the right conditions for fertilisation roughly once a month. In some women this cycle works like clockwork, but in many it is less predictable. Although the hormones produced in your ovaries and pituitary gland control the cycle, they are influenced by your physical health and mental wellbeing. Illness, poor nourishment, changes in diet, periods of stress, excitement or grief can all alter the timing of the release of an egg. That is why many women who are trying to conceive aim to create the optimum conditions with a balanced lifestyle. The average number of menstrual cycles in a woman's life is 500, each one lasting between 21 and 35 days from the first day of menstruation.

The release of an egg

You and your potential baby work together and communicate from the earliest days – the egg has a life or presence of its own even before conception and contributes to boost its own chances of survival before and after fertilisation. In the first half of the cycle – that is, in the first 14 or so days following the first day of bleeding – the pituitary gland in your brain releases a follicle stimulating hormone (FSH) and luteinising hormone (LH), which urge the ripening of eggs inside your ovary. Between 10 and 50 eggs begin to ripen in fluid-filled sacks called follicles, which begin to produce increasing amounts of oestrogen. This hormone stimulates your cervix to release a slippery mucus to aid the journey of the sperm, helps your womb prepare for pregnancy and prompts more production of LH and FSH.

About half-way through your cycle, hormone levels create optimal conditions for ovulation. One mature egg (or occasionally more than one) rises to the surface of its protective follicle and is released into the adjacent fallopian tube. The other stimulated follicles gradually disappear. Though the size of a pinhead, your egg is 100 times bigger than the sperm it is about to meet; it contains nutrients that will sustain it as it is wafted towards your uterus by tiny hairs in the cells lining the fallopian tube.

When your egg has departed, the ruptured follicle takes up fatty cholesterol from your bloodstream that turns it yellow – hence its name, corpus luteum ('yellow body'). It continues to produce oestrogen and the hormone progesterone, which brings about changes that will support the egg if it is fertilised. The endometrial lining of your uterus becomes thicker, ready for implantation; glands in the fallopian tube and uterus produce a nourishing fluid, and the cervical mucus thickens to stop further sperm entering. If conception does not occur, the corpus luteum disintegrates about 10 days after ovulation and is absorbed, hormone levels drop and the womb lining is shed as menstruation begins and a new cycle starts.

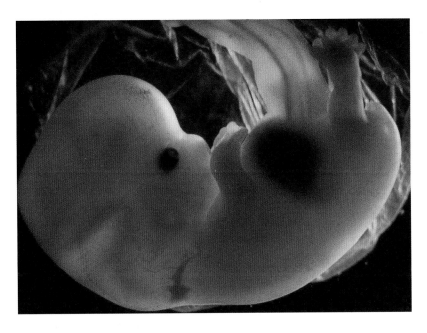

In the first trimester your baby is an embryo. In a matter of weeks he has developed limb buds and the beginnings of fingers and toes, a characteristic face and rudimentary organs – the dark patch in the abdomen is the liver.

An average menstrual cycle is 28 days, where day 1 is the first day of menstruation. During the cycle the hormone levels alter to promote the changes that sustain a pregnancy, should fertilisation occur.

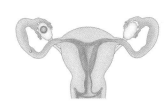

The corpus luteum in the ovary produces progesterone to sustain the pregnancy. The endometrial lining thickens in readiness for the fertilised egg to implant.

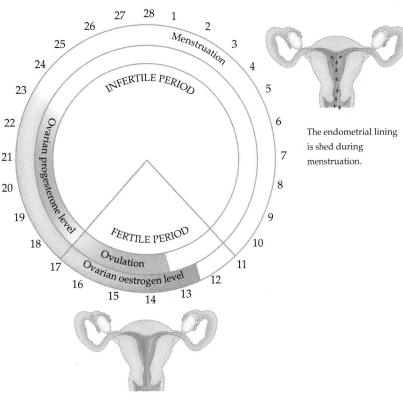

26 27 28 1 2 3 4 5 6 7 8 9 10 11 12 13 14 15 16 17 18 19 20 21 22 23 24 25

Menstruation

INFERTILE PERIOD

Ovarian progesterone level

FERTILE PERIOD

Ovulation

Ovarian oestrogen level

The endometrial lining is shed during menstruation.

At ovulation an egg is released from the ovary and the cervix produces mucus to assist fertilisation.

What's in an egg?

An egg is called an ovum. At its centre is a nucleus containing 46 chromosomes. This is protected by a protein membrane, like an egg shell, called the zona pellucida. Between the shell and the nucleus is a layer containing nutrients to nourish the embryo during the first few days after conception. All the eggs in your ovaries have been present since you were an embryo in your mother's womb. They remain dormant until ripening, one by one, with each menstrual cycle.

At the start of your menstrual cycle the maturing egg that is ready to be released becomes very active and its chromosomes divide. Of these, 23 are retained in the ovum while the other 23 are stored in a tiny envelope within the egg shell. When conception occurs, the 23 chromosomes from the egg meet the 23 chromosomes from the sperm, giving the full complement of 46 (the number in every adult body cell except sperm), and it has a mixture of DNA from each parent. The egg shell remains intact for a few days but is shed before the embryo implants in the wall of the uterus about 5 days after fertilisation.

The sperm factor

In the 16th century western scientists believed that the male ejaculation contained miniscule embryos. It wasn't until the 19th century that the woman's part in conception was acknowledged, and yet later that the equal role of male and female was accepted. With great advances in fertility treatment it is now possible for a woman to become pregnant without having sexual intercourse. Yet even test tube babies rely on the male sperm: without the sperm, there can be no baby unless human cloning becomes a reality.

The journey of a sperm

The male reproductive system manufactures sperm and transports them through the penis. It also produces male sex hormones. It is aided by a continuous production of LSH and FH by the pituitary gland – the same ones produced by women. Sperm are made inside the testicles in seminiferous tubules and then sent to the epididymis at the back of the testes, where they mature over several weeks at an optimum temperature 1–2°C (1.8–3.6°F) below body temperature. Sperm need to be transported in a fluid, which is known as semen. When a man is sexually aroused, contractions in his muscles force sperm up from the epididymis to join the semen. The mixture passes along the penis and is ejaculated during orgasm. Each ejaculation produces just under a teaspoon of fluid, within which are between 20 and 40 million sperm. Only three-quarters of these will be fully formed and mobile.

During love making the semen and sperm are projected towards the cervix. Usually the mucus in the cervix forms an impenetrable mesh but for 3 or 4 days around ovulation the mucus alters to nourish and protect sperm for several days.

The sperm face a long and perilous journey; of the hundreds of millions ejaculated only a few hundred will make it as far as the fallopian tube and the egg. Acidic fluids in the vagina actually slow progress and do destroy many sperm. Once past the cervix, sperm can swim faster in the alkaline environment of the uterus but many will be killed off by 'cleansing cells'. At the top of the uterus they then enter the fallopian tubes. Because ovulation usually occurs from only one ovary at a time, some sperm will swim fruitlessly along a tube and find nothing. Others will swim along the tube that leads to the released egg. Many will die before they reach it.

What is a sperm?

From the age of puberty male testes produce several hundred million sperm each day. Each tadpole-shaped sperm is about .05 mm long. Much of its length is made up of a thin, strong tail, which enables it to swim. The head is dark in colour and contains all the sperm's genetic materials – 23 chromosomes to join with the 23 chromosomes contained in the egg – as well as enzymes that allow it to penetrate a receptive egg. The head is attached to the tail by a short central section or body, which contains mitochondria, special structures that produce energy to sustain the sperm on its journey.

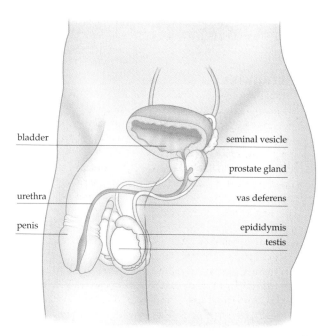

bladder

urethra

penis

seminal vesicle

prostate gland

vas deferens

epididymis

testis

The male reproductive system.

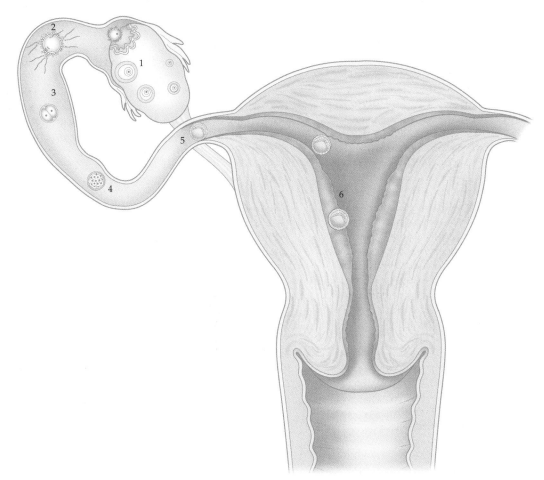

The journey of an egg from release, to fertilisation and implantation. An egg ripens in the ovary and is released into the fallopian tube during ovulation (1). Fertilisation occurs when one sperm penetrates the egg and the two nuclei fuse (2). The single cell divides (3). Cell division continues and forms a morula, which travels towards the uterine cavity (4). The fertilised egg becomes a blastocyst (5). The blastocyst implants in the endometrial lining of the uterus (6).

Fertilisation

Although it is essential for the man to have an orgasm, female orgasm is not necessary for conception. Nevertheless, the contractions of the uterus at the moment of orgasm do help the process by drawing sperm into the cavity of the uterus. The sperm that reach the fallopian tubes are likely to meet the fertile egg about a third of the way along one tube. When they do, a chemical reaction in the egg attracts them. The sperm release enzymes that allow one to penetrate the tough outer membrane of the egg. Once one sperm has succeeded, the outer membrane immediately changes to bar other sperm. The single sperm continues its journey and passes through a thin inner membrane to arrive inside the body of the egg, at which point the head of the sperm sheds its body and tail. Fertilisation takes place when the head of the sperm reaches the egg's nucleus. The two fuse to form one cell, the zygote.

Implantation

The zygote immediately divides into two, each of these two cells divide again and division continues. Some cells will form the embryo and others will become the placenta. The cluster of cells – the morula – looks rather like a mulberry. The fallopian tube is lined by cells that waft the morula towards the uterus. It takes about 4 days to get to the uterus, by which time the cluster contains around 100 cells grouped around a fluid-filled centre. At this stage your baby-to-be is known as a blastocyst, and floats in nourishing liquid produced by the endometrial lining of your uterus. Around 5 days after fertilisation the blastocyst loses its outer membrane. It is ready for implantation in the uterine wall.

As the blastocyst lands on the spongy endometrium its placental cells are arranged as tiny projections called villi, which burrow through the endometrium, connect with your bloodstream and absorb oxygen, protein, sugars, minerals, vitamins and other essential nutrients. On implantation your baby (an embryo) grows rapidly: spine, nervous system, limbs, face and organs are formed. The placental cells produce the hormone human choronic gonadotrophin (HCG), which signals the corpus luteum to continue producing progesterone and oestrogen to nourish the uterine lining. As it grows, the placenta progressively produces these hormones and the corpus luteum gradually shrinks until it is no longer needed, around Week 10 of pregnancy. Your embryonic baby has developed into a foetus, and looks like a miniature human.

If the blastocyst implants in the fallopian tube, an ectopic pregnancy results (p.457). If the fertilised egg doesn't implant, it is an early miscarriage; there may be no sign of conception or a slightly late period. Pregnancy is at highest risk in the stage between fertilisation and implantation and up to Week 10. In fact, less than a third of all human conceptions continue until a baby is born; compared to other animals, human beings are not good reproducers. We do, however, excel in nurturing our babies for an unusually long period after birth.

Your baby's genes

Every human being has a unique genetic make-up. There's an enthusiastic drive among scientists working on the human genome project to map the DNA sequence in cells and define their constituents – with around 30,000 genes inside each of the 46 chromosomes in each body cell, this is a huge task. The facts that are being revealed have uncovered the tip of a huge iceberg and are beginning to shed light on the way human beings work, and the reasons for individuality. This subject will be the basis for many medical advances as your baby grows to become an adult.

Your baby's unique DNA is created within minutes of the egg and the sperm fusing. The DNA at the time of conception comprise the formulae for his complete development and contain a genetic heritage supplied by you and your partner. Every cell of his body will contain all his genes, but not all genes will be active in every cell – different sets of genes are active in muscle cells than in blood cells, for example.

DNA is like a spiralling ladder (the famous double helix) and the genetic code can be read in the rungs of this ladder. The same genes, with little adjustments, have probably been used throughout the 3.8 billion-year story of evolution, and as we evolved from single-cell creatures additional genes allowed increased control. Most of the DNA is 'junk' – for example, as your baby develops in the womb, he passes through an evolutionary phase relating to the past when his ancestors had tails.

Your baby's genetic make-up determines his gender, colouring, stature, features and propensity to suffer from certain illnesses. Other features such as intelligence and temperament are also genetically influenced. The delicate balance between nature and nurture begins in pregnancy and is crucial in childhood when the environment and the input from family and carers will shape who your baby becomes in the years that follow.

The argument that human beings are little more than robots controlled by their genes is not true: we have great potential and our environment makes a huge difference to who we become. Although some people postulate that genes could be responsible for moods, genetic scientists may never totally explain spiritual and emotional dimensions. It is amazing that humans across the world share more than 99.9% of their DNA.

A boy or a girl?

Gender is determined by the presence of X and Y chromosomes. Physically, a woman can do little to influence the gender of her child because each of her eggs contains a single X chromosome. A man's sperm, however, can contain either an X or a Y chromosome. If an X sperm penetrates the egg, the baby created will have XX sex chromosomes and will be a girl. If the sperm is carrying a Y chromosome, the baby will have XY chromosomes and will be a boy. It is believed that Y sperm swim faster than X sperm, but that they are are smaller and live less long. On this basis some people believe that it is possible to influence a baby's sex by carefully timing intercourse with respect to ovulation.

One, two or more?

If you produce two eggs at the same time and they are fertilised by separate sperm, non-identical twin babies are conceived (p.548). Non-identical twins can be the same or different genders and are no more alike than any other siblings. The propensity to release two eggs at ovulation is passed on genetically and is more common if you are older than 35 years. Where identical twins occur, they develop from a single sperm and a single egg. During early divisions of the fertilised egg, the cells split to develop into two separate embryos sharing the same DNA. The two babies are genetically identical, so they are the same sex and look exactly the same. There seems to be no obvious cause for the conception of identical twins – their incidence is thought to be completely random.

Life beginning

Even in the case of identical twins and an identical string of DNA, two entirely different people will grow in the womb and show distinct personalities as babies, children and adults. This is evidence of the amazing life force and combination of our genes and our environment that makes us all so different. When conception occurs, this intangible power flows through new channels – as parents, you will witness at first hand this feeling of creation and momentous change.

Amazing baby

Three weeks after conception, the cluster of cells resulting from the union of egg and sperm have developed into an embryo, and the foundations of the brain and nervous system appear as your baby begins her voyage of development. Her journey over the next 18 months is staggering – an intense period of growth, learning and communication.

	Your baby's body	Your baby's brain
By Week 8 of pregnancy	The embryo consists of 10,000 cells, and already has rudimentary organs, eyes, ears and limb buds and a nervous system. It has passed through the 'evolutionary' stages of tadpole, fish and primitive mammal, and now resembles a human. Your baby's heart beats from Week 5 at about 150 beats per minute – it is the size of a poppy seed. By Week 8 she has developed the startle reflex.	The brain develops rapidly: millions of new cells are produced every minute. The proto-reptilian part, the oldest in evolutionary terms, contains the brain stem and the spinal cord. This is the seat of instinctive reactions and commands body function.
By Week 12 of pregnancy	With all her body parts present, your baby (now a 'foetus') can roll, somersault and swallow and is developing her sucking reflex. She has the beginnings of fingernails, has downy hair all over her body and her organs are functional. She practises breathing movements as her lungs fill with fluid and then empty.	Neurones (nerve cells in the brain) continue to appear and are forging links with one another that conduct body functions including circulation, sucking, swallowing and urinating. This is her genetic potential, but she also learns according to the hormonal and emotional environment.
By Week 16 of pregnancy	By Week 15 your baby has heard her first sounds – lots of noises echo in the amniotic fluid – and later she will recognise your voice. She can taste and smell the amniotic fluid and will respond if a light is shone on your abdomen, though her eyelids remain fused. She is more relaxed, perhaps sucking her thumb while floating. Genitals have formed – if she is female she already has up to 3 million eggs in her ovaries. Buds for teeth and vocal cords are growing, and a creamy moisturiser (vernix) covers her skin. Her unique fingerprints are mapped out, yet her body is only as long as an adult's hand.	Neurones in the brain continue to form at the rate of 580,000 a minute and create links with other neurones. The cortex now begins to connect with the thalamus, where emotions are processed. Your baby is able to feel pain.
By Week 22 of pregnancy	Bones are beginning to harden as the rest of your baby's body continues to grow. She develops the reflex to root and is becoming more co-ordinated – she can now reach for, grasp and stroke the umbilical cord, just as she will grasp your finger at birth. Her skin is sensitive to touch all over her body, except for the scalp (desensitised for labour). A baby born after Week 23 can survive.	Millions of links are formed between neurones and at this stage there is heightened activity in specialised areas while the brain organises sensory information. Feelings of touch, warmth, light, sound and taste are processed and stored. Your baby can feel emotions and already dreams. She is building foundations for new experiences after birth.
By Week 28 of pregnancy	Your baby has been opening her eyes for around 2 weeks now. She is laying down fat as energy stores, which will sustain her through labour and the few days before she feeds on milk. She reacts as you touch your abdomen and her heartbeat increases when she hears a noise.	All the brain's neurones (100 billion) are now formed, providing a firm foundation for learning and recognition. Hearing and speech centres mature. Up to one million chemical reactions occur in the brain each second. Many of these result in the ability to feel emotions.

Your baby's body

Your baby's brain

By Week 32 of pregnancy

Fully formed, your baby concentrates energy into maturing. A girl's labia are still small, and a boy's testicles are just beginning to move down from the kidney region to the scrotum. Your baby has waking and sleeping patterns but will be disturbed by loud noises, bright lights and your movements. By Week 32 she can recognise familiar music.

As it receives and processes information, the brain expands and your baby's head continues to elongate. It is busy even in sleep: rapid eye movement/dream sleep (REM) takes up 80% of sleep time. More and more cells are linked by connections that form as a result of activity and experience.

The last weeks in the womb

Your baby gains up to a third of her total birth weight in the last 7 weeks in the womb. Her organs continue to mature, her fingernails grow to the end of her fingertips and her bones harden (except for the skull bones, which remain pliable and will overlap during the birth). Lanugo (fine body hair) and vernix are shed into the fluid and swallowed. Her lungs produce surfactant, a liquid that reduces the surface tension in the passages lining the entire respiratory tract so that the lungs can expand in air and your baby can breathe after the birth.

The brain continues to grow at a faster rate than the rest of the body as connections are formed between the neurones. When the time comes, it triggers the release of hormones that interact with the placental hormones and stimulate the onset of your contractions.

Your birthing baby

During labour your baby might wriggle and actively move down the birth canal or stay calm and leave most of the work to your body. The scalp, protected by amniotic fluid, pushes on the cervix with each contraction and the skull bones overlap to make the head smaller. Her head rotates and when the cervix is fully dilated her head and flexible body pass through your vagina and into the world outside.

Babies sleep off and on during labour, but when awake do sense pressure and the powerful pushing force. Babies react in different ways to being born. Some feel pain, particularly with instrumental deliveries, some show high levels of stress hormones and seem afraid. The majority handle labour with ease and appear calm.

Your new baby

Your baby adapts rapidly to breathing air. This is accompanied by a cry – the first time you hear her voice. Her eyes open and her body will gradually unfurl. After practising in the womb, she will root and suck when held to your breast, and has a number of other reflexes – to grab, to step and to startle when shocked. She can focus on your face while you hold her in your arms, and will look at you and communicate on a subtle yet powerful level.

Physically and emotionally birth is a huge experience. There may be shock, but your baby can sense the security of loving arms. Within minutes her brain has processed countless pieces of information. Phase two of her learning begins: she is able to communicate and focus on you and she will know your voice.

1 month old

In just a month your baby becomes smiley and confident, with some head and neck control. Her belly button is neatly formed, she sucks and cries eagerly, and is busy using her senses to decode her environment. Her sense of smell is acute – at 5 days she can recognise your breast milk – and she still relishes the feeling of being gently stroked as she was by the fluid in the womb. She is beginning to focus beyond your face and can see a wider range of colour. Her hands are usually clenched in tight fists, but her legs and arms wriggle whenever they can.

Your baby is driven to communicate, to learn and to mimic. All the lessons learnt and the emotions felt in the womb act as reference for new information. She recognises your voice and can now connect it to the sight of your mouth moving – she may rock in time to it. She senses feelings sharply, and she often reflects your emotions. By now, your baby has no sense of being separate and feels that she and you are one.

3 months old

By 3 months your baby eats between six and ten times the quantity she did at 2 days old. She smiles and laughs, uses her hands to strike things and turns towards sounds. She can focus well and may be able to sit up when supported. Her language is developing and she has a range of gurgles. She's getting stronger – she may push herself up when lying on her tummy.

Your baby's brain expands greatly as connections multiply and create a map for interpreting information. Each experience is integrated and the brain then changes. The more an experience is repeated (e.g. the sight of your face), the stronger the link becomes. Your baby can feel happiness, fear, love and anger, and is constantly curious.

Your baby's body

Your baby's brain

6 months old

Between 6 and 9 months most babies can sit unsupported and have mastered the technique of rolling, and some have started to crawl. Your baby will know her hands well, and play with them curiously. She can reach and touch her toes, and bring them to her mouth. The teeth buds that developed in the womb may have resulted in at least one tooth and eating solid-ish food may be a regular part of her day. Her language may sound something like yours and she may already have a specific sound for her favourite object. She can now resist the urge to sleep if she's having too much fun or feels insecure.

Your baby is becoming increasingly sociable. She can choose who she smiles at, may be flirtatious, and object if she does not want to do what you suggest. She knows that her body does have limits. While her brain still reacts to all information with an instant emotional response (as an adult's brain does), it is now calculating how to give a physical response: it is beginning to rationalise with the logical brain, and can inhibit certain responses and override some reflexes.

9 months old

Nine months before birth, your baby was just one cell. Now she is 64–76 cm (25–30 in) tall and talking in her own language of dada, baba, goo and coo. She thinks she controls her world, and can reach, grasp and drop objects, put toys into a bucket and retrieve them, and pick up a tiny pea, all from a steady sitting position. She will probably be crawling – or bum-shuffling – with confidence, and may pull herself up on furniture. Her eyes see almost as clearly as they will as an adult. Her drive to explore is limitless, and she is evolving out of her baby stage and turning into a toddler, ready and eager to find out what she can do. She will use you for physical and emotional support as she experiments.

When her brain receives a stimulus, it triggers a reaction – laughter, a faster heartbeat, the urge to scream or strike out. If she laughs a lot, enjoys the feeling and getting a response from another person, she will want to laugh more – a happy baby is inclined to become happier, and it's largely down to the brain's natural development. Her memory is improving and she can hold a thought (she will probably expect you to reappear from behind the curtain when you play peek-a-boo). She knows that she's separate from you but feels uncertain; she fears being left alone and needs you to guide her through the next stage.

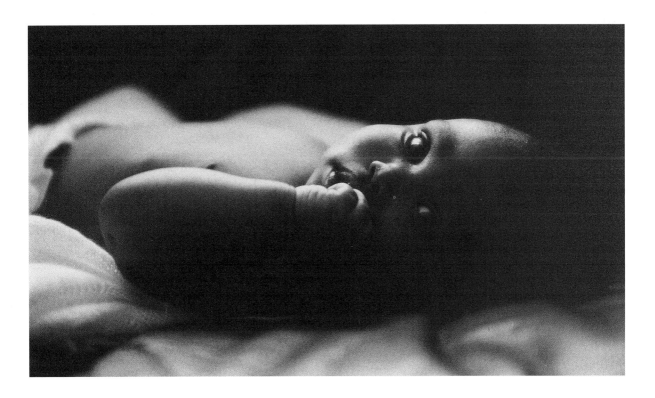

Your baby's amazing body

Your baby is amazing. It's incredible that in just 9 months, from a single miniscule cell, a little human has evolved. It's even more staggering that he learns, even before birth, to recognise, communicate and actively influence his environment. Nature has set the scene for you and him so efficiently that he can do everything he needs to strengthen his body and mind and become a social being. In the first 9 months after birth your child grows and learns more than he will in any other decade of his life. So exactly how is it that your amazing baby achieves so much between the moment of conception and the time he pulls himself up or takes his first, wobbly steps?

Your powerful baby

Generations ago scientists believed that a baby's life was passive; there could be no learning in the womb and, without language, there could be little learning in the first year. Physical development was considered more or less pre-ordained. Yet recent research paints a different picture, which is based on solid facts gleaned from experiments and close observation. Your baby learns in the womb, where he prepares to cope with life outside, and he learns during every waking moment after birth through persistent communication and experimentation. Cognitive scientific researchers reveal that babies are inclined to learn certain things at certain times, and to engage help and support from their carers. In other words, although your baby's growth follows a predictable framework, he actually helps himself to reach each milestone and persuades you to help him as he does, even when he is only days old. Inside his top-heavy head every movement is stored in his brain, everything he senses is registered, and a map of reality is created. It is no mistake that one of his greatest gifts is the ability to flirt and communicate – he needs you because he needs someone to copy, he needs to feel loved as he learns, and he wants praise and encouragement. Without these props his debut into the world would be dull and even anti-climatic; functional rather than fun.

Growth and development

Your baby journeys through the most incredible transformation as he evolves from a single fertilised egg. Inside the womb, cells divide and his body takes shape. He develops a nervous system and a brain and byWeek 8 his essential organs are in place inside a body with limbs and skin, and he has eyes, a nose, lips and cheeks, giving his face distinction. Growth continues as his skeleton hardens, his skin strengthens and his brain becomes more refined and efficient. He uses his full range of senses in the womb, and is ready for the next stage of his journey.

As a newborn, your baby seems physically helpless because, although he can suck to gain food, he cannot sit, stand or even hold up his head, and relies fully on you. Just 9 months later, body strength and dexterity enable him to control his immediate environment physically. This change is as astounding as the leap from conception to birth, and more fun for you because you can watch him develop, help him on his way, and delight in all his new-found achievements.

All babies learn basic motor skills in a similar sequence, but the age at which these are mastered depends on genetics and environment and varies widely. Some will be fast in one area, but not another: for example, one baby may never crawl yet walk at 12 months, another may be crawling by 6 months and not walk until 16 months. Babies usually learn in spurts and can master a skill in days – wobbly attempts to sit on Monday are replaced by confident sitting on Friday. As a parent you can make learning fun and encourage your baby to be physically active. Nature sets the scene for you to nurture because your baby communicates and gives the signals for you to provide the right stimulation at each stage of his amazing development.

The temptation to compare your baby to others ('Is he sitting yet?', 'When did yours roll over?', 'Is he holding his bottle?') is almost irresistible and although curiosity and parental pride are natural, try not to take the timing of developmental stepping-stones too seriously. Early achievement is not an indication of greater intelligence or co-ordination, nor of better parenting, and delayed achievement of one motor skill may correspond with early achievement in another area. For instance, some babies are good at crawling and others have a different emphasis, such as talking.

There is no need to worry about delays unless your baby is months behind, in which case your GP or health visitor will help you determine the cause of any problems. Finding a balance between being relaxed and being alert to potential problems is a challenge for every parent. The best way to prepare yourself is to learn about your baby's development.

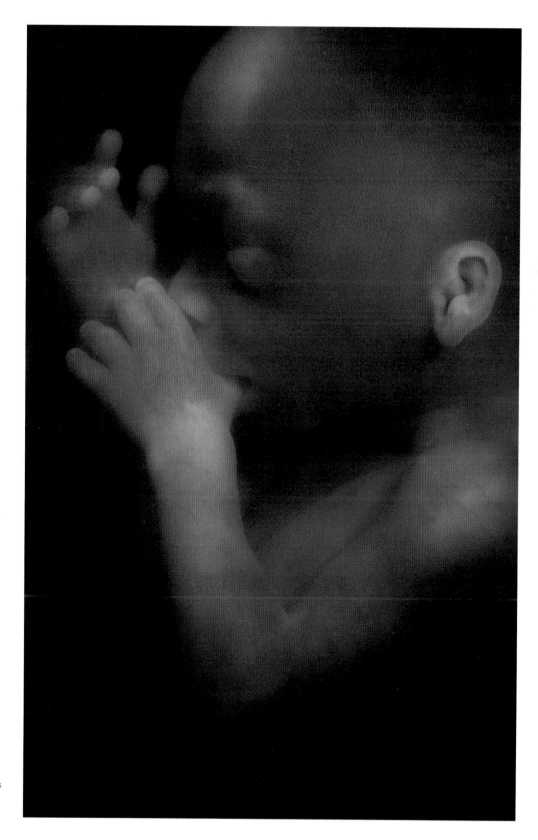

Many babies enjoy sucking their thumbs months before they are born.

How your baby hears

Just 15 weeks after conception, when your baby is less than 15 cm (6 in) long and weighs a mere 100 g (3½ oz), he can hear. Inside your womb noises are muffled but loud: your heartbeat, blood pumping, food being digested and placental activity, and he hears your voice resonating each time you speak. Already he follows your conversations as your tone rises and falls and stress shifts from word to word. The wealth of information available to him helps his hearing capacity develop. By 6 months' gestation, a number of pathways in the auditory cortex of his brain have formed and he has the capacity to hear a complex range of pitches and intensities and has learnt the first lessons about speech.

By around Week 32 your baby not only recognises your voice, but will recognise music that you often play and may respond similarly each time he hears it by kicking, moving rhythmically or resting. He is doing more than keeping step or relaxing to a tune: in his brain a complicated set of links is forming, associating what he hears with what he does, learning about sound patterns, remembering what he is experiencing and using these memories to respond similarly to future events. Some sounds he hears will be associated with the way he feels: if you are relaxed each time you listen to Bach's Violin Sonata in D Minor or become excited and energetic when you dance to The Prodigy, he'll feel it too; if you are tense and afraid when someone shouts at you, he will feel the effects of adrenalin. After birth he is likely to become similarly relaxed, excited or tense in response to these noises and sound patterns.

There is no evidence to prove that babies who are played classical music in the womb grow into especially intelligent children. Classical music, however, can be heard more clearly than pop music above the everyday noises of womb life; in addition, piano and choral pieces have sound patterns that are similar to the human voice and are therefore particularly comforting. You may choose to play more classical works for this reason, but it really doesn't matter to your baby – the more variety he hears, the more his brain learns about sound, rhythm and pitch. By Week 38 he will be able to distinguish different styles of music and may let you know with vigorous kicking or rolling movements that he is particularly stimulated. You will have to see how he behaves out of the womb to find out whether he was actually objecting or dancing to Country and Western.

At birth your baby's hearing is very well developed but noises will seem strangely distinct and unmuffled. He'll still recognise your voice, perhaps his daddy's or brother's voice, and certain tunes, but may also settle to the indistinct fuzzing of 'white noise', which is more relaxing, and is what he's used to. It takes less effort to listen to the whir of the washing machine or the gentle hiss of an untuned radio because his brain has less decoding to do (adults too can 'switch off' to the sound of a washing machine more easily than the sound of a voice).

Another new aspect of noise outside the womb is the way it alters after travelling over distance. Your baby needs to learn to locate sounds. Initially, he'll be able to place noises made in front of him most easily because the sound waves reach both ears at the same time, and he's helped along by his vision. Later he will turn to look for a sound made to the side of his head and lastly (at around 5–6 months) he will know how to locate a sound made from behind him. This ability coincides with head control: each exercises the other.

Though knowing where noises come from is an important aspect of hearing (alerting to danger, for instance), a far more subtle and complex skill develops gradually in the womb and at a remarkable speed after birth. Every voice your baby hears tells him something about language, and as he watches you speak he connects your facial expressions and body movements with your intonations and words to deduce how you are feeling and what your words imply. He has two ears and one mouth, and uses them proportionately. In the first 6 month he learns more about language through listening than through practising, and for months thereafter will understand much more than he can convey. His transition from a newborn baby to a babbling toddler is explored on p.32.

Your baby's vision

At around Week 25 in the womb your baby opens his eyelids to view a world that lights up occasionally if there is light on your abdomen. Everything is indistinct and close, yet he blinks and moves his eyes from side to side, strengthening his eye muscles. By Week 40 retinal surface area has doubled. The first time you hold your baby you have eye contact. He looks at your eyes, glances at your eyebrows, and scans your hairline, looks at your lips and returns his gaze to your eyes. It's as if he is casting a spell that entices you to look at him. His eyes respond only to variations in light: it is his brain that allows him to interpret light as the image of a face, and it soon learns.

> ### Your baby's hormones
> Your baby has a fully developed hormone system well before he is born. Both in the womb and after birth this allows him to respond to his environment. When he is stressed, his body releases adrenalin and he will feel anxious; when there is calm he will produce endorphins and feel meditative. Your baby also produces the love hormones (p.37), including oxytocin, that encourage feelings of love, happiness and bonding as he meets his new family.

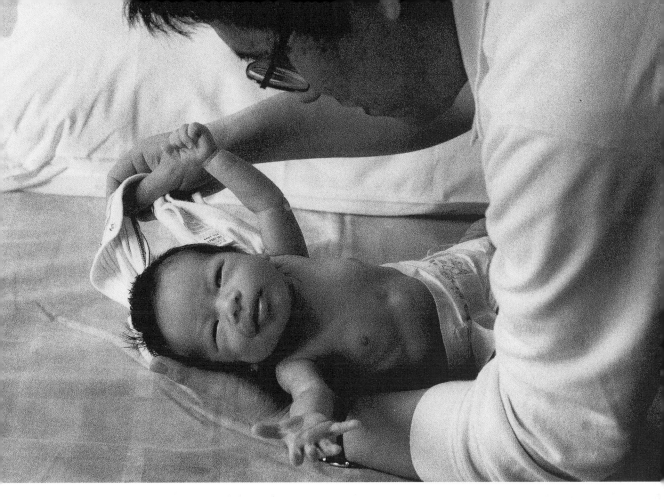

From the moment of birth your baby can focus 20–25 cm (10–12 in), which is the distance between your breast and your face. Beyond this he sees blurred, indistinct shapes. He can distinguish bold colours – black, white, red and yellow – but won't perceive blue and green for some time. The visual cortex of his brain develops in a way that inclines him to notice edges, movement, contours, symmetrical patterns and contrast, and he finds all of these in faces. For the first few weeks outside the womb, he'll look most intently at you. He is, in effect, programmed to get to know the people who care for him and invite them to join his in a dance of communication. After 10 days, and probably before, he will recognise your outline, so if you have a drastic haircut he may be confused.

At first, your baby can follow a slowly moving object with his eyes but is restricted by weak eye muscles. His visual capacity is roughly 4% of an adult's (20/500 compared to 20/20 vision). Yet already he has some amazing skills. He can perceive the world in three dimensions by noting subtle differences in shading and contours and moving his head to judge distance, and knows that your face is the same face whether it is close (large) or far away (small). Each day brings a fresh workout for his eye muscles. In just 6 or 8 weeks his brain will learn

about certain patterns of motion; his ability to anticipate an object's trajectory helps him remain focused as he tracks its movement. At around the same time, he begins to take your outline for granted and pay more attention to the details of your face: your nose and nostrils, your eye shape and colour, your cheekbones, teeth and any moles. With this added information he'll form a clearer memory of what you look like and will be able to recognise your face in a photo, if you wear a hat, have a haircut or wear glasses. He enjoys these details and will like to look at increasingly complex pictures and patterns. He also recognises his daddy, grandparents, siblings and carers, and even knows your gait and characteristic head movements. In fact, he can see details so clearly that no two faces look the same to him: even in a line of people from an unfamiliar race the faces you see as indistinguishable would be distinct in his eyes.

If you cover one eye and look at this page, and then cover the other and look with the first you see two images, but with both eyes open you see only one. At first, your baby sees the two at the same time; he is not able to integrate them into a single image until he becomes 'stereoptic' at around 10 weeks. With this, his outlook changes dramatically. Three-dimensional vision is

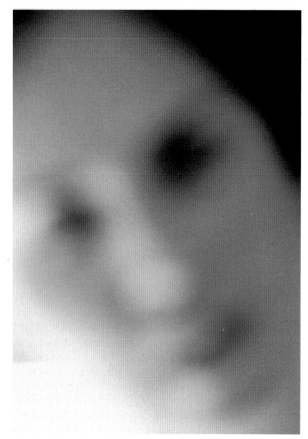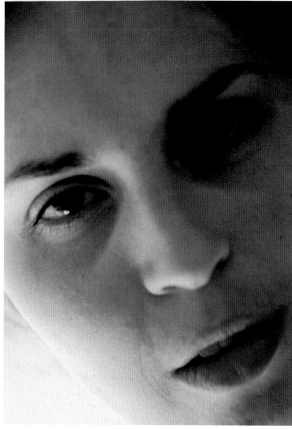

At birth, your baby sees your face clearly when you come close. If he is in your arms at the level of your breast, this is the perfect focal distance for him. As you move away, your image blurs.

established fully and he can begin to locate the position of his hands, his carers and toys more precisely. There's a great leap in development as he learns that he can reach and interact.

With the thrill of realising that he can link what he sees with what he touches, your baby will try again and again to perfect his new skill, and repetition is perfect practice. He'll show wonder at his hands and, some time around 5 months, will be distracted by them as he watches how his fingers move and link together. Once acquainted with them, and with the location of objects around him, he'll reach out with accuracy, and have his hand positioned ready to grasp what he sees. In just a few months his brain learns to judge texture, size and distance from a single image and instruct his hands to respond accordingly.

As he gains increasing postural control your baby improves his visual skills. Since birth, when he could move his head from side to side as he lay down and focus only a short distance ahead, he develops to the point when he can check out his adult companions from his perch at your shoulder by 6–8 weeks. Later, from 6 or 7 months, he can

scan the entire room as he sits up proudly. He knows he can't touch a mobile hanging from the ceiling, but can reach his toes, and can recognise a range of faces, toys and pictures. His visual capability has increased to 10% of an adult's (20/200) and he will look at you as he waits for a reply to his attempts at conversation: if he makes sounds or kicks as he looks at you, you stare blankly instead of moving your face or talking, he may try even harder. If you keep a straight face, he'll soon become upset or turn away, bored.

By the end of his ninth month he will be able to detect depth, which is important as he needs to learn about steps and other potentially dangerous drops. Yet he has lost the ability to see distinguishing features in faces that are not familiar to him (such as in a group of people from a race that he's never encountered). This is because development of links in the visual cortex of the brain has peaked, and already a 'pruning' process has begun to allow the brain to operate efficiently. It has learnt that it needs to distinguish between faces of familiar race(s), and no longer exercises its ability to notice differences in types of faces your baby never sees. He is tuned to see exactly what he needs to suit his stage of learning. His vision still needs to mature though, and focal range and muscular control continue to develop. Your baby practises during every waking moment and forms increasingly strong associations between what he sees and what he smells, hears and feels, and creates a visual map of his world.

Your baby's sense of smell

When your baby's face is formed in the womb, it is not a rounded lump that becomes sculpted. Each section is formed separately, combines facial tissue with neural (brain) tissue and then merges so it functions optimally. Like his eyes and ears, his nose is a connection of brain, bone and skin. In the womb your baby is able to smell the amniotic fluid for at least 3 months. Once born he is bombarded with a stream of novel fragrances and senses each one acutely; his sense of smell makes up for poor vision. It is so acute that if he's placed on your tummy within an hour of birth, he can wriggle up to your breast, seek out your nipple and suck. In his strange new world he will settle best when he's held against your skin; your personal aroma plays a large part in calming him. It may be that your natural scent is similar to the smell of the amniotic fluid.

A sense of smell is a key element in survival. It tells him whether you have entered the room and lets him know when a stranger is around. Five days after birth he can recognise your smell above other people's, and quickly learns to recognise the smell of his bedroom, the kitchen, the car, his blankets and other familiar people; he may nuzzle his face into his daddy's shoulder to drink in his pleasurable scent. He may cry or become tense if he smells someone unknown or someone he believes to be threatening. His sense of smell is governed by a part of his brain that forms strong associations with other parts and enables experiences to be placed in context; years later a smell may trigger a memory and rekindle an emotion long forgotten.

Your baby's mouth

One of the most sensitive areas of the body, your baby's mouth, is his first tool for exploration as he sucks on his hands in the womb, and on your nipple or a bottle-teat after birth. Although sucking is a reflex, he does need to practise: combined with yawning, grimacing and pouting, this exercises the muscles of his mouth and his tongue as well. Over the next few months his tongue will gradually separate from the floor of his mouth, growing from the tip and lengthening considerably. As it does, he has increasing control over the sounds he makes and the food he can play with in his mouth. He will use his mouth to explore his world as soon as he is able to put things in there with his hands. Although taste sensitivity is limited to the back third of the tongue, the nerve endings around his mouth are some of the most sensitive in his tiny body; in his brain the pathways relating to the tongue, mouth and lips are among the first to develop.

After 6 months in the womb your baby's taste buds have developed and he can taste the amniotic fluid in which he floats. The fluid is strongly influenced by whatever you have eaten, so your baby experiences bitter, sweet, salty and sour tastes. Some flavours are accompanied by a physical response; for example, you eat chocolate, your blood sugar rises and you feel temporarily energised, and your baby mirrors these reactions.

Taste associations continue beyond birth, which is why it is unwise to change your diet dramatically after childbirth if you are breastfeeding. Your baby's palate will already be influenced and he'll be accustomed to certain flavours. That's not to say he'll like everything you eat, though. There is some evidence that babies whose mothers eat spicy food in pregnancy don't mind hints of spice in breast milk, while those who are never exposed to it find it unpalatable. But there are also centuries of experience to suggest that every baby has his own preferences, which includes the flavours that come through in breast milk, formula milk and, of course, solid foods.

In the early months of life your baby is open to new tastes, and, in the brain, connections are made between taste, texture and how his body feels after eating. Although there's a tendency to enjoy sweet flavours, your baby can grow to like bitter or sour flavours as well. But it's not true that all babies can grow to like all flavours – there are genetic dispositions, such as a repulsion to bitterness, and your baby's temperament will play a part in his acceptance of food when he is weaned. As with all aspects of development, his taste preferences will reflect both his personality and his physiology.

Becoming mobile

Your baby is rarely still unless he is asleep. In the womb he rolls and turns, hiccups, stretches his arms and legs, and moves his tongue, lips and eyes. He pushes and presses on the walls around him, and brings his hands to his mouth as part of his busy womb exploration. As you watch him in the first few days following birth you'll see him move as he continues to exercise and explore. Almost all early movement is involuntary or a reflex, yet it is essential for his development, and even the slightest twitch strengthens muscles and helps him process information. Inside his head, his brain fires messages between its many areas, linking cells in the visual cortex, for instance, with cells that govern hand movement.

Your baby's journey to relative independence may appear easy or even passive. But these formative months allow time and opportunity for a staggering amount of development. First of all, your baby needs to adjust from

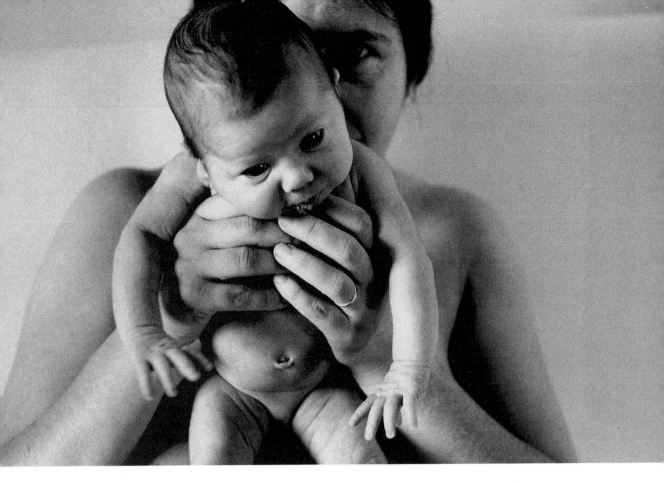

the blissful feeling of floating in warm fluid to the sense of gravity and weight. Uncurling from a secure foetal position and stretching his limbs takes a lot of muscular effort and the huge achievement of rolling is the result of a complex set of actions and judgement. Surprised by his co-ordination and a drastic change in outlook, he'll want to do it again, and again, each time building strength and control. His next milestone, staying in an upright sitting position, is a challenge that will occupy him for weeks from around the fourth month, and when he decides that it's time to crawl, he'll persevere until he masters it, however many bumps he has on the way. It may not be until you have your own baby to watch that you realise just how much practice lies behind each bodily movement, from forming an 'ooo' sound with his lips, tongue and voice box, to placing one foot in front of the other so that he can actually move forward without falling over.

Head and neck control

Your baby can control his head and neck before he can make accurate movements with his arms or legs. As a newborn he can move his head, but rarely with much control. From birth it rests to one side whether he lies on his back or front. When he's held in your arms he can make very small head movements, and uses them to help him judge distances, but most of the time his head will rest on your shoulder or in the nape of your neck. Yet curiosity to watch your face and track movement encourages him to use his head. By around 6 weeks he'll begin to hold up his head for moments, and then minutes, and gradually build the control to move it as he wishes.

Head control and the power in the neck that underpins it mark the beginning of a strengthening spine and spark further development throughout the body. Your baby strains to look up as he lies on his tummy, and begins to help himself by pushing up with his hands, thus exercising his neck and shoulder muscles. By around 3 months he'll be pretty confident at holding up his head – with a head that's four times bigger in proportion to his body than an adult's, this is a real achievement.

Spinal strength continues to develop and by 6 months, if he's pulled from lying to sitting position by his arms, his head is likely to stay in line with his back as he rises, and he'll be adept at turning her head from left to right. From then on the problem is not balancing or controlling his heavy head (though this still requires considerable effort) but co-ordinating the rest of his body. If he is lying and tries to lift his head and his arm at the same time, both will drop. As he tries to sit up he may wobble or fall when he turns his head to watch something but, with practice, he'll master the skills that you take for granted. By 7 months head movements get larger and more confident, and by 9 months barely affect his balance. This is the foundation he needs to begin walking.

Arms and hands

When you hold your new baby, how he uses his hands may be the last thing you think of as you explore his delightful face. Yet even in the first days outside the womb, when he rests for most of the time with his arms held to his chest, his hands are important. Instinctively, he grips anything that comes into contact with his palms – as he closes his tiny fingers around your single giant finger, the two of you form a connection. This body contact gives you the feeling that he is holding on to you, and gives him a sense of being loved and protected. Babies who are cared for in incubators from the start of their life and miss out on cuddles still receive love and communicate by use of this simple yet powerful gesture. This instinct to grasp is strong but there's no instinct to let go: your baby's determined and strong grip ensures that your attention and the flow of loving energy between you are sustained.

Your baby can move his shoulders and arms with precision before he can confidently manipulate his hands. Early swiping movements are gradually refined and at around 3 or 4 weeks he will sometimes reach for things. Incredibly, he will only reach for what is within arm's length, because his brain uses visual and sound information to calculate distance and sends appropriate commands to the muscles. When he extends his arm towards an object that is out of his reach he is actually pointing it out to you – it will be months before he can command a single finger to point. Reaching is slow and thoughtful, but swiping gets more vigorous (and often

includes feet as well) until he occasionally hits his target. Amazed at his achievement he tries again and again, and gets so accurate that he can, by around 12 or 14 weeks, grab the object within his reach. Each time he tries he is exercising and his muscles strengthen quickly. Meanwhile in his brain associations are made: what is seen is linked with what is felt, and both are connected with arm and hand movements. He learns not only that the moving hand belongs to him, but also that he can control it.

At 3 months your baby still relies on a certain degree of chance since he cannot judge shape or depth. The more he grabs, though, the more he learns. By around 4 months he can bring his hands together and hold something and a few weeks later he learns to reach accurately and will prepare the position of his hand to clasp an object. He will start to shake things to find out what noise they make, bring them to his mouth for further exploration and hold a different object in each hand.

Once your baby is sitting up and has more freedom to reach, obtain and explore things, he can bang and throw things, see how they interact and feel in his hands and mouth. One day he will bring his open hands together and clap. This seemingly simple gesture takes a lot of control, and is only possible on a foundation of intense practice, and he'll do it again and again if you encourage him by copying him and letting him feel that he has started a game. Now he can open his hands he'll begin to use the palms more and more, and by around 9 months he can stroke as well as pat, and use a pincer grasp to pick up raisins, pins and beads that he can then hold in an outstretched hand. Combined with his ability to move by crawling or shuffling he can conduct all kinds of experiments, and will reach almost anything he fixes her attention on.

Legs and feet

Your baby's legs come under control later than his arms, and his ankles and feet develop much later than his wrists and hands. That's not to say, though, that they don't move. On the contrary, your baby will enthusiastically exercise his legs and feet by kicking. In the first week this may be gentle, but becomes increasingly vigorous, especially if his actions produce a result, like making a bell ring on a toy. He'll kick in excitement, as a way of saying hello, and he'll kick when he cries too: it's an important part of a baby's body language.

Kicking is also essential exercise to build up the muscles needed for bearing body weight and, eventually, walking; something that your baby is genetically inclined to learn. Even as a newborn baby he exhibits a stepping reflex and will take a few determined steps if held upright with his feet flat on the floor. The reason is something of a mystery, but it does show that the brain is already sending messages about leg movements and these may be the same messages that fire up when walking begins: the instinctive stepping movement appears once again when you hold your older baby in a standing position and he tries to march forward.

Your baby is extremely flexible because of elasticity in his ligaments and tissues, and when young can curl up tightly. He may touch his toes around 4 or 5 months, and then bring his feet all the way to his mouth a month later, perhaps sucking thoughtfully on them. Now a truly bendy baby, he lies down and grabs a toy and can bring his feet up to help, and his toes may curl as he aims to grip it. He's also learning how to reach with his hands without his legs moving involuntarily, and to kick something with one foot instead of two. All this kicking provides the best workout his legs could have.

Babies who stand within the first 9 months have strong leg muscles, and their brains have mastered how to control the fine motor skills and balance needed to get, and stay, upright. As your baby gets stronger and the joints become less floppy, he acquires a better sense of his position in space. This is associated with improved balance and allows him to pull himself up to stand and finally let go of support and take his first steps. Getting upright involves many complex elements, which need to be synchronised if independent standing and even walking are to be achieved. Little wonder this takes most babies more than a year.

Your baby's skin

Soon after conception the outer layer of the embryonic cell cluster develops into the brain, nervous system and the skin that covers your baby's growing body. In the womb his skin is moisturised by a protective layer of white, creamy vernix. After birth it will recover surprisingly quickly from the transition to dry air and varied temperatures, and your baby's skin remains an efficient barrier against invasion by bacteria. Throughout his life, the way your baby's skin looks will reflect how he feels: goose-pimply with cold or excitement, glowing with warmth and health, flushed with too much heat or with frustration, or reddened due to some allergy, illness or sensitivity.

Your baby's beautifully soft skin, like your own, replenishes itself constantly. It is the body's largest organ and is stunningly powerful. It stores water, sugar and calcium, aids the essential production of vitamin D and has millions of sweat glands, which open through pores to eliminate waste and control body temperature. In every square inch it has 2000 oil-secreting glands that make it a resilient yet supple and waterproof shield, and many metres of blood vessels that help it function as a super thermostat. The skin also has around five million sensory cells that send messages to the brain about the nature of objects or the feeling of the environment.

The power of touch

There can never be a feeling of touching nothing. In the womb, your baby constantly senses his environment with his body. He feels the caress of fluid and the amniotic membrane lining the uterus walls, kicks his feet and flexes his arms and grasps the umbilical cord. He feels the sensation of skin against skin as parts of his body collide or rest against each other, feels fluid passing over his tongue and down his throat as he swallows, and experiences the sensation of sucking as he 'mouths' his hands.

In the womb and after birth his brain forges connections to link what he sees and smells with what he can feel, and his view of the world becomes richer and more complex. Each time he touches something, or is touched, his nervous system develops further and his relation to other people and things becomes clearer. Resting in one another's embrace is probably the most powerful way to tune into one another, and the way you touch can communicate love, sensitivity, tension, upset and anger, indifference and excitement. A tactile relationship offers many lessons in human nature and interaction, and when your touch is loving he will feel protected and valued. Being held and stroked is not only emotionally nourishing, it is physically beneficial because it stimulates the skin and encourages a healthy condition; one reason why baby massage features strongly in many families.

The way in which your baby feels touched and held can have a marked impact on his development. Babies who are consistently deprived of loving human contact grow to be emotionally closed and nervous and may even be slow to develop physically. Those who are welcomed with open arms, held close, stroked and kissed – like most babies are – generally go on to develop a strong emotional life and a confidence based on security; they have been welcomed and guided with the intimate language of touch. Babies who are massaged enjoy the benefit of loving touch and the healing properties of the stimulation massage gives to skin, tissues and muscles deep in the body (p.365).

It is through touch that your baby first communicates with you: in your womb he wriggles and kicks in response to your voice, some music, or the feelings of your hands massaging your abdomen. As he grows, the way he touches you is part of his language. As a newborn, he may rest against your face to feel your cheek touch his cheek or stroke or pat your breast as he feeds. Soon he grips your shoulder or arms as you hold him, reciprocating supportive contact, and will kick against you when he lies down for a nappy change. When he gains control of his hands, from 5 or 6 months onwards, he will begin to reach out and touch your mouth, cheek and hair, and explore with his palms and fingertips. Before he has this control you can bring his hands to your face and help him feel you, and let him brush his lips and tongue against your face, for they are even more sensitive than his skin.

Your baby's amazing brain

Your baby's brain is infinitely more complex and powerful than the most advanced computer. It is the control centre for the body, a store for memories, a home for emotions and an incredibly powerful learning mechanism. Its nature is to explore and learn, and it thrives on activity. The way the brain works ensures that your baby is not a passive pupil – she is an active experimenter and a systematic learner. Neuroscientists have discovered much that explains babies' behaviour and the learning that takes place in the 18 months following conception. This knowledge may have a real impact in the way you relate to and teach your baby.

Ready for action

The brain is very well ordered, and little depends on chance. Certain cells are geared up to respond to certain things, and do so at certain stages of development. For instance, some cells are ready to be stimulated by faces and because they are ready for action at birth, your baby is inclined to watch faces above all else. As she watches faces, her eyes and the cells in her visual cortex get precisely the exercise they need to develop and her desire to communicate is immediately satisfied. Watch your newborn scan your face, follow your movements, shift her gaze to a new visitor: she is checking you out and communicating with you through eye contact and body language. Just seconds after birth, she is ready, and this powerful capacity is down to an astounding brain.

Making sense of the world

Your baby's brain is made up of hundreds of millions of neurones, or nerve cells, that begin to develop in a protective layer of tissue 6 weeks after conception. Every minute for the next 21 weeks 580,000 neurones form, and around 13 weeks before birth your baby's brain has 100 billion neurones; that's as many stars as there are in the universe. There is activity between the neurones, which make links with one another, and between neurones and other cells in the body. Growth is rapid in the weeks before birth as more and more links form. Think of the number of radio waves that pass through the ether every minute of every day – activity between the neurones of the brain is much, much more complex. Each neurone has a trunk (axon), which sends messages in the form of electrical impulses to other neurones, and a number of branches (dendrites), which receive signals. Each neurone can send and receive several hundred messages a second and many millions of neurones fire at one time. This process never stops, even in deep sleep and is active long before birth.

From the first moment outside the womb new neurone connections form at an astonishing rate (a million a second) as stimulated cells fire impulses and send messages, making links that give extra bulk to the brain. It will

quadruple in size between birth and 3 years, and most of this growth takes place in the first year. The links between neurones fire across spaces called synapses where electrical impulses are converted to chemical reactions. As neurones fire together repeatedly, the connections between them become permanent and are known as hard wiring: 'Neurones that fire together wire together.' The axon and dendrites are protected by a fatty sheath known as myelin, just as a plastic casing protects the wires that run from the back of a television to the socket in the wall, and this is laid down progressively after birth as strong links are formed.

Your baby's genetic make-up predetermines many of the basic connections – cells in the ear are destined to be linked to cells in the auditory cortex, for example – as well as a number of reflex actions that are present in the womb and exhibited from birth. But beyond the basic make-up, connections between brain cells depend upon activity and stimulation. This is most significant: your baby's development and learning relies on repeated stimulation and input. The world is naturally full of colours, shapes, noises, objects and movement, and you can really help your baby explore them. In the cerebral cortex, where information is assessed and actions are considered, links depend on action and experience. By holding her, bringing objects within your baby's focal range, letting her watch your face and helping her touch different things, you will provide her with the tools she needs in order to learn.

Plasticity and pruning; becoming efficient

The rate of brain growth in the first 9 months after birth accounts for the fact that your baby's head remains, rather endearingly, out of proportion. It will seem large for her body until she's around 3 years old, by which time activity and growth in many regions has peaked, even though learning never stops. Each time a new stimulus is received, neurones fire electrical impulses, and each time one connects with another for the first time, a new link is made and the property of each neurone changes slightly. Brain function follows a number of basic rules. The brain is able to grow and form connections and strengthens those

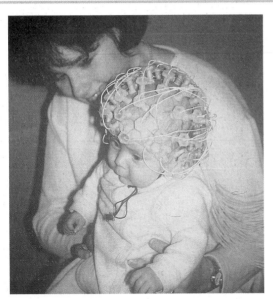

Baby Sarah at the Babylab at Birkbeck College, London. Sarah is wearing the Geodesic Sensor Net, which allows measurement of the spontaneous electrical activity of the brain in a totally non-invasive way. Studies using this system provide a window into the workings of the infant brain.

The brain

Your baby's brain comprises three sections. The oldest in evolutionary terms is the proto-reptilian part, which has been around for 500 million years. It is the first to form around the top of the spinal cord and the brain stem, and is believed to be the seat of instinctive reactions. It commands bodily functions such as heartbeat, blood pressure, digestion, breathing and sleeping, and is the seat of the hypothalamus and the pituitary gland, which activates many hormones needed to release oxytocin, adrenalin and endorphins to help your baby respond to life.

The second section, known as the mammalian brain or the old cortex, contains the thalamus and is the storehouse for emotions; it evolved 200 million years ago. The newest and largest part of the brain, the neo- or cerebral cortex, evolved 50,000 years ago. It comprises interconnected, specialised areas that evaluate information received by the senses and weigh it up against memories and expectations; this is the part of the brain that allows humans to think, and multiple areas of the cerebral cortex may fire in unison to form consciousness.

Most sensations pass through the thalamus on the way to the cerebral cortex and every thought formed in the cerebral cortex passes through the thalamus before stimulating a physical response. Every experience is therefore acutely emotional and because your baby's ability to rationalise is at best rudimentary, her experience is based on the way she feels. She's a very sensitive individual.

that are needed because they are repeated. It ignores those that aren't essential because lack of stimulation means that links are weak. In the first 9 months of life, however, it takes on board more than it actually needs to learn: every stimulation results in a link between neurones, and there is much more activity in your baby's brain than there will be in later life. Because the brain forms so many links, it can operate effectively and stores many reference points as it makes sense of the world. After 9 months, however, a process of pruning begins: connections that have been strengthened through repeated stimulation remain and frail connections formed after one or two experiences fade. What is significant is the brain's ability to adapt to its environment, and to change as a result of learning: in effect to become culturally and socially conditioned while retaining the ability to relearn. Experience alters the brain and this alters the way the brain processes each new experience: this is known as plasticity.

A good example for illustrating 'over' learning and subsequent pruning is the auditory cortex, which interprets sounds. At birth, all babies can recognise all the phonetic sounds that occur in all the world's languages but by the ninth month they lose the ability to 'hear' unfamiliar sounds in foreign languages because, without experience, connections in the brain are not reinforced. Every baby focuses on her mother tongue and this helps her to fit into her family. Before 9 months, however, a French baby, for instance, can distinguish between 'that' and 'fat' and a Japanese baby will hear the difference between 'race' and 'lace', even though their respective mother tongues don't contain the phenomes and their parents cannot tell the difference. An English baby can tell apart the French vowel sounds 'ou' and 'u', but her mother can't: an adult will hear 'beaucoup ' (a lot) and 'beau cul' (nice arse) as the same words. Yet over the months as babies repeatedly hear the sounds made in their native tongue, cells in the auditory cortex become selectively sensitive. At the end of the year the French baby will hear 'fat' when an English person says 'that', the Japanese baby will hear the word 'lace' if she's told about a 'race'. Activity in the visual cortex gives a similar pattern, so that your baby can notice subtle distinctions between a group of people of unfamiliar race at 4 months, but not at 10 months. This learning and unlearning process of building and pruning is what makes the brain plastic, and it is never more pliable than it is in childhood.

Ignoring the background and getting bored

The brain is inclined to learn, integrate and expect certain things. It becomes familiar with what it senses and begins to take things for granted. Think about how you become accustomed to your surroundings; you spend so long in your own house that you hardly notice the change of scenery as you walk from the kitchen to the bathroom.

Often your attention is only caught by something out of the ordinary. Known as habituation, this acceptance of things that are familiar begins to take effect at a very early age. It has two spin-offs: one is that your baby learns quickly by focusing on new information, the other is that she can easily become bored. You can tell if she is losing interest in something when she looks around the room for something different, stops wriggling with excitement or starts crying, but responds with joy and interest when you show her something new or take her to a different room. When her attention span is at its shortest, in the first few months, she may want a new sight, smell or other sensation regularly. As she grows, she'll be happier in one place, doing one thing, for longer. When she's grabbing things with curiosity, you may be able to take advantage of her tendency to reach for something novel: if you want to get your address book out of her hands show her something different and she'll almost certainly drop the book and reach out for the new object.

Habituation doesn't mean your baby gets bored by your face, though: she loves it because she trusts you, is fascinated by the way it moves, and it is your face that teaches her about language and human expression. Nor does habituation mean that she needs a constant supply of new stimuli. Although she will always be eager to encounter and learn new things, she will appreciate the security offered by being with familiar people, being held and interacting with them and may take time to accommodate changes of location. Her personality will determine her dependence on familiarity, but she will value it most in the first 2 months, when she is 'settling' and then again between the ages of 6 and 9 months, when she is realising that she is independent.

How your baby remembers

Only one thought can be held, and focused upon, at any one time, and this moment lasts for little more than one-ten-thousandth of a second. Everything that precedes it, in the other nine-thousand-nine-hundred-and-ninety-nine-thousandths of a second, is a memory. The process of remembering has many different strands. On one level, your baby's brain continually forms memories in relation to physical action: it learns how to orchestrate bodily functions, such as breathing, heartbeat and limb control, and does not forget unless it is severely harmed. This 'procedural' memory operates automatically and becomes more and more efficient. On another level, her brain learns to recognise familiar things. Recognition occurs before birth – when your baby is able to recognise your voice – and increases rapidly afterwards – she can soon recognise your face. Both of these memory systems, then, are up and working when you first hold your baby and get that strange feeling that so many parents experience: 'Have you been here before?'

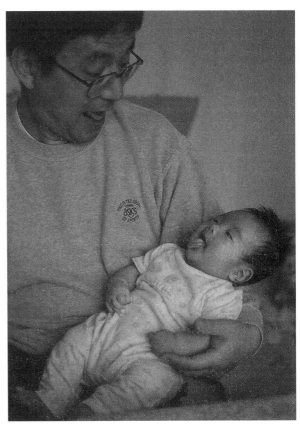

From birth, your baby is inclined to mimic you. It is a natural learning tool as well as an important method of communication, and when you mirror her, she will feel good.

Your baby recognises you, without doubt. But she's not yet very good at recalling you: the mechanisms that allow her to recall what happened to her yesterday, or half an hour ago, take around 2 months to swing into action, and rely on experience and on repeated activity in the brain. Once she begins to recall things she learns more facts (for example, 'My favourite blanket is blue.'). This more specific knowledge allows her to categorise her world. As memory comes into play in all its guises, it influences the way your baby acts and what she expects: what she experiences colours her outlook on life.

How does memory work?

Memory is the collection of links between neurones that forms a network that can be accessed in a split second. The stronger the network, the more easily it can be brought to mind. When a set of connections becomes weak (if it hasn't been used for a long time) a memory may fade. Each element of every network can trigger another related network, so memory can go on and on, often in quite unexpected ways. Like an orchestra that follows the

Object permanence

Leaving philosophical quibbles to one side, it's fair enough to say that adults believe that their friends and family exist when they're not in sight. Your baby, however, doesn't assume any such thing until she is approaching 9 months of age, and she won't take it for granted until she's at least a year old. The only world that exists is the one which she can sense – what she sees, hears, touches, smells and tastes (and what she dreams) keeps her occupied, and she's not concerned with what's out of sensory range. Out of sight is out of mind. Life for your new baby has been likened to a magic show, where objects appear and disappear and she does not question where they came from or went to. It is natural for your baby to live absolutely in the moment; something many adults who practise meditation strive to do.

Scientists have discovered babies' understanding of permanence using experiments that you could easily carry out. Show your 4-month-old baby a toy and wait until she notices it and kicks or babbles with excitement. Then take it out of sight (beneath a table, behind your back, under a blanket) and watch as her face goes blank. The same thing happens if you play peek-a-boo: hide your face behind your hands so you can watch your baby through the cracks in your fingers and you'll see that she doesn't look for you when you're gone, even though you're right in front of her. At around 6 months you might notice her waiting eagerly for you to reappear, or she may giggle in anticipation. Even at this age, if you hide her toy beneath a blanket she may shift her attention almost instantly to something else. She won't seem surprised when her toy reappears from the blanket, but she won't waste time looking for it when it's not there. She has no concept of what scientists call object permanence.

Her ability to grasp the idea that things exist when she can't see them is related to the capacity of her short-term memory. In the first year, her short-term memory is very short indeed: she moves quickly from one thing to the next. By 9 months she may look for a hidden object, but only momentarily: after anything between 1 and 5 seconds she'll move her attention elsewhere. At a year she may look for longer but even then the existence of something that's out of sight only continues for as long as she can

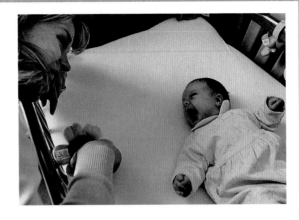

hold it in her short-term memory. She hasn't forgotten what the object is, though – she will recognise it when she sees it again – but she cannot understand space. In her brain, the area that governs spatial awareness is still developing.

Scientists have observed babies as young as 3 months who watch a toy train disappear behind a screen and look to the other side of the screen as if expecting it to reappear. The babies are not surprised if a duck emerges, but if nothing reappears they are a little confused, and watch the space for longer. Try it with your baby. What's happening is not a realisation that the toy still exists. In fact, because the visual cortex is more mature than the area responsible for spatial awareness, your baby follows the trajectory of a moving object with her eyes: she is expecting the result of natural movement, not the permanent existence of an object. She won't look behind the screen for the toy that never emerged until she's around 9 months old; roughly the same time that she begins to panic when you leave her because she can now hold you in her mind when you are gone.

It's not until she really takes object permanence for granted, as much as 12 or 18 months later, that she believes that you will come back. As she accepts that people are separate, she suspects that they can have different thoughts: she'll test the difference between her 'Yes' and your 'No' in the period that's known as the terrible twos.

conductor's baton, your brain fires up in response to a single cue (a smell, for instance, or the word 'birthday') and many related areas are aroused as all the 'instruments' join together to produce the next melody. Tens of millions of nerve cells fire in a few seconds: the word 'birthday' may bring to memory the sounds of 'Happy Birthday', the sight and taste of a cake, the smell of candles and feelings of love and happiness. The brain completes its symphony in a tiny fraction of a second and before this milli-second has passed, another symphony has been triggered by another cue. In a single second, the activity in your brain is similar to the notes an orchestra makes playing a concert ten thousand times.

The way it works can be simplified by looking at two different memory systems: long-term memory and short-term memory. The long-term memory can be likened to the unconscious mind, and the short-term memory to the conscious mind. Just as no one knows the capacity of the unconscious mind but knows it is infinitely larger than the conscious mind, so no one knows just how much can be stored in the long-term memory. The less mysterious short-term memory operates in an area of the brain called the prefrontal cortex and its capacity is very limited, like a wipe-on wipe-off shopping list. It is where something is held in focus or brought to mind, and where a conscious thought dwells for a moment before it is replaced by the next. The capacity of the short-term memory relates to attention span. An adult's short-term memory can hold one or two thoughts consecutively, and is able to store no more than seven numbers without rehearsal, although the average is nearer five (that is why UK telephone numbers are broken into sets when they're made up of more than six digits). Your baby's short-term memory is limited and cannot retain as much information: until the end of the ninth month she can only remember two or three objects or pictures (she doesn't know about digits yet) at a time.

Experiments have shown that at just a few days of age babies can remember something (a new sight or sound) for 1 minute. By the age of 2 months they may remember something for up to 2 weeks. By the age of 9 months your baby will have the capacity to store information and remember it months later. You may be amazed by her expectations. For example, a friend may stay with you for a few days and play the same game with your baby over and over again. If he returns a few months later, your baby may go to her toy box and retrieve the toy they played with the last time he was staying with you.

Your baby will remember things more quickly if she encounters them with more than one sense. This is one reason for her keen sucking and chewing of everything she grabs at around 5 months: if she can see, touch, smell and taste something, she can form a more complete memory. As she gets more active she learns yet more and regularly draws on her memory: she'll know that the red soft ball bounces, but the harder blue ball is better for rolling, or that hitting a plastic duck produces a quack. Before she recalls these facts, however, she'll show a flair for remembering faces and the people behind them. She recognises her parents from days after birth and expects certain things. She acts differently with each of you, and you have your own way of talking to and holding her. She has expectations about others too: if her uncle always tickles her she may giggle each time they meet even before the tickles begin; if Granny has a habit of wrinkling her nose in greeting, she'll try to copy her and by 3 months, with regular contact, she'll wrinkle her nose to say 'Hello'.

As you spend time with your baby, you'll realise that all her memories, from recognition of her little brother to activation of a musical box, are formed perfectly without the need for verbal language. She can't say 'mum' but knows exactly who you are; she can't say 'hello' but will have her own forms of greeting, which depend on who she meets. Today's neuroscientists, with sophisticated recording equipment, have proven that memory begins in the womb.

Emotions and self-esteem

Your baby spends a lot of time absorbing a plethora of information. Her brain is learning and maturing, and some parts take longer to mature than others. It's significant that while the rational and emotional parts of her brain work together, the links in the rational part take longer to form: unlike you, she doesn't decide whether or not to show her feelings, she just does. With the absence of verbal language, and a small capacity for rationalisation, your baby experiences everything through an emotional filter.

Emotions form the backbone of her early learning experiences and may be the most enduring aspect of her memory: the first thing she learns is to trust or mistrust her environment and carers. Early memories fuel instinctive reactions or 'gut' feelings that are often difficult to explain in later life, and this is because the emotional area of the brain stores memories for a long time and is more resistant to change than the more rational cerebral cortex.

If your baby grows from a foundation of love and positivity, she has a good start: no smile or cuddle is wasted and no praise inconsequential. What she perceives in your face is the way she will perceive herself. Mirroring is an essential aspect of her experience and exerts a powerful influence over the way in which she begins to develop her sense of self.

A baby looked at with love and joy, for example, experiences those feelings. To feel loved and valued is the most valuable foundation for your baby as she tries to work out life's challenges: how to make herself understood, how to sit and stand, how to cope when things go wrong, and how to come to terms with the feeling that she is separate from you.

Life is life, however, and no baby or family grows in an emotional bed of roses. By their nature, emotions vary, and it's important that you let your negative feelings show and acknowledge your baby's feelings of anger, frustration and sadness. Many people find it hard to deal with strong emotions, but the more comfortable you can be as you acknowledge and express your own, the more comfortable you may be with your baby's, which she'll express in raw form. And because so much of her learning depends on emotions, the more she is able to express herself, the more fully she will develop.

Many people do not acknowledge that a healthy emotional life is as important as a healthy physical, mental or spiritual life. Yet emotions are not odd things that get in the way – they are fundamental aspects of being alive. Humans have them in order to 'feel' what is happening and respond with an action that ensures survival and, as you'll discover with your baby, the emotions that are linked with communication and socialising are crucial. Any child who grows up feeling loved, respected, affirmed and accepted for who she is will almost certainly enjoy enhanced emotional health, physical health, higher levels of intelligence and wellbeing. Armed with a little awareness and understanding, every parent has a wonderful opportunity to help create this experience for their children.

Your baby's amazing communication

Your baby is an expert communicator and uses his skills to remarkable effect, even when he has little voluntary control over his body. Every aspect of his brain is geared up at birth to help him communicate with the people who care for him. He can recognise voices that he heard in the womb and notices familiar melodies of speech, he recognises people by sight and smell, and he makes no secret of his urge to interact.

Building relationships

Like all babies, yours is driven to imitate. Within hours of birth he can move his lips and poke out his tongue, copying an adult face doing the same, even though he has never seen a mirror. When he's older he'll smile as you smile, try to move his mouth in the way you do as you slowly say his name, shake a toy if he sees you do it, copy the way you eat and, later, clap and wave his hands, in just the same way as you do. He needs to copy if he is to learn, and he takes advantage of the fact that you're a natural copy-cat as well. When he smiles, you smile back, when he giggles, you laugh too.

Despite being the more experienced person, you follow his most of the time: he sets an agenda for play and communication that suits his moods and abilities long before he is able to talk. Though there may be frustrating moments of misunderstanding between you for years to come, the more often your baby feels understood, the better he will feel about himself, and he'll be spurred on to make more gestures and noises as he masters one of the most basic and important skills of his life.

Your unborn baby hears your voice every time you speak, sing or shout, he feels your movements and senses your moods as hormones in your blood pass through the placenta. It may seem that you are an extension of him (you are one and the same) or that he is constantly accompanied by someone else. Whatever his perception, there is no doubt that he has a close relationship with you that goes beyond your physical connection. He recognises your heartbeat and your voice and knows your rhythms of sleeping and waking. He can feel pressure as you touch or stroke your abdomen, and in the last couple of months will respond to your touch or voice with a movement, nudge or kick. This gives you and your partner plenty of opportunities to engage him in a playful dance. As you do, you are building a bond, preparing yourself to meet him and helping him to recognise what he'll soon encounter. Studies have shown, for instance, that babies whose fathers have spoken regularly through the walls of the abdomen recognise their voices above those of other men.

Interaction between you and your baby also takes place on a more subtle level. Many people believe that there is a psychic connection that makes your relationship unique. Just as he knows your rhythms, so he tells you his,

and these reveal something about his personality. After Week 30 he may settle into a waking and sleeping pattern in the womb – the length of his naps, the erratic or stable nature of his timetable and the vigour of his movements are all a reflection of his unique tendencies. Taking time during your pregnancy to be still, listen and feel is a great way to tune in to your baby and internalise your attention in preparation for labour.

When he is born he establishes eye contact with you and flirts seductively with nothing more complex than a twitch of the nose, or a tiny bubble blown from pouting lips. Within minutes he can imitate a simple gesture and reveals the key to his favourite games: he loves to copy, and loves to be copied. He tenses and relaxes his body to let you know how he feels, cries with pain or hunger and may pat your breast to stimulate milk flow. The small touches he makes with outstretched hands tell you he wants to be close, and even the timing between feeding or sleeping conveys his personality. As he gains more control of his body, he gets better at communicating. A smile, he knows, will win you over, so he repeats it again and again, first in response to your smile and then in an attempt to make you smile and come over for a chat. Listen, watch and let yourself be drawn into his conversations and you will give your baby just what he needs to fulfil his physical and mental potential.

In the first few days after birth your baby will snuffle, gasp, cough and grunt endearingly, and cry with pitches that range over several octaves. Within 2 weeks he'll make other noises that are a cross between crying, shouting and singing. All of these early noises, including crying, are rehearsals for more distinct open vowel sounds – 'aa . . . eeh . . . uh'– that he will make at around 4 or 5 weeks. It's a moment of wonder and celebration; immediately the way you interact changes. Following your instincts, you'll talk to him in a different way and he'll get better at copying you. Try repeating his name or a simple, two-syllable word like 'teddy' and see what he does. He will probably produce something like 'eh-ih'. By between 8 and 10 weeks, he'll experiment with the harder sound of a consonant, and begin to 'coo' and 'goo'. He will naturally expect his noises to be respected as part of conversations; he'll wait for replies and when you talk, he will respond if you leave a gap.

By around 4 or 6 months your baby will begin to experiment and mix sounds that are made deep in the throat with those that are formed by the tongue and lips, which is how he comes out with 'raspberries' and throaty 'grrrr' noises. These transitional sounds, possible because his voice box has descended and he can delay his out-breath, are known as 'marginal babbling'. Each day you'll notice advances, and you'll probably find him talking away to himself even when you're not in the room. The urge to join in may be almost irresistible. Each time you do, and whenever you give positive feedback, he'll enjoy being talkative and practise more.

By 7 months he'll be linking sounds and will babble, with intonation that reflects your own. In another month he may show that he understands some of the words you use (particularly 'no' and his name), and can grasp what you are talking about. And at around 9 months, as he emerges from the primal period, he'll be able to point to some of the things you name and shake his head if something you suggest is not to his liking. He will have abandoned the sounds he used months earlier that found no match in your language, and will have started to use words such as 'baba' or 'pada' as if he expects you to know what he's talking about. Follow his gaze or his pointing hand and if you can figure it out, let him know. Meanwhile, give him lots of chances to talk using games, books, songs and chats, and offer lots of praise and encouragement, and he'll eventually combine everything he has learnt and utter his first word. Just to warn you, this probably won't be 'mummy' or 'daddy': most children begin with something more obscure like 'truck', 'moon', 'car' or 'apple'.

Language and the brain behind it

There's no single area of the brain responsible for deciphering language: a word or sentence is never simple. Even the short sentence 'He is running' refers to an activity, a person and a sensation. Each piece of information is processed by a different part of the brain. On hearing this sentence, your brain will link up these areas in a milli-second, and in another milli-second will answer questions to provide a context: 'Who is running?', 'Where is he?', 'How does he feel?'. It will also process the tone of voice: different regions of the brain are sensitive to different tones and stimulate an appropriate response to panic, sarcasm, humour or sincerity. It's a complex procedure that your brain completes before you can say, 'Boo!'

Focusing on the context first may seem obvious to you, but things are different from your new baby's point of view. How can he break up the sounds that flow into his ears as 'whatwouldyoulikefordinnermylovelylittleboy'? In his brain there is a specific area that deciphers sounds and breaks them up. It is able to do this because it already knows a certain amount about intonation and word flow, since it has been processing voices since 15 weeks'

gestation, and works intensively after birth to get better at judging tiny differences between language sounds.

As your baby listens, he also watches. In his brain links are made between what he sees and what he hears. Everyone has an inherent reflex to communicate with a baby in melodic, exaggerated tones using a sing-song lilt, elongating your vowels, repeating words and smiling, which emphasises your lip movements. This helps your baby distinguish between words and connect mouth shapes with sounds – a tight circle for 'oooh', a wide mouth for 'aaah' and a tight, thin grin for 'eeee'. He also follows your gaze to see what you're talking about and links your expression with your intention. So as he puzzles out how to make sounds, he also learns about meaning. If you watch the television with the volume turned off, you may still be able to grasp the plot, particularly if it's a comedy where actions and expressions are exaggerated. Your baby's decoding of your conversations is similarly perceptive and he has two advantages. First, he is a much faster learner because his brain forms links many times faster than yours; second, he is more sensitive to emotions, so can deduce meaning by detecting currents of feeling that you would probably miss. He will continue to understand much more than he can convey for years to come.

Understanding what is said is only half of the language game. The other half is making yourself understood. Your baby communicates through expressions, body language, cries, gurgles and habits, yet won't be in a position to express everything he feels until he can speak or, if he has problems hearing, until he can use complex sign language. Joining in conversations is a skill he needs if he is to learn, socialise, imagine, argue and reason.

Learning to speak begins with learning to make sounds, progresses to joining sounds and using a conversational tone, moves on to making actual words and then to making sentences. In the first 9 months your baby will probably achieve the first two stages on the speech ladder and he will certainly begin to make signs, for example by raising his arms as he asks to be picked up.

Non-verbal communication

While your baby is progressing towards articulate speech, and long before he even makes his first sounds, there is communication on a deeper and more constant level. For him, this may be more direct than words. In large part it relates simply to the time you spend together, in the same room, in the embrace of feeding or sleeping in bed, when you share one another's space and can 'feel' each other. Parents and their babies are linked in a unique and powerful way, and babies can tell if they are emotionally 'held' and loved. The sound and rhythm of your breath and your heartbeat, your smell and temperature, the touch you offer and the looks you exchange communicate as much as a thousand words.

Your baby's environment in the womb

At conception a single cell is formed as the nuclei of egg and sperm fuse. This cell is the source for your baby's entire body as well as the placenta that will nourish her for the next 9 months. About 7 days after conception a cell cluster has formed. The inner layer forms the embryo and the outer layer forms the placenta, amniotic sac and umbilical cord, which will provide nourishment until your baby is born.

The placenta and umbilical cord

The placenta is your baby's lifeline. It acts as a go-between for your two separate but closely linked circulations, and breathes, excretes and digests for your baby. Via the placenta she receives the best of everything – a constant source of oxygen and a flow of substances, including antibodies, amino acids, essential fatty acids, sugar, iron and other minerals and vitamins. Your nutrition, health and the constituents of your blood influence placental function and although the placenta does have a filtering mechanism to prevent the majority of harmful substances and most infections getting to your baby, most of what is in your bloodstream will be shared for the whole of your pregnancy.

Remarkably, despite the efficient partnership between your two separate circulations (see box opposite) your blood does not pass to your baby and only very tiny numbers of foetal blood cells pass into your system. The placenta is formed as cells burrow into the endometrial lining of your uterus and form finger-like tissues called villi that implant like roots in the uterine wall. Each of the villi consists of a core of fine foetal blood vessels encased in connective tissue and enclosed by a membrane coated with placental cells. The placental cells enter the wall of your uterine blood vessels and your blood bathes them: without allowing your blood cells through, they pass nutrients and oxygen into the blood vessels inside the villi and into your baby's circulation. The villi should be deeply implanted by Week 10, enabling the placenta to function optimally throughout pregnancy.

The umbilical cord

Blood vessels from thousands of villi unite to form the two foetal arteries and the foetal vein that are contained within the cord, which runs between your baby's navel and the centre of the placenta. The foetal vein carries blood containing oxygen, nutrients and antibodies from the placenta to your baby. The arteries carry waste products from your baby to the placenta, from where they are passed into your bloodstream and excreted through your kidneys. The relationship between the placenta, your baby and your system is incredibly complex and ensures that your baby receives both maximum protection and maximum nutrition.

Substances such as oxygen flow easily into your baby's blood where the concentration is lower in a process of simple diffusion. Where your blood contains a low concentration of the substances your baby needs, such as iron, they will be transferred through facilitated diffusion. The villi filter out large substances, such as potentially harmful bacteria, but can transport the large protective antibodies that your baby needs by wrapping them in miniscule bubbles. This is called active transport.

Both placenta and cord grow as your baby develops. In early pregnancy, the placental villi and tissues entirely surround your baby and her amniotic sac. During Weeks 8–12 some of the villi disappear and others become concentrated in one circular-shaped area on the wall of your uterus to form the placenta. By Week 12 the placenta is fully developed, but it still has a lot of growing to do – from 3 to 20 cm (1 to 8 in) in diameter. By the end of pregnancy it will weigh around 0.45 kg (1 lb). Attached to the circumference of the placenta are the membranes that line the uterus.

The umbilical cord is implanted near the centre of the placenta and it grows to around 1 m (3 ft) so you can hold your baby as soon as she is born even though her placenta will still be embedded in your uterus. After your baby's birth the placenta is in a spongy layer attached to the wall of your uterus; as your uterus contracts and shrinks, the placenta shears off and is born. It looks like fresh liver and it is flat and circular, resembling the shape of a pizza.

The placenta and hormones

Your baby has a complete endocrine system and produces her own hormones, just as you do. The placenta also produces hormones that pass into your circulation and help you adapt to pregnancy. Through the placenta your baby also receives hormones that come directly from your system. Some reflect your moods, such as the 'feel good' endorphins that are released when you exercise or dance or the adrenalin buzz of fear or excitement. This mood sharing is part of your baby's in-utero development and integral to the communication between you.

Placental human chorionic gonadotrophin (HCG) has the effect of stimulating the corpus luteum in your ovary to produce progesterone and oestrogen until, by Weeks 8 or 10, the placental production takes over. Progesterone is

Inside her bubble of warm fluid your baby is in her own little world. While reliant on you, she creates and maintains her own supply of blood and keeps this circulating around her body and to and from the placenta. The rate of circulation is rapid. After Week 5 her heart begins to beat at between 110 and 170 beats per minute, a count that is lower when she is asleep, rises when she's awake and active, and averages at around 140 beats per minute. This takes blood through her vessels at roughly 6.4 km (4 miles) an hour, and around her entire body in just 30 seconds.

There is a significant difference between the way your baby's blood travels around her body in the womb and the way it will circulate after birth. The oxygen she needs is transferred from your bloodstream across the placenta, along the umbilical vein and into her heart. In adults all the blood comes to the right side of the heart, passes to the lungs, receives oxygen and then goes to the left side of heart and out to the aorta and the rest of the body. But in the womb blood passes through a physiological hole in the heart, an opening in one of the interior walls, to bypass the lungs and travel via the left side of the heart to the rest of the body via the large aorta. The umbilical arteries branch off the aorta and transfer blood back to the placenta to be re-oxygenated.

At birth the opening in your baby's heart closes as she takes her first breath and air enters her lungs. Blood is redirected from the right side of the heart to the lungs before coming back to the left ventricle to circulate to her body via the aorta. There is another bypass channel, the ductus arteriosus, which also closes at birth when your baby releases the hormone prostaglandin. After birth pulsation in the umbilical arteries diminishes over 2–15 minutes as the prostaglandin causes the wall of the umbilical arteries to contract.

essential to maintain the pregnancy and allow the muscle of the uterus to expand.

Throughout pregnancy the placenta continues to produce hormones. Together with hormones released by your baby and your body they ready you and your baby for labour and birth. They also affect your moods and emotions, encouraging mothering feelings. There are details overleaf.

The placenta also produces a number of growth factors to stimulate the ovary, affect glucose and insulin levels and stimulate your connective tissue and the production of interferon, which affects the way your immune system functions.

The amniotic sac and fluid

The placenta is only part of your baby's gestational world. She also lies within the protective waters of amniotic fluid, which is held securely within the amniotic sac. This sac is made up of two separate membranes. The outer is the chorion – which began life as placental villi that were gradually replaced with membranous tissue – which extends to the placental edge. It lines the entire womb. Inside this is the amnion, which develops from your baby's cells. Together, the membranes form a strong and protective boundary.

The amniotic fluid is clear and colourless and has a subtle, sweet scent. In the early stage of pregnancy it enters the membranes via your tissues and the fluid also seeps in and out of your tiny baby's permeable skin. Later, most of the fluid comes from your baby, who swallows it, absorbs it into her bloodstream and excretes it via her kidneys. Although she is urinating, the fluid remains sterile because the urine is free of bacteria and all of her waste products are expelled via the placenta. Amniotic fluid contains salts, minerals, sugars and proteins. Like an internal sea, it is constantly replenished and re-circulated in its entirety every 4–6 hours. It maintains a constant temperature and acts as a shield against the impact of any blows to your abdomen, e.g. if you fall.

In early pregnancy the volume of fluid is high and your floating baby probably feels weightless, as if she's in unlimited space. In it she can wriggle and somersault: she's doing regular workouts that allow her to build muscle strength and co-ordination. As she grows, fluid volume also increases, but at a slower rate, so that by the eighth month there is much more baby than fluid occupying your uterus and she is less likely to somersault, although she can still roll from side to side and kick.

Your ultrasonographer will be able to monitor the amount of fluid at a regular scan. By the time your baby is ready to be born she'll be sharing the amniotic sac with between 500 and 1500 ml of fluid (1 and 2½ pints). Before birth the membranes will break and your baby's head and body emerge through the gap. When the placenta is delivered the membranes are also born as they are attached to it.

Health in the womb and beyond

The relationship between what happens in the womb and the health of a baby has been known for centuries and there is no doubt that a healthy gestational environment is preferable. Scientific research indicates that conditions during pregnancy, ranging from maternal hormones and nutrients to placental function, can influence health in adulthood. The original studies on this subject were done by Dr D Barker in Hertfordshire, based on birth records from 1911 to 1945: 'The health we enjoy as adults is determined to a large extent by the conditions in which we developed, that can programme how our heart, liver, kidneys and our brain function.' The insight from scientific research, which becomes more sophisticated each year, may increase your urge to do the best for your baby in pregnancy by keeping healthy.

Amazing mum

You're going to be a mum. Through pregnancy and birth and the months following, your body performs physical feats that are little short of miracles as you expand and then contract, and you'll experience a wide range of emotions as you move into a new life stage. You are taking on an important role and in many respects becoming a new person. As you experience what may be the most magical, mystical and mirthful time of your life, your amazing body and mind work together to cope with the transition.

Amazing body

From the moment of conception your body adapts to carrying and sustaining your growing baby. Your hormone levels alter and your physiology changes in the first of a string of transformations. Your body will nurture your growing baby and prepare for labour. During birth the process of change will reach its apex, allowing you to go through the momentous event of labour in the best possible way. After birth your body heals itself and supports and nourishes your baby.

You may 'blossom' throughout pregnancy, but it is just as likely that you will, at some stages, feel uncomfortable. This chapter covers the most common changes; variations from the norm are listed in the A–Z Health Guide at the appropriate places. If you are aware of your changing body and care for yourself with a healthy diet and a balance of exercise and rest, you may be able to reduce the less pleasant symptoms. Even so, you can never have ultimate control over the way your body adapts to pregnancy. You'll be kind to yourself if you keep your expectations both realistic and flexible.

Hormones in pregnancy and birth

Hormones play a vital part in the smooth operation of every human. Hundreds of hormones produced by your body are transported by your bloodstream to act on your organs. Some travel a few millimetres and others travel metres before they reach their target. During pregnancy, hormones produced by your brain and endocrine glands, the placenta and your developing baby urge your body to make vital adjustments to maintain the pregnancy, nourish your baby and give birth.

- **Oestrogen and progesterone,** produced by the corpus luteum in the ovary and by the placenta, are secreted into your system in increasing amounts as pregnancy progresses. They relax the smooth muscles of the uterus, bladder and digestive tract, along with the ligaments and joints, to help abdominal and pelvic expansion and promote suppleness for labour. At the same time they influence your moods and emotions. Their negative effects may extend to constipation, varicose veins and fluid retention (pp.437, 559 and 539).

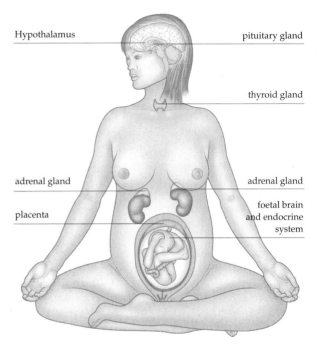

Hormones from the mother, the placenta and the foetus help to nurture the pregnancy, trigger and regulate labour and birth, and promote breastfeeding and mothering.

- **Relaxin,** produced by the placenta, further increases elasticity of your connective tissues and ligaments and contributes to flexibility in the pelvis and spine and to the softening and ripening of your cervix.
- Your adrenal glands produce extra **cortisone,** whose far-reaching effects can include a reduction in allergies (p.391) such as asthma and eczema.
- Hormones produced by your baby's brain and the placenta stimulate your uterine lining to release **prostaglandin** hormones at the onset of labour and cause the uterus to contract powerfully.
- The action of the prostaglandin is boosted by the release of **oxytocin** from your and your baby's pituitary glands. Oxytocin is one of the feel-good 'love hormones' and acts in conjunction with endorphins to guide the onset of

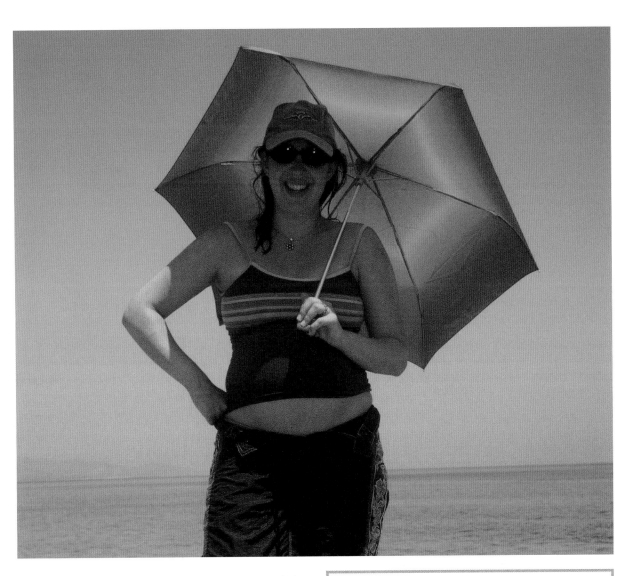

labour and keep contractions going; it flows particularly strongly if you feel warm and secure. Love hormones encourage the mothering instinct to nest and prepare for birth. After birth the flow of these hormones promotes bonding, feeding and mothering.

- **Endorphins, adrenalin** and **nor-adrenalin** form a complex of hormones that are part of your autonomic nervous system that maintains your body's involuntary functions, which include the workings of your heart, blood pressure, digestion and uterine activity. They also affect moods and emotions. Endorphins act as natural painkillers, tranquillisers and 'bliss hormones'. Laughter, meditation and exercise all raise endorphin levels, generally making you feel healthy and positive. Endorphin production increases throughout pregnancy and reaches its peak in labour when you need it most; your baby produces endorphins through the birth as

Love hormones

The French obstetrician Michel Odent coined the term 'love hormones' to describe the release of oxytocin and endorphins that make you feel good and perhaps 'high'. They are released during love making and orgasm, during labour and after the birth and during breastfeeding. Oxytocin is also the mothering hormone and promotes an intense, even overwhelming, desire to bond with your baby. Prolactin, the hormone released during breastfeeding, also promotes the mothering instinct. These hormones, together with the oestrogen and progesterone from the placenta, have a profound effect on all your organs and tissues and on your mind and your brain. They are in high concentrations and they inhibit the rational parts of your mind and stimulate the emotional and mothering aspects.

well. Adrenalin stimulates the 'fight or flight' mechanism but can also give rise to fear and anxiety or bursts of energy. At the end of labour the release of adrenalin causes the 'foetal ejection reflex' as you bear down to give birth.

Hormones after the birth

Levels of the dominant hormones oestrogen and progesterone drop quickly, and within just 2 days of giving birth the levels in your bodily tissues revert almost to their non-pregnant state. With such rapid hormonal change, most women feel unusually emotional, often weepy and sometimes suffer from the 'third-day blues'. Yet love hormones are still strong and help calm you and reduce pain. Close contact with your baby, particularly skin-to-skin, boosts the levels of these hormones, as does breastfeeding, when oxytocin also stimulates milk to flow to your nipples.

The actual production of breast milk is stimulated by prolactin, a pituitary hormone. Prolactin is essential in the menstrual cycle, but levels rise so much during breastfeeding that they have the effect of suppressing ovulation and acting as a natural contraceptive. Its production is enhanced by frequent contact between you and your baby. Prolactin levels drop gradually in the months after birth.

Body fluid in pregnancy and birth

You could think about pregnancy as life within a large sea sponge. A number of changes help you absorb water. Blood volume is doubled by Week 28 and your body produces a cup of amniotic fluid every hour. From early pregnancy hormones soften blood vessel walls, allowing them to accommodate an increased volume of fluid. This increase amounts to a staggering 7 litres (12 pints) of water – half of this is in your uterus, your baby and amniotic fluid, and the other half is distributed in your bloodstream and the cells and soft tissues of your body. This extra fluid, which accounts for a large proportion of natural weight gain during pregnancy, performs essential functions:

- The amniotic fluid provides a supporting, protective environment for your baby.
- Increased blood flow to the uterus supplies the placenta and nourishes your baby.
- Your muscles and joints become pliable so they can accommodate your growing baby and facilitate the opening of pelvic joints during labour and birth.

Excess fluid may collect in some of your tissues and give rise to swelling (p.391), which is usually most noticeable in the fingers, ankles and feet.

Body fluid after the birth

At birth a proportion of extra pregnancy fluid is lost as your baby is born and the amniotic fluid is expelled. Other retained fluid is excreted through the kidneys and there's an increased urine flow for a few days. As fluids redistribute, your ankles may swell, though this usually disappears within 5 days. Meanwhile fluid content in your breasts increases. Fluid in the abdominal wall and the subcutaneous tissue gradually recedes but extra fatty tissue may take months to disappear.

Blood in pregnancy and birth

Volume and haemoglobin: The volume of blood in your circulation rises from around 3 litres (5 pints) before pregnancy to 4–4.5 litres (7–8 pints) at Week 20 and then to, at Week 40, roughly 5.2 litres (9 pints). This increase in blood is mainly due to fluid but there is a rise in the number of red blood cells. These cells contain haemoglobin, which contains iron, and it carries oxygen, which is essential for the increased activity in your pregnant body and for your baby's wellbeing. Your baby absorbs a third of your iron stores.

Despite this increase in blood oxygen level, there is an apparent reduction in haemoglobin because the fluid component increases to a greater degree and dilutes the haemoglobin concentration: this is known as 'physiological anaemia of pregnancy'. A healthy diet and additional vitamin and mineral supplements (p.345) will replace the iron and other minerals used by your baby.

However, if the haemoglobin content of your blood is low, this indicates that your red blood cell count is also low, and oxygen in your body may be reduced. If you have anaemia (p.398) you will be advised to take supplementation.

Hyper-dynamic circulation: During pregnancy the placenta and the uterus act as an extra organ and are served by increased output of blood from your heart. Each minute your heart pumps an extra 30% more blood around your body, giving 'hyper-dynamic circulation'; your heart rate rises a little and with every beat more blood is ejected. Output increases until the third trimester, plateaus before labour and peaks when the placenta separates. The increase is noticeable by Week 8. General circulation may improve (no cold toes and fingers in winter) and skin commonly feels warmer to the touch. Your heart is working much harder. If you are fit and have a typically good cardiac function, the increased demands will be easily accommodated but you may sometimes feel a little breathless.

Veins and arteries: Hormones cause the muscular walls of your veins and arteries to widen, thus helping blood to circulate more rapidly around your body. The valves in larger veins also soften and the internal pressure rises, and in some cases can give rise to varicose veins (p.559), most commonly in the legs or vulva, or to haemorrhoids (p.523) in the anus.

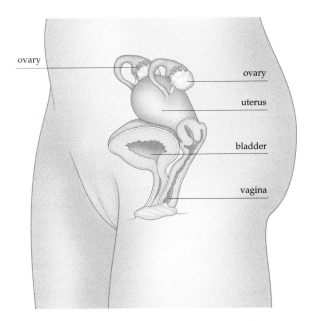

ovary

ovary
uterus
bladder
vagina

Blood pressure: In a healthy pregnancy blood pressure is similar to the non-pregnant level, but in mid-pregnancy it may fall slightly. A large fall in pressure with a feeling of faintness may occur if blood pools in your legs, perhaps if you're standing or lying on your back. High blood pressure needs to be closely monitored and it must be kept in check (p.410).

Blood loss and bleeding: During pregnancy vaginal bleeding (p.406) may indicate a problem and it must be investigated urgently.

Blood after the birth

Volume and haemoglobin: The volume of blood falls after birth, mainly because of the fluid excreted within the first week. Your extra red cells, however, are retained, so the haemoglobin concentration in your blood rises. This gives a boost after blood loss during the birth. Attention to nutrition and intake of supplements will also increase levels.

Circulation: Hyper-dynamic circulation peaks in the first few hours after the birth. Within a few days circulation returns to normal.

Veins and arteries: Following birth the elasticity of your veins and arteries gradually returns to normal. If you have varicose veins they should recede, though leg veins may not disappear completely. During the first few days, when the blood-clotting system is at maximum coagulation, there is a risk of thrombosis (p.560). Postnatal exercise and support stockings can prevent this.

Blood loss and bleeding: After birth you will lose blood, whether the birth has been vaginal or caesarean, as your uterus sheds its lining and contracts. This is like a very heavy period to begin with. Bright red for the first few

weeks, it should turn reddish-brown and reduce in quantity, and finally turn pale pink or yellow. Loss usually continues for around 4–6 weeks after birth, but may last up to 9 weeks. If you pass clots after birth, blood loss continues to be very heavy after the first week or the discharge has an unpleasant odour, consult your doctor. Heavy blood flow or clots may indicate retained placental tissue (p.407).

Uterus and ovaries in pregnancy and birth

The uterus (womb): Your uterus is shaped like a pear and is situated between your bladder and rectum. During pregnancy it expands into the abdominal cavity and reaches from the pelvis to the ribs. The upper part, the body of the uterus, is linked to the ovaries and the fallopian tubes; the lower part is the cervix. Your uterus is supplied with an abundant source of blood throughout pregnancy to nourish your placenta and baby.

The ovaries: Two almond-sized ovaries are located on each side of your uterus, deep in the pelvis and safe from injury. As you developed in your mother's womb, around four million eggs were produced and stored in your tiny ovaries. By the time you began menstruating, this number had dropped to five hundred thousand and of these, about five hundred will ovulate before menopause.

As well as harbouring eggs, your ovaries act as an endocrine gland and produce some of the hormones, including oestrogen and progesterone, that are essential for ovulation and conception. For 6–10 weeks after fertilisation, ovarian hormones maintain your tiny but rapidly growing foetus. Low levels of progesterone from the ovary may lead to miscarriage at this early stage of pregnancy.

Fallopian tubes: The fallopian tubes extend from your uterus towards the ovaries. During ovulation the egg is released from your ovary into one tube: when this meets a sperm and the two fuse, the tiny cell cluster that will later grow into your baby is nourished by cells lining the tube as it is wafted along to your uterus (p.13).

The uterine body: The upper two-thirds of the uterine body contain most of the smooth muscle fibres, which move and contract involuntarily, much like the walls of blood vessels and the intestines. Inside, the inner cavity of the uterus is lined by the endometrium with mucus-producing glands that nourish the embryo; as the placenta forms and grows it remains embedded in the endometrium. The superficial layer is shed each month during menstruation.

During pregnancy individual muscle fibres increase massively in size and continually contract (as indeed they do during menstruation), but you probably won't feel this until the last weeks when they are known as 'Braxton-Hicks' contractions, named after the gynaecologist who first identified them. In labour, contractions (p.120) are at their most intense and provide the power that is required to dilate the cervix and to deliver your baby. At birth the placenta detaches from the endometrium as the uterine muscles shorten, thereby constricting the blood vessels to stop the bleeding.

The cervix: The cervix leads from the vagina into the uterine body. It consists of a hollow passage around 4 cm (1½ in) long, known as the cervical canal, surrounded by a criss-cross of interlacing fibrous, elastic and muscle tissue. It can be touched by the penis in intercourse but the uterus is mobile and it moves out of the way.

The glands lining the cervix secrete mucus; during ovulation this becomes watery to assist movement of sperm. In pregnancy the cervical canal remains shut and a mucus plug forms between the vagina and the uterus, preventing bacteria from reaching the membranes that enclose the amniotic fluid surrounding your baby. Throughout pregnancy mucus glands remain active and secrete a sticky fluid. In some cases the mucus plug, tinged with blood, may be passed in the days or hours before labour – it is called a 'show'. In the weeks before labour, hormonal changes and uterine contractions cause the tissue in the wall of cervix to thin and shorten, which is called effacing or 'ripening'.

During labour, the cervix opens as the uterus contracts. The first stage of labour ends when the cervix has opened and reached a 'full' dilation, a diameter of 10 cm (4 in), which creates space for your baby's head to pass.

The uterus after birth

After your baby is born, the placenta shears off and is delivered. The endometrial lining of the uterus, called the decidua, sheds away during the next few weeks. The muscle fibres retract and shorten and the uterus then shrinks significantly within minutes of the birth of the placenta – within 6 weeks of birth it will have returned to its pre-pregnant size.

Considering it took the uterus 9 months to expand, reducing so rapidly is quite miraculous, but it can be uncomfortable too. Contractions feel obvious as this shrinking process occurs and they may be more acute during breastfeeding, which helps the process, and with second and subsequent babies. The cervix often tears during birth and the external opening changes shape from round to oblong for ever. It is rare that the tear needs to be stitched (p.494).

The vagina in pregnancy and birth

The vagina extends from the cervix to the labia and is around 10 cm (4 in) long. It is supported by ligaments attached to the side walls of the pelvis, and by the muscles of the pelvic floor below. The walls touch one another and stretch during sexual intercourse and birth. During pregnancy the vagina has an increase in discharge caused

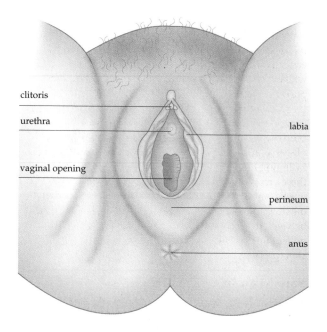

by secretion from the cervix; this may be quite profuse and is usually white or yellowish in colour but it does not have an offensive odour. If the discharge changes colour, becomes more profuse or causes an itch or irritation, vaginal infection (p.556) may be present and should be investigated by your GP.

The vulva: The vulva is the entrance or opening of the vagina. The outer lips (labia majora) and the inner lips (labia minora) form the entrance, with the clitoris in front. The clitoris is the most sensitive area and its stimulation has a major contribution to orgasm. The back of the vulva extends on to the perineum, a fleshy area between the vagina and anus where muscles protecting the vaginal entrance and the anus meet muscles running from the side walls of the pelvis. During pregnancy and birth the labia tend to soften and become fuller and more sensitive and the clitoris may become more sensitive.

The vagina after birth

Tears to the vagina, perineum and vulva are reasonably common in birth (p.494) and may need to be stitched. Discomfort ranging from slight burning sensations when passing urine to a feeling of bruising usually passes within 2 weeks. During birth the vagina's supporting ligaments expand and the vagina stretches as your baby is born. Sometimes the ligaments may tear and this can lead to postnatal laxity, but they usually heal effectively. After the birth sex may be uncomfortable until the area heals.

Your abdomen in pregnancy and birth

Your abdomen covers the middle section of your body and

contains many of your vital organs – the liver, stomach, intestines, bladder and kidneys as well as your uterus. It is encircled by protective muscles, which provide power for walking, sitting and breathing and, during labour, for pushing.

During pregnancy these muscles and ligaments expand to accommodate the growing uterus and help to protect the vertebrae of the spine. Hormones alter the physiological function of many of the abdominal organs, including the stomach, the intestines and the bladder, and these organs come under increasing pressure. By the later weeks of pregnancy this can cause discomfort. From the outside you will see your abdomen getting larger from between the second and fourth months and you may also notice stretchmarks and dark coloration forming on the skin (p.43).

Your abdomen after birth

Your abdomen won't return to normal overnight. In fact, you may look 3 or 4 months pregnant for some weeks after birth: your abdomen will only gradually shrink and the skin around your middle may remain floppy for a long time. Breastfeeding, good nutrition and gentle postnatal exercises will help you tone up.

Some women regain their shape remarkably quickly, but it usually takes 6 months, or even a year, to return to normal. Remember that exercise is better than dieting, and your newly rounded figure is natural and becoming for a new mother.

Your breasts

One of the first things you may notice when you become pregnant is a change in your breasts – they will probably become fuller and feel warm and heavy, and may be more sensitive. Your nipples may enlarge and the areola (the skin around the nipple) may become darker. Small glands – Montgomery's tubercles – may become noticeable in the areolae; these glands secrete oils to keep the skin soft and supple. As blood supply increases, you may also notice more prominent veins in your breasts and stretchmarks might appear.

Beneath the surface milk ducts and milk-producing cells increase and growth is quite dramatic. Towards the end of pregnancy, colostrum may appear in droplets on your nipples; it is a yellowish fluid that will be the first food for your baby. Although your breasts need support as they grow – you may jump a few sizes – they'll also benefit from being open to fresh air, so spend some time each day naked if possible.

After birth your breasts are ready to feed your baby with milk that is perfectly suited to his needs (p.186). Your breast milk is produced in mammary glands in response to your baby: his sucking indicates how much he wants to drink and when. In the first days after birth your breasts

produce colostrum, which is loaded with antibodies and is extremely rich in protein and sugar for energy. The colostrum also has a laxative effect that helps your baby expel the mucus and fluid that have built up in his digestive tract as meconium.

Frequent sucking stimulates your breasts to produce the transitional milk that comes in 1 or 2 days after the colostrum and is rich and creamy. Gradually the protein and antibody content of this milk reduce and after around 2 weeks your breasts begin to produce mature milk. This still varies in constituency and rate of flow that is determined by how often and for how long your baby sucks. Breastfeeding may feel uncomfortable from engorgement or sore nipples: these difficulties are, on the whole, easily remedied (p.412).

Breathing and lungs

During pregnancy extra oxygen is required to supply the increased number of red blood cells. You may notice breathlessness, particularly in late pregnancy when the enlarged uterus presses on the diaphragm and reduces space for lung expansion. You will tend to compensate by increasing how often you breathe. Exercise or regular breathing practice linked with yoga postures will help you to breathe deeply, give plenty of oxygen to your baby, and eliminate carbon dioxide effectively. Occasionally, the uterus may cause pain in the lower ribs – more common if your baby's limbs are under this area. During birth you will be guided to focus on your breath as you ride through contractions (p.154). After the birth your chest will regain its full range of movement and infections usually clear up. If you have been carrying twins or a very large baby, your ribs may feel slightly tender over the next few days when you breathe deeply.

Your spine in pregnancy and birth

The spine extends from the neck to the pelvis and is protected by muscles and ligaments. It consists of 24 bones (vertebrae) linked by spongy inter-vertebral discs that allow it to flex and move without jarring. At the base the vertebrae are fused to form the strong wedge-shaped sacrum, which forms the back wall of the pelvis and ends in the coccyx, or tailbone. The weight of the upper body is transmitted down the spine through the sacrum to the hips and legs. The spinal column protects the spinal cord and the nervous system – if the vertebrae are out of alignment the nerves may be irritated, causing pain and poor function of the muscle or organs supplied. Everyone's spine is naturally curved. During pregnancy this curvature becomes more pronounced to support the weight of the growing uterus.

Your spine after birth

After birth the curvature of your spine gradually becomes

less pronounced and the vertebrae are realigned in a process that may take from 6 to 12 weeks. Take it easy, remember your posture when sitting, feeding, lying, walking, lifting and feeding your baby, and do gentle exercise (p.357).

Your pelvis in pregnancy and birth

Your pelvis is a very strong and uniquely expandable support for your body and for your growing baby. Shaped like a funnel, it connects with the bottom of the spine and houses the lower part of your abdomen. The sacrum and coccyx sit at the back between the two hip bones. All these bones meet at joints, the two sacro-iliacs at the back and the pubis in the front, which are bound together by ligaments.

The pelvic area also contains around 36 pairs of muscles and is a crucial meeting point for most of your body's major muscles – they run up to the neck and head, around the abdominal wall, down through the thighs and legs and around the base of the pelvis, which is known as the pelvic outlet.

During and after pregnancy you will be particularly in touch with your pelvic floor muscles, which run across the base of the pelvis and meet at the perineum, midway between the anus and vagina. These muscles give support

and also help to keep the openings of the vagina, urethra, which runs from your bladder, and anus, which runs from your bowel, closed during normal activity.

The curved pelvic canal protects your uterus until about Week 12 of pregnancy, after which your uterus emerges from the pelvic cavity, although it is still supported from below. Your pelvis tilts forwards so the weight of your growing baby presses on your abdomen rather than on your pelvic area. Hormones soften and stretch muscles and ligaments so that the joints become flexible enough for your baby to pass through the birth canal – these changes may cause pelvic pain (p.519). The most important movement that becomes possible during birth is the pivotal action of the sacrum, which can move backwards, and in an upright position (squatting) the outlet of the pelvis can increase in area by up to 30%. If you are lying down, your weight on the sacrum reduces the space within the canal and your baby's journey may be more difficult.

Before birth your baby's head may 'engage', or enter into, the pelvic inlet with the widest diameter of the head lying below the widest part of the inlet. During birth the pelvic floor muscles relax and, as your baby's head passes through, they are pushed against the side walls of the pelvis.

Your pelvis after birth

Within 24 hours hormone levels alter so that ligaments and muscles around the pelvic region begin to firm up, joints become less flexible and your pelvis closes over the next few weeks. If you had pelvic pain in pregnancy, it usually disappears soon after birth. However, it is common for ligaments and muscles, particularly those in the pelvic floor, to be stretched during birth, and the nerves that run on the side wall of the pelvis can be bruised. These may take months to heal and strengthen, during which time bladder control may be reduced; pelvic floor exercises help improve muscle tone and healing (p.98).

Muscles, ligaments and joints

The body has two types of muscles – voluntary and involuntary. The internal organs, including the digestive system, the bladder and the uterus, consist of involuntary smooth muscle that is not under conscious control – it is not possible, for example, to make the uterus contract. By contrast, the pelvic, back and abdominal wall muscles are under voluntary control.

Pregnancy hormones relax the muscle fibres, which stretch as ligaments stretch. The expanding uterus and curving vertebral column stretch and alter the tension in the muscles of the back, abdomen and pelvis. These profound changes mean the body alters every day – some pregnant women feel discomfort in the muscles or adjacent joints.

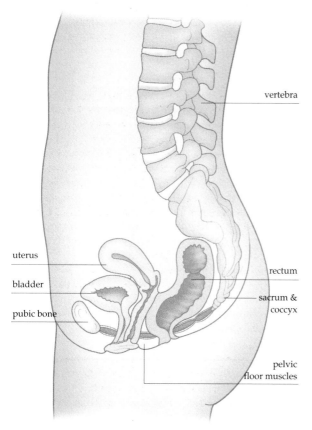

vertebra

uterus

bladder

pubic bone

rectum

sacrum & coccyx

pelvic floor muscles

Soon after birth a reduction in hormonal levels stops the ligament-softening process and aids a return to normal tension. You may feel temporary discomfort in the joints of your back and pelvis and even around the rib cage. Persistent pain suggests that yoga or osteopathic treatment is needed; this will be most effective in the first few weeks before ligaments toughen.

Muscles soften during pregnancy, and some stretch during labour and birth – most notably the vaginal and pelvic floor muscles. If the rectus or strap muscles, which run from the lower ribs to the top of the pelvic bone on either side of the navel, stretch they may take months to come together once again: in some cases they remain separated.

After birth you will need to protect your lower back and shoulder muscles, which worked hard during pregnancy and may be under too much tension from feeding and carrying. Try to sit and walk upright, change your baby's nappy and clothes without curving your back, stretch frequently and perform regular back-relaxing postures (p.357). Use a papoose to carry your baby and in time your strength will increase: bearing your baby's weight makes your bones strong.

Bladder, urine and kidney function
Your kidneys filter waste products from the blood that are transferred down the ureters as urine and passed into the bladder. The increase in blood during pregnancy means that the kidneys have more to filter, and urination becomes more frequent, particularly in the first 12 weeks and in the last 6 weeks as your enlarging uterus presses on the sensitive base of the bladder. Extra body fluid that accumulates in the tissues during the day is absorbed into the bloodstream and processed at night, which may make you need to urinate more when you'd rather sleep undisturbed. While increased urination is to be expected, feelings of burning on passing urine are not, and often indicate infection (p.552). After the birth urine flow will gradually diminish, becoming normal after about 10 days.

Due to softened tissues and ligaments, urinary leakage and incontinence (p.557) may increase in pregnancy: you may experience this when you sneeze, cough or laugh, or find that you can't hold on as long as you used to. Urinary leakage may continue after the birth if the ligaments are stretched.

Digestion during pregnancy
Pregnancy affects the entire digestive tract, from the mouth to the oesophagus, the stomach, the small and large intestines (colon and rectum) and the anus. Hormones relax the smooth muscle in the wall of the intestine, muscle tone is reduced and activity is slowed throughout the system, so you will probably feel full for longer. It may be more comfortable to eat smaller amounts.

Nausea (p.513) may occur at any time of day, though it is not experienced by all women. Changes in food and roughage intake and slow bowel activity may affect digestion (leading to indigestion [p.487]) and bowel movement (giving rise to constipation [p.437]).

Heartburn (p.487), an uncomfortable burning sensation behind the breastbone, is quite common due to the relaxed valve between the oesophagus and the stomach or to the increasing pressure of the uterus on the stomach, which allows acid from the stomach to leak back. At the lower end of the digestive tract pregnancy may cause distended rectal veins, which can lead to piles (haemorrhoids) (p.523), usually worse in late pregnancy and in the days after birth.

Digestion after birth
After birth any heartburn or indigestion usually disappears. The greatest effect of giving birth is felt around the anus and vaginal area. Combined with fresh memories of giving birth, many women are nervous about opening the bowels. There is, however, no danger of stitches breaking, and it is a relief when the first stool has passed without pain; it's normal for this to happen around 3 days after birth. If you pass excessive wind your anal sphincter muscle may have stretched excessively during labour and should regain its strength within a few weeks.

Mouth, nose and eyes
During pregnancy you may go off food you previously loved, or love food you never liked. Many women describe a metallic taste on the tongue, which may be relieved by taking mineral supplements. If you find yourself salivating profusely in pregnancy, rest assured that this will stop after you have given birth.

The increased blood flow of pregnancy may cause your gums to swell and they may bleed easily during brushing. Brushing releases food trapped between teeth and gums, which can cause inflammation and gingivitis (p.540). A high-fibre diet also helps.

Many women enjoy a heightened sense of smell during pregnancy. Pregnancy can also cause an increase in mucus production and swelling of the nasal membranes – stuffiness can begin from conception and it may be very difficult to treat. Coughs, colds and sinusitis often take longer to resolve (p.442).

The lens of the eye can swell with fluid during pregnancy and this may alter the quality of vision. This effect disappears after the birth and new spectacles are not necessary. The cornea on the outside of the eye may also swell and make contact lenses difficult to wear until after the birth.

Skin during and after pregnancy

Colour and fullness: As a result of increased blood volume your skin may take on a ruddy glow. Sometimes blood vessels become visible as red spots or as flushes, particularly in the cheeks, and you might get minor acne (p.534). Extra fluid gives your skin fullness and your face may appear rounder. As production of melanin increases, it is common for skin to darken in places – most noticeably down the centre of the abdominal wall, in a line from the pubis to the belly button. Your face may appear suntanned, particularly around the mouth (called a 'pregnancy mask' or cloasma), and nipple skin will darken. Freckles and moles may darken and enlarge. Discoloration takes a few months to fade, but traces may remain.

Warmth: Your skin acts as a radiator of heat and is one of the ways your body maintains a regular internal temperature. During pregnancy the blood flowing to the skin increases sixfold. You'll probably feel warmer, but your body temperature is maintained by an increase in perspiration. The pores in your skin that allow heat to pass away from your body are also able to absorb creams and you may want to check the contents of any lotions you use.

Stretchmarks: Not everyone gets stretchmarks – whether you do depends on your physiology. Although massage is soothing it probably does not help, but natural oils do have nourishing properties. Reddish streaks may appear on your breasts, abdomen and buttocks. The stretched skin may take many months to recede as the elastic tissue is reorganised and some stretchmarks will remain, although they fade considerably.

Hair during and after pregnancy

During pregnancy the condition of your hair may change, probably exaggerating your normal state (greasy or dry). Avoid perming and colouring with chemical products; if you want to liven yourself up, use natural henna for colour. Your hair may darken, and its growth may slow down, but baldness is not a result of pregnancy. After birth or perhaps when you stop breastfeeding, your hair may thin and more than usual may fall out when you brush or wash it. This is because growth slows during pregnancy and when the follicles resume growth, new hair develops from the roots and old hair comes out. Provided you are adequately nourished with vitamins, minerals and iron, your hair will return to normal.

Your weight

Weight increase is inevitable and important during pregnancy and will reflect your baby's size, your own physiology and the way you eat. After birth many women do find it difficult to return to their pre-pregnant weight, but with close attention to nutrition and exercise this is usually possible. There is an overview of weight gain on p.332 and a close look at eating and weight problems in the A–Z Health Guide on p.455.

Energy

Many women bloom throughout pregnancy, shine with health and feel better than ever before. Most women experience fluctuations and it's common to feel most energetic in the middle 3 months and in the last days before labour.

Many pregnant women discover amazing stamina: walking and swimming may become easier. During labour the additional fat stores in your body help to maintain your energy for a long time, particularly if you are physically fit.

Pregnancy can, however, cause fatigue (p.544), particularly during the early months and in the last few weeks as birth draws near, and you are likely to become more tired if you are emotionally stressed or confused. Spurts of get-up-and-go may be followed by fatigue and early nights. Altered sleeping habits are universal. You may go to bed earlier, have vivid or disturbing dreams or sleep for fewer hours at a stretch, although the quality of sleep may improve. In late pregnancy pressure of your growing uterus, breathlessness, heartburn and urinary frequency can all lead to broken sleep – perhaps this is nature's way of preparing you for the first months of infancy.

After the birth you'll need to rest and recover. Breastfeeding can be tiring, as can broken sleep, and most mothers underestimate how the emotional demands of parenting affect energy levels. Despite cumulative tiredness many women find reserves of energy and an unexpected tolerance to lack of sleep. You can help yourself to get more sleep by asking others to help out with some babycare: every bit of rest you get will have a positive effect on your moods and on your baby. You may also feel more energetic if you eat well, exercise regularly, rest well and attend to your emotional needs: in short, care for yourself (p.51).

Amazing mind and feelings

The way the physical and emotional aspects of your life are entwined is exaggerated during the primal period: your body affects your feelings, and your feelings affect how your body functions. The hormones of pregnancy and feeding affect the way your brain functions and your emotions alter.

The changes in your mind are as normal as the more visible changes to your body. The rational aspect of your personality recedes and the emotional aspect strengthens, as part of nature's preparation for becoming a parent. The 'love hormones' exert a profound effect on the way you mother your baby. The feelings may be wonderful or they may be difficult to live with, and sometimes can be quite confusing. Unexplained tears, intense joy, nesting urges, sadness, disturbing dreams, feelings of fear and anger may come and go with no rational pattern. Your emotional ride is an essential aspect of your pregnancy, however, as it helps you to care for both your baby and yourself with self-awareness and confidence. Pregnancy often brings change and you may find that you become less rational and forgetful: this 'cheese brain' is transient and memory always returns to normal.

During labour and birth your state of mind may help you act instinctively. In the moments and days after birth you may enter a state of euphoria. As well as the joy at seeing your very own baby, and the relief of having completed pregnancy and birth, your body is flooded with the hormones that promote this loving, maternal frame of mind. When hormone levels drop in the first week, you may feel blue and tearful. If you are breastfeeding, some of the hormones will remain at higher levels and you may feel more emotional than rational until feeding comes to an end. Caring for a new baby is extremely demanding and women vary in their response; you may drift along, you may feel normal and energised or you may feel low. Changes to your mind may be more lasting than bodily changes. Part of the magic of the primal period is that you are stepping from one phase of life to another, leaving the 'old' you behind and taking on the 'new' mantle of motherhood. How you see the world will continue to change and mature as you learn more and more about yourself and about your child.

Your body image

Every woman is different and body image comes from the inside as much as from the outside, and the emotions of pregnancy and parenthood, both positive and negative, can have a significant impact. During pregnancy the presence of a baby in your womb may make you feel loved and cared for. At birth many women feel they have lost part of themselves. If you feel upset or have a sense that you've 'lost' your identity, your self-image could fall.

An expanding body upsets other women and some worry that they will never be the same again, perhaps imagining that a flabby housewife will replace a sexy woman. Your physique may never return to the exact state it was in before your bore a child: this may mean that there's a marked improvement in your figure and stature

or that there are new curves that could take time to get used to.

Physical factors that contribute to shifts in body image include changes in shape and weight, tiredness and less time available for looking after yourself. Many women enjoy having larger breasts, and most adore breastfeeding their babies, whether this is for a few days or several months. Even so, there's often an underlying worry that breasts will be small or droopy when feeding is over, and it's common to feel that they are not sexual while being used for feeding. Weight changes, which can sometimes be extreme, can completely change your view of yourself and if gain is large, body image can be badly effected.

Sometimes a woman's partner may affect her body image with his reaction: some men love a full and voluptuous child-bearing woman, some miss the slimmer version. Stretchmarks, varicosities or skin flabbiness may make you upset. Less visible, but not necessarily less important, are changes to the genitals. Your vagina may be sore or stretched after birth and while the physical effect is usually temporary the emotional ripples may last much longer, and it may feel like the return to normal will never happen.

Becoming a mother has a huge affect on the way you perceive yourself regardless of physical change. Feeling tired or in pain can leave you feeling upset and if you haven't found time for a shower, your clothes are stained with baby sick or you've nothing flattering to wear you may not feel good about yourself. Luckily there are many ways to keep you, your body-image – and your self-esteem – more up than down and throughout the book there are tips on caring for yourself.

Amazing spirit

You might find that pregnancy, birth and mothering bring much deeper changes to your life than those evident in your body and moods. The feeling of a new being growing within can bring awe and respect for the miracle of life and a wonder at the way nature works. Birth and life, along with dying and death, are among the most mysterious and most oft discussed issues in human history and form the basis for beliefs and rituals all over the world. Humans can often be complacent about being alive, but it's harder to remain distanced when new life is flowing through you and appears before your very eyes with a power far beyond touch, vision or speech.

The side of you that cannot be explained by scientists or doctors may undergo a significant transformation, ranging from renewed devotion in your own faith to an exploration of philosophies and myths that you may never otherwise have noticed or enrichment through meditation (p.370). The curiosity nurtured by pregnancy and the connection to the power of birth and renewal could open doors to an interesting and exciting spiritual journey.

Amazing dad

There's hardly a man on the planet who doesn't feel a sense of pride when he learns he's 'got what it takes' to get his woman pregnant. After making love your sperm has fertilised an egg and you join your partner on the journey of pregnancy and birth, meet your very own child and become part of a new family.

Being a father

It's actually very common for men to develop symptoms during the months of their partner's pregnancy, ranging from backache to insomnia, that resemble those of a pregnant woman. This is called the 'couvade' and reflects the psychic connection a father can have with his baby and his partner. It's even more common for new dads to become besotted and fall deeply in love with their newborn babies, and to play a very active role in babycare.

It may seem that the spotlight rests solely on your partner and your baby. Yet your part can be central to your family's balance and happiness. In the dawn of the 21st century, many western fathers are becoming more closely involved in all aspects of family life, from antenatal care to nappy changing, and this hands-on contact helps many forge a lasting and loving bond with their children. Nevertheless, society is changing and you, in common with many other men, may find parenthood difficult as the traditional role of supporter and provider mixes with the diminishing power of the father in society. Depending on your circumstances and your relationship, you may feel stressed and isolated or optimistic and supported. You may be full of confidence and enthusiasm or you may feel reluctant and daunted.

You and your partner

Although there are some parts of the world where a father-to-be steps back from everyday activities and is cared for during his partner's pregnancy, in most cases men are expected to support their partners as their growing baby is nurtured. If you are living with your partner you will almost certainly be called upon to fulfil this role, whether it be as a masseur at the end of the day, a messenger to find food late at night or an entertainer to talk to, cuddle and soothe your baby after the birth. You may be a house parent when your partner returns to work.

Your relationship with your partner may give you security and you might both discover new aspects to your friendship, your sex life and your family values as you travel through the primal period. At times the balance will swing and your partner will offer you support, love and guidance as you contemplate your future as a father. If you encounter difficult challenges or rocky patches, we hope that you will find some guidance from the relevant chapters in Part IV of this book.

You and your baby

Though you do not carry your growing child inside you, your role as an essential player in your baby's life begins in pregnancy. From the fourth month onwards she will be able to hear and recognise your voice, and you can soothe her in the womb as you talk and let her feel the pressure of your touch as you stroke your partner's abdomen. As you give your partner love and support through the pregnancy, your baby will also feel the benefits. She learns a great deal while she is in the womb and will become accustomed to your presence and moods.

If you choose to be at your baby's birth, you may be the first person to see her face and hold and rock her as your partner recovers from labour. She will recognise you by sight within the first 2 weeks of her life after birth and will know your smell even sooner than that. She will communicate with you in the way that she looks at you, as she relaxes or tenses in your arms and vocalises her needs with a cry. As the weeks and months pass, you and she may become more and more in tune with one another. The early months and years of your baby's life are very important and will affect how close your relationship is in the future.

Your amazing body

During this period, your partner and your baby undergo bodily changes that are little short of miraculous. Your input into pregnancy does not end with the donation of one strong sperm that races against more than one hundred million others to fertilise a waiting egg. During pregnancy you will be able to do more physical chores than your partner is capable of, particularly in the later months, and during birth you may incur strains and even bruises as you support her.

After the birth your bodily strength will once again be called upon. Whether or not you carry your baby, lift and bathe her, the changes to your life and an altered sleep pattern may demand a great deal of energy and stability, and you could be impressed by your own staying power. You may choose to join your partner in eating well and exercising as you embark on family life.

You and yourself

Coming to terms with being a father is a process that unfolds in stages. As you await the birth you will have

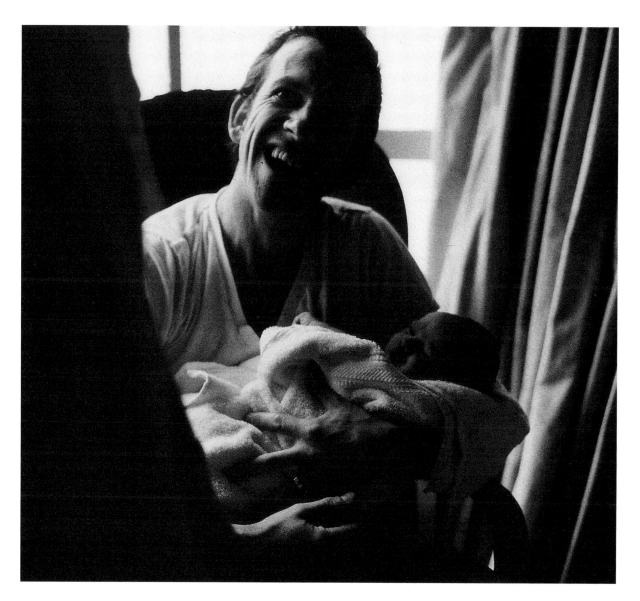

many decisions to make: How can you support your partner throughout her pregnancy? How can you give your best at work? How can you balance the demands of work and family? Will you be at the birth? What is your hands-on commitment after the birth? Each decision may add to the pride and strength you feel or deepen the pressure that mounts as you approach the unknown. This is all part of becoming a father.

You may also find that your relationship with your own father alters as you enter the ranks of parenthood. You will always be yourself, but inevitably there will be changes that alter your view of relationships, priorities, loyalties and commitment and enhance your wisdom. All of this you will pass on to your baby because you are one of her key role models.

The early days of your baby's life are precious, brief, magical and emotionally charged. Over the next 9 months you will watch as she learns to hold up her head, sits up, points and crawls, and at the same time she will also develop a broad range of vocabulary that initially only you and her mother will understand. On this road of development you will also grow because your baby is an amazing teacher. With her help, you will learn how to enjoy each moment and you will learn about the incredible power of love.

Although much of this book speaks primarily to women, you may be equally interested in your baby's development and care, and in the emotional aspects of parenting. This book is also for you, and has a special section on fatherhood (p.292).

Becoming a parent

Every situation, every partnership and every parent–child relationship is different. Some men and women become parents when they are in a stable relationship, and remain together. Some separate, some choose to parent alone, some plan their pregnancy, some become pregnant completely by surprise, some adopt. Every person comes from a different family background, and there is a rich tapestry of religious and racial cultures that gets more elaborate each time a baby is born and the next generation comes into being.

You and your baby

Whatever you and your partner's cultural, financial and social backgrounds, whatever your ages, when you have a baby you enter one of the most special and lasting relationships you will ever have. A parent's love for his or her child is multi-faceted – deep and beautiful, fierce and protective and without limit. This love may creep up gradually or it may knock you sideways the minute you lay eyes on your baby. It's difficult to imagine, and it's an amazing and indescribable experience.

Loving and feeling loved are two aspects of becoming a parent. Others are fear or anxiety as you worry about the future and you anticipate some of the trials and difficulties that lie ahead. Even if you planned to conceive and have looked forward to having a child, the realisation that you are to become a parent can be daunting.

Enjoying life with your baby is an ongoing process that depends on many factors including your baby's character and health, your personality and your reaction to the huge transition to parenthood, and the interaction between you. The message of this book is all about choice and commitment. Questions continually arise and there is no absolute truth 'out there' that defines how you should and should not behave as parents. Nor is there an absolute truth about how your baby should behave. There are simply a continued series of choices for you to make. When your decision seems right, you may repeat it; if not, you can try an alternative.

21st-century parents

In the past women had the role of bearing and raising children and were dependent on men; men were, by and large, the main earners and kept an emotional distance from their children. Childbirth was the domain of women and few men attended the birth of their own children.

Today more women have the benefit of education, independent careers, freedom to manage their own finances and control over their own reproductive cycles. Many see themselves as equals in partnership with men. Women mix work and parenthood more than ever before, and though they often take on the lion's share of childcare more men are joining in the daily running of the household

and many men attend the birth of their children. Some take on the role of primary carer and most turn their hands to nappy changing, bottle feeding and aspects of housework that barely any men would have considered doing 30 or 40 years ago. In the same few decades, single parenting has become less of a taboo.

The battle for equality has in one sense been won. Yet although many gender-specific roles have been overturned, new difficulties have been uncovered. The close-knit extended family is less common as both women and men tend to follow their dreams or their career choice and move away from their family base. When they have their own baby, at least one parent often misses the support his or her family might provide if they were closer. The juggling act between work, family, time for yourself and time for others can be tricky. More couples separate and it is now common for children not to live with both their parents and it is usually the father who leaves.

Role models

Whether real or imaginary, mythical figures can put pressure on you to structure your family and relationships. There are many mythical images of 'mother' around the world: Mother Earth, the Wicked Stepmother, the Fairy Godmother might represent the past ideas, while anyone from Anita Roddick to Madonna could represent current values. In the future popular myths will change again. Will women choose to mother without a partner, will babies be designed with the help of complex gene therapy, and how prevalent will be the idea that career is important, mothering is less valued? In your mind, is a man a saviour like Atlas, invincible like Vishnu or more of a David Beckham figure? Do the myths that you know portray men with feelings, as emotionally cut-off business types, or as stoical survivors or bullies? Do they value a father's involvement in family life?

You may see pictures of happy couples – famous or not – looking superb, feeling happy and energetic, emerging from hospital with huge grins and settling into parenthood without a hitch; breastfeeding is easy, the woman's body soon loses excess curves, the man loves being a daddy and still does fabulously at work, and both

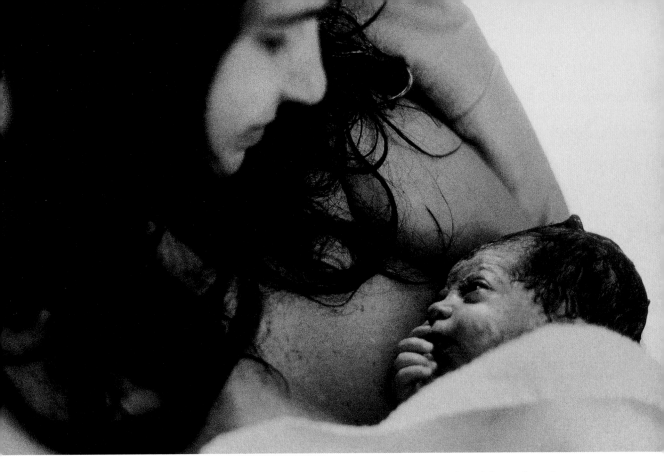

parents have time to enjoy lots of socialising and exercising . . . the myth is selective and ignores the more real aspects of life. Though the memories of pregnancy and early parenthood may be mainly positive, there may be upsets too. Almost all pregnant women have days when they resent their swelling body and lack of mobility. All births are painful at times. All newborn babies cry. All fathers can feel pressurised. All families have their sleep disrupted. All parents have to adapt their relationship as life gets busier.

Most people have an idea of how they want to parent. The role models who influence your hopes for your own family may be people you know or have heard about. Significantly, your parents, the way they cared for you and the way you feel about this could become increasingly relevant, whether you seek to imitate them or aim to avoid their mistakes. It can be fascinating to watch yourself evolve as you experience many of the things your mother and father went through when you were a baby.

Learning on the job

No one can teach you how to parent. There are countless guidelines, but no rules: what works for you and your baby may not work for someone else. Your greatest source of guidance will be your baby, who has many ways of letting you know how he feels and what he wants, and helps you to learn his language. Your relationship is not static and as

he develops and his needs and demands evolve, so you are always learning, just as he is.

Holding, soothing, feeding, dressing and washing your baby are skills you, like every parent, will learn through experience, and you may find valuable guidance from books, classes, your mother and friends, or professionals. After a few months you will have the equivalent mastery of a martial art black belt in these basic areas, and when it comes to assessing your baby's mood or calming his wails, there is no expert like you.

The learning that takes place inside may be more stirring, more exciting, and less predictable. Having your first baby means that you'll do a lot of things for the first time as you live in the moment, cope easily or with difficulty, and carry on. Your baby may help or sometimes frustrate you. His personality influences your pregnancy, the birth and the way he behaves every day of his life. He can be a great teacher and give you the most enjoyable or demanding lessons you've ever had in laughing, crying, listening, watching and loving.

Your feelings and the child in you

Everybody has a deep and private part – you might call it 'the real you' or 'your true self', your inner being, core or spirit. No one except you knows your every memory, fantasy, reflection, reaction and thought nor will ever know exactly how you feel about being a parent. Your mind is a mystery to others – even those who know you best – but, interestingly, much of it is also a mystery to you. Your unconscious mind takes up a staggering 99%, or more, of your brain. Here lie memories, emotions, assumptions, expectations and predictions that influence almost every decision you make without you even noticing. Unconsciously, you act in a way that reflects the culture of your family and the history of your race and, no less significantly, your experiences as an infant, as a child at school and an adult at work and at play. Your attitudes to discipline, eating, loving, intimacy, truth, flattery, anger and loyalty are all part of this.

Now that you're embarking on the road of parenthood, meeting a new person who is your son or daughter, protecting, guiding and loving him or her, this inheritance takes on a new significance. Knowing what it's like to be pregnant, to give birth and to hold your baby in your arms brings about a shift in consciousness that could make the unconscious more easily accessible. The hormonal changes of the primal period also have a profound effect in bringing feelings and emotions to the surface. Many people have glimpses in the form of feelings or memories of themselves being nursed or cuddled or disciplined by their own mother or father, and see their own parents in a different light. Some remember lullabies they thought they'd forgotten. Many people act like their mother or father did, even though they can't put their finger on any specific memory that confirms this.

As you welcome your baby, deep feelings may bubble to the surface, perhaps slowly and intermittently, or in a powerful torrent. Some may be vivid and wonderful, others may be frightening and upsetting and your emotions may move from profound love and tenderness to intense anger and upset, then incredible joy and sadness or longing. The feelings come and go, rise and fall like waves on the ocean.

At this important time nature provides you with a wonderful opportunity to get to know yourself better, revisit memories and see how your childhood and inheritance colour the way you live. These inner revelations may affect decisions about how you care for your baby and your approach to your family, other relationships and your work options. They can be truly empowering, and they can be confronting and frightening.

Becoming a parent carries an invitation to do what many of us may have resisted up to this point – to become aware of some personal emotional issues, and accept them. You may find it helps to see this as the first of many gifts your baby brings you: as you begin to acknowledge and deal with old issues you'll experience greater freedom and enhanced vitality. Not everyone does this easily. One of the roles of this book is to help you with advice and guidance to create and use a support network around you.

Your emotional awareness corresponds with your baby's own 'primal period', which comes to a close at 9 months when he begins to realise that he is a separate individual. This is one of the most impressionable times in his life when he looks to you for love and guidance and you look to him for lessons in life. It's a neat symmetry, an integral part of the magical parent–baby dance that continues to evolve for the rest of your life together.

The birth of your family

Your family is unique, and has an energy and life of its own that come from the way you all interact, with your baby revealing his personality more and more each day. Your family energy can be incredibly powerful – it can affect your decisions, your happiness and your future and will certainly affect your child's development. It offers rewards and can have its down sides. For some people the first 9 months are the most magical; others find it difficult and life gets easier and more fun when these months have passed. The first year after birth is a time when many couples feel their ability to communicate with each other becomes more difficult. We take a close look at how families develop and evolve in the chapter Families (p.276).

The birth of your first child could bring a dramatic shift in all your key relationships. A good way to start thinking about this can be to look at your partnership as parents. Before your baby was conceived, there was one relationship. With the arrival of your baby, the dynamics change completely. Now there are not one but four relationships: mother–baby, father–baby, mother–father and parents–baby. At the same time, your relationship with your parents may alter. Whether planned or not, having a baby is a declaration of independence as you change from being the child of one family to being the head of another.

Having a baby may help you to be more intimate and honest with others, or it may take up so much of your time and energy that other relationships become squeezed out. Some relationships may flounder and some may be rekindled. The most important for your growing baby and for your new family are those you have with yourself, your baby and your partner. Sometimes you may need to take a step back and ask if each is getting the time it deserves – this could prompt you to build a support network so that you can find the time you need.

You and your partner may have different expectations – you may come from different family models of thinking and backgrounds, possibly from different religious, racial or cultural environments, and you are individuals. Men and women often see things from a different perspective and they are subjected to different hormonal influences. Having a new baby highlights agreements and differences and one of the most exciting challenges is taking note, at times changing your own ideas and at times integrating the differences as your new family evolves (p.288).

Caring for yourself

From the moment pregnancy is confirmed, or earlier, you are caring for two. The way you care for yourself – physically and emotionally – has a direct effect on the child growing within you, and will continue to affect her after the birth. She will feel your hormonal shifts and physical changes just as you will feel the impact of her demands. For everything to go as smoothly as possible for both of you, in pregnancy and beyond, caring for yourself is top priority. All you need is a feeling that you're ready to enrich your life, and want to commit, little by little, to being kind to yourself.

Your physical health

It has been proved through countless personal experiences and intensive research that a woman's health and wellbeing benefit her growing baby while illness or physical neglect can have detrimental effects. Most women visit their doctor or a midwife when they discover they are pregnant and from this first appointment onwards their health is closely monitored. In pregnancy women who feel ill go to their doctor sooner than they would have before and many turn to complementary therapists in addition to their GPs. Minor complaints, such as coughs and colds, are extremely unlikely to affect your growing baby, but it's always worth discussing any worrying symptoms with a professional.

Terms used by your midwife, obstetrician or ultrasonographer or written on your records may confuse you. In Part II and the A–Z Health Guide medical reference terms for your baby's health are explained. In pregnancy you might be unsure as to whether your physical symptoms are normal or not. Remember that you can ask questions and if you go armed with some background knowledge you will find out more.

It's important that attention to your health continues after birth and you give yourself the best chances of remaining healthy through eating well, taking vitamin and mineral supplements (for suitable amounts to take during pregnancy and after birth see p.345) and exercising within your capacity (p.357). While most women do tune in to their bodies at this time, it's often dads-to-be who unwittingly neglect their own physical wellbeing. Men can find the pressure of parenthood quite intense, and traditionally view themselves as the supporters and providers in their new family. It is quite common for fathers to become overweight and lose their fitness, and for their self-esteem and body image to drop if they feel stressed, isolated and tired (p.292).

Emotional health

The way you feel on an emotional level affects your physical health and all your relationships. During one of the largest transitions in your life, emotional fluctuations are hardly surprising, nor are the new emotions that will surface. Even though having a baby may be the happiest period of your life, caring for yourself does not mean that you should aim to dwell constantly on cloud nine like a rosy-cheeked mum in a glossy magazine advert. You will be caring for yourself superbly if you take time and space to listen to your heart, to tune into your feelings, however powerful, unsettling or strange they may be. Some you may wish to keep to yourself, some you might share with your partner, friends or family.

Pregnancy and parenting are not easy rides for everyone. In fact, many women feel blue at some point in pregnancy, the vast majority feel upset after birth and some women find it hard to express or accept their feelings. If you feel down, reach out for support and a listening ear and remember that you are entitled to feel just how you feel, and you are not alone.

Your awareness

Travelling through pregnancy and parenthood is a new experience for all first-time parents. Suddenly your ears will prick up when you hear people talking about births and breastfeeding and you'll have a new awareness. Everybody learns differently and information is available in all kinds of guises: books, videos, novels, personal stories and first-hand experience.

Awareness in a meditation sense is being aware of your thoughts and feelings and still remaining calm, even if there is a storm. This can be hard to attain when, as new parents, you do sometimes feel overwhelmed and can find it difficult to remain aware of your own needs on top of everything else that's going on.

Listening

Listening is the most powerful thing you can do. As you focus on what is communicated, you then have the choice whether you wish to act on it. Information will come from many different sources. Primarily it will come from you. Often bodily symptoms reflect emotional feelings: when you are happy and optimistic, you glow with energy; when you are sad, melancholy or confused, you look wan and

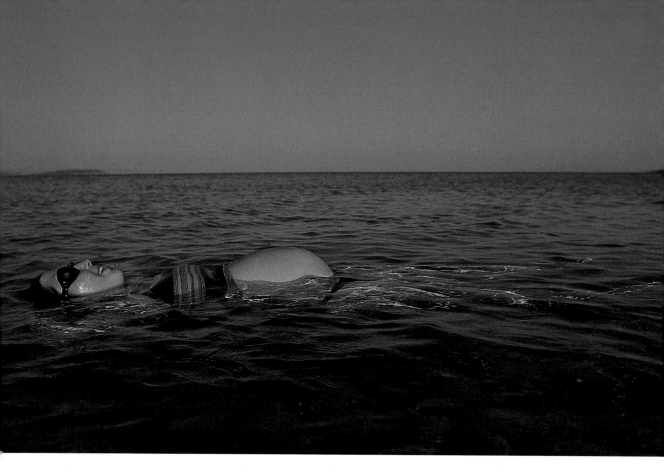

feel lethargic. The way you feel reflects whether you need to rest or exercise, and illnesses can often be triggered or exacerbated by feelings of sadness or dissatisfaction. One important aspect of caring for yourself during and after pregnancy is choosing to listen to the small voice within you. Some people find it easy to tune into their emotions and others find it hard.

It may be simple to go through life blocking your innermost thoughts and feelings until, that is, you reach a crossroads. Parenthood may be one such crossroads and at this time the more you listen to yourself, the more open you become to your inner strength and to new possibilities. What you discover about yourself is part of you, and being honest about your strengths and weaknesses is a good place to start.

There's a very important person in your life who makes her voice heard from early in your pregnancy: your baby. She sends messages through movement and hormones which induce a response in you, both conscious and unconscious. After birth she can communicate with you even more powerfully. Her cries are easy to hear but not always easy to decipher, and listening by tuning into her – her eye movement, body language, smiles and squeaks and patterns of sleeping, waking and hunger – is a crucial part of the learning process for your both. Her voice, opinions and inclinations, from the very first day of her life, are important and will influence the way you and your family settle down.

Listening to your baby is just a part of the whole, for it expands to your partner, your family and the other people in your life. The process is ongoing – it never stops evolving as all of your relationships evolve. For ways of effective listening, turn to p.290.

Eating

In pregnancy you may feel the need to eat well because you wish to care for the baby growing inside you. If your diet needs improvement it could take time to put nutritional principles into practice but every small change will give results.

Changing your diet for the better does not mean giving up everything you like and only eating bland food. The reality is quite different: a good diet (p.332) can be both delicious and indulgent, support a healthy weight gain during pregnancy and benefit your baby.

Once your baby is with you, the timing of shopping, cooking and eating will change, but continuing to eat well can aid your recovery and is a powerful way to get through tiredness. If you are breastfeeding, everything you consume is passed to your baby, and you will need to be as vigilant as you were in pregnancy as you monitor what and when you eat.

Smoking, drugs and alcohol

There's little dispute that smoking (p.535) in pregnancy can have a variety of detrimental affects on a growing baby, and that drugs (p.450) are harmful for both mother and baby. Drinking alcohol (p.391) is also inadvisable and heavy drinking can put your baby at risk of developing foetal alcohol syndrome. The occasional drink probably does no harm – it is ongoing consumption that is dangerous. Other toxins that are best avoided or reduced include caffeine and tannin (found in coffee and tea), insecticides and chemical additives (found in many processed and non-organic foods).

Exercise and rest

The human body thrives on exercise. It is designed to be active and activity maintains health. Movement and stretching also contribute to feelings of wellbeing: the buzz you feel when you dance, swim, go to the gym, walk or cycle is the result of endorphin hormones. Your unborn baby also feels these effects and exercise improves your circulation, promotes a healthy immune system and keeps the body's muscles, ligaments, bones and joints in good working order.

During pregnancy it may be difficult to find enthusiasm but even a short and gentle walk or swim can lift your spirits. Simple yoga stretches can powerfully energise you, even in a short space of time, and help you to relax and let go of tension. Yoga can also help you prepare for birth and focus on your baby. After birth, exercise and yoga will both help you to regain body tone and work gently towards your pre-pregnancy weight, and find time for yourself and a little balance in your day.

While your body is undergoing changes, it is vulnerable and while you are pregnant, so is your baby: heavy physical exertion is not appropriate nor is pushing yourself beyond your comfortable tolerance level. After birth, load bearing by walking with your baby in a sling is an excellent way to encourage your bones to lay down calcium and prevent osteoporosis (p.517).

Rest is the balance to activity. It is possible to get the most out of resting, just as it is possible to rest in a way that doesn't really give your body and mind the chance to recuperate. Resting at night is important, and if you find your sleep is troubled or broken, there are many simple things you could try to improve it (p.544). During the day, regular breaks can considerably boost your energy levels and your moods.

Remember that gentle activity can often be restful – a walk in the fresh air, a very gentle series of yoga postures or a calm swim are all good ways to give your mind a break and release bodily tension. You could combine these with visualisation (p.370) as you take your imagination away to a beautiful place or connect with your baby within, or practise some quieter meditations. These can bring

Relax while exercising

To enhance your sense of wellbeing, consider practising any of the following. Each of these areas is expanded later in the book, as indicated by the page references. As your body relaxes the mind follows – letting go of worries and anxiety and feeling healthy and supported are all part of relaxation.

- One of the gentlest ways to increase flexibility and bodily awareness is to practise yoga, a collection of positions and movements that gradually stretch and relax. The intention of a Yoga routine, whatever your standard, is to bring the body and the mind to relaxation, and you may find the philosophy of peace and acceptance is just what you need when you're in the midst of motherhood (p.346).
- Explore relaxation through cranial osteopathy, aromatherapy and other therapies (pp.376 and 378).
- You may find your thoughts wander more than usual in pregnancy and you begin to look more deeply inside yourself. A good way to focus on this is to spend a little time each day or each week stilling your mind through meditation or following a visualisation that calms you or brings you in touch with your baby (p.370).

about a state of mind that brings rest and makes you open to changing your view or overcoming anxiety. Like most things, the more often you try them, the more effective they become. Some women who practise visualisation during pregnancy slip easily into a relaxed and positive frame of mind in labour.

When you rest through watching television, socialising or reading, remember to keep an eye on your posture (p.346). If you sit or lie with balance, your body tires less and you are likely to relax more: slouching or slumping, on the other hand, may make you feel stiff, heavy and lethargic, and during pregnancy does not encourage your baby into a good position for birth (p.349). If you take power naps, your posture is equally important – a good firm mattress is ideal.

Complementary therapies

Complementary therapies may be used to enhance your sense of wellbeing and contribute to relaxation and a feeling of balance. As your body relaxes, your mind follows; as you let go of physical tension your worries may seem smaller. Massage is a wonderful way to relax, and in combination with aromatherapy oils (p.378) can address specific symptoms. For instance, some oils may relieve insomnia, some relieve nausea, and others can be truly revitalising. You could also use the essential oils in a vaporiser in the home.

Other therapies (see Part V) can also improve your energy levels, release tension and help you to rest well. These include acupuncture, reflexology, osteopathy and homeopathy. Each of these can work with physical and emotional causes of tension and as you work with another person you may feel supported and encouraged – this is also part of relaxation.

Your image

Many women form a new relationship with their bodies that lasts through pregnancy and persists for months or years afterwards. It is extremely common for women to alter their views of themselves at this time. Some feel admiration for the miraculous nurturing properties of the body and gain a new confidence and pride, fulfilled and empowered by the role and responsibility of parenting. Some women feel that their body has been overtaken and after birth it may be hard to regain a feeling of control. There are a wide range of physical changes that contribute to the way you feel about yourself and these are explored in Amazing mum on p.36.

It is very common for women to be unhappy about their own body image. If your self-esteem begins to fall, you may need to remind yourself that you are worth spending time on, and focus on things that can put you in touch with the positive aspects of your body. Exercise and healthy eating are an important step towards feeling good physically, from the inside out. You can help yourself feel good from the outside in by assessing your appearance. You may find it easy to do this alone, or need the honesty and objectivity of a good friend who can pick out the most flattering clothes for you and help you with your hair and make-up. Some people find it helpful to spend time looking at themselves in a mirror and trying to view their bodies without criticism.

Dressing up yourself and your self-esteem

Everybody has to change the way they dress in pregnancy, and most for months afterwards. The fashion you choose will depend on your preferences and the trend in your social circle, yet you can follow a few guidelines. Resist the temptation to swamp yourself in tent-like dresses or squeeze into things that are too small. Until the last few months you may be able to wear non-maternity drawstring trousers and tunics or buttoned shirts in your normal size. As soon as these get too tight, it's time to move into maternity clothes: non-maternity clothes two sizes larger than you used to wear will not flatter.

After birth many mothers stick with maternity wear and keep good clothes for special days – a new baby brings spills, stains and reduced ironing time, so comfortable and easily-washed clothes are best. Enjoy wearing your baggiest tracksuit pants at home. When you're feeling more lively or want to lift your spirits try things that emphasise your good bits and draw attention away from your less attractive features. For instance, tops with low necklines accentuate the face. If you have long, thin legs, an indistinct waist and flat chest, wear a short skirt or closely fitting trousers and a tunic top with a lazy neck line. If you have a pear-shaped bottom, large thighs and smaller waist, try tops cropped at the waist and loosely hanging trousers or knee-length skirts. If you have a large chest, vertical stripes across your top will make it seem smaller.

Sex and intimacy

Throughout pregnancy and the postnatal months it is safe to have sexual intercourse (except in early pregnancy if you have a history of miscarriage) but you may not always feel comfortable or energetic enough to relax into it; sex does become less frequent for many couples. But frequent or infrequent, sex is important in a relationship, and one aspect of caring for yourself and your relationship is acknowledging the role that sex plays and the changes that are taking place.

The level of intimacy in your life contributes to your self-esteem and confidence and is linked with romance, friendship, honesty and self-expression. Talking about sex is not always easy, though. The subject is explored in more detail on p.285.

Time to enjoy

Knowing that you'll soon have less time and more responsibility may spur you on to make the most of your relative freedom and in pregnancy parties, trips away, reading, videos or a new hobby can take a renewed appeal. The 9 months of pregnancy also present a good chance to practise organising your days and weeks. If you are already an expert at organising, then you need read no further. If you find that days run away with you, the spaces between seeing close friends and family get wider or there seems no end to work, you could probably do with a re-assessment.

Assessing your days

Let out a relaxed breath and take a look at your days. Consider whether your lifestyle gives time for indulging, perhaps treating yourself to a walk, a hair cut or a weekend away. Do you have time to be with your partner as much as you would like, or to meet up with your family and friends regularly? And how much time can you afford to sit quietly and focus on the baby in your womb?

It can be helpful to consider what is most important: a tidy house, a walk in the fresh air, a full fridge, a fun evening out, a good book, a completed work project or a visit to your relatives. Your priorities will change: in early pregnancy you may feel too tired to go out in the evenings; in late pregnancy you might want tidiness and order above everything else as you follow your nesting instinct; and with your newborn baby, time to sleep may be most important. And sometimes matters of urgency will dislodge all plans.

A weekly plan

A plan for your week or day can actually free up time, almost magically. By beginning with a list of things you need or want to do, you can see how you can fit them in over the week. Not everyone is a 'list' person, but you can do this in your head or talk to someone. Set realistic goals as this will reduce a build-up of unfinished tasks and ensure that you find space for things that often get delayed. Moreover, if you are easily able to meet your goals, you will feel relaxed and under less pressure, your self-confidence will be boosted and you can then be more adventurous. Allotting time accurately is a skill; many people are inclined to underestimate the amount of time they require to do something and some are so used to feeling pressured, they fill every moment and more. Consider making it easy for yourself by deliberately over-estimating how much time you need and only using phrases such as 'morning' and 'afternoon' rather than 10am and 2pm.

If something can't be fitted in, move it to another day; if something else seems to take up all your time, think about getting help or delegating. Once you are looking at the whole picture, you may notice that you're neglecting some key areas; very often these involve play and relaxation. On a positive note, your plan may show that you have more spare time than you imagined, and this can feel good.

Pregnant women and new mothers often tune into their feelings and their instincts very powerfully and can direct their energy well. It's equally common, however, to find it hard to concentrate, remember or see things through to completion. If you are disorganised – 'cheese brain' can strike at any time, and last for days, weeks or months – you'll need to take things at at least half the pace you normally would.

Quality time

You may have heard the phrase 'quality time' and perhaps you will wonder, 'How can time not be quality time?' During pregnancy there is a lot to think about and a lot to prepare, and after the birth you may feel pulled in many different directions. If you focus on one thing at a time, then you are giving yourself quality time. Having quality time is to enjoy the experience of doing what you are doing, from moment to moment.

If you are stressed you may find it hard to let go of anxiety over what you are not doing, and this can be made even more difficult if you are distracted by thoughts. Yet it is usually more efficient and more enjoyable to give full attention to one thing at one time. This is particularly the case when your attention is on another person and your communication with them.

Time for you, your baby, your relationships

While you are pregnant, quality time for yourself, which helps you to work, rest, play, dream and plan, also directly benefits your baby. Time for your relationship with your partner is also a really positive step towards a secure family base for all three of you. Pregnancy hormones and the impending shift to parenthood often inspire this, and it may come perfectly naturally. If you need to make a conscious effort, the practice will reap rewards after birth when you are even busier. Feeling loved will also prepare you to focus on your baby, who will respond to energy rather than words and know when you are distracted by other thoughts. One of the most important gifts you can give her is quality time to feel the emotions that teach her so much about life. It will give her a great start. You cannot give yourself to your baby completely and neglect your own needs, yet it is surprising how she'll respond to even half an hour of really focused time with you (p.178).

Time for work

The months of pregnancy provide opportunities for talking about short- and long-term work goals, financial requirements and the possibilities that may lie ahead of you. When your baby arrives there's little time to go over these issues, so bringing a few ideas to mind in advance is good preparation. The key is to aim for a balance between family life and work. Sometimes nothing needs to change, except for preparations for childcare. Sometimes a dramatic change in career direction can enhance the family energy and bring exciting, unforeseen opportunities. You may find useful guidance on p.320.

Time for relaxation and play

Playing is an essential part of life. But all too often this is the last area to receive attention, either because life gets busier after you've had a child or because play is not seen as a priority. Yet babies learn best through fun and play and this also applies to adults. Your baby will make you laugh on many occasions and she will prompt you to play with her and hear her own rippling laughter. All this will get your 'feel-good' endorphin hormones flowing around your body and consequently release your inhibitions – great ways to unwind.

Apart from playing with your baby, there are many opportunities for fun in other areas – at home as a family, with other mothers and babies, on your own and as a couple. You may need a strong commitment to fit playtime into your schedule, but playing often contributes more to happiness and optimism than rest and sleep. Life is sweeter when it has quiet and frivolous moments.

Your community

Some people never find themselves short of company or help. Others rely on a small group of friends and family, and those who have recently moved house may feel alone. Whatever your current situation, your community is potentially large. Think of friends and family, colleagues or neighbours, your midwife, health visitor or GP. Keep going – how about other expectant parents or new parents who go to antenatal and postnatal classes? Then there are people who share your interests and meet regularly at clubs, societies or courses; people who play games or exercise in your area.

You may crave company most when those in your close community aren't available, perhaps because they are working. Branching out and meeting new people is not always easy, but you will probably find that early parenthood is, in fact, a great time for this. You may meet other parents at classes or groups in your community or nearby and, if you think you'll get on, you could arrange to meet them again – perhaps at your house or theirs. Some of you may become close friends.

If going out with the intention of finding friends puts you under pressure, try to go to a class or meeting for what it offers and treat any friendships that develop from it as a bonus to enjoy. Many of the other women in the class may be in the same position as you and would value your friendship and support, particularly in the months following the birth.

Sharing your load

It takes many years to make good friends, but it doesn't take long to extend your community. Though you don't know exactly what help you'll most value until you have your baby, you can safely assume that your own burden will be lightened if you have support in some areas. Even help with the smallest things can make a lot of difference to what you can get done and how emotionally supported you feel. And for those who support you, whether it's your partner, your mother, your sister, a best mate, neighbour or paid helper, lending a hand may be a pleasure rather than an imposition. The very act of asking for support or advice can bring you closer to a friend or relative and give them a practical way to express their love for you.

When friends or family are around and willing to help, take them up on their offer, particularly after the birth. Many parents find it difficult to ask for help but there is no need to feel apologetic – most people fully appreciate what it's like to have a new baby and find that they enjoy giving and sharing. Helping out could make someone feel good, particularly when they are in the presence of a beautiful new baby.

There is a difference between inviting and enrolling someone to help you and coercing him or her to do so. It is best to ask people clearly and to accept that they may be unable or unwilling to help. Even if you feel disappointed, the seed may germinate and they may feel better about doing something for you later.

Before you ask, consider what other options are available, and this could relieve your anxiety about being turned down. When you are open to a 'no' answer, your tone and body language will convey this and you won't sound too forceful. If you are coercive, the person may feel upset or obliged and may find it difficult to do the task with a good heart.

Sharing your load is not just about coping practically – it's also about sharing your emotions; it can be a relief for you and a chance for someone to help if you talk about your feelings. Your mum or your oldest friend may not be at hand to change a nappy, and could be on the end of the phone to encourage you and listen to the daily run-down of your baby's development.

Knowledge into action

As a parent you will find that your natural skills shine. You'll also find that you have to learn a huge amount in a very short time and sometimes you may feel unsure about what to do or confused by a variety of advice. Transforming what you know into action, with and without the help of others, is a life-enriching tool that can help you to make lasting changes.

There is a difference between thinking positively and acting positively. For example, if you know that exercising makes you feel better, the next effective step would be to commit yourself to regular exercise. If you notice that too much caffeine gives you a headache, you'll know that cutting down on tea, coffee and chocolate will relieve stress; actually cutting down, and continuing to do so, requires commitment.

Every day you will make choices as new situations arise, both trivial and significant. Choices that concern your baby may bring remarkable and positive change to the way you interact in some of your key relationships. Learning about yourself, your baby and new aspects of practical life, and acting upon what you learn can, little by little, bring tangible results. Each small result may increase your – and your family's – comfort and happiness. Turn to the Wheel for Living overleaf for a practical application of tackling any areas of your life that may require help.

Dreams, expectations and reality

Awaiting the birth of your baby is a time for dreaming, and every parent has hopes and fears about what is to come. Expectations can be helpful as goals and as principles that guide your choices and decision. When the expectations become stubborn or inappropriate, however, or are pressed on you by others, they can become a hindrance.

As you enter parenthood, it could help to take a look at your expectations and accept that in reality there may be aspects that fit your dream, and you will also be taken by surprise. You might be optimistic, and feel an anticlimax if things don't work out as you hoped, or you may be apprehensive yet find that instead of hardship and problems, pregnancy and birth bring love and joy, and parenting is wonderful.

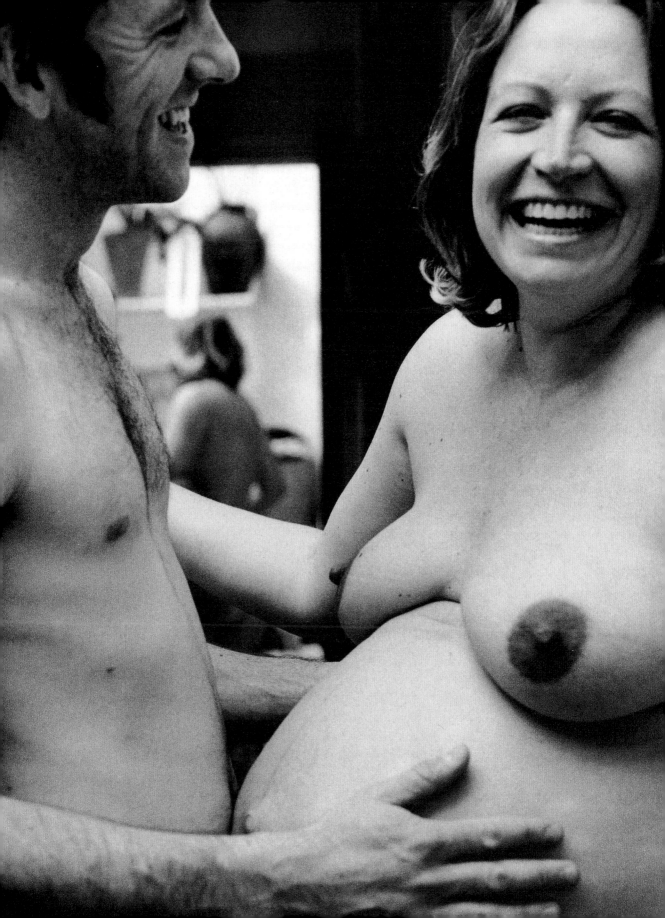

The Wheel for Living

Everybody needs different things to help them deal with a problem and there is no 'right way' to move on. The Wheel for Living illustrates a process whereby you can identify an issue and take steps to improve a situation, and takes account of practical, emotional and spiritual aspects. Progressing through all five stages may help you to find a range of new possibilities and realise positive change. As you do, this will help your confidence and you might reappraise how you use time. It is a practical guide and recognises there is always more than one way to solve a problem. Everyone faces problematic situations – from difficulties at work to coping with your crying baby, from unforeseen illnesses to conflict in a relationship.

Being realistic

It is best to start small and build up gradually. If you aim to do more than you can manage you will begin with a burst of energy but if you can't keep it up you may feel upset and abandon your attempts altogether. Small changes can and do have a big effect. It may be best to write down your commitment and review it, making alterations to suit your circumstances. It may suit you to begin in one area or to make small changes in a number of areas – for example, starting gentle exercise and learning about yoga or massage.

Be patient and bear in mind that all change has a growing time and some changes are easier to make than others. Feeling confronted or 'stuck' is inevitable occasionally. Sometimes implementing the solution takes years, yet each small step can enrich your life and in ways you may never have imagined.

It may take time and commitment to recognise the behaviour patterns that you have fallen into and to alter them where they are no longer appropriate. Sometimes this may require great courage as well as love and help from your friends and family, particularly if stepping out of your usual pattern means you acknowledge some difficult truths you usually prefer to ignore. The Wheel is neither exhaustive nor compulsory – simply choose what appeals to you and add your own spokes if you wish.

What's wrong ?

It helps to take time out to see how you are feeling and objectively look at what is wrong. This enables a problem to be broken down into smaller parts that are easier to approach. Use these questions to try to identify your problem and the possibility of change.
- *What is the situation that you are not happy with?*
- *What feels uncomfortable or wrong?*
- *How is your baby behaving?*
- *Is your problem related to your partner?*
- *Is the problem related to other people?*

Have time

Everyone has 24 hours in each day, and 7 days a week, yet time has a habit of stretching out when things are monotonous and flying past when you are busy or having fun. As a parent, the key issues are to be organised and remain flexible. Quality time implies being present with a good heart. To improve the quality, you may require support to reduce your feelings of anxiety about leaving things incomplete.
- *How can you organise your days and weeks to balance time with your baby, work, family and yourself?*
- *Could you make a regular commitment to your partner so you can go out together?*
- *Would it be useful if someone could help and free up time for you?*

Enrol support

Everyone benefits from practical and emotional support. Feeling supported is to feel loved and acknowledged and sometimes a new parent may need almost as much love and attention as a new baby. The person helping will also feel loved and needed, even if they are paid to assist. Your baby will get used to being in an environment with other people and will pick up on the benefits of loving and sharing. There are many sources of support – your partner, friends and family, work colleagues, community and professionals.
- *Who is available when you need company?*
- *Can you arrange a schedule for childcare with other parents?*
- *What does your partner need and how can you help one another?*
- *Who in your family is willing to help?*
- *Can colleagues at work help, perhaps by re-ordering their schedules or sharing tasks?*
- *Is there a friend or neighbour who might come to a class or start a group with you?*
- *Is now a good time to see a health visitor and ask about home help or childcare?*
- *Will your doctor help obtain emotional support or counselling?*
- *Can you find advice and answers from books, magazines, videos and/or the Internet?*

Eat well and exercise

There are many things you can do to improve your health and vitality, many boiling down to a good diet and exercise.
- *How does your body feel?*
- *Are you getting enough vitamins and minerals?*
- *Are you enjoying what you eat?*
- *Have you noticed the effect of exercising on your energy levels?*
- *What is the current balance between rest and activity?*
- *Can you improve the quality of your sleep?*
- *Where can you explore new ways of looking after your body or join exercise classes?*

Let go, take leisure and lie down

At the end of a busy day remember the ancient Maori saying 'What's done is done, what's not done is not done – let it be.' There are many ways to relax your mind and body. As you do so, consider that at this moment, everything is fine just as it is – there is nowhere to go because being here is perfect. When you start again you will have benefited from the break.
- *How do you most enjoy relaxing? It could be television, reading, meditating, cooking or listening to music.*
- *Are you finding time to let go and not think about all the things that need to be done?*
- *Have you tried some of the techniques in Part V (massage, yoga or meditation and visualisation)?*
- *Are there any complementary therapies that might suit you (e.g. acupuncture, homeopathy)?*
- *Are you giving your baby quality time to relax and enjoy playing with you?*
- *Does your partner have time and space to enjoy himself?*
- *Can you create the time and space to pamper each other?*

Jane's problem and action plan

It may help to follow an example of how the wheel might be put to use. It can be used in stages but the choice about which areas to pursue are personal. These are only guidelines and you would probably use different approaches within each stage if you had the same problem.

'I feel angry and tired. I'm jealous of my husband. I resent the fact that he goes to work and socialises like he always did, and he doesn't get up in the night with our baby. He thinks I have the "easy" job of caring for our baby. What can I do to make things better?'

What's wrong?

'I want to be acknowledged for the time and effort I put in. Looking after our baby and the house is difficult when I am not having much sleep. I need time to do things that are for me. I don't want to be like my mum – she always complained that she did all the work for the family, and my dad never seemed to help or compliment her. My husband and I are not communicating well. I want him to understand me and I'd like to plan things as a couple.'

Have time

'I have made a list of things I have to do, and allotted times – like sorting out bottles and feeds each morning, and washing clothes every other morning. My mum is going to help on two afternoons and I've arranged a Wednesday babysitter so I can have at least one evening out with my husband. I'll review how this is going in 2 weeks' time and see if I can make space for a yoga class.'

Enrol support

'I have spent time talking to my husband and he has told me how he feels. He would like to look after our baby on his own for at least one afternoon at the weekend and one evening so I can go out. I went to the parenting group that meets once a week. Already I feel less isolated. I'm letting go of blaming my husband for my lack of time.'

Eat well and exercise

'I have begun sleeping more, often when my baby naps and I walk most days with her. We are starting a swimming class and I have begun doing stretches at home – she plays beside me happily. I am asking about an exercise class geared towards mums with babies. I often forget to eat well so I am cooking larger meals and freezing half.'

Let go, take leisure and lie down

'I have decided that 7.30pm is my cut-off point when I have done what I could for the day, even if I haven't done all I planned to do. I am more relaxed in the evenings now and time with my husband is more enjoyable. Letting go at the end of each day helps me start the next day with a lighter feeling.'

The problem was: I was jealous of my husband's life outside the family and I felt trapped.
The possibility now is: I am no longer jealous, feel fulfilled by my own life and have a loving partnership with my husband where we communicate well.

W   **What's wrong**

H   **Have the time**

E   **Enrol support**

E   **Eat well and exercise**

L   **Let go, take leisure and lie down**

Russell's problem and action plan

'My baby is 3 months old. I feel he is being spoilt because my wife and her mother believe it is best for him to be fed whenever he cries. I feel discipline should start early.'

What's wrong?

'I want to have a say in how my son Aidan learns and I do not want him to be spoilt. My wife and I have different opinions and I'd like to reach an agreement – who is correct? I want to find out why my baby cries and whether it is right to feed him so frequently.'

Have time

'I spend an hour with Aidan every morning before work, and again each evening while Donna has a bath. I am really getting to know him. Sometimes I can't soothe his cries, but when I do I feel great. Donna and I have been out alone and it was really good – we're going to try and do it every Saturday night.'

Enrol support

'I spoke to some dads at work and read a bit about baby development. There are lots of reasons for crying, and no quick solutions but it helped me see that a baby is a complex thing, and so are parents! I now know that babies can't be naughty and crying is just part of their language. I am beginning to worry less about his crying and about him being spoilt, and enjoying learning about how we communicate with one another. I still feel that children need strong boundaries and discipline but I also want to talk to the health visitor and to my parents.'

Eat well and exercise

'My frustration made my body tense. Exercise helps me vent my feelings and I feel physically better now that I'm running regularly. I find eating little and often does not help very much – I prefer to eat widely spaced meals.'

Let go, take leisure and lie down

'I am finding home more relaxing because understanding Aidan better has made me worry less, and I'm no longer angry towards my wife. We have spent some nice evenings together, and I'm going out with my friends regularly.'

The problem was: I was troubled by my baby's crying and did not agree with my wife's view of discipline.
The possibility now is: My wife and I can talk about discipline and enjoy our baby to the full.

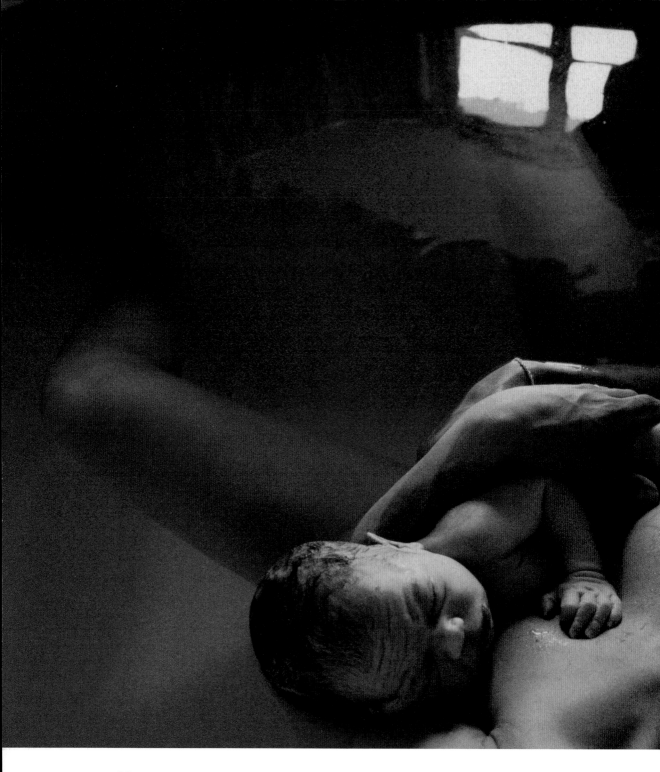

part ii **pregnancy and birth**

A new life within

The time has come: you and your partner have shared in creating a new life. How long can you wait before doing a pregnancy test? Who will you tell, and when? In the early days of suspecting and then confirming pregnancy you'll feel your heart beat strongly, through anticipation, surprise, excitement or disbelief, and your head will be giddy with thoughts. Whatever your hopes or fears, these early weeks will be an unforgettable start to your journey.

Symptoms of pregnancy

You may 'just know' that you are pregnant. Some women have powerful dreams and some men are the first to sense that something is different about their partner. Although you may have very few physical symptoms, it's likely that you'll feel different from around 2 weeks following conception. The first and most obvious sign is usually a late period. As the days add up, your suspicion will increase and other signs will probably become apparent.

Physical and emotional signs

Depending on your physiology, you may notice changes in the way your body looks, feels and behaves within days or weeks of conception. Your breasts may feel swollen, heavy or tender and already your bra might feel tight. You may find it hard to button trousers surprisingly early and within a month you may see a new softer, fuller shape. Pregnancy hormones can bring other changes like unusual or intense mood swings, the need to urinate more often, food preferences or nausea and changes to skin and hair.

Also common is a draining tiredness. Early nights will probably be the norm at this stage. Sometimes tiredness can be accompanied by light-headedness or weakness and a strong urge to sit down. This won't be made any better if you suffer from the dreaded morning sickness: nausea (p.513), often followed by vomiting, can strike at any time of day although it's most common first thing. This may be due to your body's reaction to pregnancy hormones, to underlying anxiety or a predisposition to nausea. Whether you feel sick or not, you might notice quite dramatic changes in your appetite, disliking some things and craving others – stories of pickled onion and jam sandwiches could begin to ring true.

If you have unpleasant symptoms you'll want to do something about them. It's true that not all nausea or tiredness can be eliminated, but a combination of small lifestyle changes could make a huge difference to the way you feel. Each pregnancy symptom, along with its underlying causes and various treatments, is covered in detail in the A–Z Health Guide.

Even if you feel physically fine you may be emotionally volatile. Early signs of pregnancy can be similar to premenstrual tension, with capricious moods and unexplained melancholy. You may also find that your dreams take strange pathways as your unconscious mind processes the news.

Testing for pregnancy

Today home-testing kits are extremely accurate. Within 7 days of conception, placental cells secrete the hormone human chorionic gonadotrophin (HCG) into your bloodstream and urine. All pregnancy tests detect the presence or absence of HCG.

Urine tests are able to detect pregnancy by the first day of a missed period. Depending on the type of kit you have bought, you will look for a spot, a line or a colour that confirms pregnancy. You can do the test at home and choose whether to be alone or with your partner or a friend. As you absorb the evidence, you can embrace the news in private, and feel free to leap with excitement or weep with disbelief.

I am really sure that I am pregnant, because I have several symptoms and my period is late. But the test is negative. What can it mean?

While positive results have over 95% accuracy, a negative result is more likely to be incorrect, particularly if you conceived late in your cycle and HCG levels are still low. If you are experiencing signs of pregnancy or feel strongly that you are pregnant, ask your doctor to do another test, preferably a blood test. You may be advised to wait another week before retesting.

Your doctor may do an examination but this is not as accurate as other means of testing. Your doctor will feel for subtle changes in your uterus, which will be larger and softer.

If your tests continue to be negative but your period still doesn't come, ask your doctor to rule out other conditions that could cause delay. She may advise an ultrasound scan as an important investigation. If you have an ectopic pregnancy (a pregnancy that takes place outside the womb, p.457), you will probably have symptoms such as a tender abdomen and spotting or bleeding. Although it is rare, an egg may have been fertilised, but HCG levels are low and the text is negative.

However carefully you perform a test, you might find it tempting to repeat it. You may want your doctor to confirm the news; some surgeries are happy to do this. If you need early confirmation of your pregnancy (after fertility treatment, for example), your doctor is likely to recommend a blood test, which is the most accurate method of detecting HCG but will take some time and expense to be processed by the laboratory.

Dating pregnancy and birth

Across the world women's cycles have been likened to the phases of the moon, and dates of conception and birth calculated according to its waxing and waning. The word 'menstrual' comes from the old English word *mona*, meaning 'moon'. Pregnancy usually lasts 40 weeks or 10 lunar months, each of 28 days; this is the equivalent of 9 calendar months.

You are experiencing a new partnership in which you and your baby share control: the date of conception relied on the release of your egg and its union with your partner's sperm, and the date of birth depends mainly on your baby. Even an expectant mother who can pinpoint the date and time of conception cannot be sure when her baby will arrive. It is now understood that although over 80% of babies arrive within 2 weeks of their due date, only 4% arrive on the appointed day and 2–5% arrive more than 14 days beyond the due date. The time of birth is determined by when you conceived and how your baby develops.

Using your menstrual cycle to predict birth

The usual system for establishing a baby's due date measures pregnancy according to a 28-day menstrual cycle. The first day of the last bleed is taken as Day 1 of pregnancy, and ovulation is set at Day 14. The date of expected delivery is 38 weeks after ovulation, which is 40 weeks after the first day of the last period. Of course, cycles vary widely: some women have shorter 3-week cycles, some bleed every 5 or 6 weeks, and others are very irregular. Thus to estimate your baby's due date you need to consider the date your last period began and the usual length of your cycle.

- For a 4-week cycle, add 40 weeks (or 280 days) to the first day of your last period.
- If your cycle lasts 3 weeks, add 39 weeks (or 273 days) to the first day of your last period.
- In a 5-week cycle, ovulation is likely to have taken place later, so add 41 weeks (or 287 days).
- If you know the date of conception, your estimated due date will be 38 weeks (266 days) after this.

Ultrasound scans to date pregnancy

Scans (p.80) are the most accurate way to date pregnancy and monitor the development and wellbeing of your baby. Dating is most accurate during the first 12 weeks when the prediction is reliable to within 3 days. As your pregnancy continues, scan dating becomes less precise because your baby's growth is determined by many factors. In the last 12 weeks the reliability widens from 3 days to 3 weeks. If there is a discrepancy between your dates and the scan, it is best to repeat the scan a few weeks later to get a more accurate prediction.

Absorbing the news

However much you've planned, hoped for or feared pregnancy, when it becomes a reality you may react in unexpected ways. Some women are surprised by the powerful joy that they feel, some don't feel the ecstasy they had anticipated, and some feel as if the wind has been knocked out of them.

Your feelings may change from day to day, not least because your hormones change rapidly and colour your reaction to the news. One moment you may want to jump for joy and sing to the rooftops, the next you may be weepy and feel a child-like vulnerability. Your relationship with your baby's father and his reaction will also be important. Some men experience an immediate attachment to their unborn child and embark on the road of pregnancy with vigour; others find it hard to believe. If you are both pleased and feel ready for the change, you will be able to celebrate together and plan excitedly for your future as a family. If one of you is happy and the other is not, you may feel upset. In the event that you and he are not getting on well, the idea of living together with a baby, or coping alone, will no doubt occupy your thoughts. The chapters in Part IV explore such concerns.

Sharing the news

It is quite usual for women to wait until Weeks 10 or 12 before sharing their news with any but the closest of friends because of the higher risk of miscarriage in early pregnancy, particularly if there has been a previous miscarriage. This can be a good and a bad thing: if you feel unwell or refuse alcohol, it's hard to explain without giving the game away. When you do reveal the truth, others can accommodate your needs; they'll be in a position to help you out and pamper you.

Pregnancy brings excitement and hope, and people may act as if you and your baby are up for public discussion. This can be a wonderfully sociable aspect of pregnancy but some women do not enjoy it.

It might be appropriate to tell your boss or work partner long before you tell your best friend, so that any altered performance or nausea can be explained. You may find support in the workplace, and once your news is out having a short rest each day could be respected. You may also wish to discuss maternity leave. Alternatively, you may be anxious that your job will be affected and attitudes will change or conditions be made difficult. You are not

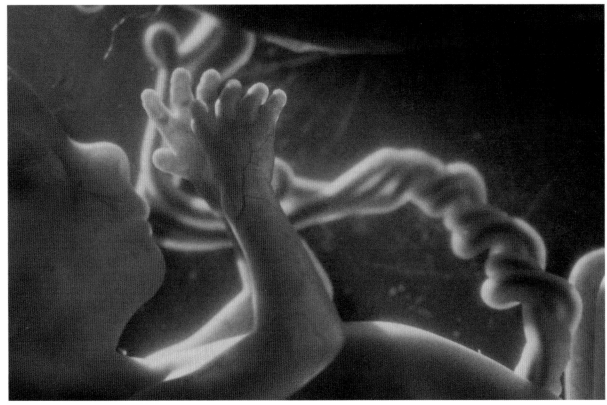

The whoosh of blood through the placenta and the umbilical cord is a constant companion throughout pregnancy.

Two weeks ago I went to an all-night party and got drunk on red wine and smoked quite heavily. Now I know that I was pregnant at the time I am worried that I may have harmed my baby. Is this possible?

You are not the first person to have partied in the early stage of pregnancy, and you certainly won't be the last. Although it gave you a hangover, your one-off binge is unlikely to have had an effect your baby. The risks associated with the use of alcohol, cigarettes and recreational drugs depend not only on how much you consume but how often (p.450). It is more hazardous to use small amounts for a long time than to have a single over-indulgence.

If you are very concerned about the wellbeing of your baby you may be able to book an early ultrasound scan to check his development. For yourself and your baby's wellbeing at this early stage, the best thing you can do is relax and wait. From now on, though, you do need to watch what you consume. The usual advice is to eat well, stop smoking, drinking alcohol and taking any recreational drugs during pregnancy. If you have long-established habits, you could be motivated to change now you are aware of the risks. A good example of this is requesting a smoke-free office at work.

obliged to tell your employers about your pregnancy during the first trimester although you do need to inform them as soon as possible if you are doing work that could be hazardous to your pregnancy (p.388). If you sense that your employer will be unsupportive, or even hostile, talk to other mothers or fathers at work and see what advice and support they can offer. You do have entitlements (p.323) and can make inquiries by talking to your human resources manager or your midwife or GP. If you have problems, visit your Citizens' Advice Bureau.

On the road of pregnancy

While your baby's genetic make-up is not in your control, there is plenty you can do to keep yourself well and fit during pregnancy, and optimise your baby's womb environment. It is important to start caring for yourself, emotionally as well as physically and, as soon as pregnancy is confirmed, caring for your growing baby, too. In the next few weeks you will become increasingly aware of your baby's power to determine your wellbeing, to reshape your body and your life. Little by little, you can introduce new ways to care for yourself and your family through pregnancy that will enhance your health and wellbeing in the long term.

Childbirth philosophers

Every woman inherits ideas, beliefs and advice from her friends and her family, which may have been passed down through many generations. There are also several dominant figures whose approaches continue to help women as they give birth and influence attitudes and preparations throughout pregnancy.

Robert Bradley
Developed in the 1940s, the Bradley approach emphasises a healthy active pregnancy, a natural intervention-free labour and the role of a 'coach' who guides a mother through the pain of labour. This may not be right for all couples; some women need pain relief and some fathers become over-focused on their coaching role.

Ferdinand Lamaze
In many parts of the world the name of the French obstetrician Ferdinand Lamaze is the most recognised in childbirth education. Lamaze believed that before birth mothers need to develop techniques to help them cope with labour pain. A trip to Russia showed him the value of psychoprophylaxis techniques, through which women are conditioned to cope with pain.

Lamaze childbirth preparation courses, popular in France and America, focus on: teaching about labour and birth, so women feel less afraid and participate in decision-making; learning to relax and use pain-relief techniques like massage and heat and cold, and rhythmic breathing to distract from the pain of contractions.

Frederick Leboyer
Another French obstetrician, Frederick Leboyer, focused on the baby's experience of birth. Responding to the belief that distress at birth will result in problems in later life, Leboyer developed an approach that minimises trauma for the baby. His 1975 book *Birth Without Violence* proposes that birthing rooms be welcoming places with soft lighting and minimal noise or movement. To comfort the baby after birth, he recommends that baby and mother have immediate skin-to-skin contact and that the baby be bathed in warm water to recreate the soothing watery environment of the uterus. Leboyer advocates the massage of babies and his ideas of gentle birth resonate with many mothers and health professionals.

Michel Odent
Michel Odent has played a key role in refocusing obstetric care. He believes that labouring mothers should be helped to release themselves from conscious thought and focus on their inner, primal self – a self that instinctively knows how to labour and which benefits from the body's natural pain relief, endorphins. He termed the hormonal release in labour 'love hormones' because

their effect is similar to that produced when making love. Together with Igor Tcharkovsky in Russia, Odent is the pioneer in water birth. At his unit in Pithiviers, France, Odent created a birth environment that encouraged women to labour without inhibition, using water for pain relief and birth and delivering in upright positions. Pithiviers enjoyed low rates of intervention. But Odent's views have often attracted controversy and despite increasingly clear evidence of the safety of water births, opponents remain unconvinced. Others find Odent's ideas challenging – he has suggested, for example, that women are able to labour more freely without men present.

Sheila Kitzinger
The British social anthropologist Sheila Kitzinger sees birth as a wholly natural and personal process, not a medical one to be managed by professionals. She believes that birth need not be painful, and has likened delivery to orgasm – when women surrender to the force of their body and abandon control. Kitzinger has campaigned vigorously for women's right to choose the kind of birth they want and their right to give birth at home if they wish and participate fully in decision-making. Kitzinger's passionate views have at times provoked heated debate; in particular, women who have suffered painful labours question her attitude to pain. Nonetheless, her contribution to the reform of childbirth services in the UK and elsewhere continues to be enormous.

Janet Balaskas and Yehudi Gordon
Responding to the highly medicalised approaches to childbirth in 1970s Britain, Balaskas, a mother and author and childbirth educator, and Gordon, an author and obstetrician, began to campaign on behalf of mothers. Balaskas introduced the phrase 'active birth' to express the belief that women need freedom to move about in labour and participate fully in decisions. Balaskas is the founder of the Active Birth movement and Gordon is the pioneer active birth obstetrician. Because western mothers face powerful pressure to accept a medical model of birth and are bombarded with frightening images, Balaskas and Gordon believe that women need support and education to recover their primal, instinctive ability to give birth. Janet Balaskas, together with Lolly Stirk and Meloma Huxley, initiated innovative use of yoga to help women focus on their calm inner self and strengthen and open their bodies in preparation for birth in upright positions. Gordon has demonstrated that active and water birth approaches can work in hospital settings as well as the home. Together with a group of like-minded colleagues, he founded a birth unit, now based in the hospital of St John and St Elizabeth in north London, which aims to provide integrated holistic care and a supportive environment for women to give birth as they choose.

The first trimester: Weeks 1–13

Feeling a child within you, hearing her heartbeat and sensing her spirit is a truly moving experience. You will feel your body change as nature performs one of its most fundamental and miraculous functions, and inside you your baby rapidly develops. This first trimester marks the beginning of momentous changes. You are totally connected with your baby every day and night, and your body nurtures this new life. Meanwhile, you will be thinking about practical issues that will face you throughout pregnancy.

Your baby and you

Your baby: Weeks 1–4

Two weeks into your cycle your partner's sperm reaches the centre of your egg, their nuclei fuse, and a single cell is created. This is conception. This tiny cell contains the genetic imprint of you and your partner and already your baby's gender, hair and eye colour and physical features as well as aspects of personality and intelligence are established.

Over the next week this cell divides and multiplies and travels towards your uterus. In the first week after conception as the cells divide, the embryo travels down the fallopian tube. The cluster of cells then embeds into the wall of your uterus by the end of the first month, 2 weeks after conception. The tiny embryo evolves into a flat disc no bigger than a pinhead, with three layers of cells. The outer layer forms the neural tube from which the brain, backbone, nervous system, skin, ears and eyes will develop, the middle layer will form bones, muscle and heart and blood vessels, and the inner layer will form the organs, digestive and urinary systems. Your baby has made an incredible journey from a single cell to an embryo. In some respects, this can be regarded as the most hazardous journey in her life.

You: Weeks 1–4

As you ovulate, hormones change mucus in your cervix, helping sperm travel towards your ripened egg and aiding passage of the embryo to your uterus after fertilisation. Outward signs of ovulation may be the effect of hormones on your moods, a heightened sex-drive and a clear or whitish discharge or slight pain. Your body temperature may drop slightly, rising again when ovulation has passed.

Despite fertilisation, your body releases menstrual cycle hormones as normal. But about 7 days before your period is due, additional hormones released from the developing embryo make oestrogen and progesterone levels from the ovary rise. These are responsible for the intense premenstrual symptoms that many women experience in early pregnancy.

Every woman's body reacts slightly differently to the physical and hormonal changes. You may have unmistakeable symptoms, sense that a period is due or feel nothing abnormal. Some people feel 'different' before the first day of a missed period, some suspect nothing. Common signs of pregnancy include swollen or tender breasts, feelings of tiredness and heightened emotions. You may need to urinate more frequently and you might feel nauseous, although 'morning sickness' is more common from the second month onwards. Some women begin to notice altered taste preferences very early in pregnancy.

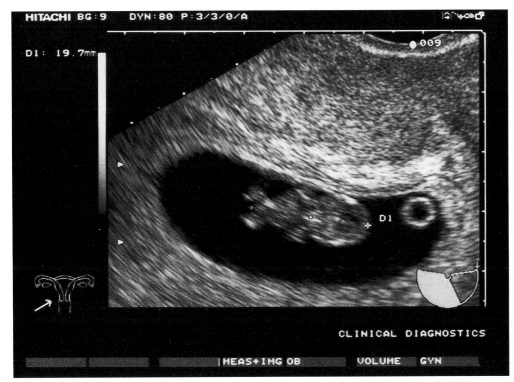

An 8-week ultrasound scan showing the baby's head to the right and early development of the arms and legs.

Your baby: Weeks 5–9

By the end of Week 5 your baby's brain and the rest of the nervous system have started to develop, a heart is beating and blood vessels have formed; and there is a connection to the developing placenta via a tiny umbilical cord.

Over the month, the embryo bends and curls and then straightens in stages that resemble the phases of human evolution. Initially it is the shape of a tadpole with a tail-like prominence at the base of the spine, later it resembles a fish and then a primitive mammal. Then facial features begin to appear: the ears begin as folds on either side of the head, there are openings for the mouth and nostrils and the retinas of the eyes begin to form. The limbs appear as buds tipped with nodules that will form hands and feet. The tail becomes less and less prominent until, by Week 8 of pregnancy when bones begin to form, the embryo is discernible as a tiny human being. At around 13 mm (½ in) long your baby is 10,000 times larger than the fertilised cell that floated in your uterus only 6 weeks ago.

You: Weeks 5–9

Inside your body, ligaments have begun to soften in preparing your body to bear weight and to expand and give birth. Your heart's output has increased by up to 40% to meet the additional demands of your pregnancy. One sign of this is the expanded network of veins supplying your breasts and abdomen. Your weight rises because you retain fluid in your bloodstream and in your tissues. Your breathing may be faster and you may feel breathless at times. Despite the tiny size of your baby, your body is extremely busy, and you may feel tired in the second month. This is one of the most common complaints in early pregnancy.

Increased levels of progesterone affect your digestion and you may experience indigestion, nausea, wind or constipation. Due to hormones and extra energy expenditure, your metabolic rate might have increased by up to 25%, causing you to sweat more than previously and feel hungry more often. You could feel tempted to eat constantly or you may feel nauseous and rarely enjoy eating. On top of this, hormone and chemical changes affecting your saliva may change your taste and you might go off, or crave, certain foods.

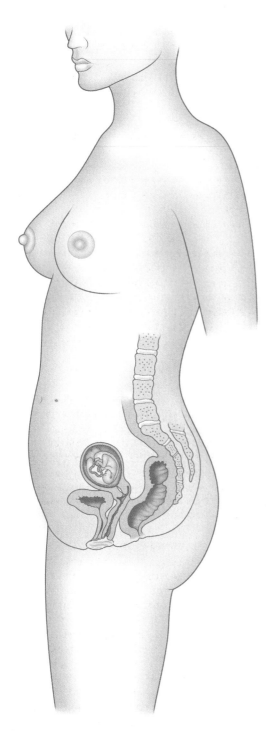
Week 12 of pregnancy

Your baby: Weeks 10–13

By Week 10 your baby has completely lost her embryonic tail and straightened out. She has well-formed limbs, fingers and toes with the beginning of nails, and facial features giving a profile with a large forehead and tiny nose. In medical terminology, she has made the transition from an embryo to a foetus. All of her internal organs are fully formed now, and will mature over the pregnancy. Her skeleton is also complete but is still in the form of cartilage. By the birth much of it will have ossified and become bone, but parts will not harden until adolescence.

In this rapid period of development your baby grows from around 2.5 cm (1 in) and 8 g (⅓ oz) to 12 cm (4¾ in) and 110 g (4 oz). The placenta, which initially surrounded the embryo and the amniotic sac completely, now occupies one area of the uterus and the chorion membrane, which remains after the placental villi shrink, lines the rest of the cavity of the uterus, enclosing the amniotic fluid. You may have an ultrasound scan and see your baby for the very first time. She kicks and punches, and arches her body and moves her lips and head while wrinkling her forehead as part of the swallowing and sucking reflex that will allow her to feed as soon as she is born. You will be able to hear her heartbeat while you are being scanned.

Her skeleton is also complete, moulding into shape on a base of cartilage (as in the spine and bones of the limbs) or matrix bone cells (the flat bones of the skull, jaw, face and collarbone). For the rest of pregnancy her bones ossify (grow and strengthen) and they will be strong at birth, although ossification continues into adolescence.

You: Weeks 10–13

By the end of the first trimester your uterus will have emerged from the space within your pelvis and your doctor will be able to feel it above your pubic bone. You may feel a release of pressure on your bladder. Your waist is probably thickening and your belly beginning to round gently, but the changes may only be obvious to you and your partner. The uncomfortable symptoms of early pregnancy might make life difficult, but take heart: nausea, vomiting and tiredness tend to diminish as the first trimester comes to a close.

The production of oils in your skin may lead to spots, or alternatively you may experience dryness. Your hair may thicken and become shinier or become limp and greasy. Your breasts may remain tender and are already preparing for feeding: new milk glands grow, the tissue around them swells, the dark area around the nipple (the areola) darkens further and may expand, the bumps around the nipple (Montgomery's tubercles) enlarge and imperceptibly secrete lubrication. Well-fitting and supportive bras can make a big difference to your comfort.

What's special

The first trimester brings changes in every area of your life as you deal with physical symptoms, absorb the news and feel the effect of emotional changes.

Your feelings

If you welcome this pregnancy, these first 3 months will be euphoric times, when thoughts of motherhood and images of your baby will seldom leave your mind. Indeed, you may find it surprisingly difficult to concentrate on any other subject.

You may also experience moments of confusion, doubt or anxiety. With the joys of becoming a mother come responsibility and compromise; neither are easy to imagine at this early stage. And if you are feeling unwell or tired – which many women do – it can be hard to keep optimistic. However, the coming months will give you time to mull over your thoughts and make practical plans. If you don't feel like doing either in the first trimester, don't worry – there is plenty of time ahead for this. Your priority now is to care for yourself.

Some women feel strangely numb in early pregnancy and it may take many weeks for the news to hit home. You may be surprised that you feel depressed but, coupled with the hormonal changes if you are uncertain about how you can accommodate a baby, this may affect your mood. It is likely that feeling low will pass when nausea and fatigue disappear and your plans for the future evolve, but some women do suffer from depression (p.462) during pregnancy.

Your relationships

The most obvious relationship that will feel the impact of pregnancy is your partnership. Your commitment to one another may deepen and planning for the future as a family might be really enjoyable. However, if one of you is more excited than the other – and the balance may swing from day to day – or one of you is not happy, things could be less rosy.

If you clash, remember that hormonal changes can be very powerful, and you may shift from feeling vulnerable to being controlling, short-tempered and quite irrational. Your partner's moods may also go up and down like a yo-yo and the strength of your relationship may be put to the test. Where your moods are opposite or in conflict, it will help to listen to one another even though the honest truth may be challenging. Planning practical issues may help you work as a team.

Ideally, your friends and family will share your joy and offer support, though it may be disheartening if they are worried or give the impression that they lack confidence in your ability to be a mother. Occasionally, where your moods are taken personally rather than as part of pregnancy, friendships go 'off the boil' and it may take

time to pick up the pieces. In your close family you and your brothers and sisters may begin to relate to one another differently: sometimes jealousy arises or disappears and sometimes love deepens. Most notably your parents, particularly your mother, will now treat you differently, and this may bring you much closer.

Time to enjoy

In the early stages of pregnancy if you are feeling tired or unwell, your social life may quieten down. This may be a good excuse for curling up in front of the fire or watching a video, or perhaps having soothing massages, but you may feel saddened by restrictions to your fun. In most cases, lethargy and sickness pass after the first trimester and many women bounce back with vigorous energy and a real lust for life after the third or fourth month.

During this period some women slow down a lot and have to space commitments widely. If you feel out of sorts you will probably need more rest than usual, and benefit from a bit of pampering – perhaps a quiet walk or swim. You could introduce some moments of relaxation, perhaps go to an antenatal yoga class or try some simple visualisations (p.371). A few minutes of quiet time with yourself, each day, may give you more energy to enjoy your pregnancy.

This stage of pregnancy is a good time to consider your network of friends and supporters. If you are feeling low or want to take time off work, you will already be calling on your colleagues. If you haven't the energy to keep up with household chores, there are people who can help – your partner, your mum, a friend or paid help could all assist with cooking, cleaning or DIY. This will free up your time and could reduce anxiety about how much you need to do. Your support network could continue through your pregnancy, and remain after birth.

Your body and body image

As your stomach begins to round and your breasts swell, your body takes on the beauty of pregnancy, undergoing a transformation that is little short of miraculous. Many women find this exciting, and so do their partners; you might enjoy taking regular photos and documenting the changes. You may feel radiant or the changes could be uncomfortable and you may feel out of control, perhaps if you expand sooner than you had anticipated, if you have an underlying weight problem that is exacerbated by pregnancy, or if you feel unwell.

If you care for your body through eating, exercise, dressing well and looking after your skin and you feel healthy, you will automatically adopt a positive stance and have the 'glow' often associated with pregnancy. If your body changes shape quickly, don't delay in buying clothes that fit comfortably – a couple of new outfits may give you a great outward image and boost your confidence.

If your body image is low, you may find mutual support among other expectant mothers or women who have been pregnant. It can be soothing to feel heard and acknowledged and they may offer you some great tips as well as a host of compliments: you might be the last to recognise how beautiful you really look.

Eating and weight gain

How you eat will probably take on new significance when you know that what you eat will be passed to your baby. Changes in what you eat and your weight are inevitable. Try to concentrate on eating healthy food and obtaining the nutrients, vitamins and minerals you and your growing baby need (p.332). At the same time it is good to be cautious about putting on excessive weight. Unfortunately, being pregnant can make it difficult to eat well: many women feel constantly hungry, many have cravings for unsuitable food (like crisps or chocolate) and many who feel nauseous find it hard to keep down meals or want only sugary foods. Smoking is also a part of what is consumed. If you smoke, do all you can to stop. This also applies to alcohol and drugs. Quitting tips are on p.451.

If you are craving sweet or fatty things, you may be lacking some vitamins or minerals, and taking a supplement (p.345) could make a difference. Another change that could help you is the spacing of meals. Eating small amounts of slow-burning foods and snacks roughly every 4 hours will help your blood sugar levels remain stable. Remember that fast-burning sugary foods, including fruit juice and colas, push your blood sugar level up, bringing a high followed by a hypoglycaemic slump, and your baby will feel the same highs and lows. The section on sugar highs and lows and its accompanying chart relating to the glycaemic index on p.334 is well worth having an understanding of at this stage of your pregnancy.

Even when you know just what's good for you and what isn't, you're bound to slip up from time to time. The occasional treat could be just what's needed to lift your mood and isn't a problem unless unhealthy food becomes a regular part of each day. Try to focus on positives and experiment with delicious healthy foods.

Everyone gains weight differently, but the average gain in these early months is 1.4–1.8 kg (3–4 lb). These are guidelines and there is a lot of individual variation (p.332).

Exercising and relaxing

If you are struggling to cope with morning sickness or feel exhausted, it will be hard to focus on exercise. But regular exercise or yoga, even if it is very gentle, is probably the most powerful route to feeling good. If you keep up the exercise you enjoyed before becoming pregnant or begin to exercise now, you should be able to stay agile and fit, have a better chance of an active birth, and more easily regain your figure afterwards. The object is to maintain fitness.

Throughout pregnancy your baby will benefit from your increased circulation and good spirits, just as long as you take a few precautions: warm up, and don't overheat; work out gently; stop as soon as your body tells you to; be aware of how pregnancy is altering your concentration and balance. Check with your doctor and refer to p.357 so you know that the exercise you choose will not put you or your baby at risk.

Try out a few options. Choices include taking walks, swimming, cycling and doing floor exercises either at home or in a group. Many sports centres offer antenatal classes of gentle aerobics, sometimes in water ('aqua natal') that stretch and relax to build suppleness. Or try antenatal yoga (p.350), which exercises and relaxes your body and introduces ways of breathing and meditating that can help any nausea and tiredness you may suffer and be invaluable for birth and beyond.

Dad's issues

As a man you will experience the early weeks of pregnancy quite differently from your partner. You may be bubbling with excitement and delight or perturbed by the changes to your life. In the early stages you might find it hard to believe the pregnancy is real; seeing your baby on a scan could make it more tangible.

You may rush into a protective, caring role with enthusiasm and do as much as you can to care for your partner, staying positive as you imagine your new family and celebrate your creation of another human being. Some men find it easier to get used to the reality by plunging into DIY, giving up smoking, experimenting with a new diet or taking up regular exercise, choices that have positive results and could be part of the bigger change of becoming a family.

Whatever your practical response to pregnancy, inside you could feel confronted by difficult questions concerning your relationship, responsibility, work, money and time (p.292). It would be quite normal for you to worry about your ability to be a good father or be concerned about the birth. Doubts are part of the reality of parenting and sharing them with your partner or friends can be one of the most constructive parts of pregnancy.

Even though pregnancy does not affect your body, you may have some surprising symptoms. It's actually quite common for men to experience weight gain, backache and even nausea, as if in sympathy. If you're worried, talk to your GP. Physical symptoms may be manifestations of deeper anxieties if you are dealing with challenging emotional issues.

Your emotions could be changeable and you might feel confused or depressed, particularly if you have ambivalent feelings about having a baby. Depression strikes many men both during and after pregnancy. As you contemplate the future you may reflect on your own upbringing, too, and the relationship with your parents could take on a whole new significance (p.298). In terms of keeping up your social life, you might find that you are even more daunted than your partner about the coming restrictions because, unlike her, your body isn't being flooded with mothering hormones.

Sex and intimacy

Joy at the miracle of conception can bring oneness and physical intimacy, and you may feel liberated from the pressure to conceive (or not to conceive). You might have new enjoyment with your sex life – your breasts may bring positive changes and vaginal lubrication may increase. Sex is perfectly OK throughout pregnancy, unless you have a history of miscarriage and have been advised against it by your doctor. Oral sex is safe.

Though sex may be great, not everyone experiences a leap in activity and pleasure as soon as pregnancy is confirmed. In fact, a combination of physical symptoms and new emotions often bring a reduction. Tiredness, nausea and sensitive breasts can reduce libido, and you may need time to adjust to your baby's presence. If either or both of you do not feel sexy it is important to maintain intimacy in other ways, which could range from going out for a meal to taking a shower together and massaging one another. Keeping physical closeness, whether or not this involves sexual stimulation, will reinforce your love and help you communicate and support each other through the coming months (p.285).

Work and finances

The early days of pregnancy need not involve large costs and some people manage pregnancy without great expense. You will, however, need funds for maternity wear, gentle body-care products and healthy food and you may plan to move or redecorate or to upgrade your car. Financial considerations are an extremely common cause of stress so it's worth doing all you can to be clear about your options as well as your restrictions. You may need to begin saving or cutting back, and make some concrete plans concerning work and maternity leave.

If you are working, your comfort will be as important as your finances (p.320). Work can be very enjoyable and sociable and take your mind off any unpleasant symptoms and your colleagues may be excited and supportive. Yet coping with nausea and tiredness can be more difficult if you cannot explain the reasons for reduced performance. If you are feeling ill and need time off then it may be wise to tell your employers. You are entitled to time out for antenatal checks.

In the morning have a good relaxed breakfast or a nutritious snack if you can't hold down a full breakfast, and make your journey to work as easy as possible – getting a lift with a colleague may be an option. At work try to do what you can to ease strain on your back, try to put your feet up during breaks and lie down or even sleep at lunchtime if possible. Plan ahead to eat well to keep your energy up. If your work involves exposure to hazards (p.388) you will need to reduce risks or step into a safer role. Your employer has legal responsibilities for ensuring your safety at work.

Medical checks

Once you have confirmed your pregnancy, it's up to you to visit your GP or book an appointment with a midwife. Here begins a series of visits and checks that continues through the next 9 months and beyond. Together you will estimate a date for the birth of your baby and discuss preferences about where you want to give birth. You will probably have two or three appointments in the first trimester during which you can address your hopes and fears and physical symptoms. Your midwife will record your weight, blood pressure and urine, and consider your pregnancy against the background of your personal family and medical history.

You will be offered a number of tests to monitor pregnancy and determine the health of your baby (p.78). You may also have your first ultrasound scan around Week 12. This allows you to see your tiny dancing baby, toes, fingers and all, and can reliably detect the presence of twins and confirm your dates. The other purpose of the ultrasound scan is to check for markers of foetal abnormalities and for normal development. Fortunately the vast majority of pregnancies are normal and tests provide confirmation that all is well.

You may find it difficult to make choices about which tests to have. Your medical team is there to guide and support you and will answer any questions. The tests are designed to diagnose, protect and treat you and your unborn baby in pregnancy and at birth, and to plan for specialist care if it is needed. Receiving good news is never difficult, but awaiting results can bring anxiety, and hearing about potential difficulties can be very worrying indeed (p.434).

Holistic care

Pregnancy brings many women in touch with their bodies in a new way, and it also places restrictions on drugs and chemicals because many can have detrimental effects on a growing baby. It's unfortunate that early pregnancy also brings uncomfortable symptoms such as backache, headache, nausea and fatigue. There are forms of health care that offer a range of safe possibilities to treat illnesses and physical discomfort, and to strengthen the body's natural balance, many of which are covered in Part V. You might find that homeopathic remedies or acupuncture are very helpful for nausea (p.513), as are herbal teas and massage with gentle essential oils.

Common concerns

The vast majority of concerns are easy to sort out because all you really want to know is: 'What is going on?,' 'Is it normal?,' and 'Will it have an adverse effect on me or my baby?' Some issues cause greater worry. The most common queries are listed briefly here. If you would like to have more details, many issues are explored in more depth in the A–Z Health Guide, which covers prevention, emotional and physical healing and complementary techniques that may be used in conjunction with medical assistance.

Why do I feel down and depressed?

Many women are taken aback if they do not feel happy and elated during the first trimester. A combination of factors comes into play here. If you are affected by premenstrual syndrome then you may feel similar now because levels of oestrogen and progesterone hormones continue to rise; nausea and vomiting, a change of diet and eating only small amounts may also affect your moods. If your family relationship or financial circumstances are difficult, you may be anxious about how things will turn out; where depression has been an issue in the past you may worry that the strain of having a new baby will affect you.

It is usually possible to tide yourself over the first 3 months until your energy improves and you may find that optimism returns. If you have persistent underlying worries then you may need to find help – antenatal depression (p.412) is a real issue for men and women alike and postnatal depression can be reduced or avoided by approaching concerns before the birth.

I'm feeling incredibly tired and need to sleep a lot. How do I deal with this?

Being tired is often significant in early pregnancy and it usually improves as the second trimester approaches. It is caused by a combination of hormonal changes, nausea and eating patterns and emotions (p.544). There is no need to fight your tiredness – in fact, doing so may add an extra stress and exacerbate it. Listen to your body, rest and sleep and don't overdo things – you may be happier about relaxing if you feel supported by your partner, friends, family and work. The best advice is to eat well and exercise, however gently. If you are working and cannot find enough energy there may be ways to cut down your load, share some tasks or take time off. At home, getting help with household chores could make time for you to rest.

How can I cope with peeing every few minutes?

Many women have to pass water very frequently because the kidneys increase urine production, and the enlarging uterus puts pressure on the bladder. After Week 12 your uterus will rise and pressure may be relieved. Occasionally, urinary frequency is due to cystitis (p.552), an infection in the bladder. Get your urine checked for infection and reduce your fluid intake at night to help you to sleep, but continue to drink plenty of water during the day.

How can I deal with nausea?

If your nausea is mild, ensure you eat slow-burning foods every 3–4 hours to preserve your energy and drink well. If it is severe there is a range of conventional and complementary methods that can bring relief (p.513). If you are vomiting frequently and feel dehydrated and weak then visit your doctor urgently.

I have noticed a little blood stain on my pants. What does this mean?

Slight spotting is very common in Weeks 6–8 and is usually caused by an implantation bleed as the placenta burrows into the lining of the uterus. When implantation is completed the bleeding usually stops. Occasionally bleeding (p.406), particularly if there is a lot of blood, indicates a threatened miscarriage but even if this is the case pregnancy may continue normally. A bleed is not a sign that your baby will show a developmental problem later in pregnancy. It is a good idea to tell your doctor and if the bleeding continues, an ultrasound scan will help assess your pregnancy, define the cause and reassure you that all is going well.

Why do I have pain in my tummy?

Stomach pain is very common in the first trimester and in most instances pregnancy continues normally. If you feel pain in your lower abdomen or your pelvis (pp.518 and 519) it is probably stemming from the corpus luteum in your ovary, which produces the hormones needed to maintain the pregnancy for around the first 10 weeks. If you are constipated or nauseous, pain may arise from your intestines. More serious but rarer causes giving discomfort may be a threatened miscarriage if a period-like pain is accompanied by vaginal bleeding (p.512), or an ectopic pregnancy if pelvic pain originates from the fallopian tube (p.457). If your pain is severe see your doctor urgently to be examined and an ultrasound scan may help to define the cause and reassure you.

When should we tell other people that I am pregnant?

The timing is very individual. You may decide to tell everyone as soon as your pregnancy test is positive if you do not mind people knowing if a miscarriage happens or tell a select few people and keep the news from the majority until later. Many couples feel that it is better to wait until the first scan confirms that everything is normal at 12 weeks. There may be other reasons to delay the announcement and these include work deadlines and not wanting your pregnancy to affect a deal or contract.

I am constipated. What can I do about it?

Constipation (p.437) is common and arises from the effect of pregnancy hormones on the movement of the bowel and from a change in eating habits. Ensure that you have a normal intake of fluid of 1.5–2 litres (2½–3½ pints) a day, eat fibre-rich vegetables and brown bread and rice and try adding whole linseeds to your food two or three times a day. If it is still a problem try a bulk laxative like lactulose. In the rare instance that this does not work you may need a stronger laxative.

Why do I have a chronic headache?

Headaches are often related to hormonal changes, altered eating patterns or poor posture. If you are seated at work for long hours, examine how you sit because shoulder and head pain may be caused by muscle tension. Towards the end of this trimester your ligaments soften and your spine curves to accommodate your growing baby, which may cause discomfort. Emotional stress also increases tension and may lead to a headache. There are a number of ways to ease headaches without using painkillers and these are covered on p.521.

My breasts are painful and hurt when I walk or knock them accidentally. Is this normal?
Your breasts may change and become uncomfortable before you even miss a period, particularly if you experience premenstrual breast pain. As your pregnancy progresses, the hormonal effect increases as the breast tissue prepares to secrete milk but towards the end of this trimester your body may have accommodated the changes. Breast pain sometimes sparks anxiety about cancer but fortunately it is very rare in pregnancy and discomfort is not a symptom. Wearing a well-fitting and supportive bra will help and you may feel better wearing a sports bra at night. Sometimes gentle massage (p.195) is soothing.

I am vegetarian. Will my baby get the nutrients that he needs from my diet?
If your diet is well balanced then your baby can get just what he needs in order to grow. The main factors to consider are whether you are obtaining sufficient protein, essential fatty acids, vitamins and minerals. You'll find tips in the eating and weight chapter (p.332), and you will also find information for vegans there.

I have severe indigestion – why is that?
Indigestion (p.487) in early pregnancy is caused by the way hormones affect your stomach and intestines and perhaps by changes in your eating pattern. If you are observant you may be able to reduce the foods that make you sensitive. If you are vomiting, acidity may make you uncomfortable and you may find that a mild antacid is helpful. Homeopathic remedies can be very useful.

I find that there are many things I cannot eat. Is this okay?
It is very common for appetite to alter during the first few months and you may feel turned off by some foods to the extent that you can't look at or smell them without feeling sick. You can make changes so that if you are missing nutrients you can get them in another way. If most foods make you feel unwell, continue supplementation and eat little and often the foods you can stomach. When the nausea of the first trimester has settled you will be able to expand your diet. Beware of too many sugary foods.

During the first trimester your baby's organs are forming and it is a sensitive development time. Even so, your baby is still small and for nourishment he can use the reserves of minerals and vitamins that were stored in your body before pregnancy.

My skin and hair have gone really greasy, which is not usual for me. What can I do?
Having greasy hair, acne and oily skin can make you feel unattractive. You could try a variety of facemasks, which will leave you feeling fresh and give you an excuse to sit down and relax for 5 minutes, or some new cleansers. You might find that drinking plenty of water and cutting down on tea and coffee, dairy products, fried foods and wheat makes quite a difference too. For your hair, you could consider trying different shampoos or conditioners, but the solution to the problem may be simply washing your hair more frequently. Once the hormonal changes have disappeared after birth, your skin and hair should return to their former state. Sometimes facial skin is greasy but elsewhere there is dryness – a few drops of pure oil (almond or grapeseed) in the bath and a light body moisturiser can help.

Shall I start eating organic food?
The most important thing about nutrition is to eat a well-balanced diet. If you have the financial resources, eating organic food is the best option because you can avoid insecticides, chemical additives and hormones and some organic food may also have a higher mineral and vitamin content than mass-produced food. A growing number of people are eating more organic produce and the variety of foods available in the supermarkets is increasing rapidly. Remember, however, that organic food is not necessarily always nutritious – some organic snacks are very sugary and laden with 'empty calories'.

When will I show?
There's a possibility that hormonal changes will affect your body very soon and the increase in breast size and abdominal bloating can make you show within 2 weeks of missing a period. There's an equal chance that your pregnancy may not be obvious until the end of this trimester. Women who are overweight tend to show later but even thin women may not be obviously pregnant for months. You will no doubt start noticing that every woman changes shape differently and carries her pregnancy in a different way.

What about the microwave and my portable phone? Can they be dangerous in pregnancy?
Every decade new advances in technology bring unknown risks. At the moment there is no evidence to suggest that a modern, well-functioning microwave isn't safe. The best you can do is to make sure that yours has no leaks or other problems, and for your own peace of mind you may wish to use it sparingly. In the same way, there is no scientific proof of danger associated with mobile phones, even though there have been scares relating to microwave radiation. It takes at least 10 years for research and evidence-based results to give solid facts. It may be best to use neither your microwave nor your mobile phone in excess while you are pregnant.

I take medication. Can I continue?
If you need medical treatment for an underlying condition it is best for your specialist doctor to check the effects on the development of your baby. There is a wealth of information available about the effects of medication on foetal development. Essential medication will need to continue and there may be an option to choose the type that is safer for foetal development. If you take occasional medication for pain or allergies or mild infection, the general rule is to take as little as possible particularly during the first trimester as the foetal organs develop.

I'm worried that I will miscarry. Are my fears justified?
You are not the only pregnant woman who feels this, because the first 12 weeks are the most common time for miscarriages to occur and the incidence is around 15% (p.512). It's often hard to believe the pregnancy is fine before you can feel movements or see a swelling in your abdomen. If your personal history suggests you are at risk of miscarriage, your midwife or doctor will want to take close care of you. When you have had a normal ultrasound scan your mind may be put at rest. You can boost your own health and provide a good environment for your growing baby by caring for yourself, avoiding exposure to unnecessary risks, eating well and taking vitamins and minerals and exercising gently.

I'm 10 weeks pregnant and have a bad stomach upset and a cold. Could this harm my baby?
The vast majority of infections, whether due to a virus or to a bacteria, will have no effect on your baby because the placenta acts as an efficient filter. Among a small number that carry risks are rubella, toxoplasmosis and cytomegalovirus, none of which cause a cold or stomach upset and there are blood tests available to detect them. Your symptoms do not suggest you have anything severe: the main thing to remember is to look after yourself so you can get better – rest and keep yourself well nourished and hydrated. You may find homeopathy works well for your symptoms and there are antibiotics that are safe to use in pregnancy if you need them.

This baby will be my parent's first grandchild. What can I expect?
You will know best about your relationship with your parents and how you are all going to adapt to the transition. In some families it is easy and there is a subtle change from a child/adult relationship to the feeling of adults supporting one another. You may now have more respect and more understanding about what your parents went through when you were conceived and they may see you in a different, more 'grown-up' light. If you do not have a supportive relationship with your parents and feel they are distant or critical these feelings may be magnified and you may be lonely or upset. Fortunately there are many months ahead for all of you to repair bridges and pregnancy may be a turning point for this. It might be you who brings about changes (perhaps with the help of the Wheel for Living, p.58) or they who instigate a new approach. Some parental relationships are very tense and difficult and might now be deeply engrained in your family culture – seeing the way each of you interacts may help you to move forward with optimism (p.276).

Is my job safe?
It is illegal to fire an employee because of pregnancy. Try not to become unnecessarily anxious and remember that there is time ahead for you to make plans. Although many companies have an excellent approach to pregnant women in the workplace and sound policies regarding maternity and paternity benefits, some are not very understanding about your needs as a pregnant woman. We examine your entitlements in the chapter on work (p.323). You can make further inquiries by talking to the human resources manager at your company or to your midwife or general practitioner.

My past medical history is not straightforward. Will this affect my pregnancy?
There are a number of conditions that you may be worried about. Your concerns are natural and it is best to talk to your midwife or doctor about your particular case. You may find that your medical history will not affect pregnancy in any way. If it indicates that you or your baby are at a higher risk of complications, either in pregnancy or during or after birth, early discussions about treatment are worthwhile so that you can take the best approach to ensure safety for you both. If you are content that you are receiving adequate medical care and your carers know about your history in full, you may be less anxious and begin to enjoy pregnancy more and look forward to the birth of your child. As a first step, turn to the A–Z Health Guide for the particular medical condition(s) that relate to you, and book an appointment to see your midwife or doctor. You may feel less worried if you take another adult with you (perhaps your partner) who can help you ask questions and record the information you receive.

I have heard of an ectopic pregnancy but don't know what this means. Can you explain?
In a small number of pregnancies the placenta implants in the fallopian tube and not in the uterus. As the baby grows, the tube may rupture causing internal bleeding into the pelvis, accompanied by intense pain. If you have pain in early pregnancy it is best to see your doctor urgently and have a scan to assess your pregnancy. The ectopic may need to be removed surgically. Ectopics are more likely to occur if you have had assisted conception, previous pelvic infection or conceived on contraception with the mini pill or an IUD, and are looked at in detail on p.457.

What do I do about my smoking and occasional recreational drugs?
It is best for your health and for your baby's development if you do not smoke tobacco or marijuana, so it is best to do what you can to stop or cut the amount to a minimum. There's detailed advice about the potential harmful effects from smoking (p.535) as well as guidelines to help you stop in the A–Z Health Guide (p.451). If you are addicted you may need a lot of patience and considerable support as you go through the quitting process. Of other recreational drugs, cocaine and amphetamines (such as speed) are particularly harmful for your developing baby.

When must I take vitamins and minerals like folic acid?
It is best to begin taking vitamins and minerals – particularly folic acid – before you conceive but if you have not done so then start as soon as possible. Scientific studies show that a full multivitamin and mineral programme is preferable to taking single vitamins or minerals during pregnancy. There are full details on p.345.

I am having a great time and feel so energetic. Is it OK to really go for it?
It is really fine to enjoy yourself during this trimester. Go for it and have a great time – just listen to your body and be cautious not to get over-tired or consume anything that carries risks for you or your baby.

Care in pregnancy

During the 9 months of pregnancy and birth a range of health professionals and carers offer expertise, support and guidance. When you visit your doctor to confirm your pregnancy, you meet the first of this potentially large team where each person has something different to offer: a skill, years of experience and a certain outlook on life. You may choose who cares for you at each stage and widening your network brings diversity for you and your baby. This could make pregnancy and birth safer and more enjoyable, and establish a support network that may continue for years.

Making choices

The love, support and care you receive in pregnancy are strongly linked with your labour and birth, and also affect the way you feel when you are caring for your baby. You may be happy to let things change around you, or you may prefer to actively make decisions that suit you, your partnership and your baby. Making positive lifestyle changes and converting problems into possibilities have been discussed in Part I. Here the focus is on choices concerning care in pregnancy to assist your transition to motherhood.

Everyone who is pregnant for the first time needs guidance and support. Throughout history and across the world this has been offered by sisters, mothers, priests, nurses, doctors, spirit guides and astrologers. Like all women before you, you will benefit from others' experience: making choices involves listening to yourself, placing trust in others and choosing to delegate, and is the perfect preparation for an active birth.

If you want to be involved in keeping as fit and healthy as possible, choosing where to give birth, what level of intervention and pain relief you want and who will care for you in labour, you will begin to make choices early in pregnancy. Knowing that you have explored your options and enrolled people you trust may boost your confidence for labour and for being a mother.

Antenatal care

You could, providing you had no difficulties, get through the whole of pregnancy without attending a single antenatal visit as your body works in its own natural way to nurture your growing baby. Yet that would be far from ideal: antenatal visits can be fun and reassuring, bringing you more in touch with your baby, and carers are highly trained in supporting pregnant women, detecting complications and treating special needs. Sophisticated antenatal monitoring has significantly reduced the risks that may be faced by babies and mothers. Moreover, continuing and friendly care throughout pregnancy has been proved to reduce the likelihood of ill-health and emotional difficulties.

Antenatal care refers to everything you receive from the start of pregnancy until your baby's birth. It is a term taken from the Latin words *ante* (before) and *natalis* (to be born). Its goal is to help you and your baby to stay in optimum health and give you both the best possible start. Because all aspects of your social, mental and physical wellbeing can impact on your pregnancy (and vice versa), your carers may address health problems and social and emotional worries as they keep an eye on you.

Pregnancy is not simply a once-a-month event marked by a visit to your midwife; rather it stays with you day and night, and continues to change from day to day, so a holistic approach – nurturing your *whole* body and your *whole* lifestyle – offers the most comprehensive care package. Although visits to your midwife or doctor and undergoing standard or specialist tests are the key events, they need not be the only attention your pregnancy receives. Classes and groups are an important aspect of preparation, as are the lifestyle changes and the way you care for yourself.

There are also many other therapies that can ease your pregnancy and optimise your baby's health and you may choose to investigate these and incorporate some into your antenatal programme. New life is a cause for celebration and joy, and you're likely to find that people who have chosen to be involved with birth and babies are usually loving, supportive, positive and enthusiastic.

Your team
The core team who monitor your health may consist of three individuals – your GP, midwife and obstetrician – who care for you throughout pregnancy, or there may be more people involved. Carers work shifts and all take breaks and holidays. If you are seen by different people from week to week, you'll need to rely on yourself to keep up and ask questions and make plans. Remember, too, that if at any time you feel uncomfortable about the doctor or midwife caring for you, you are entitled to ask for an alternative.

Where you receive your antenatal care can have a big impact on how much you enjoy it. Different people like different things – some hate hospitals, others feel safe and welcomed in them, some receive prompt and considerate treatment, others are kept waiting. If you have 'shared care' you will attend your local surgery and see your GP or midwife for most visits. If you are considered high risk or a problematic condition is identified during pregnancy, you will be asked to go to hospital for most visits.

For many women a small and intimate maternity unit offers the best environment, where the team is close-knit and flexible, but you may not live in a part of the country where this is an option. Whatever your situation, you will be able to make choices about your team of supporters. If you are encouraged and well informed, you will almost certainly approach birth and parenting positively.

Your GP (General Practitioner)

Your first meeting with your GP – the traditional family doctor – will probably entail congratulations, a discussion of your gynaecological history and advice about making some lifestyle and nutrition choices.

Only a few GPs deliver babies but most continue to play a major role in their patients' pregnancies and in caring for the babies and families after the birth. A GP is trained in the care of pregnant women.

If your pregnancy goes without a hitch, you might not need to see your GP again until your 6-week check following the birth. Even so it is good to visit her once or twice so she can keep up with your progress. You may value the relationship once your baby is born; your midwives will offer support for about 6 weeks after birth, whereas your GP will probably oversee your medical care for years to come. GPs are also trained in helping women postnatally, and helping with the 'blues' or depression.

Midwives

Midwives have been at the heart of women's birthing experience for as long as history remembers, supporting, soothing, caring and sharing their experiences with the mother. Across the world they have been seen as purveyors of a sacred or even magical craft. Some are maternal or paternal, others feel like a best buddy and most are gentle and loving. Midwife means, literally, 'with woman' but the same term in other languages translates variously as 'she who holds', 'wise woman' and 'mother's adviser'. The common quality that seems to be offered by all midwives is support: their role is to reassure, encourage and guide a mother antenatally in labour and birth. They are also skilled in helping a mother care for her newborn baby. Most women have nothing but praise for the team of midwives who helped them.

Midwives are health professionals who have special training in caring for mothers and babies during pregnancy, birth and the postnatal period. Some midwives are based in hospitals whereas community midwives may be separate or part of the General Practice surgery. Independent and self-employed midwives can be hired to attend a birth, whether it happens at home or in hospital. If you choose an independent midwife it's advisable to check that she is insured.

Midwives can be female or male (though male midwives account for only a tiny percentage) and have varying degrees of expertise. They are governed by a code of conduct that allows them to provide total care for normal pregnancy and birth, which involves antenatal check-ups, delivering babies and doing procedures such as performing scans, episiotomies and stitching. They are not permitted to use forceps or perform caesarean sections. Community midwives do antenatal visits and attend home births; they visit all mothers and babies daily for around 10 days after birth.

Midwives work shifts, so it will probably be impossible to specify which midwife you want to attend your birth. The more midwives you meet, the more likely you are to be among familiar faces when you are admitted to the hospital in labour and this may make a difference to your confidence and progress.

Doulas

A doula – ancient Greek, meaning 'handmaiden' – is a support person who assists a woman in pregnancy and birth and/or in the postpartum period. You could see a doula as a modern-day supporter who fills the role once commonly held in small communities by older women who assisted mothers through pregnancy, labour and birth, eased pain through natural means and offered practical help in the newborn period.

Doulas are most common in the USA, and surveys have shown that their support can significantly reduce the length of labour and the need for epidural pain relief. A doula may have done a course in physical and emotional needs through pregnancy, labour and beyond, and in non-medical pain relief. Many doulas help women at home after the birth. Not all, however, have qualifications beyond the trust that they can inspire in a labouring mother and their sensitivity to different circumstances. A doula can be any age and will usually be a mother herself. If you want help and company in addition to the midwives and any other birth supporters who'll be with you, a doula may be a good choice.

Obstetricians

An obstetrician – from the Latin *obstetrix* (midwife) – is a specialist doctor responsible for ensuring that mother and baby are safe during pregnancy, labour and birth. In the 18th century when men first became involved in labour, they received a bad name for viewing pregnancy and birth as a condition that needed to be treated. They have been blamed for reducing the role of midwives and medicalising birth and were held responsible for advocating the reclining position for birth: this allowed them easy access to the vagina, but reduced the woman's power to push. Gradually, however, control has been reinvested in the hands of birthing women and their supporting midwives, with obstetricians providing an invaluable safety net.

Obstetricians and midwives work together and if you are planning a hospital birth, you will be booked under the care of a consultant obstetrician, who is the most senior doctor involved. Your obstetrician may also be a gynaecologist, a doctor who specialises in female reproductive health. Some hospitals book in antenatal patients for a number of visits to their consultant but you might not see your obstetrician at all if your pregnancy progresses normally, unless you have specifically requested an appointment. You may also be seen by other doctors who are at various stages in their long training programmes.

Paediatricians

A paediatrician is a doctor who specialises in the care of babies and children. If your pregnancy is complicated, the paediatrician may be involved in helping to choose the timing and method of birth. If you need assistance during labour or if your labour has been complicated, a paediatrician will examine your baby immediately and give him any help he needs. All babies are checked over by a paediatrician in the first couple of days after birth. Babies with a significant health problem will be in the care of a paediatrician until the problem is resolved.

Hospital team

The wider hospital support team who you may meet includes one or more ultrasonographers who may also be qualified as obstetricians or midwives and have experience that enables them to assess the development of your baby. Most expectant mothers meet the ultrasonographer two or three times during pregnancy.

You may also meet an anaesthetist if you choose to have an epidural during labour or if your baby is delivered by caesarean. Behind the scenes there is also a team of laboratory doctors and technicians who conduct standard and emergency tests throughout pregnancy. In addition, your hospital team may include a counsellor trained in family support to help with a broad range of issues connected with parenting.

Your extended support team

Your team may already contain many more people besides the medical professionals outlined above, and there will be potential to extend it to include anyone who could help. While you are at the centre when it comes to caring for yourself and your baby, there will be people who will be able to help with your physical and emotional health as well as with practical day-to-day chores and preparations for labour and life afterwards.

Your partner, friends and family

You may have a partner standing by you throughout pregnancy and sharing plans for the future. If so, you will probably ask him to be with you during labour when his encouragement, love and physical support will be invaluable. His genetic link and fatherly bond with the child you are carrying gives him a special place.

Beyond this centre, some of your most important supporters may be friends, family and colleagues – people who find time to ease your domestic or professional load or to nourish your mind and body. You may have a firm bond with your mother and a strong tradition of female support in your family.

You'll find more advice at antenatal and other pregnancy classes (p.94) where you may meet a teacher or a mother whose opinions you particularly respect. Your team of 'home' supporters will stay with you through your baby's early life and beyond, and may offer practical help and gems of wisdom that you may find among professional health workers.

Is there anything I can do during pregnancy to prepare for care after the birth?
In most areas a basic level of care for you and your baby will follow seamlessly after birth. You will be visited daily by one of a local team of community midwives until your baby is 10 days old. You do not have to accept this service, but most mothers find it very helpful and reassuring. The midwife who visits you may help you build practical skills with looking after your baby and offer emotional support. She will check how you are healing and weigh and monitor your baby.

Responsibility for your home care is then passed on to your health visitor, a nurse with special training in family health. She will probably be based at your GP's surgery or a local health centre and may contact you within the last month of your pregnancy, depending on policy in your area. If you want to meet her before birth where this isn't normal practice, you can request a home visit or meet her at one of the clinics she runs at your surgery. Your health visitor's role is to support you as you care for your baby and to ensure that you receive information about standard health assessments, vaccinations and checks until your child is 5 years old.

If you plan to get hired help (p.324), you will need to explore your choices well in advance of your due date and interview prospective candidates. Some are booked up in advance.

Complementary therapists

Pregnancy is a great time to enter the world of complementary therapy. Because many allopathic (conventional medical) remedies, from tetracyclines to tranquillisers, are out of bounds, you might find yourself looking for alternative ways to resolve health problems that are based on natural healing. Even if you don't feel unwell, complementary treatments can be used to improve constitution, enhance the body's immune system and prepare the body for labour. Many are effective as pain relievers and relaxants in labour. If you take some time during pregnancy to acquaint yourself with alternative therapies (p.330), you may discover remedies that suit you well and, at the same time, form lasting relationships with therapists who will care for your family in years to come.

More progressive GPs, midwives and obstetricians will encourage you to explore complementary therapies and may help you find qualified practitioners of massage, osteopathy, reflexology, homeopathy, aromatherapy, nutritional therapy, reiki, acupuncture and hypnosis, among others. The number of surgeries referring patients to such therapists is increasing, and although some treatments may be covered by the NHS, you are unlikely to receive complementary therapies free. Don't let that put you off, though. Some therapists offer a sliding scale of charges and there may be something to suit you. Take things gradually unless you have a pressing problem and want attention immediately. It may take time to build your confidence.

Dentists and counsellors

Pregnancy can impact upon your body in surprising ways. Your teeth and gums, for example, are more susceptible to problems. NHS dental care is free of charge during pregnancy and it is best to visit your dentist and brush your teeth more assiduously than usual.

You may find your pregnancy makes you acutely aware of emotional shifts, relationship difficulties or unresolved issues from your early life. If you are concerned about these, have a chat with your GP or midwife. If you need further support or opportunities for longer, more in-depth discussions, your GP can direct you to a counsellor. Opening up to someone who isn't connected to your family or circle of friends can be very helpful, but it is a difficult thing to do and you will need to trust in your counsellor.

Antenatal visits

As soon as you have confirmed pregnancy you can make a booking to see your midwife at your hospital or local surgery. Routine visits will then be spaced at monthly intervals until Week 28, then they will be every 2 weeks until Week 36 and finally every week until your baby is born. The frequency of checks ensures that problems can be identified and dealt with at the earliest opportunity. If you

have any concerns in between appointments, emergency consultations are done via your GP or directly through the maternity department of your local hospital.

Your first antenatal or 'booking visit', serves the dual purpose of assessing your health and booking you into the care of a team. If you are planning a hospital birth, you will be booked in under the care of one consultant obstetrician whose name will appear on your notes. Your midwife may also arrange your first ultrasound scan.

At this visit, which will be longer than subsequent visits, most of the time will be spent talking about your feelings, reviewing your medical history and giving an outline of what to expect over the next 9 months. Once your midwife has a picture of your circumstances, care can be tailored to meet your specific needs. She may also chat briefly about your hopes for birth, ideas about parenting education and plans for maternity leave.

Your midwife will also ask a series of questions and what you tell her will be kept in your file. If you are worried, she will give practical suggestions and emotional support to make changes. She will ask:

- About your general medical history: any incidence of pregnancy-related illness, diabetes, high blood pressure or kidney problems, any emotional problems or depression. All other information that contributes to the picture of your health, including any sexually transmitted diseases, and your family's health is helpful.
- About exercise, if you smoke, your drinking habits, your diet and any vitamins you are taking, any use of recreational drugs, medication and any sources of stress or distress in your life.
- If you are in a secure partnership, whether you work and some details about your social and financial support network.

Information about any previous pregnancies, labours and births and the health of your children is central to your medical history. If you have had an ectopic pregnancy, a miscarriage or an abortion, difficulties in a previous labour or birth or a baby with an abnormality, you may be anxious about this pregnancy. Your midwife will offer any necessary monitoring and tests and advise appropriate treatment or referral to a specialist.

Routine tests at antenatal visits

At every visit your midwife or obstetrician will perform the tests and procedures listed below.

Blood pressure

Your blood pressure measures the pressure in the arteries as your heart pumps the blood around your body. The systolic pressure shows pressure during a heartbeat. In your notes this figure is the upper of the two numbers in your blood pressure reading. The lower figure is your

Understanding your notes

Your notes record your background information and the results of all antenatal tests. Eventually they will contain a record of your birth and your postnatal care and you may be given a copy if this is hospital policy. You may also want to carry a copy with you if you are travelling.

At first glance your notes may look like a web of strange hieroglyphics. Most information is recorded in shorthand and not all doctors make records in the same way. If you're confused, don't be afraid to ask.

Common abbreviations and medical terms in notes

EDD   Estimated date of delivery

LMP   Last menstrual period

Primagravida or Para 0   Your first pregnancy

Multigravida or Para 1 or more   You have had more than one pregnancy lasting over 24 weeks

7/52   7 weeks

FMF   Foetal movements felt

FMNF   Foetal movements not felt

FHH   Foetal heart heard (usually possible from Week 14)

FHNH   Foetal heart not heard

Alb   Albumin: a protein that may be detected in your urine

BP   Blood pressure

Fe   Iron tablets (prescribed if you are at risk of anaemia)

Hb   Level of haemoglobin in your blood, which indicates whether you are at risk of anaemia (p.398)

Height of fundus or SFP (symphysis fundal height)   The height of the top of your uterus (the fundus), measured from the top of your pubic bone

MSU   Midstream urine sample

NAD or nil or a tick   Nothing abnormal detected (often related to urine sample)

Oed   Oedema: swelling of the hands, feet or face (p.539)

PET   Pre-eclamptic toxaemia (high blood pressure) (p.410)

TCA   To come again

VE   Vaginal examination

Ceph or Vx   Cephalic or Vertex – your baby has his head down

Br   Breech: your baby has his bottom down

E/Eng   Engaged: your baby's head has moved down into your pelvis

NE   Not engaged

ROA or LOA   Right occiput anterior or left occiput anterior: your baby is lying with the back of his head facing the front and pointing right or left.

ROP or LOP   Right or left occiput posterior: your baby is lying with the right or left side of the back of his head facing your back

diastolic pressure, which is the blood pressure between heartbeats. The average blood pressure for adult women is 110/70.

High blood pressure above 130/90 is known as hypertension (p.410) and needs careful monitoring. Early in pregnancy high pressure usually indicates underlying hypertension. Later in pregnancy, if your blood pressure rises and you also have swollen legs or protein in your urine, you may have developed pre-eclampsia and will need prompt treatment. If the readings are below 90/60, you have low blood pressure and you may feel faint.

Urine test

You will be asked to take a sample of urine along with you. A mid-stream sample, that is, one collected midway through emptying your bladder, will give the clearest results as it is unlikely to contain any vaginal secretions.

Your midwife will dip a strip of treated paper into your urine on which are marked several coloured lines. The colours may change on contact with your urine and reveal the presence or absence of any of the following substances.

Protein: If your test reveals protein, it is measured in + from 0 to ++++. The presence of protein can indicate a urinary tract infection (p.552) or, if you also have high blood pressure or swollen legs, pre-eclampsia. It may also indicate an underlying kidney disease that can be investigated during pregnancy.

Glucose: The presence of glucose in urine may be normal, caused by the increased blood flow through your kidneys during your pregnancy. As it may also indicate diabetes (p.444) if it is present on two occasions, a glucose tolerance test is done to exclude diabetes.

Ketones: Ketones are substances produced by your body when no carbohydrates are available and body fat is used for energy. These commonly appear if you have been vomiting and may indicate that you are not getting adequate nourishment or have developed diabetes.

Blood: Blood in urine may indicate an infection or bleeding coming from the vagina. It may very rarely be due to a problem in the kidney. If the urine culture is negative and the blood persists then kidney function will be checked using a blood test and a scan will exclude a kidney stone.

Your weight

Weighing is part of antenatal monitoring in some hospitals. Your midwife may weigh you and calculate your BMI (body mass index) to adjust your weight for your height. If you begin pregnancy under- or overweight or gain too much or too little, she will give you nutritional advice. Your weight gain is an important aspect of antenatal care; for more, see Eating and weight (p.332).

Examining you

A few generations ago all diagnoses in pregnancy were made through external examination and midwives gathered great skills in sensing a baby's age, wellbeing and position. Across the world the placing of hands on a woman's abdomen and regular massage is believed to encourage the baby into a head-down position for birth.

Your midwife may not massage you (although this could be one of her unexpected specialities), but she will be able to tell a great deal about your health from the way you look. Your expression will convey your mood while the way you walk and stand will reveal whether you have aches in your back or legs. In later pregnancy she may look closer to check your hands and ankles for swelling or puffiness (p.539) and may check your legs for varicose veins (p.559).

At each visit she will place her hands on your abdomen and will feel the size and position of your uterus. Charting its size provides a useful indication of your baby's growth. A low growth rate does not necessarily mean a small baby but it warrants increased surveillance (p.488). From around Week 26 your midwife will be able to determine if your baby is head down and facing your back or your side.

From about Week 14 your midwife will be able to hear your baby's heartbeat using a hand-held monitor that allows you to hear it too. Your baby's heart beats fast – around 140 beats per minute. Sometimes because of your baby's position the heartbeat is difficult to find, in which case your midwife may suggest using an ultrasound scan for reassurance that all is well.

Internal examinations

If you had become pregnant 10 or 20 years ago, your doctor may have examined you internally to confirm pregnancy. Today, except in France and Japan, where it is standard at most antenatal visits, an internal examination is no longer routine.

Some hospitals perform a cervical cancer smear test during early pregnancy. If there is confusion about your due dates, you and your midwife may agree that an internal examination to assess the size of your uterus may help although an early ultrasound scan is the most accurate tool. Where there is concern that your cervix may not be competent (p.426), an internal examination may be of value. Relax, focus on your breath and think of something that will distract your mind. Your doctor or midwife will insert one or two gloved fingers into your vagina. The intrusion will be over quickly and, if done sensitively, may not hurt at all.

When you go into labour, or if you have passed your due date, your midwife will be able to assess the condition of your cervix from an internal examination. This may be the first time you need an internal.

Screening in pregnancy

During pregnancy all the tests are screening procedures that assess you and your baby's health. The 21st century is the age of informed consent and choice: women have the right to know what they are being tested for and to opt out of any of the tests. Full information is not always given but it is a legal requirement that every woman gives her consent, albeit verbal, to have a test done.

From the earliest weeks you will receive information about your baby's health and be invited to use tests to identify risks or diagnose problems. The quest is to ease anxieties that an unborn baby is healthy. Below is a list of the more common tests that are carried out. Problems that occur in a minority of pregnancies are covered in detail in the A–Z Health Guide.

Ultrasound scans

Sophisticated ultrasound scanning has radically changed antenatal care. Scans are now the primary source of information about a baby's age, size and gender and are becoming increasingly reliable as tools for detecting problems relating to mother or baby. All parents now have at least one opportunity to see their baby before birth, kicking, turning or sucking his thumb. The excitement at seeing your baby for the first time may well be mixed with anticipation as you wait to hear that your baby is healthy.

Most scans are conducted through your abdomen. Your bare abdomen is smeared with a warm jelly and the ultrasound operator slowly passes a transducer or probe over your skin, pressing down slightly and moving in all directions. If the scan is carried out through your vagina (a trans-vaginal scan), you will be asked to draw up your knees with your feet flat on the bed, while the probe (like a tampon) is inserted into the vaginal entrance. Trans-vaginal scans can provide more detailed images, especially in very early pregnancy, and are becoming increasingly common.

Ultrasound scanning uses very high frequency sound waves that are beamed into your uterus from a transducer that is connected to a computer. The sound waves are then reflected by the tissues in your baby's body back to the transducer and the computer creates an image of your baby from the ultrasound echoes. While your baby is small you may see his complete body or catch a glimpse of his face and tiny fingers. Later, as the ultrasonographer zooms in on your baby you may not see everything in perspective. She will probably try to keep up a running commentary, but her chief task is to study the changing image carefully and bring into view each limb and organ to confirm that all is in order.

Your ultrasonographer may also be able to view blood flow in your baby's body and the placental blood vessels using a technique known as Doppler. This detects the movement and flow of blood, displayed by the computer as colour superimposed on the normal ultrasound image, and provides a dynamic picture of your baby's health and the function of the placenta. By examining the flow in your uterine arteries in mid-pregnancy, it can also predict the risk of pre-eclampsia (p.410).

Number of scans

Whether you are offered one or several scans will depend on your hospital and how your pregnancy proceeds. If you want early confirmation, have been undergoing fertility treatment, are concerned about an ectopic pregnancy, or have a history of miscarriage, you may have a trans-vaginal scan from Weeks 6–8.

More commonly, the first scan is given between Weeks 12 and 14. This confirms viability, number of babies and pregnancy dates and is the most important initial antenatal screening test for Down's syndrome and other chromosomal disorders (p.449).

A second-trimester scan between Weeks 16 and 22 is regarded as the main check for growth and other possible abnormalities. Ultrasound at this stage enables very close

---

If I have ultrasound is there any risk to my baby?
There is no evidence to suggest that ultrasound scanning can cause any harm to an unborn baby: the waves are very low intensity and have no impact on development. Because scans are used for diagnostic reasons, there is a strong argument that it is safer to have them than not to have them, because if a problem is discovered that can be treated or alleviated, you will be reducing risks to your baby's health.

The testing dilemma

As medical science advances, the accuracy of testing is improving: care can be customised to individual mothers and babies, so that pregnancy, labour and birth can be made as safe as possible.

Most expectant mothers and fathers opt for all the standard antenatal tests. Yet many are anxious about discovering that something might be wrong. Despite their long-term advantages, the testing procedures and the ethical and emotional issues they raise can interrupt the joy of pregnancy. Take time to talk about the tests and their implications with your midwife. You might also find it helpful to discuss your feelings with your partner or seek additional support and advice. Tests usually reassure that potential problems have been excluded.

The majority of the tests lead to clear-cut results. For example, if your haemoglobin level is low you are anaemic (p.398). Some tests are not black or white and can only indicate the need for further investigation. If this investigation reveals that the pregnancy is normal then the initial test gave a 'false positive' result. Sometimes further investigation is invasive; that is, tests involve taking samples from the amniotic fluid, umbilical cord or the placenta and such tests carry a small risk of causing miscarriage. As screening techniques improve, false positive rates diminish and invasive tests are needed less frequently.

---

examination of all parts of your baby, including the internal organs, which have now developed sufficiently for investigation. The placenta and amniotic fluid can be also be assessed more accurately as can the Doppler flow. In experienced hands, many high-risk pregnancies will be diagnosed at this stage and the parents offered counselling and clinical advice. Most couples are reassured that their baby is healthy.

You may be offered a third-trimester scan (Weeks 32–34), which will confirm how your baby is lying and growing and estimate his weight. The site and appearance of the placenta and the volume of amniotic fluid can be clearly analysed at this stage. Colour Doppler studies allow measurement of blood flow through the umbilical cord to reflect how well the placenta is working and can help assess your baby's welfare as the end of pregnancy approaches. If your baby is late you may be offered a further scan to evaluate your baby's wellbeing so you and your birth team can make informed decisions about induction (p.497).

If there is a suspicion that your baby is 'at risk', your obstetrician or midwife may advise 'serial' ultrasound scans to monitor your baby regularly and frequently. These assess your baby's rate of growth and the volume of the amniotic fluid, while Doppler studies assess health by checking the blood flow to the placenta and to the baby's brain, liver and abdominal organs.

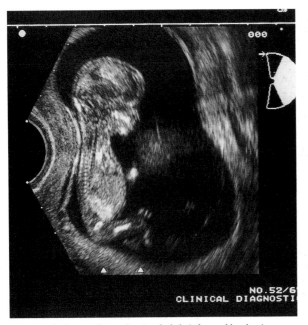

An 11-week ultrasound scan showing the baby's face and head, spine, crossed legs and one hand.

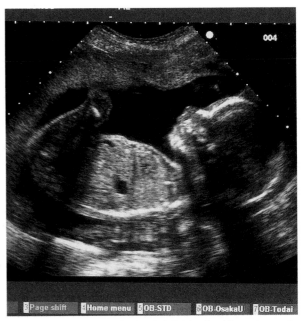

A 13-week ultrasound scan showing the baby's head and face, spine, trunk and left thigh.

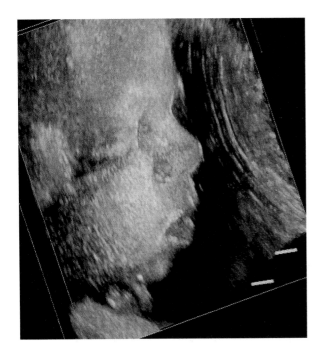

A three-dimensional ultrasound scan of the baby's face at Week 26.

Blood and bacterial tests

Information from blood tests contributes to the overall evaluation of your health and the identification of any conditions that may affect your baby. The first blood test is usually offered at an early antenatal visit. The exact analysis done on your blood depends on your medical history, the stage in your pregnancy, and the usual practice in your locality. As screening practices improve, 'false positive' results are becoming rarer.

Standard analysis

Your blood group: Identification of blood group is necessary in the rare event that you need a blood transfusion (p.412). If you have an unusual blood group, your medical team will ensure blood that matches your type is available at the time of your labour.

The rhesus factor: Your sample will reveal whether your blood contains the rhesus factor – a protein that is attached to red blood cells in the majority of people. If you lack the factor (as do 15% of the population in the USA and Europe) you are 'rhesus negative' (p.410). If your baby is rhesus positive there is a small but significant risk of incompatibility between maternal and foetal blood where you could develop antibodies that may, in subsequent pregnancies, cause an unborn baby to become anaemic. Treatment is simple using an anti rhesus-D injection during pregnancy and after birth to prevent any potential antibodies from developing.

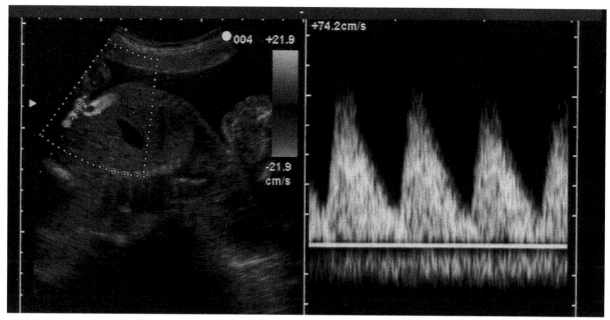

The left side of the picture shows the baby's abdomen and the umbilical cord. On the right, the same baby's Doppler blood flow image is seen from the umbilical cord artery.

Haemoglobin level: Haemoglobin is the pigment in red blood cells that transports oxygen. If your levels are low you may be anaemic (p.398). Your haemoglobin level and 'blood count' (the number of red cells in your blood) can be increased by treating the cause. Expect another routine haemoglobin test in the third trimester of your pregnancy.

Sickle cell anaemia and thalassaemia: Sickle cell anaemia and thalassaemia (p.398) are inherited conditions caused by an abnormality in the haemoglobin molecule. The anaemias are more common among certain racial groups. If you are at risk you will be tested; if the test is positive your partner's blood will be checked. If both of you are carriers you will be offered amniocentesis or chorionic villous sampling (p.395) to detect whether your baby is affected.

Tay-Sachs disease (p.540): This metabolic disorder affects fat metabolism and brain and liver function. It is more commonly found in families whose parents were of Ashkenazi Jewish origin. If you are positive, your partner will be tested. If both of you are carriers, your baby may be affected, and a check through amniocentesis will be advised because the condition is extremely debilitating and causes severe difficulties physically and mentally throughout life.

Tests for infection and immunity

Your blood may also be analysed for infections or your immunity to infections. All of these are covered in the A–Z Health Guide.

Hepatitis: If you suffer from hepatitis B, a viral infection of the liver, it could infect your baby at birth or through your breast milk. If your test is positive, your baby may be given a vaccine within 24 hours of delivery and again at 1 and 6 months to prevent infection. Your blood may also be tested for hepatitis C.

HIV virus: Screening for HIV is increasing as treatments for pregnant women and unborn babies are becoming more effective. All health authorities offer it to all pregnant women and even if you do not suspect that you have been at risk of infection, either through sex or contact with infected blood or blood products, you may wish to take the test. Discovery that you are not infected will clearly be a relief. If you find out that you are infected, you will need guidance and counselling. The reason for the test is not only so that you can begin treatment: early treatment and extra precautions during labour and birth can greatly reduce the risk of passing HIV to an unborn baby.

Rubella (German measles): Rubella is a viral infection that can seriously affect the health of an unborn child if the mother becomes infected in the first 16 weeks of pregnancy. If your blood reveals that you are not immune you cannot be vaccinated until after your baby is born, but you can be aware of your vulnerability and avoid coming into contact with people suffering from the infection.

Syphilis: Although this is an extremely rare sexually transmitted infection, it can have serious effects. The infection can pass unnoticed for years, yet it does threaten foetal and maternal health. Syphilis can be treated with antibiotics and any risk to a growing baby greatly reduced or eliminated.

Toxoplasmosis: If a mother is infected with toxoplasmosis, commonly passed on through soil, uncooked meat and cat faeces, her baby is at risk of developing the infection and suffering mild or serious damage. Testing for this infection is rare in the UK, but commonplace in France.

Vaginal infection – strep B, vaginosis and chlamydia: Screening for these bacteria is not routine but if you have previously had a vaginal or sexually transmitted infection then a swab test is taken and sent to the laboratory to be incubated. If the organism is present then you may require treatment during pregnancy or in labour.

Down's syndrome testing

Down's syndrome is a chromosomal abnormality, usually due to the occurrence of an extra chromosome 21 (trisomy 21), which has a profound effect on a baby's physical and mental development (p.449). Though its occurrence is rare, it is the most common chromosomal cause of severe learning difficulty. The possibility of a baby having Down's is indicated by a number of factors including maternal age, ultrasound assessment and a blood test. In the rare cases that these indicate a chance that is higher than 1 in 200, a sample of the baby's cells obtained through an amniocentesis or CVS (p.395) can be cultured to count the baby's chromosomes. If you want the best detection with the minimum number of false positives or misleading results, then it is best to have both an ultrasound scan and a triple blood test. The blood results are fed into a computer and combined with scan information, accurate dating of the pregnancy because the levels of the markers increase each week, facts about age, weight and height and previous history, and a single risk factor is calculated. If the risk is greater than 1:200 an amniocentesis is advised, and parents are given advice and counselling.

In an early ultrasound scan (Weeks 12–14) subtle anatomical details can be detected. The thickness of the skin behind the baby's neck is called nuchal translucency and is used to indicate Down's syndrome risk. Early ultrasounds pick up over 80% of Down's babies screened; the triple blood test identifies a further 5–10% for further confirmatory tests that are invasive (below).

For the triple test, only one blood sample is needed any time from Weeks 10–16. Between Weeks 10 and 13, it will be analysed for three substances produced by the baby or the placenta; if it is taken between Weeks 14 and 16, different marker substances will be analysed. The markers vary as new research information becomes available. As a mother's age increases the incidence of Down's rises, thus the risk is greater for a 40-year-old mother than for a 30-year-old mother. Yet it can occur to women of any age, and age alone is not a sufficient indicator. The risk is computed by analysing the scan results and levels of marker substances in the blood as well as the mother's age. The computer provides a risk factor to advise whether an invasive test is needed.

Fewer than 1% of expectant mothers are advised to have amniocentesis, CVS, or a similarly invasive procedure to check for Down's syndrome or other rare genetic problems. During the test samples of amniotic fluid (amniocentesis) or placenta (CVS) are obtained and cultured to define the chromosome or genetic content of the foetal cells.

All invasive tests carry a risk of miscarriage so there must be a significant risk of the foetal abnormality before the test is undertaken. You will need counselling from your midwife, obstetrician or a specialist geneticist and time to discuss your preferences with your partner and any other members of your family you wish to involve.

Down's syndrome risk and mother's age

Age	Risk	Age	Risk
26	1:1286	36	1:307
27	1:1208	37	1:242
28	1:1119	38	1:189
29	1:1018	39	1:146
30	1:909	40	1:112
31	1:796	41	1:85
32	1:683	42	1:65
33	1:574	43	1:49
34	1:474	44	1:37
35	1:384	45	1:28

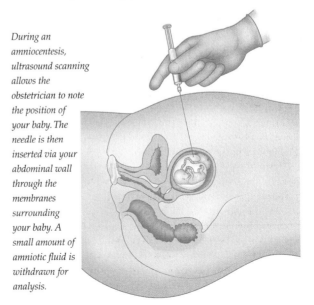

During an amniocentesis, ultrasound scanning allows the obstetrician to note the position of your baby. The needle is then inserted via your abdominal wall through the membranes surrounding your baby. A small amount of amniotic fluid is withdrawn for analysis.

Cystic fibrosis testing

Cystic fibrosis is a recessive inherited condition caused by a defect in a single gene, the CFTR. This gene allows salt and water to pass in and out of cells, and in cystic fibrosis sufferers there is an accumulation of thick mucus in the lungs and digestive tract with consequent severe digestive and respiratory problems (p.443).

Around one in 24 UK Caucasians is a carrier of the CFTR gene. The proportion of carriers is lower among Asians and people of Afro-Caribbean origin. If you choose to be tested, you will be asked to give a mouthwash sample. If you are found to be a carrier, your partner will be similarly tested. If both of you are carriers there is a likelihood that your baby may have cystic fibrosis, and you will be offered an amniocentesis or CVS (p.395).

Specialist care

If your pregnancy is thought to be at a higher than normal risk for mother or baby, specialised care by the team of midwives and obstetricians is needed.

Maternal conditions such as diabetes, asthma, heart disease, inflammatory bowel disease and multiple sclerosis and others can influence health in pregnancy and may themselves be adversely or positively affected. If you have one of these conditions you may have discussed the implications of becoming pregnant.

Depending on the severity of your condition you may need a bigger team to care for you throughout your pregnancy, and possibly in labour too. If you already receive care from a specialist team, it is best to continue with them provided they are used to dealing with pregnancy and you may play an important role in ensuring that your obstetric team is informed and maintains communication with them.

If your baby is at risk of having health problems you may require the services of a foetal medicine team geared to detecting, assessing and treating problems during pregnancy, birth and in the postnatal period. In addition, you will need emotional support from your family and friends, and perhaps from professional counsellors. Examples of when a pregnancy is high risk (p.483) may include previous recurrent miscarriages, a baby with intrauterine growth restriction, placental insufficiency or infection or the presence of a developmental abnormality. The team will establish a surveillance programme to perform the necessary tests and monitoring and treatment if it is needed. By keeping their finger on the pulse of your pregnancy, they will inform you of what is happening, and in consultation with your obstetrician and midwife you can decide on when and how your baby should be born.

If your baby needs extra attention after birth, the paediatric and obstetric teams will offer treatment, guidance and support for you both. Coping with problematic conditions during pregnancy, in birth and beyond, requires courage, effort, support and stamina, and is not easy. You may find it useful to refer to the Wheel for Living on p.58 to help you through this time or refer to the appropriate entry in the A-Z Health Guide. The general advice given here on seeking and receiving essential care and support is adapted from the Wheel for Living. You may choose to use it in part or as a whole.

What's wrong?

What support do you need medically and emotionally?

Have time

How can you organise your work, home, family and friends to make space to deal with the issue? What plans can you make for the birth and your future as a family?

Enrol support

Use the hospital team of midwives, obstetricians and paediatricians and find out about classes for parents in similar positions where you may receive loving support and understanding. Use your GP and local midwife and health visitor.

Eat well and exercise

Eat well and exercise to keep yourself fit and energised, and follow the specific medical advice of your birth team.

Let go, take leisure and lie down

Let go and do whatever you enjoy to relax as much as circumstances allow.

Positive pregnancy

The purpose of antenatal care is to allay anxiety and detect potential problems as early as possible in your pregnancy. Expectant parents do vary greatly in their desire to know about the health of mother and baby during pregnancy while the medical community is striving to find ways of making pregnancy and birth safer.

Increased awareness, heightened confidence and improved levels of care bring good news and mean that expectant women can be more involved in their care and less burdened by anxiety born from unanswered questions. While active birth was once a reality for only a few women with the right support, it is now accepted as a very real option for most mothers.

As you prepare for your baby's momentous journey into the world, you can be comforted by the knowledge that your care team are able to do a great deal to ensure both you and your baby are safe. There is less likelihood that unsuspected difficulties will arise. Hand-in-hand with centuries of wisdom and experience, science is able to support one of the most natural human processes to enhance the power of every birthing woman and the health of their baby.

The second trimester: Weeks 14–27

In the second trimester, your uterus will begin to enlarge and you will feel your baby's movements, first as tingles and then, by Week 27, you may be feeling quite forceful kicks. This is commonly the most energetic period of pregnancy and you may enjoy making practical arrangements for birth and for family life.

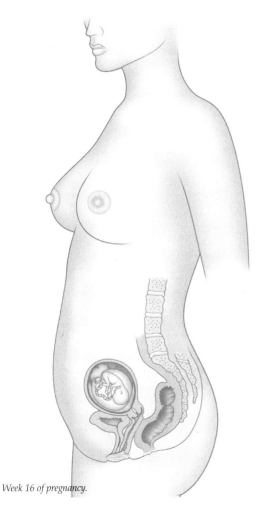

Week 16 of pregnancy.

Your baby and you

Your baby: Weeks 14–18

Your baby's face, limbs and organs are increasingly well formed; a scan would show the delicate eyes, nose and ears. Because her body is now growing more rapidly than her large head, your baby begins to look more in proportion. Her skin is translucent with her blood vessels clearly visible and she looks thin because she has no body fat yet. Over the course of the month, parts of her skeleton harden, her fingernails develop, taste buds form on her

tongue and tooth buds develop in her gums. She hears her first sounds around Week 15 and will listen to your heartbeat, digestion and voice for the rest of the pregnancy.

The amniotic sac contains around 180 ml (almost 7 fl oz) of fluid. In it your baby is constantly exercising and develops the range and intricacy of her movements. She touches the cord, sucks her fingers and makes complex facial expressions. These are involuntary reflexes that are an essential part of her genetic programming. Others include the breathing reflex, which is well established as she 'practises' passing the watery amniotic fluid through her lungs, and the swallowing and digestion reflexes that enable her to swallow the fluid, pass it through her kidneys and out via her bladder. She hasn't yet developed the blinking reflex and her eyes remain shut, but they are growing sensitive to the changes of light inside the uterus.

All your baby's movements help nerve pathways between the brain and the muscles to strengthen, and encourage development of neural pathways in the brain. The cerebral cortex, the centre for thought and feeling pain, which began to form in Week 10, matures from Week 17.

Your baby will be growing at a rate determined by her genetic potential and the nutrition she receives via the placenta. By Week 18 she'll be around 19 cm (7½ in) long and weigh about 170 g (6 oz). You and your midwife can now hear her heartbeat using a monitor.

You: Weeks 14–18

Between Weeks 13 and 16 most women who have suffered from nausea or extreme tiredness begin to feel better and energy levels improve. The change may be instant or happen over a number of days or weeks. Your muscles and ligaments will be softening to help you feel relaxed yet strong, and you may feel increasingly supple. Your bump will probably be noticeable and you may feel internal flutters, at first like butterfly tickles and then getting stronger. These are your baby's movements. Don't worry if you feel nothing – in first pregnancies, movement is often not felt until Week 20.

Pregnancy hormones may bring bodily changes that progress from the first trimester, and you may notice differences to the tone and quality of your skin and hair or changes in your breathing. Nausea lessens and some women experience excessive weight gain from now on.

Your baby: Weeks 19–23

By the end of this stage your baby is roughly 20–25 cm (8–10 in) long and may weigh about 340 g (12 oz). Your baby's skin is now covered with fine downy hair called lanugo and a white waxy coating called vernix to keep it moisturised, and beneath it fat is being deposited. This will give her a plumper appearance and provide energy in the days following birth until feeding is well established.

The first strands of hair will be growing on your baby's head, and eyebrows and white eyelashes are also forming. Beneath her eyelids your baby's eyes move from side to side and eye muscles strengthen. Much of this movement is during REM or dream sleep. Her sexual organs will be fully formed by now and clearly visible on an ultrasound scan. If you are carrying a daughter, her mammary glands will have formed, as have her ovaries, which hold millions of eggs carrying the genetic imprint for your future grandchildren.

Learning is rapid. The connections between the cerebral cortex and the rest of the brain are expanding and the number of synapses between the neurones in different parts increases rapidly; there is crucial development in the areas of the brain processing sensory information. Your baby begins to recognise your voice and your heartbeat, may respond to loud noises and music and will feel touch if you massage your abdomen.

You: Weeks 19–23

You will have felt your baby move, even if only a few times. The flutters will have no regularity or pattern and may be quite faint. These feelings will probably be very exciting, and a cause for celebration that boosts what is usually a positive and energetic time in pregnancy. Your abdomen will also expand, though just how you look will depend on your build, your baby's size and the amount of amniotic fluid. Some women carry their baby high, others low; some look wide, others compact.

Your muscles and ligaments continue to soften to ease your weight bearing, and your spine curves a little more. And as your shape changes, your balance does too. You may take this in your stride, or feel discomfort, most likely around the pelvic area and lower back or as a headache. Relaxation exercises and yoga, along with attention to posture and care when lifting, may reduce these. Your legs or feet may also be uncomfortable – you might need to go up a size or wear open sandals if your feet swell.

You may occasionally feel faint, particularly if you get up suddenly or stand for a long time and your blood pressure drops (p.411). Fainting is less likely to happen if you eat regularly and if you are not anaemic.

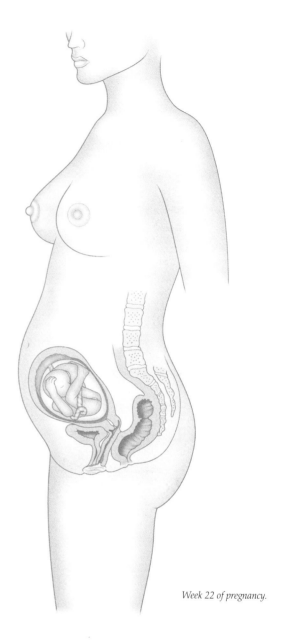

Week 22 of pregnancy.

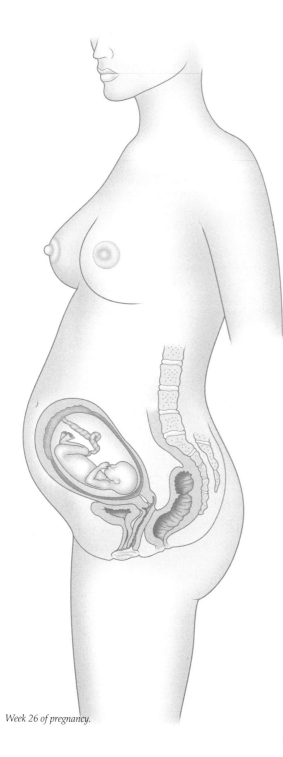

Week 26 of pregnancy.

Your baby: Weeks 24–27

Your baby is already capable of survival outside if intensive care is available, although it is best for her to remain protected and continue her development in the optimal environment in your womb. Her lungs are still immature. Ideally they need many more weeks to breathe optimally in air. Her body matures as her muscles, organs, limbs, eyes, ears and mouth exercise and develop. The connection between the thalamus, the part of her brain responsible for pain and emotional perception, and the cerebral cortex, which is where thinking occurs, becomes more established during this month. She is beginning to remember and to learn from repeated experiences of hearing and feeling your activity, as well as swallowing, urinating and touching the walls of the uterus.

Around now your baby will open her eyes for the first time and glimpse her womb world whenever there is light on your abdomen to dispel the darkness. She may catch sight of her own hands or the umbilical cord, but will have no idea what is part of her body. Her skin is now opaque and reddish and quite wrinkly.

Although she has grown significantly – by Week 27 your baby will be around 33 cm (13 in) long and weigh about 500 g (1 lb) – she still has lots of room to move around. This is her most active period as she turns and twists, somersaults, kicks and punches, and grabs and strokes the umbilical cord.

You: Weeks 24–27

Your baby's movements will by now be an accepted part of your day and night. Her strong kicks will be much more than flutters, and others will be able to feel them by placing a hand on your abdomen; you may see the kicks as well. Although movements may still be erratic, you might notice things that influence your baby's activity – she may move more when you rest, after you have had a meal or if you are feeling excited. You might also feel her moving rhythmically as she hiccups.

As your baby grows, your body needs to work harder to pump blood and maintain circulation (your growing uterus needs five times more blood supplied to it than before pregnancy). Aches and pains related to increased weight may appear or heighten now, and there is a chance that varicose veins (p.559) may appear in your legs, labia or anus (where they are called piles). You will probably begin to feel more thoughtful and mentally relaxed, which is a natural prompt for you to rest as your body accommodates all these changes, but it is also important to exercise within your capacity and, of course, to eat well – you and your baby need a good supply of nutrients.

What's special

The second trimester commonly brings the least discomfort, and many women feel energised and physically fit in this middle stage. Your growing baby has also passed her most vulnerable phase and you may find it easier to believe that everything's OK and make realistic plans for the birth and for the future. By Week 16, if not before, your enlarged abdomen will be quite easily visible.

Your feelings

During the second trimester you may just be beginning to accept that you will be a mother, and by the end of this period you will be two-thirds of the way through your pregnancy. The heightened emotions and extra sensitivity continue and you may begin to feel anxiety and excitement about the birth.

You might wonder how you'll treat your baby, what makes a good parent and how you can do your best. This is natural and fun and can be constructive. Some expectations may be realistic while others may not – you still have plenty of time to think over them, discuss them and prepare yourself. Towards the end of this trimester it's common to begin to focus inwards on yourself and your growing baby, and you may dream and daydream frequently. It is normal to have horrific dreams about birth or death or injury and this is your unconscious mind processing fears that the forthcoming birth brings to the surface.

If you still feel ambivalent or unsure, you may feel guilty when everyone is saying how lucky you are and how wonderful life is – this is just one of the common emotions at this time (p.300). Confide in others – it may help increase your inner strength and free you of some emotional weights in time for you to greet your baby.

Your relationships

Generally speaking, even if there are some continuing physical symptoms such as backache and tiredness, most women have an optimistic outlook in the second trimester and you might begin to feel more gregarious. In your relationships, too, you may feel more positive and spend time looking to the future. If you had a rocky start to pregnancy and your relationship with your partner reflected this, you may now feel closer and enjoy planning together.

There may also be days when you wonder or perhaps worry about the changes that await you. You may worry about being different or holding different views from your mothers or feel strongly about family issues, such as discipline, sleeping or diet, and discover that your partner doesn't have the same outlook. This may bring conflict yet presents a chance to go over things that seem important and to look back on your own childhoods to trace the origins of your own priorities (p.276). One of you may

decide to compromise or you may reach agreement, and although the reality of family life may differ from your ideal, bringing these issues to light now can help to open a discussion for the months ahead.

Time to enjoy

The middle period of pregnancy may be a lively time. Providing you have no medical complications there is no reason not to travel, party, eat out, go to the theatre and cinema or do whatever makes you feel good and feels right for your baby. You can add to your comfort by taking things at your own pace and making adjustments from having a cushion to make sitting more comfortable, keeping a bottle of water to hand or requesting a healthy choice of restaurant.

The second trimester is a great time to take a break away from home (p.545) because it's free of early pregnancy problems and not overshadowed by the prospect of an early labour. Wherever you go, take your antenatal card with you in case you need to visit a doctor. If you are travelling to a remote country, you may choose to have an ultrasound scan before you leave to ensure that the pregnancy is developing normally. When you are abroad, eat food and drink water that you know has been carefully prepared and won't carry a risk of stomach infection. If you need inoculations or anti-malarial prophylaxis, it may be best to postpone your trip. You can fly with most airlines until Weeks 32 or 34. Holidays will never be the same once you have a baby with you.

Your body and body image

The physical change between Weeks 14 and 27 will be considerable: from an almost flat abdomen you will round out and your breasts may also continue to get larger. Your body may be a source of tremendous pride and pleasure, especially if your partner is attracted to the new curves. The more you pamper and nurture your body, the more likely you are to feel good about its transformation. If you are not enjoying the changes, it may help to remember that they are temporary and will regress in a few months. You will probably feel better and stand taller if you do not drape yourself in baggy clothes. Shop around for clothes that will let you revel in your new shape. Every compliment you receive will make you feel more resplendent.

More subtle physical changes that can affect your body image may include a linea nigra, a dark line down your abdomen, thicker or darker body hair, or darker pigmentation around your face (a 'mask' known as cloasma). And while some women do positively glow, it's just as common to notice less flattering changes. If you feel uncomfortable about blotchy skin, try some face powder or cream: chemical-free is best while you're pregnant and your skin is extra sensitive.

Eating and weight gain

If you felt nauseous, off your food or inclined to gorge yourself in the first trimester, things will probably have settled down now. You may now feel calm and be ready to take a more measured approach to your diet. If you don't have time to cook, try to stock up weekly on healthy foods like fresh vegetables, washed salad, fresh soups, baking potatoes, live yoghurt and sliced wholemeal bread. When you do cook, make double quantities and freeze half to eat another time. If you don't enjoy cooking, ask friends or family to help and investigate healthy restaurants or take-away outlets.

Beware of sugary foods and drinks, including fruit juices and colas, they contain more calories than you need. It is preferable to continue your vitamin and mineral supplement programme. Your baby's rate of growth means that you will continue to gain weight steadily (p.332). Though the exact gain varies enormously, about 500 g (1 lb) per week is average, giving a total gain of 3–6 kg (6½–13 lb) from Weeks 14–27.

Exercising and relaxing

As your pregnancy progresses you will probably notice that after a few hours without movement you begin to feel stiff. Taking appropriate exercise will keep you feeling vitalised and may be easier to contemplate now that weariness and any sickness you may have suffered have passed. Any strength and fitness you develop will stand you in good stead both in labour and as you look after your new baby. Even without a directed routine you can improve overall body condition, circulation and flexibility with regular swimming or walking, and the fresh air will help you feel good.

A home exercise routine will help you stay supple and is particularly useful if you prefer to exercise in private or can't make it to a class. Include gentle warm-up and cool-down exercises as well as movements that stretch all your body, strengthen your back and legs and your pelvic floor and increase your mobility (p.357).

Rest and sleep are precious and as your body becomes heavier and less agile you may need to adjust your sleeping arrangements. Try sleeping on your side with your upper leg bent at the knee and resting on a pillow or two, or put a pillow between your legs. An extra pillow under your bump might be comfortable. If you suffer from indigestion (p.487) make a back rest with pillows so you can sleep semi-upright. Ensure you have a good mattress as this will give firm support to your back.

Your mind also needs rest from the many thoughts that buzz round it all day. Breathing practice, visualisation and meditation (p.370) can be restful and bring you in touch with your baby. You might enjoy doing them with your partner and/or mix them with gentle stretches, yoga or massage (pp.346 and 365).

Dad's issues

Now that you can see your partner's abdomen and feel her enlarging body in your arms, things seem more real and you'll probably share more intimacy with your baby, when you feel kicking from the outside. Some of your practical plans may also swing into action.

As you pursue your work, exercise and social commitments, your partner may need to help you make time for everything and she could also help you have space and feel supported. Pressure from her adds to your other daily concerns and it may help to sit down and discuss both your needs. Together you may come up with an acceptable balance.

Some days you may be put out if your partner is introspective or seems obsessively focused on the baby – many men already ask, 'What about me?' If you feel left out, make time for the two of you to indulge one another. Feelings of exclusion can peak soon after birth and it may help you to express them now. There are a number of ways of getting your needs met, ranging from talking about your feelings, dreams and concerns to making love to organising extra help before the birth. If you find it difficult to express your feelings the advice on active listening and the YES system on p.290 might help you.

Issues concerning work, money and time may need confronting, and your feelings about fathering or attending the birth will still be present. This may be the easiest time for thinking over your concerns, your needs and those of your partner and new family.

The last few months of pregnancy pass all too quickly so this trimester is a good time in which to learn about labour, birth and babies. If you are nervous about attending the labour or being with a small baby, the knowledge you gather now will be invaluable and increase your confidence.

If you have the time, join your partner at an antenatal class or find out about couples' or fathers' groups where you can chat with other men and see how they view life with a new baby. If you have concerns about the birth or don't feel happy about attending, you could visit your doctor or the midwife for a chat – they may help you make up your mind.

Sex and intimacy

As your body becomes increasingly voluptuous and any fears of miscarriage that you may have diminish, you may find your thoughts turn easily to making love. Already your shape may make the traditional 'missionary' position uncomfortable, and you could have fun – and pleasure – with other positions. Some parts of your body may be much more sensitive than usual, for better or for worse, and telling your partner about these might herald a new openness in your sexual relationship. When you make love your baby can feel movement and hear sounds but she does not interpret them as an adult would. After orgasm the release of 'love hormones' will make your baby feel good too.

Some women enjoy sex less in pregnancy, some love it – there's a similar variation among men. Many women experience intense or multiple orgasms and often orgasm is followed by 'aftershocks'. These are contractions in the uterus, which takes a while to relax after orgasm, and are completely harmless. If you find it very uncomfortable you may prefer to concentrate on your partner's orgasm or enjoy forms of intimacy that aren't so arousing. Indeed, there will be days when this is preferable for both of you.

Some women and men cannot think of a mother-to-be as a lover and this feeling becomes stronger when the baby's physical presence becomes unmistakeable. Doing intimate things together that don't involve sexual intimacy – a night out, a candle-lit dinner or a good video – can keep the bond between you strong.

Work and finances

In these middle 3 months you'll need to make some definite plans for taking maternity leave and investigate benefits and allowances (p.320). You can backdate some, but it's better to claim in advance and this will make financial planning easier.

You may start feeling tired at work, too. If this is the case, the first thing to do is to improve the quality of your sleep, make sure you are taking the time to eat well throughout the day and do some exercise. You could consider talking to your colleagues and devising ways to ease the pressure on you. It may be enough to create time and space to rest, or you may need to reduce your hours or revise your dates for maternity leave. Work commitments are often very stressful – emotional tension is exhausting – and you will need to take time away from work to relax your mind and reduce tension in your body, perhaps through going out, yoga, exercise, meditation or visualisation.

There are also decisions to be made for the father-to-be, who may need to increase hours or arrange time off. Some jobs need weeks' or months' notice. If a career change is on the horizon, do as much planning as you can now – time to focus on this clearly after the birth may be scarce.

Many couples find this time financially stressful as they consider the costs of childcare and preparing their home. If you keep your worries to yourself this will increase your feeling of pressure, and because your partner may have similar concerns it could be better to share them.

Medical checks

Until Week 28 you'll be invited to visit your midwife every 4 weeks for standard checks. Your midwife will assess your baby's growth and wellbeing and if she has a hand-held heart monitor, you may be able to hear your baby's heartbeat from around Week 14. Some midwives guess at the sex of a baby from the way it feels or from the speed of the heartbeat; if you don't want to know the gender of your baby, be sure to say.

Most hospitals offer an ultrasound scan at around Week 20. This allows a detailed look at your baby's size, position and organs, the volume of amniotic fluid and the blood flow in your uterine arteries. You will see your baby in more detail and might be lucky enough to see her face. At this stage the sex can be fairly reliably determined. Very occasionally this second scan reveals signs of problems that were not previously visible.

Holistic care

You may now feel more in touch with your body and your feelings. If you did the detective work and found therapists in your area last trimester, now's the time to meet them and try things out.

Exploring the world of aromatherapy can be great fun in pregnancy, particularly if you involve your partner or a good friend in soothing massages using oils that are safe and relaxing (p.378). You could make a trip to a masseur or aromatherapist to find out more about oils or simply to relax under a professional's touch.

As your baby grows, you may feel added pressure to your pelvis; a cranial osteopath may be able to sort out this problem for you. A yoga class might invigorate you.

Even if you don't use any alternative therapies now, it will be worth reading about them: many can alleviate pain in labour, assist birth, promote the body's natural healing ability and aid comfort in breastfeeding. Turn to Part V for information and advice. The main areas that are covered there are homeopathy, osteopathy, acupuncture, aromatherapy and herbal medicine.

Antenatal classes

Some women do not begin to attend antenatal classes (p.94) until the third trimester, but it might be worth enroling earlier as classes can get booked up. Some classes, for instance labour preparation, are geared towards couples or women who are in late pregnancy, but others, such as yoga or exercise sessions, are useful earlier. It is never too soon to start yoga.

Antenatal classes vary enormously – if you have a wide choice, find out about the philosophy and content. Those that deal exclusively with labour and birth have a clear focus but it is helpful to address wider issues and look into the months beyond the birth. Some classes are directed only to women, others welcome men. The majority welcome single mothers. There may be a class in your area where couples are invited to tell their own birth story and you could get some tips, a chance to see and hold a young baby and advice on making the most of life after birth.

Common concerns

Extended information on these concerns, and a range of other antenatal health issues, are covered in the A–Z Health Guide.

There's no mistaking that I'm pregnant. What can I do about strangers in the street thinking that my belly is public property and offering advice on all kinds of issues?

Second only to a woman with a new baby, pregnant women are magnets for attention. The idea of a new baby brings excitement and curiosity, and some people can't resist the temptation to find out how far pregnancy is advanced and whether you hope for a boy or a girl. Some go further and rest a hand on your abdomen before asking if it's OK and offer uninvited advice. This will increase when your baby is born. Try your best to reduce any tension this gives: listen and then let their advice flow away like water off a duck's back and do not feel guilty about making your own decisions. But remember that sometimes an unasked for suggestion could be a very handy hint.

I am nervous that I will not be able to learn how to care for my new baby. Does it come naturally?

You are designed to mother and nurture your baby, and pregnancy prepares you for this. Tuning into your own baby will come easily if you take time to be with him, listen to him and watch him. Everyone learns at a different rate and you may need a lot of time to feel confident and put what you learn into practice. If you do physical things easily then mastery of basic babycare will come quickly with hands-on practice. If you feel clumsy then practising before your baby is born will be very useful. Many things you do, from feeding and changing nappies to understanding your baby's sleeping preferences, will require some learning. The best way to help your confidence is to spend time with a mother and new baby. Consider visiting a friend or join a postnatal class to get the feel of what it is like to hold and change a baby. Even if you feel embarrassed at first, you may be surprised how quickly you learn.

I feel so good and have lots of energy, whereas before I wanted to do nothing but sleep. Does this mean everything is OK?

This is often the most relaxed trimester and it is lovely that you are feeling good. These feelings are worth enjoying. There is nothing wrong, and while you're feeling this way your baby will receive the effect of your feel-good hormones. It is a good time to keep fit and well.

I feel OK but my partner says I am not attractive. Could this continue?

It's not uncommon for a man to feel less attracted to his partner in pregnancy. He may feel that the stresses on him of a new baby are being ignored or he might be upset or jealous that you have been 'taken away' by the pregnancy. His feelings could change or intensify when your baby is born.

Although you may feel that he is selfish and unsupportive, both of you will benefit if you bring your feelings into the open. While pregnancy is temporary and your physical changes will revert, it is worth acknowledging that this will take many months. You may be able to talk through his concerns and both feel happier. Alternatively, you could agree to separate sex and friendship, at least for the time being, as a way of avoiding an undercurrent of upset or dissatisfaction in your relationship. Although it is very hard to accept his feelings, this is potentially an optimistic time and it may be a turning point in exploring new possibilities in your physical relationship.

My mum disagrees with my plan to have an epidural. Who is right?

Because obstetric practice has changed since you were born both you and your mother are on a learning curve about what is on offer. You may have different ideas of benefits and disadvantages, and indeed how to approach birth. An epidural is only one of the issues that will come up now and in the near future (p.159). Other possible points of difference include how to feed your baby and routines around sleep and illnesses.

Your disagreement about an epidural may simply be a difference of opinion where there is no right answer. Alternatively, it might reveal a pattern in your communication. If your mum sees you as a child then she may be driven to influence or even dominate your decisions: if you feel that she interferes, your gut reaction may be to disagree with or defy her. It may be useful to explore the epidural question when you don't feel rushed so you both have time to air your views and to listen. You may find a new way of communicating where you both feel respected and heard (p.290). In the end it is your choice to decide on your style of labour and how you care for your baby.

I am always hungry and feel so restless because of it. What can I do?

Hunger arises from the physical need to nourish. It also stems from an emotional need to feel comforted, and in this case while eating makes you feel better for a while it does not resolve the underlying feelings.

If you try to satisfy your hunger with sugary snacks your body will absorb them rapidly but within 90 minutes your blood sugar level will plummet and you will be hypoglycaemic and feel low and hungry again. You can avoid this by eating balanced meals and slow-burning snacks every 3–4 hours. It is a discipline that needs practice but soon pays off. Even if you don't have a history of an eating disorder (p.455) it's best to look at your feelings and perhaps attend to them, rather than leaving it until after the birth. Hunger may be a symptom of depression. The way you eat in pregnancy is the first lesson your baby learns about food and the sugar highs and lows are shared by both of you.

I want to go to a music and dance festival. Can the noise levels hurt my baby?

Don't worry about the noise level hurting your baby's ears. Your baby may wake up and move quite vigorously, but this isn't a sign of distress. Though it isn't advisable to stand right next to the speakers, your body provides ample cushioning against sound.

I am worried about being restricted. Should I feel guilty about wanting to go out a lot before I become a father?

Fathers often feel enclosed and want to go out while the going is good. It may be important for you to continue to socialise. It may be best for you to have a night out with your friends although going out every night could mean that you neglect your partnership. As a couple, you could change the way you party – earlier starting and ending times in smoke-free places may be easy to arrange and allow you to have fun together, particularly if your friends join in.

My back and pelvis are really sore. I find it difficult to walk and even turning over in bed is difficult. What can I do?
As the weeks pass, backache becomes very common and there are thousands of pregnant women who sympathise with you. The hormonal and joint changes of pregnancy cause the pain, and the way you sit, walk and sleep can make it worse. Emotional stress can also affect it. Ways to help overcome it are given on p.459.

I feel fat and unattractive. What can I do to make me feel better about myself and look more attractive?
Feeling attractive begins from within. Your feeling about your own body has evolved since you were a little girl and it probably changed as a teenager and as an adult, and is part of your self-esteem. Your perception of yourself may not reflect your true figure – though you feel fat, you may look dazzling. Changing your clothing and your make-up may make a big difference to how you feel, and talking to other women will show you that many of them have similar feelings about themselves. Remember that it is important for you to gain weight during pregnancy. Some of the gain is simply fluid retained in your body and you can tell this by your face rounding and your legs swelling.

If you are gaining excessively then this trimester is an opportunity to put the brakes on. For some women pregnancy is the time when a weight problem begins and it often comes as a surprise. The sooner you approach any weight issue the better it will be for you (p.332).

My feet hurt. What should I do about them?
Sore feet are very common in pregnancy: your weight has increased, your centre of gravity, posture and walk have altered, your feet may be swollen and your ligaments are softer. Consider buying trainers or very comfortable shoes, possibly a size larger than usual, and if it is the summer, choose open shoes that allow your feet to breathe. Watch how you walk, particularly if you waddle because your pelvic joints may become sore. Reduce the time you stand at work, and put your feet up when you get home. Antenatal yoga poses and calf stretches (p.350) can release foot tension, and a massage will feel good and may help a lot.

My gums bleed when I brush my teeth. This has never happened before – is it due to pregnancy?
The increased blood supply to your gums during pregnancy can lead to swelling, and inflammation or bleeding if particles of undigested food become trapped. The major cause of bleeding is oral hygiene. Try to take special care of your teeth by brushing and flossing well two or three times a day and taking up the free dental care available to all pregnant women in the UK. Good dental care is important and pregnancy increases vulnerability to gum disease (p.540).

My skin is itchy and I have a rash. Is it serious?
An itchy skin is very common in pregnancy (p.534), and is sometimes due to stretching. If you are prone to dermatitis, acne, allergic reactions or other conditions that affect your skin, they may now flare up. There are also skin disorders that are specific to pregnancy and may be very uncomfortable – some cause a rash, redness or an eruption.

If you have an intense itch with minimal rash it is worthwhile being checked out for cholestasis (p.429). This is a rare condition that affects the liver and is related to oestrogen hormone levels. It is important to diagnose this condition because cholestasis may affect your baby and necessitate early induction of labour.

I feel faint and my midwife says I have low blood pressure. What effect could this have?
Low blood pressure (p.411) is usually a sign of good health and is common among athletes. The only disadvantage is that you may feel faint when you stand up or after you have stood still for a while. Try to avoid sitting or standing in one position for long periods, and remember that exercise and movement encourage good circulation.

I'm not sleeping very well, which I expected, but I'm also waking up with leg cramps. Why is this?
Leg cramps (p.522) are due to tightness and spasm in the calf muscles, and stretching them during the day helps to release the tension. Additional vitamin and minerals, including calcium, may help. Many women find it difficult to sleep through the night and disturbances become more frequent as labour approaches. There are a variety of things you can do to improve sleep: attend to any back and pelvic pain, don't drink much at night, make sure your mattress is supportive and use cushions to make yourself more comfortable. Talking over your anxieties and feeling loved can help you to sleep more soundly. A yoga stretch with breathing or a visualisation before going to bed may help you connect with your baby and calm your thoughts.

My mother had varicose veins and piles. What can I do to prevent them?
In some families there is a tendency to dilated veins during pregnancy: if you have inherited this then there is not much you can do. If you have a job that involves a lot of standing then you could investigate whether it is possible to alter your type of work and rest more. For varicose veins (p.559) in your legs you could wear support tights and put your feet up at night, and avoid gaining too much weight. To guard against bad piles (p.523), prevent constipation by altering your diet to decrease the pressure when your bowels open.

My scan shows that I have a low placenta. Is this a problem?
A low-lying placenta, also called placenta praevia (p.524), can cause bleeding during pregnancy. Many placentas detected as low in this trimester will appear to move up to a normal position by Week 34 when the ultrasound scan is repeated. If your placenta remains low in the third trimester, you may be advised to give birth by caesarean section (p.419) to avoid the risk of dangerously heavy bleeding from your uterus.

Looking ahead

From the moment pregnancy is confirmed, every expectant parent thinks about the actual birth. You may conjure up images of power and mystery, or you may think of pain and fear; you might dwell on thoughts of the birth for months or push the idea to the back of your mind. Anticipation brings up a range of feelings that are a part of the journey into parenthood. You may feel anxious about the unknown. Tapping into these feelings and finding out about how a birth may unfold are some of the ways you can prepare yourself. It is easier to gather confidence if you prepare in advance. This is what this chapter is about.

Active birth

Active birth is a term that can be applied to the whole of pregnancy and to the months beyond, involving active preparation for labour and birth, choices about how best to care for yourself during pregnancy and looking ahead to family life. There is a continuum from conception through to the first months after birth.

In terms of labour and birth, in an active birth you will aim to be physically active during labour so that you can follow the rhythm of your contractions, choose the most comfortable positions and harness your natural power and the force of gravity. Your supporting team can help you feel empowered and make choices that might include pain relief or intervention. After an active birth, it is likely that you will go forward into the early days of parenting with positivity and confidence.

The direct opposite of active birth is 'managed' labour, where you are advised to lie on a bed throughout labour and an obstetric team makes decisions about when and how to intervene. Thankfully, managed labours are becoming less common, but some hospitals are still constrained by poor resources and a lack of open-mindedness.

You have months to read, chat to other parents, go to classes, watch videos or talk to your midwife to decide how and where you want to give birth. During this time you have the opportunity to ready your body and mind. Informed, prepared and aware of your options you can then take an active role in your care, whether you give birth with or without painkillers, in water, on land or have a caesarean.

Natural birth

A 'natural birth' is one where no medical pain relief is used. Many women do manage without any medication: the female body is designed to give birth and cope with a certain level of pain, and there are many natural ways to encourage smooth progress, maintain energy and minimise discomfort. For some people 'natural' represents the holy grail. But medical pain relief or assistance to ensure safety may outweigh the commitment to natural birth. This integrated approach combines the benefit of modern medicine with the best of traditional birthing wisdom and is a very positive way to give mothers a fuller range of options and enjoyment. The selection can combine the best of both worlds.

Classes, groups and workshops

Classes offer information, professional guidance, mutual support and companionship – for many women they are one of the most positive elements of antenatal preparation. In your area there will be an NHS antenatal class that you can attend from Weeks 20–30. It will probably be held in a meeting room in the surgery or hospital. Topics covered include labour, pain relief and medical assistance for birth, plus breastfeeding and basic babycare. It may also focus on the reality of having a new baby and the effect this can have on partnerships.

Some classes are like workshops, with chances for mothers or couples to get involved; some are more like lectures. Some of the meetings may be held at the maternity unit, where you and your partner can visit the labour suites and mothers' ward.

Another popular choice is to attend a series of National Childbirth Trust (NCT) classes, for which there is a fee. Women more often bring their partners along. Topics covered are similar to those in NHS classes. In many areas there are active birth classes with yoga. Meetings are sometimes held in a private house and may continue after the birth. There may be other groups that suit you. Ask your midwife, GP and health visitor, check your leisure centre or contact the organisation concerned.

If you have specific needs, for example if you are expecting twins or you have a medical condition such as diabetes or your baby has a problem such as Down's syndrome, there may be a support group in your area where you can meet other parents who face similar issues.

Although your future appears to be focused almost exclusively on labour and birth, it can be empowering to look beyond. Some classes for parents include meeting babies and listening to first-hand birth and parenting stories and first aid instruction.

Tuning into your baby

In early pregnancy, before you can feel your baby moving, it can be difficult to focus on the tiny being inside you. As pregnancy advances, you will become constantly aware of your baby's presence, which will change the way you walk, bend over, tie your shoelaces, get into the car, sleep and eat. You might notice that he moves boisterously when you play certain music, kicks with extra vigour when you're in the bath or sleeps when your body rocks as you walk. From the womb he'll be showing some of his personal traits and, in his own subtle way, communicating with you. Many women enjoy massaging their abdomen and feeling the responsive movements. You may absent-mindedly place your hand on your belly and your baby will get to know this feeling of pressure. For your partner, stroking or resting a hand on your abdomen or singing to your tummy are powerful ways to get in touch with his baby.

Some women feel intimately connected to their baby long before birth, but it's also common to feel distanced and some women are unable to 'tune in' until they see their baby after birth. The best place to start may be by focusing on yourself in a quiet moment with few distractions. You could consider a few methods of relaxation: breathing exercises, visualisations or yoga (Part V) are effective ways of quietening thoughts and directing energy inwards. With practice, alone or using the visualisation on p.372, you may experience a profound love and connection that boosts your confidence.

Optimal foetal positioning

A baby can take an optimal position: facing down with his head tucked in, arms and legs crossed and spine facing the mother's abdominal wall, he is least likely to have difficulties during birth. This is the most commonly assumed position, known as 'occipito anterior' (the occiput is the name for the back of the baby's head) (p.120). This position will encourage the head to engage when the widest diameter has entered your pelvic cavity.

The way your baby lies affects your comfort, particularly around your back or pelvic regions. Keeping your mind on your posture may come naturally if you exercise regularly and practise a simple yoga routine as part of antenatal care. Your posture affects your energy levels and moods and, with guidance and attention, maintaining good posture can be easy (p.346).

The position your baby chooses in the womb may relate to the location of the placenta, the size and shape of your pelvis and his own size and shape. It may also be determined by your own posture and activity during pregnancy. If you habitually slouch, stoop your shoulders and curve your abdomen, you may hinder your baby from taking a good position. Poor posture reduces space for your abdominal organs, including your uterus, and might make you feel uncomfortable. It could also encourage your baby's spine to fall towards your own spine and take the occipito posterior position (p.149), which may hinder progress in labour.

Your baby will have maximum space and may be more inclined to take the optimal position if you sit and walk straight, extend your spine and support your lower back. A few adjustments could make a significant difference. Check your chair at work and how it fits the table or desk. Beware of couches and soft armchairs – they look cosy but it is best to sit on the carpet with your back upright and well supported. Your posture when lying down is also important – use a supportive mattress and during the day take 5 minutes once or twice to lie flat and relax your spine. Practising squatting is excellent because it helps to lengthen and release the muscles and ligaments in your lower lumbar spine, encouraging good posture while you stand and sit. This is one of a number of useful yoga postures (p.350).

Preparing your body

Your body is designed to birth a baby and inherently knows what to do. With freedom and privacy, you will probably follow your instincts. Although one of the most powerful ways to help your labour progress well is to 'go with the flow', you can prepare by building flexibility and stamina and by learning to relax. Even if you have a caesarean section and don't experience contractions, this will help you feel centred and recover. Preparations during pregnancy aid postnatal healing and they may also contribute to successful breastfeeding and enjoyment of your newborn baby.

I have had two antenatal visits with my community midwife, and I don't feel very comfortable. We have very different views on birth. What can I do?

It is unfortunate that you don't get on and also unusual because in most areas midwives are friendly and open-minded. They are in their job because they love mums and babies. Usually if you have a particular wish they will try to meet it, unless it is in conflict with hospital policy or is something about which they have no experience.

You have found yourself in a difficult position. It is reassuring and safe to have the support of one or more midwives yet it is not easy to live with differences of opinion. If you can, ask about the network of midwives to see whether there is anyone else who is closer to your perspective. You will need to be gentle but firm; you may resolve the issue, or she may agree to hand your care to a colleague. You might find it easier to talk things through with your GP or you could approach the supervisor of midwives attached to your local hospital who may have different possibilities to offer. You may also investigate independent midwifery care.

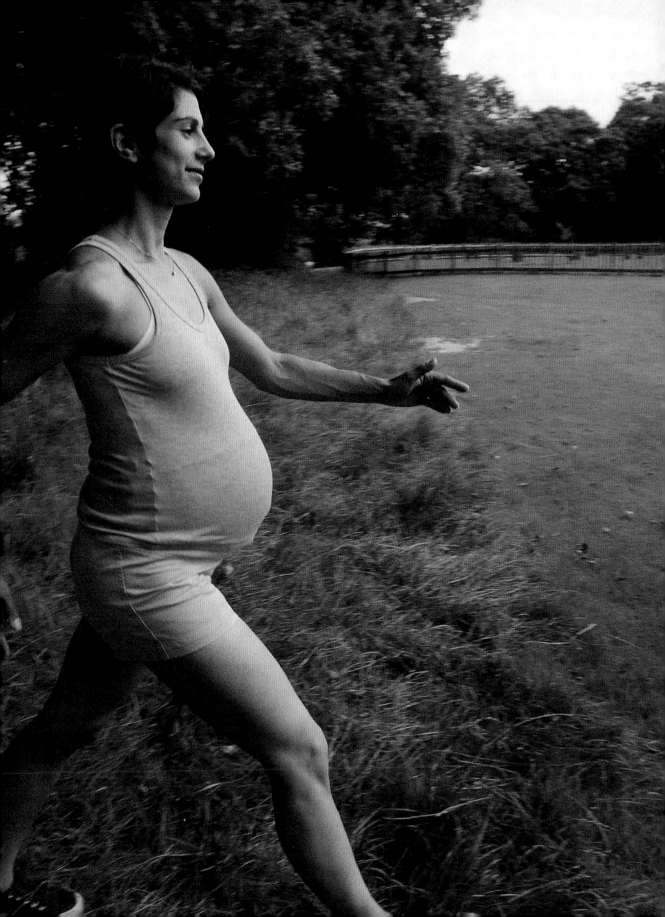

Improving flexibility, fitness and stamina

While it is important to listen to your body and take adequate rest, taking the term 'period of confinement' literally and resting exclusively is not appropriate unless you have a medical condition (such as high blood pressure). On the contrary, regular exercise and stretching are important during pregnancy and there are certain yoga, aerobic and anaerobic exercises geared specifically towards labour and birth (Part V). Any improvement in flexibility, power and balance will assist your intuitive sense of using movement to enhance the progress of birth.

It is common to be in labour for between 10 and 20 hours, during which time you may find it impossible to sleep. Many women tap into exceptional energy reserves, but anyone using physical energy for this amount of time will tire. You can boost your staying power by exercising in pregnancy. An important part of stamina is being able to let go when effort isn't needed, which may come naturally. Letting go is part of any yoga stretch. In labour your birth partner or midwife will encourage you to relax.

Discovering the power of breath

If you feel nervous or in pain, your body reacts by taking short and shallow breaths or you may hold your breath. Taking longer, deeper breaths and slowing the outbreaths can reduce heart rate and blood pressure and bring you back to your centre, calming your body and helping your mind relax too. Getting into the habit of observing your breath and practising controlled breathing will equip you for labour where the breath is a powerful tool for riding the waves of contractions and bearing down. You will find techniques to practise on p.152 and at antenatal classes.

Practising positions for labour

Most antenatal classes give guidance on labour positions and some encourage birth partners to get involved. With practice comes confidence in using and moving your body, and some postures or attention to balance may be second nature by the time you go into labour. Some women draw on their practice, some cope by following their instincts while some need to be reminded. You could try out the postures suggested on p.152 and do any yoga you enjoy. Through practice you'll discover which positions need support (squatting, for example), which help you breathe freely and practice will reduce stiffness.

Being upright for labour and birth

The practice of giving birth while lying down was introduced as 'standard' by western medicine in the 18th century. For centuries before this, women followed the natural instinct to be upright for a large part of labour and when the urge came to bear down and give birth. It is the best way for a mother to harness her power, help the pelvis to open for birth and aid her baby through the birth canal

The benefits of being upright

During labour

You are free to move and express yourself. This boosts confidence and encourages the secretion of hormones that are natural pain relievers.

- Gravity helps your baby's head to be well applied to the cervix, so contractions are more effective – this may result in faster dilation and a shorter labour.
- Forward tilting of the uterus helps modify pain, and may reduce the need for an epidural. You can have a mobile epidural to take away your pain while you continue to use the upright position.
- Blood flow to the placenta is optimal, because there is no compression of your internal blood vessels as there may be in a lying or semi-reclining position. This provides your baby with maximum oxygen flow and reduces the risk of foetal distress.

For birth

- Being upright maximises the natural pushing force of your body.
- The pelvic joints are not constricted as they would be if you were lying down. This increases the pelvic capacity by up to 25% and maximises the space available for your baby's head.
- The entire vaginal opening stretches more efficiently and tears are less frequent.
- If the position helps you to progress well, your baby will have a minimal risk of side effects from drugs or interventions and is likely to be born in an optimal condition.
- If your partner is actively involved in supporting you he will feel the power and magic of birth.

After birth

- Gravity helps the separation of the placenta once your baby is born and sitting upright will help you to hold and welcome your baby.
- Hormone secretions are maximised – these include the 'love hormones' to encourage mothering and breastfeeding.
- Mothers who have given birth in an active upright posture generally feel good – this makes caring for a newborn easier.

and is still favoured in many parts of the world. If you are keen to remain active during labour, it is worth practising upright and squatting positions with your partner or birth attendant. You can change positions during labour and be upright when you actually give birth.

You may need to rest between contractions and it is important to preserve energy. When it comes to it, you may be more comfortable sitting, standing, lying on your side, or floating in water. While being upright is a central part of active birth, the most crucial element of remaining active is to listen to your body, do what feels right and keep safe and comfortable.

Repeat the exercises in sets of five to ten at least five times a day. You can do them anywhere, at any time – no one will know what you're up to. Think of a trigger to remind you: perhaps you could do a set each time you are in the car or waiting at traffic lights or when you watch a regular television programme. After the birth a useful connection is to do a set each time you feed your baby. Walking and exercising are powerful ways to strengthen the pelvic floor, as are some yoga postures.

- Tighten the pelvic floor muscles as if you are holding urine in or tightening your vagina around a penis.
- To begin with you might find it easier to start at the anus and tighten the area gradually, moving towards your vagina.
- Tighten, count to five, and consciously release and relax. Do this five times and then do five sets of tightening without holding the tension.
- As you build up strength and control, practise on your partner during intercourse and see how many tightenings he can count – the extra squeeze for him is guaranteed to thrill.

Perineal massage

A light and gentle massage of your perineum can improve its ability to stretch. From 6 weeks before birth, begin to massage your perineum, three to four times a week, for 2–4 minutes at a time. Massage after a bath or shower, ensure your bladder is empty and relax your pelvic floor as you do it. In the beginning you will feel tight, but with time and practice the tissues will relax and stretch. The massage shouldn't hurt.

- Lubricate your thumb or fingers with olive, almond or grapeseed oil and squat or rest one foot on a chair or bath.
- Place two fingers or a thumb about 5 cm (2 in) into the vagina (up to the second knuckle) and move rhythmically from 3 o'clock to 9 o'clock and back again, using a sweeping motion with downward pressure.
- If there is a tender area, breathe in, hold the pressure lightly on the area and breathe out very slowly while relaxing your abdominal and back muscles and your pelvic floor. You may repeat this two or three times and you will feel the area relax.
- You can also massage the perineal skin between your fingers and thumb. Apply steady pressure downwards towards the back passage until you feel a tingling sensation, which is in fact like the feeling of your baby's head crowning before birth.

Preparing your vagina and perineum

When you give birth to your baby, there is pressure on your vagina and perineum (the area of skin and muscle stretching between your vaginal opening and your anus). Your body prepares for this as hormones soften muscles and ligaments to encourage stretching; you may notice the effect of this during pregnancy if your vagina feels 'loose' or you experience slight incontinence. Active preparation of your vaginal area can improve strength and increase flexibility, reducing the likelihood of you needing a cut to widen the entrance (episiotomy, p.494) or tearing when you give birth. It also has long-term benefits that may improve urinary continence, sex and body image. In addition, attention to perineal strength in your first pregnancy can reduce feelings of looseness in your next. Massage and pelvic floor exercises practised each day can have huge results. Once discovered, these exercises should never be abandoned.

Preparing your mind

Being in touch with what is happening to you emotionally is an important aspect of an active birth and it is valuable to take time to listen to yourself as you wait to meet your baby. You may find it helpful to confide in your friends and family, talk to your midwife or counsellor or explore your thoughts through meditation (p.370). Part IV explores many of the emotions that parents commonly feel before and after birth.

Very few women approach labour without some trepidation. It's perfectly natural to fear pain and to fear the unknown – for all women, giving birth will be a new and powerful experience. Even if your baby is delivered by caesarean, the experience will be one of the most moving you have ever had. Depending on your feelings, you may need to quieten excitement and introduce calm, or dispel fear through relaxation and trust. The two chief ways to prepare for labour are to become informed of your choices and the possibilities ahead of you, accept them and then to learn to relax.

Knowing your choices

Whatever your state of mind, you will be better equipped if you know what can happen. Knowing your choices at each stage is a powerful way to prepare yourself for enjoying labour and birth, and making decisions when you need to.

This preparation begins when you choose a place of birth and talk to your birth team about your options (overleaf). The next level involves classes or reading about labour and acquainting yourself with its stages. To inform yourself one step further, it is helpful to know about the variety of pain relief and the ways that birth may be given a helping hand. This could bring your attention to a range of natural pain relievers (p.156) and medical help (p.164). Often knowing about assistance can make the difference between being afraid of intervention and welcoming support if it is needed.

Preparing your birth partner

Who you have with you during labour, and how confident they feel, can have an impact on your progress. If you feel physically and emotionally supported you are likely to relax, going with the power of contractions. If your partner is afraid, you may pick up on his energy, becoming tense

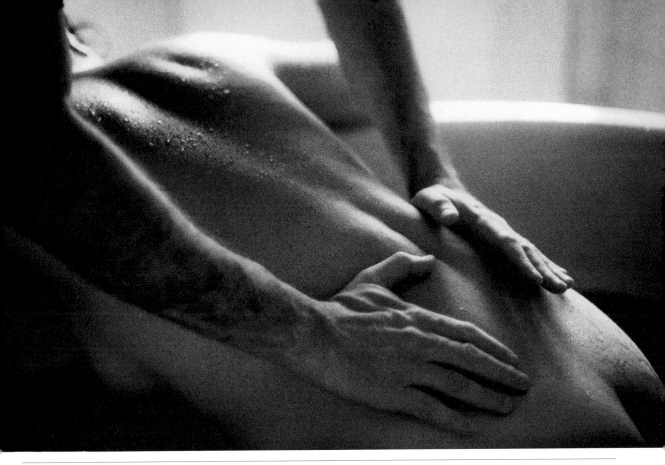

I am nervous about the birth because I fear being in pain. What can I do to feel more confident?

It is not surprising that you are anxious, and quite understandable that your main fear is pain. If you can quell your fear in advance of labour, the later stages of your pregnancy will be more enjoyable. Many women gain more confidence and trust in their own strength when they have acknowledged their fears. If you have a phobia of hospitals or needles there are ways of accepting and reducing these feelings.

Labour does involve discomfort. Yet your body is naturally tuned to give birth and hormones released during labour act as natural painkillers – their release is maximised if you remain mobile and feel loved and supported. You will be able to choose from a broad range of pain relief at each stage of labour. If you are aware of what is available (it is not the same in every hospital), you may feel more at ease. You may also like to explore the possibility of using a water pool: for some women this offers exactly the right level of relief.

Try not to feel guilty for having fears. Most women do. Some worries relate to birth and some to the days beyond – both can interfere with confidence and it helps to talk them through. Your midwife is used to expectant mothers' worries and may be able to reassure you or direct you towards further help if you need. If you are very anxious about something you may find some of the advice on p.461 helps you to feel calmer.

- I don't think I'm strong enough.
- I am afraid of needles and an epidural. I don't know what will happen if I panic.
- I'm worried I won't know how and when to push.
- I'm afraid of bleeding and tearing.
- I have a deep-seated fear of dying, and of my baby dying.
- I worry that my baby will struggle to breathe or be damaged.
- I have heard terrible stories.
- Say my baby is damaged or disabled in some way I'm not sure we'll know what to do.
- I hate the thought of making a wee or pooing in public.
- I'm worried that my partner will faint – he's really squeamish.
- Say I can't breastfeed, I'm concerned my baby miss out on the best start in life.

Making a birth plan

A birth plan ensures that everyone, including your partner and birth team, knows what your view is. You might find the frame below helpful. Remember that while it is encouraging to be committed to a plan, it's good to remain flexible. You cannot take complete control and it is best to prepare in advance and then accept how birth unfolds for you and your baby. If you remain present for what happens you will feel the exhilaration of birth and feel proud of what you achieve.

Considering your options

Who would you like to be with you in labour?
Your partner, a friend, your sister?

What are your preferences when in labour at home?
Bathing, music, massage, homeopathy, pain relief?

At what stage do you want to go to hospital?
When contractions are 5 or 15 minutes apart?

What would you like to have with you during labour?
Healthy snacks and water, favourite pillow, night shirt, music, homeopathic remedies, aromatherapy oils, photographs.

What pain relief are you happy to consider?
Epidural, water pool, massage, homeopathy, visualisation?

Would you like to use the water pool?
In early or late labour? When you want to bear down?

Do you have a preference about boosting contractions?
Oxytocin drip, rupturing of the membranes, massage?

What about cutting the umbilical cord?
After it has stopped pulsating? Your partner wishes to cut it?

How would you like to give birth to the placenta?
After an injection of oxytocin? In your own time?

How soon would you like to hold your baby?
Straight away? After he is washed?

How soon would you like to bring your baby to your breast?
As soon as possible or after you have both been washed? Not at all – bottle feeding?

How long do you wish to stay in hospital?
As short or long as possible? According to baby's health?

Who would you like to support you following birth?
Your partner only? Your mum and your family? A range of friends? A doula, maternity nurse or nanny?

and nervous. Sometimes fathers can be uneasy among a group of women who seem to know more about labour than they do.

You may both decide that it is appropriate to have a friend or a family member with you instead of your partner or as a back-up in case he needs to take a break. Some people choose to have a family gathering through labour.

Preparations for your partner begin with becoming informed about the stages of labour, pain relief and medical assistance. He may want to read up on the subject, go to classes or join you for antenatal appointments or you can go over the basics with him. He may help you make decisions on the day. If he has strong expectations surrounding the birth, it is helpful for you to reach an understanding before labour arrives.

Your partner may spend time massaging you, practising positions for labour or joining in breathing practice. He will probably find that keeping fit and eating well help him to feel strong, centred and confident. Like you, he may be less nervous if he feels supported by friends and family; arranging this may be a central part of his preparation.

Accessing your power

There are many ways to tap into your energy during labour and birth (p.156). In pregnancy, you can begin to access your power to birth and care for your baby in a number of ways, and this may help you look forward to the birth with confidence. This involves trust in your partner and other helpers, and in the natural process of birth. Knowing that you will be supported can be very empowering.

Although there is no way of knowing what will happen on the day that you go into labour and give birth, you can practise relaxation techniques, movements and breathing and try some visualisations that could help you relax and go with the flow. This practice will also make you feel good in pregnancy.

You may find it most empowering to tune into your baby, imagining that he is taking the optimum position for birth, and reminding yourself that he plays an important part in labour (see the visualisation overleaf). He can work in unison with your body as you give birth, and has strength and stamina and an inherent drive to be born so that he can meet you, face to face.

Where do you want to give birth?

Your comfort during labour and the level of trust you feel when you give birth are central to your experience. Feelings of support and love can assist progress, reduce inhibitions and allow you to move and express yourself freely to maximise the efficiency of your contractions. While who is with you is more significant than where you are, your physical environment will play a part in inspiring

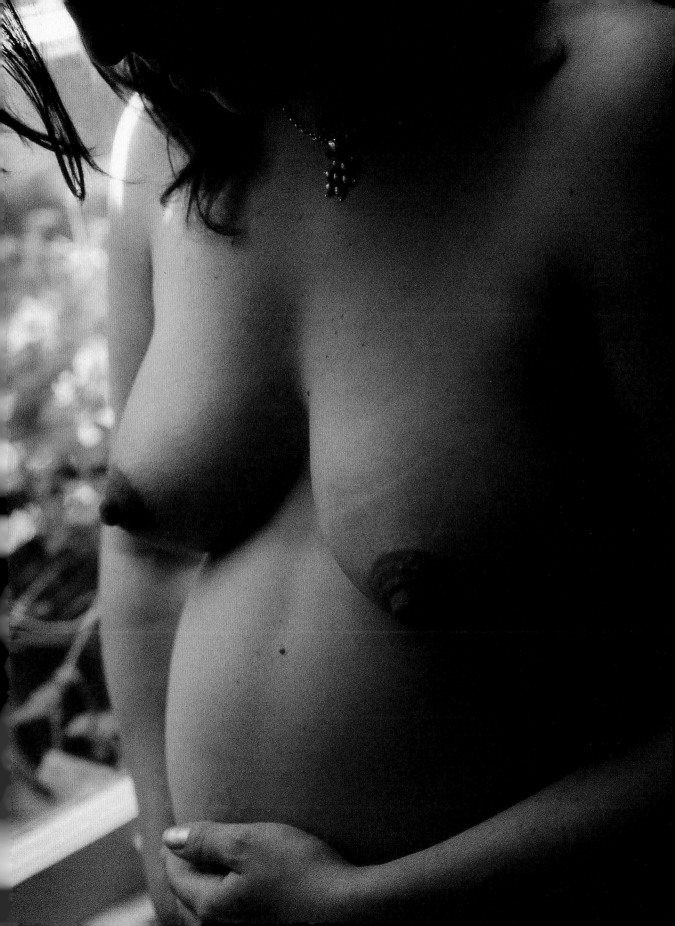

A visualisation for gentle birth

Focus on the birthing part of your body. Take your inner eyes into the deepest part of your abdomen and locate your pelvic circle of bones, which provides the frame on which the muscles of your abdomen, lower back and thighs are attached. Just as your muscles have the ability to move, know that the bones in your pelvis can expand at the joints and ligaments. Between now and the birth, visualise the inner diameters of your pelvic space becoming wider every day. Imagine your baby's head moving down into the lowest part of your uterus and coming into contact with the inner opening of your cervix, the neck of your womb, and encourage your baby to find the optimum position for birth.

Flex your head so your chin is tucked on to your breastbone. Ask your baby to adopt this position and to face towards your spine so that the smallest diameter of his head sinks into your pelvic space. From Week 36, visualise your pelvis and your baby's head moulding comfortably and your placenta producing generous quantities of hormones to prepare your birthing spaces for gentle opening and release at birth.

Encourage your baby to feel calm and nurtured so the placenta produces generous quantities of all the hormones to prepare your birthing spaces for a gentle open-release at birth.

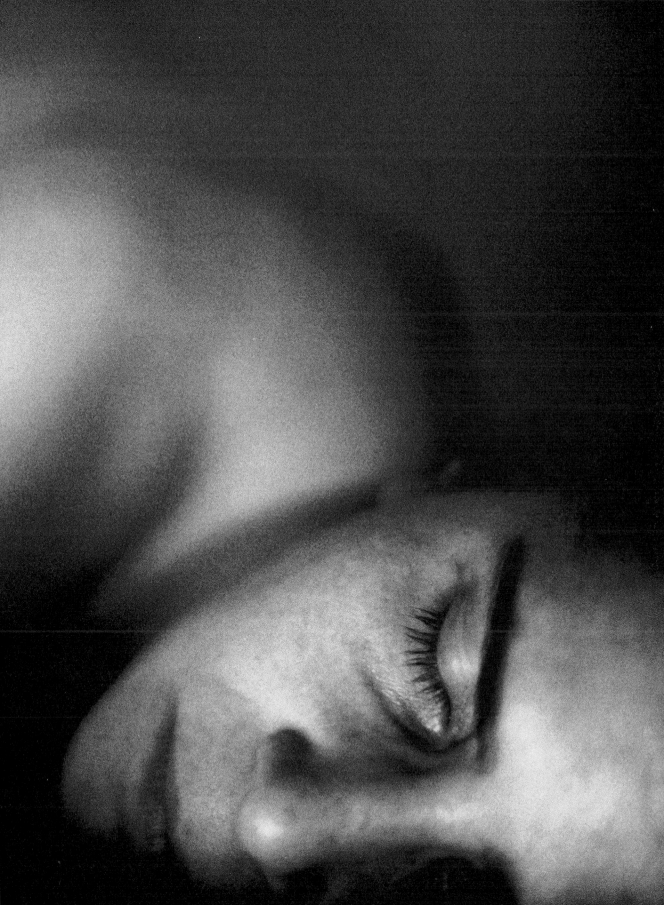

you to tune into your birthing power. It can also offer reassurance if assistance is needed and provide a welcoming environment for your newborn baby.

The most obvious choice exists between a home birth and a hospital birth. Beyond this are options that can contribute to the best possible environment. There may be more than one hospital in your area. The sooner you choose, the better, as you can then get to know the location and the birthing team, and enrol any additional support.

Your kind of birth

The kind of birth you want will determine where you choose to give birth. If you have your heart set on a water birth, for instance, you'll need to find a maternity unit where this will be supported. If you are keen to have an obstetrician, paediatrician and anaesthetist on hand, you will need to book into a main district or teaching hospital. If you want a home birth you may have choices about the midwife and doctors who can assist you.

In any location you can aim for an active birth. Whether this becomes a reality will depend largely on you, your baby and your team of supporters; but the environment matters too. At home you are free to create the ambience you like. A hospital is different and although many still have an unmistakeably clinical feeling, more and more are aiming for a home-like environment.

Hospitals

Most women opt to give birth in hospital, particularly in the first pregnancy. The main reason is that a hospital offers amenities and a skilled medical team, giving a sense of security and trust. Another reason is the company a hospital offers. You may feel encouraged by the team of midwives and refreshed by new faces and energy that comes with each shift change. Some women enjoy the special world of womanly power and new life: sharing stories and feelings, laughter and tears, with other mothers. This may provide a good environment for settling into life with a baby. A comfortable stay in hospital gives the space and time for relaxation, for focusing exclusively on your baby and for postnatal recovery.

Some hospitals offer more disadvantages than benefits and this is well-known locally or obvious when you visit. If the throughput is high, women can feel as if they are part of a production line. In a large, busy hospital you may be looked after by a midwife you have never met and there may be few facilities to meet other mums. In such places women may not relax with their babies until they're home.

What to look for

Hospitals come in many shapes and sizes. Once common, small and intimate maternity homes are rare today. In their place are self-contained maternity departments in community hospitals, district hospitals and large teaching hospitals. Although there are many qualities that combine to make the 'perfect' place, some are more important than others. Loving and considerate midwives more than make up for uninspiring food, for instance. Your choice will be influenced by your own views and your baby's health. If you or your baby require extra surveillances you may need to book into a larger hospital.

Your local hospital may have a maternity unit that suits you well, relieving you of the need to search further. You may, however, be less fortunate: not all hospitals offer the comfort and the level of care that will suit you. Many delivery rooms still look like operating theatres but things are changing. More progressive maternity units provide a home-like environment with soft furniture and lighting and facilities for playing music, should you desire to hear some during or after labour. In some units you may be in one room from admission until the birth is over.

Often a change in a hospital's physical environment is accompanied by new organisation and a shift in attitude. In many comfortable, mother-centred units midwives run the unit, drawing upon the skills of obstetricians when they identify a problem: these are often praised by mothers for creating a conducive environment and midwives feel valued and empowered. For example, they may encourage dads to visit frequently or even stay for a few days after the birth. Midwives here are likely to encourage you to stay

---

What if I change my mind and don't give birth in the way I have planned?
During pregnancy you can prepare but when you enter labour you leave the preparation behind and enter the unknown. What's done is done: in labour it is time to let go and 'be' in what is happening. You cannot control everything and labour involves your baby, too, his size and position and whether his head is tucked in; it also involves the power of your uterus and the size of your pelvis. Your mind and spirit and the free release of love hormones are also important. Because so many different variables combine it is best to have a broad view: if it is too rigid you are likely to be disappointed or even guilty you did not provide the 'perfect' or 'only' start for your baby.

A good way to prepare yourself for enjoying the natural birth of your dreams and for minimising your anxiety if things don't go according to plan is to have faith in your birth partner and the team. They will bring extra support during labour and boost your self-confidence.

Bear in mind that the way we are born is important but human babies are resilient and their brains have the power of plasticity to adapt to what happens in their lives and learn from experiences. What happens in pregnancy and how your baby is mothered after the birth is probably as or more important than the birth itself. Your baby also plays an important role in labour and birth.

How do you choose the place for you?

There are three chief ways of finding out about hospitals: talk to your GP or midwife, talk to other parents and visit each maternity unit. Try to talk to more than one mother who's been to the unit, because everyone will have had a unique experience.

When you go to the hospital, see if you can look at a delivery room as well as the wards or rooms where you would stay after the birth, and chat to the midwives to get an idea of the unit's attitude. Your visit will be most fruitful if you ask questions. You may find some that are important to you in the list below, and others will come to mind as you read more about labour and birth.

Antenatal care

- During your antenatal visits will you be cared for by the team of midwifes who will attend your birth?
- What range of classes does the unit offer?
- Will you be seen by the same midwife or doctor throughout pregnancy?

Care in labour

Many decisions are made according to the way you feel and how labour is progressing, and may depend on the number of women in labour at any one time.

- Will a midwife be with you throughout labour?
- Will you be moved to the delivery room late in labour, or will you be allowed in the delivery room as soon as you are admitted?
- If you have a separate room, will you be able to give birth here rather than in the delivery room?
- Are beanbags, cushions and birthing stools provided?
- Will the midwives encourage and support you if you want to move about during labour?
- Will you be able to dim the lights and bring objects from home to create a more familiar environment?
- Is there a tape or CD machine? If not, can you bring your own?
- Will you be allowed to eat and drink during labour? How much food is provided and when?
- Can you bring aromatherapy ointments, essential oils or homeopathic remedies into the labour room?

Medical assistance

Most maternity units have statistics to show how many births proceed without intervention and what percentage need forceps or episiotomies or caesareans. If a water pool is available, there will also be a record of how many women give birth in water.

- What is the policy on induction? Is it routinely recommended after your waters break or a certain number of days after your due date? Does the hospital prefer to induce mid-week?
- If the hospital has a birth pool, are you able to use it at any stage during labour and birth or after the birth?
- Is it hospital practice to conduct foetal monitoring in labour with you lying still on the bed or is it more common to use a hand-held monitor, which interferes less with your movement?
- If your waters do not break are they artificially broken and at what stage of labour does it happen?
- What pain relief is available? Will an anaesthetist be available to give you an epidural any time of day or night?
- Where in the room do most women give birth (on the bed or squatting on a mat on the floor)?
- Will an obstetrician be available to care for you and a paediatrician to care for your baby should you need them?
- What is the hospital's policy on caesareans?
- Is the umbilical cord cut immediately after birth, or only after it has stopped pulsating? Will your partner have the option of cutting it?
- Is the birth of the placenta encouraged with a hormone injection?
- If you have an episiotomy or tear, can a midwife stitch you or must you wait for a doctor to arrive?
- Is there a special care unit, should your baby need it?

Your stay in hospital

Time in hospital can be a great opportunity to learn about feeding and caring for your baby, provided the midwives in the unit have time to support you.

- How long can you expect to stay in hospital if your birth is straightforward?
- Will your baby be able to sleep in or beside your hospital bed?
- Is there a nursery where the midwives can care for your baby while you sleep?
- Can your partner stay, or visit freely?
- Are there any single rooms?
- Is a breastfeeding counsellor available?
- What kind of meals are served? Is there a facility for storing and preparing your own food?

close to your baby as you learn to breastfeed. Many prefer women to stay until 2 or 3 days after the birth so they are satisfied that feeding has started well.

Independent maternity units

In the UK there are very few free-standing birthing units but these are more common in other countries throughout the world. In general the advantage of the birth units is the low intervention rate but because there are no facilities for caesarean section the issue of safety for mother and baby is the one most frequently discussed. A birthing unit must have a well-defined booking policy to exclude women with a high risk of needing intervention and if difficulties arise during the pregnancy or birth then it is essential to arrange for a transfer to a larger facility. Women who give birth in a birthing unit are usually very happy that the atmosphere was close to having a baby at home, unless they needed to be transferred urgently.

The importance of your environment

Being familiar and happy with your surroundings is important because when you're at ease and feel safe, your body will release labour and birth hormones more effectively. Some of these help you to feel loving and relieve pain. If you visit your birth location in pregnancy you can plan to make it cosy, perhaps by bringing personal possessions with you or altering the lighting. When in labour all of your senses may be heightened and some things to keep you comfortable and secure could help.

If you can't find the perfect hospital

Like any professional group, midwives and doctors encompass a wide range of perspectives. If no unit fulfils your preferences, you may compromise and still be confident that you will be supported well.

I am only 6 weeks pregnant but I already know that I really want to give birth to my baby in my own home. But my GP has told me that it's not the best option for my first baby. Why is this?

If you had already given birth without difficulty, your GP might support your choice more readily. The first birth is a new experience and subsequent births tend, in general, to be easier. At this early stage in your pregnancy your antenatal care has only just begun. Your medical team will be in a better position to agree to a home birth once they have formed a fuller picture of your pregnancy.

You do have the right to choose birth at home and it is up to you to weigh up the risks. The list below gives some of the more common conditions that make a hospital birth advisable.

- If you suffer from a health problem such as heart disease or epilepsy, you will benefit from close monitoring and access to specialists. If you are suffering from pregnancy-related problems such as anaemia, high blood pressure or signs of pre-eclampsia or if your placenta is not working effectively and your baby has intrauterine growth restriction, or a placenta is covering your cervix in late pregnancy, a hospital birth is vital.
- If your pregnancy has lasted less than 36 weeks, your baby may need assistance to breathe. If your pregnancy lasts more than 42 weeks, there is a higher chance of foetal distress.
- If your baby is lying in a breech position you will require more assistance and your birth team may strongly advise a caesarean section (p.419). If your baby is large at the end of pregnancy the birth may need assistance.
- If you have had a caesarean section previously there is a small risk of the scar rupturing in labour.
- If you are carrying twins (or more babies) complications are more likely to arise.

If the hospital cannot dim its lights, ask if you could bring a small lamp or even burn candles and essential oils. If the midwives are not confident about guiding you into different positions, you may be able to find classes where you can practise with your partner. If the midwives are overstretched, an arrangement for a breastfeeding counsellor to visit after your baby's birth may help you get off to a good start. And finally, if the maternity ward has a reputation for being noisy at night, making sleep difficult, you could buy ear plugs or request to be discharged soon if your birth is straightforward and you have support at home.

Home birth

In many parts of the world giving birth at home is the obvious choice, perhaps because it is tradition, a woman lives far from a hospital or hospital care is not reliable. In fact, 80% of the world's children are born at home or in a birthing room used by the local community. In the UK around 1 in a 100 babies are born at home, but the figure has not always been so low – in the mid-1960s, around 1 in 3 births happened at home. Since then there has been a progressive trend towards hospital birth because of the safety it offers.

When a mother chooses her home as the birthing environment, she and her friends and family are able to prepare in the way that suits them. The idea of nesting takes on a new meaning as towels and sheets are washed, ironed and readied, furniture is moved and the bathroom cleaned to welcome the baby.

In your own space, you may feel more in control of your choices and your other children may enjoy being part of the experience. You may want to hire a birth pool. You can decide who is present and what happens in the sacred moments following birth.

If you decide to stay at home, you will need to think about your decision carefully, and take responsibility for several aspects. You will need to be aware that birth does have risks: there is a chance that a complication may arise that necessitates the move to hospital and one of the safety issues to consider is the distance to hospital. A home birth is usually only sanctioned when mother and baby are known to be low risk.

Organising a home birth

The first people to talk to if you are considering a home birth are your midwife, who can fill you in on the practical details, and your GP, who is in a position to give you the go-ahead. Your GP may be an integral part of your birth team. In most areas there is a team of community midwives who can attend home births. You may prefer to hire an independent midwife who will care for you throughout pregnancy and birth and might have a more flexible approach to childbirth.

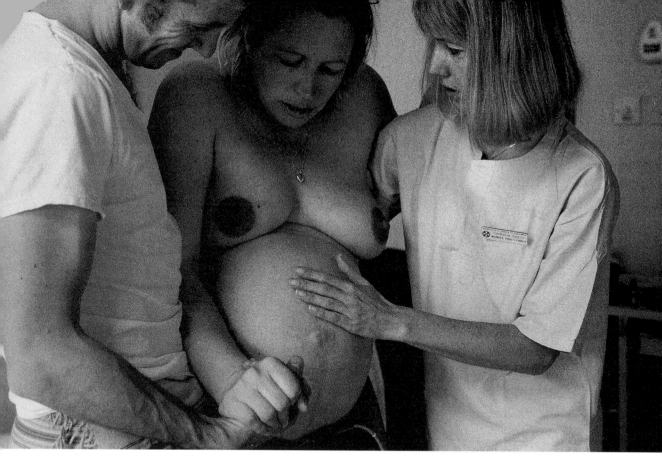

Your midwife supports and encourages you during labour. She plays an important role in helping you to feel relaxed and confident.

You will have many questions to ask the midwife who will attend your birth. Many of the questions on p.105 concerning care in labour and medical assistance will be relevant. Ask also about her back-up team and how she will handle any complications; what emergency equipment will she bring to assist you and your baby and under what circumstances will she arrange a transfer to hospital?

Home labour, hospital delivery

While the environment at home and the loving support of your family may increase the likelihood that birth will go smoothly, there may be unforeseen events that interrupt the flow. A midwife attending a home birth may have several reasons to believe that transfer to hospital is the safest option. If you or your baby needs assistance for which she is not qualified, she is obliged to enrol the appropriate medical support.

In a small number of cases, labour and birth proceed without any cause for concern but the baby needs assistance at birth. Midwives carry equipment to encourage breathing and are trained to administer neonatal resuscitation until a transfer can be arranged. They also carry injections and gas and air (Entonox, p.158) to help painful contractions and equipment to stop bleeding from the uterus and to provide intravenous fluid to prevent or treat blood loss. In an emergency the midwife will summon help from the paramedics in the local ambulance service and from the nearest hospital maternity unit.

If your midwife feels you need to be transferred, she will call the maternity unit and arrange transport. You will go directly to the labour ward, not to accident and emergency, and your midwife may accompany you as well as your birth partner. When you arrive, your care will be taken over by a hospital midwife and doctor, and after they have assessed you and your baby, they will recommend a course of action.

What happens on the day

There are high chances that you will give birth in the location you have chosen, but something may happen that prevents this. As you make plans, it is best to keep an open mind. You do not have sole control over what happens during labour – your baby has an equally strong influence. The way things turn out on the day, even if you could never have imagined them, may barely affect the pride you feel as a mother, or the love you feel towards your baby.

The third trimester: Weeks 28–40

This final trimester of pregnancy carries the most visible changes as you grow, and ends as you meet your baby at birth. There may be changes at work as well as at home, and inside you, your baby matures so that she is ready for birth and life outside the womb and the next stage of your journey as a family.

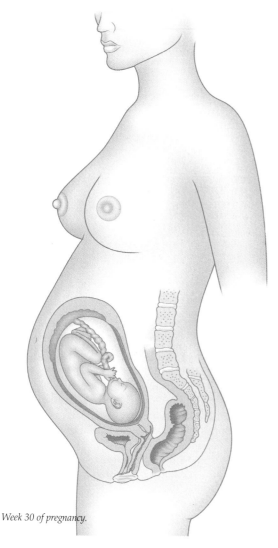

Week 30 of pregnancy.

Your baby and you

Your baby: Weeks 28–32

In this period your baby will nearly double in weight from around 900 g (2 lb) to 1800 g (4 lb), by which time she will be around 40 cm (16 in) long. She opens her eyes often and begins to assume a rhythm of waking and sleeping. She recognises patterns in your speech, the voices of people you're often with and music you play regularly. She dreams a lot – in fact, up to 80% of her sleeping time is REM dream sleep.

All the neurones in her brain are now in place and she already has billions more than there are stars in the universe. From now on, each neurone is forming up to 15,000 links with other neurones as she receives and responds to signals and information.

Rapidly filling the available space in your uterus, she rolls and turns less but will still kick vigorously. As her fat reserves increase, her skin appears less wrinkled. If you are carrying a baby girl, her clitoris will appear prominent because her labia are still forming; if it's a boy, his testicles are just beginning to make their journey towards the groin from their location near the kidneys.

You: Weeks 28–32

The beginning of the third trimester marks a change in your pregnancy as your body gears up to give birth and nurture your baby afterwards. Your breasts may begin to leak colostrum and you may notice tightening in your lower abdomen as contractions in your uterus, which are always occurring, become stronger. These 'practice' contractions are known as Braxton-Hicks and will become stronger in the coming weeks. They are not a sign of labour, and nor is an increased vaginal discharge, which is quite normal at this time. It's also common to feel warm (or too hot if it's summer) most of the time. You may become more distracted and forgetful, and rely on mental lists of everything from purse to keys each time you leave the house.

You may notice new stretchmarks on your breasts, stomach, bottom or thighs. You'll probably also become less mobile, even though you may be more flexible. Getting in and out of the bath, for instance, may be quite difficult; remember to move slowly and try not to take all the pressure of movement on your pelvis or lower back. These are not the only areas under strain: your internal organs are also becoming increasingly compromised. You may need to catch your breath more often than usual, and because there's less room for your stomach it might be more comfortable to eat smaller meals. Physical discomfort may contribute to patchy sleep, which may also be due to vivid or troubling dreams that result from your unconscious mind processing your fears and fantasies about your baby, the birth, and your role as a mother.

Your baby: Weeks 33–36

Your baby will weigh about 2800 g (6 lb) by Week 35, after which she continues to gain around 280 g (10 oz) per week. She is becoming more mature and less wrinkled as the weeks pass. By Week 34 her fingernails will have grown to reach the tips of her fingers and the hearing and speech centres of her brain mature so she's ready to respond to your language at birth. The link between the feeling of moving the mouth and its location is forged, which is one reason why she can imitate your tongue movements within hours of birth.

She swallows, urinates and makes breathing movements. In preparation for breathing your baby's lungs secrete a surfactant, which will help them to remain expanded after the birth and allow oxygen to enter from the air. Meanwhile, a store of glycogen is building in her liver. She will draw on this and her fat reserves for energy during labour and in the following days while feeding is established.

She's still moving and exercising despite decreasing space, and may hiccup regularly. Her eyes are blue and scan her environment as she turns her head from side to side, and she may have wisps of hair on her head. Protected by her still flexible skull bones, her brain expands rapidly as the sensory and motor connections increase and her head grows more than the rest of her body to accommodate it. The sleep cycle varies from baby to baby but at this stage babies usually sleep and wake in 30–50-minute cycles.

You: Weeks 33–36

With the increasing weight of your baby and the final softening of your ligaments in preparation for birth, your pelvis may be tender. If you have had pelvic or back discomfort, it may get more painful now. You may have less control over urinary leakage. Water retention may increase, giving swelling in your feet and hands, particularly if it's hot, so rest regularly with your feet up. Braxton-Hicks contractions can become quite strong at times. If the feeling of tightening becomes regular and is accompanied by pain, you may be in early labour.

You will, of course, feel larger. It's usual to gain around 570 g (1¼ lb) a week in this penultimate month. Your days may already be tinged with nostalgia as you know that pregnancy will soon be over, as well as excitement as birth gets closer. You may feel calmer and more centred, move slowly and spend more time than usual being quiet. You may be anxious about the labour.

You will feel your baby moving and kicking, and her actions may have fallen into a recognisable pattern. Perhaps she sleeps more in the morning, and then wriggles on and off until the evening before quietening down again. It is usual to feel at least 10 kicks per day.

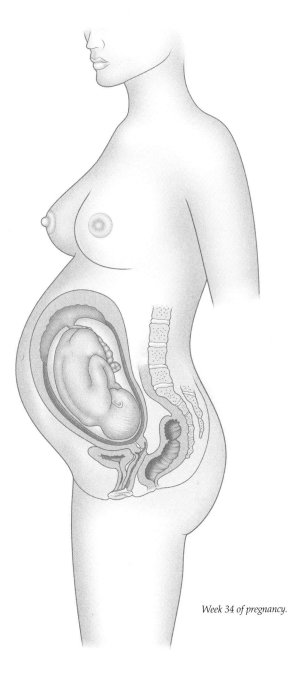

Week 34 of pregnancy.

Your baby: Weeks 37–40

Your baby gets ready for her arduous journey. The amniotic fluid diminishes and your baby grows to fill the available space: a typical baby at Week 37 weighs almost 3 kg (6 lb 8 oz). If she has not settled with her head down and her tummy facing your back (occipito anterior, p.120), you can encourage her to turn.

By full term, which depending on your cycle and your baby may be anything between Weeks 38 and 42, your baby's lungs will be mature enough to breathe air, her brain cells will be highly organised and her hearing will be excellent. Her vision is not great, but already good enough to allow her to focus on your face when you hold her at your breast. As links in her brain become established, the size of the brain increases rapidly. By term her cerebral cortex has grown so much that it no longer appears smooth but has formed the creases that give it the appearance of a walnut.

If this is your first pregnancy, your baby's head will move down and 'engage' in your pelvis, probably around Week 36, although this may be delayed until labour has started. In second and subsequent pregnancies it is common for engagement to occur in labour. Her full weight – averaging 3.2 kg (7 lb) at full term – will now be bearing down on your pelvis. When the time comes, her brain instigates the production of hormones, which stimulate the placenta and uterus to send chemical messages that trigger contractions. The wait is over and the passage to the outside world begins.

You: Weeks 37–40

As you get closer to birth, you may feel calm but tire easily. It's just as usual, though, to feel a burst of energy, even though your sleep may be disturbed or you are fed up. As your body prepares for labour your ligaments reach maximum softness to allow your pelvic and sacro-iliac joints to expand.

Your cervix softens and thins (ripens). As it does, the mucus plug that sealed off the uterus from the vagina may be dislodged, resulting in a 'show', which may be tinged with blood. This is one sign that labour may start within a few hours or days. Other signs are described on p.120.

In the last days, pressure on your pelvis intensifies. Walking and even standing may be uncomfortable, but resting well and regularly keeping upright and moving can help. If you go beyond Week 40 (which is common with first babies) you might find the extra days tedious – it may be nice to have a little more time, but you're probably ready for labour by now.

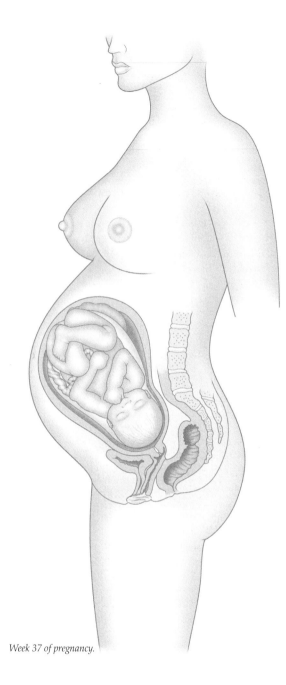

Week 37 of pregnancy.

What's special

For some women this last trimester flies past, but for others, often those who've given up work or for whom mobility is a problem, it drags on. The prize at the end – labour, birth and a baby – can seem exciting, terrifying, delightful and dreadful all at once. Your baby will grow a lot and while you may start off this trimester feeling quite sprightly, by the end you may feel much heavier and be greatly looking forwards to being lighter and fitting through doorways with less trouble.

The physical changes are just part of the picture; you are bound to think about the birth and the days, weeks and months that follow, and may talk about this often with your partner and friends. You may have incontrollable urges to wash the floor, sweep the cobwebs, tidy the kitchen cupboards and organise your house. This nesting instinct is extremely common, and it's natural to be concerned that everything is in order for the arrival of your baby. In fact, frantic tidying can be a sign that labour is imminent.

Your feelings

There will be moments or days of excitement about meeting your baby, feelings of love and wonder, and some meditative contemplation, particularly in the last month as you naturally become more introspective. You might also be laughably forgetful or scatty, which is very common in late pregnancy. At times you may feel fed up – this boredom is quite normal.

You won't be alone if you begin to worry about childbirth or balancing life as a mother. You may often ask, 'Will I be a good mother?' Such thoughts are a vital part of your preparation, and every mother-to-be has them. Take time to tune into yourself and share your thoughts with people you trust.

The first signs of labour may trigger a buzz of excitement, or they may frighten you. Although antenatal preparation can suggest what it may be like, when the reality dawns, you may be happier or more energetic than you had imagined you would. Equally, you may feel overwhelmed and nervous. Call in your supporters as soon as you feel the need, and don't worry about expressing yourself. Joy and excitement or pain and fear are essential ingredients in labour and arise in part from the special blend of hormones in your body.

Your relationships

As the big day approaches, you and your partner may feel closer. You will rely on him for practical support and he may relish being the protector. He may also need emotional support from you. Being there for one another can bring balance and understanding. Furthermore, enjoying time alone together is a lovely way of celebrating your partnership before beginning to deal with life with a baby.

On the other hand, you may both feel pressured and find that you tend to fly into a rage much more easily than you did before.

Whether or not your partner has chosen to be with you in labour, accentuating the positive and strong aspects of your relationship now will bring strength, trust and intimacy as you welcome your baby. If there are difficult issues, some immediate things may need to be resolved before the birth, and some may be better left: often conflicts arise because you are both anxious about the unknown, and some disagreements may disappear completely once you have your baby.

Your relationship with your parents may get stronger now, and your mum may want to spend lots of time with you preparing your baby's room or going through baby clothes. For her these scenes may be very emotional because she is watching you change from being her baby to being a mother. You might end up sharing knowledge and secrets about childbirth, babies, husbands and a lot more. She may be very supportive and want to be there to empower you and tell you how highly she rates you. Your mum may not be in the same town and you may feel sad and miss her strength and support.

If your relationship with your mum is less close and her views differ from yours then you will need the courage to listen to her and make your own decisions. If you find that by trial and error her view is correct for you then give in gracefully and acknowledge her experience. If your mother is around more than you would like, be gentle as you let her know that you need time to yourself and with your partner. Alternatively, if she does not want to be involved, you may need to draw on the love and support of other family members and friends.

Time to enjoy

If you're uncomfortable you will have a very different concept of enjoyment from someone who has boundless energy. You have one thing in common, though, and that is more time to yourself than you will have after the birth. If you do things that make you feel good, it will lift your spirits and send positive hormones racing round your body and to your baby.

A little conscious time-management could help you find time for yourself, with your partner, family, friends and possibly for work too (p.51). In this last stage of pregnancy you may find that everyone wants a piece of you. Remember not to put yourself under pressure; if you don't feel good, cancel an engagement; if you feel like company but are tired, ask friends to bring food and a video to your house.

You may continue to be sociable or find large gatherings difficult when your mind is distracted. If you enjoy being solitary don't forget your wider network of friends who will be wondering how you are and probably very excited about your baby. Women who've been through it all before will be particularly empathetic, and if you are worried, they will almost certainly help you see the lighter side.

Your due date may sometimes feel like a looming deadline. Before you pack too much into your days and sacrifice rest and relaxation, remember that time is not stopping at the birth; things may change, but life and enjoyment goes on.

Your body and body image

As you get bigger and feel heavier, body image can go one of two ways – up if you feel gorgeously glowing, or down if you feel like a hippo squeezed into a boob tube. In these last months you may feel less and less control over your growing body, particularly if you're swollen or in some discomfort.

If you're feeling low, try not to turn to food for comfort. Your mood may improve if you take a bath with relaxing oils, meet a friend for tea, go for a haircut or simply relax. Perhaps a massage or osteopathy session could ease strains, or gentle exercise, yoga or a swim revitalise you.

Even if you've only a few weeks of pregnancy left, treat yourself to something that makes you feel good – it may be underwear or a warm cardigan. Tuning into your baby could also lift your spirits and bring your bodily changes into perspective. Try not to take it to heart when everyone you meet in the street says, 'You *must* be due soon!' or 'What, still here?'

Labour is likely to go most smoothly if you don't feel inhibited, and if you are nervous about being naked it may be difficult to express yourself or move freely during labour as a way of relieving pain. Consider taking time to focus on your body, now in the fullest flush of pregnancy, as a vehicle for your baby. It might help to do antenatal exercises or yoga movements at home in front of a mirror, or go to pregnancy classes where you will see the many shapes of pregnancy.

Eating and weight gain

Your growing uterus is taking up more and more of your abdomen, so you'll find it easier to eat small amounts frequently – every 3 hours is best. While you wait for labour, though, you may have time on your hands and be tempted to eat too much or turn to sugary foods: avoid these and fruit juices and colas or foods that cause heartburn. Plan in advance for labour – stock up on healthy snacks for you and your partner that can be easily taken to hospital. You might also want to prepare meals for freezing to eat after the birth.

Your baby is laying down calcium in the bones and you need to get enough: in addition to milk and cheese you could eat nuts, seeds and green vegetables. As your baby lays down iron stores it is best to eat iron rich foods and take a supplement (p.345).

If you haven't already explored herbal and fruit teas, try some now. When you are breastfeeding it is best to take caffeine-free drinks, and some herbal teas can refresh, aid the success of feeding or help you to sleep, so discovering what you enjoy drinking might be a helpful thing to do now. Raspberry-leaf tea is a good uterine tonic that may improve your contractions.

Inside your body the weight of your baby is increasing but the placenta stops enlarging and the amniotic fluid levels drop slightly. It's usual for weight gain to continue as in the second trimester and level out after Week 38 (p.332). The average gain for the last trimester is between 3.6 and 4.5 kg (8 and 10 lb).

Exercising and relaxing

Many women spend these last 3 months getting physically ready. It is common in the last trimester to tire easily, so avoid over-exertion. Yoga postures and exercise classes can be energising, increase flexibility and bring you in touch with your body as it prepares for birth, and they may help you sleep better (pp.346 and 357). Good postures to focus on include squatting for bearing down and upright kneeling or sitting positions for relaxation. Swimming and walking are great for loosening up and improving circulation. The way you move and sit could encourage your baby to take a good position for birth and it's important to remember to do regular pelvic floor exercises and perineal massage (p.98).

Now at the height of pregnancy, you will tend to be more emotional than rational, a shift reflected in your own thoughtfulness. The breathing aspect of yoga may help you to feel centred and calm. You may dwell on your vision of the future with your baby but it could also help to practise visualisations (p.370) that help you welcome birth.

Dad's issues

The final stages of pregnancy may be a mix of fun and frivolity and a muddle of nerves and anticipation. Practical preparations will now include being ready for the trip to hospital, and you may want to learn more about labour so you'll understand what's going on for your partner. If she is making a birth plan, your input will be valuable and you may be able to practise postures or breathing techniques together.

Many antenatal classes will include you and there may be a group visit to the maternity ward. Pack your own bag for labour: you'll need snacks to keep your energy up, perhaps a change of clothes or some comfortable shoes, phone numbers and other personal items such as your favourite music. Don't forget a camera loaded with film.

As the due date approaches, sort out your plans concerning work and make sure you and your boss are clear about what happens if you have to leave suddenly. As your partner gets more uncomfortable, you may need to help around the house more than usual, which can add a few hours to your working week. Take time for yourself too and meet up with your friends while you can.

You may wonder about long-term changes to your relationship and the effects they may have. This is quite common and it's best if you can talk about it with your partner or a friend. You will need to consider your feelings about labour too. Are you afraid of things that you haven't yet shared? Do you have anything you wish to discuss to do with babycare or breastfeeding?

Sex and intimacy

Every woman and man is different when it comes to sex late in pregnancy. Some feel really sexy, find it great fun or laugh a lot, others are turned off. Some women have reduced feeling in their vagina but a really sensitive clitoris. Men often feel the difference as the vagina alters in preparation for birth, and both partners may get more satisfaction from mutual masturbation or oral sex. Risk to the baby is negligible unless you have an underlying condition like a placenta praevia (p.524) or the membranes have ruptured, in which case it is best to abstain.

The old wives' tale about stimulating labour through love making may be fun to put to the test, but is unlikely to do much unless the prostaglandin hormones in the semen reach your cervix when it's on the verge of ripening. Another way of encouraging the onset of labour may be through nipple stimulation, which releases oxytocin hormones.

Work and finances

If you are working, take things easy. Eat well to keep your energy levels high, take regular rests and if you're getting swollen ankles or varicosities, support stockings may ease discomfort. Where your work involves a lot of sitting down you may feel lethargic and tired because you're not actually moving enough – get up, walk around and have a stretch every 40 minutes, and keep an eye on your posture. If you feel tired, move about or have a lie down before you reach for a chocolate bar to tide you over, and make sure that you drink enough water.

Leaving work is one of the big transitions you will make in your journey to becoming a mother. You may have more friends at work than at home and once you have left, the reality of parenting will be very real. Talk to other mothers who've been through maternity leave. Isolation has been a problem for expectant and new mothers for generations and you may worry if you do not feel close to the people who live near you. But there are always ways to extend your friendships and your community (p.51). You may enjoy being at home and getting ready for your baby, and meeting work colleagues socially could bring new richness to your friendships. You could also meet people through groups and classes that are geared towards pregnancy or newborn babies. Ask your midwife, GP and health visitor; check your leisure centre or contact local organisations. If you're used to physical work, put your energies into gardening, walking and exercising, cooking or making things for the nursery, and if you prefer mental stimulation, set aside some time for reading or filling in a pregnancy journal.

If you haven't already completed the paperwork to do with receiving maternity or paternity benefits, you'll need to act before the birth (p.320). Once you've made arrangements you might consider the implications of not returning to work, or returning part time. Whatever your plans now, remember that you may change your mind once your baby is born.

Medical checks

After Week 36 your doctor or midwife will assess you and your baby each week. You will have a blood test for anaemia around Weeks 32–34 and may be offered a late pregnancy scan depending on local practice. Enrol in an antenatal class if you haven't already done so, and gear yourself up for the birth; this may help you finalise your birth plan. Take these last weeks to think over your hopes and go through your preferences with your birth partner and your doctor or midwife. You may feel more confident about the approaching birth if you find out how to recognise labour and pre-labour signals (p.120), and make sure you always have the phone numbers of your hospital or midwife to hand. You may be responsible for taking your own maternity notes to hospital.

If your labour has not started on your due date, the birth team will assess your baby's wellbeing and you will be checked more frequently in the days that follow using foetal heart monitoring combined with ultrasound.

Holistic care

It's time to make firm plans if you want to use complementary therapies for labour and/or for postnatal healing. You'll need to rely on your birth partner to remember your wishes or to pick the right essential oil or homeopathic remedy during labour, so take time to get this clear. The chapter Complementary therapies for labour and birth (p.162) provides ways to use homeopathic remedies together with aromatherapy, massage and acupuncture during this time. If you become familiar with remedies during pregnancy, integrating them into your labour care will be much easier when the time comes.

If you are uncomfortable or not sleeping well in late pregnancy or your baby is a breech presentation, complementary therapies may also be very useful. Appropriate treatments are provided in relevant entries of the A–Z Health Guide.

Common concerns

Extended information on these concerns, and a range of other antenatal health issues, are covered in the A–Z Health Guide.

I feel the need for some kind of ritual to prepare for my baby and my own transition into motherhood. What could I do?

The easiest ritual is a dinner party or a day out with friends or family. In many countries mums-to-be throw a 'baby shower' where friends (usually female) gather round and give presents. This often leaves the mum with all her baby paraphernalia from car seat to cot, vests to wallpaper. It also provides the opportunity for chatting about pregnancy and birth experiences and celebrating friendship. In other parts of the world women meet to embellish the birthing room or the expectant mother's house with decorations that may be symbolic and protective as well as beautiful.

Can my doctor predict how labour will be?

Birth depends on many factors and is notoriously difficult to predict. If you and your baby have been well during the pregnancy, your baby's position is good and your pelvic shape and size don't conflict with your baby's size, you are off to a good start. If your cervix is effaced and soft and ripe and your uterus contracts well, labour is likely to progress easily. These are only physical aspects of labour; if you feel confident and have faith in your own ability and your baby's contribution, you will increase the chances of an uncomplicated birth.

I am afraid of hospitals and needles and exposing my body. What will I do when I go into labour?

Many people have these fears. Sometimes they are irrational and intense, and they often prevent relaxation whether at a simple consultation or on admittance for labour. It is similar to the fear of flying. Talk about this with your midwife, who may ask you to visit the labour suite because acclimatising to the reality may reduce your fantasy. In many hospitals maternity wings are welcoming and homely, and midwives are used to women's fears. It may help to know that your midwife will help you keep covered as much as possible and during the birth your vagina can be discreetly visible. As a way of accepting your fears and building positivity, you might find visualisations help. Your antenatal preparation classes may also dispel your doubts. If your fear is still intense, you may need counselling or hypnotherapy, particularly if you have had a previous bad personal experience in hospital (p.461).

Will I have the stamina to get through the birth?

How much stamina you need will depend on the length and intensity of your labour. Your stamina will be greater if you are physically fit, well supported by people you trust, well nourished as labour progresses and free to move around. Complementary therapies like homeopathy and massage and water can extend your staying power, while staying calm and breathing and visualisations can preserve energy as you relax between contractions. If your energy dips, an epidural anaesthetic could bring relief and give you time to build your reserves.

I am so excited I feel bonded with my baby. Could this help my labour?

As this trimester progresses you have probably found it easier to tune into your baby and notice his movements and his wake/sleep rhythm. By the time labour begins you may be counting the minutes to see and cuddle him, and already feel that you know him. It is great to feel bonded and he will sense your love now and as soon as he sets eyes on you and feels your embrace after birth. It is lovely that he has already been welcomed as part of your family. Feeling connected may indeed help your confidence in labour, but remember that there are many other factors involved.

What do my partner and I need to do before the birth?

The main thing is a feeling of trust and love between you. Your partner will probably be brilliant even without instruction but it is best to attend antenatal classes together and practise massage, breathing and positions for labour. He may feel more confident if he knows some basic medical facts about birth and he may represent your views and your birth plan to the midwives in labour. You could talk about what happens if you are difficult or demanding and how he can be there for you and not take things you say or do personally. If labour is long or he takes on a very physical role, he'll need time out to rest, eat and nourish himself, and you need to be OK about him leaving the birthing suite from time to time. If he is squeamish or nervous, you may agree in advance that there are some aspects of labour he'd rather not witness.

Who is around for my baby and me after the birth?

In terms of medical care a midwife will visit you for 10 days, and then your health visitor will make regular calls or you can visit a local clinic and your GP acts as backup. If you have a strong family network they will be around for you and your partner might take time off for a few days or weeks. If you feel nervous about babycare or don't want to spend time doing domestic chores, you might want a paid helper and you'll need to sort this out before the birth. You may also find great support and good friends at local couples groups or mother-and-baby meetings. You will always have people to speak to, and, over time, the friendships you form will thrive.

If my labour is late my family will pester me. My mother only has 2 weeks off work from the time of my due date. Should I induce for her sake?

It is very difficult to avoid feeling under pressure if you are close to your parents. The onset of labour is mainly triggered by your baby. Your family may be anxious for your baby to be born not only for convenience but because they're anxious that something may go wrong. Many parents have heard that the placenta does not function as well after Week 40. Provided your medical checks and ultrasound scan indicate your baby is healthy, your decision about induction is best based on your own feelings. If you choose to wait you may feel stressed by family pressure but this is one of the times when you will hear advice about your child and have to make your own choice.

I can't stand this extra weight. Can dieting help now?

Dieting in pregnancy is not a good idea, and dieting in the third trimester is definitely inadvisable – your baby is building up his body and needs a full quota of nutrients. He requires a range of vitamins and minerals, particularly calcium and iron, proteins and essential fatty acids. If you are concerned that you're gaining too much pay attention to your diet. You can get everything to nourish yourself and your baby without taking surplus calories. If you eat well (p.332) you will get the fuel your body needs, keep your energy levels stable, avoid excessive gain and be preparing for labour and your recovery after birth.

I am concerned by how much discomfort my wife is having but I feel redundant. How could I help?
It is very common for men to want to protect and support their partners and your concern will be appreciated. You could help practically around the house to give her more rest time, and your wife may feel really supported if you share your feelings. It is not long before the discomfort of late pregnancy will pass.

I feel very anxious about the birth and how we will manage financially – when I'm a dad I'll be the sole breadwinner. Could I do anything to feel better?
It is very common to feel nervous about the birth, and also about life with a new baby. Prepare as much as you can, through reading, going to classes and relaxing, and find out how you can help practically during labour. Your worries about money may be magnifying your anxiety about the birth – before the big day consider spending time to go over your finances. You may be able to take practical steps to boost your income or cut down expenses, or it might be better to look at the possibilities for achieving a balance between time at home with your baby and time earning money.

My partner wants sex a lot but I feel too close to the baby, and her vagina feels different. What can I do?
Do talk about this. She may be buzzing with excitement about the birth and feeling really good in her body but she needs to know if you're not turned on. If you tell her gently and are honest, you can avoid hurting or insulting her – it is extremely common in late pregnancy for men to feel strange about sex. It could help your intimacy and reduce her feelings of rejection if you can be close in other ways, perhaps through oral sex or without any sex at all. When your baby is here you may find it hard to steal undisturbed moments to watch videos, eat a meal or go out together, and full sex may not resume for weeks or months after birth.

What do I need to take to hospital?
As labour approaches, you may want to pack a bag. The contents will depend on what your hospital provides and they may give you a list. The main things are personal items for labour to make the room feel friendly, drinks or snacks for you and your partner, clothes for yourself and something for your baby to travel home. It is important to remember your notes and records and your birth plan. There's a fuller list on p.126.

What can I do to prepare to breastfeed my baby?
If you are keen to breastfeed, it is useful to find out about it during your antenatal classes. If you know anyone currently feeding, talk to her and even arrange to spend a few hours in her home to see at first hand what is involved. You will also see other aspects of caring for a new baby. Your breasts have been preparing themselves throughout pregnancy and it is not essential to do anything. If it makes you feel more in touch or

confident about feeding, you might enjoy breast massage (p.195) and nourishing the skin of your nipples with pure oil (almond or grapeseed). You also need to buy feeding bras, which are best fitted after Week 36.

My nausea and indigestion have come back. What can I do about it?
Your nausea may be due to a number of factors: the pregnancy hormones are still flowing, your uterus is pressing on your diaphragm, your diet may have altered and the valve in the entrance to your stomach may not hold the food in. Many of the issues that are relevant to nausea (p.513) also apply to indigestion and heartburn (p.487). There is a very small possibility that you may need anti-nausea medication.

My feet are swelling and it is difficult to get my shoes on. It looks as if I'm gaining a lot of weight. Can I reduce this?
Fluid retention is very common in the second half of pregnancy and it is an integral part of the hormonal changes that allow the tissues to expand and open your joints during birth. It is normal for your feet to swell in late pregnancy because your body retains fluid. Sometimes the swelling may warrant an extra shoe size.
There is a chance that swelling may be caused by excess weight gain, and you may label fat deposits as fluid. If you press on your leg for 30 seconds and it makes an indentation it is fluid. Even so, fat and fluid can coexist. Ask your doctor or midwife to help if you are in doubt. There is little you can do for the excess fluid retention (p.397), although you may try eating fewer sugary foods to reduce the fat gain component. Diuretic pills to increase urine flow are considered harmful and are no longer used. Homeopathy can be useful. If your blood pressure is normal and there is no protein in the urine, you do not have pre-eclampsia (p.410).

My doctor says that my blood pressure is high. Need I worry?
High blood pressure is a cause for concern. You require intensive surveillance because it is a sign of pre-eclampsia (p.410), a condition that can affect both you and your baby adversely. If the blood pressure levels remain mildly elevated, you will need monitoring and examinations. If the levels are severely high and you have protein in your urine, you will require admission to hospital and early birth for your baby.

Why do my hands feel numb?
Many women find that their hands and fingers are numb or tingling with pins and needles. This is often because the ulnar nerve in the carpel tunnel on the front of the wrist joint becomes compressed by retained fluid (p.397). Yoga-based stretching exercises combined with a wrist support worn at night tend to help, and the compression and the symptoms usually disappear after birth. Sometimes fluid retention affects the other joints in the fingers, and they may be painful. If you feel a tingling sensation in your lips as well as your hands and feet, it may be caused by hyperventilation – slowing your breathing will stop it.

I'm 34 weeks pregnant and I have terrible rib pain. Is this usual?
Pain in the lower ribs is very common as the growing uterus pushes the ribs upwards. If you sit stooped the effect worsens, but when you're aware of your posture you can minimise the

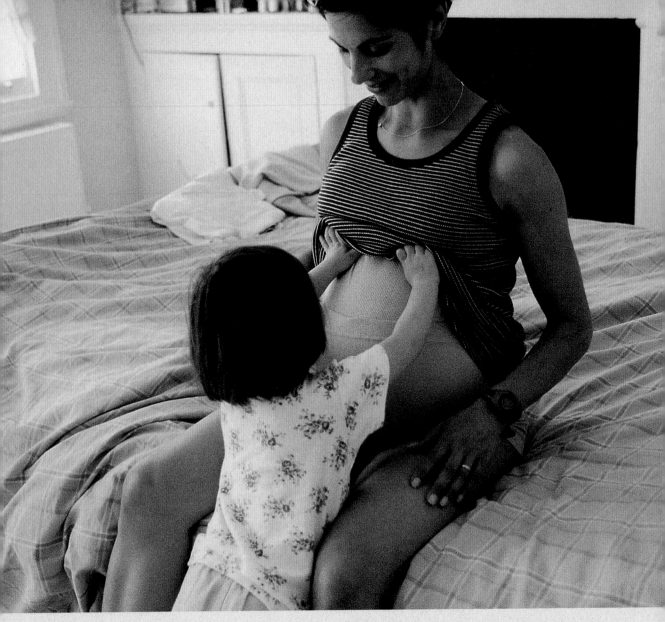

pressure. Yoga stretches and massage may reduce tension, as may osteopathy. When you tell your doctor he may examine you and recommend investigation to rule out the possibility that pain is arising from problems in your kidneys, gall bladder or lungs.

I am small-framed. Could this make birth difficult?
You are fortunate because the size of your baby is probably in proportion to your own size. Your midwife and doctor will estimate the size of your baby and they may also use an ultrasound scan to predict the weight. If your baby is very big you may need help with the birth but it is difficult to predict in advance how all the factors will combine in labour. The birth also depends on your baby's position and how his head is flexed as well as the size and shape of your pelvis and the intensity of your contractions. If everything is normal and your uterus contracts well, then the birth is likely to go smoothly.

I'm 30 weeks pregnant and my GP says my uterus is low. What does this mean?
There are two main reasons for a low uterus. The first is that your baby is engaged in your pelvis and the top of the uterus feels low but your uterus and baby are normal in size. Using the example of an elevator: when you descend you do not become smaller as you go lower. The second reason for a low uterus is that your baby is small. In this instance your baby may be healthy but small; a scan will determine your baby's size and the Doppler blood flow will show how well the placenta is functioning. If the scan shows a potential problem, your doctor may suggest follow-up examinations and scans to keep a check on your baby's development. The majority of babies who are small are very healthy and have developed normally both physically and mentally. Sometimes a small baby has intrauterine growth restriction (p.488) and may need extra surveillance in pregnancy and in labour. If the scan

reveals that there is a low volume of amniotic fluid (p.397) this will also be taken into account during labour.

I'm 38 weeks pregnant and can't feel my baby moving as actively. Could there be something wrong?
Each baby has a different rhythm and women often say that one of their children moved less than the others. Some women, particularly those that are very active, may be less aware of their baby's movements. If you have noticed a reduction in movements you need to see your doctor or midwife soon. They will examine you and check your baby's size and listen to the heartbeat, and may take a continuous heartbeat trace (CTG) for 15–30 minutes. The other test is an ultrasound scan to check for normal growth, amniotic fluid levels and placental function. Provided the checks show that your baby is well, you will be asked to observe the movements and report back if you are worried between regular visits. Many babies quieten before birth but if labour has not begun, it is wise to be examined if this happens. Usually the baby moves more than 10 times in 24 hours. If your midwife or doctor is concerned they will arrange for your baby to be assessed frequently.

Is there any way of predicting if I will give birth late?
One of the most common questions women ask is when labour will begin. It is easy to use statistics to say that fewer than 5% of first births will occur 14 days or more after the due date predicted by an ultrasound scan, but no one can predict precisely for you. It is true that first pregnancies more often last beyond the due date, and if you have had two late labours or if your cervix is not effaced (ripe) at term then you are more likely to be late. Early engagement of your baby's head is not a signal that birth will be early. Labour will not begin of its own accord until both you and your baby produce the hormones to stimulate the process. There is no absolute way to know when this will happen.

My underclothes are wet. Could I be incontinent?
It is common for small amounts of urine to leak late in pregnancy but wetness may also arise from a profuse amount of mucus produced by your cervix in preparation for labour. A vaginal discharge is virtually universal in late pregnancy. If your membranes have ruptured, there may be a small leak producing a trickle rather than a gush of fluid. If the wetness is due to amniotic fluid, it will smell different from urine. Contact your midwife or doctor who will check for ruptured membranes and may investigate you for a vaginal or urinary infection (p.123).

What happens if something goes wrong in labour?
Your labour may flow smoothly, you may need a little help and encouragement or you may need active assistance, all to ensure that you and your baby have the best possible outcome and experience. Simple intervention may offer a boost to your energy and guide you as you give birth naturally. Where intervention is greater it may interfere with 'natural' birth but still enhance the positive experience of giving birth. When maximum intervention is needed, for example a caesarean section, most women are extremely grateful and relieved that their baby has arrived safely. If you are very worried about something going wrong, it's best to talk to your midwife who

may provide information and quell your fears so that you are less likely to feel tense on the day.

Is there any way I can prevent needing stitches?
Your vagina is naturally able to stretch during childbirth. If you massage your perineum consistently during the last 6 weeks of pregnancy, you may increase elasticity and strength and reduce the likelihood of tearing (p.98). Pelvic floor exercises are also effective (p.98), and giving birth in water makes tears less likely. If you give birth upright, kneeling or squatting, the force of your baby's head is evenly distributed around the vagina, and this helps the outlet to stretch evenly. Bear in mind that preparation is useful but cannot have guaranteed results – your baby's head may be large or come at an awkward angle. If you do tear, the stitching process is painless using a local anaesthetic injection and healing is usually rapid (p.494).

I feel so loved up and happy. I can't wait to give birth and meet my baby, but I'm also loving my life now. It's like having the last few days of a brilliant holiday. Is it normal to have a last fling with single life?
Many women enjoy the third trimester and as term approaches feel very peaceful and happy. The last few days before labour can be very calm and loving and couples have talked about the feeling of being on honeymoon or revisiting the weeks when they first met. You may feel the energy of new life very strongly at this time, though your baby is not yet visible, and your mothering hormones are probably flowing strongly.

I am so afraid of labour and birth that I want a caesarean. Can I insist?
Many (but not all) hospitals support women who choose to have a caesarean section where there is no medical necessity, yet this is still an issue of heated debate. Attitudes are altering with the increasing safety of the procedure and changing fashions, and the likelihood that your request will be granted depends largely on your own reasons and on your hospital's policy. Because a caesarean is a major operation it carries risks and recovery after a caesarean is generally more protracted than after a vaginal birth. Discuss your wishes with your midwife and obstetrician: you may decide to give a vaginal birth a go. Alternatively, booking an elective caesarean (p.419) could quell your anxiety for the remainder of your pregnancy.

How will I know if my labour is established?
In most instances the onset of labour is very obvious and you will be having regular painful contractions that increase in intensity as time goes by. Sometimes the diagnosis is less clear if your waters have broken early, you have a show of mucus or blood or you are having runs of irregular pre-labour contractions. When you become aware that something is happening then contact your midwife or doctor and discuss your situation. They may choose to examine you to discover whether your cervix has begun to dilate. If you are likely to have a fast labour because you have previously been quick or you are early it's best to contact your midwife early on. The same applies if your baby is small, if your doctor has been concerned about your baby's health or if you bleed. There's more detail about the onset of labour on p.120.

Labour begins

The miracle of birth is amazing and exciting, a process that is powerful and unpredictable. The weeks and days leading up to your due date will be coloured with expectancy: you wait for what you know will be an unforgettable and life-changing event, yet you don't know quite how it will unfold. You may experience a variety of feelings as your mind and body ready themselves and you wait to meet your baby.

The approach of labour

By the end of pregnancy your abdomen will be at its largest and the pressure this places on the rest of your body will be at its height. At the same time, your body is also at its most flexible and is naturally capable of relaxing. If your baby's head has engaged and settled into your pelvic inlet, you may feel more pressure on your pelvis and hips, but slightly less under your ribs so that feelings of breathlessness or indigestion may be reduced. Your baby's movements, however, may be quite uncomfortable by now. You may also have discomfort arising from needing to pass water frequently and have difficulty sleeping; these feelings are shared by most heavily pregnant women.

Your body prepares

Although the muscle wall of your uterus does contract frequently throughout pregnancy contractions are neither well synchronised nor very powerful. For most of your pregnancy your body inhibits the intensity of uterine contractions while allowing the uterus to expand and protect your baby. It does this by releasing a number of hormones (including progesterone, relaxin and prostacyclin) and nitric oxide, which is produced in the foetal membranes and the decidual lining of the uterus. Nitric oxide acts in conjunction with the hormone progesterone to inhibit the contractions of the uterus. Relaxin also aids the connective tissue in your cervix to soften as it ripens and prepares to open.

Late in pregnancy, over a number of weeks, your baby helps to activate contractions in your uterus: he plays a crucial role in determining the date of birth. He responds to an innate genetic mechanism and produces proteins that progressively enhance the sensitivity and power of your uterine muscle. At the same time, he gets larger and larger, and it is believed that the way he stretches your uterus also boosts the power of contractions. This may be why twins are likely to be born early.

The production and release of hormones depends on the complex inter-relation between you and your baby. Both of you produce oxytocin and inside your baby's brain signals are sent via his pituitary gland to the adrenal glands near his kidneys, which release cortisol. This cortisol stimulates the foetal membranes to produce prostaglandins and will only be released when your baby

has reached maturity. When it reaches the lining of your uterus, prostaglandin triggers the muscle in the uterine wall to contract and feelings of tightening get stronger. These contractions are known as Braxton-Hicks. Over a period of weeks Braxton-Hicks contractions become more powerful and begin to fall into a pattern.

You're less likely to be aware of your changing cervix, which is ripening so that it can open ('dilate'). The lower part of your uterus is connected to the cervix, which becomes progressively thinner as the powerful muscle in the upper part thickens and strengthens. As labour draws nearer, hormones stimulate the connective tissue and muscle of the cervix to soften: its wall is progressively pulled up into the uterus so that it shortens and then begins to open. This change, called effacement or ripening, occurs gradually during the last 6 weeks and is more obvious in subsequent pregnancies. In some pregnancies the cervix remains long and hard and unripe until the onset of labour, in which case labour usually takes longer.

Though the process can be explained to a certain extent through hormone release, it is clear that the onset of labour can be affected by wider emotional and physical circumstances. Your own wellbeing, your confidence and state of mind, your nutrition and your fitness all have an impact, and it is likely that your baby's emotional state is also influential, as it may be during birth.

Your mind prepares

During labour and birth your energy is focused on your abdomen where your baby and your uterus are working together. You will be drawn to follow your instincts as your body takes over. In the days leading up to labour this may be reflected in your moods and energy levels.

It is likely, then, that you will feel quiet and calm and become thoughtful or meditative as you rest or sleep more than usual. You may also be concerned for your welfare and for your baby during the birth. Don't be surprised if you also have powerful urges to clean and tidy, to ready your baby's environment and even to bake.

Your baby gets into position

If this is your first pregnancy, in the last 4 weeks your baby will probably move down in the uterus and the widest diameter of his head (at the level of the top of his ears) will

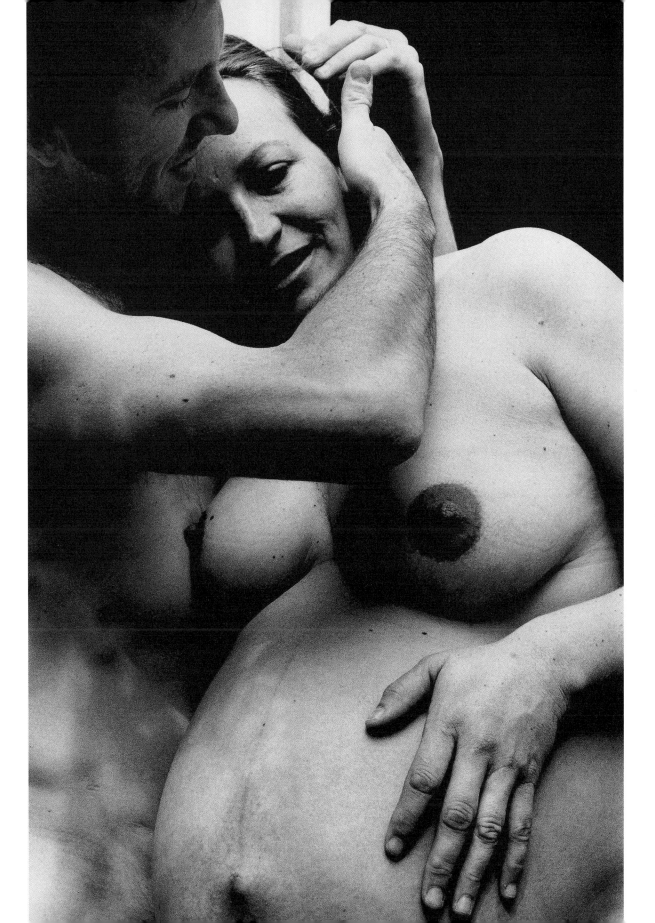

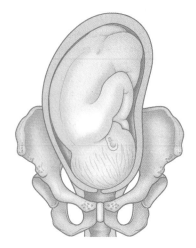

Occipito anterior position: The most efficient for birth. The baby lies with his head down and his back towards the mother's abdomen.

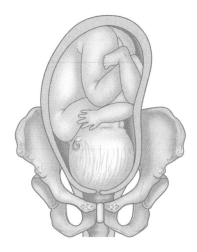

Occipito posterior position: The baby has his back towards the mother's spine and his head down. This may give back pain in labour.

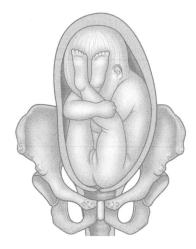

Breech position: The baby has his buttocks down towards the cervix. Caesarean section is usually advised for birth.

pass the inlet of your pelvis. This is a process of engagement (or lightening), and you may notice when your baby 'drops' down. When your baby's head is not engaged in your pelvis there are a number of possible explanations (p.499). Engagement doesn't always happen before labour starts: its delay is more common among African and Afro-Caribbean women, and in second and subsequent pregnancies.

Your baby also assumes his position for birth. Most babies tuck the head into the chin and face down towards the cervix, with the back facing their mum's belly button. This position, occipito anterior (OA), is the most conducive to a smooth journey through the pelvis and is most likely to result in an unassisted vaginal birth. Some babies are not comfortable like this, however, and your baby will adapt his position to suit the match between his shape and size and the shape and size of your uterus and your pelvis, and also the situation of the placenta. Malpresentation (p.498) could interfere with your baby's descent or necessitate a caesarean section (e.g. if he is a breech baby).

Rarely, a baby may choose to lie sideways, in a transverse lie, with a hand or shoulder or the umbilical cord nearest the cervix. Sometimes this position can be changed but if it persists, delivery by caesarean section is commonly advised (p.419).

The signs that labour is coming

For a few women labour begins with contractions at maximum intensity, and comes with very little warning. It's more common to have advance notice, which may be as much as 3 or 4 days, or as little as a few hours. You may experience one or more of the common signs and know that it's time, feeling a mix of excitement and anxiety.

Contractions

Regular painful contractions are the most common sign that labour is beginning. The experience can be compared to sailing on the sea: you start in a calm, flat and peaceful surface, begin to feel the light rocking of waves following one another with a gentle rhythm, and then become tossed

---

How do I know if I'm having Braxton-Hicks contractions? Are they like the real thing?
Pre-labour Braxton-Hicks contractions can be quite strong, and while everyone feels them differently they are seldom accompanied by any pain. Your abdomen will feel tight while each contraction lasts 30–60 seconds then relaxes and runs of contractions may last for 10 or 60 minutes. With each contraction, the muscle wall of your uterus tightens as the fibres shorten, beginning at the top and working towards the cervix, reaches a peak where it may feel really tight, and then relaxes from the top down. The difference in tone can be felt by anyone placing a hand on your abdomen. Occasionally Braxton-Hicks contractions may be painful and then it is difficult to distinguish them from labour.

With your first baby it may be hard to believe that they aren't the real thing, but Braxton-Hicks come in runs and do not continue regularly for more than 60 minutes. The muscles of your abdominal wall or your bowel may also contract and mimic labour. In true labour, the runs of contractions continue and the time between each one diminishes to less than 5 minutes and discomfort increases. If you are in doubt, you are probably not in labour. Even so, your midwife will be happy to see you if you would like her advice.

---

around and buffeted by winds and squalls. Sometimes labour begins in high seas within minutes of starting. In some labours it's as if a storm is circling, becoming intense and insistent and then dying away for a time before returning with renewed vigour. In others the sea remains calm with an occasional wave and contractions may need to be boosted.

Each contraction is a tightening of the muscle wall of your uterus beginning at the fundus (top) and spreading down towards the cervix. Pain usually begins when the uterus has begun to tighten, reaches a peak at the height of the contraction and disappears completely when the muscle wall relaxes. You may feel little more than slight discomfort and then deep and even blissful relaxation, or intense and overpowering pain with barely any respite. There may be menstrual-like cramp in your lower belly or back, your thighs, or all three. As your uterus contracts and the muscle fibres shorten, the blood flowing to the placenta is reduced; the rest period between tightenings allows your blood to flow strongly to nourish your baby with oxygen and gives you a chance to relax and gather inner strength. Contractions may make you feel nauseous.

In early labour it can be difficult to see a pattern. Contractions are usually spaced between 10 and 30 minutes apart. It is common but not universal for them to come forcefully in runs and then to have times when they are slight or even disappear altogether. Timing your contractions is an obvious way of gauging how labour is progressing. The time is measured from the beginning of one contraction to the beginning of the next. Although it's useful to know about timing, try not to become a slave to the clock. It is much more helpful to relax or move gently rather than to become apprehensive about the next tightening. Some women feel happy to get on with something like cooking or walking or cleaning while things are relatively calm.

More frequent and powerful contractions indicate a progressively dilating (opening) cervix and usually begin at spaces of 15 or 20 minutes and gradually become more frequent. Each contraction is over within 30–60 seconds and then you relax.

The pattern varies from woman to woman. The contractions may be spaced closely, far apart or irregularly, and may drop off altogether for an hour or two, or they may be intense from the outset. The feeling of tightening, and how strong it seems, is a very personal thing because pain perception varies widely.

Very sensitive people may experience pre-labour contractions as being painful while others describe their contractions as being a source of discomfort rather than pain. If you feel anxious, this may increase your sensitivity. At the other end of the scale, as the cervix dilates some women feel very few contractions and no pain at all, though this is rare.

'False' or 'pre-labour' and 'true' labour

The distinction between pre-labour and true labour is medical: labour is 'progressive dilation of the cervix', a process usually accompanied by regular contractions, and can only be verified by an internal examination. Some women experience strong contractions long before the cervix dilates, in a phase known as pre-labour. Others begin to dilate with few contractions and don't go through pre-labour. Pre-labour may be marked by a strong shift in mood or altered consciousness with intense mental preparation. True labour is said to be present if the cervix is 3-cm dilated.

Before true labour commences you may experience pain over a few hours or a few days, often with runs of contractions at certain times of the day or night. For some women the sensations of pre-labour are intense and difficult to cope with, while for others they are mild with Braxton-Hicks contractions or persistent discomfort in the back. It is important to remain calm and restful when you begin to feel contractions, for if you are in pre-labour there may be some time to go before your cervix begins to dilate and you will need to preserve your energy. Feeling the first contractions can be exciting, especially in the stillness of night when they may seem stronger.

A minority of women, particularly in their first pregnancy, have runs of strong Braxton-Hicks contractions that are not accompanied by a ripening of the cervix, so they feel as if they are in labour but they are not progressing. This is 'false labour'. Occasionally, these early contractions die away, and it may be hours or days before pre-labour begins once again.

The onset of labour is triggered by a number of factors. Runs of 'false labour' indicate that all the ingredients are not in place to allow true labour to continue. If contractions have been going on for a number of days a mother can become very tired and her doctor will consider induction to initiate cervical dilation while she still has sufficient energy. If you are unsure whether or not you are experiencing false labour, the information on p.500 may help you identify the source of your 'labour' sensations and decide on the best course of action.

A show

As your cervix ripens and effaces, it changes shape. As it does, the plug of mucus that acts as a barrier between the uterine membranes and the vagina may come away and be discharged as a jelly-like substance. It is often brown, pink or stained with blood because tiny blood vessels in your cervix may bleed as it opens. If it is accompanied by heavier bleeding or blood clots, you should contact your maternity unit immediately. A show does not indicate that labour will start immediately – it may occur hours or days before labour, and is not always a feature of labour.

Provided the membranes have not ruptured, your baby is not at higher risk of infection. It is safe to bathe because the vaginal walls touch one another and prevent

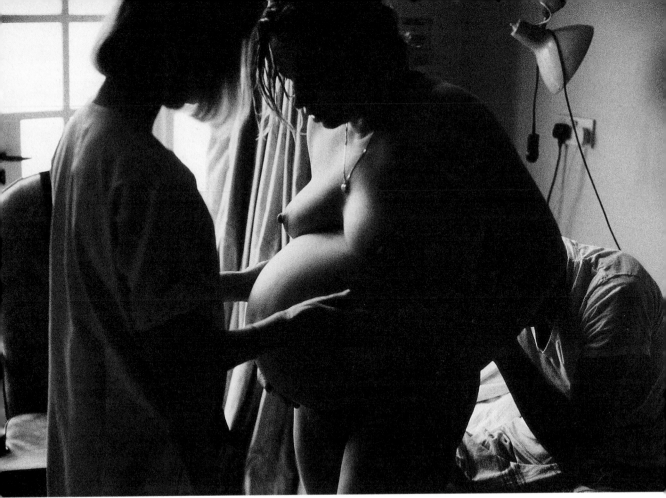

Midwives are endowed with the instinct and experience to sooth a mother by gently massaging, while assessing the power of contractions and the progress of labour.

Your midwife and your contractions

If this is your first baby you will probably value a professional opinion. Most labours in first-time pregnancies begin with a gradual dilation of the cervix, which is usually accompanied by widely spaced contractions. If yours begins like this it is fine to delay calling your midwife until the contractions are roughly 5 minutes apart and each lasts for more than 30 seconds, unless your membranes have ruptured in which case you should call her straightaway (see box opposite). If your midwife or obstetrician has extra medical concerns about you or your baby, or you live a long way from hospital, she may have asked you to call earlier – perhaps when contractions are 10 minutes apart.

When you first talk to your midwife, you will probably have a contraction. Don't hang up! Your tone of voice, or the length of your silence as you breathe, can tell your midwife a lot about you. If you are having a hospital birth she will advise you when you should come in. If you are planning to give birth at home, your midwife will decide when to come and see you.

the entry of water to the level of the cervix. Sexual intercourse is also safe. In fact, the prostaglandin content of semen may stimulate your uterus to contract and expedite labour. Remember that there may be a delay before the onset of labour. If the discharge persists, it is worth asking your midwife to check because the symptoms may indicate a vaginal infection.

Ruptured membranes

At some point before birth, the membranes surrounding your baby and the protective sac of fluid will break. If the waters do not break until your baby's head has emerged from the vagina, this is known as being 'born in a caul'. The waters usually break during labour. This most commonly happens in the first stage but can occur in advance of contractions when it is called premature rupture of the membranes (p.501). You might want to protect your mattress with a waterproof under-sheet in case your waters break at night. Some women think they have wet themselves if their waters break early. But you can tell the difference from the smell: amniotic fluid is urine coloured, but has a slightly sweet smell that is easy to distinguish from urine.

Sometimes when the waters break there is a puddle but if your baby's head is sitting snugly in your pelvic inlet, you will experience only a dribble. Your baby's urine and the placenta replace the fluid up to six times a day and the volume remains more or less constant, so your baby is not at risk of becoming dry, unless there was reduced amniotic fluid (p.397). Usually, contractions begin within 24 hours of the waters breaking but the leak can continue for longer.

Other signs of labour

The prostaglandin hormone released by the lining of your uterus may stimulate your bowels to empty more frequently, and it's common for movements to become loose when labour is imminent. Other common signs are backache and abdominal pain.

Caring for yourself in pre-labour

A sign of labour may trigger a rush of adrenalin and you may be tempted to become active and do a lot physically. But because pre-labour can last some time, it's good to combine physical activity with relaxation. While it is important to rest at this time, this doesn't suit all women: some sleep easily through their contractions, and some stay awake for 20–40 hours and still feel elated when their labour is all over.

Pre-labour can be scary, particularly at night. It's good to know that your midwife and doctor are available 24 hours a day. Women do worry that they could run out of energy for the birth or that a long pre-labour is a sign that the baby wants to be born but there is something hindering

the process. Fortunately, your baby can be monitored to ensure that all is well. If you have a sensitive personality, a long pre-labour is more likely: knowing this in advance may help you relax.

Caring for yourself in pre-labour mainly consists of preserving energy for labour. You may feel calmly in touch with yourself now, or anxious and need support to help you through the coming hours.

- Eat and drink well: small portions and light snacks will probably be most easily digested. Avoid fatty foods and sweets. Drink water or herbal teas and drop a spoonful of honey in for some extra energy.
- Rest as much as possible. Sleep if you can. If not, lie in a relaxed pose, do some yoga stretches or move gently with the rhythm of your contractions. Some women find a slow flowing dance or massage relieves pain and helps progress.
- Carry on everyday activities as usual but don't set yourself any difficult tasks. If you want to cook, do something simple.
- Go for a walk, either indoors or outside.
- Try relaxing in a bath (marjoram, clary sage or lavender oils may suit you), but do not make it too hot or you will sap your energy.
- Concentrating on your breath can be very relaxing. If you have learnt breathing techniques or visualisations for calming yourself, try them now.
- Exclude visitors and telephone calls if you need a rest, but ask for company if you need it.
- Try homeopathic remedies or aromatherapy oils that have been recommended to you.
- Fears and anxieties may surface; your partner or birth attendant may offer great support. Remember you can always call your midwife.
- If you are at home, keep in touch with your midwife to arrange when to be checked.

Once labour has started

Unless you are in hospital your labour will start at home where you can begin to use postures and relaxing techniques to ease the pain of contractions. Your midwife will talk to you on the phone and assess your progress (see box on p.122).

When you go to hospital will depend on the spacing between contractions, on your state of mind and how supported you feel at home, as well as on the policy of the hospital you are attending. Some hospitals will encourage women to come in and make themselves comfortable in early labour, others prefer to admit them when active labour is fully established. If you are planning a home birth, your midwife will come to be with you when you both agree that you need her presence.

The progress of your labour is unpredictable: it may take anything from 2 to 12 hours of contractions, or

When you're in hospital

Call the hospital to let them know you are on your way so they can be ready for you. Once you have made the journey you will be admitted by a midwife. Your partner will support you if you need help walking or want to rest while a contraction passes.

Moving from your home to the hospital may alter your state of mind considerably and you may take time to adjust. Contractions may diminish when you move (particularly if you dislike hospitals) and could take an hour or two to speed up. Your birth partner will be with you to help you remain calm and talk you through your breathing and contractions while you acclimatise and have the necessary checks.

Your assessment on arrival

The midwife who greets you will find out how you and your partner are feeling and will examine you. By feeling your abdomen she can tell how strong your contractions are and assess the volume of amniotic fluid and the position and size of your baby. She'll also want to check your pulse, temperature and blood pressure and will compare these with the information in your notes.

To assess whether your cervix has begun to dilate, she will do a vaginal examination. Though she will prefer to do this while you lie on the bed, she may be happy to do it while you kneel on all fours, if you are more comfortable. During the short examination she checks the softness, stretchability, length (ripeness) and dilation of your cervix. She can detect the position of your baby's head, and how far it has descended into the pelvic cavity, and she will also check the shape of your pelvis to ensure that there is adequate room for your baby to pass through. If you relax and breathe gently any discomfort will be minimised. It may hurt a little if you are tense or if your baby's head or your cervix is high and the midwife has to reach up. It may be possible to have the examination between tightenings although it could help your midwife to check during a contraction to see how your baby's head moves down.

If you have made a birth plan, now is a good time to show your midwife so she can see your preferences about

I wonder about whether I will be shaved or be on an intravenous drip. Are these procedures common?

In a labour without complications neither are necessary. In modern birth practice, women are no longer routinely shaved. Only if you need a caesarean will you be shaved, and then only a thin sliver of pubic hair at the top of the hairline, approximately 2 cm (¾ in) wide, will be removed. There is never any need to shave around the area of the labia or perineum. You will only be put on an intravenous drip if there is a clinical need, such as the administration of an epidural.

sometimes even more. It is safest for you and your baby to be in hospital before you reach full dilation, because by that stage you will be in transition and getting ready to push and give birth.

Your baby's heartbeat (CTG) – the details

Monitoring a baby's heartbeat (CTG) is one of the cornerstones of obstetric and midwifery care. Heartbeat patterns are a very good indication of a baby's wellbeing. An abnormal heartbeat pattern may suggest foetal distress arising from a fall in oxygen supply to your baby. It will prompt your medical team to investigate the possible cause and consider the best course of action to ensure your baby's safe delivery.

Heart rate

The normal heart rate of a baby falls between 110 and 160 beats per minute, about twice as fast as an adult's. A very rapid or slow rate may indicate foetal distress (p.472).

Variation

In health, the baby's autonomic nervous system causes the heart rate to vary by more than 10 beats per minute. During sleep, the variation is reduced and it returns when the baby awakens. Normal variation is a sign of health.

Acceleration

When your baby moves, his heart rate speeds up by 10–20 beats per minute, in the same way as an adult's heart rate reacts to exercise. On the graph, an acceleration is marked by a peak and is a sign of good health.

Deceleration

Deceleration is marked by dips on the graph.
- Early deceleration occurs when the heart rate drops at the beginning of a contraction and rises by the end. It indicates pressure on the head of the baby and is not usually a sign of distress.
- Late deceleration occurring after a contraction may indicate a reduced flow of blood (and oxygen) to your baby.
- Variable deceleration between contractions may indicate umbilical cord compression.
- Variable and late deceleration suggests foetal distress.

There may be more than one explanation for deceleration. To correct the pattern it may be a simple case of moving from your back to your side or changing to an upright position to increase blood flow to the placenta. Alternatively, your midwife may increase your fluids, particularly if you have been given an epidural, or reduce the dose of oxytocin if this is being administered to boost your contractions. You may have an internal examination to exclude a cord prolapse.

Your medical team may be concerned that the deceleration pattern indicates foetal distress and asphyxia resulting from low oxygen. If your baby was healthy in pregnancy and is born soon his condition at birth will be normal because he can draw on his glucose stores for energy. If your pregnancy was considered high risk, your team may be keen to expedite the birth, because your baby's reserve energy stores may be low. Your obstetrician will assess the degree of risk to your baby. She may check your baby's pH and oxygen levels by taking a blood sample from the scalp. Where readings continue to cause concern, a caesarean (p.419) or assistance with forceps or ventouse (p.496) may be advised to ensure that your baby is delivered safely. If there has been foetal distress your baby may require assistance at birth.

No reading or very high and very low numbers

This usually indicates that the transducer placed on your abdomen has slipped. If this happens your midwife will adjust it and reassure you that your baby's heart is still beating normally.

Accuracy of monitoring

Your baby's heart rate pattern provides an indication of health but it is only one index, so it is assessed in conjunction with other factors that have affected your pregnancy. Monitoring the heartbeat is not 100% reliable. Sometimes there are variations but a baby is born fit and well (a false positive) or, occasionally, a monitor can give a false reading and a baby without variations requires breathing assistance after birth. For the many advantages offered by detection of a baby's heartbeat there is a price to pay: some extra caesarean sections are performed.

---

pain relief and advise you what is best depending on how far you have progressed. In early labour TENS is generally recommended. This and other methods of pain relief are detailed on p.158.

If labour is well established you may be invited into the labour suite; alternatively, you may be left in a separate room with your partner. If you are in the early phase you may enjoy this privacy but when your contractions become strong you will almost certainly want a midwife present to support and monitor you and your baby.

Monitoring your baby

Your midwife will confirm your baby's size, position and the volume of amniotic fluid when she examines you. If the membranes have ruptured, the volume and colour of the amniotic fluid are noted. She will also note previous scan and blood test results.

If the initial assessment confirms that your baby is healthy and at low risk of problems, your midwife will reassess the situation intermittently throughout labour. If there is an increased risk of problems, your baby will be monitored more intensively.

Foetal heart monitoring (CTG)

An electronic foetal heart monitor, also known as a cardiotocograph or CTG, assesses your baby's heartbeat and shows the pattern and intensity of your contractions. While you are lying or sitting, your midwife will strap an

What to bring to hospital

Have a chat with the midwives during pregnancy and find out what personal possessions and natural or complementary remedies for pain relief you can bring. When you pack your hospital bag, you'll also need things for your baby. For the first of countless occasions, it's time to pack nappies and clothes. Find out what your hospital offers: some provide washable but not disposable nappies, some provide babygros and most provide blankets. Most hospitals are warm so you and your baby won't need thick clothes except for going home.

For you: essentials
- Your maternity notes
- Your birth plan
- Nightshirt or T-shirt (a shirt with buttons makes feeding your baby simple after birth)
- Several pairs of maternity pants
- 2 pairs socks
- 1 pair slippers
- 1 dressing gown
- 2–3 supportive bras with drop-down cups for feeding
- Breast pads (for after your milk comes in, around day 2 or 3)
- 1 pack sanitary towels: 'heavy flow', 'night-time' or 'maternity'
- 1 pack sanitary towels: 'medium flow'
- Clean set of comfortable clothes
- Toiletries
- Towel
- Snacks to keep up your energy
- Camera and film

- List of phone numbers for calls to friends and family after birth, and loose change

Optional
- Disposable pants for after the birth
- Herbal or homeopathic remedies
- Herbal teas
- Mineral water, fruit juice or cordials
- Book
- Diary
- Atomizer or water spray for cooling yourself in labour
- Blanket, pillow or photographs
- Tapes or CDs
- Ear plugs for quieter sleep on the ward

For your baby
- 2–3 babygros: average size 3 kg (7 lb) or 'newborn'
- 2–3 vests
- 1 cotton hat
- 2 lightweight cardigans
- 1 pair scratch mitts, in case your baby scratches his face
- 1 pack nappies: 'newborn'
- 3–4 muslin cloths to protect your clothes from your baby's dribble

For the journey home
- 1 warm suit/coat/jumper for your baby to wear
- 1 car seat for travelling home, tested to fit in your car

---

external transducer on your abdomen and monitoring will continue for around 20 minutes. The monitor measures your baby's heartbeat using ultrasound and it gives a numerical read-out and traces a graph on paper. The belt holding the microphone rarely causes discomfort and doesn't impede kneeling or squatting.

There are also small hand-held monitors that allow you to hear the heart rate without a graphic record. These are ideal during an active birth and they're also designed for use under water in the birth pool. Your midwife will check the heartbeat every 30–60 minutes early in labour.

As you bear down in the second stage your midwife may listen after most contractions because if the umbilical cord is around your baby's neck, it may tighten. The tones of a normal heartbeat are reassuring while you enjoy the natural force of labour. For more information about monitoring your baby's heartbeat and understanding the CTG graph, see the box on p.125.

Internal monitoring
Very rarely, when the external monitor cannot detect the

heartbeat accurately (usually in women with a thick abdominal wall), an electrode needs to be placed on a baby's scalp to obtain an electrical signal of the heartbeat. The insertion probably causes a baby momentary pain similar to the discomfort from a blood test.

If the membranes have not already ruptured to allow access to the head, they will have to be broken. Internal monitoring should not be done if you carry the hepatitis or HIV virus because viral particles may be transferred to your baby.

Getting into the swing of labour
The transition from home to hospital could cause a natural hiatus in your labour, although if you are already having intense contractions their flow may remain uninterrupted. Once the preliminary assessments have passed you will be settled into a labour suite, a ward or room. With your birth partner's help you might want to make your space more cosy and get to know the midwives on shift. They will help you to keep balanced and on course as your body and your baby respond to the waves of labour.

Birth: a natural process

You and your baby are ready and together you both will work towards birth. Giving birth is arguably one of the toughest things a woman ever has to do; at the same time it can be one of the most fulfilling and liberating experiences of a lifetime. The physical energy required has been likened to that needed to run a marathon (backwards) and the mental journey compared to an otherworldly experience or an hallucinatory trip. Time seems to lose relevance, you respond to the birth energy and follow your instincts as you would in a moment of sheer joy or sudden fear. Once it starts, there's no turning back: the peaks and troughs of joy, excitement, fear, pain and bliss ahead will be a dramatic prelude to the arrival of your baby and the delicious calm that follows.

The environment for birth

When the environment is safe and comfortable it is common for labour to progress naturally in its own time and rhythm. Labour and birth are involuntary, or automatic; the uterus contracts spontaneously to open the womb and prepare for birth.

Hormones initiate the process and are also responsible for stimulating and maintaining contractions, aiding relaxation, providing natural pain relief and, when the time comes, encouraging bonding between mother and baby. In common with all other mammals, like the cat who seeks her own private birth space, women need to feel safe and protected in order to secrete these 'love hormones' freely and easily.

It is ideal if the birthing room gives a feeling of comfort and privacy. You may choose to make your surroundings soft and gentle like a nest and perhaps dark or give yourself a feeling of light and space. In the environment of your choice you'll feel free to move, breathe, change positions, use the birth pool, make as much noise as you need, have your own music to listen to, use homeopathy and be supported by your birth partner. You may choose to use aromatherapy or take a herbal pillow with you. Smell is a deeply engrained sense and making use of herbs in this way makes a huge contribution to your feeling of calm, confidence and comfort.

When you feel welcomed and cosy you can more easily relax and give in to the power of the birth process. You will be supported by midwives, the traditional guardians of active birth, who have the skills and intuition to guide you and create the right environment for a physiological birth.

Feelings of loving and being loved, coupled with comfort and confidence in labour, are known to reduce potential complications and the need for medical intervention. In the event of you needing medical help, the motherly presence of midwives continues alongside an obstetrician's guidance.

The stages of labour and birth

Labour is a continuous process but it has been divided into stages by medics to make it easier to understand. Most women experience it as a continuum that increases in intensity to the moment of birth but there are many different patterns. Progress may be rapid and incessant, it may be slow and calm or variable. The range of times here relate to a first labour.

The first stage: 2–20 hours
The first stage of labour is marked by progressive dilation of the cervix so that the diameter of its opening enlarges from 0 cm to 10 cm. There are two phases but in most births they merge imperceptibly into one another as the contractions gather momentum.
Latent phase (up to 3 cm dilation): 1–12 hours
The latent phase, while the cervix opens to a diameter of 3 cm, is called pre-labour. Usually, but not always, contractions are mild, building up in intensity and frequency. Sometimes the cervix begins to dilate before labour; this is more common in second or subsequent labours.
Active phase (from 5 cm–10 cm dilation): 1–6 hours
Contractions usually become more frequent. This is commonly the most intense part of the process.
Transition: 5 minutes–2 hours
The transition phase follows full dilation and precedes the urge to bear down and give birth. At the end of transition descent of your baby's head on to your pelvic floor and powerful contractions stimulate the reflex urge to bear down.

The second stage: 5 minutes–2 hours
The second stage involves bearing down and pushing and culminates with the birth of your baby.

The third stage: 5–60 minutes
The third stage is a time for the first contact and welcoming your new baby and ends as the placenta and membranes are born.

Visualisation for birth

Today is the day I will see my baby face to face. I can feel my contractions come and go. They are like the practice contractions but are stronger and regular. Each is a firm tightening that begins at the top of my uterus and travels down to my cervix like a wave that helps my baby down. I am pleased and surprised that I feel so calm. I know that with every contraction there is relaxation, and each one helps my cervix to open.

I feel my baby is able to drop easily through tissues that have softened in my pelvis and vagina. My baby's head moulds comfortably into my pelvis and snuggles onto my cervix, helping it to open easily.

I can feel the energy of birth flowing through me and from my baby. I can sense the lower part of my body becoming very soft and warm, silky and elastic.

Soon I will feel an urge to help my baby to birth. I will confidently push, knowing there is a lot of space around my baby's head and my vagina can expand. I will feel my body powerfully open to release my baby.

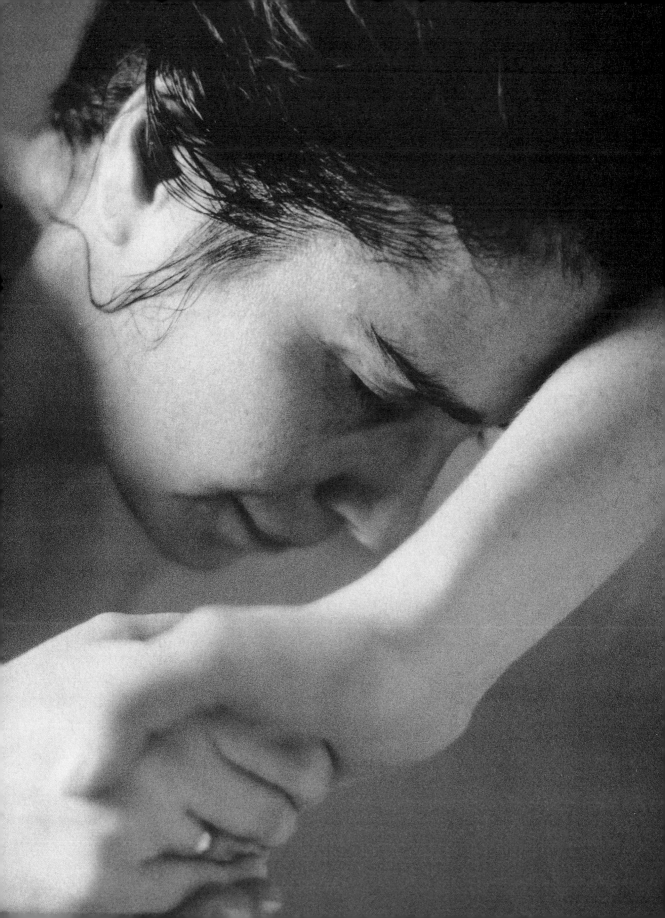

The first stage: to full dilation

The first stage of labour is that in which your cervix dilates enough to let your baby's head pass through, and is usually the longest. It is characterised by your uterus tightening involuntarily, but you may be able to enhance its power by moving with the rhythm of your body, by relaxing, singing or shouting, or by feeling the security of your partner's embrace or the soothing touch of massage or water: every woman needs a different level of support.

Each labour has its own rhythm and within one labour there are many possible variations: if the first stage lasts 12 or more hours, which is often the case in a first labour, it is likely your energy will fluctuate. You may progress from moderate tightenings to full-blown contractions or have mild tightenings that lead to slow, progressive dilation.

The latent phase

The latent phase is often characterised by contractions that are experienced as part of pre-labour (p.120) when discomfort is usually, but not always, mild. You may feel pain in your uterus, lower back or thighs, or all over this region. Sometimes contractions follow one another relentlessly, but it's more common for them to be widely spaced and you may have intervals where you can rest, catch your breath and recoup your energy. However, this stage progresses, it will help to focus on each contraction, one at a time, without putting too much thought into what is to come.

Contractions will be spaced anywhere from 3 to 20 minutes apart and last for between 30 and 45 seconds. If they become very calm your midwife may check to see how you are progressing and assess whether you and your baby need a little help.

The active phase

Although you are unlikely to notice the moment your cervix reaches 4 cm dilation, you will probably experience contractions that get closer and may become more painful. In most first labours and subsequent labours, contractions only reach full intensity in the active phase. There is great variation, but you could expect contractions now to be 3–4 minutes apart, and lasting for between 40 and 60 seconds.

This is where you can move your body to get through each surge of pain by 'riding' the waves, use your breathing to give you the energy and courage – and visualisations to help you believe that you can be stronger than the waves that are testing you beyond your limits. Your partner will be able to help. You may feel a greater need for pain relief now (p.156).

In transition

When your cervix has dilated to 10 cm, you will pass into the transition phase. Your contractions may change completely, and will probably become longer and more intense. They may be spaced as close together as every 2 minutes and if they last for 60 seconds you'll only get a short space of time to relax. You may feel particularly exhausted not only because of the pain but also because your body's muscles in the uterus and elsewhere have been working and consuming energy. In the throes of transition, women often roar like a lioness or moan as they breathe out. Your 'birth song' may become really loud while your contractions last and you access your power and then soften or become silent as you rest and breathe.

Emotionally, the transition phase is often the toughest. It's common to feel open and vulnerable, weak and fed up, confused, overwhelmed by pain, irritable and ready to quit. This is a natural reaction and prompts an adrenalin release that can boost energy and confidence and stimulates the foetal ejection reflex to help birth. When you are through this, you have done most of the hard work.

You may feel that you have been taken over by a force beyond your imagination and cry out that you can't go on or that you are dying. 'I can't do it, I can't go on,' followed by a midwife saying, 'Yes you can, you are doing it! You're doing great!' is one of the most common choruses heard in the birth room. This intense transition phase is the most

---

How can I make my labour shorter?
Every labour is different, and will progress in its own time. You can help your labour to progress well by doing what you can to create a secure environment with people you trust. This will encourage your body to release hormones that may speed progress. Remember, though, that a short labour is not necessarily a 'good' labour, and a long labour is not necessarily 'bad'. Sometimes a short labour may be painfully intense, while a long labour can be more mellow.

When you are in labour, your perception of time may change considerably and you are unlikely to be counting the minutes and hours. Your birth team will tell you if they feel your progress is unusually slow (p.502). As part of your birth plan, you may wish to talk to them about their time limits and your preferences for assistance and intervention.

Labour may be shorter if:
- You have already had a baby.
- Your baby is small.
- Your baby is in a good position, with her head well flexed and her chin tucked in.
- Your cervix is effaced and soft during pregnancy.
- Your pelvis is large and the shape is optimal.
- Your uterus contracts strongly: this may be aided by an upright position.
- You are fit and well nourished.
- You are in a positive frame of mind and feel secure in your environment.

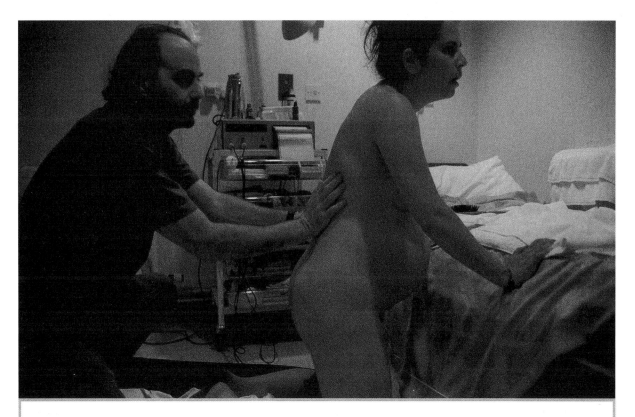

As a birth partner: first stage

If contractions are mild or widely spaced you may be able to help in a calm and relaxed way.

- You could make a cup of tea or give a soothing massage wherever your partner feels the need – her back, hands, thighs, shoulders, face or feet. She may appreciate the feeling of a cool damp cloth on her forehead.
- You could walk or sway gently with your partner as she leans on you.
- To help yourself, eat and drink well to keep up your energy.

It may help to breathe with your partner. When you focus on her breath and on your own, you may become centred and calm.

- If you have practised visualisations you may be able to talk her into a peaceful place.
- If it's appropriate, take a break and have a stretch or a short burst of exercise or a shower.

Towards the end of this stage it's common for women to become frightened and many show anger or struggle to carry on. You'll need to summon all your stamina and energy. Try not to take any abuse personally – you are a vehicle to help your partner to release her tension. The whole experience may be intense, and can be most difficult when you see your partner expressing pain or crying out.

- Breathe with your partner, encourage her and let her know she's doing well, and help her to let go of all her tension so she can relax fully between contractions.
- If she does not want to be touched or has put her trust in one of the midwives, try not to take it personally.
- Now may be a time to dim the lights, change the essential oils you are burning, wet the cloth you are using to stroke her forehead or replenish a jug with fresh cold water.
- It may be difficult just to be there, especially if you are used to being active and doing things, but your presence, love and commitment are immensely powerful.
- If you are overwhelmed or freaked out you'll need support from the midwives who will probably encourage you to take a break, perhaps to have a drink and something to eat, so you can return with new energy. When your partner looks at you she'll feel energised.

common time for women to request pain relief but before it is given a midwife will check if the birth is imminent and she may encourage you to go on, because relief will come very soon when your baby is born, much sooner perhaps than the time it could take for pain relief to kick in. Many women vomit during the active phase of labour, particularly during transition. This is a good sign that birth is imminent and often signals the foetal ejection reflex.

Because of the force of your descending baby and the feeling of pressure on your vagina and rectum, you may feel like pushing. Even in the midst of pressure, noise, fear and pain, you will need to do all you can to resist this urge until your midwife says you are fully dilated. If you push on the cervix before that, it will become swollen and interfere with the passage of your baby's head. The front of the cervix closest to your bladder is often the last part to open – gentle massage by your midwife may help if it is taking a long time. If she is concerned you are pushing too much too soon and your cervix is not fully dilated, she may advise you to kneel with your head on the bed and your bottom in the air to use gravity to slow it down, or she may suggest an epidural. When you are fully dilated, your contractions will change once again and your body will exert a natural pushing force. You have entered the second stage. Go with your body and rely on those supporting you if you do not feel strong enough to support yourself.

I've heard that some women do a poo in labour and I am nervous that this may happen to me. I'm also afraid of vomiting, which I really hate.

When your baby's head is descending you will feel pressure in your rectum and if there is any excreta there it will be forced out: your midwives will clear it away in an instant and ensure the area is sterile. It happens with virtually every birth and no one will mind, not even you because you'll be much too busy. You might not even be aware of it happening. For your midwives it is an exciting and a positive sign that labour is progressing well and birth is near.

As for vomiting, this is also quite common. However unpleasant, retching may actually help your contractions because it causes your diaphragm to push against your uterus. It often signals the end of transition and the arrival of the second stage. If you feel sick, the chances are that your midwife will be there to soothe you and wipe your face to relax you and before you know it you'll be on to the next contraction. If you were a Mayan woman you might have little choice: one tradition is to crack a raw egg into the mother's mouth to make her retch.

If you have been given an opiate drug for pain relief you may feel sick, though these are often administered with an anti-nausea drug. Vomiting in labour usually stops soon and is followed by relief and new energy.

The second stage: giving birth

When your cervix has fully dilated and your baby's head is descending, you have left transition behind and entered the stage of labour that culminates in the birth of your baby. This can take anything from 20 minutes to 2 hours. Contractions may vary and be intense or widely spaced and involve your whole body as your muscles tense when you push. You may feel new optimism and wake from the despair of transition with a sense of purpose and power that's in part stimulated by your body's release of adrenalin and endorphin hormones.

It is also common to feel scared by the unbelievably strong desire to push and the strange and uncomfortable feeling of a baby's head ready to emerge. But if you are encouraged by your supporters, your reservations may disappear as you give yourself over completely to the birth. Letting go of your rational mind and going off to 'another planet' helps you rise and fall with the waves of energy that are now urging your baby downwards: it might help to visualise her on her journey towards your vaginal entrance (p.128). At this stage you may enter an almost mystical state as you hover on the threshold of birth and let the power of new life flow through you.

The urge to push arises from the descent of your baby's head on to the muscular pelvic floor, when there is pressure on your bowel and sometimes on your bladder. If the urge is weak or absent it may be because your baby's head has not descended far enough and you are still in transition or because you have had an epidural anaesthetic that has not worn off. Sometimes a very strong fear of tearing or stretching can inhibit the pushing reflex. Providing she is happy that your baby's heartbeat is fine and you are feeling OK your midwife will let you progress in your own time. Her decision will rest on her observations and on hospital policy about 'acceptable' time for each stage.

Pushing or bearing down

When you have left the transition stage you will probably feel yourself bearing down as each contraction rises: pushing often happens naturally. If you feel able to surrender to the power of contractions and focus on your breathing you can let your body do the work, and if your baby is descending quickly you may need to do little but focus on being gentle. More commonly, at least in a first birth, you will need to help the power of your uterus. If you are upright, the process should be less strenuous, for gravity encourages your baby's head on to your pelvic floor and aids her descent, enabling you to breathe spontaneously, directing your energy and relaxing between contractions. Try to bear down towards your vagina, rather than 'push' noisily from your throat or face. It is often best to focus on bearing down rather than on shouting or groaning, which directs a considerable part of the energy

As a birth partner: second stage

You may become almost as focused on the birth as your partner is. It is surprising how many people dread the idea of labour and end up totally engrossed, discarding inhibitions and finding hidden reserves of energy, love and support. Some partners, men or women, do find it very difficult and it may be frightening to watch someone overcome by the forces of birth. When your baby's head becomes visible you may be overcome with joy and relief, and shout out instantly to let her know that you can see her baby. Your congratulations and encouragement will help her find the energy for the final pushes, and you will be the first to see the baby's face and then the rest of the body.

When your partner is pushing she'll probably rely on you for maximum physical support, particularly if she is giving birth upright. At times you may need to bear most of her weight: if you're worried about this or have a back problem, let the midwives know so that they can help you. Even if you're not sure about massage, your partner will tell you where she needs to feel pressure.

- If you feel yourself panicking, hand over your role to a midwife or another birth partner and take a break – this could refresh you.
- If you don't want to witness the actual birth you could stay close to her head.
- Even if you are very exhausted you will probably feel a surge of energy when you meet your baby.
- You may wish to cut the umbilical cord.
- Once your baby is born you may be the one to pass her to her mother, or your partner may ask you to cuddle your baby while she recovers. You begin communicating through touch, talking and eye contact.
- If there's room in the bed, or your partner is in the water pool, you could join them both.
- If any difficulties arise during labour your love and support will mean a lot. You may be a valuable go-between for your partner and the midwives. If intervention is recommended she may need your help to make a decision.

When the time is right, you can tell the world what you (and your partner, of course) have accomplished. But it may be best to delay phone calls until you have had time to sit quietly with your wonderful newborn baby.

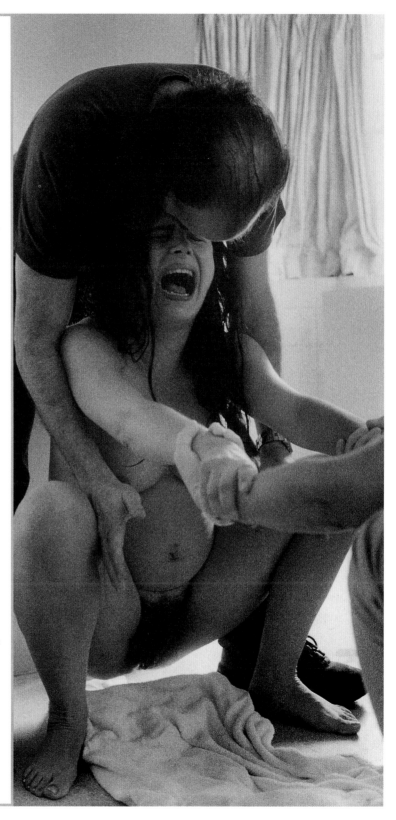

upwards. At the end of the second stage you may feel the desire to push between contractions – this is when your midwife will guide you.

As you bear down it will help if you can relax your vagina and perineum: if they are tense, the efficiency of your pushing may be reduced. It's similar to passing a stool when you automatically push to help the bowel to empty, but your pelvic floor and anus relax at the same time. If you do not enjoy the feeling of being watched or you are afraid of tearing, you may unconsciously hold your pelvic floor, anus and vaginal muscles tight. This reduces the space for your baby to emerge and it means your uterus has to work harder and you will need to put more effort into your pushing.

If you are getting exhausted and have feelings of, 'I can't do it', resting for a few contractions can help you muster strength. If you feel like crying, swearing, shouting or wishing the whole experience away, let it all out. Releasing these feelings may unblock any resistance that is counteracting your pushing power and make space for renewed energy, and it may be necessary now to consciously let go of your preconceptions for birth, which may be inhibiting you. In many labours a temporary letting-go, both mental and physical, is needed to break through the resistance, let go of tension and move on to the next stage. The power that rises after a break can be

---

When my baby arrives I want to hold her close, and smell her before she has been washed. I want the whole experience to be as natural as possible. Will my birth team agree?
It is now well accepted that mothers and babies need time together soon after the birth. How this is achieved varies from hospital to hospital. If the umbilical cord is not cut immediately you have an opportunity to hold your baby in the first few minutes after birth. Minimum fuss is needed apart from wiping amniotic fluid off your baby's skin, which often stimulates the first breath. If she doesn't breathe your midwife may stimulate the soles of her feet or blow gently on her face.

You can stay skin to skin because your body is the perfect temperature for your baby: her belly can rest on your body and your two hands will provide cover for her back. She may have traces of blood and vernix on her skin and will have a very special smell. If you give birth in water then your baby will be automatically bathed.

It will not be necessary to suction fluid from the mouth because any amniotic fluid she swallows will be absorbed into her circulation, unless your baby has breathing difficulties or has passed meconium in the womb. Depending on the policy of your hospital, weighing and measuring and clothing your baby can be delayed until you have gazed into one another's eyes in welcome and you are ready to have a cup of tea.

momentous. When you sense the pressure of your baby's head coming closer to your vaginal entrance you may feel exhilaration and excitement: it won't be long until you meet one another, face to face.

Your baby's head crowns

As your baby's head descends you will notice a stretching and burning sensation in your vagina and perineum. It can be daunting, particularly if you are afraid of tearing. Many women find it easiest to direct their energy by willing their baby down into the burning sensation and relaxing the anus at the same time. This gives the direction for pushing and utilises the power from above.

When your baby reaches the opening of your vagina the burning becomes really intense as his head 'crowns' – this can be one of the most painful parts of labour. Your birth partner will be able to see the top of the head through your vaginal opening, and you may want to touch it. Now your baby is ready to be born, although birth may not follow immediately. Sometimes only one or two contractions pass from the moment the head becomes visible to the birth, but it may take longer. At this point your body and your baby work naturally together. You may not need to push; alternatively, your baby may need you to direct your energy downwards.

Some women are overtaken by a deep-seated, primitive instinct to bear down and give birth and remain oblivious to everything and everyone else while their contractions follow one another like waves. Others have tranquil, widely spaced contractions and an intermittent pushing urge and need more encouragement. Some have strong contractions but still need encouragement to push through the sensation of stinging. You may need the entire birth team saying, 'You can do it, we can see your baby's head, one more push and it's over, big push now, your baby's coming, you are nearly there, well done.'

At the moment of birth your midwives will encourage you to take gentle short breaths or pant and let go of any desire to push to give your perineum time to stretch gradually. Your midwife may help by massaging it, and will gently guide out your baby's head. With the next contraction she will help first one shoulder emerge, then the other, after which the body follows easily with one final push from you.

The chorus of sounds in the birth room may vary from quiet meditation to loud encouragement and, at the moment of birth, women commonly let out a loud groan or yell known as the 'primal scream'. It has a characteristic sound that has accompanied birth for centuries and your midwife would know when your baby was born even if she was not looking. You'll probably feel a surge of energy as untold emotions rush out of you in your scream and your baby's head emerges in one exhilarating, relieving and magical moment.

Your baby is here

After your pushing, your patience and your perseverance, your baby will finally emerge and you will feel a range of emotions beyond words. At birth there is a moment when tension is replaced by relief and wonder. The sound changes from your primal scream and the encouragement of the birth team to quiet murmurs. 'Look at your wonderful baby, here she is, how soft her skin is, isn't she beautiful? . . . You're my baby, I love you, you are gorgeous.' The smell also changes, as the slightly sweet aroma of baby and amniotic fluid permeates the room.

The initial feeling in the birth – 'she did it, she actually gave birth' – is replaced soon by a focus on your baby. Your birth partner and midwife immediately look at her with different eyes: your partner amazed that this person could emerge so complete and your midwife checking to see whether your baby looks normal, has a pink colour and is ready to cry. Within seconds she will feel the touch of human hands for the first time and take her first breath.

If you feel strong enough to hold her on your abdomen or chest and feel her tiny body in your arms, your midwife will pass her to you. Your baby is still attached to the placenta by the umbilical cord, which is usually long enough to allow her to be placed on your tummy. The midwife may wrap your baby in a towel or wrap a blanket around the pair of you once you are embraced, because her skin will be moist and she may lose heat rapidly if left uncovered. If you have given birth in a kneeling position she will be passed between your legs. If your baby is born into water the midwife will bring her gently to the surface and into your arms.

If the lights are not already dimmed, ask for them to be softened so your baby isn't dazzled by bright light and she can be welcomed into the family in an intimate atmosphere. Your first contact, preferably skin to skin, is blissful, as you stroke her delicate body, let her fingers curl around yours, smell her unique scent and hear her snuffles and cries for the first time. The sight and smell of your delicious baby may be enough to make your heart melt: seeing her is the culmination of 9 months waiting, and being close to her stimulates your body to release oxytocin and endorphins, the 'love hormones'. You will be mimicking one another as you gaze into one another's eyes and touch for the first time. Even if you are exhausted a new energy will probably well up in you. You may want to continue holding your baby and might try breastfeeding. But you will have been through a lot and may need to rest and hand your baby over to her dad or the midwife for loving cuddles.

The initial meeting between you and your baby may not be as romantic if you feel exhausted, overwhelmed, tearful or upset. You may also be shocked if you baby looks very pink or wrinkled, or has an odd-shaped head, all of which are normal newborn characteristics. If feelings of love, joy and connection don't come to you immediately and you do not want to hold your baby, don't worry: they may take time to surface and you don't have to feel them instantly to be a good mother. You have just completed one of the most challenging and miraculous feats of your life, and it can be difficult to absorb the reality of a new baby if you feel physically and emotionally exhausted.

The third stage

Once your baby is born you may feel that it's all over and be totally absorbed in her. Yet labour has not quite finished. Your baby's protector in the womb, the placenta, still needs to be born. It won't follow your baby instantly so you'll have plenty of time to change position. You may want to remain squatting or kneeling or, if you are keen to hold your baby, you can move to a supported sitting position. After a water birth, you may want to relax in the water with your baby and wait peacefully.

The placenta is born

In a natural labour within 5–15 minutes your uterus will begin to contract with afterpains that are much gentler than former contractions, although in third or fourth births they can be as strong. These encourage separation of the placenta, which is embedded in a layer of spongy decidual tissue lining the cavity enclosed by the wall of your uterus. The muscle fibres in the wall shorten after the baby is out, a process called retraction, and the placenta shears off. It may take anything between 15 and 30 minutes.

If contractions are not strong enough to deliver the placenta, you may stimulate them by bringing your baby to your breast: her sucking will prompt the release of the hormone oxytocin, which powers contractions. Your midwife can also help by gently massaging your uterus via your abdominal wall.

When the placenta emerges you will need to push a little. There is no stretching, just a warm, slippery feeling. If you like, you can see and touch the organ that has nourished your baby. Your midwives will examine it to check that no part of it has come away.

What will happen to my placenta? I've heard that placentas are used in the manufacture of beauty products. Is this true? In western births the placenta is rarely valued by parents, although they may be interested in the way it looks and feels. It was once used to make a variety of cosmetic products but because of the risk of spreading infection it is now discarded. In some cultures the placenta is valued as a baby's womb-friend and as a symbol for the baby's future. In Sudan, where it is believed to be the baby's spirit double, it is buried in a place that symbolises the parents' hopes for their child, and in Hawaii it is traditional to bury it under a tree that becomes the child's tree.

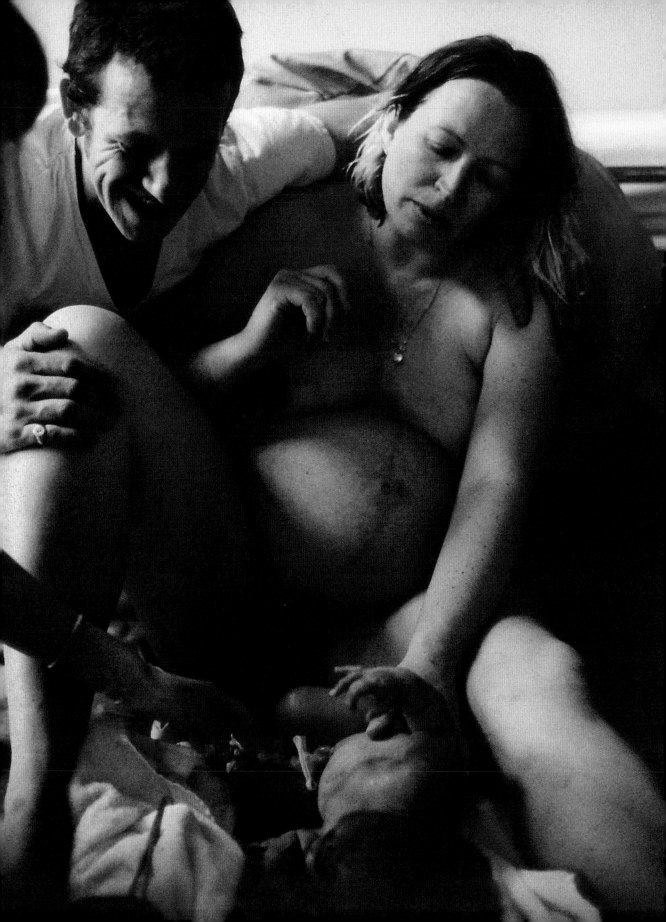

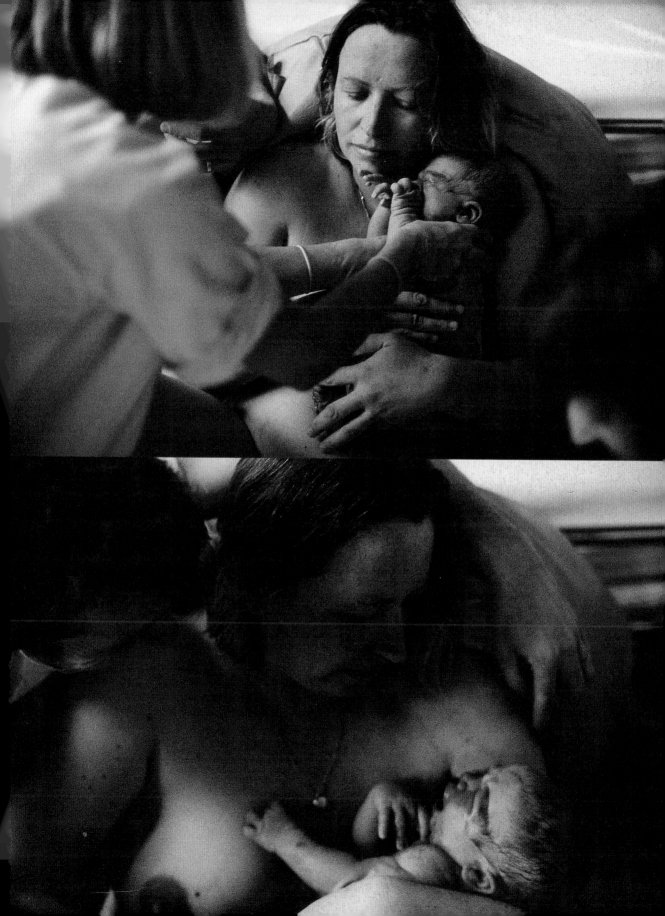

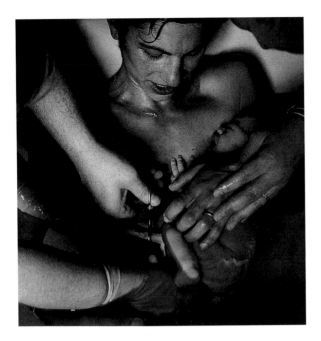

Swapping lifelines

The umbilical cord that your baby has been gripping and stroking in the womb pulsates after birth, providing her with both a lifeline and a source of oxygen while breathing is established. Your midwife can quickly assess your baby's wellbeing by feeling the blood's pulsation in the cord. It is safe to hold your baby in your arms or on your tummy without cutting it.

Prostaglandin hormones released when your baby's lungs expand cause the umbilical arteries to contract and the flow of blood gradually decreases, leaving the cord white and flaccid. It is no longer needed to transfer oxygen or nutrients and can be clamped and cut about 2.5 cm (1 in) from your baby's body.

She will be totally unaware of the process since there are no nerve endings in the cord and the site will heal naturally over the next 10 days. All that will remain is a neat belly button. Whether your baby's belly button faces inwards or outwards has nothing to do with the way the cord is cut.

Looking at your baby

Glossy images of smooth-skinned babies with delicate tufts of soft hair and flawless chubby cheeks don't actually convey the reality. These cherub-like characteristics appear after a few days or even weeks. In the first minutes of life your baby, while quite probably the most amazing and beautiful thing you have ever seen, will still possess

Usually the umbilical cord will be clamped and cut when it has stopped beating and before the birth of the placenta. Your uterus will continue to contract as the muscle fibres shorten and constrict the blood vessels that fed the placenta, thereby stemming the bleeding. Your uterus subsequently shrinks back to the size of a pear in the weeks following the birth.

In some hospitals midwives recommend the injection of a synthetic oxytocin hormone, Syntocinon, to encourage the birth of the placenta and as a precaution against excessive blood loss. Sometimes Syntometrine is used, which consists of the hormone oxytocin and the drug ergometrine. Many units use Syntocinon alone because of the side effects of ergometrine (nausea and vomiting, hypertension and headache) and reserve the ergometrine if bleeding occurs.

If Syntocinon is given as a routine then the third stage is shortened. Your midwife only need pull lightly on the umbilical cord and the placenta will be born within 5 minutes. The cord will be clamped before or very soon after the injection, to prevent the drug from entering your baby's circulation.

On balance, if your pregnancy has been normal and your baby is not excessively large then there is no need to speed up the third stage. If your hospital routinely uses an injection you may be able to request Syntocinon alone. Some hospitals have a selective policy of administering oxytocin if there is a risk of extra bleeding. If you begin to bleed excessively following the birth of the placenta your midwife will massage your uterus to help it to contract and you may also be given Syntocinon or ergometrine to help it remain contracted.

Is it best to cut the cord soon after birth?
For years there was some concern that leaving the cord unclamped could carry a risk of blood draining from the placental pool into the baby and causing a high haemoglobin level, or draining out of the baby into the placenta and causing anaemia. It's now known that a baby's hormonal system equilibrates the blood volume and there is no danger of loss or gain of blood. Cutting the cord when pulsation has stopped is the most natural thing to do. Very early clamping of the cord within seconds of the birth may trap extra blood in the placenta and less remains in your baby's circulation.

Very early cutting of the cord may increase a baby's need to be given oxygen because the placental reserve supply is cut off. In hospitals that practise routine administration of Syntocinon to reduce bleeding after the birth the cord must be clamped soon to prevent the drug from reaching the baby. In a small percentage of births the birth team may decide that a baby would benefit from resuscitation with external oxygen under pressure rather than cord oxygen. If the cord is wound tightly round the baby's neck or breathing does not begin soon then the cord will be clamped and cut soon so that she can be taken to the oxygen on the resuscitaire.

in-utero features. Her skin will be covered or dabbed with vernix, the white creamy substance that protects and moisturises her in the womb, and there may be traces of blood. She may also appear wrinkled and very pink. Some babies are born with spotty faces, a neonatal acne resulting from blocked sebaceous glands. And because your baby's skull bones are soft and overlap during birth and the scalp skin may be swollen, her head may appear squeezed or even conical in shape.

You may notice that your baby's breasts seem a little puffy: this is a minor stimulation resulting from hormones and soon recedes. Her or his genitals may also appear swollen. Again this is a hormonal effect, and in girls may result in a small amount of blood or vaginal discharge for a few days.

All these features will begin to recede in the first hours, and after a few days and a bath her hair will fluff up. Gradually, skin becomes less wrinkled, even though there may be slight peeling in reaction to the new airy environment and her conical head shape will alter noticeably within a day.

The birth is over

As soon as you feel ready, either before or after the birth of the placenta, you and your baby can enjoy close skin-to-skin contact and this may be a perfect opportunity to bring your baby to your breast for her first sucks. This is not to feed, because your baby can go for hours without food, but it offers a loving welcome and helps you to tune into one another; feeling, smelling and looking at each other. Within a few minutes the baby–mother dance begins and you respond to one another's embrace, calmness and unique scent. With low lights and little noise in the room you can indulge in one another in an intimate space and your partner may join you.

Your midwife will check your vagina and perineum for tears, and will be able to give you stitches in a quick and painless process using a local anaesthetic while you hold your baby or relax.

What follows depends on hospital practice. The midwives may bring you a cup of tea and a small snack and a phone so that you can call your friends and family. You may be offered a bath or be given a gentle wash as you lie in bed. If there is a birth pool you may be welcome to bathe with your baby (and your partner if he wishes). Then when you are ready it will be time to go to your ward or room together as a family.

As you sit with your partner, you will marvel at your baby before welcoming your friends and your baby's grandparents, uncles and aunts to celebrate the birth. Soon it will be time to break open the champagne and toast your new arrival and your success.

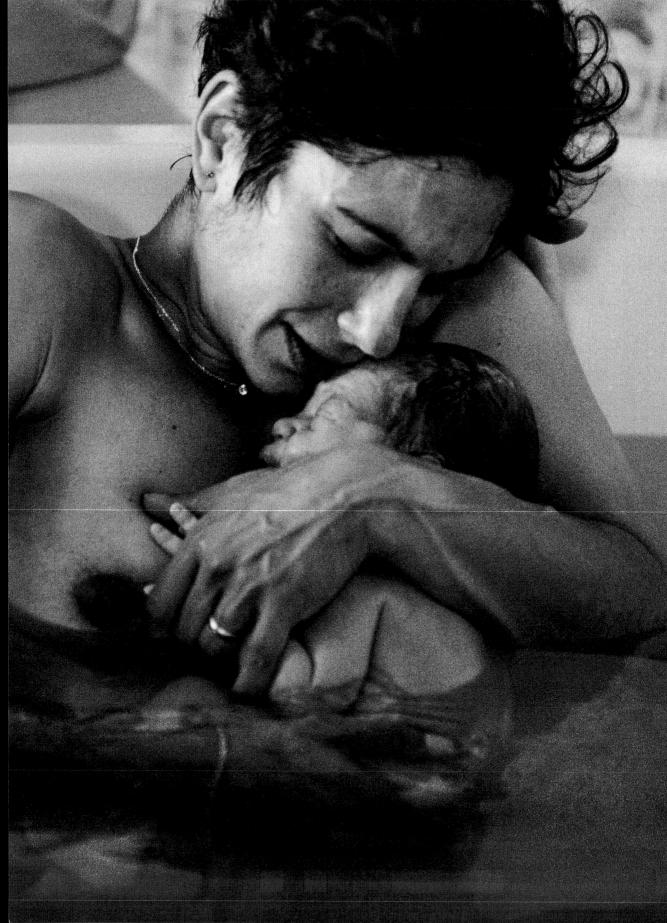

Climbing a mountain

There's nothing quite like going through labour and giving birth, and no two are the same, so even if you've done it once, your second experience will be totally new. In some ways the experience can be compared to climbing a mountain. No two mountains are the same and each climb is unique.

There will be times when the going's easy and you progress at a steady pace with time to enjoy your surroundings. There'll be other times when it's tough and you focus completely on the task in hand, and still others when it seems impossible – 'I'll never reach the top. How can I ever push hard enough?'

Most climbers experience feelings of despair at some point and want to turn back, but the draw of the summit is very powerful. There's no turning back in labour: like a climber, you need physical strength, you need to maximise your energy and seek out your deepest reserves, keep nourished and keep up your emotional stamina. Sometimes the next phase is aided by relaxing and going with the natural flow and at other times you work hard to progress and keep going despite the pain. You need to trust and rely on your partner, sometimes handing him the ropes and sometimes taking the lead yourself. Each time you negotiate an obstacle and your baby descends further you get a power surge and a feeling of accomplishment – as if you've reached a higher stage of the mountain. As your baby's head crowns you are so near completion that your adrenalin keeps you going and birth – or the top of the mountain – is marked by the 'primal scream' as your body generates the final rush of energy. You can now rest, sink down in relief, relish the incomparable view, congratulate yourself and marvel at your reward.

Using water for labour and birth

A warm bath takes away the stresses of the day and helps relaxation. In labour, water may have a similar effect, reducing anxiety and helping you to focus, but its influence is even more powerful: it can help relieve pain, encourage dilation of the cervix, aid stretching of the vaginal opening and offer your baby a smooth and calm entry into the world. While it is a relatively recent feature in the birthing world tens of thousands of women have used it.

The properties of water

A baby's transition from womb to water of the same temperature is thought by many to be gentler and less shocking than birth into air. Some natural birth advocates believe that this calm birth experience can positively colour a person's early life, although this has never been proven. There is no doubt, though, that birth in water receives the highest satisfaction ratings from the mothers. Midwives are also calmed by the presence of water and by the relaxation of mother and baby.

The power that water has to relax a labouring woman, enhance the release of the body's natural pain-relieving hormones and encourage dilation of the cervix has been witnessed over the last 30 years but remains something of an enigma to scientists. Yet everyone knows that water relieves aches and pains and women in labour are attracted to water: running a shower or a bath and letting the water caress you may help you withdraw from distractions.

During the 1970s, Michel Odent in France and Igor Tcharkovsky in Russia pioneered the use of water in labour. The trend of using water for labour and birth has increased since the early 1980s. Yehudi Gordon was one of the first obstetricians to use it in England. It is now widely accepted as a gentle way for a baby to be born.

Water in labour

When you enter the pool in labour you may take a few minutes to settle. Your birth team may have props, or you may have brought some – a stool, towels or a plastic pillow – and your partner may join you. There will be room to sit, kneel, squat or float with your legs straight out. In the pool you may use the same techniques during labour as you might do on land, with the added support of the water.

It is best to use the pool after your cervix has dilated to 5 cm. Before this, the relaxing effect of water may reduce the power of contractions, but after this your contractions are more likely to retain their power and the water can help your body to relax. You are less likely to need synthetic oxytocin to boost the power of contractions (p.164) or epidural anaesthesia for pain relief (p.159). It has been suggested that this is because immersion in water lowers levels of stress hormones and increases the body's natural

release of endorphins and oxytocin, the hormone that stimulates the uterus to contract. Water also relieves pain because it stimulates the skin's sensitive nerve endings. As they send messages of sensation into the brain, they occupy nerve pathways and effectively 'gate out' some messages from the nerve pain fibres supplying the uterus.

Immersion in water below the maternal body temperature (under 37°C/98.6°F) tends to aid labour for up to 4 hours: longer than this and progress may be slowed. If you do not feel secure and comfortable or if your midwife senses that you or your baby is in difficulty, you will be asked to leave the pool. Though it has many benefits, water is not a substitute for good midwifery and obstetric care.

Water for birth

When you begin to push, you may feel more confident to harness your power on dry land. If you choose to stay in the water, you can lie and float, squat or kneel; perhaps only your legs and pelvic region will be in the water. You can use the pool side to support whatever position you choose. When your baby's head has crowned, the water takes the edge off the stinging and gives some lubrication to encourage stretching, making tears less likely.

Your midwife will gently help the birth of your baby's head if this is needed, and the body will follow with the next contraction. Your baby has a diving reflex and will not inhale water. He will be stimulated to take a breath when he senses cool air on his skin. In less than 30 seconds your midwife will lift him out of the water and on to your tummy or chest. You may then gently blow on your baby's skin to stimulate breathing if he has not already taken his first breath. Water babies are often calm at birth but many still need to cry to expand their lungs. When your baby is breathing well, you or your partner can hold him in the water with his head above the surface and wait for the birth of the placenta, which can be born in water safely.

Water pools

As water births become more popular many more hospitals are equipped with birth pools. If your hospital has a pool the midwives will be trained to use it for labour and birth. For a water birth at home you will need to hire an approved birth pool and ensure that there is someone with you who can keep the temperature below 37°C (98.6°F).

You will need to check that your community midwife will support your choice. Make the room you have chosen intimate and make sure the floor supports the weight of the full pool. It is a good idea to fill the pool and use it with your partner before labour as a trial.

Safety of water birth

Concerns about safety are common among parents-to-be yet research and experience have proved that water is safe when there is appropriate care.

The dive reflex

Your baby won't draw breath until there's contact with the cooler air above the water. In the rare occurrence of even a single drop of water reaching the back of his throat, receptors stimulate the diving reflex to prevent breathing. A tiny risk of inhaling water only occurs if a baby has had foetal distress, lacked oxygen during the labour and birth and the reflex to gasp overrides the diving reflex. This is where midwifery skills come into play and by listening to your baby's heartbeat while he is still in the womb your midwife will be aware of foetal distress and you will be asked to leave the pool.

Sterility

The birth pool in a hospital will be cleansed thoroughly before use and your baby is protected from organisms that pass from your body into the water by your natural antibody immunity that crosses the placenta. You or your partner will need to be responsible for ensuring the pool is sterile if you hire one for use at home.

Protection from infection

HIV and hepatitis can be transmitted if there is a crack in the midwife's skin and blood from the mother is in the pool. Midwives are able to take extra precautions by wearing long gloves and ensuring that their skin has no cuts or abrasions. It may be preferable for you to be tested for HIV and hepatitis.

Under what circumstances would I be advised to leave the birth pool?
- If you do not feel comfortable or happy in the water.
- If you choose to have an epidural anaesthetic.
- If your contractions are ineffective or if your baby's heart rate suggests foetal distress.
- If your midwife is concerned about either you or your baby and needs to monitor you more closely.
- If labour is prolonged or complicated and you or your baby need help.

Water temperature

Your baby will be very sensitive to a rise in your body temperature because he uses your blood to maintain his temperature. To ensure you remain comfortable, your midwife will maintain the water below your body temperature (37°C/98.6°F). If you stay in the pool after birth the temperature of the water will ensure that your baby does not become cold.

Comfort and support

Your birth attendants will be easily able to touch, massage and assist you by leaning over the sides of the pool. Extra support, such as towels, pillows or a stool helps with comfortable positioning and the pool sides are strong and easy to grip if you are kneeling or squatting. Your birth partner can give you maximum support from either in or outside the pool.

Maximum power

Being in water makes it easy to squat and harness some of the power of the upright position. If you need more energy and the birth is delayed, it's best to leave the pool and give birth on land in an upright position. You may want to return to the water and bathe with your newborn. In spite of being in strong labour it is very simple to leave the pool within 20 seconds between contractions. It is the same as stepping out of a bath.

Safety

The most recent research studies in England Wales concluded that babies who were born in water to women with low-risk pregnancies did not have an increase in major complications or deaths directly attributable to the use of water.

Your choice

Despite its many advantages, the use of water for birth is not for everyone. Many women feel much happier on dry land and, for some, water instils fear rather than confidence. After chatting with your midwife you may decide that a water birth could offer you a natural method of pain relief, even if you do not go on to give birth in the pool. You will know on the day what feels right for you and whether you want to use it.

Michel Odent himself warns that being attached to water can make some women become 'prisoners of their projects'. They may inhibit their own labour by clinging to hopes and goals when it would be better for them to be out of water, or they may become disappointed, angry or guilty if they don't stay in the pool. If the pushing stage of your labour requires maximum power it is preferable to be upright on dry land. The best thing for you and for your baby is that you are comfortable and that you are able to go with your instincts.

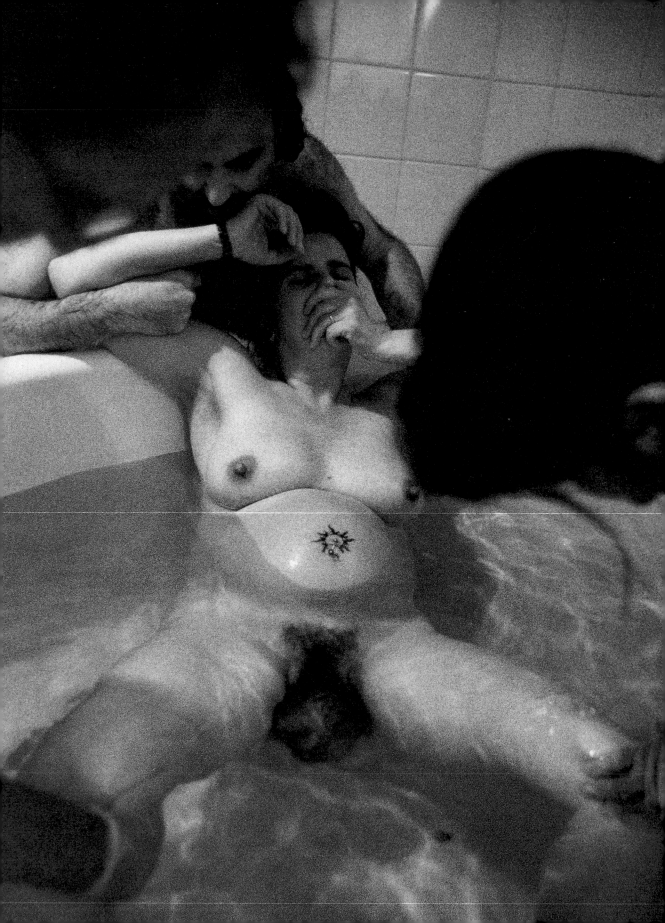

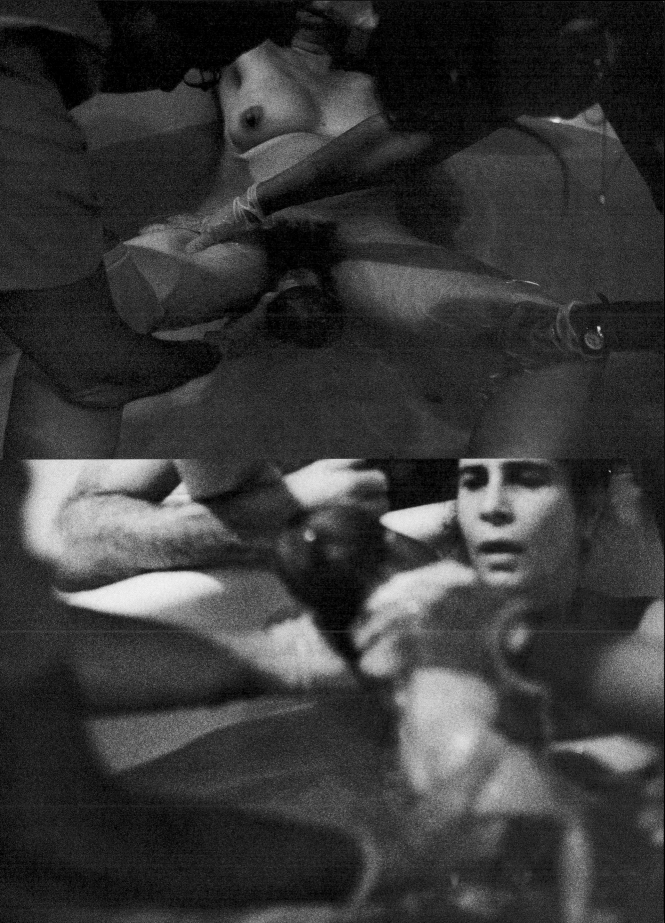

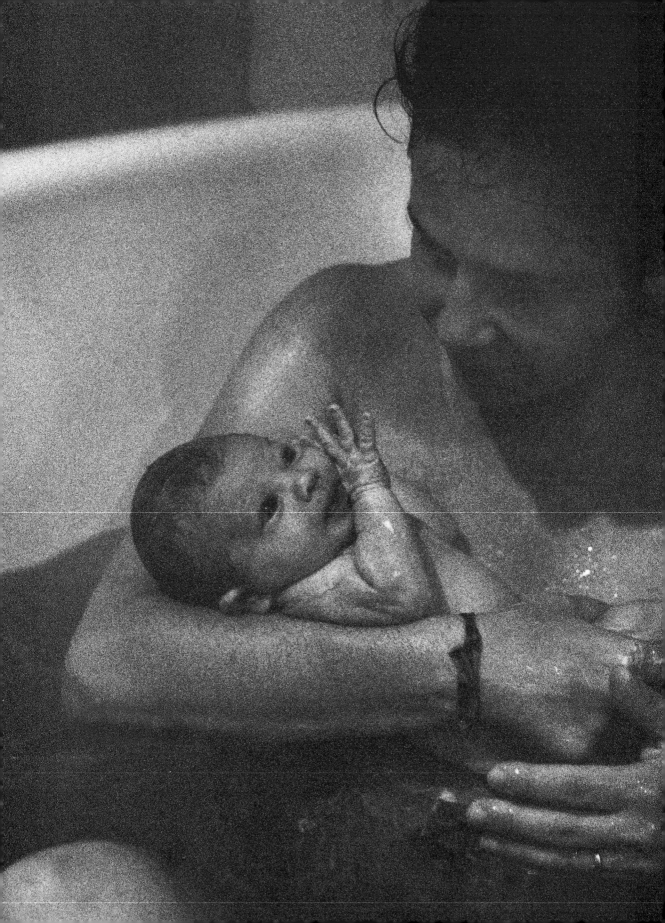

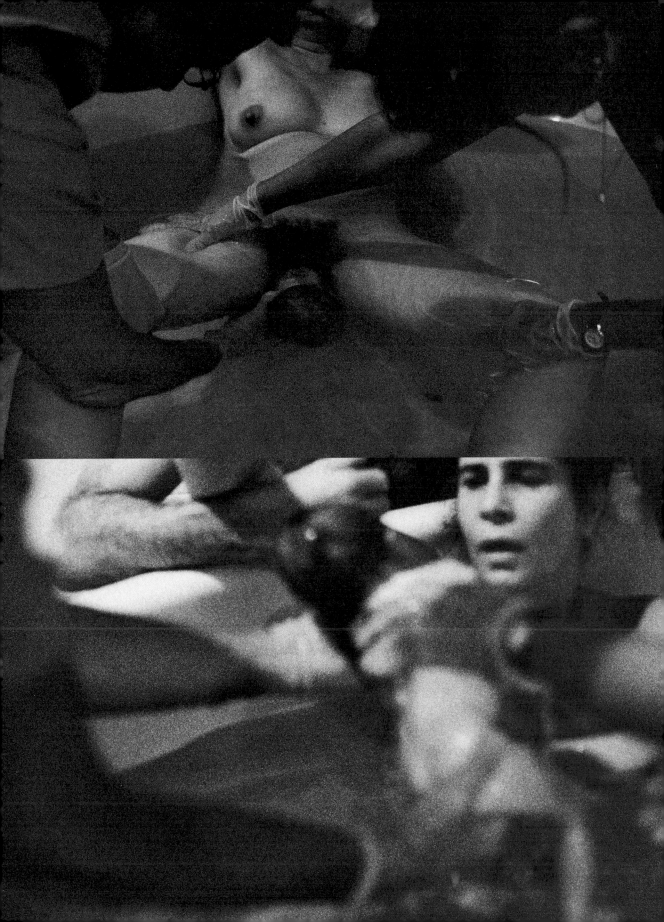

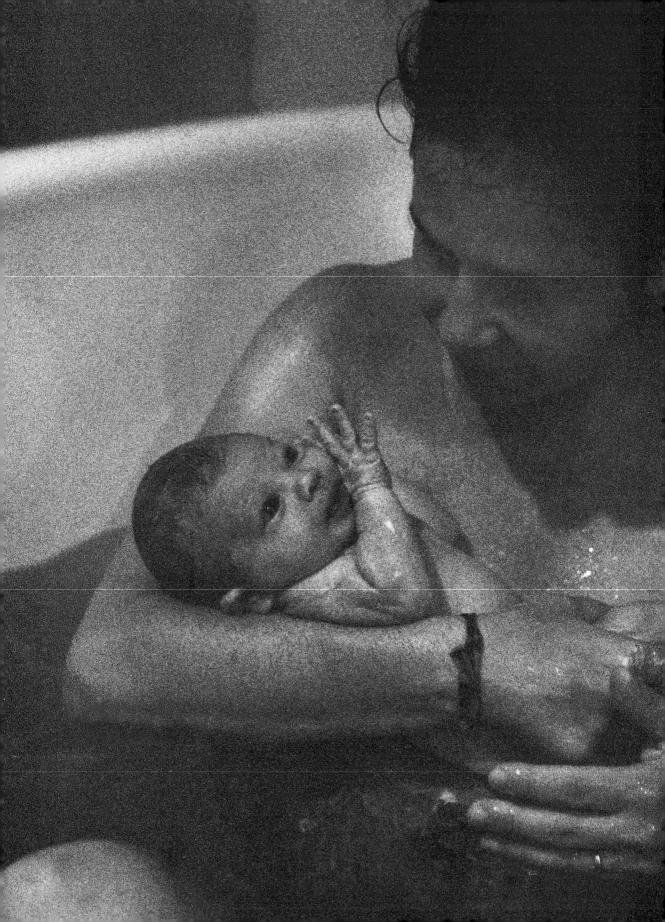

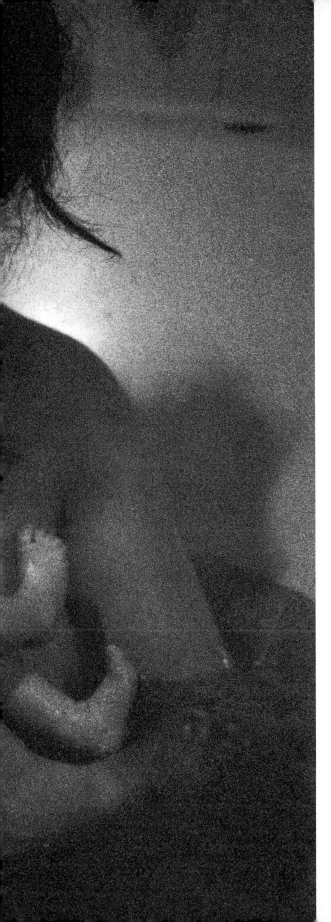

A water baby

There is something poignant about the moment a baby is brought to the surface of the water. He is greeted by his ecstatic mother, who is relaxed and supported in the pool, and a contented father who also feels the calming properties of the water.

It is easy to hold your tiny baby in your hands with his face out and his body warmed by the water, and also simple to bring him to your chest.

As you look into one another's eyes he may remain calm and dreamy before he opens his mouth and makes his first cry. If all is well you will be able to stay together, embraced in the warm water, until you are ready to leave the pool.

Your baby in labour and birth

Your baby prepares for birth in the weeks leading up to labour, and influences progress through her position and release of hormones, as well as her movements and her emotions. After birth, when she gazes at you for the first time, smells your skin and hears your voice, your baby plays an even more important role as she invites you to fall in love.

Natural timing

Hormones released by your baby's body stimulate your cervix to ripen and your uterus to contract: she has a shared but central role in deciding when labour commences. Although she does not consciously know what lies ahead, biologically she has reached the stage of development when it is appropriate to move from the security of your womb into the larger world. Nature genetically endows your baby's brain and hormonal system with the ability to detect what is happening in her body. In a superbly orchestrated way, at different stages your baby's system switches on different proteins and enzymes that not only stimulate labour but ensure that her development is appropriate for the week of pregnancy, for labour and birth and then for breathing in air and for the months beyond.

Your baby's body is adapted for birth, particularly the head and neck. Her skull bones overlap, her head rotates as it passes through the birth canal and her neck bends and flexes freely. The rest of her body may aid the process by moving or she may remain passive and be guided by your contractions. If she is afraid, her body will secrete endorphins to combat it, and she may also feel fear with a rush of adrenalin and cortisol if she is stressed or shocked.

How your baby may feel

Trying to ascertain how a baby feels during labour is an ongoing study with results that are partly based on observation with scans and heartbeat patterns, and partly speculative. Labour may be easy or difficult – a lot depends on the size and shape of your baby's head, its position as it descends and the shape of your pelvis. The intensity of your contractions and the oxygen from the placenta also exert an effect. At times your baby may be calmed by the rhythmic contractions of the uterine walls that massage and stroke her skin through the amniotic fluid and at times she may be frightened by the intensity of the waves or sudden changes in rhythm.

Each time your uterus contracts, the cervix is drawn up and presses on her head. Your baby may move slightly or wriggle in response: as she presses on the cervix, she encourages it to open but it is unlikely to be painful, for a cushion of amniotic fluid lies between her head and the cervix until the waters break. The top of her head is not very sensitive to pain and the skin may become filled with fluid, called a caput, giving extra protection. But the rest of her body is extremely sensitive, and each time the walls of your uterus press on her, cells in her skin send messages through her nervous system readying her body for life outside the womb.

If you are upright, there will be more room for her to negotiate the birth canal during the second stage because it enlarges. As she emerges, the soft tissues of your vagina surround her face and she feels none of the urgency or burning that you feel. Because she gets oxygen via the placenta, she will not feel suffocated or restricted by the vaginal walls pressed around her head: they are more likely to be comforting and muffle the noise in the room where her arrival is awaited.

Although your baby does not experience the world like a mini adult, she will sense your moods because hormones in your blood filter into her system and she will be aware of your movements and heartbeat and know when your voice sounds calm or fraught. She has the special 'something' that makes her a unique individual and she will not mimic your feelings: she will react to the messages in many ways. Sometimes she may fall into a deep and pleasant sleep, even during the intense part of labour, or wriggle and kick and try to move with the downward pressure. Her mood immediately after birth will reflect her experience and reaction to labour. Every baby, and every labour, is different.

Entering the world

Not long before the moment of birth, the top of your baby's head becomes visible as it crowns. She will feel your contractions as your body's expulsive force and the pressure of your pelvic tissues reach their height, and as her head is born the lips of your vagina will pass smoothly over her face, perhaps with a feeling of tightness.

Your baby will sense the difference in temperature as she gets her first experience of air. This is a natural stimulus for her to take a breath, although this may not come until her body is born. She might remain quiet and calm for a few seconds or open her mouth wide as the reflex to gasp for air kicks in, then utter a cry. She will feel hands on her head and her body will continue to rotate so that it's in the best position to be born with the next

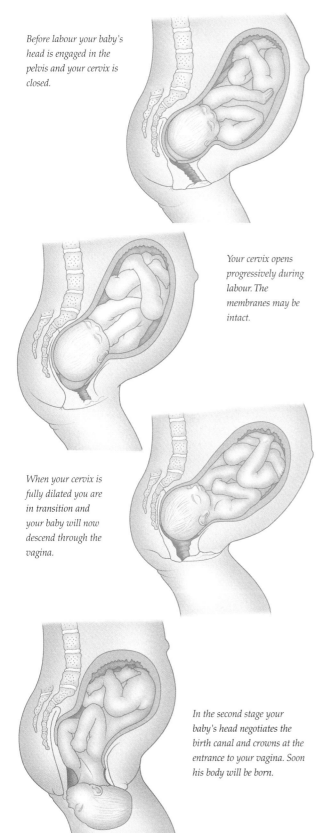

Before labour your baby's head is engaged in the pelvis and your cervix is closed.

Your cervix opens progressively during labour. The membranes may be intact.

When your cervix is fully dilated you are in transition and your baby will now descend through the vagina.

In the second stage your baby's head negotiates the birth canal and crowns at the entrance to your vagina. Soon his body will be born.

contraction. First one shoulder, then the other, and then the rest of the body emerge, feeling the air. If your baby is born in water she will sense a different feeling on her skin. When she is brought to the surface she will register her new airy environment and draw a breath.

Outside the womb

At birth your baby feels the cold air on her skin. At first her eyes are closed and her hands clenched. Then in the first minute breathing begins, perhaps with a gasp, a pause, another gasp and then regular breaths, or with a cry and each breath heralded by another cry so that crying and breathing are one. In the early minutes, crying is a reflex and does not imply that your baby is upset. The pressure of crying opens her lungs to their full extent, but she may do this by breathing gently. A small number of babies require help with breathing. When breathing is easy your baby opens her eyes and watches you with a profound look as if the wisdom of the ages is inherent in her gaze. This happens within minutes, sooner if the room is darkened. After this her hands relax and she opens her arms in a gesture that says, 'I'm here.'

She is likely to be awake and alert for an hour or two, exploring you with her eyes and keen sense of smell. She can focus on your face immediately. The feeling of your touch, which will be most exquisite and warming if it is skin-to-skin, will communicate welcome and love and take over from the closeness of the womb she has just left. The temperature of your skin is the same as that of the amniotic fluid. Your baby will be fully conscious and flooded by new feelings, including the force of gravity, the texture of your skin, the sight of shapes and colours and the sound of unmuffled noise.

Her spine will stretch and extend fully for the first time and her body will gradually unfurl. She'll be comforted by loving surroundings, the sound of your familiar heartbeat and voice, the smell of your body and the warmth and protection of your embrace. If she enjoys stretching she may like to lie naked on you, with her body touching yours and her spine stretched out. Some babies prefer to flex and draw in their hands and feet and enjoy being swaddled or clothed and held tightly.

Crying and breathing for life

Crying at birth expands the lungs and allows air to displace the liquid that filled them in the womb. Internally, your baby's physiology is undergoing the most remarkable transformation. Contact with the cooler temperature of the outside air stimulates the breathing reflex, opening and inflating the air sacs in her lungs for the first time. The liquid they did contain is either coughed out or absorbed and any excess is passed out as urine. As your baby's lungs expand, the pressure changes within them and there is a release of prostaglandin hormones: this combination closes channels in her heart that bypassed the lungs in favour of the placenta to obtain oxygen from your blood while she was in the womb. Now she can derive oxygen from the air.

Your baby's lips change from blue to pink and the rest of her body takes on a pink colour within a few minutes. Her hands and feet may remain a little blue, not because there is any lack of oxygen, but because circulation is naturally sluggish.

If you have been in an upright position your baby will have been born head downwards, which helps clear her passages for breathing. To help this process your midwife may lay your baby face down on a towel immediately after birth, or you may feel strong enough to lay her on her belly over your thigh and stroke her back gently. It is not necessary to routinely apply suction to the nose and mouth but if your baby needs assistance to establish breathing, it will be at hand.

What if labour is difficult? Will my baby become stressed?
Babies who feel stress are in the minority: oxytocin and endorphin hormones are a natural antidote and human babies secrete them and are biologically geared to being born. They have an incredible ability to move from one frame of mind to another and are usually able to relax more rapidly than adults. Because nature is on the side of mother and baby, the vast majority of births end well. And with increasingly adept obstetric skills, most stressful situations can either be avoided or dealt with rapidly.

If there is stress, your baby will release adrenalin and cortisol, stress hormones that may lead to anxiety, and feel emotions connected with this inherent fight or flight reaction. Her heartbeat will also change.

There are a number of things that may make labour stressful. If your baby's head is stuck and takes a long time to negotiate your birth canal she will be aware of pressure. If forceps or ventouse are used, she can experience pain. When there is a fall in oxygen she will use energy from glucose stored in her body – if she uses all the stores she will find it difficult to cope and her body will produce high concentrations of stress hormones. Prolonged low oxygen levels may make her shocked and she may need breathing assistance at birth. She might be irritable and upset for hours, days or weeks as she recovers.

Not all babies appear stressed following intervention and many handle a forceps or caesarean with ease. Sometimes a baby may seem tense after a relatively smooth labour: feeling upset may be a part of personality and not to do with the birth. Skin-to-skin contact, a loving welcome and early breastfeeding can reduce anxiety and replace it with calm. Some babies also benefit from massage or cranial osteopathy that realigns the body after the twisting and turning of birth.

What your baby can do
As you gaze at your baby, talk to and touch her she will respond gently with a changing expression in her eyes and by moving her mouth and tongue. She is able to see, albeit with vision that is a little blurred, at a distance of 25–30 cm (10–12 in), so she can watch your face as you hold her in your arms. This is comforting – newborn babies like to focus on soft, rounded objects.

Although your baby's movements are involuntary, she will be fully aware of your presence and of other movements and noises in the room. As her arms and hands stretch they will collide with her face and also with your skin and help her assess her environment. She has powerful intuition that prompts her to focus on your face and smell, as if she is programmed by nature to get to know her mother. She can sense your emotions and with her winning eyes and perfect body will ease your anxiety and kindle love and contentment. If she is held by a midwife or your partner for a while after birth, she will find security in their embrace, but once she feels your body, smells your motherly scent and hears the heartbeat and voice she has listened to for almost 9 months, she will know she's with you and feel the baby–mother bond.

Your baby will also recognise her daddy's voice and may relax to the familiar deep tones. She may spend time in the arms of her father while you rest, and this is hugely significant for he has never had the chance to feel his baby before. The baby–father dance may sway to a different tempo, but certainly begins the instant the two smell, see and touch one another.

Feeding
With her acute sense of smell and touch, your baby may follow her rooting reflex if you hold her to your breast and with a little guidance take your nipple in her mouth and begin to suck. In the womb she practised sucking and swallowing, and she intuitively knows what to do. Some parents have noted that within minutes or hours of birth if their baby is lying on their chest she wriggles towards the breast – even fathers have had this happen to them. Your body, stimulated by her presence and as a natural follow-up to birth, releases the love hormones that help you feel motherly and happy, and one of them, oxytocin, encourages colostrum to flow from your nipples.

Some babies turn very soon to the breast but most need to establish breathing before sucking. If you are both well and relaxed, you can try the first feed within minutes of giving birth. This may last for an hour or more and after this you and your baby may fall into a deep sleep for several hours. Unless she is very small she does not need the calories from food so soon, but connecting with you brings intimacy and trust that is as significant as food. If she is crying lustily, this is because she needs to expand her lungs: the calmer moments for sucking will come later.

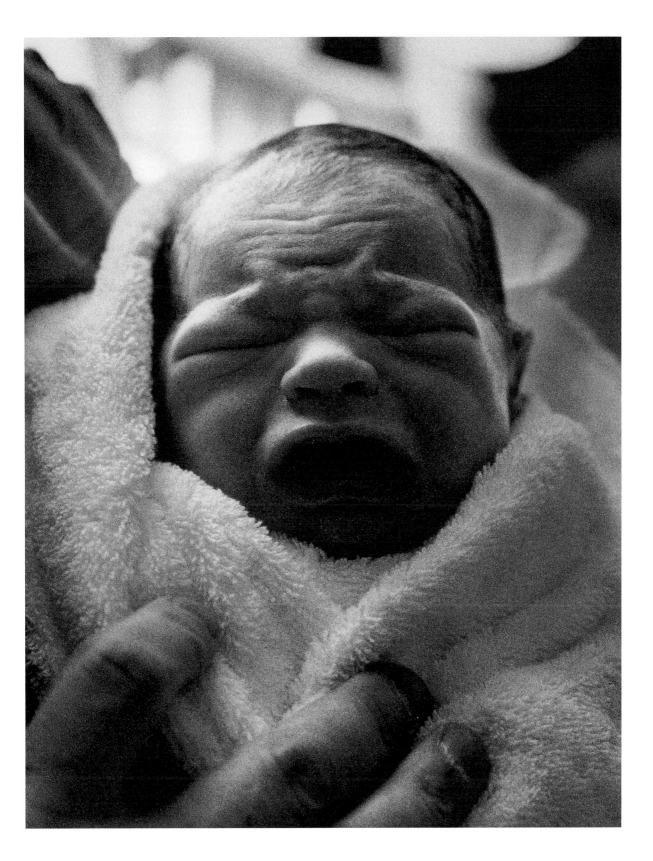

Movement and breathing for birth

The idea that a woman should lie on a bed for labour and birth is, thankfully, dying out. Today there is far more encouragement for you to move with the rhythm of labour, use your breath and harness the force of gravity for birth. This can reduce discomfort, lift your spirits and encourage progress.

Movement for the first stage

Sometimes you will naturally do what is best for you and your baby; at other times, your midwives will guide you. Letting your body move in response to the flow and intensity of your labour helps you to use your breath, takes your mind off pain and encourages the release of contraction-stimulating and pain-relieving hormones. You may intuitively begin a labour 'dance'. If the room is lit by a dim lamp and there is the soothing sound of music you might relax more easily.

Walking, dancing and standing

In a gentle dance, where you sway or rotate your hips, contractions are very effective and movement helps carry you through the pain. Walking has a similar effect. Try not to tense up during a contraction; instead move and ask your body to open. Alternatively, lean on your partner or a wall for support and rest with your feet flat and shoulder-width apart, gently bending your knees.

Kneeling

A good position if you are feeling contractions most strongly in your back or if your baby is in a back-to-back position (occipito posterior). There is a choice of postures: kneel upright with cushions under your knees and your hands on your hips, or hold on to a chair or a low table. Kneel on one knee and place the other foot to the side; gently rock back and forth. Kneel forwards with your hands and head resting on a beanbag or supported by a birth partner so you can block out distractions.

All fours

In this position you can move your lower back and hips and maximise the opening of your pelvis. Use cushions under your hands and knees and let your head hang forwards. Close your eyes and try to relax your shoulders, elbows, feet, back and pelvis, which releases tightness from your lower back, tummy and thighs. Don't arch your lower spine as it reduces the effect of gravity.

Squatting with support

Squatting is most useful in the second stage, but may help in the first stage if you are comfortable doing it. It gives a feeling of space and assists deep breathing. Place your feet flat on the floor with your weight on your heels, which will reduce tension in your thighs, knees and calf muscles. You'll need support from a partner behind, who can hold you and let you lean back. You might want to hold on in front. Don't hold a squat for too long, as it can be tiring.

Resting

You might rest between contractions or for a series of contractions to gather strength. Some women doze for a power-nap of 3–5 minutes. You could rest on all fours or kneel or sit with cushions under your buttocks or facing a beanbag or a chair with your feet flat on the ground so your legs are open and you can rest your arms and head. In the birth pool, water gives extra support in all these positions but the pool is best saved for use once you are in the active phase.

Lying down

If you are lying flat, gravity is not acting to help your baby down on to the cervix, back pain may feel more intense and your pelvis will have least room to open. Lying on your back may reduce the flow of blood to the placenta and make you feel faint, and you may also feel heavier. When you need to recline, rest your head and upper body on raised pillows, and lie on your side. An extra pillow

---

As a birth partner

- You may need to hook your arms under hers as she squats or let her wrap her arms around your neck.
- Keep yourself grounded with your feet widely spaced or sit so you can be balanced and conserve energy. If you are standing, then bend your knees a little to protect your back from strain. If you have a back problem sit on a bed while supporting her. Be patient: she may need to change positions frequently or stay in one for a long time.
- She might ask you to join her in the pool.
- At times it may be best for you to sit and hold her hand or give a gentle massage.
- If you get stiff or uncomfortable, a midwife can take over while you stretch or take a break.
- If you have practised different positions together, you may be able to give suggestions: but don't take it personally if they are ignored!

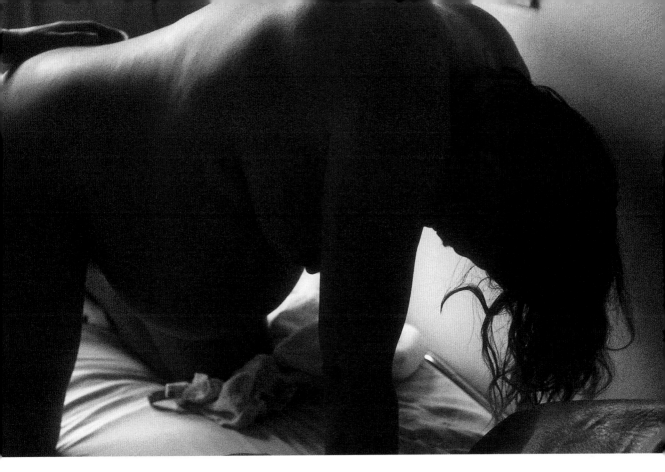

between your legs will keep your thighs apart. Sitting very nearly upright with lots of pillows to support your back will encourage your baby to descend.

Transition
During transition, kneeling or resting on all fours is a good position to use: you can rest your head, move your body through contractions and keep your bottom high. Keeping your bottom high helps to reduce downward pressure and also your urge to push before your cervix is fully dilated. If you find that you need to rest, lie on your side with your upper body raised.

Breathing for the first stage
Your breath is your most natural aid. It helps you focus on contractions and relax between them. It also takes your mind away from pain and energises your body – your muscles need oxygen to work. Deep breathing also nourishes your baby with oxygen.

You will have a strong instinct to breathe deeply, and if you have practised during pregnancy (e.g. with yoga, p.346) your learnt response will kick in. If you breathe well while contractions are mild, you will be in the swing of things and automatically keep your mind on your breath when they intensify. Singing or sighing with the out-breath is a powerful way to prolong the breath and relax.

If you become tired or panic or lose touch with the rhythm of your contractions, your birth partner and midwives can help you come back to yourself and breathe gently. Don't worry – you are never more than a few seconds from the next breath.

Breathing through your contractions
Begin to inhale as you feel the first tension: relax your shoulders and breathe slowly and deeply as if you are filling your abdomen with air. The slow inhalation keeps you steady and supple. Imagine the breath taking energy throughout your body, to your uterus, and to your baby. Your exhalation is a long, continuous release of tension. Think of sending the pain out of your body as the breath flows up your throat and past your lips. Let all the air out before you take the next inhalation, as if you're making as much space as possible for the next dose of energy.

Keep breathing deep breaths, one after another, until the end of the contraction. When your contractions get stronger you may need to pay more attention to your out-breath, which is likely to be short or too fast if you are tense and is easier to control than the in-breath.

Don't hold your breath. As a human your instinctive reaction to pain and fear is to tense up, bring your shoulders around your ears and hold your breath. As a woman, you are also designed to cope with the pain of labour, providing it is not too severe. Holding your breath or breathing shallowly and rapidly creates tension throughout your body and deprives you and your baby of oxygen, causes energy to drop and fear and pain to rise.

Rapid breathing is called hyperventilation and you will feel light headed, weak and afraid, with tingling lips; your muscles lose their power and twitch out of your control. If this happens you can counteract it by slowing your breathing: your birth partner and midwives will help.

Talking yourself through your breath

It can help to focus or meditate on a positive thought, like a mantra that you say to yourself with a rhythm that matches your breath. Use one phrase for each set of breaths through a contraction. Try declaring, 'I am fine, I am fine, I am fine', 'My body knows how to give birth to my baby, my body knows what to do', 'My baby is helping me, my baby knows what to do', 'Be soft, open gently, be soft, open gently.' Visualise with the breath or picture your baby travelling towards your vagina (p.128).

Another way of focusing is to count. On the inhalation say to yourself, 'I am breathing in one, I am breathing in two, I am breathing in three,' and as you exhale, 'I'm breathing out one, I'm breathing out two, I'm breathing out three,' etc. If this suits you, it may give a sense of rhythm and help you ride contractions.

Transition

Moving and making a noise are very powerful ways to keep breathing steadily: counting or talking silently to yourself may help you stay with the raft of your breath in the storm of transition. If you have the urge to push before your cervix has fully dilated, breathe lightly through the contraction with slow gentle pants – hoo, hoo, haa, haa. A partner or midwife may need to accompany you, as it is difficult to switch from deep breathing to panting.

As a birth partner
- You don't need to coach your partner constantly, for her breath and movement will be most effective when they are natural and instinctive.
- If she loses her rhythm, you can gently guide her back. Bring your face close to hers and say her name, and 'Breathe with me.' Then inhale fully and exhale long and slow, until she begins to mirror your rhythm. Establish eye contact if you can.
- Affirmations in time with her breathing can encourage her. Talk to her by name: 'You are doing fine, you are doing well . . . our baby is coming down gently, everything's going well . . . I'm with you, I'm here.'
- If you have practised visualisations use hypnotic language as you guide her.

Movement for giving birth

You will not know until the moment comes whether you will choose one of the following positions, or simply follow your body's natural inclinations. The most important thing is that you feel comfortable. If you have been pushing for a long time a different position may help conserve energy, free up spaces in your pelvic region and help your baby to rotate. In water you can float on your back, kneel or squat.

Supported squatting

Place your heels on the floor with your weight on your heels, as far apart and as far in front of you as is comfortable. Avoid resting on your toes or the balls of your feet because this will make your thigh muscles tighten and your vaginal muscles will follow, making the outlet smaller. You'll need support from a partner behind, to hold you and let you lean back and relax between contractions. You might want to hold on to someone else's hands as he or she kneels facing you. Another person may apply very gentle pressure to your knees to help you hold them open.

When your baby's head is visible you might want to lean forwards and see it. A slight lift from the person behind you will allow your sacrum to open fully. Your midwife will guide and protect your baby as he emerges and you can see him as soon as he is born. Then you can relax and sit on the floor with your baby on a towel between your legs as he takes his first breath.

The supported sitting position has many of the advantages of a squat, and may be easier if you are very tired or do not feel strong enough to balance on your legs. The alternative is to use a birthing stool designed to support your thighs with your vaginal outlet open.

Kneeling

Kneeling with your bottom raised well above your heels and your hands and head resting on a higher surface directs the pressure of your baby's descent towards the clitoris and away from your perineum. It can help slow down the birth and give your vagina and perineum a chance to stretch and open gradually. It is most commonly used in subsequent births when the birth force is stronger.

Reclining

Lying down may be comfortable if your contractions are strong and your baby is descending well, and you may find it easier to relax when your spine and shoulders are supported by the bed. But if you are lying flat the birth is likely to be more difficult and there will be more pressure on your perineum, so it's best to be propped up on a bank of pillows or with the head of the bed raised. With a cushion beneath your buttocks you could lean against your partner in a semi-upright sitting position, and at the moment of birth he may be able to lift you slightly to give maximum space for the head.

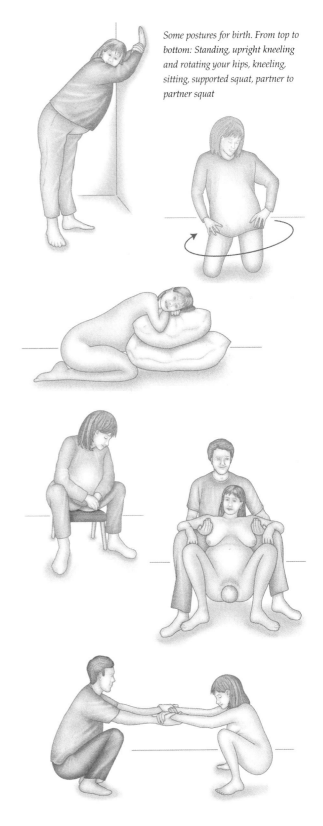

Some postures for birth. From top to bottom: Standing, upright kneeling and rotating your hips, kneeling, sitting, supported squat, partner to partner squat

As a birth partner

- If your partner is holding her breath for short periods while she bears down she may want to grip your hand or bite on a cloth, which you can hold for her. Help to bring her back to a calm state between contractions.
- If she is finding it hard to slow her breath talk to her gently: 'Breathe in, breathe out, breathe with me, breathe in, breathe out. . .' If this does not help, massage may be more effective.
- She may be so focused that she does not need active help and just wants you to be there quietly.
- Try not to mirror her breathing – if you can breathe regularly you'll preserve your own energy.
- As your baby emerges, your encouragement and praise will help your partner summon her power.

Breathing while giving birth

In the second stage your contractions change and your breathing will alter to follow your pushing urge. Instinctively, you will take in sharper breaths and push with a powerful downward movement, which incorporates the diaphragm and abdominal muscle. It is best to push for short bursts while you hold your breath briefly for 15–25 seconds. Then breathe out and take another breath and hold again and push a second time and perhaps once more in the same contraction. If you hold your breath and push throughout the contraction, you may reduce oxygen intake.

Between contractions your body will relax as your muscles release tension. You may feel the need to breathe rapidly to recover but there will be time to slow down your breath, relax and recoup energy. As you feel the next contraction mount, try to wait for it to build and breathe in calmly and deeply before you bear down.

Crowning

When your baby's head crowns and you feel a stinging sensation, try to focus away from the feeling between your legs and back to your breath and keep it even so you are energised for the next contraction. At this stage your uterus can usually push your baby out of its own accord or you may need to push gently. Concentrating on regular breathing can reduce fear and relax your vagina and perineum so they can open without tearing.

Birth

When your midwife sees the moment of birth approaching she will ask you to breathe in fast short breaths, or pant ('hoo, hoo, haa, haa'). This helps your contractions and stops you from pushing hard, causing your baby to emerge too quickly. As your baby's head is born you will probably give a loud moan or scream. After the head is born, the final contraction will give birth to your baby's body.

Accessing energy

In every city and village across the world, a woman's experience in labour is characterised by energy and pain. The two are intertwined: positive energy can significantly reduce pain, being in pain saps energy. Many methods for relieving pain also improve energy. You may feel happy to draw exclusively on your own birthing powers and a range of natural techniques, or you may want to combine these with medical pain relief. Your choice on the day will be coloured by the length and intensity of your labour, your stamina and pain threshold, and the support of your attendants. Your attitude will also play a part: some women accept pain as an essential part of the experience, others want to keep pain to a minimum from the outset.

The best choice for you

Everyone responds differently to labour and to techniques for improving energy. You may find that some give you a boost, others reduce the intensity of your sensations and there are some that alter the way your mind responds to pain. It is hard to know what you will do in advance because your priorities might shift on the day. The best thing is to know what's available and how you can prepare yourself, and then go with the flow of labour. Remember, there are no rules about how much or how little pain you need to feel. Every woman and every labour is unique.

You can do more than one thing at a time. For instance, you can be in water with dimmed lighting, move around freely and focus on your breath during a contraction, and you can visualise your baby moving down your pelvis while your midwife gives you a massage. One thing, like moving around, may help you do another, perhaps voicing your feelings or finding your courage. And your needs will alter – something that suits you at one stage may be inappropriate later on.

One contraction at a time: The concept of taking one contraction at a time is very powerful. It helps you to be confident rather than worrying about what is to come. Allow each contraction to take over, to surrender and breathe through it, moving your body and making sounds in whatever way is natural. Ride the wave as it rises to its peak, then relax as it recedes. Feel but don't fight the pain, and use the pain-free space between contractions to rest.

Create the the environment: Use the lighting and furniture, some music or some aromatherapy oils to make the room feel comfortable and safe – this helps your body release hormones that encourage birth, love and optimism. Your midwives and partner are there as the guardians of your birth to protect you and your baby.

Breathe and relax: Use your breath as your anchor in contractions and your raft as you rest and float between them (p.153).

Let yourself be touched: Touch can be healing and reassuring, whether you hold someone's hand, feel the stroke and pressure of massage or have your nipples stimulated. The touch you respond to will vary with the stage of labour.

Find your courage: Your birthing hormones are a potent source of courage, make you feel positive, reduce pain and encourage you to surrender to your birth energy. They'll flow better if you move and express yourself freely and if you're with people who believe in you and your natural power: it is wonderful to be surrounded by the love from people with positive energy.

Feel the feelings: Your feelings are part of the experience of labour and birth. Whatever they are, it is most helpful to acknowledge and express them so your supporting team can help in the best way. If you resist them, you are more likely to become tense and distanced, and this could hinder the birthing process. Try not to feel guilty if you feel something you did not expect. If you are calm, this helps you to surrender to labour's natural rhythm. If you are excited, this keeps you going. A feeling of despair can help you let go of the urge to make things better and result in relaxation, and is also a useful signal that you need support and encouragement.

If you feel afraid in the first stage it is good to let your supporters know so that they can reassure you, because fear may hinder your contractions if you become tense. Fear in the second stage, however, can help progress because the adrenalin release boosts the power your body needs to bear down.

Express yourself: Just as you feel your feelings, express them. If you are not inhibited your labouring rhythm will flow well. You may cry, laugh, curse, moan or roar. You may remain quiet and focused internally as if you are the only one in the room. At the moment of birth you will involuntarily utter the 'primal scream' that wells up from the centre of your being and is released with your breath.

Visualisation: If you visualise a beautiful outcome you may help it come about: your faith strengthens, you can avoid feeling overwhelmed and take yourself into a private world. Your energy is focused and your labour flows, even in the most intense moments.

Choose your charm: You may want to pray or chant, hold a charm or icon, look at a picture, bring a poem for your partner to read, or play a tape; any of these may increase your belief that you and your baby will be fine and the birth is not far away.

Move freely and use gravity: Moving freely helps labour progress and will help you to go with your contractions. It can help you express yourself and get in touch with your inherent birthing and mothering energy, lifting your confidence. Being upright is beneficial.

Rest in water: The soothing properties of water not only relax but can also help you to gather your energy, and may reduce your pain and help the uterine muscles to contract.

Eat and drink: You will probably get thirsty, so have lots of water to hand or a selection of sweet (but not fizzy) drinks. If you feel like eating, small snacks can boost your energy levels. This depends on hospital policy.

Keep warm: If you get cold, throw on some clothes or a blanket or turn up the heating: your body's muscles relax more easily when they are warm. Be careful not to get too hot, particularly if you are in water, as this will sap your energy and can be dangerous for your baby.

Homeopathy: Remedies may reduce pain and fear, increase energy, and stimulate hormone release, boosting strength and reducing the need for intervention (p.162).

Aromatherapy: Your sense of smell is at its height in labour. The scent of oils used during massage or in a burner could soothe or energise you (p.163).

Acupuncture: Acupuncture can increase energy, reduce tiredness and pain and enhance contractions. Not many women have a skilled practitioner for labour, but you may have a treatment earlier to realign your energy. You may be fortunate to meet a midwife practitioner in labour.

Feel free to make choices about pain relief: Part of being active and feeling confident is being involved in choice. Even if you have intended not to have medical relief, your level of pain may take you by surprise. Find out what's available so you can decide when the time comes, and let your partner know your preferences in case you need him to communicate on your behalf.

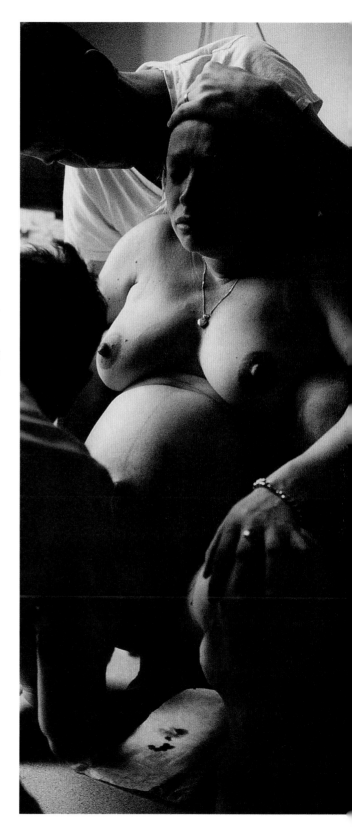

Medical pain relief

Pain relief has always been available, ranging from emotional support and herbal remedies to the sophisticated anaesthetics of today. With the advent of safer anaesthesia, women have more options, many of which barely interfere with a normal vaginal birth. It is easy now to incorporate natural methods with medical technology.

Using pain relief

Every form of pain relief has risks and benefits. As you choose the best course you will weigh these up with the needs of you and your baby. The general principle is to use the option that ensures you have a rewarding experience and your baby has a safe birth.

You may request pain relief, or your midwife or obstetrician may suggest it. It is always your choice and the birth team can advise but not insist if:

- Pain is distressing you.
- Pain is reducing the efficiency of your contractions.
- You have an uncontrollable urge to bear down and your cervix is not fully dilated.
- Your pain is so intense that you are inhibited from pushing in the second stage.
- You require assistance such as ventouse or forceps.
- Your baby needs to be delivered by caesarean.
- Progress is slow and you need a rest to relax your muscles and reduce resistance to your baby's descent.

You might let the pain relief wear off before giving birth. In early labour you will probably have time to talk over your options. When you are in strong labour if you have 'gone off to another planet' it will not be appropriate to have a long discussion. The key is to trust in your partner and the birth team so you know your needs are heard and you do not feel coerced. If birth is likely to occur soon your midwife may encourage you to wait, breathe and take contractions one at a time as you enter the intense stage that culminates in birth.

Most women are happy with the pain relief they receive, even if it was not planned, and are elated to give birth and finally meet their baby. Often relief makes way for renewed energy and a feeling of involvement. For others, there is a compromise between relinquishing control and being in pain. Some feel disappointed if the presiding memories of labour and birth are of pain and distress that could have been avoided, others are upset if they 'opt out' of experiencing all the sensations of birth.

If you have set your heart on a natural birth you may be disappointed or feel that you did not try hard enough, or that if your baby had been in a better position it would have been different. It helps to be open to the possibility that you may need pain relief and that your need may be much stronger than your birth plan. If you feel resentful it's important to talk about your feelings with your partner and with a midwife or doctor who was at your birth. If you tried pain relief that didn't have the desired effect or you experienced a complication, discussing it may be reassuring and help to clarify the medical circumstances.

TENS

'Transcutaneous Electrical Nerve Stimulation' works in a way that is similar to acupuncture. A TENS set contains sticky pads (usually two or four) each containing electrodes linked to a battery-powered unit. You place the pads over specific spots in your lower back and switch on the unit, which sends impulses to the nerve endings in your skin and helps to prevent pain signals travelling from your womb to your brain.

When it might be used: TENS is best used in early labour but cannot be used in water. Try it out before you go into labour. You can adjust the level of electrical impulse and maximise the stimulation during a contraction.

The benefits and risks:

- It operates from outside the body and does not affect the baby or alter the mother's chemical balance.
- TENS is available at some birth units and can be hired for use at home from a range of chemists and suppliers.
- It may be sufficient to control pain throughout labour and has the advantage of being very safe.

Gas and air (Entonox)

Entonox is a mixture of 50% nitrous oxide (an anaesthetic gas) and 50% oxygen (30% more than in normal air). The gas is inhaled from a mouthpiece linked to a cylinder on a mobile support so you can breathe whatever your position or if you are in the pool. Your midwife will help you to combine inhalation with effective breathing.

When it might be used: It is seldom used early in labour but may be helpful when contractions become more insistent. Rather than relieve pain completely it takes the edge off, or takes your mind away from the pain. Some women find it very helpful, others find it less useful than focusing on breathing.

The benefits and risks:

- Entonox may make you nauseous but has no long-term side effects for mother or baby.

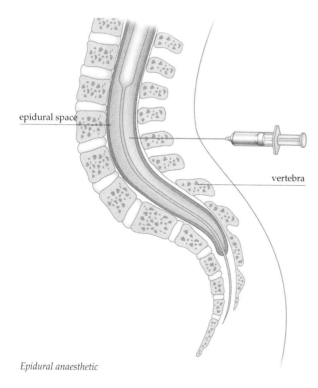

epidural space

vertebra

Epidural anaesthetic

block nerve fibres and an analgesic to reduce the pain sensation in the spinal cord. When an epidural is working effectively you will not feel pain, but can still feel touch and your baby being born.

A drip is inserted into a vein in your arm to provide extra fluid and keep your blood pressure stable. This is because a fall in blood pressure occurs when the anaesthetic relaxes the blood vessels in your legs and the blood flowing back to your heart is reduced. You will be asked to lie on your side while the skin on your back is numbed with local anaesthetic. Then a needle is placed into the epidural space in the lumbar vertebra of the spine and a fine polythene tube is inserted before the needle is withdrawn. The tube is taped to your back so the anaesthetic solution can be topped up painlessly when needed. Your wellbeing, blood pressure and your baby's heartbeat are monitored frequently.

When it might be used: Many hospitals prefer to use mobile epidurals, which do not block the nerves supplying the bladder, abdominal and leg muscles and therefore allow movement, upright positions and vaginal birth. You are less likely to need Syntocinon to stimulate uterine contractions, and it is less likely to distress your baby. It takes 20–30 minutes to become effective. The anaesthetic solution can be topped up every 1–2 hours.

A full epidural uses a more concentrated anaesthetic, which usually inhibits abdominal and leg muscle movement and sensation from the waist down, often affecting control of urine flow, in which case a catheter is used. You'll be on your side or sitting up in bed to maximise blood flow to the placenta. The anaesthetic remains effective for between 4 and 6 hours.

A mobile epidural is most easily administered in early labour, although it is available at any stage. The full epidural is the favoured choice when obstetric intervention such as a caesarean section or a forceps or ventouse is needed.

Many women use an epidural for a respite during labour, have a sleep and then allow it to wear off to summon maximum power to give birth. Alternatively, an epidural can be left to work during the birth, whether or not intervention is required. The epidural can be left in place for 36 hours for pain relief following an operative delivery.

The benefits:
- Pain is relieved without altering consciousness or inducing drowsiness.
- It may help rest or sleep and assist dilation of the cervix.
- It aids a doctor who needs to intervene (ventouse, forceps or caesarean) and allows the mother to remain awake and alert to greet the baby.
- It is much safer than general anaesthesia for both mother and baby.
- It reduces high blood pressure.

- You may enjoy feeling light-headed and even laughing (nitrous oxide is 'laughing gas') but it could take a few moments to regain control so you have less time to relax between contractions.
- The gas is most useful at the end of the first stage of labour. During the second stage using the mouthpiece may hinder you while you bear down and you may have to stop the inhalation to find your full power to push. It is usually a less powerful pain reliever than being in water or using an epidural.

Epidural anaesthesia

Epidural anaesthesia alters the conduction of pain impulses from the uterus, abdomen and vagina to the spinal cord by using a combination of a local anaesthetic to

---

Regional anaesthesia

Regional anaesthesia are special anaesthetic agents that can be injected alongside nerves to block the nerve fibres that conduct pain impulses travelling to your spinal cord and brain. These agents were originally derived from cocaine. As the agents improve they selectively block pain fibres without interfering with the motor fibres so muscle and bladder function are less affected. Regional anaesthesia may be administered as an epidural, a spinal block or a pudendal block.

- An epidural counteracts the fear of pain and may relax pelvic muscles sufficiently to encourage the baby's descent.
- It can transform a traumatic experience into one of pleasure and joy.

The risks:
- The incidence of side effects is low and epidurals have become progressively safer as the dose of local anaesthetic is reduced. Side effects are less likely to happen when skilled anaesthetists, obstetricians and midwives manage labour.
- Bladder numbness is less frequent with mobile epidurals but a catheter may be needed to pass urine.
- Occasionally one of the nerves leaving the spinal cord is not fully blocked and the contraction pain is still present in one area. This may be due to the anatomy of the nerve in the epidural space. If the pain is severe it may be overcome by re-siting the epidural.
- Contractions may become less powerful, particularly if you are lying flat. It may then be necessary to use oxytocin to stimulate contractions.
- With a full epidural your pelvic muscles may be paralysed and your baby's head is less likely to rotate forward so a forceps or ventouse delivery may be needed. If there is no sign of foetal distress it is preferable to wait until your baby's head rotates and descends through your pelvis before you begin to bear down. This will increase the likelihood of a normal birth.
- The epidural may lead to foetal distress and urgent delivery. Anaesthetic may transfer to your baby, causing a slowing of heartbeat. Your blood pressure may fall and a reduced flow of blood to the placenta may cause foetal distress. If you are repositioned on your side and the fluid from the drip is increased that is usually sufficient to bring the heartbeat back to normal. Foetal distress is much less common with a mobile epidural.
- After an epidural, back pain may occur at the site of the injection and persist for weeks or months. It may respond to osteopathic treatment.
- When the epidural is set up the needle may enter the dural space (a dural tap), which could cause a drop in cerebrospinal fluid pressure, leading to a headache that can persist for days. Lying flat in bed for 2–4 days until the fluid pressure readjusts is the treatment. You will be able to breastfeed if you lie on your side.
- Occasional serious and dangerous side effects have been reported following an epidural. Nerve damage from the needle to one of the lumbar nerve trunks is a very rare complication. With a high dose of anaesthetic the nerves that control chest movement and breathing and blood pressure may be affected and you may need artificial ventilation for a few hours until the nerves recover. Fortunately, with the low-dose mobile epidurals this is now very rare.

Spinal block

This may be used in place of an epidural for operative delivery. A very fine needle is inserted between the vertebrae in the same way as for an epidural but the cerebrospinal fluid is entered and a mixture of local anaesthetic and analgesic painkilling solution is injected before the needle is withdrawn.

When it might be used: In an emergency it is quicker to administer and some anaesthetists use it routinely for caesarean sections.

The benefits and risks:
- Anaesthesia is usually excellent and it is equivalent to a full epidural, giving pain relief for 4–6 hours.
- The main disadvantage is that top-ups are not possible and a low-pressure headache is more likely.

Pudendal block

The pudendal nerves supply sensation to the lower half of the vagina and they can be blocked for low forceps or ventouse deliveries or to repair an episiotomy. A needle is inserted via the vagina and the local anaesthetic is injected into the pudendal nerves by your obstetrician while you lie on your back.

When it might be used: A pudendal block does not affect the sensation from the uterus so it is only useful during the late second stage of labour.

The benefits and risks:
- This form of regional anaesthesia is useful if an anaesthetist is not immediately available to administer an epidural or spinal anaesthetic.
- The pain relief is less reliable than with an epidural anaesthetic.

Local anaesthesia

This is injected using a fine needle into the tissues around a tear so the repair is pain free. Most women feel the injection as a sharp sensation that lasts for 20–30 seconds before the area is numbed.

When it might be used: Often used before an episiotomy is performed or before a tear is stitched after the birth.

The benefits and risks:
- The benefit is a pain-free stitching.
- The risks are minimal and include bruising at the injection site.

General anaesthesia

This is now used much less often as regional techniques improve. During the anaesthetic, sleep is induced by administering an intravenous injection and it is maintained with muscle-relaxing injections. Analgesic gases are administered via a tube inserted into your airway to give pain relief. Following a general anaesthetic you will be able to hold your baby within 30 minutes to 1 hour of birth and you will be encouraged to breastfeed as soon as you wish.

The benefits and risks:
- The main advantages are speed in an acute emergency or if you are anxious and want to be asleep during a caesarean section.
- The major knock-on effect for a baby is that he may receive gases or drugs via the placenta and become sluggish and sleepy, particularly if he is premature. However, modern anaesthetic agents and a skilled anaesthetist ensure that the baby receives the minimum amount of anaesthetic agents and is unlikely to be severely affected.
- You may feel groggy and nauseous and may have a sore throat from the endotracheal tube.
- The most serious complication of general anaesthesia is inhaling vomit into the lungs, which has the potential to trigger severe aspiration pneumonia due to the acidity of gastric juices. This risk is minimised with the use of a fluid-tight endotracheal tube to prevent fluid from tracking into the lungs. It helps if the anaesthetic is given on an empty stomach; even so, an antacid is given to neutralise the acidity of the stomach contents before the operation.

Analgesics: pethidine and morphine

Pethidine is derived from morphine and is the most commonly used opiate for analgesia-pain relief. Other morphine derivatives include omnopon. Morphine itself may sometimes be used depending on hospital policy and the standpoint of obstetricians and midwives.

Pethidine is usually given by an intramuscular injection in labour but it may occasionally be administered via a slow intravenous infusion. The effect of pethidine wears off with time and the injection may be repeated after 3–4 hours.

When it might be used: It is preferable to administer a morphine injection when labour is clearly established and the birth is at least 3 hours away.

The benefits and risks:
- It does not usually slow down uterine contractions and it may actually help a dysfunctional labour.
- The degree of pain relief from pethidine varies from slight to very effective.
- This powerful narcotic can induce nausea and vomiting, drowsiness and lack of control, and a feeling of being anxious or spaced out and not really involved in the labour and birth.
- Many women feel they have missed out because they cannot remember the birth. It is impossible to predict, in advance, whether you will be susceptible to the side effects of pethidine but they may be more pronounced than the pain relief.
- It may also exert a significant effect on the baby, particularly if it is given within 3 hours of the birth. Premature infants with immature brains are very

susceptible to the drug and the effects increase the younger they are.
- The most serious effect is depression of breathing and the need for an intravenous injection of an antidote and resuscitation with oxygen administration at birth.
- It also affects the alertness of the baby who may be sleepy and unable to suck.

Fortunately these effects usually wear off within 24 hours except in cases of prematurity. There is some information to suggest that giving high doses in labour may increase a baby's susceptibility to drug addiction as a young adult.

Tranquillisers and sedatives

Hospitals and midwives vary in how much they administer sedatives and tranquillisers and it's worth discussing this during your antenatal preparation. These drugs are often used to enhance the effects of opiates and reduce the side effects of nausea and vomiting.

When they might be used: They may help you relax if you are very anxious or having false labour. It is important not to administer sedatives or tranquillisers close to birth or during premature labour because they cross the placenta into a baby's circulation and take 4 hours or longer to leave his system.

The benefits and risks:
- Women vary in their reaction: some enjoy the relief from anxiety whereas others do not like being out of control.
- A large dose may interfere with your hard work in preparing for breathing and you may be too sedated to breathe rhythmically and to enjoy the birth of your baby.
- If your baby is born when he is under the effect of a sedative he may have difficulty breathing and be drowsy and unresponsive, and this will be accentuated for days if birth is premature.

A history of pain relief

1847: chloroform was used for the first time during birth.

1950s: the first use of epidural anaesthesia.

1950s: suspicion that anaesthetics may have an adverse effect on the baby before and after birth.

1960s and 1970s: evidence that some anaesthetics increased the number of forceps and caesarean sections.

1970s: introduction of water as a means of pain relief.

1980s: natural childbirth proponents lauded labour without pain relief as 'the best way to give birth and to bond optimally with the baby'. This led to many mothers feeling disappointed and guilty if they needed help.

1990s: epidurals widely available.

2000s: safer low dose mobile epidurals became more commonplace.

Complementary therapies for labour and birth

Complementary therapies can work well when used alone or in combination with medical assistance. For some women they alter the need for intervention, significantly reduce pain and enhance the power of contractions. Many can augment slow progress in labour.

Homeopathy for labour and birth

Homeopathy can powerfully support you in labour, assisting progress, reducing physical tension, or lifting your spirits. The way you feel emotionally is very significant, and a remedy may help you overcome fear and relax into your natural rhythm. The way to choose a remedy is to look at your symptoms: what is the problem; what is your state of mind; are you hot or cold; are you in pain, and if so, where is it and how does it feel? More information about finding a remedy is provided on p.374.

Self-prescribing during labour can be difficult, and you will probably have to rely on your partner. It is extremely helpful for both of you to become acquainted with the different remedy pictures in advance of labour, so that you can make choices on the day.

When you have chosen a remedy, take one tablet in 200c potency. If it's suitable, it is likely to take effect within a matter of minutes. Only repeat the remedy if the same symptoms reappear. If there has been no change within 10 minutes, you may need a different remedy. A quick reassessment may bring a subtle but important point to your attention – for instance, if you want fresh air and feel hot, *Pulsatilla* is good, but if you want fresh air and feel cold, *Caulophyllum* is more suitable.

For the first and second stages

If your birth partner or midwife can pinpoint the reason for difficulties this will help enormously in finding the correct remedy: the cause could range from you being afraid or uncomfortably cold to contractions weakening or your baby being in an awkward position.

If labour is slow and you are fearful of being touched or worry that your baby will die, you feel better for fresh air and have intense contractions without dilation, use *Aconite*.

When contractions slow down or stop entirely due to exhaustion, they are short, irregular, feeble or feel sharp and you feel them low in the pelvis or groin; you are shaking and trembling, perhaps irritable too, and you feel chilly but want fresh air, use *Caulophyllum*. It is not advisable to take this remedy routinely in the last few weeks of pregnancy with the intention of promoting a faster labour. This is a question asked by many pregnant women.

If the rhythm of labour is interrupted, for example, on arrival in hospital, your symptoms are changeable and your contractions feeble, irregular or too short with no cervical dilation; you become clingy and apologetic, have a dry mouth but don't want to drink; feel hot and want fresh air and feel better for sympathy and encouragement, try *Pulsatilla*. This may have the effect of kick-starting your labour and you could then have a dose of *Caulophyllum* 10 minutes later.

For slow progress in the first stage (particularly if your baby is in posterior position), if you feel labour in your back with sharp pains radiating into the buttocks, relieved by pressure or massage; you are over-sensitive, obstinate, bossy and irritable and feel bloated, possibly flatulent, try *Kali Carb*.

When you are hypersensitive – to pain, light and/or noise – and become irritable and irrational; pain tears you apart; contractions are irregular and there's no dilation, you're frustrated and become rude; feel dizzy, faint and nauseous and need to urinate frequently; you look hot and want to strip off, try *Chamomilla*.

For transition or slow progress (anticipatory anxiety) when you doubt your ability to carry on, feel anxious, exhausted, dizzy and faint, and you tremble, you have pains in your joints and muscle; contractions hurt your back with pain that travels up so it seems your baby is ascending rather than descending; you don't want to be examined and feel better for moving around, try *Gelsemium*. This may work well when *Caulophyllum* seems appropriate but fails to act.

If you feel stuck, self-conscious and exposed, want to be left alone; have a headache; crave fresh air and feel thirsty for gulps of water, try *Natrum Mur*. This works well if you are holding back emotionally. After taking the remedy it may be like flicking a switch as labour begins to progress rhythmically.

If you are spaced out, and look terrified, like a glassy-eyed, scared rabbit; your breathing is irregular; your skin is clammy and sweaty and contractions slow right down or cease, try the remedy *Opium*.

If you want to be in control, and cannot be; your labour pains are in your back, exhausting and violent and give you the urge to pass a stool or urinate (although nothing comes); you are not making progress; you feel sick and may retch, with no result; become irritable and rude and feel worse from cool air, try *Nux Vomica*. This can help you let go of the desire to be in the driving seat.

If labour lacks rhythm and there are changeable emotional and physical symptoms and there may be failure to dilate; some contractions feel like electric shocks; you may be excitable, but worse from noise, cry out in agony or claim you cannot go on, become mistrusting and gloomy and feel cold, try *Cimicifuga*.

For fatigue and exhaustion *Kali Phos* is useful at any stage, particularly when there are very few other symptoms. It is best to give the remedy between contractions until energy picks up. This is useful for partners or attendants whose energy is also flagging.

For nausea and vomiting throughout labour, with hot-cold feelings, pale appearance with blue-black rings under your eyes, use *Ipecac*.

For the third stage
Homeopathic remedies can aid this last stage to progress smoothly and effectively, leaving you free to rest and concentrate on your baby. If you react well to a remedy it may be necessary to repeat the dose (200 potency). If there is no change, then try a different remedy as may be indicated here.

To boost contractions and energy, *Caulophyllum* is the number one remedy and *Arnica* may help after a long, tiring labour.

For encouragement and relief, when the placenta seems to be high, contractions seem ineffective, you have urine retention, your lower abdomen feels hot and tender and you are tearful, hot and bothered, try *Pulsatilla*. This is best taken as your baby is being born, or very soon after.

To calm emotions, if you have tearing pains but your contractions are absent or lazy, you are very afraid of going crazy, feel chilly and tremble, try *Cimicifuga*.

If you feel indifferent towards your baby, you have bearing down pains but the placenta is slow to descend, and you have pains in the cervix and rectum, try *Sepia*.

If Syntometrine has been given *Secale* helps to counter side effects and is indicated if you feel hot and distressed and have strong, constant contractions.

Aromatherapy and massage
All of these can be blended with a carrier oil, such as almond or grapeseed, and used for massage in a mix of 10 drops to 100 ml (3 fl oz) of oil. Or you could put 2 drops in water and heat gently in a burner or vapouriser or in a bowl placed on a radiator so the scent fills the room. If you need a strong boost you could sniff a few drops on a tissue.

Camomile: Reduces sensitivity and calms you.

Clary sage: Can be euphoric – good in times of stress and anxiety. It may act as a mild painkiller that relaxes and aids breathing, and can boost contractions.

Frankincense: This may help you to overcome fear and has the power to cut links with the past and quash memories of bad experiences. It also encourages slow and regular breathing.

Jasmine: Known as the king of oils, it is a uterine tonic and its relaxing properties help to relieve pain and cramps. It also helps to strengthen contractions.

Lavender: A good all-rounder that calms and stimulates circulation and healing. It is also a good painkiller and can reduce headaches and feelings of faintness. It is the oil most commonly used in labour.

Marjoram: Helps with breathing and acts as a mild sedative. It can help to lower blood pressure, has a warming effect and helps with pain relief, particularly for muscular pain, e.g. in the back. It has antispasmotic properties, aids blood flow and is a uterine tonic.

Neroli: Good for calming the nerves, it reduces anxiety and tension, is good for shock and is an antidepressant and antispasmodic.

Acupuncture in labour
While contractions are relatively mild in the passive first stage of labour, you or your birth partner can use finger pressure to decrease pain.

Locate the acupuncture point 'Bladder 60' midway between your Achilles tendon and your outer ankle bone. Press the point quite firmly with the thumb at the beginning of each contraction, and continue with this pressure until the contraction has finished. Repeat with each contraction for as long as it remains effective.

As labour progresses and contractions become stronger, the relief provided by finger pressure alone on Bladder 60 will diminish. Advanced acupuncture can alleviate labour pain considerably but can only be done by a fully trained acupuncturist.

When a helping hand is needed

Very few women give birth without help: being among a supportive team is the first ingredient and around the world traditional support includes the use of oils, herbs, massage and guidance with movement and breathing. These traditional methods are complemented by a range of obstetric practices that maximise safety. Basic intervention aids the natural process of labour and birth and often increases a woman's sense of involvement. Where intervention is greater it may interfere with 'natural' birth but be welcomed and even enhance the birth experience. Although some women feel out of control or disappointed, the majority of women needing maximum intervention, for example a caesarean, are extremely grateful and relieved that the birth has ended safely.

Choices and hospital policies

In an ideal birthing situation the midwifery and obstetric team will be sensitive to your needs, your emotional response to pain, your fitness and stamina levels and your baby's safety. Different hospitals, midwives and obstetricians have different opinions about when labour needs a helping hand, and this is reflected in their records showing the number and type of interventions performed each year. For instance, measurement of 'slow progress' varies widely. For one woman, 40 minutes of pushing in the second stage may feel too long, while for another, 2 hours may be acceptable: a midwife may aid progress in the first case and in the second case offer encouragement and support without intervention.

Your obstetrician or midwife may believe that medical assistance could help your labour and reduce stress. It may be that you want intervention even though they have not suggested it. As you discuss the options, perhaps with the involvement of your partner, the strongest deciding factors will be your feelings and comfort and your baby's safety. Sometimes a midwife advises against intervention if her experience shows that the difficulty will resolve soon and easily. If she recommends intervention and you refuse, then she cannot insist, even if you or your baby is in danger. It is always your choice.

Except in an acute emergency you will have the time to delay your decision, see how labour progresses and then discuss your options once more. Your obstetrician will be involved in every major decision because midwives have a statutory obligation to report any labour that has become significantly abnormal.

If you need assistance

If labour is not progressing optimally, and providing the situation is not urgent, you may have several options. You might wish to try non-medical methods first. The following situations where intervention will be advised are listed briefly. Each is explored more in the A–Z Health Guide.

If labour needs to be activated: 'induction'

Of the many indications to induce (p.497) the most common is going beyond your due date. If there is no urgent need for your baby to be born, you could try helping labour to start by making love, nipple stimulation, homeopathy or herbal remedies, each of which may take a few hours or days to have effect. If the need is semi-urgent, labour may be induced using prostaglandin gel placed in the vagina to stimulate contractions. In urgent cases it may be more effective to have your waters broken or receive the hormone oxytocin to encourage contractions. The same hormone is used if labour has begun but progress is slow.

If your energy levels are dropping

As in pre-labour, eating nutritious snacks, moving your body and taking periods of rest can help boost or stabilise energy, as can homeopathy, aromatherapy and visualisation. A comforting environment and loving encouragement may also help. You may choose an epidural to allow you to rest (p.159) or an infusion of fluid and electrolytes to correct dehydration and boost your energy. Oxytocin may also be used to boost contractions.

If progress is slow

Ideally, your delivery team will follow broad guidelines but there are no rigid time limits for the progression of labour. If your birth team is concerned about your baby's safety or think you are at risk of becoming too tired they may help to advance the process, or if you feel exhausted or the pain is too great you may want assistance to get you through. Movement and breathing techniques can help focus your energy (p.152) and using homeopathy or essential oils for massage or inhalation can rekindle progress (p.162).

Medical assistance (p.158) includes breaking the waters (ARM) to encourage the cervix to reach full dilation, intravenous infusion of oxytocin (Syntocinon) to enhance contractions or using ventouse or forceps or even a

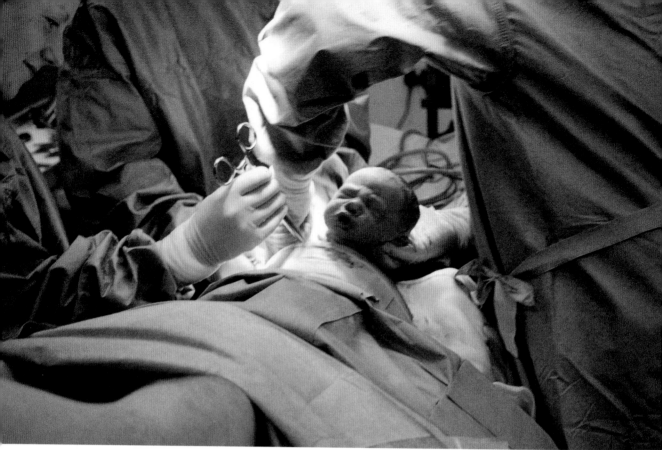

The midwife is greeting this baby as his head is born during a caesarean section operation.

caesarean to aid delivery (pp.496 and 419). In the third stage, an injection of oxytocin possibly combined with ergometrine will help quicken the birth of the placenta or it may have to be removed manually if it is retained.

If your vaginal entrance needs an episiotomy

If your baby's head has crowned but birth is delayed, your midwife will help your vaginal entrance and perineum to widen by using perineal massage or altering your posture. If there is undue delay, foetal distress or if it is excessively painful or if your tissues cannot stretch sufficiently to accommodate your baby's head, you may require an episiotomy (p.494), or cut, which enlarges the vaginal entrance. After a local anaesthetic is injected, the cutting process is painless. It allows room for the head to leave the vagina with the next contraction, or for your midwife to give further assistance. The cut is stitched under local anaesthetic and usually heals well.

If you bleed excessively

Before birth, heavy bleeding could be an emergency needing immediate assessment and delivery by caesarean section. Early bleeding may indicate a low lying placenta (p.524) or placental abruption (p.525) where there is

separation from the uterine wall: both need urgent medical assessment. After birth excessive bleeding will be assessed and if it stems from retained placental fragments (p.407) these may be removed by your obstetrician.

If your baby needs assistance

The object of care antenatally and during labour is to monitor your baby's wellbeing and detect problems as early as possible so long-term effects can be minimised or prevented. If a problem is detected with your baby, you will naturally become concerned: these are sensitive times for any parent. In most cases everything goes smoothly and a baby thought to be at risk is born healthy. In high-risk pregnancies where difficulties during labour or following birth can be predicted, the medical team will do all they can to ensure safety. Situations where intervention will be advised are listed briefly here. If you would like to know more, each is explored in the A–Z Health Guide.

Assistance before labour

Surveillance in pregnancy allows your medical team to assess your baby's health and detect events that may give cause for concern during labour. For instance, babies who have intrauterine growth restriction (IUGR) or are premature may be monitored more closely because small babies are more susceptible to foetal distress (see below). When the environment in the uterus is less safe than the outside world (for example, severe IUGR) there may be persuasive reasons for intervention to induce labour early or if the baby does not have sufficient energy reserves, to deliver by caesarean section. An operative delivery may also be advised if a baby is positioned awkwardly, most commonly in the breech position. Emergencies, such as bleeding (p.406) or placental abruption, need immediate attention – fortunately these are rare.

Assistance in labour

It is helpful to remember that the progress of labour and birth belongs to and is influenced by both you and your baby. Slow progress, for instance, may be due to your physiology and power of your uterine contractions, your state of mind or energy levels and the size and shape of your pelvis. It may also be significantly influenced by the size and shape of your baby's head and the position that your baby takes in the womb. Intervention to speed up labour also speeds up the birth.

If your baby shows signs of distress in labour – foetal distress: While in the womb, your baby derives oxygen from your blood. The flow reduces during contractions but your baby can cope with this, deriving energy from glycogen sugar reserves stored in the liver. During and after birth he is able to use this energy to survive unharmed without oxygen for up to 10 minutes.

There are a number of reasons for a baby's heart rate to become abnormal (p.125) and one may indicate that he is not receiving enough oxygen. This may be referred to by

your medical team as foetal distress or asphyxia (p.472). Because there is a risk of cerebral damage when oxygen deprivation is prolonged, particularly if a baby is small and therefore has low sugar reserves, the obstetrician may be keen to expedite the birth.

Another sign of possible distress is greenish meconium staining of the amniotic fluid, apparent when the waters break, which indicates that your baby has passed his first bowel motion. This sign is not significant unless the baby's heart rate is abnormal. In the majority of cases where there are signs of distress in labour and the birth team intervenes, the baby is born safely and has no long-term difficulties. Close monitoring during labour in high-risk pregnancies (p.483) enables midwives and obstetricians to intervene at the most appropriate time.

If your baby needs help to be born – forceps and ventouse extraction: Most women would prefer not to have forceps (p.496) either for themselves or for their baby's comfort, but sometimes a baby may become stuck or the heart rate shows that he needs to be delivered as quickly as possible. The forceps, like a wide pair of spoons, are eased around the baby's head and used to exert a pulling force when the mother pushes. An episiotomy is often performed. The use of a ventouse suction cup applied to the baby's head is becoming more popular because it tends to be gentler for the mother and is equally efficient at assisting birth, and may not require an episiotomy.

Problems with the umbilical cord: If the umbilical cord is wound very tightly around the neck it can cause foetal distress, which will usually be detected through heartbeat monitoring. If this unusual event causes a reduction in oxygen flow, an urgent delivery is essential.

When it lies between the baby's head and the cervix, cord prolapse (p.550) can occur very rarely. When the membranes rupture there is a risk that the cord may prolapse and become compressed as the baby's head enters the pelvis, thus restricting blood and oxygen flow. A prolapsed cord can be detected by a vaginal examination and requires urgent delivery by caesarean section.

If a caesarean section is needed: Caesarean section is the most serious intervention at birth (p.419). Some women elect to have a caesarean section, perhaps following a previously traumatic birth experience, and some know in advance that it is the safest option, for example if they are carrying twins or a breech baby. Unplanned delivery by emergency caesarean section is usually prompted by concerns about a baby's wellbeing, and can be positive because the baby is safe but the procedure may also be stressful. Many parents are relieved that everything has worked out well but may need continued physical and emotional support in the weeks and months that follow.

Is an episiotomy offered as a matter of course?
There was a trend to offer an episiotomy in all first births, and in some countries it became the most commonly performed operation on women. But because research studies have failed to show that there is any advantage in giving an episiotomy where there is no medical indication (p.494), they are no longer given as routine practice in the UK where the incidence is around 20% of births. It is a good idea to check your own hospital's figures and talk to your midwife and obstetrician about their preferences, as rates do vary.

If you want an episiotomy, you may be able to request it. If you want to reduce the chance that you'll need one, antenatal preparations and an upright position for birth can help, but cannot guarantee prevention. An episiotomy can be useful if your baby must be born soon because of foetal distress, if your vaginal opening is too small or if your baby needs to be assisted with forceps. If a ventouse is used, an episiotomy is not always necessary.

Assistance after birth

The majority of babies adapt immediately to their new environment at birth but some do need help. The most common problems at birth are caused by minor breathing difficulties and can be resolved within moments. During labour if there is concern that your baby is in distress the birth team will prepare to give close attention at birth. Baby resuscitation equipment is routinely at hand in all hospital and home births.

In the rare case of a baby needing emergency care, the midwives, obstetricians and paediatricians will give immediate assistance. A very small percentage of babies have problems that require intensive care. Maternity units that lack facilities have links with larger hospitals with special care baby units (SCBU) (p.536) and can arrange for a rapid transfer for mother and baby by ambulance.

If your baby has breathing difficulties: It is remarkable that so few babies have difficulty making the incredible effort needed to take their first breath. Of the small percentage who do, most establish breathing after a warming rub or once their mouth and nose have been cleared of mucus and birth fluids.

If your baby needs help, suction is first applied to the nose and mouth. If this is insufficient, the umbilical cord may be cut before it has stopped pulsating so he can be carried to the resuscitation equipment in the birth room and be given oxygen via a face mask or through a tube passed into the larynx and trachea. As soon as breathing begins, he will be handed back to you. If the problem continues, he may require admission to a SCBU for respirator support until the problem resolves.

Problems with the circulation: Foetal distress may be associated with a drop in blood pressure and reduced blood flow in a baby's circulation. When oxygen is given during resuscitation it is often enough to correct the problem but occasionally a baby may need intravenous fluids. Sometimes circulation problems are associated with heart or lung disorders and these need to be treated on a SCBU. Usually a congenital heart or lung problem is detected by scanning in pregnancy.

Birth injuries: With modern obstetric care, injuries to babies at birth are extremely rare – where they do occur the baby usually recovers because of the human body's natural healing capacity. Most common is bruising, particularly among premature babies or those delivered with forceps or ventouse. Occasionally a large bruise with a raised lump on the head called a cephal-haematoma results from pressure during birth, and this usually disappears in a few days. Injuries to the shoulders, neck or collarbones are rare and may occur with shoulder dystocia (p.502) when a baby is big and there is difficulty delivering the shoulders. The risk of all birth injuries is reduced with good midwifery and obstetric care and the use of an upright or squatting position.

Small baby with intrauterine growth restriction (IUGR): A small for dates baby with IUGR (p.488) usually has no breathing problems unless it has been necessary to deliver very early, when there is a combination of IUGR and prematurity. The main problems are low levels of blood sugar (hypoglycaemia) and low body temperature. Your baby can stay warm if he is on your body and hypoglycaemia can be usually prevented by early feeding.

Small baby born early – prematurity: If your baby is born before 36 completed weeks, he is said to be premature or pre-term (p.526) and because he is still maturing there is a chance that some of his organs or bodily systems may not function optimally. Most commonly these are the lungs, liver and immune and nervous systems. All babies born early require special attention and some are more resilient and self-sufficient than others. It is usual practice for a woman who goes into premature labour to be cared for in a hospital where there is a SCBU. Because of advanced neonatal care, babies born early have increasingly good chances of survival without long-term health problems, though difficulties are more likely the earlier a baby is born. A very young baby often needs high-tech treatment in an incubator but can benefit from skin-to-skin contact and his parents' presence.

Moving on

Although most women are relieved that their baby has arrived safely, it is equally OK to feel upset if you need intervention. The issue during labour is to get on with it, be pragmatic and deliver your baby safely. In the days following birth when hormones change dramatically and weepiness is common, feelings about intervention, choices and consequences may be very strong. You may feel guilt or wonder if you could have done something 'better' and it might help to talk over the birth with your midwifery and obstetric team who have detailed notes of your progress. If necessary, you will be able to talk further with any obstetrician or paediatrician who was involved.

If you have negative feelings after the birth acknowledging them, voicing them and doing what you can to work through them is a powerful way to begin the next part of your journey and welcome your baby with an open heart. Often a father may require more clarification or reassurance than the mother, and coming to terms with the way birth unfolded may be a vital part of the transition into family life. In the days following birth your new family comes together and you will become increasingly absorbed in your baby. If he has arrived safe and well this may be thanks to the intervention you received.

The first 24 hours

The first day is often a romantic time when mother, father and baby meet for the first time and rest after the marathon of birth. It involves contact and exquisite sensations. For many parents, and certainly for many babies, the first day has a dream-like quality. The pregnancy has disappeared, and there is instead an amazing baby gazing at the wide world, and the family welcome begins. Your baby brings wonder to the moment, and there may be a few thoughts of the future.

Mum

The first 24 hours, and probably beyond, are primarily for resting, recuperating and meeting your baby. If you are in hospital, the midwives will be on call should you need anything, and you may spend most of the day in bed. At home your family and other supporters will make you comfortable.

Nature does play the right cards: labour is hard and forces you to rest and then focus your energy on your baby and on yourself. If you feel exhilarated and energetic, you will be off to a great start, but it is still worth taking things slowly. An adrenalin burst may drive you at first but cannot sustain you: you need rest and sleep and nutritious food for this.

If you are exhausted or upset following labour you may feel stunned for the first day but your hormones will draw you to your baby. You and your baby may both sleep for hours and have eye-to-eye contact from time to time. It is important for you to begin the process of recovery and use the support of your partner or the birth team. As soon as you feel able they will pass your baby to you and support you as you cuddle her, or they will help you both with some early attempts at feeding. She may either be in your bed or beside it where you can watch her peaceful sleeping face.

The hormones that flooded your body during pregnancy and reached their peak during labour and birth take time to recede. The oestrogen and progesterone will be gone in a few days but you will still feel the effects of the 'love hormones' that make you feel happy and loving, because every time your baby sucks from your breast they flood your body. The hormones help you tune in and initiate or augment a powerful bonding process. At the same time, the oestrogen and progresterone encourage your breasts to produce colostrum and your uterus to contract to its pre-pregnant size.

There is no right or best way to be with your baby after birth. The partnership between you and your baby may be like gunpowder, igniting a spark immediately you see one another. Or it may be more like a charcoal fire, taking concentration and time to bring to flame. If you take it more slowly, it might be compared to a fire of dense coal, whose ignition needs lots of kindling, but nevertheless brings sustained warmth and light.

How much pain will I feel after the birth? I believe it can be quite bad.
Discomfort after birth is almost universal, although it is often very mild and being with your baby may take your attention away from it. You'll feel afterpains as your uterus contracts, most strongly while you breastfeed, which become lighter within a few days. You may be able to breathe through these or ease them with homeopathy. Painkillers are occasionally needed, more often after second or subsequent births.

Your vagina may feel stretched and bruised, and tender for a few days if you had stitches, with a stinging feeling when you pass urine. This can be eased by pouring lukewarm water on the area as you urinate and bathing in a warm bath; perhaps scented with the healing herbs comfrey, calendula or marigold. You may have a sore throat from shouting and stiff muscles as if you have run a marathon.

Pelvic pain (p.519) may arise if the bones and joints were under strain during birth. Ligaments are still soft so the joints are still wide but they will close over the next weeks. Rest, along with gentle postnatal exercises and yoga and osteopathy, can help. If you have had a caesarean or vaginal stitches the area will feel very tender.

Dad

Many fathers walk around in a daze after labour. Usually the arrival of a new baby gives incredible feelings of pride and joy, though this may be tinged with disbelief and shock if intervention was needed. Fathers who go home soon after the birth have time to come to terms with their experience of the miracle of birth and their first encounter with their baby, but they often also feel sad to leave their new family.

In some hospitals the father is welcome to stay as long as he wants. This gives wonderful 'bed-in' time. Often a father helps out by making tea, preparing food and changing nappies.

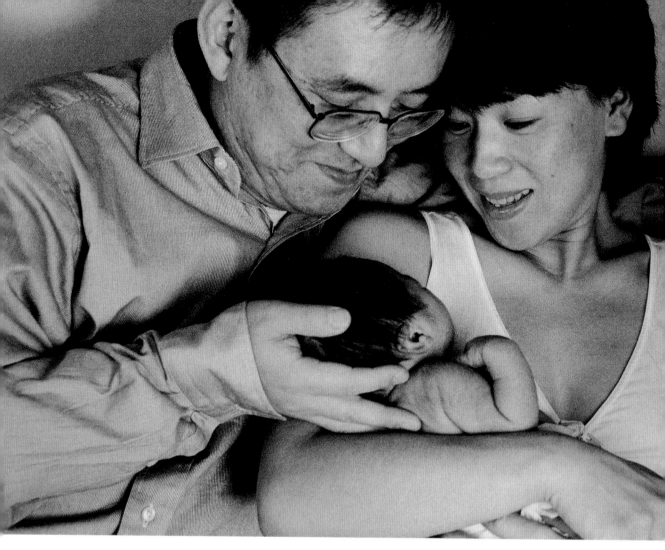

Your baby

The two most important things for your baby in the first 24 hours are a loving welcome and her health. At birth, the midwives will check her (p.139) and she'll then be given a more thorough paediatric examination. She is all yours and will relish being with you.

It takes time for your baby to 'land'. Initially she may be calm when there is comfort, company and human touch. She will probably sleep for most of the first 24 hours, but not at a single stretch. Each time she wakes she will look for your embrace, and may root for your breast and ask to suck. She will also cry – sometimes for comfort, sometimes for food and sometimes just to have a good bawl.

Some babies don't cry much until day 2 or 3 when there's the new experience of digestion. Some cry with gusto from birth, announcing their presence and their need for comfort and food. However your baby responds to her great transition, let her snuggle into you and take the chance to let her sleep peacefully on your chest – a great privilege that comforts you both and passes all too soon.

Massage is a lovely way to smooth out tension for both of you, and can be effective from the earliest days as your baby lies on your chest and you stroke your hands over her back. If you want to explore the potential of baby massage further turn to p.365.

Feeding your baby

Early in the first 24 hours, and perhaps as soon as 10 minutes after birth, you will bring your baby to your breast (unless you have chosen to bottle feed). She follows her powerful sense of smell and her reflex to root and suck and will help start the process even if you are unsure just now how to hold her.

Feeding is the most intimate contact you will have with one another, and as your baby sucks, your body releases hormones that will produce milk and will also help you bond and find peace after labour. Your midwives will help you both find a good position and it's good to feed her frequently: sucking can release tension in her head and neck and helps you to relax.

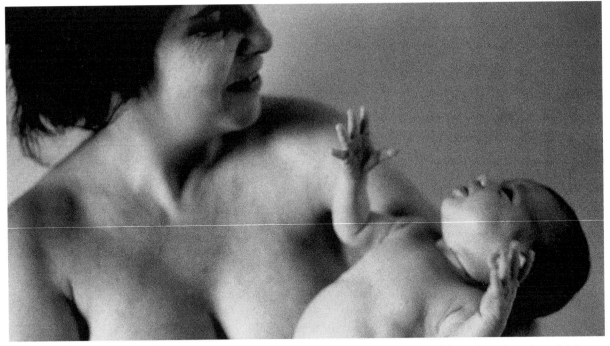

When a baby is startled, the Moro or 'startle' reflex causes her to throw her arms wide. It may be an evolutionary left-over from primate days: a baby's instinct to cling to her mother when there was a sign of danger (see box opposite).

Your baby's reflexes

At birth a lot of activity is reflexive and follows a theme of survival and learning. Many – like the unstoppable urge to kick, wriggle and swipe – are essential for building muscle strength and neural links that lead to bodily control. Some reflexes don't serve much obvious purpose but were probably useful a few rungs down on the evolutionary ladder. Reflexes that are apparent after birth are already evident in the womb: for instance, babies as young as 8 weeks gestational age have been observed through ultrasound throwing their legs and arms wide in the Moro reflex (above and opposite).

Being on the receiving end of your baby's reflex actions – as she grips your fingers, sucks at your breast, or her limbs splay out like a star fish's when you turn on the radio at maximum volume – is one of the many endearing sides of early parenthood. Your baby's reflexes also give valuable medical information: any variations from the norm can be assessed and approached as part of her general health care.

Over time most reflexes disappear because muscular strength and conscious control improve and your baby's brain develops so that it can over-ride and 'unlearn' unconscious reactions. Some, like blinking in response to a sudden bright light or an approaching object, will persist, and still have their uses in adulthood. There are a number of reflexes that won't become apparent until your baby is older; for instance, the righting reflex that helps her locate her centre of gravity as she sits, or her instinctive use of her hands to break her fall as she topples.

Family and friends

As the generation gap is bridged and your baby is lovingly held by her granny or grandpa, aunt or uncle there may be a feeling of completion and family bonding. Your brothers and sisters and your friends will also want to welcome your baby to the world, and each person will bring their own particular energy into the room. It can feel incredibly special when your sister, brother or close friend holds your baby for the first time and you see a lifelong friendship begin. Becoming a grandparent, even for the second, third or tenth time, can be an uplifting event bringing joy and much celebration.

As you beam at your visitors and agree that your baby is indeed beautiful you will be feeling proud and also exhausted and sore. You may need to specify some time after birth when you can be alone with your baby and partner, and create visiting schedules so that you have time to rest and indulge in motherhood without distraction. Visiting hours are great if you want lots of rest. If you are embarrassed to feed in public it's particularly important that you create space for both you and your baby: right now security and comfort are the most important things for both of you.

Newborn reflexes

Babinski's reflex: If you stroke the sole of your baby's foot from heel to toe, her big toe bends backwards and the others spread out. This will disappear when she starts to walk.

Breathing reflex: As soon as she feels cold air on her skin, your baby automatically begins to breathe. Her breathing rhythm may not become completely regular for around 6 months, but it is always an involuntary activity that she doesn't need to think about.

Diving reflex: Your baby has a strong instinct to survive: the diving reflex makes her throat close as soon as there is a sensation of water. This is a natural response that means that water birth does not present a risk, and also allows your baby to swim. There is no scientific confirmation of how long this reflex lasts: it may disappear by 6 months but if activated could last longer.

Grasp reflex: If you place your finger or a small object against the palm of your baby's hand, her fingers will curl tightly around it. This reflex is an evolutionary leftover: in primates the baby needs to cling to its mother. It is not redundant for your baby: it increases the information she can glean about objects. Between 2 and 4 months she begins to grasp deliberately – by 9 months she can over-ride the reflex and grip and release objects at will.

Moro or startle reflex: If a loud noise, a sudden bright light or a sudden touch startles your baby, or support of her head is dropped suddenly, she will throw her arms and legs wide, extend her hands and fingers and open her eyes wide. This is a response to danger and will be less pronounced after 3 months, disappearing completely by 8 months. It may be an echo of the primate's urge to cling to its mother's body for security. The startle reflex is generally more pronounced in boys.

Plantar and palmar reflexes: If you put gentle pressure on the base of your baby's toes they will bend inwards – a kiss here may make them curl around your lips. The same happens if you put pressure at the base of your baby's fingers (palmar – of the hand). A practical application of this reflex is your baby's response to open her mouth if the palm of her hand is gently squeezed. If she is reluctant to suck on your nipple or a teat, you could try this gentle encouragement when she's awake and calm.

Rooting reflex: If you stroke your baby's cheek with your finger or breast, she will turn towards the sensation. When she is held to your breast she'll turn towards your nipple and her source of food and comfort. This reflex commonly disappears by 4 months, although she may still turn towards contact in sleep.

Stepping or walking reflex: When your newborn baby is held upright with her feet touching a hard surface she will make stepping movements with precision and determination, feet flat and knees raised high for up to four or five steps. Her ability to do this will fade after a few weeks as she gains more voluntary control over her legs. Its function is unclear – would it have helped a primate wriggle up its mother's body? Or might it, as some neuro-scientists suggest, help the brain form pathways associated with walking that can be built on many months later?

Sucking and swallowing reflexes: Your baby practises sucking in the womb and has a powerful grip and sucking motion. She may take time to learn about the shape of your nipple and the strength with which she needs to suck to obtain milk. She may splutter as she gets used to regulating breathing with swallowing.

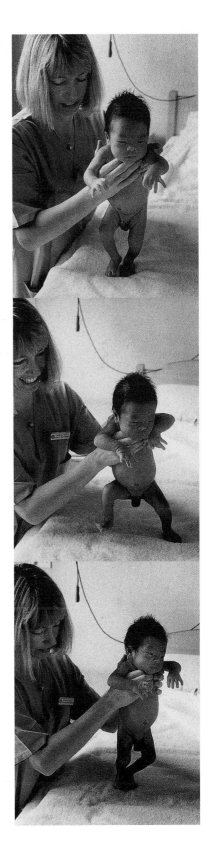

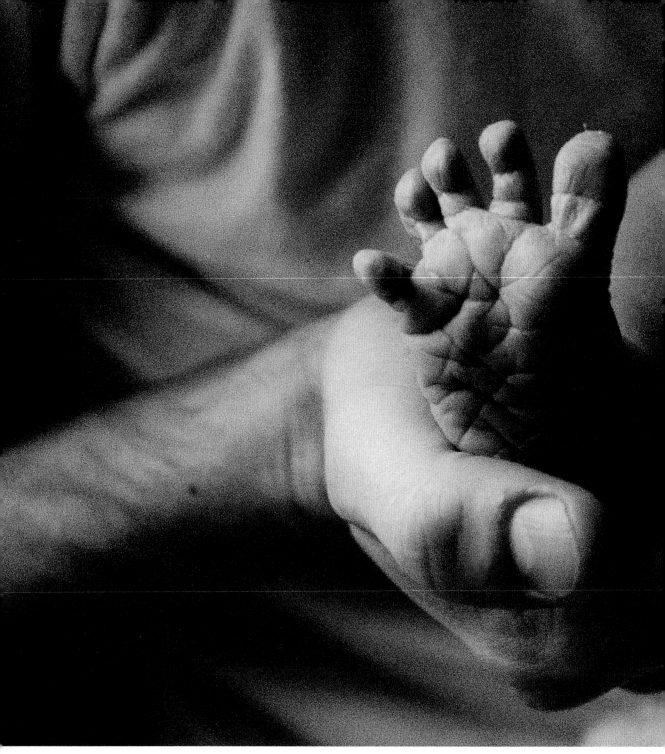

part iii **your baby and family**

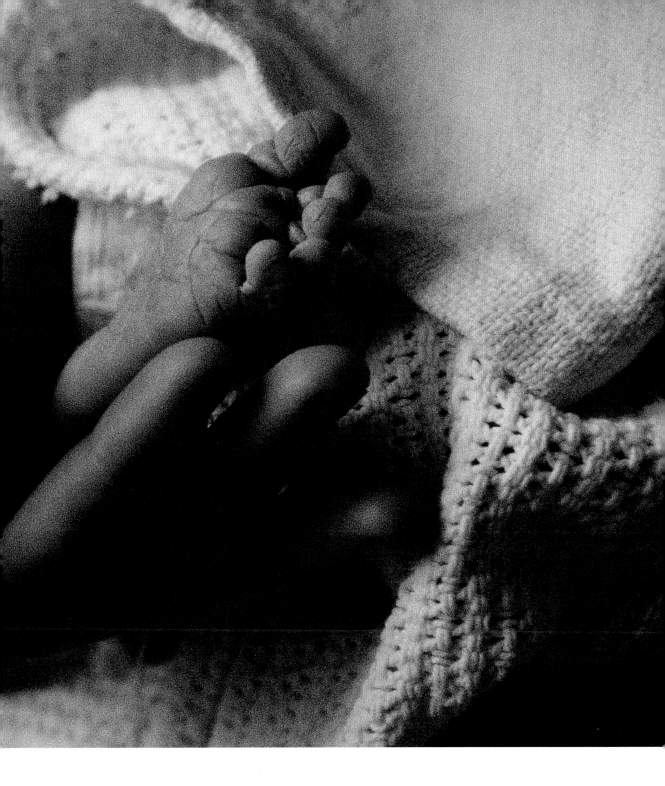

Hello baby, hello family

Your baby begins life outside the womb with no control of his head, and no understanding that he is separate from others. You begin parenting with curiosity and wonder, and perhaps some anxiety. You both have hormones and reflexes that help you tune into one another. With your protection and loving guidance, your baby learns and adapts perfectly. And with his encouragement, you will form one of your most precious friendships as you settle into life as a parent, and as a family.

Hello baby

As you touch and feel touched, smell one another, listen to one another's voices and join in the wordless, curious exploration that comes with eye contact, you and your baby experience a sensory explosion. As the days pass you come to know one another more and extend your mutual greeting, picking up on one another's moods and rhythms. You may be physically further apart than you were in pregnancy, but because communication between you is natural and direct, you are drawn back together.

Your baby is ready to communicate and has an amazing capacity for learning. He recognises your voice at birth and knows your smell just a few days later. He engages you with his beautiful eyes, endearing stretches and newborn body to make sure you'll be there as his teacher and supporter. He flirts similarly with his daddy, and many others who are pulled into his tempting aura of wonder and intimacy. Even in the hours and days after birth, he has strong body language, and subtle movements show his feelings: he may be calm, letting his arms and legs hang loose, excited and fidgety or scared and tense. As he fixes his stare on your face and moves his lips and his face as he mirrors you, he plays a central role in the conversation between you.

The baby–parent dance

The two-way relationship never stops. In pregnancy you respond to one another's movements and energies, and from birth you mirror one another: moments of eye contact in a still and quiet embrace bring you close and your moods and energies often merge or reflect one another. As he cries for food, your instinct is to offer him milk; as he stretches his tongue and lips, you unconsciously move your mouth in imitation: you answer his request for comfort with a cuddle; he answers your desire for laughter with an amusing grimace and quells your anxiety with his calm presence and beautiful face.

You don't need to be a child psychologist, a telepathic magician or a paediatric wizard: you will parent well without consciously trying because it is a natural part of you. Your body may miss the baby that was inside your womb but you can already do what is part of your human nature. As you learn the practicalities of care your baby will help you – not only physically, but with his powerful communication. If he screams when he's bathed, he's telling you he doesn't like it. If he wants to pause for a chat and a tickle when his nappy's changed, the look in his eyes will stir you to smile and join in.

Your baby's rhythms

Your baby's rhythms are a reflection of his unique personality as well as his physical make-up, and will affect the development of your family. You will look to him for clues about what he needs, and he will rely on you to guide him. By his very nature your baby may love sleeping, or he may prefer to gaze into your face as you carry him around the house and rock him to sleep. He may want to be held in a certain way when he's tired. There is so much in between sleeping and feeding – new smells, sights and sounds and limitless learning. Some days your baby may be calm and on other days he may be unsettled and ask for almost constant comforting.

States of consciousness

Your baby's states of consciousness alternate from deep sleep to dream sleep and light sleep, to awake and meditative, calm and alert, restless and crying. He can shift from one state to another quickly and will go through each stage many times during each 24-hour period. There will be repetitive patterns of sleeping, crying, eating and contented wakefulness. His brain and body need to alternate between these phases of rest and activity and it is an essential part of his development.

When your baby stares into space with a calm expression, his brain waves show he is in a state of meditation. This occurs spontaneously many times a day and may not last long. If you are aware it may happen and you have a chance to join him in that calm space.

The time he spends in each state will not be the same in the first week as it is in the second, and his patterns at 3 months may hardly resemble his rhythm at 4 weeks. Yet even from the first week you will be aware of his unique character.

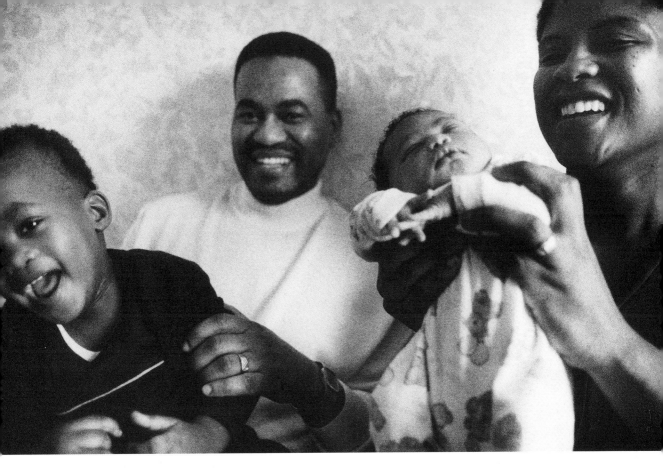

Crying and more

There's a common myth that newborn babies do little except cry, eat and sleep. Happily, this is untrue and there are many other sweet and delightful sounds: grunts, gurgles, hums, squeaks, sniffs, sneezes (several in a row is not uncommon), loud, wide-mouthed yawns, sucking sounds and even loud pops as the lips smack in readiness for a nipple.

Crying is a mixture of excellent programming for your baby and heartache – and headaches – for you. It is a reflex and an expression of both physical and emotional needs; it is just as likely to signal a heartfelt desire for body contact as for milk. Often, your baby may cry when he doesn't actually need something, it is quite simply an expression of his feelings, and he'll need to 'let it all out' not just in the early days, but for months and years to come. He may also enjoy making noise for its own sake, and there will be days when he cries more or less than usual. Some babies who cry a lot turn out to be very talkative toddlers; perhaps they loved the sound of their own voices even in their earliest days.

Sometimes crying sounds almost tuneful, sometimes it seems incessant and it can sound desperate. You will have a natural response to these noises: you may feel loving, angry or worried. These reactions help you to do what's necessary and without realising it you are learning to understand your baby's language. Because crying is such an important issue, there is a chapter devoted to it for each 3-month period of your baby's first 9 months outside the womb (pp.208, 240 and 262).

Joining in the conversation

At birth your baby has the ability to hear the basic sounds of every language on earth (p.32). In the second month he begins to make the coos and gurgles that are made by all babies his own age the world over and as time goes by and you relax with one another you will begin to understand his language. Naturally, he'll entice you to give the stimulation he needs, and he'll have an increasing role in your conversations. He tunes into everything around him, listens intently and watches your facial expressions, gauging your intentions. These months of listening are very important; he is busy learning his 'mother tongue', the language he will eventually use.

By 8 or 10 weeks, your baby can sit on your lap and listen as you chat in company, looking from one person to another. He may interrupt, and will already expect to be part of your conversations. Talk to him, leave a pause, and wait for his reply.

What your baby can vocalise at the end of 3 months is the result of an incredible amount of learning and practice. What he hears is as important as what he says, and he

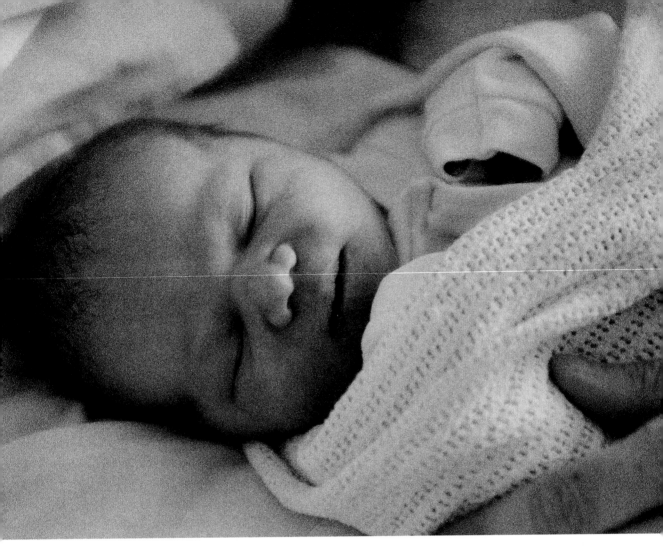

understands more than you may realise. He can sense the emotional background to your words from your expression, tone, body language and energy.

If you feel silly talking to a newborn baby, don't worry; lots of people have the same experience. Try to let go of your inhibitions and talk to him: it is great to begin talking from or before birth so that you continue and get used to communicating personal or difficult things aloud. It is also great for your baby to have space in the conversation so he can join in.

Hello family

When you and your baby meet one another for the first time at birth you take your first step as a family. The hours and days that follow may be filled with love and tinged with wonder, awe, disbelief and relief, interspersed with anxiety and confusion. Often referred to as a 'babymoon' these days can be almost unreal: everything is new and exciting and you may feel almost oblivious to things going on outside your private space.

Soon, however, the outside world will come into focus, whether it is in the form of visitors, work commitments or an empty fridge that needs filling, and gradually your new lifestyle establishes itself. As it does you'll begin to see how your personalities balance and how you all communicate and work as a team.

The first few days

When it's time to go home from the hospital you might all have a butterfly feeling in your stomachs. Many mothers feel a sense of loss at leaving the security and friendship of the maternity ward, and slight trepidation at leaping into the future. You may also feel sad and miss your pregnancy. Alternatively, you may be confident and all too eager to get home. Fathers, too, are usually excited to bring the new family home and curious or anxious about what the future will bring.

At home it is obvious that your space will never again be the same. You arrive with your hospital bag, your baby, a car seat, armfuls of presents and flowers, and suddenly

Cosy safe corners

It will be lovely for your baby if he is comfortable, can be near you and has interesting things to look at and do. He will appreciate feeling included in your world and while he is young you'll spend most of your time together. You can make it as comfortable as possible for both of you by creating cosy corners.

To avoid having to be in two places at one time you could set aside a space in each room for him and while he is tiny this only needs to be 1 square metre. Decorate it with bold pictures, a mobile or some hanging ribbons and use a mat or blanket for him to lie on. You might have one favourite rug that you move from room to room. In the kitchen you could hang something interesting from a cupboard door handle, so it's at the right height for your baby to focus on and, when he's able, to hit; in the bathroom you could set up an engaging scene with empty shampoo bottles or toothbrushes lined up on a low shelf. The possibilities are limitless: from your baby's viewpoint everything new is an object of curiosity, and he won't much mind if it's a 'toy' as long as it's visually stimulating. If it moves, or makes a noise, all the better, and as he grows he'll get more curious about textures. As part of your cosy corners you could also store changing equipment on each floor or in the rooms you most often use.

Your baby's attention span is very short, and regular changes in stimulation and scene will stem boredom. He'll enjoy moving from room to room and adjust more easily when he recognises his cosy space. In later months your baby will get better at spending time in a room by himself when the value of having a safe and cosy corner continues.

Your own 'cosy corners' may involve anything from a favourite chair within easy reach of entertainment systems or bookshelves to new gentle lighting for your bedroom. Consider investing in a cordless phone or fitting extensions and setting up an answer phone if you don't already have one. There are lots of small touches that can help you relax. Creating cosy corners is a very practical way of marking physical boundaries; you know where your baby's space ends and adult space begins.

the place is cluttered. If you are well organised, you may soon have everything in its place; alternatively, you could sit down and wonder just how one extra tiny person could possibly take up so much room. For the first hours, though, the most important space you need is emotional – some time to sit down, cuddle your baby, gaze at his amazing face and hands, and take it all in. You are a family, and you are at home.

A day with your baby may start at 4 in the morning, 7 or 9am. It might follow a night of peaceful rest, or a series of troubled naps. In the early weeks the whole concept of 'a day' can seem foreign, as your life is broken into 2- or 4-hourly stretches and you share your baby's routine of waking, feeding and sleeping. It may seem hard to believe, but in time your family will settle into a rhythm that takes account of each individual's needs.

Different parents, different babies

Your baby has his own character and you have yours. The chances are that you will have many similarities and many differences, just as you resemble and differ from your own parents. Your baby leads you as he signals his need for food, comfort, sleep and learning, and he can control the situation because he is naturally flirtatious. Even the most placid of babies leads the way in the relationship that he forms with his mother, father and wider family. How smoothly these relationships form and settle, though, depends on the people involved.

Within each relationship certain roles are played. You may be happy to follow your baby's tune, you may want to lay down rules or be inclined to compromise. There is no right or wrong way to parent and the way that works best for you will depend on how your baby's personality matches yours. If he responds well to what you do, you will get on fine, and this is the most likely scenario because your instincts and human nature set you up to do the best for him.

Some things you do may not suit your baby's personality, causing difficulties and prompting you to rethink your approach. For instance, you may try to stick to a routine that doesn't correspond to his natural rhythms, you may want cuddles when he wants space, he might want to feed more often than you expect or you may both have strong, conflicting personalities.

As you dance together, sometimes you will alter the tempo, sometimes it will be your baby who calls for a break or a change. Going with the dance is a good way to have fun, experiment with balance and build on your natural abilities as you find a daily structure that suits you both. It is important to be flexible, because things change from day to day, and it's also important to be consistent and assertive: you are both his carer and his guide. This apparent contradiction between flexibility and consistency is one of the challenges of parenting, and may be best approached by listening with an open mind – to your baby, to yourself and to your family.

One of the first things a baby learns is to trust (or mistrust) his environment, in which his mother is, of course, the prime focus. He has been in tune with your feelings for months before his birth and the imprints of his reactions to your feelings are part of his personality. He cannot be fooled, even if you try to hide your feelings. Honesty is the greatest gift you can give your child. Your baby reacts to your smiling face by smiling and, seeing the other face respond, believes he has made it happen. His understanding is: 'You look at me with warmth and love, I can trust that you will keep me safe and know what I need.

I feel valued – and therefore I value myself.' Think how crucial this message may be in enhancing your baby's sense of self-esteem. If your face does not respond, your baby may become anxious.

Dynamic boundaries

It's very common for new parents or parents-to-be to wonder how days will be structured with a baby. Your opinion about routine may be influenced by your own upbringing and by what your friends and family have done. There is so much to learn when you start out as a new family and it is not appropriate to structure your baby's day until you know more about him and how to care for him.

At first it is important to put your energy into getting to know your baby. You will learn by following your instincts and through a process of trial and error. At the same time he will receive a powerful message that you listen to him and value him for who he is rather than for how you expect him to behave. This foundation is important for his self-esteem. It may also mean that your relationship does not hinge on you being in control but instead is based on respect and trust.

The following chapters give details about feeding, sleeping, crying and daily babycare. Once you have experience of these basics you will feel clearer about what suits your baby and your family. By the second or third month you may find it easier to create boundaries around your space and time that can stretch and alter when necessary, and still provide a structure to help your baby to feel settled. Within these boundaries – for instance, bedtime – you can build patterns by encouraging your baby to form habits that suit your family boundaries. If you repeatedly give the same cue for a certain event, his brain will connect the two and over time the response becomes almost automatic.

Put simply, this works when he smells milk and turns to your breast or his bottle in search of a drink. In relation to bedtime, if you give your baby a bath and a feed in a certain place, or play a specific piece of music before bed, and repeat it over 10 days, his reaction (sleep/tiredness) will almost certainly follow the cues.

When a boundary is dynamic, it is created according to everyone's needs and can flex as these needs change. Dynamic boundaries provide a framework but not a cage, guidance without coercion. Simple examples include giving your baby ice cream – inappropriate at 2 months but fun at 9 months – or setting mealtimes that need to change as your baby grows.

Boundaries may need to be most flexible around sleeping times, when they may be challenged if your baby is not tired when you expect him to be, and around adult time, because your needs will alter. Reassessing your boundaries at regular intervals (p.276) helps to keep them

appropriate, so that each member of the family has space in which to enjoy themselves and thrive.

Quality time and love

Your child needs to feel loved – with the emphasis on feel. The best way you can let him know what you're feeling is by spending time with him. If you cannot take time off work, you can still spend 'quality time' with your baby. This is time when you focus solely on him and on the connection between you as you enter his world. Through time spent with him he will feel loved and respected, and be encouraged to express himself.

Time spent with your child but waiting for the next phone call or being anxious about the week ahead is not quality time, and he may react to this with disruptive behaviour that is a cry for attention. Creating space for quality time with your baby – and time with yourself that is away from him – is an important part of setting boundaries. Space and time help him to grow and benefit the whole family.

From newborn to settled baby

The newborn period is precious and all too brief. There's no set time for a baby to pass out of this stage. As a parent you will sense when your baby is more used to life outside the womb, a little more comfortable as he lies out of your embrace and more obviously responsive to you. Some babies seem settled in the first 2 weeks while others take 8 or 12 weeks – a lot depends on their personality, their birth experience and the family environment that surrounds them. When you feel your baby settle, you will mirror him and you will also relax.

Your child, your teacher

He can teach you to . . .

- Enjoy the moment.
- Love.
- Hear your inner voice and be patient.
- Laugh and feel overwhelmed with joy.
- Cry and feel low, and rise again into happiness.
- Prioritise, placing love and happiness at the top of the scale.
- Trust your instincts and be open, yet boundaried.
- See the influence of your own childhood on your present life.
- Respect your body as a life source for you and your child.
- Manage your time efficiently, value your community and delegate.
- Enjoy your feminine aspect.
- Share and give time to your relationship with your partner.
- See your parents in a new light, and transform your relationship with them.
- Believe that you are a wonderful, powerful human being.

Your developing baby: weeks 1–12

After 9 months of development and learning in the womb, your baby emerges not as a 'blank slate' but as someone equipped with skills and abilities and immeasurable potential. Inside you she wriggled, kicked, sucked, tasted, smelled, heard noises, explored her environment through touch, blinked and looked upon a dim reddish landscape. Your baby has instincts and yearnings, inclinations and reflexes and, so scientific research suggests, an innate understanding that she is human, and very, very similar to the people she sees and smells. Her genetic make-up contains ingredients selectively evolved over hundreds of thousands of years and her experiences from her environment affect her greatly. This mix of nature and nurture combine to make her a unique person.

Your baby's perception

For your baby the world is a sensual banquet: she has an acute sense of smell, excellent hearing, sufficient but still developing vision and a body that's very sensitive to touch and movement. In these first 3 months she encounters an incredible amount and learns to link what she sees with what she hears, smells and feels as body co-ordination improves and her brain develops (p.27). Yet your baby remains vulnerable and totally reliant on others for survival and development. Humans are alone in the world of mammals in needing such a long period of parental support and guidance – without stimulation your baby's senses cannot develop their full potential.

Your baby lives purely in each moment: she sees a movement, notices it and becomes interested, then the movement stops and she fixes her attention on something else. As in a magic show, things appear and disappear, and there is rapid change. An adult ponders about where things come from and what happens to them when they are not visible, but a baby accepts them. She can be excited, wriggling and kicking one minute, and the next look blank even though she's still interested. Her mind is like a sponge absorbing information – she needs periods of activity as well as calm and safety to integrate what she learns.

Being in your baby's moccasins

As you play with your baby, look around and imagine seeing through her eyes. What does she see, hear, smell and feel? Does she like to feel protected in your arms, or lie on her mat as she explores the room with her eyes? Will she like familiar things that reassure or novel things that intrigue? If she's bored with an unchanging scene, she may fall asleep, or simply go quiet until something new arouses her interest, or she might get frustrated and complain. On some days she will need to calm down and absorb what she has learnt, on others she will want to pass quickly from exciting moment to exciting moment and will demand constant entertainment.

Talking to your baby: Motherese

Like adults across the world, when you talk to a baby you automatically use 'Motherese': you speak slowly and prolong words, the pitch of your voice rises by nearly an octave, your sentences are melodic and you accentuate all the vowels. As sounds reach your baby's ears, her brain receives signals that help her to interpret the noise; these signals are stronger as you elongate, stress and repeat words. The stronger the signals, the more connections her brain is able to wire and the more she learns. If she was never spoken to in this way, her understanding of language and her own speech development might be delayed. And Motherese also makes you feel good: it's easy to smile as you talk and, because you're speaking slowly, you have time to listen to her reaction.

Talking like this can seem very strange at first, and many parents need practice although adults and children have a natural tendency to do it. What's important to your baby is that you talk to her, make eye contact and let her feel included in your conversation. Come in close to her face so she can focus on you. You will notice that she watches your eyes and the way your lips move. Often your voice will provide familiarity in a noisy or strange place.

Don't worry about what to say. If you're changing her nappy, give a commentary. If you're thinking about your mum's visit tomorrow, talk about that. If nothing comes to mind, mention the colour of the walls, the kitchen or the curtains, your baby's hands, her nose or her hair. If you feel happier talking 'baby' language ('ooh . . . aah . . . ba ba ba'), that's fine too. These 'non-words' help her learn to distinguish between one sound and another and they are fine for you to use too.

As you get used to talking to your baby, ask her questions ('Do you like that?', 'Does that feel nice?', 'What's going on?') and give her praise ('Well done, wasn't that a lovely bath!'). The tones and spaces that you use teach her a lot about the art of conversation, and she'll soon begin to talk back to you with her own sweet sounds.

As the weeks pass, regularly change your baby's toys and pictures, introduce different noises and smells to her world, hang jingling, colourful toys in her pram and let her hear music, voices, songs and chit-chat. Keep her with you and invite her to join you in a game of discovery as you cook, take a shower, drive the car, fold the washing, and take her out of the house every day if possible. When you play together, follow her gaze or respond to her kicks. In that way you will take her lead and go at a pace that suits her best. There is no need to be obsessive, though – play can be a part of daily life.

Developmental range

This section and each of those that follow on p.232 and p.254 focus on the normal range of development in healthy babies. Of course, there are some who achieve some things much earlier than others, and some who tend to be slow in one area but not in another. If you are concerned that your baby is lagging behind, arrange to visit your GP or a paediatrician for a thorough check.

Communication

Though your newborn baby may not know who she is, from birth she recognises you by the sound of your voice and heartbeat and soon knows your smell. She relaxes when she's content and cries when she is not. She is sociable from day one and lures her parents and carers into her bubble of sweetness, helps them relax and makes them respond to her. She has strong innate instincts.

Weeks 1–4

Your baby has no concept that she is separate from people around her, especially her mother. This is a psychological feeling of being linked: without consciously thinking, she expects that she is attached to you as she was in the womb, and at a deep reflex level she expects to receive everything she wants and is unaware that you cannot understand her. She will almost certainly appreciate being close to you. Her brain processes most new experiences via its emotional centre in the thalamus, so what she learns has a significant emotional component (p.27).

With a strong instinct to communicate, your baby loves to copy and entices others to come close, talk to her and fall in love: from the moment of birth she begins to form relationships. By 4 weeks she has learnt to predict certain things such as your face when she hears your voice or a feed when she smells a breast or sees a bottle. Even though she doesn't have the bodily control to communicate this with arms or hands, she may let you know by tensing, relaxing or crying.

Weeks 5–8

After a matter of weeks your baby can remember specific greetings made by different friends or family members and

Communicating games

- Some babies are more outgoing than others but all are naturally sociable. In the early months your baby spends a lot of energy asking for things so that she is comfortable, warm and well fed. If these needs are met, she'll feel emotionally secure and can use energy to explore and interact: babies who are ignored or left to cry have less social confidence and are slower to learn than those who have their basic needs met without question or delay.
- When you include your baby in your conversations and tell her what you're doing or where you are going, you help her feel part of your life. This is the best basis you can give to help her develop the confidence to be sociable and to learn about language. Being in the company of other parents and babies is an excellent way to socialise and older children are great teachers.

may even smile in anticipation of a sloppy wet kiss or a tickle from someone she sees every day. She'll remember certain favourite toys and know that some, if kicked, make an exciting noise. At around 6 weeks she utters her first open vowel sounds – 'ooo's and 'aaa's – and play becomes more exciting and interactive as adults join her conversations. She'll enjoy feeling the physical limits of her body, but does not yet know she is separate.

Weeks 9–12

Your baby is most open and entertaining with those she is familiar with – her parents, siblings, and any other carers – and if she feels secure she'll probably have wide grins for everybody she meets. She knows that smiling brings smiles, and it makes her feel good (partly through the release of 'feel good' endorphin hormones), so she'll do it again and again. She'll give glimpses of her sense of humour and laugh now and then completely out of the blue, as if enjoying the sound and the feeling. She'll also get lots of enjoyment from making sounds and practising as she moves her lips and tongue to see if she can make noises like you.

Vision

What your baby sees is very different from what you see. Her eyes perceive light and send electrical impulses to the brain where signals are interpreted. At first, there's no experience on which to base interpretation, but she has an innate interest and drive to study her world.

By the end of the third month, development in her eyes and the visual cortex of her brain enables her to see objects where at first she only saw light, smiles where she once saw blurred shapes and hands that she suspects may be her own. Her ability to perceive colours is also refined throughout this time.

Weeks 1–4

From the seventh month of pregnancy, when sunshine or a light shines on your belly, your baby can sense the change in light. She may blink and sees her womb environment and closes her eyes to sleep; they flicker as she dreams. When your baby opens her eyes at birth she can focus clearly for up to 20–25 cm (8–10 in), just the right distance to see your face as she nestles at your breast or relaxes in your arms. Beyond this she sees muted shapes and colours and it's hard for her to determine where one thing ends and another begins, although she is aware that patterns of human movement belong to people.

A specific area of your baby's brain gives her a preference for faces, and she'll explore yours slowly and thoroughly, settling on points of contrast or movement – your hairline, eyes and eyebrows and your lips. In a matter of days the shape of your face will have become 'imprinted' in her brain, and it's this that she'll favour above any other visual stimuli for the next 12 weeks. Soon she will link the way her mouth, tongue and eyelids feel with the way yours look, and you may notice her imitating the movements of your mouth.

Your baby is also inclined to notice moving objects and anything that has contrast or shadows, or is coloured black, white, yellow or red – the things that will improve her vision. Looking at these gives her eyes and brain practice at noticing borders and edges and she'll learn to distinguish between one object and another.

Weeks 5–8

By 6 weeks your baby can track a slowly moving object and will begin to move her head so she can follow it further. She focuses more quickly on objects that are close, and some time around the eighth week she may begin to fix on one object even though something else is moving. From now on when she turns to look at something it's because she wants to – the reflex to turn towards movement can be suppressed for the rest of her life.

Once she is smiling and gets a response, your baby will look keenly at your face and wait for your smile. She notices tiny details within the familiar outline and begins to learn what many of your expressions mean. By around 8 weeks she may begin to reach towards what she sees, if it is close, and the challenge of making contact is huge. If she does, albeit by chance, she makes an important discovery about her body and other objects. In the weeks to come she'll repeat this experience again and again as her hand–eye co-ordination improves.

Weeks 9–12

With stronger eye muscles and good head and neck control, your baby's eyesight continues to improve (although it's still only around 7% of perfect adult vision). She can now focus further and her eyes begin to work

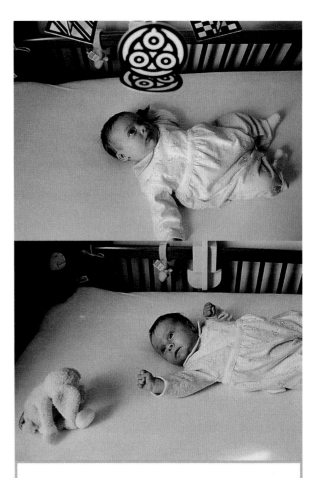

Visual games

- From birth, show your baby pictures of contrasting images – black and white lines, stripes or spirals will probably elicit an enthusiastic wriggle, as will drawings of faces. She'll prefer colours to grey. Fasten pictures like this to the side of her cot.

- Once she begins to lie with her head straight and look upwards (around 4 or 5 weeks), the bobbing figures of a mobile or toys on a baby gym may fascinate her. She'll soon begin reaching for pictures or toys. At first she may be able to touch objects placed to the side of her face most easily.

- Change the pictures in her cot every few days: a sad clown with a top hat followed by a happy clown with a peaked hat, or a black cat followed by a striped cat, and increase the level of detail as she gets older. Use crinkled tin foil or holographic wrapping paper fastened above her cot or to the underside of the table for some really exciting visuals.

- Don't forget that she shares your visual world and almost everything in it is new and begging to be explored. Show her the books on your shelves and pictures on your wall, light switches, curtains and leaves. She'll be intrigued by the banana you're eating and the magazine you're reading, and interested to hear what you have to say about them.

together: the two scenes they send to the visual cortex in her brain are integrated into a single image and she no longer has to move her head to judge distance. All this means that she finds it easier to co-ordinate her hands and eyes. By the end of this month your baby recognises the movements of the people she's often with, and will turn her head to locate you if she hears or smells you approaching.

As for colours, she will prefer long-wave colours, red, orange and yellow, over short-wave (blue and green) and all colours over grey. What's more important than her colour perception, however, is her experience: visual development depends on lots of stimulation.

Hearing

Sounds heard outside the womb may be confusing for your newborn baby. At first her brain receives messages from her ears without being able to make sense of them: the words you speak flow into one another and collide with other noises – a door closing, traffic passing, music, footfalls or the stroke of your hand on her head. Gradually she learns to locate where a sound is made and filter out

background noise. By the end of the third month your baby not only responds to different tones and speech patterns, but also begins to copy you.

Weeks 1–8

Your baby has been hearing sounds from around Week 15 in your womb and is born with fully developed hearing. In the open air noise is no longer muffled and reaches her ears with a wider range of intensity but some sounds are familiar – your voice, your partner's voice and possibly music you listened to frequently in late pregnancy.

A natural tendency to tune into voices helps her to develop listening skills. She pays particular attention to the lilting high-pitched tone called 'Motherese' (previous page) that you naturally use. At first, she can locate a sound made in front of her, and will look towards it. Without thinking, you respond to her natural development: you'll spend most of your time talking to her while you're looking at her, and some time talking from the side as you cradle her in your arms. By the end of the second month she looks to sounds made from the sides. Even though she can't locate you when you're behind, she'll hear you and wait for you to come close, and may signal her anticipation with a kick, wriggle or cry.

Weeks 9–12

By around 8 or 12 weeks your baby will respond to your voice with a smile, even before she sees you. Now that she can 'coo' she will spend more time playing with the sounds she can make and she is beginning to connect mouth shapes with the sounds she hears – for example, when she sees your mouth make a tight circle she'll anticipate an 'ooo' sound. This is just one step in her ongoing lesson in language.

She may realise that if she hits a bell on the side of her pram it makes a noise. She may do it again deliberately, although efforts to make a noise from a toy don't usually appear until at least 4 months, and often not until 6 months.

Smell and taste

What your baby tastes is closely linked with what she smells. Together these two acute senses help her orientate herself in what may otherwise be an overwhelming world of blurred images and incessant sounds. And the experience of taste is closely linked with texture – she uses her mouth to touch and feel and it is more sensitive than her hands and fingers.

Weeks 1–4

In the brain neural pathways relating to the mouth, tongue and lips develop early and your baby is born with an acute sense of smell. In the womb her taste buds were alerted to a full range of tastes (bitter, sour, salt and sweet) by the

---

Listening games

- Your baby loves listening to your voice when you talk and when you sing. She'll be curious about many noises, though, so take her out of the house where she can hear wind rustling the leaves of trees, flowing water, the voices of passers-by or traffic.

- In the house, washing machines and vacuum cleaners are often great favourites and, almost definitely, she'll like music. Hold and rock her as you listen to your favourite tunes or give her a musical toy.

- Some children (and adults) are better listeners than others. You can encourage listening and keep boredom at bay with simple sounds – anything from 'woo' to 'sshhh' – and with objects – rattles, a spoon on a tea cup, your hands clapping, crumpled paper, bells . . . the list is endless. In the first weeks, your baby will respond by moving, kicking or wriggling. As she masters body and voice control, her response will turn to coos, smiles and gurgles.

- She'll also love rhymes and songs and by 12 weeks may recognise and expect certain sounds – she's never too young for 'This Little Piggy.' Being bounced on your knee can be great fun, particularly if accompanied by a high 'wheeee' or a low 'booo'. After three or four goes she may let out a smile with the 'wheee', and giggle as she lands and you 'booo': as she waits for the noises her listening skills are developing well. This foundation will prove invaluable – those who listen well learn well, and listening is a valuable tool for building friendships.

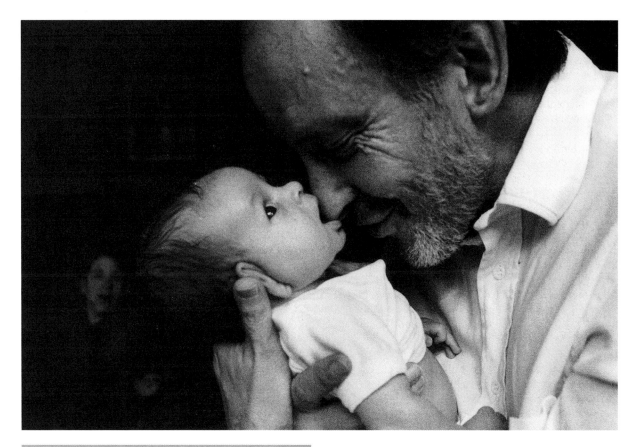

Smelling and tasting games

- As often as possible, hold her naked body against yours: skin-to-skin contact is uniquely intimate.
- Your baby relies on her sense of smell to identify you and to work out whether something is friendly or hostile, familiar or novel. When you're with her, be aware that she notices smells more than you do.
- In new places hold her close to you. Take a familiar blanket in her pram.
- If you're cooking a strong-smelling meal open a few windows because it will smell even stronger to her. But don't shy away from introducing her to new smells – every object and person has a scent as well as a sound and image, and she'll love discovering it and piecing together the puzzle of identification.
- Introduce her to aromas – she can smell the wind in autumn trees; take her close so she can smell the bark. As you walk past a cake shop, take her in and let her smell a fresh scone; as you hang the washing, let her smell the wet clothes.
- When she starts putting things in her mouth give her a range of safe objects with which to play. You could let her suck a variety of materials in your house: a wooden spoon, a velvet or silk cushion, denim or corduroy trousers, a cotton or wool top or a piece of cardboard.

variation in the amniotic fluid and at birth she loves the sweet flavour of colostrum. She uses her sense of smell to find her way to your nipple and to identify you. She finds your smell deeply reassuring. She'll settle most comfortably if she's held against your body; being cuddled by her daddy comes a very close second. In just 5 days your baby can recognise your scents, and will already be using smell to recognise familiar places.

Weeks 5–8

The range of smells your baby has experienced is already vast, and plays an important role in her identification of people and things and in her developing memory. You might notice that she may turn away from unpleasant smells, and sometimes she might startle in a new place because of strange aromas that your less sensitive nose cannot detect.

Weeks 9–12

Your baby's tongue has grown considerably and if she has started putting toys or blankets in her mouth, she is using her lips, tongue and mouth as an extra sense organ to define textures as well as tastes. Her digestive system is not yet ready for solid food, so resist the temptation to let her taste your dinner or ice cream.

Touch

There is a theory that hundreds of thousands of years ago babies were born after 12 months of development in the womb but then the hominid brain evolved, heads grew larger in gestation and babies needed to be born earlier to fit through the bones of the pelvis. Whether or not it is true that human babies complete gestational development outside the womb, it is indisputable that babies need and indeed thrive upon close contact with another body. The skin develops from ectoderm – the same layer of embryonic tissue as the brain and nerves – and there is an established link between stimulating the skin and stimulating the brain.

The first 1–3 months is commonly a 'babe-in-arms' period and the feeling of being embraced is important. Touch is essential for normal development and ensures that intimacy continues. Your baby is extremely responsive to massage, which soothes, aids development and encourages her to trust you (p.365). And it's not just a matter of comfort and stimulation – you pick up bacteria from your baby's skin and take these into your system and develop antibodies so that your milk will help her to ward off infection.

Weeks 1–4

Your womb provided a constant all-over-body massage and comfortable rocking and there was never a moment when your baby did not feel embraced. Touch is the most developed of all the senses at birth – and the nervous system ensures that she feels every stroke and caress, the softness and warmth of a blanket and the intensely pleasurable feeling of skin on skin. As she searches for your nipple and feels the skin of your breast on her cheek, your baby knows where she is, feels good about it and starts to suck; she may explore your body in an instinctive way as her hands move and knock on your skin. Even as a newborn, your baby may love a massage.

Weeks 5–8

Your baby has already learnt a lot through touch. She learns most from how others touch her, but also takes in a lot of detail about textures – your skin, her blanket, her clothes, your hair – and links this with the shades and contrasts she sees, building up knowledge that will later help her guess how something will feel before she touches it. She still has the grasp reflex: if you place your finger or a toy against the palm of her hand, her fingers will curl around it and she'll grip it strongly. She will even do the same with her feet. She can't let go on purpose yet: that takes another 3 months.

Weeks 9–12

With a little more freedom of movement and experience of touching and gripping, your baby has linked information about familiar objects and people: what she feels with her hands and skin relates closely to what she sees and smells. She may be reaching out to brush your chin or mouth with her fist or fingers. She is beginning to use her power of touch to explore and may start to play with her own fingers and marvel at how they seem to respond to her commands.

Body development

Your baby is unable to use her body to support herself. Yet, clothed in skin and wired with an extensive network of sensory nerves, it is a powerful learning tool. At birth many movements are controlled by the oldest (proto-reptilian) part of her brain where the connections governing reflexes are already hard-wired. As the months

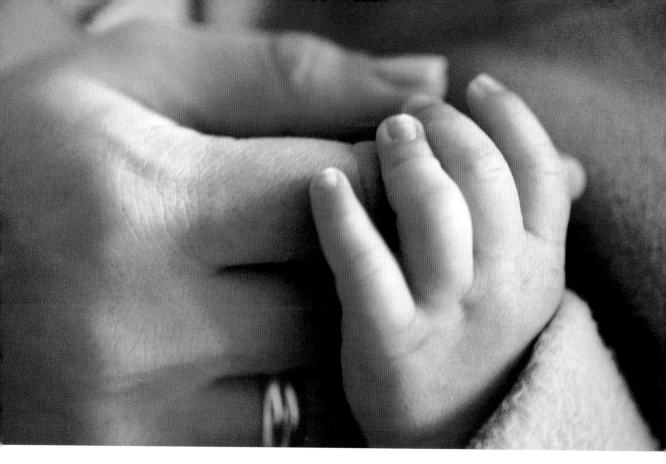

go by, the newer part called the neo-cortex gradually matures and conscious control improves, allowing her to communicate more clearly and put some of her intentions into action. By a process of trial and success as the nervous pathways are used, the connections become organised. Your baby's body control develops from her head towards her hands and feet and from the centre outwards.

Weeks 1–4

Your baby's body is miraculous. If you lie your newborn baby on your tummy, she is able to wriggle up towards your breast where she will instinctively suck. As she sleeps, her head naturally falls to the side so she breathes easily and mucus, vomit or dribble flows from her mouth so there's no danger of choking. She sneezes a lot to expel the mucus that built up in the womb, and she may suck her hand or fingers for comfort. From birth, her reflex to suck gives her a great foundation, and with each passing day she learns more about how her mouth and tongue move.

She will often put her hands to her mouth, usually with clenched fists, and sometimes they'll collide with or scratch her face. These reflexive movements help her develop strength and control. By 4 weeks she may swipe at a picture or toy, especially if it makes a noise. Her legs kick when she's excited, and rest in a bent position, often with her ankles crossed.

Weeks 5–8

Already your baby has a little more control over her heavy head. When she lies on her back it doesn't fall to one side any more and she can lift it momentarily as you hold her, and raise it for up to 45 degrees while she's lying on her tummy. Some time around 6 weeks she is just becoming aware that she has some influence on her own body, and that sometimes she can make other objects move. She swipes with her arms but is not yet in command of her fingers. She's gaining control of her legs and kicks higher each day: your baby is already enjoying kicking something to produce a noise.

Weeks 9–12

When she's lying on her back your baby can kick up her legs and bring her feet to waist level, and may already be strong enough to bear her weight momentarily when held in a standing position on your lap. She'll eagerly bring things to her mouth. As early as 10 weeks, or not until 14 weeks, she will master control of her head and hold it up proudly when you hold her. Around 2 weeks after this achievement she will be able to sit with support for a few minutes, and will just be mastering control of her arms so she can hit more accurately. She's also beginning to release her clenched fists and is ready to take on the world with open hands.

Breastfeeding your baby

Each time you feed your baby, you also give him warmth and comfort and stimulate his senses: he smells you, he hears your voice, he sees your face, and from this loving security he'll begin to explore his world with eager hands. Breastfeeding gives your baby the ultimate start.

The feeding partnership

Breastfeeding is the ideal way to feed your baby from birth, and for as long as suits you both. It has many dimensions: it is a perfect and natural source of nutrition and brings you together in the most intimate way possible. It prompts your body to release hormones that make you feel good and the sucking that helps your baby release tension is all the more soothing when he can feel his whole body pressed warmly against yours.

You and your baby may take to breastfeeding quickly and easily, or it may take a number of days before it becomes easy and enjoyable. Breastfeeding can be tiring or difficult but most problems can be overcome with a combination of perseverance, patience and love.

Breast milk goodness

The first taste your baby gets from your breasts is colostrum containing sugar and protein for energy, plus protective antibodies and hormones to stimulate digestion. It usually looks clear yellow. In 2–3 days, rich and creamy transitional milk flows before the mature milk gradually comes in – this has a white or bluey-white fore milk and thicker hind milk that completes the feed.

Breast milk is primarily made up of water, in which are dissolved or suspended the other ingredients. Its composition changes according to your baby's age and the time of day, and its flow alters throughout each feed. Your milk is a living substance. In many ways it resembles your blood, without the red blood cells.

Calories: The calorie content if the milk is flowing normally encourages your baby to thrive.

Fat: On average, fat accounts for 4% of breast milk volume and 50% of its calories, giving energy for growth. Babies need fat for energy and to provide heat. Your baby also uses fat for coating and protecting the fibres connecting nerve cells (p.15).

Breastfeeding – the healthy option

- Your milk nourishes your baby from birth, continuing the nutrition you provided in pregnancy.
- Your breast milk is tailored to your baby's needs and changes from day to day. It is by far the best food and it contains everything your baby needs to thrive.
- The many hours of skin-to-skin contact make for close bonding.
- Your milk contains antibodies to help your baby resist infection.
- Exclusive breastfeeding for at least 4 months offers significant protection against illnesses during the first year of life. The incidence of gastro-intestinal illnesses is 40% lower in breast-fed than formula-fed infants, while respiratory illnesses are 30% lower. In general, infections in the baby are less frequent and less severe when they occur.
- A baby who is genetically prone to allergies including eczema and asthma may avoid them or manifest allergic reactions later if breastfed, and they may be of a reduced severity.
- Breast milk may reduce the risk of infant death.
- Exclusive breastfeeding for at least 4 months may reduce the incidence of serious childhood disease including diabetes, leukaemia, bowel and liver disease.
- Infant obesity and excess weight gain is unlikely; a breastfed baby is expected to gain weight normally.

- Breastfeeding reduces the air your baby swallows and colic is less likely.
- Breastfeeding may reduce maternal disease such as diabetes, multiple sclerosis, thyroid and breast and ovarian cancer.
- It stimulates your uterus to shrink following birth.
- It is a natural contraceptive.
- Breastfeeding may be great for dads, who know their baby is getting the best start.

Breastfeeding – the downsides

- On a day-to-day basis, breastfeeding may be harder for mums than bottle feeding. Even taking the downsides into consideration you may remain keen: the long-term effects on mothering and on a baby's health are extremely significant.
- Breastfeeding may make you feel tied down.
- It can be difficult, with sore nipples, mastitis and engorgement as possible problems.
- Your baby receives whatever you consume, and there will be restrictions on your diet, e.g. alcohol consumption.
- Breastfeeding can be a very emotional business and it influences your hormonal balance.
- It may interfere with libido and sex life.
- Some fathers feel left out and upset while feeding continues.

Fatty acids: These are essential building blocks for cell function and assist the absorption of calcium, which your baby needs for developing strong bones and teeth.

Protein: Proteins are essential for the normal function of the body. Breast milk contains a special protein that is broken down easily and quickly absorbed: breastfed babies rarely get constipated and they also need to feed often. Breast milk also contains unique proteins, the protective antibodies that increase your baby's resistance to infection and allergies.

Leucocytes: These protective white blood cells flow into breast milk and help your baby to fight infectious diseases.

Lactose: Sugar in the form of lactose is a source of quick energy. Only a proportion of the lactose in your milk is digested and the rest passes into your baby's large bowel where it promotes the growth of helpful bacteria known as lactobacilli, which reduce the incidence of diarrhoea and contribute to the slightly sweet smell of stools.

Vitamins: If your nutrition is good your baby will receive the vitamins he needs from your milk, in the right proportions. Breast milk contains larger quantities of vitamins A, B, C and E than cow's milk, but less vitamin K. Babies are routinely given vitamin K after birth (p.266).

Minerals: The mineral content of your milk depends on your nutrition. In general breast milk has minerals and salts in just the right quantities.

Getting started

Soon after birth if you hold him close or lie him on your chest your baby follows his rooting reflex, turns towards your nipple and follows his reflex to suck. He may suckle within minutes of birth. Every mother starts as a novice, and so does every baby and you may both need practice. The midwives will guide you: you may both settle well after as little as a day or as long as 2 weeks.

Setting the scene and making quality time

It's important for you and for your baby to get the atmosphere right for your feeds. Try to remain quiet and focused. If the room or ward is noisy, keep your face within your baby's vision and speak softly to him. Turn down the television or radio and consider unplugging the phone. Choose a comfortable chair or nestle quietly in bed as you begin. Once he is sucking he may close his eyes or gaze up at you, his arms tucked into his chest or spread out so he can pat your breast with his tiny hands.

For the first days you could choose to climb into bed and hibernate with your baby to encourage your milk to flow and make the most of being close. Within 3–4 days your colostrum will be replaced by milk. Breastfeeding needs quality time to become established and thrives on this for the weeks or months that follow. You may need to ask friends or family to help with some daily tasks so you have the space to feed without rushing.

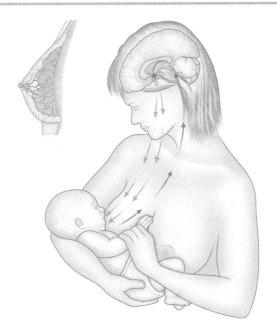

How breast milk flows

Your breasts are made up of 15–25 segments, or lobes, each of which consists of several clusters of glands called alveoli. Each gland is lined with milk producing cells and surrounded by muscle cells. As your baby sucks he stimulates nerve endings in your nipple that transmit messages to the pituitary gland in your brain. This triggers the release of two hormones: prolactin stimulates milk production and oxytocin activates the 'let-down' reflex. This stimulates the muscles around the alveoli to contract and force the milk into tiny canals that converge to form a milk duct. Each lobe has its own milk duct, and each duct travels to your nipple. If your baby stops sucking, or if his cry stimulates milk flow before you bring him to your breast, your milk may flow with such speed that it sprays out in fine jets from your nipple. Oxytocin also helps you feel loving and tune into your baby.

Your baby gets 90% of his milk in the first 5–10 minutes of a feed. You might notice him gulping large mouthfuls and then settling into a mellower suck. The slower sucking coaxes the fattier hind milk to travel from the milk ducts to the nipple, and gives him the other 10% of milk that makes up a complete feed. Getting this last 10% means that he receives essential calories, sends messages to your body to produce the amount of milk he needs and prolongs each feed so you can both enjoy extended contact. He might suck for anything from 10 to 40 minutes.

Your milk flow will be encouraged through regular and frequent feeding and lots of physical contact. Offer your baby your breast whenever he seems hungry, or whenever you want to give it a try, and, if it's warm enough, take off your top and dress him in nothing but a nappy so you can lie close, skin-to-skin. Information on positioning and latching on is given overleaf.

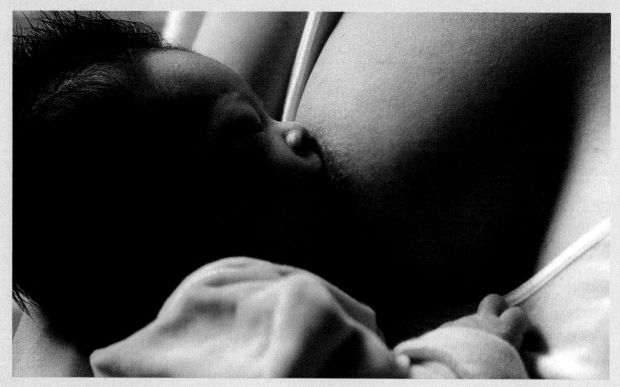

Positioning and latching on

The key to successful breastfeeding is latching on (attachment). Latching on well rests on two factors: your position and your baby's position. You are more likely to get a good position, and enjoy the feeds, if you are relaxed and well nourished – don't forget that what you eat and drink, and how you feel emotionally, all contribute to feeding success.

When your baby latches on well your milk will flow freely and he won't tug on your nipple and make it sore or cracked. He needs to take your nipple and the whole of the areola (the brownish area surrounding it) into his mouth, with your nipple touching the roof of his mouth and his lower lip covering the areola beneath the nipple. His bottom lip will roll out and down, pressing against his chin – if it is held against his teeth he cannot suck so efficiently. In a good position he will squeeze your breast and produce a strong, rhythmic sucking motion, which won't be painful. If you feel pain, ease him off by gently breaking his suction with your finger, reposition and try again.

Achieving the perfect latched-on position may be tricky when your milk 'comes in' and your breasts swell around the third day, making it difficult for your baby to get a grip. If you cup your areola between your thumb and forefinger you can make it protrude a little, so it's easier for him, or you may need to soften the areola by expressing a little milk. Your breasts will settle down once your baby starts sucking. If they become full and heavy later on, they may be engorged.

Tips for successfully latching on

• Bring your baby to your breast as if in a straight line running from behind your nipple to the back of your baby's head.

• Whichever position you choose, allow his head to tip back slightly. Support his head with your fingers rather than your forearm, which will restrict him.

• As he comes towards the nipple, his mouth needs to be wide open – more than 100 degrees. At the correct angle his nose will face your nipple before you begin and as his head tilts back slightly his chin, bottom lip and tongue will meet your breast first: his nose will stay clear, or no more than its tip will touch your breast.

• Your baby needs to take the areola into his mouth as well as the nipple. If you can see any of the areola while he is feeding, this should be above, not below, the nipple.

• He must not suck on the nipple alone. If he does, break the suction by inserting your finger into the side of his mouth, and reposition. The 'mouthful' should be two-thirds areola and one-third nipple. The nipple will be far back in his mouth and will not be compressed after the feed.

• If your baby is reluctant to open his mouth, squeeze the palm of his hand and stroke his top lip or nose with your nipple. Expressing a little milk may give him a tempting smell. When your baby is quiet and alert, try to teach him to open wide by showing him your wide open mouth: he is naturally inclined to mimic you and this is possible from birth. When he gapes, move him quickly and gently very slightly upwards so he takes the bulk of the areola below the nipple into his mouth.

• If you try to place him on your breast when he opens wide during crying, his tongue will be too far back in his mouth and he may find it hard to latch on. You may need to calm him before feeding or he may calm quickly when he feels your nipple and tastes the milk.

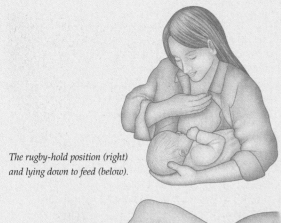

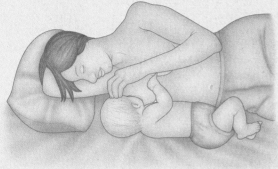

The rugby-hold position (right) and lying down to feed (below).

Place your baby so that your nipple is just above his upper lip and, as he opens wide, guide him up on to your breast. Once he is settled you can rest his head in the crook of the arm on the side he is feeding from (illustration on p.187). A cushion under this arm, and sitting upright with back support, will reduce strain on your shoulder.

If you have very large breasts it might help to support the breast your baby is feeding from with your hand. Place your flat hand against your ribs with the side of your index finger on your breast. This will lift it slightly without changing its shape or obstructing your baby's mouth. If your breasts are very heavy, move your hand forwards slightly or make a 'sling' with a scarf or bandage that fits around your neck and beneath your breast. Keep the cloth around 7.5 cm (3 in) wide for good support.

The rugby-hold position: This is a good position for beginners or to slow down your flow. Sit down, rest your baby on a pillow under the arm on the side you will be feeding from with his feet tucked by your side, pointing behind you, and his nose to your nipple. Cradle him close to your body, using your hand to hold his neck. Put your spare hand on your breast in a 'C' hold. Babies often latch themselves without much assistance in this position. Make sure that he has at least as much of your areola in his mouth below the nipple as above it.

Lying down and in the bath: Lie on the side you are going to feed from, with your baby's feet facing your waist. Prop yourself up on your elbow, with your hand in a 'C' hold on your breast. With your supporting hand on his neck, place your baby's nose to your nipple and guide him on to your breast. When he is securely latched, slide your arm down flat so that you are lying comfortably on your side. You can feed in a semi-reclined position with your baby lying on your belly when you are in the bath – this is beautifully intimate.

If your flow is very fast: Try the rugby position with your baby sitting fairly upright. Alternatively, control a very fast flow by feeding with your baby on your tummy while you lie on your back so gravity is in his favour. When you're sitting up, limit the flow by applying pressure to your breast by pressing and releasing on the areola with two fingers.

Signs that your baby is not latching on well:
• Breastfeeding hurts.
• Your nipples are painful, feel stretched and may be cracked.
• Your breasts do not feel fully emptied after a feed and begin to feel engorged.
• You need to press your breast away from your baby so his nose is not blocked.
• Your baby gulps noisily or sucks very fast without falling into a slow, steady rhythm.
• Your baby does not appear relaxed while he feeds.
• Your baby seems hungry even after a long feed.
• Your baby is reluctant to end a feed, even after 40 minutes – with good latching on he will let go spontaneously.
• Your baby is not gaining weight as you would expect.
• If you are at all uncomfortable, turn to the advice for breast pain in the A–Z Health Guide.

• If your baby's nose is blocked by your breast, do not press your breast away from his nose as this may plug a breast duct. Instead, take him off and reposition him.
• If your baby is sleepy, undress him and he will be more willing to latch on.

Your position

One of the most important aspects of feeding is your posture and comfort. Sit in an upright chair and bring your baby to your breast, rather than leaning over to give your breast to your baby, and always ensure your back is well supported. Leaning back tends to compress the breast and makes it more difficult for your baby to find and grasp your nipple. As you settle into one or more favourite positions, try not to compare yourself to other mothers – everyone does it differently and the most important thing is that you are comfortable and your baby is latching on well. If one part of your breast is tender or inflamed, changing position from feed to feed will encourage the milk in the inflamed area to flow freely. If you do get stiff or sore, focus on your posture and try yoga exercises, which can ease tension (p.346). Breastfeeding need not cause pain, strain or discomfort.

The traditional breastfeeding position: Sit upright and hold your baby with his belly towards your belly, using a pillow or two to bring him to breast height. With his face at one breast and his feet towards the other, support him with your arm along his back. Hold his neck with your hand and don't restrict his head, so that he can flex it and tilt back. Your other hand (the one on the same side as the breast you are feeding from) can be positioned in a 'C' and cup your breast.

Burping

For nearly every baby getting wind up is part of feeding time, either at the end of the feed, half-way through or at intervals throughout the feed. Some babies are particularly windy, some less so, some need lots of help and others do it themselves. Often babies who have difficulty burping get better at it after the first 2 weeks when their system is used to digesting milk and they've learnt to drink without taking down too much air.

In the early days if your baby is crying and you're sure he's not hungry, he may be bothered by wind. He might root for your breast, instinctively seeking comfort to ease his pain, yet not feed. To bring the wind up he may need propping up for a few moments, or like to be held against your shoulder and have his back rubbed. Another effective position is to hold your baby on your lap in a sitting position, with the palm of one hand against his chest, his chin cupped between your thumb and forefinger, and your other hand rubbing and patting his back.

If your baby seems to be in pain with wind, drawing his knees up to his chest and grimacing, he may be swallowing air as he feeds. Watch his position: keep his head higher than his stomach and if your flow is fast help him pace himself (there are tips on p.189). If your baby cries a lot he may swallow more air as he feeds. Feeding him before he is really upset may help him avoid this self-perpetuating cycle.

Possetting and vomiting

After feeding, all babies posset or regurgitate small amounts of milk mixed with saliva. The most common reason for this is reflux, where stomach contents effortlessly come back up the oesophagus (food tube). Drape a muslin nappy or cloth over your shoulder to catch this while you wind your baby.

Vomiting is also common with newborn babies, bringing up what may look like the whole feed with the milk curdled rather than clear and liquid. Sometimes this is caused by trapped wind that forces up milk. If you are concerned about your baby's vomiting, particularly if it's accompanied by diarrhoea or your baby has projectile vomits frequently, refer to p.561 in the A–Z Health Guide and talk to your health visitor or GP.

Timing feeds

In the first week your baby needs to suck little and often. This helps you both get used to feeding and his frequent sucking gives him plenty of colostrum and establishes your milk supply. From the second or third week, providing he sucks for long enough to benefit from the rich, calorific hind milk (at least 20 minutes), he may then have longer periods between feeds.

Because breast milk is easily digested, a gap of around 2–2½ hours between feeds is the average but some babies eat as often as every hour, and some can go for as long as 4 hours without a feed.

Aim to feed for at least 20 minutes on one breast, but remember that all breasts and all babies are different. Some babies get a full feed within 10 minutes, others need 40–60 minutes to get the milk and comfort they need. Your breasts will respond to your baby: if he needs lots of thirst-quenching fore milk, your breasts will produce this, and if he needs more calories, his extra sucking will encourage more hind milk to flow.

Initially your baby will probably feed at only one breast. You need to stimulate both, however, so at the next feed, offer the other. If you have difficulty remembering which breast to feed from, wear a ring, a ribbon or a brooch as a marker. When your baby needs more milk he will no longer be satisfied after one breast. Offer him the second and let him suck as long as he likes. At the next feed, begin with this breast.

Babies generally fall into two groups: 'stuffers' who feed actively every few hours, stuff themselves full and then go off to sleep; and 'grazers' who snack regularly, sleep for short periods and overall seem to be feeding constantly. Both are normal. Your body will create the right milk for your baby to satisfy both his thirst and his hunger.

Schedules

In the early days it is best to let your baby suck as often and for as long as he likes. Your baby will let you know if he is full because he will come off the breast himself or show no further interest in sucking. There's no need to force it: breastfed babies usually eat just what they need, and rarely eat too much.

As feeding takes up so much time each day (second only to sleeping), it forms the backbone to daily structure. Some 20 or 30 years ago it was common to feed babies according to a timetable set by the parents, and this meant feeding every 3 or 4 hours, often to the minute. Some parents still choose to do this but it is more appropriate to feed on demand. Just like an adult, a baby's appetite varies from day to day and meal to meal and only he knows what he needs. Breastfeeding works on a supply-and-demand basis. If your baby is hungry or needs extra calories during or after a growth spurt, he'll eat more and your body will respond by making more milk. If he's not allowed to suck when he wants, your body doesn't receive the message that it needs to make more. When you feed on demand, trust that your baby will establish the feeding routine best suited to his nutritional needs.

After a number of weeks – as little as 3 or as many as 8 – you may recognise a pattern for when your baby wants to feed. If you want to feed at particular intervals you can gradually merge his pattern and your timetable by postponing or prolonging feeds by a few minutes each day, guiding him while acknowledging his needs.

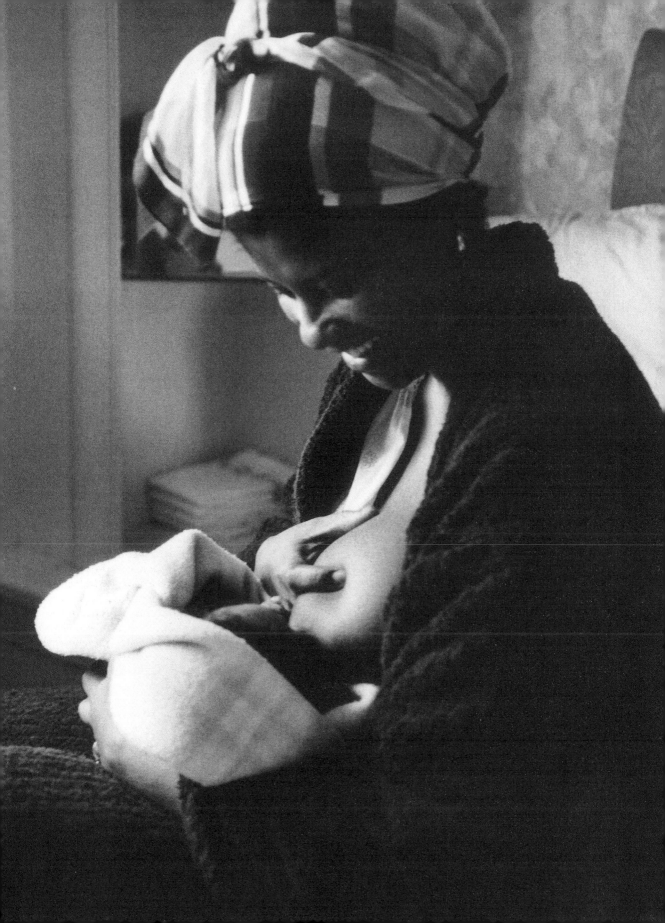

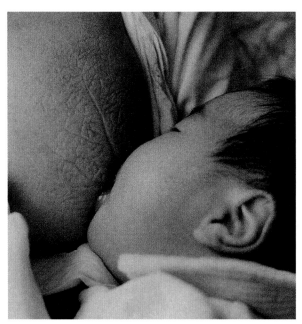

A cabbage leaf, chilled in the fridge and then placed on the breast for 10–20 minutes every 4 hours, is a long-tested remedy to relieve pain from engorgement or sore nipples.

Even if you are keen to set up a routine, it is unrealistic to expect one to fall into place instantly. If your baby eats at certain times but spends a lot of time crying, you will both be unhappy. Some mother–baby partnerships achieve structured days and nights by 6 weeks, some by 4 or 6 months. Some mothers are not interested in a routine and let things flow. Whatever your 'routine', there will be upsets: illness, teething, bad dreams and growth spurts can all cause your baby to ask for more food, more cuddles or more sleep. Let him have his say and keep the boundaries dynamic. Remember, every baby is different and every mother–baby partnership unique.

I have very small breasts. Does this mean they cannot produce enough milk?

The size of your breasts, nipples and areolae bears no relation to their capacity to feed your baby: whatever their size, all breasts contain roughly the same number of milk-producing cells and function equally effectively. Much of the bulk comes from fat tissue between the milk cells. What might be significant is the extent to which your nipples protrude – if they are inverted your baby will find it hard to latch on and stimulate the nerve endings to encourage milk production and flow but it is usually possible to remedy the problem with massage and/or nipple shields (p.195).

Growth spurts

Some babies have a 'growth spurt' (or at least an appetite spurt) every fourth day, others every fourth week. Just before he enters a spurt, your baby may seem more settled, demand less food and sleep better. He's channelling his energy into growing. A day or two later he'll start asking for more food – your baby has grown, he's bigger and hungrier, and now needs extra calories so he'll want to suck at your breast more frequently. Soon after he'll settle down again, and may go back to his original feeding times but the cycle will repeat itself – next week or next month, depending on your baby's rhythm.

Night feeds

Night feeds can be magical when all is calm and quiet and you and your baby sit or lie close together, completely uninterrupted. Because they will be part of life for weeks or months, you may find ways of making the most of them – some women like to meditate or focus on their breathing. Problems arise not because your baby needs to feed, but if he or you have difficulty going back to sleep after a feed.

From the earliest days, provide a different atmosphere at night – help your baby to learn that these dark hours are not daytime – and make it as comfortable yet as boring as possible. Give him his last feed in the dimly lit bedroom and when he wakes for a feed don't offer any distractions. Stay in the quiet room, don't turn the lights on, talk as little as possible and wind him fully before putting him back to sleep. If you stay with him so he doesn't feel left alone, he will feel secure enough to drift back to sleep, although it may take a few days or weeks before he settles without fuss. If you are sharing your bed with your baby or choose to feed in bed at night, you can doze while your baby feeds and he may fall asleep without any complaints when he has had enough. Many mothers prefer to do this, not least because they get less disturbance and don't have to get up in the cold night.

Feeding in public

Whether you start to go out after 6 days or 6 weeks, you'll soon find yourself in public places at feeding times. If this makes you feel exposed or nervous, start feeding with other mums or close friends, which will help to build your confidence. Wear clothes that allow easy access for your baby without revealing your entire chest. Anything from a T-shirt to a cardigan will do, and there are special maternity shirts with modest side slits.

Breastfeeding rooms are available in many public places. A number of breastfeeding and maternity support groups have been busy lobbying on behalf of women so that barriers to breastfeeding are diminishing and feeding in public is, on the whole, now more widely accepted. If you have a problem when feeding in public, you can contact these groups for advice and support.

Problems with feeding

Although breastfeeding is nature's way, it is not always plain sailing for mothers and some babies also find it hard to get settled. Problems are usually easy to remedy with attention to latching on and position and to your own wellbeing. Starting on p.412, there is a comprehensive section in the A–Z Health Guide advising on the causes and remedies for common breastfeeding difficulties. The entries include information on engorgement (where there is a build-up of milk, leaving your breasts heavy and sore), low milk flow, painful nipples, and blocked ducts, mastitis and abscesses. If you have any discomfort at all, this advice together with support from your health visitor or midwife may help you enjoy feeding and feel happy that you are nurturing your baby well.

Breast rejection

Sometimes a baby favours one breast more than the other, and the reason for this isn't always clear. It may be the shape of nipple or the milk flow. It may also be a pattern that started very early on, perhaps because it was instinctive or more comfortable for you to feed from one side, or you need to have one hand free for drinking tea or holding a book.

If your baby feeds from just one breast he can still get adequate nutrition but it is not preferable. You can try to resume feeding from the other by starting each feed there and by expressing milk regularly on that side. If this doesn't work, you may have uneven breasts for a time and will need to be careful not to develop mastitis (p.413) in the underused breast.

If your baby rejects both breasts, the first thing to ask yourself is how your baby is behaving – is he crying a lot, and apparently in pain, or is he quiet and withdrawn, or even unresponsive? If the answer is yes or you are concerned that he may be ill, call your doctor. If he seems fretful but not unwell, he may have earache, a cold or discomfort from colic (p.431).

Your baby may not be keen to suck because of the flavour of your milk or the smell of your breasts, for example if you have eaten food that alters the taste of your milk or changed soap or perfume. Alternatively, if you are feeling tired or anxious your milk flow could be low as a result or your baby may be picking up on your moods. If this is the case some relaxation techniques or a soothing bath with or without your baby may help you to unwind, and plenty of body contact between you and your baby will stimulate your breasts to make milk.

Your baby's food sensitivity

What you eat not only passes to your baby, it also determines your own energy levels and wellbeing, yet the two of you may or may not have the same food sensitivities. Sometimes your baby may not like the taste of your milk and if he refuses milk when he is obviously hungry, cries while feeding, gets a rash, an upset stomach, constipation or excess wind, something you have eaten may be upsetting him. All babies are different, but there are some foods that more commonly cause problems when they are eaten in excess:

- Wheat gives a feeling of bloating or reduced energy.
- Dairy products may cause or aggravate a stuffy nose.
- Carbonated drinks, beans and brussels sprouts can cause wind.
- Alcohol may sedate or over-stimulate a baby.

Be wary of sugar as well, as too much can upset a sensitive tummy: things to watch out for include chocolate and cakes, but also large quantities of fruit, including grapes or strawberries. Heavily spiced food may also be off the menu, as may any foods that trigger allergies or bad reactions in you or your family. Try to reduce or eliminate any food you suspect by being vigilant and noticing your baby's reaction to different meals.

My baby seems to fall asleep each time he eats, after just a few minutes of sucking. Is this normal?
In the first few days your baby will almost certainly fall asleep on your breast at most feeds. Sucking is intensely pleasurable and has a relaxing effect, and it's also an energetic task that can be tiring. Think of his sleepiness as a good sign because the feed and cuddle have calmed and satisfied him.

However, if he continues to fall asleep after every feed you may want to help him stay awake with gentle distractions. Feed him undressed, stroke his cheek, blow on his skin, rub his toes or move your arm as he lies on it, but don't force him to stay awake. All babies are different and there is no 'right' length of time to feed: the important thing is that he sucks long enough to get the calorie-laden hind milk (slow sucking and an 'ummm' sound as he swallows). If you are worried about his intake, look for signs: if he is thriving and settles between feeds, he is probably getting enough. You can check for sure by asking your health visitor to weigh him.

A habit of falling asleep at the breast can lead to difficulties with night sleeping. If, by 8 or 10 weeks, your baby is still falling asleep at every feed, gently break his association with your breast and sleep. Start during daytime feeds. By the end of the third month, try putting your baby in his cot or bed after a feed before he drifts off. You can gently break the suction with your finger when you know he has had his fill of hind milk and notice that he's swallowing less. Helping him to fall asleep without the comfort of your breast may take a bit of work to start with but in the long term it can prevent him needing a suck every time he wakes.

Looking after yourself

Breastfeeding nourishess your baby directly from your body and looking after yourself (p.51) is the best way to ensure that he gets the milk he needs, and your body copes well. Give yourself time to enjoy feeds, and time to relax between them. Throughout the day take care to eat well, and regularly, to maintain your energy levels; this is particularly important around the middle of the day to maintain milk quality and reduce crying in the evening.

Caring for your breasts

When feeding goes well, your breasts will care for themselves. There's no need to clean your nipples. Your baby needs the natural bacteria carried on your skin to populate his bowel, help his digestion and to boost his immune system. Montgomery tubercles in the areolae secrete lubricating moisture, so there is no need to use any creams or lotions on healthy breast skin. Nevertheless, gentle massage with a pure oil, e.g. almond, is good for your skin and may help you to get used to the feel of your breasts. It may also feel good to expose your breasts to the air for 20–30 minutes a couple of times a day.

Between feeds, your breasts gradually fill up and become heavy, so a well-fitting and supportive bra is essential, preferably made from cotton, with comfortable, thick shoulder straps. When you're trying on a bra, test it by opening and closing each cup with just one hand. Avoid underwires as these may cause pinching and could block a duct under the breast.

Before, between or after feeds one or both of your breasts may leak and you can absorb this excess with washable or disposable breast pads. Leakage varies from woman to woman and over time excess production usually diminishes. Plastic-backed nipple shells and plastic-lined pads are not recommended as they stop air getting to the nipple and encourage the skin to crack.

You can help your breasts stay comfortable, by keeping them dry and tending to any problems as soon as they arise. The important thing to remember is to keep feeding when your breasts become sore. If your milk builds up you will probably feel more uncomfortable, and there is a risk that mastitis may develop.

Medication and feeding

A number of drugs and medicines are contraindicated when you are breastfeeding, so ask your doctor what is suitable if you do need medication. There are antibiotics that can safely be used and the progesterone-only 'mini' contraceptive pill is also reputed to be safe. Although it is best to take as few medicines as possible, if you are in pain it is better to take something to relieve it, checking first with your doctor. Some of the constituents from the medicine will pass into your milk, but when appropriately prescribed, the effect on your baby will be minimal. If you

Do I have enough milk?

This is perhaps the most commonly asked question among breastfeeding mothers. One reason for your doubt is that you cannot see how much milk your baby is drinking, another is that you are naturally inspired to want the best for your baby. Your concerns may stem from your baby's crying, and in the early days it can be difficult to know just what makes him cry. Because a warming suck at the breast so often calms, many mothers believe that their babies cry because they are hungry, and mistakenly draw the conclusion that there is something wrong with their milk. Try not to worry. Your milk flow is probably fine and it is perfectly natural for babies to cry. Here are some ways you can help yourself.

- The best way to get reassurance is to visit your health visitor, who can weigh your baby. If he is gaining weight as expected, this is a sign that your milk flow is fine and he is drinking enough. She will also consider whether his crying and feeding patterns give any cause for concern. If he seems happy and is gaining weight, there is nothing to worry about.
- If, however, he is gaining weight but still seems troubled, there may be a number of causes that your health visitor can help you explore. Among these are colic (p.431) and oral thrush (p.423). If you are feeling anxious or depressed, your baby may reflect this with unsettled behaviour. These emotions can also affect milk flow and quality.
- Your milk flow will be optimal if you are well-nourished and rested, and care of yourself physically and emotionally. If your breasts leak this is a sign that you have enough milk. If they squirt milk across the room, you definitely have enough. There are guidelines on boosting milk flow on p.415.

If your baby is not gaining weight as expected, your health visitor or doctor may recommend regular checks on his weight and give you some advice on feeding. Inadequate intake of calories is the most common cause of slow weight gain, and can usually be simply rectified with attention to feeding positions and your own nutrition. You need to feed for long enough for your baby to get the calorie-rich hind milk. If these measures are not effective, you may be advised to use supplemental bottles of formula for a short period to help your baby catch up. Your doctor will want to investigate further if your baby is regularly vomiting or if she suspects a problem with your baby's digestive system, although this is rare. Failure to thrive is explored in detail on p.563.

Wondering about your milk flow may reflect low confidence: perhaps you sometimes ask yourself, 'Am I good enough?' This question can be extended to many aspects of baby care. 'Is my milk good enough?' is just one concern that may disappear as you get used to mothering and to feeding, get to know your baby and understand his signals, and feel supported by the other adults in your life.

take painkillers with a small amount of food you can avoid stomach upset.

The emotions of feeding

Breastfeeding may make you brim with pleasure. Nourishing your baby can feel intensely satisfying, and many fathers enjoy seeing their loved ones being so intimate and their baby so well nourished. Yet hormones encourage feelings to surface, and they may be stronger if you are tired and feel vulnerable. You can use the quiet feeding time to focus on your emotions, to help you on your journey into motherhood. Your partner's emotions are also important. He may feel envious that your baby has pushed him out (p.292). If your partner is upset it may interfere with the rhythm you and your baby have established.

There may be times when your feelings are negative or even painful, and the cumulative effect of being on duty 24 hours a day becomes tiring. If you are not happy feeding, your emotional struggle may leave you exhausted, your milk flow may decrease and your baby might become unsettled. Admitting your feelings, and sharing them with someone – your friends, partner, breastfeeding counsellor or health visitor – is usually helpful and feeling less upset could improve your milk flow. If breastfeeding does not work for you, it could be better to introduce a bottle and to share feeds.

Body image and sexuality

The intimate bond between you and your baby redefines the role of your breasts. It is natural for each woman to have her own views on this issue and her own feelings of pride or anxiety – enjoying a full bosom is common, and so are concerns about sagging, larger or smaller breasts. The way you feel about your breasts and about feeding will affect your own body image and self-esteem after birth.

Breastfeeding also has a strong influence on sexuality. While your baby is feeding, your breasts are primarily for him, and though some women find them sexual they often remain numb to loving touch. The hormones that are designed to make you feel maternal combined with everything else in your life could lower your libido, and vaginal lubrication can be reduced until periods begin months later. Your partner will have his own reaction too: men often worry about causing pain or stimulating milk flow if they touch lactating breasts.

Combining breast and bottle

If you decide to introduce bottles, whether they contain formula milk or expressed breast milk, avoid doing so for the first few weeks until you feel your feeding is fully established. Supplemental feeds are only advisable at this early stage if your doctor or paediatrician recommends them because your baby is not gaining weight adequately.

Massaging your breasts

You can begin to massage your breasts gently in pregnancy. Once your milk begins to flow there may be occasions when you feel discomfort, particularly if you miss a feed. When you feel pain, massage can bring relief and help prevent milk-duct blockage and mastitis.

Massage should be gentle, and the purpose is to soothe your breasts rather than encourage milk flow. Begin at the periphery of the breast (covering the whole area from collarbone to armpit) and massage gently towards the nipple. This mimics the direction of milk flow through the ducts. Focus on any sore patches. Use the palm of your hand and stroke your breast firmly but gently – you should not feel pain. Start at the top of the breast (12 o'clock) and massage towards the nipple and then move on to the next segment at 1 o'clock and massage from the periphery towards the nipple. Go through the stages of the clock so that each segment receives attention, and each stroke ends at the nipple. You may find it easier to massage after warming your breast in the bath or shower and with a gentle natural oil, such as grapeseed or almond.

When you begin to mix breast and bottle your breasts may respond by reducing milk production. If you introduce the bottle at the same time(s) each day, it's likely you'll have an adequate supply to continue giving full breastfeeds at other times. Some babies take from both bottle and breast equally well, but your baby might find the bottle easier and favour it.

If you are returning to work and miss feeds, your breasts may leak or feel full and uncomfortable. After a couple of weeks your body will settle into a new pattern. Many women express in their lunch hour to maintain their milk supply so they can revert to breastfeeding on days when they don't work. Employers in the UK are required by European Union Law to provide time and appropriate facilities for women to express breast milk.

Expressing milk

During the first 6 weeks your baby will need all the milk you produce and your body will be adapting supply to demand. You should therefore not express milk until later. Expressing stimulates the breasts and urges them to produce milk. Thus the more you express, the more milk you will produce. If your midwife has suggested your flow may be low, you can express a little after each feed to increase supply.

You may feel comfortable feeding with one breast while expressing from the other, or prefer to express when your baby has finished. If you are expressing while you are feeding, choose a time of day when your milk flow is strong and you think that there is more than enough for your baby. Express at this same time each day. Often this is after the morning feed. If you are expressing because you are missing a feed, perhaps while you're out at work, express from the breast(s) from which your baby would otherwise drink.

Some women find expressing unappealing or difficult. It can by-pass the let-down phase so the small amount of milk produced can be disappointing. Because it is not the same as sucking, the quantity expressed doesn't indicate the quantity your baby can extract. As you express, continue until the heaviness in your breast subsides or the flow drops. Expressing too much, particularly between 6 and 8 weeks after birth, may over-stimulate your breasts, which can lead to discomfort or mastitis (p.413).

Expressed milk will keep in the fridge for 24 hours, and in the freezer for a month (you can freeze two or three sets of milk in a single bottle). Sterilise your expressing device and the bottles for storage (p.201), and reheat milk as you would formula milk.

Technique for expressing

As with learning any new skill, hand expressing your breasts may take patience and practice. However, mastering hand expressing is worth it. It may maintain your milk supply better than breast pumps. As you are learning, take your time and try a few times before you need the milk. If you rush, your urgency will almost surely interfere with milk flow and make the whole event a frustrating waste of time. Expressing in a warm bath or shower is often easier, or using a warm cloth on your breast and gently stroking it towards the nipple to encourage your milk flow before beginning. It may help to have your baby with you, or something that smells of him.

Wash your hands, place your thumb flat against the upper edge of your areola and cup the rest of your hand

---

I switched to bottle-feeding formula 8 days ago, when my baby was 4 weeks old, because I had sore breasts. My breasts no longer hurt, and have got smaller, but I've changed my mind. Can I resume breastfeeding, or is it too late?

Yes, by all means resume feeding at the breast although you will need to re-build your milk supply. You will find it easier with the help of your health visitor or breastfeeding counsellor. The process should go as follows: breastfeed your baby at the beginning of each feed, then express that breast for 10 minutes and give this expressed milk to your baby. Follow with a further top-up of formula. The idea is that your baby will gradually require less formula as your breasts produce more milk. Be aware that your baby may resist the switch back to the breast, as bottle feeding is often easier and faster. You could switch to cup feeding the expressed milk and formula to minimise the bottle/breast nipple confusion. It is worthwhile persevering but it is not always successful.

under your breast. Gently push your breast back against the chest wall then gently squeeze your thumb and forefinger together again without sliding them over your skin. Release the pressure on your fingers and then repeat, building into a rhythm. Let your milk flow into a bowl that you have sterilised. Don't be rough – it shouldn't hurt. Remember your posture – sit at a table or stand over a high worktop so you don't have to stoop over the bowl.

If you are expressing on a regular basis you may opt for a hand- or battery-operated breast pump. You may need to try a few before you find one that is comfortable. All pumps should have intermittent pressure to avoid breast trauma. When using the pump, take care that your nipple is well centred in the milk-collection funnel to prevent harming your nipple.

When breastfeeding ends

Knowing when to stop breastfeeding is not always easy. Your baby may lead the way and seem happier on bottles or it may be your choice. Whatever the reason, most mothers feel the loss of a very special intimacy. It is usual to go through feelings of guilt and grieving, which can be particularly intense if your breasts continue to produce trickles of milk or if you feel rejected by your baby.

Suckling from your breast may be the most satisfying thing in your baby's day. Yet you may have other demands – another child, a relationship, a job or activities – that make you want to reduce or stop the feeds. It is up to you to weigh the benefits of breastfeeding and your attachment to it against the advantages of being less restricted and perhaps less tired. If a strain in your relationship is swaying your decision, talk and listen to your partner. If he feels excluded, you may think of a solution by taking time out to be together without your baby on a regular basis or by including him in more aspects of your baby's care.

If you want to continue but it is time to stop, your baby may pick up on your anxiety at feeding time so his time to relax can instead be unsettled. If this happens, it may be better for you both if you wean your baby on to bottles. Some mothers continue to mix-feed for a long time, often by giving the breast at the night and morning feeds and a bottle or cup in between, but this doesn't work for everyone.

When you make the break, leave your breasts well alone. Don't express and don't massage, avoid getting hot water on your breasts when you shower or bath, and wear a tight bra. Begin by substituting one breastfeed a day with a bottle. Then substitute one more feed each day, leaving the morning feed until last. Your breasts may adjust after days, although it can take weeks until the milk completely stops and hormones return to normal. It will take longer still for your breasts to reduce to their pre-pregnant size. As you adjust, particularly if you find it difficult, remind yourself that you have given your baby the best start in life.

Bottle feeding your baby

When you bottle feed your baby, you give her good nutrition as well as loving comfort and attention, and she can get these from you, your partner and other members of your family or circle of friends – an advantage that can give many opportunities for firm friendships to begin. Although formula milk cannot supply the antibodies that are present in breast milk, it does contain essential ingredients for growth, and sucking on a bottle is soothing and pleasurable. Whether you bottle feed from birth or switch to bottles after days, weeks or months, the formula will give her the calories, vitamins and minerals that she needs.

Formula milk nutrition

Formula milk is specially prepared to make it digestible and ensure it contains the necessary nutrients. When untreated, cow's milk has too much sodium and protein and not enough fat (calories) or vitamins for a baby and may cause allergies and digestive difficulties. Formula milks contain added unsaturated vegetable oils, to make the fat content more like that of breast milk, and a number of added vitamins. And because breast milk contains almost twice as much sugar as cow's milk, manufacturers usually add other types of sugars. Commonly these are sucrose (table sugar) or fructose (fruit sugar). Cow's milk must also be treated to reduce dangerously high quantities of sodium and potassium (salts), which contribute to the body's fluid balance. Goat's milk contains even higher levels of minerals and must also be treated.

Different brand names tend to contain the same, or very similar, components, but your baby may find some brands easier to digest than others and you may wish to exclude some ingredients if you have a special diet (vegetarian or kosher, for instance). For your first feeds buy a small tin of milk powder until you feel confident that it is suitable. If you are switching from breastfeeding, your baby may seem unhappy while her digestive system adjusts to the formula.

Many baby-milk formulae can contain genetically modified products and these may not be labelled. If you want to avoid GM products, opt for organic formula milk. Until your baby is 6 months old, do not use 'follow-on' milk, whose constituents are not suitable for her digestive system.

Alternatives to cow's milk

Cow's milk-based formula is the most appropriate for a baby. A small number of babies show an adverse reaction to their formula and this may reflect an allergy or intolerance (p.391). If your baby develops diarrhoea or fails to gain weight, take her to the doctor, who will consider the possible causes and monitor your baby regularly.

You may be advised to try formula based on modified goat's milk or soya, which can be bought in chemists and supermarkets or prescribed. Like cow's milk formula, they require no supplementation. Unmodified soya milk or goat's milk should never be given as they do not provide sufficient nourishment and the sodium content may be dangerously high. The plant oestrogens (phyto-oestrogens) in soya formula have not been shown to have any harmful effects.

Bottle feeding from birth

Born with the instinct to suck, your baby will probably take to a bottle teat without any fuss. When you settle for your first feed, hold her to your chest so she can feel your skin. This intimate contact gives her security. You may find a bit of privacy goes a long way, so choose a quiet place or, if you are in hospital, draw the curtains around your bed. If she frets, take it gently. Help her to feel relaxed and comfortable in your arms, perhaps with some soft singing or gentle whispers, and wrap or swaddle her snugly if her hands get in the way. Let her look into your eyes and take as long as she needs. If she's crying, do your best to calm her down before offering her the teat.

Take advantage of any help that is on hand while you're in hospital, and ask the midwives if you need support. Formula and bottles may be supplied and a midwife may mix them so you can concentrate on your baby for the first feeds. Your partner might enjoy making these early feeds.

If you bottle feed from birth, your breasts will take time to settle down because they'll be ready for feeding, but without the stimulation of sucking, milk production gradually stops. This can take a few days and you may feel uncomfortable if the milk builds up.

If your breasts leak, wear a good bra with firm support and use pads. If you need more support, try wrapping a towel or large cloth around your upper body so that extra pressure is applied to your breasts. If your breasts feel uncomfortably heavy and tight they may have become engorged and using cold cabbage leaves under your bra will be of great help (p.414). The hormonal effects of starting to lactate and stopping so soon may leave you feeling emotional.

Comfort and positioning

Your baby will enjoy being close to you and cuddled as she feeds and when she's finished, so the more comfortable you both are, the better. Find a chair that supports your back and allows you to place both feet flat on the floor (or on a foot rest). Rest your baby with her head in the crook of your arm so that you are facing one another, and her body presses against you. Use a cushion to support your baby if this helps.

As you hold the bottle, tilt it so the milk flows smoothly and air doesn't settle in the teat, as this could contribute to wind. If your baby's head is higher than her stomach, digestion will be easier. Watch her progress and wind her (p.190) when she needs it – this may be mid-feed or when she has finished altogether.

Never leave your baby alone with a bottle propped up; not only is there a very real danger that she could choke and suffocate, but this deprives her of physical contact, caresses and a sense of security.

How much to feed your baby

In the first few days your baby needs to eat little and often; she may be hungry every 1 or 2 hours, and drink only 50 ml (1½ fl oz) at a time. By 2 or 3 weeks, the gaps between feeds may stretch to 3 hours, and she may take 100 ml (3 fl oz) per feed. Gradually you will begin to recognise her hunger cries. As you are learning you might mistake a tired cry for hunger, and watch her fall asleep after her third suck on the bottle. You may have lost a bottle but you'll have learnt a bit more about her language, and the two of you will gradually work things out as you get to know each other better and better. In the early days, feeding on demand (p.190) ensures that your baby will be fed when she is hungry.

A pattern for mealtimes often falls into place naturally with bottle-fed babies usually with feeds about every 3 hours for a total of six to eight feeds a day. As your baby grows, the number of feeds she has each day may not change, but the amount of each feed will increase: 60 ml (2 fl oz) in the first week may rise to 125 ml (4 fl oz) by

My baby guzzles her feed and half of it seems to drip down her chin, then she gets windy and often throws up. What can I do about this?

It's quite likely that the flow of milk is simply too fast for your baby. Try a new shape of teat with a slower rate of flow and see if it suits her better. You might also find that tilting the bottle at a different angle helps – holding it in a less upright position puts less pressure on the milk and helps decrease the flow. Try it out on your hand: is the milk dripping slowly or squirting out? Finally, give your baby plenty of time to feed at her own pace, and break off as often as she wants.

4 weeks, and by 12 weeks your baby may be happily drinking 210 ml (7 fl oz), although there's no need to worry if she still only takes 125 ml (4 fl oz) as long as she is gaining weight adequately.

Even the most predictable baby, however, has unexpected hunger in the middle of the night or a voracious appetite one day and wants less the next. Like all babies, yours will be affected by growth spurts and may have unsettled or hungry patches, so keep your routine flexible and always make one more bottle than you need – there is nothing worse than rushing to make up a bottle with a crying baby in tow.

Formula feed must be always mixed accurately according to the manufacturer's instructions: adding more than stated will make your baby overweight and can be dangerous. It cannot help her sleep through the night. If formula is mixed with too little water, high sodium content will make a baby thirsty and a damaging cycle could begin – if she is given more incorrectly mixed milk she will continue to be thirsty and ask for more and her kidneys will strain to cope.

Night feeds

For the first 8 weeks your baby will usually need a bottle of milk in the early hours of the morning (between midnight and 6 or 7am) as well as last thing at night (around 10 or 11pm). Do what you can to keep the night feeds as uninteresting as possible (p.192). Some time after the eighth week she might drop the early morning feed, although it is

How do I know when to increase the number of ounces my baby needs at each feed? I'm anxious that I may give her too much to eat and make her sick, or fat, or both.

If you 'feed on demand' and listen to your baby's cues, she will eat the amount that suits her. Watch her and listen to the signs she makes. If she's still hungry, she will cry. If she has had enough, she'll show her lack of interest by crying or turning her head, or even hitting the bottle with her hands. She may continue sucking if you press her, even though she doesn't actually need to. If you give her what she needs, rather than what you think she should eat, you will avoid having a hungry baby, or a baby who is gaining weight too quickly.

When you make up a bottle, make 30 ml (1 fl oz) more than she usually drinks so that she generally leaves a little. When she begins to drain the whole bottle, increase the amount by a further 30 ml (1 fl oz), and continue to do this in stages.

Your baby may bring up a little milk at the end of every feed as she possets (p.190). If she vomits because she has eaten too much, this will only happen occasionally. If it happens more often and if it is projectile, you should consult your doctor (p.561).

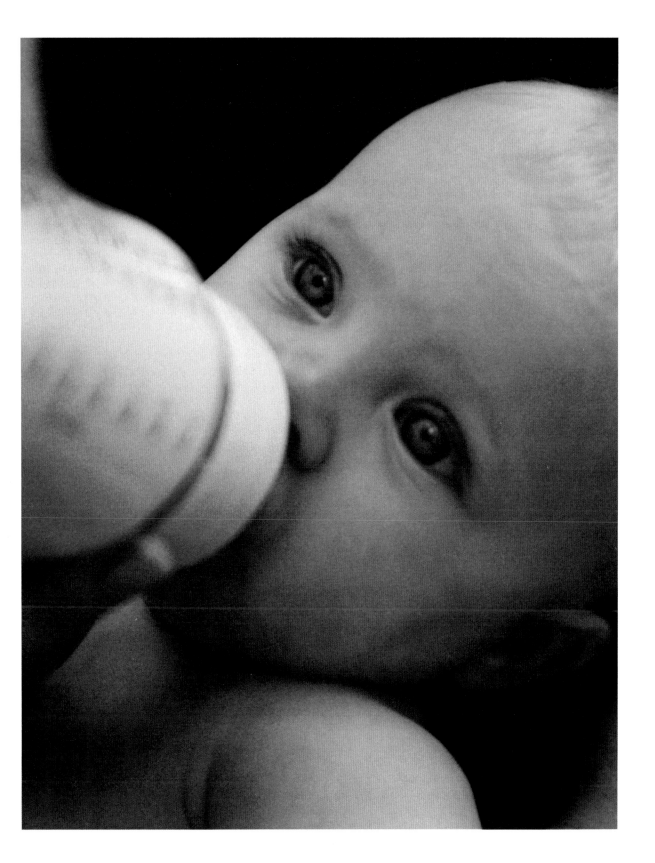

just as usual for a baby to continue to ask for it for longer. Her preferences depend in part on her own digestive system and how peacefully she sleeps, and in part on how you guide her. Whether she wakes for a feed during the night may also depend on how she eats and sleeps during the day (p.205).

If your baby is waking frequently and drinks only 30 ml (1 fl oz) before falling asleep, you could assume that she is waking for comfort rather than hunger. If she is in the habit of 'grazing' during the day this might continue through the night and can be a hard habit to break, so start to extend periods between bottles during the day: in general, if she gets the calories she needs, she is less likely to wake from hunger at night. That is not to say that she will not wake at all if she is not hungry, but if you know that she does not need a feed you can encourage her to sleep soundly in other ways. There is advice in the next chapter, Sleeping like a baby (overleaf).

Never resort to adding extra formula to a bottle or mixing it with baby cereal in an attempt to get your baby to sleep for longer. Adding solid food to her diet before 4 months affects her digestion and contributes to excessive weight gain.

Feeding away from home

If you're feeding away from home, carry warm water and make up the feeds when they are needed, or take cooled bottles in a cooler bag and heat them using a special bottle heater or in a jug of hot water. Don't keep warm milk in a flask, as this is a prime breeding ground for germs. You can also buy ready-made formula milk in sealed cartons. Although it's unlikely in the first 6 weeks, your baby may be quite happy to take her milk at room temperature – this is a great help when you're on the move.

Sharing night feeds

If you are sharing night feeds with your partner, for the first few nights you may both wake, sharing the wonder of

your baby's presence as well as the feeding and soothing. But beyond the first week there is little point in having two tired parents. It's best to decide in advance who will do the feeding and keep it as simple as possible:

- Have a bottle made and stored in the fridge.
- You could keep water hot in a thermos so you can quickly fill a bowl for heating the bottle if you don't want to go to the kitchen.
- Keep the lights dim.

You may be woken by your baby's sniffles before she breaks into a cry, even when it's not your turn to do the night feed. This is common, and mothers usually have an acute awareness of their baby.

If you can't sleep while your partner does the feeding, it might be best for you to carry on feeding in the night and get to bed early or have an extra patch of sleep during the day if night duty is making you tired. Alternatively, you could sleep in a separate room, or even use ear plugs. Just one full night's sleep every now and then can make a real difference to your energy.

The emotions of bottle feeding

Bottle feeding brings you and your baby close for at least half an hour, several times a day. Your baby gets one-to-one attention, enjoys feeling your body, smelling you and hearing your heartbeat and voice. This quiet time gives you space as well. It gives you time to explore your baby and to relax, and to dwell on nothing else other than the thoughts that pass through your head.

Feeding times are often the moments in a busy day when you and your baby can sit quietly and mirror one another. As you look into her eyes and feel her relaxed body in your arms, you may be overwhelmed and buzzing with love, or feeling overstretched or exhausted because of the physical and the emotional demands of mothering; or a mixture of both.

If you have changed to bottle feeding sooner than you planned because you or your baby found breastfeeding difficult, you may feel relieved if stopping breastfeeding leaves you and your baby less stressed, particularly if she had difficulty gaining weight. Alternatively, you might be upset or feel as if you have failed. In some circles there is a lot of stigma attached to bottle feeding. But it may be by far the best option for a mother and baby, and the wider family, and it is a perfectly acceptable, loving and healthy way of feeding your baby.

Defending yourself or justifying your choice can be emotionally tiring, however. So if you feel pressurised by other people's or your self-imposed expectations, remember that you are still giving your baby good nutrition for her growth and the love and contact that she enjoys so much. If you still feel criticised, talk to someone who you know supports your choice.

Water softeners

Water softeners work by replacing hard insoluble calcium with sodium (from salt). Although the water is not salty to taste it will have higher concentrations of sodium, which is dangerous for small babies' kidneys.

- Do not use domestic softened water for your baby. The manufacturer of the water softener will have advised the installer to leave at least one tap out of the system, to deliver mains water.
- It is also best to boil mains water. Mains water that has been put through a filter will still need to be boiled and cooled before you give it to your baby.

The practicalities of feeding

Essential equipment

- **Bottles:** You'll need at least six bottles: 250–280 ml (8–9 fl oz) size will last the whole year. Bottles come with teats, flat caps and tops and can be bought in sets. Try a selection of different colours, as some babies form strong habits: if you give your baby variety now, he's less likely to complain if you change bottles later.
- **Teats:** Teats come in various shapes and sizes. Some are reputed to be orthodontic friendly and teats for wide-necked bottles are slightly closer to the breast in shape. Start with newborn (slow) flow.
- **Cleaning equipment:** Buy a special bottle brush. Teat brushes are also available.

Optional extras

- **Pre-sterilised bags:** You can buy bottles with disposable pre-sterilised liners. They minimise the amount of air inside the bottle by contracting as the milk empties and are often recommended for babies suffering from colic (p.431).
- **Bottle coolers:** Use a standard picnic cool bag or buy a purpose-made bag to keep prepared bottles cool when you're on the move.
- **Bottle warmer:** Handy for warming up a bottle when you're not near a stove. Wrap a cold bottle in the thermostatically controlled warmer and it heats within minutes.
- **Mixing jugs:** You can get special jugs to prepare a whole day's feeds and pour the contents into individual bottles.
- **Bottle-drying rack:** A useful tool to keep bottle paraphernalia away from the rest of the washing-up.

Making up feeds

If you plan in advance it needn't take more than 10 minutes to make up all the feeds you need for a day.

- Wipe clean the area and wash your hands.
- Boil water in a clean pan and leave it (covered) to cool. You can use tap water, but not water that has been boiled repeatedly, as this increases its sodium content. Do not use filtered water.
- Wash and sterilise your bottles, teats and caps, and any jug you are using for mixing.
- Using the measuring scoop provided, follow the instructions for mixing precisely (usually 35 ml [1 fl oz] of water to one level scoop of powder). Always add the powder to the pre-measured boiled and cooled water. Place the cap on the bottle, beneath the teat, and shake it well so the formula dissolves. Some powders don't mix well unless the water is fully cooled.
- When you're ready to feed, take the cap out from beneath the teat and heat the bottle in a pan of water until the milk is just a little warmer than your body temperature. Shake the bottle to ensure the heat is distributed evenly, and test it by dripping a little on the inside of your wrist. If it feels hot rather than warm, cool it by standing in cold water or holding under a running tap.
- Don't use a microwave as it can heat the milk in patches so some parts are dangerously hot.
- If your baby drinks only half the milk in a bottle, do not give her the remainder later or save it for the morning; germs breed rapidly in warm milk and can lead to infection.
- Don't keep the boiled water or any made-up feeds for longer than 24 hours.

Cleaning and sterilising

Your baby has a very sensitive digestive system and for the first year is particularly susceptible to bacterial infection, so it is important that everything that she sucks and drinks is sterile.

Always clean bottles thoroughly in hot soapy water using a bottle brush that is not used for ordinary washing up, and make sure all milk deposits are cleaned off. Turn the teats inside out and squeeze them lightly to test for blockages. Everything should be thoroughly rinsed. After cleaning, sterilise everything used for preparation and feeding. If your bottles or teats become damaged or torn, throw them away as cracks trap dirt.

- **Boiling:** Immerse everything in a pan of water and boil for 10 minutes. Keep the bottles in the sealed pan until you are ready to make them up. Regular boiling can shorten the life span of teats.
- **Steaming:** Electrically operated steam units sterilise very effectively without chemicals and are large enough to hold a good quantity of bottles and accessories. The sterilisation cycle takes 10–12 minutes, turning off automatically, and it can be re-used soon after – handy when you're in a hurry or discover you're one teat short. You can also use a standard vegetable steamer, but if you do, keep it for bottle use only and watch it while it's on the heat (15 minutes); the water will evaporate if left boiling for too long.
- **Chemical sterilisers:** Sterilising units use cold water and a chemical solution or soluble tablets. This sterilises in 30 minutes and items can be left soaking for up to 24 hours. When you are ready to make up the feeds, every part of the bottle kit needs to be rinsed well with previously boiled and cooled water.
- **Microwave:** Special sterilisers are available for use in microwaves, designed to avoid any 'cold spots'. The microwave is not otherwise a suitable method for sterilising.
- **Dishwashers:** After cleaning your bottles and teats with a brush, you can run them through a dishwasher cycle that may be hot enough to sterilise them, and you'll need to make up the feeds as soon as the washing programme has finished.

Sleeping like a baby: weeks 1–12

Sleeping goes hand-in-hand with feeding and for the first 8 weeks after birth most of your baby's day will be taken up doing one of these two activities. He needs to eat little and often and will wake up regularly to make sure that he gets his fill. While he sleeps, he grows and, like his body, his brain never stops developing. Of sleep time, 80% is spent dreaming, working out the world and reliving experiences on a subconscious level.

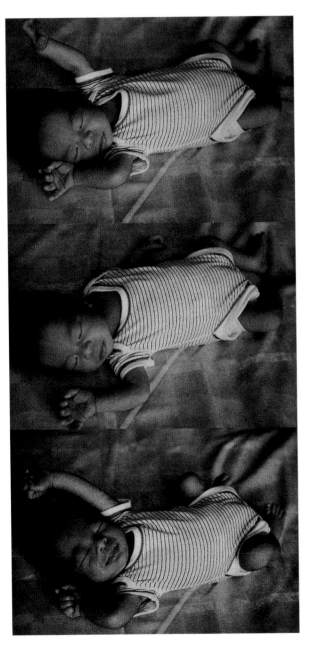

Your baby's sleeping rhythm

Babies' sleeping habits present the most common difficulties for parents. Primarily, this is because it's a huge challenge to adopt a pattern that involves very few long stretches of sleep and many parents are shocked at just how demanding it is. Waking twice or more in the night is normal in the early weeks but as your baby settles his waking will reduce. Some babies settle into an adult-like sleeping pattern by the end of their sixth week, sleeping mostly at night and having a couple of naps during the day. Many babies, however, do not. Parents are often surprised that babies need guidance.

Sleeping is as important to your baby as breathing, and as significant for his development as kicking, touching, sucking and seeing. He will sleep as much as he needs to and it is never a waste of time, it is part of his development. Growth regulatory hormones are released in larger and more frequent pulses in sleep. In the first 6–8 weeks his rhythm may suit you well and pose no difficulties: perhaps you need to wake once to feed him between the hours of midnight and 6am. Alternatively, his sleeping pattern might be out of synch with your own. By the time you both reach the end of the third month, your habits may be much more co-ordinated.

Deep sleep and light sleep

The different stages of slumber range from deep, dreamless sleep to light, dream or REM (rapid eye movement) sleep. Your baby can also seem awake but be so restful that he's almost in light sleep. Generally speaking, once he is in deep sleep he won't be stirred by noises, lights or movements. After anything from 5 to 45 minutes he'll surface to light sleep, twitch and smile as he dreams. He may then fall back into deep sleep if he's not distracted by something he can see or hear or by a feeling of hunger or discomfort. The sleep cycles get longer as he gets older.

As you pass from deep sleep to dream sleep you may wake, roll over and go back to sleep totally unaware that you have woken. This is because you have sleep clues – dark room, comfy bed, etc. Your baby may open his eyes during REM sleep and appear awake (this is a common reason for parents to say that their baby doesn't sleep well).

If you pick him up during this 'eyes open but asleep' state, he will wake up but become fractious and irritable. A baby needs to 'learn' his sleep clues. If these are being breastfed, rocked to sleep or sucking a dummy he will need these clues again when he wakes at night. You can teach him new clues, which will enable him to fall asleep on his own. A normal baby will wake up about 20 times a night and even if he gets back to sleep 90% of the time, just two or three occasions when he doesn't settle himself can be hard for him as well as his parents. Most parents who have 'problems' in fact have entirely normal babies but are striving for some ideal sleep pattern that doesn't exist.

Sleep and wake cycles start to change from birth with gradual lengthening of the wakeful period and a reduced need for sleep, with sleep periods becoming consolidated into blocks. Eventually your baby will take the longer naps and sleep overnight, as is considered 'normal'. This is a learnt process, which can take several years, and it is easily disturbed during babyhood and infancy. Little wonder that broken sleep is so significant in the first few years of life.

Comfort in sleep

Some babies adapt to sleeping in their own cot or basket quickly and others take persuasion and time to feel confident when away from their mother. You may be happy to let your baby sleep against your chest in a sling, or rest with him each time he falls asleep and share your bed at night. The bliss of having your baby sleep in your arms or on your chest is a privilege that only lasts a few weeks, and you might want to indulge in this.

Keeping your baby warm and safe

Your baby will probably be happiest if he is sleeping in your bedroom for the first 3 months or longer. He can sense you and you can hear his steady breathing and go to him easily when he cries. You might choose to share your bed or he can be in a Moses basket or crib for 3 or 4 months. If he turns out to be a very light sleeper and is woken by you snoring or moving, or you find his snores or grunts stop you from sleeping, it may be better for him to sleep in a separate room. Whenever and wherever your baby sleeps it's important that he's safe.

- To reduce the risk of sudden infant death syndrome (SIDS) (p.213) lie your baby on his back.
- Lie your baby on his back with his toes at the end of the cot in the 'feet-to-foot' position.
- Tuck blankets and sheets in well so there is no risk of him covering his face: even when he's small he can wriggle and may pull loose covers over his face.
- Use flannelette sheets and blankets made of natural fibres. Fitted sheets over the mattress are more comfortable because they don't crease or ruffle.
- An extra sheet or cloth beneath his head will catch dribbles or vomit and can be washed easily.

Swaddling
Second best to your embrace is wrapping or swaddling, a practice that has been successful for mothers and babies for thousands of years. It may help your baby sleep longer because it stops him from waking himself with the jerky body movements of light sleep. Once you have the basic technique you can swaddle your baby while he's in your arms and pass him gently into his cot or into your bed. Some babies don't like to be swaddled (and make this quite clear with angry cries), but for many it can work wonders.

After 6–8 weeks your baby will probably want more freedom of movement and may be too large to swaddle comfortably. His own body movements should no longer wake him. If you think he misses being swaddled, tuck a blanket snugly around his waist.

Lie your baby on a bed sheet (or a cellular blanket if it's cold), folded in a triangle, with his neck in the centre of the longest edge and the pointed apex beneath his feet. Gently hold his right arm by his side and pull the sheet over, tucking it under his left buttock. Then bring the other side of the sheet over his left arm and tuck it under his right side. If he sucks his fingers, bend his arms across his chest before wrapping so he has access to them. Another sheet or blanket tucked over the top of your baby will help him feel held and will keep his legs down as they twitch in light sleep; be careful, though, not to over-wrap him. Note the outside temperature, the number of layers you are wearing, and never use more than four layers of sheets or blankets to cover him. If it's hot, he may only need his swaddling sheet.

- Use up to, but no more than, four layers on the bed in addition to what your baby is wearing (which should be no more than a vest and a babygro); count any swaddling sheet or blanket as well as outer sheets and blankets and never use a quilt or duvet. If it is hot, reduce the number of layers.
- Make sure the surface is flat and supportive, without being too soft. This is best for his developing spine. Baby mattresses are designed to give the right support.
- If you are all in bed together, remember that your body heat will contribute to his warmth, so clothe him lightly. Overheating is dangerous.

Your baby may kick off blankets but won't be able to pull them back again so it will be up to you to check him and adjust the bedding according to temperature. In the first 3 months he cannot easily produce heat. If you take him out of bed for a feed or he wakes because he is cold, hold him close so he can use your heat to warm up. If he kicks off the blankets and wakes up, try a baby sleeping bag or sleep suit but remember that these are more insulating than blankets and you won't need extra coverings. If he's in your bed he's unlikely to get cold but he may get hot.

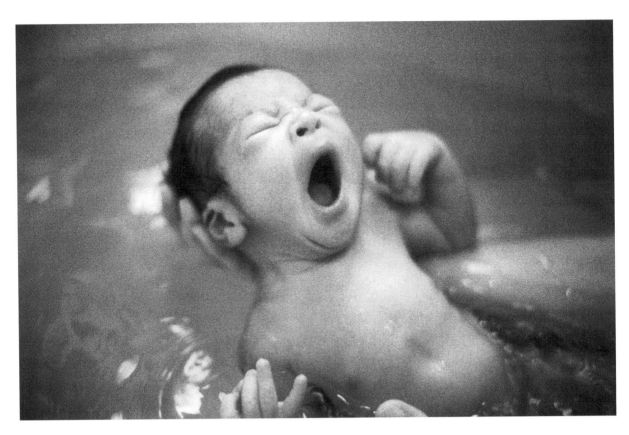

Three in a bed

In many parts of the world families sleep together for many years. There are many advantages of sharing. For your baby, there is nothing more natural than sleeping beside you, feeling your breath and heartbeat. It also encourages milk flow and night-time breastfeeding may be simple. You may, in time, welcome more children into your bed. Co-sleeping is safe for babies – you and your partner will be aware of his presence except if you are drunk or take drugs.

There may be disadvantages, however. If you do not sleep soundly tiredness may mount, and you or your partner may feel that your baby is intruding into your personal space. Safety is an issue when your baby is able to roll and crawl out of bed.

If you do share now, later you might want to give your baby his own space. You could lay his Moses basket next to your bed or use a three-sided cot level with your bed, and bring him into bed after you have had some time with your parner, or for a feed. Many children crawl into their parents' bed each morning for years and feel welcomed.

Newborn sleep patterns

A newborn baby usually sleeps between 16 and 19 hours each day, waking up every 2–3 hours to eat and sometimes napping for less than an hour at a time. It is unusual to sleep for more than 4 or 5 hours at a stretch, although some babies do sleep for more than that, maybe for up to 8 or 10 hours at night-time. This is all right providing that the baby is healthy.

There are many factors that affect sleep: the experience of being born, the need for food and the comfort of sucking, dream activity, reaction to light, noise and movement and the ability to adapt to different environments. Your baby's pattern will determine your day: no longer a division of 24 hours into day and night, but a collection of 2- or 4-hourly segments.

In the days after birth your baby will drop off to sleep after most feeds, and often mid-feed – he cannot stop himself. He may be staring at you intently one minute and drifting into dreams the next, or sucking eagerly at your breast then suddenly falling into a deep sleep. And despite his need to rest he'll be woken often by new sensations, such as hunger.

In each 24-hour period your baby will almost certainly have at least one long snooze lasting from 2 to 5 hours. He will also have at least one period when he's particularly alert – this is often early evening or first thing in the morning. As you spend time with him you will see the pattern and recognise signs of tiredness – crying, yawning, swollen eyes, drooping eyelids. When he's tired you could hold and rock him so he can sleep with you, or put him in his pram or cot. Remember that it's not good for him to sleep in his car seat on a regular basis – reserve it for use in the car.

Night-time, bedtime

In the days after birth some babies are like night owls, perky and alert when everyone else sleeps; others are larks and put all their energy into daytime, sleeping soundly at night. All, however, need to learn about sleeping more at night than during the day. You can help your baby make the distinction between day and night from an early age. In the day lie him down for naps in a pram or a basket in your living space or let him sleep on you, and don't worry about noise levels; use the cot or crib or your bed in the quiet bedroom for night-time, and perhaps for one or two long naps during the day. Keep his night sleeping environment dim and uninteresting; when he surfaces from deep sleep, which he will do as often as 20 times a night, he may open his eyes momentarily and it's best that he's not stimulated.

You can also help him recognise bedtime by giving a cue that marks it apart from any other time of day. Generations of mothers have seen how quickly a baby can form habits, and behavioural scientists have shown through studying the brain (p.27) that habits can be established early on. If you always give your baby a bath and a feed in a certain place, or play a certain piece of music before putting him to bed, and subsequently repeat it over 10 days, he will soon automatically respond by drifting to sleep.

Newborns are often alert and active between around 8 and 10pm or midnight, so it may be best to begin a bedtime routine around 9 or 10pm. It doesn't matter that your baby wakes one or two times in the night for a feed. What's important is the routine. With it, you'll find it easier to bring bedtime forwards to 7 or 8pm when your baby is older: he'll know the cues for sleep and respond to these rather than the time shown by the clock. Sometimes a familiar bedtime routine helps a baby feel settled. It may take many weeks until you establish this routine, and it is important to remember that as your baby grows his patterns may alter and the boundaries you have set need to alter accordingly.

If you can alternate with your partner or involve another person in the routine, you will have the option of relaxing or going out on some evenings.

Introducing sleep patterns

If you wish to have a routine to your day, remember it is important not to introduce this from day one (p.178) because you will need time to get to know your baby's rhythms, and he needs to feed often. Yet as early as the second week or as late as the tenth, your baby will cry less and begin to sleep more peacefully and ask for milk at regular intervals. This is a good time to follow his lead and structure the day, if you wish to.

Your baby may sleep between 9 and 10am one day, 9.30 and 10.30am the next, and 8.30 and 9.15am the next. Though the times are not the same, there is a clear pattern emerging. At night he may get tired at around 8pm (with variations between 8.30, 9 and 7pm), which suggests a point around which you can weave a familiar night-time routine. To bring some order to daytime naps, and improve sleep quality when napping, you could put him to sleep in a quiet bedroom or in his pram for a long afternoon nap. If he surfaces into light sleep and wakes, a gentle rock or stroke may help him go back into deep sleep.

When your baby is tired he may still cry if you lie him down awake – many babies need help to fall asleep. It may take him time to relax and when he's weary he'll feel more vulnerable than usual. Stay with him, stroke or rock him, talk or sing softly. If you know he is tired you may feel comfortable to step out of the room for a couple of minutes while he calms down – some babies need to cry themselves to sleep.

Depending on your approach and your baby's character, it may be a week before he begins to fall asleep without complaint, or it may take several months. Many parent and baby partnerships have to work long and hard at timing, comfort and making the separation from one another. Some never let go of falling asleep in one another's embrace.

Night-time sleeping

In the third month your baby may naturally begin to sleep for longer at night. Ideally he will only wake when he is hungry and this may be predictable, for example after 4 or 5 hours, and if he is sleeping happily during the day he is more likely to sleep peacefully at night. But he may also wake because he is uncomfortable, wants to be with you or has had a bad dream, and there will be some nights when he sleeps better than others.

To cut down on night waking, begin by working with bedtime. If you want your baby to go to sleep at 8pm each night but he is usually alert until his 10 o'clock feed, start by bringing his 10 o'clock feed forwards by 5–15 minutes every other day, winding him down beforehand with cuddles or a gentle massage. Feed him in his bedroom, reduce noise in the bedroom (television, music, other children, chatter), ensure he has a clean nappy and is comfortable, and settle him in your usual way. Continue to bring bedtime forward, bit by bit. Remember to take it easy – it may take effect in weeks but could take months.

Having gone to bed, your baby will sleep until he wakes for a feed. If he wakes before you expect him to, don't leave him to cry, for even if he cries himself back to sleep he will wake again soon, even more hungry, and you will have been denied two batches of sleep. It is best to go to him and give him comfort and reassurance and a feed if he is hungry. You could try waking him for a feed before you go to sleep (11pm or midnight) in the hope of reducing his hunger later in the night, and he may sleep for 6 or 7 hours. Loosen his blankets and let him rise into light sleep before picking him up. This works for some babies, but some cannot rouse themselves from sleep to take a proper feed and still wake in the middle of the night, directed by an internal rhythm that's more powerful than parental needs.

If you have a routine around bedtime or night feeds that is working, stick by it but keep flexible. Remember that the boundaries can be dynamic: you may aim for 8pm but settle for 8.30 if that suits your baby better, and occasionally put him to bed much earlier if he is

---

My baby is 6 weeks old, and I know when he's getting tired. He nods off in my arms but wakes as soon as I put him down. Although I love cuddling him, I don't sleep well and I'm exhausted. What can I do?

The first thing to do is to be sure your baby is nourished and gaining weight and is medically fit and well. Illness, pain or failure to thrive may disturb his sleep. He obviously needs to feel secure before he can fall asleep soundly. There are several ways you can help him. If he is falling asleep after a feed, take him off the breast or bottle as he is dozing off, so he falls asleep in your arms. When he does this, try swaddling him and lying him down awake but tired – warm his bedding so it mimics your body temperature. Slide your hands gently from beneath him and place one on his chest or head and stroke him for reassurance. He may also be comforted by your voice, smell or the sight of your face, so sit close. If he cries, resist picking him up straight away but stay close, soothing him. Gradually withdraw and leave when he is asleep.

At first you may be with him for half an hour and give him one or two cuddles before he dozes off, but if you persist, after several days he may fall asleep in 5 minutes. You are guiding him and both your lives will be easier when he manages to sleep well.

Other ways to help your baby fall asleep out of your arms include pushing him in the pram or taking him for a drive in the car. Though handy, try to phase these out – they don't give you a break and your baby is not learning that it's safe and comfortable to fall asleep in his cot at night.

particularly tired at night. If your baby is upset and crying when he 'should' be asleep, go to him and give him the comfort he needs. He is still very young and needs to know you are there.

Daytime sleeping: your settled baby

If, by 10 weeks, your baby wakes more than once between the hours of midnight and 6am and doesn't go back to sleep easily, a daytime pattern may help him sleep better at night. Regular daytime sleeps also help him keep happy and energetic. If your baby sleeps for 2 or 3 hours twice a day, shortening one nap could help him sleep longer at night. As he surfaces from deep sleep gently wake him, perhaps offering the comfort of a feed to bring him round. See how he reacts – he may feel more rested after an hour's sleep or rest sufficiently in 30 minutes. For many babies it's better to keep the longer rest in the afternoon. If your baby sleeps from 2 until 5pm, keep him awake until bedtime – a feed, a play, a massage and bath and another feed will set him up for a good sleep. If he naps between noon and 3pm, let him have a rest around 5pm for around 30 minutes if he's tired, and then work towards bedtime in your usual way.

What your baby does when awake contributes to how he sleeps. Keep daytime active and interesting, feeding his curiosity and filling his senses: play with him, let him kick and exercise, introduce him to new sights, sounds and smells, and incorporate some quiet time. Try to keep the last 30 minutes or hour quiet so he doesn't go to bed while his mind is racing. Satisfy his thirst and hunger too – well-structured feeds help stabilise energy levels and lead to calmer sleep.

If your baby falls asleep outside nap times it's because he needs to – you can alter the rest of the day's structure accordingly and go back to your routine the next day or make changes if his needs have altered. He will have sleepy days and wakeful days and as he grows he'll need less sleep during the day. Remember, too, that your baby may not be ready to slot into a timed routine and in the first weeks your routines alter as the baby grows.

Your influence

The needs and sleeping patterns of individual babies vary enormously. As you help your own baby learn about day and night, remember that your influence can be very strong. Sometimes a baby needs guidance, and his parents create a framework, but sometimes a baby is expected to slot into a routine that is not suitable for him. Very often, a parent's expectations reflect his or her childhood experiences more strongly than they reflect their own baby's character ('I hated being told when to sleep, so I won't do that to my son', 'Babies need to have 12 hours sleep a night and that's the way I was brought up'). Another common pattern is that a mother enjoys touching

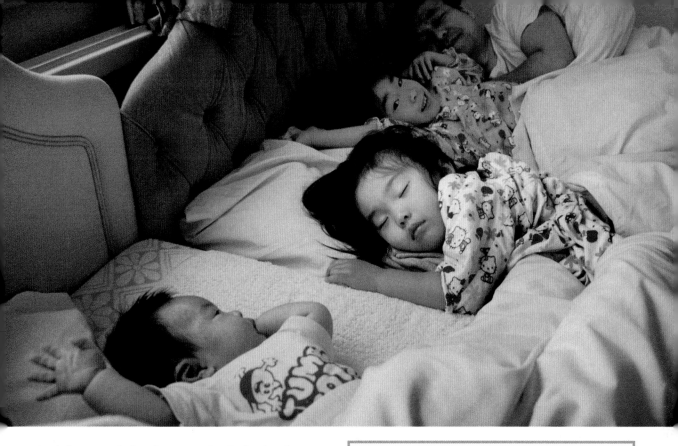

her baby so much that she unconsciously deprives her baby of long and undisturbed sleep – sometimes this reflects a deep longing to feel needed. With similar effect, parents who desperately want their baby to go to sleep may actually hinder it, because their baby senses anxiety and becomes tense.

If lack of sleep is a problem

Sometimes sleeping difficulties reflect a medical condition, and it is worth visiting your doctor or health visitor if you are worried. Yet concerns about sleeping are extremely common and most parents are tired at this early stage. Although persistence and consistency usually reap rewards not all babies respond to guidance. If your baby continues to wake frequently you need faith that things will get better and support to help you enjoy these early months.

The immediate priority is to look after yourself. If you get out of the house or take exercise, talk to others about your feelings and ask a friend or relative to babysit while you get some sleep; you may then catch up and feel more in control of your life. Your health visitor may offer good advice or run a sleep clinic and you may find a range of tips and complementary therapies suit your baby (p.535). It's usually the case that when a mother is less tired and lets go of her anxiety about sleep, her baby responds well, but it is also true that the first 3 months are for settling in. After this, it usually becomes easier to break the habit of night waking.

Sleeping easy

- Newborn babies wake every 2–3 hours for food – it's physiological and normal.
- It is normal for babies to surface from sleep 20 times at night.
- Keep your baby's night-time sleeping environment dim, quiet and unexciting.
- When you recognise signs of tiredness, encourage your baby to sleep.
- Warm up blankets and sheets on a radiator, so they are welcoming.
- Use daytime naps and bedtimes to learn what sends your baby to sleep, and then apply the techniques in the middle of the night if you need to.
- A baby who seems frustrated and won't sleep may need more stimulation during the day – play with him and let him kick and move his body. He might enjoy swimming or massage and stretching (p.365), which are known to promote good sleep.
- Occasionally, sleeping difficulties relate to a medical problem: consult your doctor or health visitor if you are concerned. Make sure his hunger and thirst are being satisfied and that he does not have pain or a food allergy or intolerance (p.391).
- If you are tired, ask for help so you can catch up on sleep.
- Aim to have at least one fixed point by the end of the third month – bedtime is best. This will help you order your days and have time to yourself and gives your baby orientation.
- Sleeping on the back is safest.

When your baby cries: weeks 1–12

Your baby's cry is her loudest way of letting you know how she feels and what she wants. When she cries, you can't ignore it and that's the way nature intends it to be: her cry can speed up your heart rate, sets off your mothering hormones, making you feel attentive and protective, and may bring milk to your nipples if you are breastfeeding. Like her cry, your response is instinctive.

What your baby is telling you

Like every other aspect of your baby's behaviour, crying is both a reflex and a reflection of her personality. In general, newborn babies cry for a total of between 2 and 4 hours in a day in short bursts with the odd prolonged bout. Usually crying signals, 'I'm hungry', 'I need to sleep', 'I need a cuddle', but at times it may be a means of self-expression. Sometimes you may be able to soothe your baby quickly, sometimes it will take half an hour or more. Some babies are mellow and seldom cry for long, while others are very vocal and there may be days when the parents wonder if crying ever stops.

Crying is the most urgent method of communication because it forces you to take notice. This is what your baby wants you to do – whether she's hungry, tired, upset, angry or bored, she needs you to organise her environment to suit her. When she does cry she shows you what she likes and doesn't like, what she can tolerate, what makes her tired, and how much she values your love and comfort. If she needs to feel secure she may ask you to tend to her constantly and if she's having an easy-going day your baby may be happy with things the way they are and communicate mainly through touch, movement and her loving eye contact.

In time, you will begin to recognise different cries. Your baby is capable of covering a staggering five octaves in pitch (that's half a piano) and she may have a huge repertoire. Depending on what she wants – food, games, cuddles, etc. – she will leave certain pauses and vary the intensity or loudness of the cry. If she's bored, for instance, she may cry intermittently, pausing as she waits to see if you're coming to be with her. But her cries do not necessarily express negativity – she may simply be expressing herself and in the first 6 months crying will be the most common and frequent sound she produces.

You may often be surprised by new expressions and learning her language will be an ongoing process. Unfamiliar wails and persistent crying may really worry you (as they do most parents at some stage). When you're worried, watch the clock – what may seem like an hour may only be 5 minutes. Use the checklist on this page and think about possible triggers that apply to your baby. If you are still worried, or think your baby is sick, call your doctor or health visitor and ask for medical advice. If your gut reaction is one of fear or panic there may be something in your baby's cry that signals danger: your parenting instinct will drive you to act quickly and find help.

As your baby becomes more settled she will cry less often, although there will be days (and nights) when she cries much more than usual. She is expressing her emotions and can switch from inconsolable crying to joy in an instant: she may yell in your arms for 20 minutes yet smile and flirt the minute she's passed to her daddy, or giggle as she plays on her mat then in the blink of an eye screw up her face and start screaming.

Why does your baby cry?

Communication
- All babies cry – it is a method of communication.
- It may be a request to be held – in the womb she was constantly held.
- It may signal tiredness.
- It may be a release of fear: this may have arisen during birth.

Hunger and digestion
- Hunger is the most common trigger.
- She may be uncomfortable from digestion, prior to opening her bowels or from wind.
- Colic is a potent cause.

What's happening
- Your baby may cry if she is too hot or cold, has a wet or dirty nappy, or clothes wet from dribbled milk.
- She may reflect tension anxiety or unhappiness in her family.
- She may be bored and want stimulation.
- She may need to release pent-up energy – a swim or massage may help.
- Many babies cry at a particular time (often in the evening).

Illness
- Crying when ill may seem whimpery and distraught: you may need medical help.
- If your baby is in severe pain, your instinctive response will be urgency or panic.

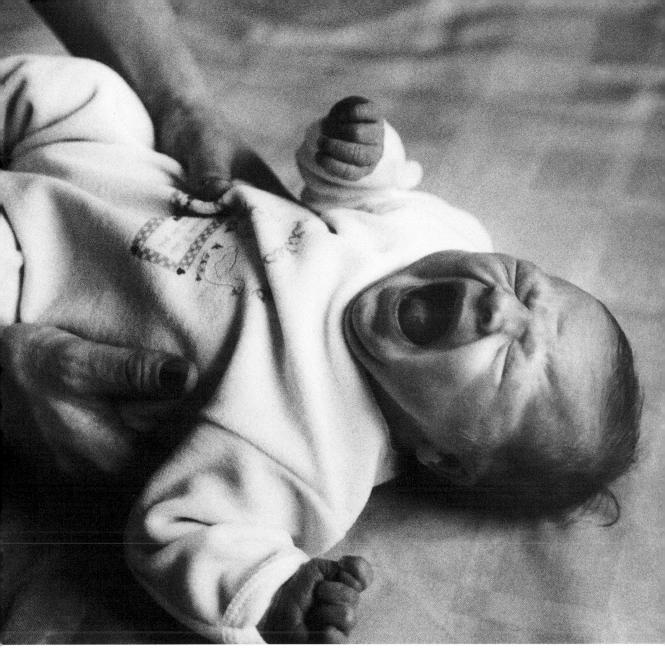

Soothing your baby

When your baby cries you'll have a gut feeling and may automatically go through the possible reasons. Your strongest instinct will be to pick her up and cuddle her, and often this alone will work as she feels your touch, hears your voice and smells your scent. If you stroke or massage her, her body will respond to the sensation of touch by slowing her heartbeat, regulating her breath and relaxing her muscles. Of course, when she's hungry, nothing but milk will do.

Your baby is in a new world – soothing her may be easier if you try to see things from her point of view. Is she angry or upset? Is her digestion troubling her? Think of the causes and talk to her gently, responding to her feelings: 'I know you're angry, and I can hear you', 'Does your tummy hurt? I will try and comfort you now', 'I know that so much is new and I will hold you.' She will not understand the words but she will hear your tone and know that you are there for her If she is not hungry, her nappy is clean and she has been winded, and you don't think that her crying indicates pain, the best thing may be to stick with her as a companion, listening to her as you hold her, and giving her love: 'There now, have a good cry, let it all out.' Accepting her bad times as well as her good times is an integral part of parenting. Between them, over the years, mothers, fathers and carers have devised countless ways to soothe babies, and you will find your own methods. Although it may be difficult, try to relax and let go of your own tension so that you can feel your instincts and be objective. You might find a walk in the pram or papoose does the trick, or a drive in the car soothes instantly. She may be calmed if you walk with her, dance or sing, and hold her in a certain way (on your shoulder with her ear by your cheek, or lying in your arms and looking at your face). Music, the sound of running water or the washing machine can have calming effects, or your baby may relax in a bath, or in a cosy bed with a familiar blanket or a dummy. When her crying is a request for attention and stimulation, she'll enjoy company, chit-chat, laughter and games and may be happier if you start off while you are holding her.

Evening fretting

Although not every baby has fretful times in the evening, most do, and few parents know why. Even health visitors and midwives often find it hard to explain. Your baby is likely to have an hour or two (or three, or four) when she cries almost non-stop and wants to do little else except suck at your breast or her bottle and doze in your arms. This may last for the first week or for as long as 5 or 6 weeks, between 4pm and 8pm, or later, between 8pm and midnight. What could cause this evening fretting?

- Your baby might find the busy life of the bright, wide world overwhelming and by the end of the day want to be bathed and held in a loving embrace, and have a constant supply of delicious warm milk. Darkening the room and reducing the stimuli often helps.
- Sometimes your baby may need to exercise or be actively massaged to use up any extra energy.
- If you are breastfeeding she may be crying because your milk supply has dipped because you are tired or haven't eaten well (p.186).
- Your baby may be extra hungry at a particular time of the evening, and a long feeding session may precede a long stretch of sleep at night.
- Another explanation for evening crying sessions is colic, a condition related to painful wind that strikes at the same times each day, often the evening (p.431).
- If you are tired and feel over-stretched your baby may reflect your anxiety with her own tension.
- Whatever the reason, you can be confident that unsettled evenings usually pass by around 10–16 weeks.

Coping with unsettled behaviour every evening can be very difficult, particularly if you need to make dinner for the rest of the family and care for other children. It can also be hard on your partner, particularly if you are on edge and feeling vulnerable, perhaps quick to snap at him. This is a common flashpoint between couples and by being aware of it you may avoid an argument when your partner returns from work. This will further deplete your energy.

You might find it less trying if you have support so you can preserve energy for later.

When your baby's crying time arrives, it often helps to go with it. Find a comfortable position – lying down is perfect if she wants to feed – and use the time to relax. Accepting that your baby needs to be comforted and probably needs to feed will probably minimise stress for you, whereas trying to stop her crying and get on with other things will be exhausting and ineffective. If you have a toddler you might be able to read him a story while feeding your baby.

While difficult evenings persist, write off any chance of doing anything else and get to sleep yourself as soon as your baby finally drops off. Put the answer phone on and don't worry about the washing-up. In several weeks, this stage of your baby's life will almost certainly have passed.

Leaving your baby to cry

In the late 20th century there was a prevailing opinion that tending to a crying baby instantly was a sure route to having a spoilt child. Attitudes have changed, however, and this is partly due to scientific research indicating that a baby actually cries less throughout the following 24 hours when her cries are answered promptly. In the early months your baby has the reflex to cry and as she gets older she will get better at over-riding her reflexive cry. Babies under 3 months of age do not cry because they are naughty.

As a mother, you are instinctively compelled to soothe her. This is quite natural and, while she is very young, it is exactly what she needs. If you want to pick her up and cuddle her, go ahead, because if you resist this loving contact you won't be happy, and nor will your baby. As she grows, she still needs to feel loved and supported but you will be able to communicate more clearly with her and introduce boundaries.

When she cries she is asking for something, and learns quickly whether she has been understood. If she regularly gets the result she's looking for she will trust you and feel comfortable to explore other means of communication – using her body, her eyes and her hands, and practise making speech-like sounds. If, on the other hand, her cries are persistently ignored, she may withdraw and she could find it hard to trust other people and be less vocal.

In your days and nights together, though, there will be times when you feel it's fine to put your needs before hers. Leaving your baby to cry is the first step you make as you define your individual spaces. There are several ways to 'leave your baby to cry' that needn't be soul-destroying, although cries for food or complaints of discomfort are best answered. At its most gentle, leaving your baby to cry means holding her and accepting that she needs to vent her emotions – crying is her language and you don't always need to 'fix'. With this view you may talk to her as she cries when she's not in your arms, for instance if you are getting dressed, making dinner or getting her pram ready – as you chat to her she'll feel that you're relaxed instead of worried, and may herself relax.

The most common time that you will leave your baby to cry is at night, when you wait to see if she will comfort herself or go back to sleep of her own accord. How long you wait before going in to her will be a very personal thing. At first 1 minute can seem like 10, and 5 minutes may seem like an eternity. Sometimes leaving her to cry for a few minutes is the most effective way for her to go back to sleep, but when you have waited as long as you want to, it's time to go to her. Give her a cuddle then put her down and sit with her and stroke or pat her so she knows you are there. Sing, talk or whisper if you like, and gradually withdraw. When you have left the room if she is still crying, watch the clock. Return to her as soon as you feel the need. You may need to return several times before she relaxes and settles. If this is a regular event, which it may be if she cries at bedtime, leave her for a minute longer each day. As the days pass you may return to her three and then two times, then once, and finally she may settle of her own accord.

Your baby is unlikely to suffer any psychological damage if she is left to cry for short periods now and then. Acknowledging her but delaying a cuddle for a few minutes gives her an early lesson in sharing time and space and may actually help her vent her emotions freely. If you think you cannot cope, you will certainly not be the first mother to feel this. It is an indication that you could benefit from support.

Soothing yourself

Alongside sleep deprivation, almost all parents find dealing with crying one of the toughest challenges of life with a baby. Crying can stimulate all kinds of feelings, and can be very draining – as well as creating noise, it pulls on your heart strings and can make you feel frustrated, guilty, inadequate or upset. When you've been up half the night, your baby's cry can render you angry, or tearful, or both.

You might find it easy to combine your attempts to soothe your baby with something that's relaxing for you: try bathing together with some lavender oil, massage your baby half an hour before her regular crying time, or play your favourite music and dance to it. Be honest with her too. You may be surprised how easy and relieving it is to admit how you feel: 'I feel trapped and frustrated, tired and unkempt, but I know you can't help it.' For you both this is more positive than saying, 'Shut up! I can't take any more crying.' Even while she is young, it's good for her to experience your negative as well as your positive emotions. When she is crying and you want to step aside, take yourself to a quiet room or into the garden for a few minutes before returning. It might help to have a cup of tea and sit down, or do a short burst of exercise or stretches or

have a good scream and hit some pillows to vent your feelings. Ear plugs may help to turn down the volume to a level that does not upset you.

The sound of your own baby crying and the flame of your parental instinct may bring up memories from childhood. If you had a troubled infancy the cries can put you in touch with these long-forgotten feelings. It might be worth asking your parents how you were as a baby and you may then understand why you respond to your baby's crying very intensely. This could soften your reaction to crying and help you soothe your baby more easily.

Remember that there is support around you, perhaps from your partner, mother, other relations or friends. At mother and baby groups or baby clinics you will meet others who are having a similar experience. If you are ready, let someone give you a break so you can recharge your batteries. If days pass and things don't get better, call your health visitor or doctor and let them know how you are feeling. Having a crying baby can contribute to depression and there are several ways of alleviating the stress, as outlined in the box below.

If your baby cries a lot

- It can be disheartening looking after a baby who doesn't seem happy, but most start to settle by the end of the first month. Have faith that crying is likely to diminish as your baby grows older. Take comfort that crying is usual and prolonged periods each day are common.

- Excessive crying may be due to a medical problem – seek advice, and consider complementary therapies (p.442).

- The fact that your baby cries does not mean that you are not a good enough parent. Accept as much help as you can, and try to meet other parents regularly. You may find tips and support from your local baby clinic or mother–baby group, or your GP, health visitor or paediatrician or from a support group.

- Although it can be embarrassing if your baby cries in public, try not to stay in because being isolated is worse than being embarrassed. Many of the adults you meet are parents themselves and know that it's natural for babies to cry.

- Look after yourself by eating well and rest as much as possible to keep milk levels high – sit quietly and focus on your breath or try a visualisation if you can't sleep. Even when you are bottle feeding, your own wellbeing is vital. Your own wellbeing is equally important if you are bottle feeding. Acknowledge that tension you or your partner feels may affect your baby.

- Some babies do cry more than others, and many find adjusting to the experience of birth and being in the world unsettling. A baby like this needs to be introduced to new objects and people gradually with the feeling of being emotionally and physically held and protected. Some are very active and need lots of stimulation plus plenty of time to unwind.

Daily babycare

The care of a tiny human being brings with it wonder and joy, loving embraces, and surprising surges of instinct and insight, as well as confusion and questions; yet, like every parent, you learn quickly. To being with checking for a dirty nappy may be the last thing that occurs to you when your baby won't stop crying, and bathing him may be daunting, but soon his presence in your arms or at your breast will feel 'right' rather than strange, and caring for him will be second nature. As the weeks pass and you and your baby get to know one another you'll go about the daily business of dressing, feeding and changing him with little thought for the details that might have thrown you at first.

Comfort at home

Most first-time mothers spend a great deal of time in their bedroom with their baby in the first week or for longer. Some mums are on the move and visiting with their baby after a week while others need to stay at home and settle in fully before they show their baby the big outside world. Everyone is different. In your home, make the most of 'cosy corners' (p.177) and, when you're out, take everything with you that you and your baby may need.

In your arms

How your baby likes to be carried may vary from hour to hour, day to day. Sometimes he may want to be held close and secure so he can doze, perhaps on your chest, or cradled in your arms where he can hear the familiar beat of your heart and feel the rocking motion of your body as you walk. At other times he may want to look around – holding him against your shoulder where his ear is close to your voice is good for this, or under his arms with his back against your chest.

Your baby will guide you as you learn. Something he enjoys when he has just fed may not suit him when he's ready for a play, and he may love lying across your chest in the first week but not by 3 months. Sometimes a change of position might settle a bout of crying or soothe colicky pains.

Lifting your baby

As your baby is lifted from the floor to your shoulder he passes through a space that is nine or ten times his own body length. He will rely on you and it won't take long before you both feel at ease. Holding his head is most important. With your hands and arms, large compared to his body, you can offer perfectly moulded support. Take it slowly. Slip one hand gently beneath his head and neck, and the other under his back. When your arms have taken his weight, lift him gently to your chest. Bend your knees if you are picking him up from the floor to avoid straining your back and to cut down his journey through space.

When you're putting him back down, don't take your hands away from under him until he feels supported where you have laid him down. If you tell him what you're planning to do and talk as you lift him, he'll know by your tone that change is coming and feel reassured as he is moved.

Lying and sitting

When he's not lying in your arms, the most comfortable position for your baby is to be lying down flat on his back. It's good for his spinal development and allows him to

---

My 2-week-old baby won't settle in my arms, whichever position I choose. He doesn't like being cuddled by anyone. Why not?

With trial and error, and what may be days of practice, you should soon find it easier to calm your baby and he will find it easier to settle in your arms. Some newborn babies, however, just don't like being cuddled. If you think this describes your little cherub, try not to take it to heart and do what you can to block out the little voice inside your head that may be saying, 'I'm not good enough'. It may be that he just doesn't like feeling enclosed, and could take some time (days, weeks or even months) to get used to being held.

For now you'll need to find alternative ways to be close, because if cuddling means crying, it's no fun for either of you. Your baby may love having his legs stroked and his toes tickled as he lies down on a rug and might love gentle massage. Let him see your face close up and give him long enough to study it while you talk softly to him. He may feel secure when he's swaddled. When his preferences change – and they almost certainly will – he'll enjoy being cuddled and your frustration will be firmly in the past.

If your baby is crying excessively you may need to see your doctor and ensure that he is not in pain or ill with colic (p.431) or another complaint.

kick, wriggle and punch the air with the reflex movements that help him to build up strength and get to know his body. He may not enjoy lying down alone at first; indeed, some babies take a few days or a couple of weeks before they feel confident enough to relax out of an adult's comforting arms.

When he does settle, make lying down interesting for him by staying close so he can explore your face, and giving him other things to look at (p.180). Give him time on his tummy so that he can strengthen his neck and shoulders as he strains to peer at the world. Now that sleeping on the tummy is warned against for safety reasons, this position is often forgotten or neglected and babies are not given the chance to exercise their upper bodies or develop their crawling reflex. He will be safe if you are with him and he is awake. Also try lying your baby face down across your knees so his face is unobstructed and he can kick freely.

After a couple of weeks your baby will be able to sit up in the reclined, supported position offered by a proper baby chair with safety straps. Car seats are not appropriate and do not offer good support. If the chair rocks or swings, he will love making this happen with vigorous kicking. You can prop up your baby with your hands and let him sit with you on the sofa or other comfortable chair, or use cushions to support him, but he will topple easily and should never be left unattended.

Dressing your baby

Before your baby arrives your preoccupations with dressing will probably be the number, size and colour of clothes. When you have your baby, your first concern quickly becomes dressing and undressing, something you may have to do several times a day. When he is still very young you may not wish to make a distinction between day and night clothes, but from the second month on the change into nightwear can be a useful part of a bedtime routine.

Most babies object to being undressed, as their warm outer coating is exchanged for cooler air and their hands and legs are pulled and squeezed into clothes. Make it less of an ordeal by laying your baby on a warm surface and being gentle but quick. As you pull a vest over his head, stretch it between your thumbs, put your thumbs inside it so they protrude through the neck, and lever the vest over his face keeping it clear of his forehead and nose as you cup his head with your fingers. Use front-opening overclothes as often as possible so you can lie your baby on them and button or popper them together easily. When you're trying to get his arms into sleeves, put your fingers through the sleeves, take his hand between your fingers and thumb, and ease the sleeve gently over his arm. With babygros, start matching the poppers from the top and there's less chance of getting it wrong.

Protection against cot death or SIDS

The tragic occurrence of death where no cause can be found, once commonly known as cot death, is now more often referred to as sudden infant death syndrome (SIDS) (p.510). Research over the years has pointed to a variety of possible causes, including overheating, yet the reasons remain elusive.

While it is important that you do what you can to protect your child, try not to let your worries cloud the wonderful days of your baby's early life: only one in 3000 babies a year die from SIDS (although the risk increases for premature babies). All babies are at reduced risk after 6 months, when their breathing systems have matured, and are considered to be out of risk by the age of 2 years.

What you can do to reduce the risk

• Place your baby on his back in the 'feet-to-foot' position to sleep (p.203).

• Not all babies settle in this position. If your baby is not comfortable on his back, lay him on his side, making sure that the underneath arm is brought forward to prevent him from rolling on to his tummy. In rare cases a baby will only settle on his tummy.

• Wall thermometers are widely available if you want to check room temperature: the optimum is between 18°C (64.4°F) and 22°C (71.6°F). If this is not comfortable for you, particularly through the night if you are sleeping in the same room, keep the room cooler and be aware of your baby's comfort, dressing him sensibly. Use lightweight, natural fibres because synthetic fabrics increase risks of overheating.

• Make sure that no blankets can cover your baby's head – he needs to lose heat from here – and also avoid using cot bumpers.

• Never over-wrap your baby. A useful rule of thumb is that he will feel comfortable in whatever you feel comfortable in, e.g. if you have one or two layers, this will suit him. This is especially true at night, when babies are frequently over-dressed.

• Check how warm your baby is by feeling his chest – not his hands and feet, which will often be cold.

• Do not put your baby to sleep beside a radiator or fire, or with a hot water bottle or electric blanket.

• Do not smoke in pregnancy. Do not smoke after you have given birth. Do not let anyone smoke near your baby.

• If you share your bed with your baby, make sure that heat loss from his head cannot be obstructed with a pillow and he is not overdressed under the covers (your body heat will warm him too).

• Do not let your baby sleep in your bed if you have drunk alcohol or taken drugs, are unwell or a very deep sleeper. You may unwittingly suffocate him.

• If your baby is unwell, seek advice immediately.

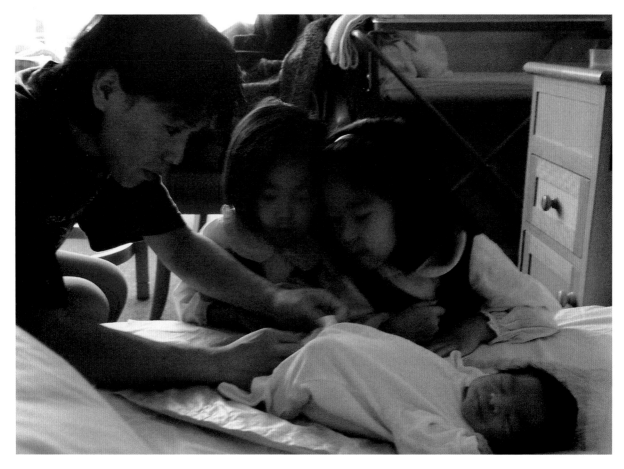

Keeping your baby warm

In the womb your baby never needed to accommodate to a change in temperature. As a newborn he finds it difficult to produce heat and may lose excessive heat if he is not wearing enough layers of clothing. Small babies have low fat stores and are particularly vulnerable to fluctuations in temperature. In the first month be wary of temperature changes inside and outside, and protect him from cold winds and hot environments.

After about 4 weeks your baby will be a little better at conserving heat, but he still won't cool down easily if he does get hot. Until he is around 12 weeks old, or over 5.4 kg (12 lb) in weight, he'll rely on you to regulate his temperature.

When he falls into a deep sleep, think ahead and add or remove covers before his body temperature changes rather than waiting until he is too hot or too cold. Remember to remove hats, along with coats and other extra clothing as soon as you enter warm buildings. At night-time don't use cot bumpers, pillows or duvets, and make sure that the bedclothes won't accidentally cover your baby's head. When it's hot outside, it's fine to leave your baby's skin exposed.

Don't let your baby get too hot

Your baby will let you know if he's too hot – he will have flushed cheeks, may sweat and will probably cry. Sometimes overheating is due to a combination of body contact, warm room temperature and excessive clothing, and sometimes to too much bedding. To cool him, remove clothing or a blanket, or take him to a cooler room, but be careful not to let him cool too much.

On a very hot day strip your baby down to his vest and make use of cool spots such as the shade beneath trees – keep exposure to direct sunlight to a minimum, and always use sun block. If you're travelling in a hot car, keep him shaded and try hanging a wet towel or cloth over a slightly opened window to give an instant air-cooling effect. You can also cool him by fanning him with your hand or a book, or bathe him gently with a warm sponge or wet cotton wool and help him lose the heat by evaporation.

Nor too cold

If he is chilly, pick up your baby and cuddle him before putting on extra clothes. Your body heat will help him warm up, but adding an extra blanket to his already cold body will not. Signs of coldness include unusually rapid breathing, crying, pale appearance, a cold chest and back. Shivering is very uncommon in babies under 3 months, as the mechanism is not yet established. This is one reason cool babies cannot warm up, as they are unable to activate the muscle furnace that leads to re-warming by shivering. Usually a cool baby will warm up when moved to a warmer environment.

A baby who is becoming dangerously chilled may be quiet (since he has no spare energy for crying), and lie quite still, but should respond well to a cuddle and a warm feed in a warmer place. If he's not helped to warm up he might cool down to the extent that his bodily functions slow down dangerously. If this happens, he will have pink hands and feet, seem floppy and unresponsive and remain cold to the touch. This is called neonatal cold injury (p.486) and needs to be dealt with urgently by medical professionals.

Nappies

Many mothers and fathers have never changed a nappy before they have their own baby. Don't worry if this is you – you will soon learn to do it quickly even when your baby is wriggling or you are stuck in the back of the car. This is parenthood! If you can spend time with a young baby before you give birth, you'll have a head start and a little more confidence.

How often you change your baby's nappy will depend on his diet, skin sensitivity and digestive system. If his nappy is uncomfortable, he'll let you know, and he may soon settle into a pattern. As a guide, expect to go through

---

I always try to use environmentally friendly products. What is the benefit of using washable nappies, and how convenient are they?
Disposable nappies are environmentally unfriendly and are also very costly over the years. If you use washable nappies you'll avoid adding to buried waste across the country, and although you will consume energy washing (and drying) them, there is a certain satisfaction in knowing that you can use them again and again. You will, however, have to put in a lot of work. Soiled nappies need to be soaked prior to washing and you may build a backlog of wet nappies if you don't have a drier. To ease your work, you could use a mixture of washables and disposables, or make use of a nappy service at roughly the same overall cost as using disposables. Your health visitor will be able to give you details.

There's a wide variety of washable nappies on the market. These are no more likely to give your baby nappy rash, although they do not draw urine away from the skin as effectively, and may need to be changed more frequently.

between six and ten nappies in every 24 hours over the first few weeks. You'll need to change the nappy as soon as he has passed a stool, but don't set him down on the changing mat straight away – he may take 5 minutes to complete his motion. When his nappy is wet he'll need it changed roughly every 3 hours.

During the night there's no need to disturb him with a nappy change unless it is soiled or he has sensitive skin or nappy rash. He can safely wait until morning. On the other hand, a nappy change is worthwhile if you want him to wake for a feed, or think a change when he wakes at nigh will help him go back to sleep soundly.

Changing times will often be very quick, but can also double as 'getting-to-know-you' time. Encourage nappy-free play as often as possible, giving your baby space to kick and stretch freely, and to feel air on his skin. This is particularly important if he has nappy rash. With nappy-changing equipment close to hand in the 'cosy corners' of your home, you can fit this essential task seamlessly into your day.

The details

You'll need a plastic changing mat with a flannelette covering or a towel to take away the chill, a spare nappy, a nappy-sack, plastic bag or a bin within reach, some cotton wool and lukewarm water. Your new baby's skin is very sensitive, so save baby wipes for when you're away from home or for cleaning a really messy stool. Always lie him on the floor or on a wide and secure surface, and don't forget your own wellbeing: kneel if you're using the floor, or use a changing table that is the right height so you won't strain your back.

Girls should be cleansed from front to back to prevent urinary infections. When you are changing a boy's nappy, never pull back his foreskin, and hold his penis down when you're putting on the clean nappy; if left free you or he may get a squirt in the face, and if it's pointing upwards when the nappy's on, urine may leak out of the top. Incidentally, fresh urine is sterile and will not hurt you or your baby. After each change, always wash your hands. This is particularly important if your baby has recently had a polio vaccination because the live virus can be carried in faeces.

My baby's faeces are green and very alarming. Is this normal?
Green motions are common. Most frequently they are associated with a change from breast to bottle feeding and are harmless. For some babies, more commonly breastfed, but occasionally bottle fed, the passing of a green motion is associated with insufficient feed. If green stools persist and your baby was thriving but is now gaining weight poorly, you will need to follow your doctor's advice (p.563).

To care for your baby's skin, rub a small amount of pure oil on to the nappy area after a change – almond or grapeseed oil or calendula cream are good. Some families habitually use barrier creams as prevention against nappy rash (p.531) but it's generally better for the skin to breathe. Some creams moisturise while others (petroleum based) repel liquid and can help sore skin to heal.

What goes in must come out: excreting

An unborn baby's intestines are filled with sticky, greenish-black meconium. While a few babies pass meconium in the womb, and some at birth, most have their first bowel movement within 48 hours of birth. If your baby does not have his first bowel by this time, tell your midwife who will probably recommend that your baby see a paediatrician, because there may be a blockage.

If your baby is breastfed, he will soon begin to pass stools that vary in colour from bright yellow to pale green, usually no thicker than margarine but often quite runny, and smelling little stronger than soured milk. Sometimes they may be mixed with mucus (particularly if he has a cold) or seem curdled. A bottle-fed baby's stools are usually thicker looking and stronger smelling, as well as darker in colour.

Your baby may have a soiled nappy nearly every time you change it, but it would be equally normal for him not to pass a stool for 3 or 4 days, providing he does not seem unwell. This is more common in breastfed babies. After around 6 weeks he may fall into a pattern of passing a stool at a particular time of day.

If your baby goes for several days without passing a stool, or passes a hard stool after a few days, he may be constipated. You can relieve constipation (p.435) by giving your baby more liquid (more breastfeeding or pre-boiled water in a sterilised cup or bottle, heated to body temperature), but you should also seek medical advice.

If your baby soils every nappy with unusually loose and watery stools and you're worried that he has diarrhoea (p.446), keep a soiled nappy in a plastic bag and take it to your doctor, who will check for an intestinal infection. Bowel actions in babies can vary a lot over just a few hours, and everything may return to normal soon. However, if your baby seems unusually lethargic, is feverish or is vomiting, you need to seek medical attention for him as a matter of urgency.

Urine

A healthy newborn baby will urinate frequently. If your baby has a dry nappy when you change him, and it is still dry after a couple of hours even after he has fed, watch him. If it is very hot he may be using up more fluid than usual, but he could also be starting a fever. Give him as much to drink as he wants. If he then urinates, there is no problem. If his urine is very dark and concentrated, he simply needs more to drink. One problem with the very absorbent nappies is that it can be very difficult to detect small amounts of urine.

Newborn baby girls often pass stringy white mucus, occasionally mixed with streaks of blood from their vagina. This is because of withdrawal of maternal hormones in their system and is nothing to worry about. In the first few weeks of life boys and girls may have pink staining of the nappy, with what appears to be flecks of blood mixed with urine. This is, in fact, not blood, but chemicals called urates, which glow pink.

Keeping your baby's body clean

How often you choose to bathe your baby will depend on your personal preferences, and on how dirty he gets on a particular day; some parents bathe their baby morning and night, others give a bath once a week and a gentle wipe down once a day. Your cleaning routine will also be determined by your baby: if bathtime is unpopular, reduce the frequency of baths, at least until your baby begins to enjoy the water.

Your baby's skin is finer than an adult's, with more sensory receptors and a larger number of pores, sebaceous glands and hair follicles per square centimetre. This means that it is capable of absorption to a higher degree than an adult's skin. It's important, then, to treat it gently with the purest products you can get.

If your budget allows, use clothes made from soft cotton fibres rather than nylon, which stops the skin from breathing, and oils, creams or bath preparations that are derived from plants. These enhance your baby's skin's natural cleansing and moisturising properties. Mineral-based products are derived from crude petroleum and block the skin's pores.

Bath time can be a wonderful part of the day when your baby delights in the feeling of weightlessness and warm water. It can also be a time when he screams angrily and wriggles and kicks. In the first few weeks there is no need to bath your baby every day unless he is dirty from milk, vomit, faeces or urine. If he doesn't enjoy it, a short dip will do – as little as a minute – and gradually he will be happy spending longer in the water.

It is important to keep his vital areas clean, though, with a simple 'top-to-toe' routine. Wash his bottom as you do at nappy times, and wash his face gently with cotton wool dabbed in cooled, boiled water, using a different piece of cotton wool for the mouth and nose and for each eye and ear, and paying special attention to the folds in his neck, which easily trap dribbled milk and vomit. Clean other creases where dirt can collect – under his arms, behind his ears and in the folds at the top of his legs – and his hands. Don't clean out any orifices as they are all self-cleaning, and you could cause damage by poking cotton wool in his nose or ears.

The family bath

Baby baths are not essential. In fact some parents prefer to use the large family bath from the start. You can undress you baby once you are undressed, hold him close to you and step into the bath, gradually letting him feel the water on his skin as he lies against you. When he relaxes, you can let him float with your hands for support.

It is easy to wash his hair by supporting his back on the palm of your hand, holding his head on your fingers and using your free hand to pour water over his head. Once you're confident, it can be relaxing and fulfilling for both of you, deeply intimate, fun and a good place for a feed. When you have finished, lie him on a towel beside the bath and then get out yourself. If your bath is big enough your partner may be part of regular bathtimes, or you and he may take turns.

You can also use the big bath to bathe your baby on his own. Kneeling by the side, gently lower him into the water and he can enjoy the feeling of floating and gliding – his first taste of swimming. If the water is deep enough you can sit or stand him in it. Accessories to help your confidence and keep him well supported include towelling or rubber bath seats.

Always take care: first run the cold water and then add hot water – babies can get scalded in baths. The temperature should be between 25 and 28°C (77 and 82.4°F), and the room well heated – around 29°C (84.2°F) is ideal for a naked baby. Run the water warm, and test its heat with your elbow or a bath thermometer. Use rubber bath mats on the floor and in the bath if you are concerned about slipping.

My baby, now 4 weeks old, hates being naked. I'm really disappointed because I wanted to massage and bath him regularly. How can I make him feel comfortable without clothes on?

Having known nothing but caresses and embraces before he was born, your baby is finding it difficult to relax when he can't feel anything against his skin. He's like many other newborn babies and his frightened or angry response to nakedness will pass in time. For now, let him feel protected and minimise the time he spends without clothes. Reduce the number of baths he has, cleaning him bit by bit with a sponge or cotton wool instead, and dress and undress him in stages.

He may feel comfortable when he's naked but in your arms: snuggle up in bed beneath a cover or in a warm bath and hold him against you. This skin-to-skin contact can be reassuring, intimate and warming, and if he relaxes against your body he will develop trust. With trust comes confidence, and when he's ready he'll enjoy his bath more and revel in massages. In the meantime, massage him gently through his clothes.

Using a baby bath

Baby baths give less of a chance for intimacy and for increasing a parent's confidence, and are not essential for keeping your baby clean. If you choose to use one, however, set it safely on the floor before filling it, or rest it on a special stand or across the adult bath if it is designed for this. If you have to lift a full baby bath it is better to use the adult bath.

When you and the bath are ready, take your baby's clothes off and clean his nappy area using cotton wool. Swaddle him in a towel so his arms are tucked away but his head is free. Then hold him with his head resting on one hand and his body lying on your forearm, his toes peeping out from the crook of your elbow. Kneel over the bath and use your free hand to pour water slowly and gently over his hair. This caring wash gives your baby a soothing introduction to the water. Use the towel to dry his hair lightly before unwrapping him and giving him the full bath.

The easiest position for bathing your baby is to support his head on your left forearm, bringing your hand beneath his arm and around his chest. He will probably feel more secure if he is able to grasp your finger or thumb, and can feel your right hand under his lower back. Midwives in many hospitals show new mothers how to bath their babies before they leave. If you are nervous, ask your health visitor to give you some additional tips, and try to have support or, at the very least, some adult company. You might find it much easier just to share your own bath with your baby.

Cleaning your newborn's cord stump

The brown stubby remnant of your baby's umbilical cord has no nerves so doesn't hurt, and will drop off within a couple of weeks of birth. Caring for it is not difficult – the best thing to do is to leave it well alone. It is fine to submerge the navel in bath water. The area may have a slightly rancid smell. This is normal because bacteria in the

---

I'm frightened to wash my baby's face, or even let him stay in the bath for long, as I don't want to get water in his ears. Can it harm him?

Clean bath water, even if a bit soapy, will do no harm to your baby's ears, which are protected by water-repellent waxy material that prevents water entering the outer ear canal. If you choose to clean his ears, only clean the crevices of the external ear and never use an ear bud in the ear canal.

Only very prolonged exposure to the irritant effect of swimming pool water could lead to inflammation of the lining of the outer ear canal (otitis externa or 'swimmer's ear'), a condition easily recognised by a smelly discharge. It responds to local antibiotics and antiseptics.

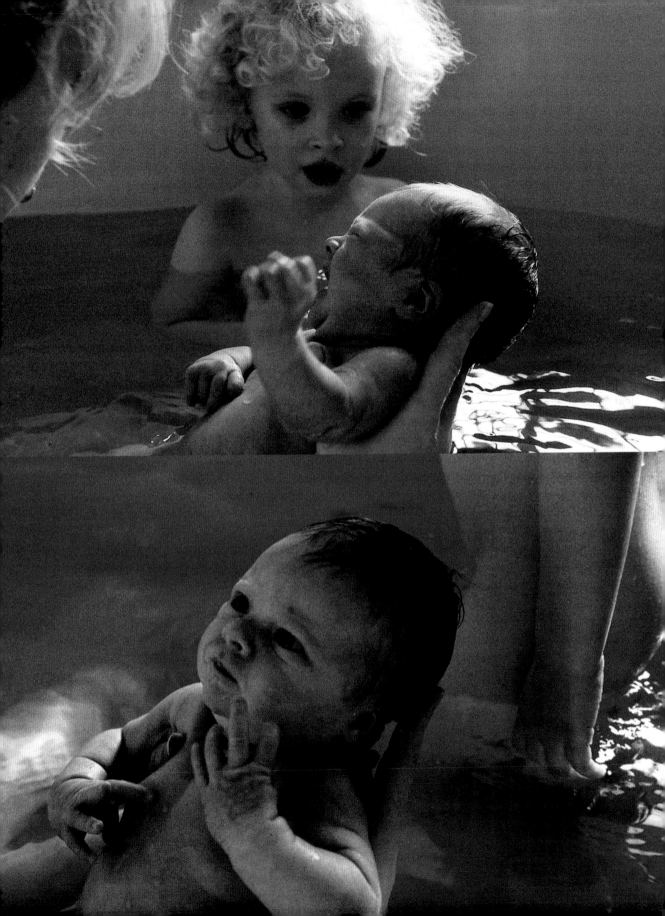

skin help the cord to separate. Signs of infection (p.551) include a strong odour, dampness or any oozing. Don't tamper with the cord, even if it seems to be hanging on by just a thread: it will fall off naturally. Fold nappies to avoid uncomfortable rubbing by the cord, and dry the area well after a bath. Clean the navel gently with cotton wool and cooled, boiled water. Before long he will have a perfect little belly button.

Your baby's nails

Your baby's nails may be quite sharp. You could use mittens, or 'scratch mitts', to protect him from scratching himself. Yet mitts prevent your baby from exploring his hands, chewing on them or feeling the intimacy of contact between his bare hands and your skin.

At first you can trim your baby's nails by nibbling them with your teeth, relying on the sensitivity of your tongue and mouth to do so safely. When his nails strengthen, special baby scissors are the safest option – adequately small and rounded at the ends.

Exercising with your baby

Your baby is designed to develop strength and control so that he will eventually sit, stand and walk, and you can help him maintain his flexibility, encouraging relaxation, confidence and intimacy. As with you, during exercise the feeling of wellbeing arises because his brain releases endorphins.

From birth he will benefit from gentle massage (p.368) and the closeness of swimming with you (in the bath to begin with) or lying on you as you work through some gentle stretches: he will feel in touch with you and with the world around him, and you are literally 'getting in touch' with him. If he gets upset, stop and cuddle him, and resume if you feel he is ready.

Swimming

Swimming develops your baby's muscle tone and co-ordination and inspires confidence, and you may be surprised by the length of time he wants to spend in the water. It is a great way to exercise together. Water allows your baby to feel weightless and cushioned by fluid, as he was in the womb, and presents no danger provided you are there to hold him.

You can start swimming with your baby as soon as you like and you can begin in the bath at home. Every newborn has a 'diving reflex', which prevents water from entering the lungs (p.171). You do, however, need to be there all the time to care for him.

A large adult bath makes a perfect bathing spot for a tiny baby, reassured and supported by her mother's hands. Elyssia is lucky enough to be able to enjoy a large family bath with her sister, Seraphina, as well as her mother.

Find out from your local health centre, sports complex or health visitor about classes for mothers and babies. As you help him 'swim', you will need to support his torso with your hands, as he won't have the physical strength to swim unsupported until 2½–3 years of age, but give him space to splash with his arms and legs as this is an essential part of swimming. You might both enjoy it when you bounce him up and down in a standing position or hold him close to your chest and over time learn to use floats and other accessories, which are great ways to build up confidence and balance. If your baby is a playful water baby, let him enjoy the feeling of being dipped beneath water. He may also teach you about confidence and fun in water. If he becomes afraid or upset take him out of the pool, dry him and comfort him, and whenever a swim has ended, give him a warming feed.

For your baby, who is naturally hedonistic, every aspect of life offers a chance to play and to learn, and to build a sense of control. During exercise the feeling of wellbeing arises as his brain releases endorphins. Help him stretch and play when he is content and well fed, and go at his pace. At 4 weeks he may find 10 minutes of stretching or massage adequate or even too much, yet by 12 weeks he may enjoy half an hour of playful exercise.

Out and about with your baby

Babies like changes of scene just as much as adults do, and they appreciate the revitalising effect of fresh air, moving trees, racing clouds or blue sky, and the smell of grass, flowers and water. They also enjoy meeting different people and being in new places. As much as possible, take your baby out for walks, or to visit friends. Useful items to take with you include:

- Spare nappies – always one or two more than you'd expect to use.
- Baby wipes.
- Changing mat.
- Nappy sacks/plastic shopping bags for dirty nappies.
- Clean vest, babygro and cardigan.
- A set of spare clothes if you're out longer than 4 hours.
- Overcoat and hat.
- Muslin square or small towel to catch dribbled milk.
- Colourful toy or rattle.
- Dummy or comfort blanket if your baby has one (plus a spare).
- If you're bottle feeding: the number of bottles you expect to use, plus one spare. Keep made-up bottles cool and heat them up for use, or carry warm, boiled water in a thermos and add the powder to sterilised bottles when you're ready.
- If you're breastfeeding: breast pads and a spare bra or T-shirt if you tend to leak profusely.
- Wholesome snacks for you, and a bottle of water (you'll be thirsty if you're feeding).

Essentials for your baby

Clothes

This list suggests the minimum requirements. Remember that before birth you don't know how big your baby will be, and he may outgrow some clothes within 2–4 weeks. Sometimes you'll need three sets of clothes in a day. If possible buy natural fabrics and check the design – avoid tight necks and check that trousers are stretchy or have poppers under the legs for easy nappy changing. All clothes and bedclothes need to be washed before use.

You may need:

- 6 vests or baby suits (no legs, short arms; long arms if it is cold).
- 6 babygros (long legs and long arms).
- 1 hat – sunhat in summer, woolly in winter.
- 3 natural-fabric cardigans (easier than jumpers).
- 2 pairs trousers or leggings.
- 2 pairs tights (optional – may be comfortable for boys as well as girls).
- 1 coat, and a snowsuit for winter.
- 3 pairs socks, and booties in winter.
- 2 pairs mitts (optional – can stop your baby scratching his face).
- 4 bibs (optional – having several can save on washing).

General equipment

When you buy baby equipment, first check that it complies with safety regulations, indicated by the kite mark of the British Standards Association (BSA). Some things are best ordered well in advance of your due date – delivery may take weeks or months, and you may want to replace things if there's a fault or you change your mind. If you buy second hand, check carefully for damage and danger spots.

Don't use cot bumpers as babies can get tangled up in the ties used to secure them to the cot. Buy a proper cot mattress, which will be designed to be safe for a baby and do not use a mattress designed for older children. If you're installing new furniture or fittings, do it with a toddler in mind – by the end of the first year your baby will almost certainly be mobile enough to reach sockets, low shelves and standing lamps.

You may need:

- Easy-to-wipe changing mat/disposable ones.
- Muslin or old cloth to put on your shoulder and to catch your baby's dribbles.
- Nappies – 12 muslin/cloth or two packs newborn size disposable nappies.
- 1–2 packets of nappy sacks (optional).
- 1 large packet of cotton wool (balls are too small and fiddly for wiping very dirty bottoms).
- Fragrance-free baby wipes (best kept for use away from home while your baby's skin is delicate).
- Formula milk, sterilising pack and bottles if you want to be prepared for bottle feeding.
- Soft rug or fleece blanket for your baby to lie on when awake.

- Bouncy chair or rocking seat (good after a couple of weeks, but only for short periods as it doesn't support the back well).
- Baby bath, unless you choose to share the family bath (p.216).
- Gentle oil to add for massage or bath.
- Breast pump for use after 8 weeks if you are breastfeeding (p.195).
- Non-biological soap powder.
- Toys (pp.179, 232 and 254).

For nappy changes: Changing mats can be large, plastic and padded (not easily portable), small, foldable and plastic backed, or disposable. Changing bags come in all shapes and sizes, with any number of pockets, zips and pull-out mats, which may or may not be easy to wash. The bag can quickly become heavy, so make sure it will not strain your back – in fact a backpack style is best. You may already have something that is perfect for carrying spare clothes, a few nappies and a bottle or two.

Toys: For your newborn baby the most entertaining thing is another face. He will also enjoy looking at pictures or patterns that are contrasting – black on white – and within easy focusing distance on the side of his cot and pram.

Newborn babies also find movement interesting: mobiles, movement of leaves on trees, curtains swaying in the breeze, or a brother or sister dancing around the room, and enjoy music, particularly if they are held and rocked.

After 3 or 4 weeks your baby may enjoy lying beneath a baby gym – a frame with colourful objects hanging from it. You can introduce other toys that suit his development and curiosity as he grows and learns to use his arms and hands. Babies also like looking at everyday objects, from door handles, tables and the pattern on cushions to necklaces, watches or glasses.

Bedroom

You may need:

- Moses basket or crib (a cot can wait for 3–5 months).
- Snugly fitting mattress.
- 4 natural fibre sheets and cellular blankets to fit the crib.
- 1 room thermometer for bedroom or nursery (optional).
- Baby intercom (optional, but handy if you are out of earshot).

Baby intercom: Baby intercoms vary greatly. Some can be powered by battery as well as mains electricity, which makes them more flexible – you can carry your unit around with you, or put the baby unit beside the pram if your baby's sleeping outside. Some show noise levels with a set of lights so you can turn the sound off or down. There are also models that monitor breathing, and beep if breathing stops, and some that provide a video link-up.

Kitchen

Buying a high chair: When you're buying a high chair, consider your baby's needs now and in 6 or 12 months time.

You will need clips for securing a baby harness while he is very small, and safety straps that will suit him when he's larger.

Some chairs are better for older babies but can be padded with a booster seat. Many have more than one height setting and some can be adjusted into a low-chair and table that will still be useful in a few years. One with a removable tray may suit your baby when he's older and can join you at your table. Whatever you choose, satisfy yourself that it is completely sturdy. For travelling or to fit in a kitchen with limited space, you can buy a chair that clips on to an adult chair or table.

Out and about
You may need:
- Pram.
- Pushchair or buggy (useful after 10 or 12 weeks).
- Changing bag, possibly with an attached changing mat.
- Sling or papoose.
- Car seat with comfortable handle and extra head support for a newborn.

Prams and pushchairs: If you have space, you may rock your baby to sleep in his pram in the house, yard or garden, and you will certainly use a pram for walking. Newborn babies need to lie flat, but most prams are adjustable so your baby may sit up when he's older. Some convert to pushchairs, useful from around 12 weeks. There are also three-in-one pram/pushchair sets that act as a frame for supporting a car seat.

The advantage of 'all-terrain' or 'off-road' three-wheeled pushchairs is lightness – they are easy to push, particularly up-hill and on rocky or sandy ground. Although designs are improving, some are large and can be awkward, some have very little room for storing baby equipment or shopping and many take up a lot of space, even when folded.

If you are considering buying a second-hand pram, check the wheel alignment and stability thoroughly and buy a new mattress. When buying a pram, new or second-hand, always consider the following:
- How difficult is it to fold and put in the car, lift and reassemble?
- Is it heavy for you, even without a baby in it?
- Will it fit in your car, and through your front door?
- How easy is it to operate the brake?
- Is its handle at a comfortable height?
- Are the covers easy to remove and wash?
- Does it come with a plastic rain cover and sunshade (both essential), and is an insect net included?
- How long will it suit your baby? Some are too small for a large 3-month-old baby to lie in comfortably; some that convert to pushchairs last for up to 4 years.
- Does it have a safety harness for a sitting 6-month-old who may be all too keen to 'escape'?
- Does it rock or have suspension (rocking/bouncing can help babies fall asleep)?
- Does it have pockets for storage?
- Does it have a tray for your shopping, and could this make it difficult to push?

A papoose or sling: A sling or papoose is the best way to transport your baby in the early weeks, whether you're walking long distances or doing chores at home. He can smell and feel you, hear your heartbeat and feel rocked just as he was in the womb. It also strengthens and tones his muscles and supports his spine, while stimulating your vertebrae to lay down calcium, thus reducing the risk of osteoporosis in later life. As your baby gets older, he'll enjoy taking in the scenery as you walk, so a papoose that has a front-facing option (viable from around 8 or 10 weeks when your baby has head control) is a good investment.
- Check the shoulder straps: are they wide and padded so they won't dig into your shoulders when you're carrying for a long time or your baby gets heavier?
- What kind of head support is there for a newborn baby?
- Can you turn it to face forward?
- Will it be comfortable for your partner to carry?
- How easy will it be to strap your baby in, for example when you're in the car or parked in a busy street?
- How easy is it to secure? Watch out for fiddly clips round the back that are impossible to fasten with one hand.
- Is the papoose adjustable to carry a newborn in the summer and a 4-month-old in a snowsuit?

Car seat: Whenever you take your baby out in a car, however short the journey, you will need a car seat: it is illegal and dangerous to travel without one. If you have air bags in the front seats you must strap the car seat into the back – in the event of a crash an air bag can cause serious injury or death.

Some seats can be secured in the car semi-permanently, usually with the seatbelt passing through the back, while others are designed so you strap your baby in first and then fasten the seat in the car. The first type is better if you don't intend to carry your baby from house to car in his seat, even when he is asleep. If you choose the second, don't use it as a seat out of the car. Car seats are designed for safety when driving and do not provide adequate support for your baby's back. Your baby's back tone and strength are stimulated by holding him or carrying him in a sling, or lying him down on a flat surface.

Extras you may need include sunshades for the car window (although it's illegal to have a shade on a front window). You may want a mirror for your windscreen that allows you to see your baby in the back.
- All seats should carry the BSA kite mark of safety.
- If you intend to use a second-hand car seat and do not know its history, check under covers and around the back for cracks.
- Watch out for danger spots like metal or even dark-coloured plastic, which can get especially hot if the car is left in the sun for any length of time.
- Check that the seatbelts go around the seat comfortably, and fitting it isn't too difficult. This is particularly crucial if you have a two-door car.
- Imagine carrying the seat from car to house – how awkward is it?
- The seat can be made more comfortable with extra head support. Is one provided?
- Are the covers removable for washing?
- How long will it suit your baby?
- Can the seat be used with a pram chassis, as part of a larger set, and does this suit you?

The learning curve: weeks 1–12

Everything has changed. You have both become parents. You've been through pregnancy, given birth to your baby and your family's future is spread before you. The first 3 months of life with your new baby will be intense – intensely loving, intensely beautiful and, at times, intensely challenging and tiring.

What's special

If you can, rest as much as possible; although it's the mother who goes through the greatest physical exertion, a father will also feel physically exhausted, and for both of you the emotional ride may have been extreme. In the days after birth your minds begin to absorb what's happened as you cuddle and stroke your baby. You will be emotionally up and down. Take time, make space and ride through what could be the one of the most bizarre and amazing times of your lives.

It may be weeks or months before the 'babymoon' passes. One day you'll wake up and feel that you're back – part of the real world – and able to expand your focus beyond your baby, although she will still be at the centre. It takes time to learn about your baby and how to care for her. By the end of the third month 'life before baby' may be a distant memory, and you are active and experienced parents, part of a family unit, and two individuals wizened by nurturing a very precious life. If you think of the postnatal period as a mirror of your pregnancy, you are one-third of the way through the next 9-month cycle.

Mum's body

Your body is undergoing huge changes as it reverts to its pre-pregnant state. Your uterus needs to contract, which may be painful for a few days, your muscles and ligaments alter, your balance, your spine, your vagina and your skin all change. It may take many weeks before you feel fully recovered and vaginal bleeding stops.

Your body also needs to support and nurture your growing baby. Your breasts will get larger and feeding may take up a considerable amount of time and energy. It is extremely important that you look after yourself so the natural processes of transition, healing and feeding can work well: if you overdo things or do not get enough sleep, you will feel the effects physically and this will be reflected in your emotions. Listen to your body, expect it to take time to heal and give it a chance to do so by resting, eating well and exercising gently and sensibly. In this way you will be doing the best you can to look after yourself and give your new family the best start.

Medical support

In hospital standard checks may include examining your uterus and stitches and checking your blood pressure and temperature and giving advice on posture and any aches and strains. Your midwives will advise on care of stitches, grazes and tears. The midwives will also discuss and help you with breastfeeding or using a bottle, if that is your preference. There may be a midwife or physiotherapist who will go through simple postnatal exercises with you and discuss long-term care of your back and pelvic floor.

When you are discharged depends on hospital policy, the birth and your baby's health. At home it is a legal requirement to be visited by a midwife for 10 days, or a little longer. She will check your baby and ensure the umbilical cord is healing well, and will assess you and advise you about care for both of you. Most midwives also give excellent moral support.

Some time in the first 14 days you may have a visit from your GP. Your health visitor will come round as well. She is trained to support families and may offer a listening ear for years to come. Although she makes just one statutory visit (at 11 or 14 days), she'll leave a phone number so you can contact her if you have any concerns.

You will be offered a 6-week check either in your GP's surgery or in the obstetric unit in the hospital. At this visit the doctor will ask you about how everything has progressed for you and your baby and discuss contraception. You will be offered an examination that includes a vaginal check (overleaf). If you have had a caesarean, your scar will also be checked. Many doctors offer a cervical smear to check for cancer but the postnatal period is not the best time to do this – it is better to wait until your menstrual cycle recommences.

You may find a number of complementary therapies extremely useful: particularly valuable are osteopathy to rebalance your body after the strain of labour, homeopathy for addressing any breastfeeding difficulties and assisting postnatal healing, and aromatherapy, massage and yoga for relaxation (see Part V).

Your feelings

The depth of love you feel for your baby may be unexpected, whether it hits you after 10 minutes, 2 days or 2 weeks, and will probably influence your entire outlook on life. In addition to the joy of meeting your very own baby, you will be flooded by the 'love hormones' that flow immediately after birth and while you breastfeed. While feeling 'loved up' is usual, it's not exclusive, however.

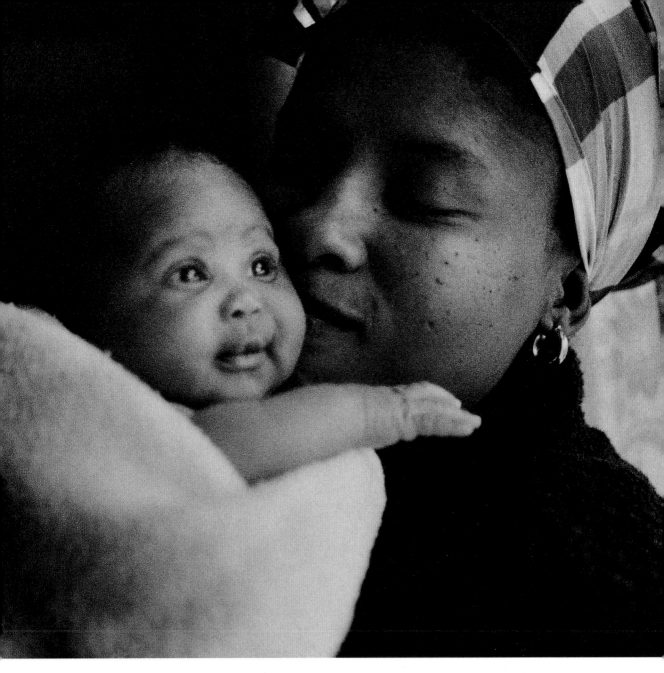

Some parents feel overwhelmed and are surprised and even guilty that they don't establish a loving bond straight away (p.302).

Mood swings are part of parenting and although they may be more intense in the mother because of hormones, fathers have them too. It's fine to feel joyful, loving or proud; it's just as fine to feel stressed, angry or confused. Some people find that the first weeks of parenthood can be confronting, so don't be surprised if you need a good cry occasionally. Crying may also be triggered by hormones or fatigue, and usually helps to release tension but if it continues for weeks it may indicate postnatal depression.

Your relationships

In the early days your baby is the most important person in your life, and the most time-consuming. Your second most important relationship – your partnership – will change. You may feel really loving and find a new depth to your love and sense of commitment. Because this is a stressful life stage there may also be less positive aspects.

When the novelty of having a new baby has faded, and perhaps one partner returns to work, tensions may arise about who spends time with whom, who works the harder, who sleeps the better, who forgot to buy the baby milk, and so on. The new and frequently difficult

Back and head

You may feel stiff from pushing but most people do not have back or head pain. If you feel pain, this may be due to incorrect posture, which is perhaps aggravated if you slouch while you feed or carry your baby. Imbalance in the pelvis may also lead to lower back pain, and if you have had an epidural there may be pain from the site of the injection. These causes may also lead to headache, which may be exacerbated if you are very tired or not drinking enough liquid. Remedies for these aches are discussed on p.521.

Bladder and bowels

For a day or two after the birth you may sting when you pass urine. Otherwise, urinary function will be as normal but there may be slight incontinence early on. If you urinate very frequently or feel a burning sensation as you do, this may indicate infection and you need to tell your midwife or doctor. Bowel movements usually resume as normal soon after birth: it is common to be slightly nervous of pain or stitches breaking, but passing the first motion is not difficult. If you do not pass a motion for more than 3 days after birth, treat constipation (p.435).

Breasts

Your breasts are likely to feel heavy and full for a day or two after birth, perhaps reaching their fullest on the third day when milk flow replaces colostrum. This is normal engorgement (p.414) and is best relieved by frequent feeding. If you have sore nipples or burning pain and your breasts are hard or tender, your midwife can help you attend to latching on your baby and she will check for blocked ducts or infection.

Infection

If you do not feel well, have a rise in body temperature, or there is an unpleasant smell to your vaginal discharge or burning and pain inside your bladder or uterus, you may have an infection. Let your doctor know because you may need antibiotics.

Your pelvis

The joints of your pelvis, including your sacrum and coccyx, may feel tender. This is normal and will progressively reduce as the ligaments harden and the spaces between the joints close. You may also feel uncomfortable if the muscles of your pelvis have stretched; these will also gradually return to normal. Postnatal exercises can relieve discomfort. If you have prolonged pelvic pain (p.519), let your midwife know.

Your uterus

The size diminishes progressively and your midwife will check this for 10 days. It will be back to pre-pregnancy size by the time your doctor examines you at 6 weeks. As your uterus shrinks you may feel afterpains. How much discomfort these give varies and is usually most intense in the first 1–3 days after the birth, and when breastfeeding.

Vaginal bleeding

Bleeding after birth is usually heavy. This is normal providing you do not pass clots, membrane or placental tissue. If you notice any of these, tell your midwife and keep a sample for her. At birth there may be some extra bleeding from vaginal tears. Bleeding remains heavy for a week and it reduces over the following weeks, changing in colour from red to brownish to pink. It may stop any time between the third and ninth week – 6 weeks is the average.

Vaginal pain

The area around your vagina, perineum and anus may feel sore after birth, perhaps with bruising and swelling. This is normal and, with stitches or a tear, you may be more uncomfortable and sting when you urinate. The tenderness and swelling often passes in a few days. Piles may also feel tender in your anus. There are many ways to soothe the pain (p.523), including regular pelvic floor exercises, which increase blood flow to the area and help healing. If the pain is intense or prolonged, tell your midwife.

---

dimension to your relationship presents the challenge of finding a balance that will depend on many factors.

Almost all new parents find it hard to get quality time together in the early months. The guidelines on active listening (p.290) may help you find the time and space to sit down together and talk about how you are feeling and how the practical arrangements for babycare, work and domestic chores are working. If you are honest with each other, you may be able to support one another during the most testing part of the first year. Your family, too, may take a while to get used to the idea that you are a parent. Your mother or mother-in-law may become your best friend and helper or your most dreaded visitor, and your relationship with her and other family members will probably change when your baby exerts her presence.

Making time to enjoy

The focus on baby and sleep does pass and by the end of the second or third month, though you may still be tired if your baby doesn't sleep well, you will be a long way from the half-awake limbo of the first weeks. As soon as you feel confident, take your baby out to visit friends or meet other parents and babies, and ask someone to join you for a walk. You could get help so that you have time to yourself and you may need forward planning so you and your partner can have time together.

Getting out and about with a baby is often easiest in the early months. Your baby sleeps more than she will later, and will probably be happy to sleep just about anywhere in her Moses basket or against your chest. Provided you are equipped, you may be able to enjoy many an evening or day out and introduce your baby to your friends. She will be fascinated watching and listening to your interactions.

Childcare and support in the home

Before the birth you might have planned to have help. If so, it's important to assess regularly how well it is working. Do your baby and the carer get on? Do you need more help? Do you need less help with your baby but more with household chores? How does your partner feel about the arrangement? Be honest about how things are working: this is a formative time for your baby and you are delegating considerable responsibility to a carer.

If you planned to care for your baby alone but you're finding it difficult, you may find support among your friends and family before looking for hired help. Small gestures can be really valuable. Could someone cook meals for you or take dirty washing and bring it back clean and ironed? Is there somebody who would help with cleaning or babysit? If you were reluctant to ask for support before the birth and you have changed your mind now, you may find people who get pleasure from helping you.

Baby groups

Socialising is great for your baby, and she will really appreciate the company of other babies from as young as 8 or 10 weeks. You might have a circle of friends with babies who already meet up regularly. If you're the first of your bunch to have a baby, try a mother and baby group.

Almost every town has a range of baby clinics (weekly or monthly) as well as mother and toddler groups. Many health visitors run weekly drop-in sessions for new mothers and babies that cover issues such as massage, first aid, feeding, weaning and postnatal depression, and provide a good environment for meeting new people; long-term friendships often begin here. Some boroughs hold swimming or baby exercise classes and also groups specially for fathers.

Your body image

Many women take weeks or months to feel comfortable as mothers. Some glow with happiness, but low body image is common in this transitional period, particularly if there is little weight loss – your belly may not lose the extra inches until well after the third month has past. How you view yourself may be most strongly affected by the way breastfeeding makes you feel – proud, beautiful and happy, or tired, tied down and moist. Your baby also becomes part of your image. You may be able to boost your body image with the clothes you wear – remember to pack a spare top when you go out so that you can change if your baby spews milk on to your shoulder or your breasts leak.

It's common for men to feel down about their bodies as well, for reasons that vary from lack of sex and exercise to uncertainty about their paternal feelings.

Eating

Even with very little time you can eat well to keep up your energy and maintain the quality of your breast milk without your weight rocketing. Few women lose weight quickly after birth, and some don't begin to shift it until they stop breastfeeding, when the extra pounds provide a store of calories and energy. Keep your goals realistic, with an overall nutrition programme including vitamins and minerals (p.345), and do not try to lose weight by dieting. Your weight will stabilise in the time that suits your own physiology and metabolism. Cook and freeze things in advance and ask a friend or relative to do some shopping and/or cooking for you.

Exercise and rest

From the first day after birth you can begin to do postnatal exercises and stretches while lying in bed: pelvic floor (p.98) and gentle pelvic tilts and abdominal tightenings (p.360). Walking is an effective yet gentle workout – opt for a stroll instead of a drive in the car and carry your baby in a sling when you can, as this helps your bones lay down calcium. At home you could do postnatal exercises on the floor while your baby lies beside you and you can use her as a weight when stretching. It's important to take your exercise programme gently: because your muscles and ligaments are adjusting, avoid strenuous aerobic exercise in the first 6 weeks, and then build up a routine gently. If you're using the gym take advice from a qualified teacher.

At first you may feel driven and energetic because your adrenalin is flowing strongly, but if you do too much you could deplete your energy reserves and become exhausted. Don't forget to balance your exercise, and all the energy you spend caring for your baby, with rest. Visualisations and breathing exercises are easy to do while you feed your baby and may help you get back to sleep after night feeds or take revitalising naps during the day. You could also do yoga with and without your baby. If you can share night-time bottle feeds you may get better sleep.

Dad's issues

Even without hormonal changes you are susceptible to mood swings, tiredness and anxiety. You need time to recover from the birth and it may help to talk. In the early days your partner will probably do most babycare, particularly if she is breastfeeding, but it is important that she rests and you may be able to give her opportunities for a sleep or a break when you are at home. This will also ensure that your extra help with household chores or extra hours at work do not rule out time to be with your baby.

If you feel left out by breastfeeding, you may be able to arrange some ways to have more time with your baby. Apart from cuddling your baby, you might enjoy bathing her, letting her sleep on your chest, changing nappies and playing. There may be a postnatal group in your area where you could get some useful tips and meet up with other fathers. Some men prefer to be hands off, however, and have more time to themselves.

One of your important roles in the early postnatal weeks may be to arrange support for your partner to rest or arrange a babysitter so that you can go out together. You may also be in charge of sorting out financial issues and the weekly shopping. If you feel pressurised consider the options for sharing your workload with colleagues and for creating time for yourself to exercise and socialise. This is discussed in the fatherhood chapter (p.292).

Sex and intimacy

Becoming a parent may mark a kind of rebirth and your sexuality may begin anew. For a woman, there is often a feeling akin to virginity, because the vagina has been used as the baby's entrance to the world and needs to take on a sexual role once again. Men feel the shift too, and it can take time to feel comfortable with the balance you both perceive between mothering and making love. Some couples resume sexual intercourse within the first 6 weeks; others prefer to focus on their baby, and it may be months before they explore the sexual aspect of their relationship again. If sex does not feature for you at first, it is still important to keep the flame of intimacy alive, particularly if one of you misses the physical side of your relationship.

It is usually, but not exclusively, harder for a woman to relax into sex after birth because vaginal healing can take time, particularly if there were stitches. The mothering hormones of breastfeeding often reduce libido and vaginal lubrication and always wearing a bra and breast pads may be a passion killer. Some women feel revitalised as they stride into motherhood, but some feel violated after birth, perhaps after a difficult or assisted delivery. If your sex-drive remains low for months, it may be an indication that one or both of you are emotionally low or even depressed.

When you are ready to make love, you may find it easy to be spontaneous. Alternatively, you might need to do some planning because your baby will take up much of your time and many of your hugs. For instance, an extra nap during the day and a bedtime routine for your baby may give you more energy to enjoy evenings together. A night away could create the space for you to get to know one another's bodies once again. Don't forget that you can conceive again, even if you are breastfeeding, so don't overlook contraception. There are a number of possibilities that include using a condom, diaphragm, IUD or the mini pill, about which your doctor or midwife will advise you.

Work and finances

In the first 3 months the costs related to your baby will include some or all of the following: nappies, extra washing, clothes, formula milk and childcare. You may also spend more if you are buying organic food. Your costs may

Medical care for your baby

Your baby is checked at birth (Apgar score, p.139) and before discharge by a paediatrician. Then for 10–14 days, depending on local practice, she will be checked in your home by a midwife. Care then passes to a health visitor and GP. You may receive one or more home visits, or take your baby to a clinic for assessment.

Every parent has moments of doubt and in these early days you may sometimes wonder if everything is all right: this is quite normal and is actually your instinct to protect and nurture. It is quite astounding how the parent–baby dance extends to picking out the normal from the abnormal, and most problems in babies and families are first noticed and acknowledged by parents. If you are concerned about anything, do turn to your doctor or health visitor or someone who can offer advice and support. Most of the illnesses small babies have are not serious.

Weight

Most babies lose 10% of their birth weight by day 3–7, and regain this by 10–14 days. More than 15% weight loss (p.563) in the first 10 days after birth usually signifies inadequate feeding and needs to be looked into. Weight loss at any time after this initial period would be concerning. Although the usual cause is inadequate intake of calories, other causes must be considered, especially urinary tract infections.

Vitamin K

Vitamin K is essential for normal blood clotting, but levels are low during the first weeks because the vitamin is made in the baby's bowel by bacteria acquired after birth. Breastfed babies are usually given additional vitamin K by mouth in 3 doses (at birth, 1 week and 4–6 weeks) or by a single injection into the muscles at birth. Bottle-fed babies require a single dose at birth, because formula contains added vitamin K, but may be given more.

Approximately 1 in 100,000 newborn babies (65 a year in the UK) suffer from bleeding related to a deficiency of vitamin K (p.407).

Heel prick (done at 6–12 days of age)

This test involves pricking the heel of your baby, and soaking up the blood on to spots on a special card. This card is then sent to a laboratory for testing. The reason for testing early is that early treatment improves the outcome for the baby.

All babies are tested for a deficiency of thyroid activity, called hypothyroidism. Its occurrence is roughly 1 in 2500. If the baby's thyroid gland is functioning at a low level, or is absent, this leads to a slow brain and body development. If the levels of thyroid hormones are low, a simple replacement tablet each day can prevent adverse effects (p.542).

All babies are tested for another rare condition called phenyl ketonuria, or PKU (p.523), which affects around 1 in 75,000 babies and may affect brain development. It is treated with a special diet and closely monitoring levels of phenylalanine in the blood by further heel prick tests. Other tests carried out depend on where you live and may include cystic fibrosis (p.443) and certain blood disorders such as sickle cell anaemia (p.398).

The 6- or 8-week check

This is part of the special service offered throughout childhood by the NHS and the purpose is to detect as many conditions as possible that may affect growth and development. Usually the surveillance is carried out by health visitors, but sometimes a GP does the tests. Initially designed to coincide with the 6-week postnatal check, the main aims of this check are to:

- Ask about any concerns you may have.
- Measure and weigh your baby and to plot these measurements on the growth charts in the parent-held record.
- Make sure growth and nutrition are proceeding normally.
- Detect any major congenital abnormalities of the heart.
- Recheck the hips for dislocation.
- Check the reflexes.
- Check the testicles are descended in boys.
- Determine parents' vaccination plans, and in 8-week-old babies to give the first vaccines if they are requested.
- Ensure that any antenatal problems have been checked after birth and arrangements for follow-up have been made.

Testing of hearing and vision is not yet routinely done at this check. Until routine newborn testing is introduced, the first hearing test is at 7 months. You will be asked whether you think your baby can hear you, how visually alert he is, whether he's moving all four limbs and if he smiles. The health visitor will check everything in the course of the visit so it is best to bring a written list of questions if you have any concerns.

Vaccinations

Vaccinations are designed to protect children against infections or diseases that may have damaging consequences. The standard programme is constantly reviewed and updated. Take the advice of your GP or paediatrician and do as much research as you wish before making a decision. Immunisations against infection are detailed in the A–Z Health Guide (p.554). The programme may begin at birth with BCG and hepatitis B vaccines. In most of Europe the schedules for vaccination begin at 8 weeks.

When to call the doctor

Babies under 1 year are the most frequent visitors to doctors and other health-care services. They are rarely seriously ill, but are frequently unwell with minor illnesses, the majority of which are viral and self-limiting – they go away in 5–10 days with no special treatment.

It is reassuring to know the average baby has eight viral infections a year. Even so, if you are worried about your baby's health, it is safest to call a doctor. Details about illnesses, including those most commonly causing concern, such as vomiting, coughs and colds and fever, are in the A–Z Health Guide.

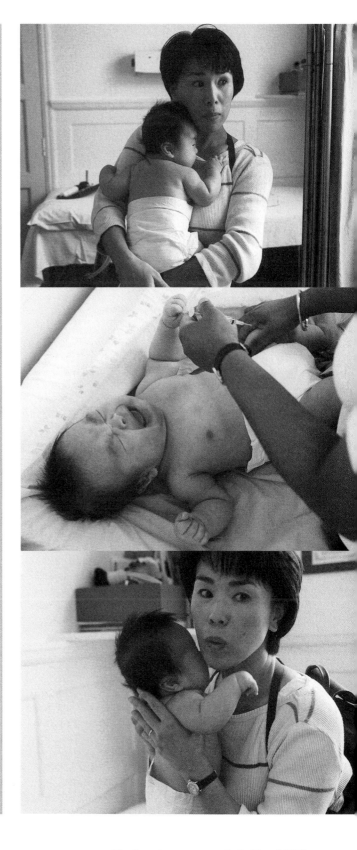

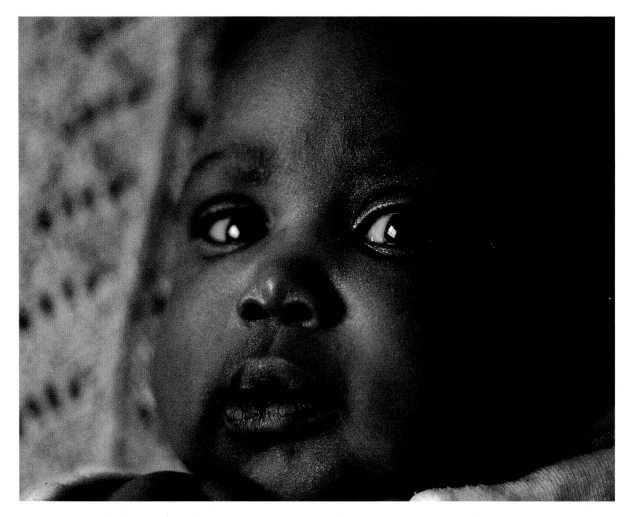

balance with what you save by staying in regularly, but you might still have to budget carefully.

There is likely to be a drop in family income unless your maternity-leave pay is unusually high. If you return to work in the first 3 months, the most important thing is to care for yourself so that you have lots of energy for your life. You have just been through a demanding 3 months. You might find some of the guidelines on p.323 helpful.

The birth certificate is filled out at the council offices nearest your baby's place of birth. You may also be entitled to maternity pay and other benefits, for which you need to apply as soon as possible. The local DHSS office will have information and your health visitor will advise you.

Going away from home

Going out for day trips or for an evening is relatively simple, though the first time you do, it may take an hour or more to get things ready. Soon packing your baby's bag will be second nature. When you're ready to make a longer trip, planning will help.

If you are happy to let go of routine you may be surprised how easily your baby integrates change. Let her sleep in her travel cot or basket for a few days before you leave so she is used to it. It might be best to share your room and perhaps your bed with your baby so she feels secure. If she is ill, abandon the trip.

On long journeys take your baby out of her car seat regularly so she can stretch and kick. If you're flying, book a seat with room for a cot. On the flight, drink plenty and feed your baby whenever she asks so that she doesn't get dehydrated, and sucking as the plane takes off and lands will help her adjust to the pressure change. Take care on long flights to prevent deep vein thrombosis in your legs by wearing support tights, drinking plenty of fluids and walking around every few hours. When you arrive if there's a small time difference, stick with your baby's usual routine according to the time at home; if the difference is large, be prepared to sleep at strange hours. Keep your goals for each day realistic and relax into it as much as possible.

Common concerns

Extended information on these concerns, and a range of other postnatal health issues, are covered in the A–Z Health Guide.

I have been bleeding for over 6 weeks. Is this usual?
It is common to bleed for at least a month but by 6 weeks the bleeding has usually stopped. This is the time when your postnatal examination is due and you can discuss the bleeding with your doctor. If the flow is diminishing and the examination is normal your doctor may advise you to wait. If your uterus is still enlarged you may be offered an ultrasound scan to ensure that fragments of the placenta or the decidual lining of your uterus have not been retained. If fragments are present and the scan shows that there are still blood vessels nourishing them, you may have to go into hospital for a dilation and curettage (D&C) to remove them (p.407). Sometimes bleeding is caused by a reaction of your vagina's lining to stitches and the healing tissue is fragile and bleeds.

My vagina is still sore after 4 weeks and I have a profuse discharge. What shall I do?
It is common for your vagina to be uncomfortable after the birth. This is caused by a variety of factors: you may have torn or needed stitches, the low levels of oestrogen associated with breastfeeding makes the lining thin and sensitive and you may have an infection that also leads to a discharge. You need to ask your midwife or doctor to examine you and to check for infection. Herbal remedies and homeopathy help stitches and cuts to heal (p.494) but antibiotics may be needed.

I cannot control the flow of urine and I leak when I cough. What can I do?
During the birth your vagina stretched and the ligaments that support the valve at the base of your bladder may have been torn or stretched. During the next few months control is likely to improve as the ligaments shrink and the normal tone is re-established. It is useful to do pelvic floor exercises and after 6 weeks you can begin to use vaginal cones, perhaps combined with gentle electrical stimulation to strengthen your pelvic floor (p.98). In approximately 6 months you will know how much your body has recovered.

I am having headaches. What can I do?
Headaches (p.521) often arise from tension patterns in your spine. Sleep deprivation and how you hold and carry your body also contribute to muscle and head pain. Massage and osteopathy or physiotherapy are useful; yoga or visualisation can reduce tension, and eating well improves your energy and relaxes muscles. If you feel low, the emotional tension may be surfacing as headache. Occasionally migraines may surface for the first time and it is worthwhile looking at your diet to exclude food allergy.

I have backache and slight sciatica – how can I reduce it?
Backache is very common after birth and it is often associated with pain in other parts of your spine: shoulder, neck and headaches (p.519). During pregnancy and birth your spinal curves were accentuated and your pelvis opened but now these changes are reverting. The way you hold your baby as you feed and care for her and how you carry her may cause or aggravate a strain pattern. If your pain radiates into your thigh or down your leg, you need to see your GP or a specialist to ensure that you do not have a prolapsed intervertebral disc. There are many things you can do, including attending to your posture and how you sleep, resting and doing gentle postnatal exercises and yoga stretches. You might find that massage and osteopathy or physiotherapy or acupuncture can also be helpful in soothing backache.

How can I make my baby's sleeping space cosy and safe?
In your room or in your baby's nursery you could have an extra chair or cushions, soft lighting for night feeds and a space set aside for storing nappies. There may be room for a clear space on the floor where you can lie your baby for playing or massage.

Give the room plenty of fresh air. As you decorate you're likely to come up with good results if you see things from a baby's point of view. Choose light and calming colour for the base and add bold contrasting decorations with some at low levels – looking at them will entertain your baby and help her eyesight develop. If you are hanging up a mobile, put it close to the cot where she can focus on it. You may find some ideas on pp.179–85.

Every evening when I get home from work my wife is pulling her hair out with stress and my baby's crying. I get the baby and have to deal with it. How can I make things smoother?
If you find your baby's crying difficult to take you could follow the advice given in the chapter on crying (p.208) as you try to soothe him and keep yourself relaxed at the same time. It may be a flashpoint that results in you feeling upset with one another and having an argument, and anger will further drain your energy and increase your tension. If you recognise the pattern you may alter it. It may help for you and your partner to have a quick chat when you meet so you can catch up on her day and she on yours and find out if your baby has made any exciting advances. Use it to plan what needs to be done in the here and now. Later in the evening is a better time to share your thoughts and feelings. If this brings about an atmosphere of relaxation, your baby may pick up on it too.

My baby, now 10 weeks old, seems to have a squint. Is this serious?
Until your baby is around 12 weeks old, she uses her eyes independently of one another, and the appearance of a squint is common. You might look at her sometimes and notice one eye moving while the other remains still. She won't develop 'binocular' vision, which is the ability to use her two eyes together, until the end of the third month. This relies on muscle strength and on her brain learning how to integrate the two images it receives. As your baby gets accustomed to using her eyes in unison, she may still seem to have a squint from time to time. If, however, her squint continues beyond the age of 4 months (p.465), it's worth taking her to the doctor or eye clinic for a check.

My baby is 3 weeks old and seemed to hear me fine until today. Is something wrong?
It's very unlikely that anything is wrong with your baby's ears. While she loves hearing your voice, she's also easily distracted if something else catches her attention. She may hear a noise

that you take for granted – a car passing or a change on the radio or television – or she may see something that sparks her curiosity and fix her attention on that. Although in some areas babies are offered hearing tests as early as 6 weeks, it is difficult to spot genuine problems in the first months. Over the next few years accurate electronic testing of all newborn babies' hearing will be universal. If you have concerns about her hearing discuss them with your health visitor and arrange testing if you are advised to do so.

Why does my baby draw up her legs and curl up so tightly?
Because your baby was curled neatly in your womb, this position may be one she finds very comfortable, although at times she'll also enjoy bending and stretching her legs. If she's crying, irritated and tense as she does it, however, this may indicate stomach pain or wind, which may be colic (p.431). Sometimes babies love to take the foetal position, with arms and legs drawn into the chest for relaxation. If your baby is disturbed, perhaps by loud noise, or uncomfortable in an unfamiliar environment, she may withdraw into this position and close her eyes without actually sleeping.

I am overwhelmed. How can I make it easier to cope?
It is very common to feel overwhelmed when you have your first baby; indeed these feelings crop up for most mums each time another baby arrives. It is hard to imagine before the birth just how long it takes to do things, how full each day can be, and how easy it is to lose time for yourself. Feeling you are always giving and seldom receiving, or being indecisive because there are so many things to learn, is normal. Have faith that things do get easier, and that it may be possible to create time for yourself by following the Wheel for Living (p.58). Your pre-pregnancy expectations may be contributing to your feeling overwhelmed – and it may be easier to let go of how you think things should be and take one day at a time. When you have difficult decisions to make, such as immunisation, talk to your medical supporters and your friends. Talking honestly with other mothers may be comforting when you discover how many share your dilemmas. You may also find useful advice on emotional support on p.459.

Is it good or bad to use a dummy?
Some babies are inclined to suck for comfort, can't find their fingers or thumbs and respond well to a dummy, or pacifier. Others have no need to be settled this way. As for good or bad, it is parents rather than babies who hold opinions and some people think they look horrible or show that the parents are 'not good enough'. Yet for the baby who finds comfort in sucking, a dummy is a part of life. Having a dummy is not detrimental to development: there is no danger of nipple confusion or breast rejection, nor will it stop a baby from practising sounds. The only risk is infection if dummies are not properly cleaned and sterilised.

If your baby already has a dummy you can try to limit his attachment to it by offering it only when he is tired, and taking it from him after he has fallen asleep. These steps do not always work in practice. A mum desperate for quiet quickly reaches for the dummy, and a baby surfacing from deep sleep in the night may cry for it. The sleeping issue can persist, leading to many months of broken nights, and weaning him off his dummy may require a lot of patience and perseverance from you.

Do I really need to buy all the latest high-tech toys?
Among the huge range of today's toys, many are designed against a background of medical and psychological research and are excellent tools for promoting development in babies. Another great advantage is that they have been tested and are guaranteed to be safe within specified age limits. Your baby uses toys and play to learn about his world and he needs stimulation to develop. But you don't have to go out and buy all the latest thing – the basic designs are simple to mimic with very little cost, if you enjoy making things yourself, and your baby will find much of the normal 'adult' world extremely interesting. You can string up wooden spoons, paper plates with faces drawn with a thick black marker, or a range of bold designs drawn on white card and suspended over the cot or play-mat on the floor. Remember, you can find novel toys at friends' houses and there may be a toy library in your area. There's more on the type of toys and games suitable for this age on pp.179–85.

My baby seems to hate the car. What can I do to make it better?
Your baby may object to being in the car for a number of reasons: perhaps he's uncomfortable in the car seat, doesn't like the smell or noise, feels a draft or is uncomfortably hot, misses close contact with you or just gets bored. He will get used to it in time. You may let him get used to his car seat by sitting him in it two or three times a day and tucking him in with a familiar blanket or an item of your clothing that smells comforting. Playing music that he likes or talking to him may help. There are also plenty of car activity sets that range from stimulating pictures and mobiles for newborns to touchy-feely scenes for the older baby. You could give your baby something interesting for car journeys without much expense – your own pictures clipped to the seat in front of him or ribbons hung on to a hook above the window are just two examples.

I am sure my baby has smiled at 2 weeks – is it wind, or is he happy?
Even the youngest of babies seem to smile at times, when waking and asleep. It is a reflex action that has been observed in the womb and is present at birth but from a parent's point of view it seems to be more than this; there may be a glint in your baby's eyes that tells you he's smiling from happiness. In sleep he may smile as he surfaces from deep sleep into dream (REM) sleep. His true, purposeful smile will come anywhere between 3 and 6 weeks of age, and after that will just get bigger and broader. He will smile at pictures and mobiles, moving trees and curtains, but his biggest smiles will come in response to smiling faces, especially yours. It won't be long before he gives his first airy chuckle. Laugh and smile back, and you'll both enjoy the new aspect to your conversations.

My baby was born prematurely and spent the first 5 weeks of her life in an incubator. How can I make up for missed time now she is home? Will she know who I am?
Although your baby may often have squeezed your finger while in her incubator, and as she became stronger enjoyed closer body contact, a lot of the touch she experienced may have had negative connections, perhaps because it involved needles or tube feeding. You now have lots of time to rectify this and to get used to holding her. Being lovingly touched and held is helpful both physically and emotionally for pre-term babies (p.527).

Your baby will know she is loved by the feel of your touch,

e sound of your voice and your body language. Within days of
ing out of her incubator she will associate your smell and feel
th love and protection. Give her as much contact as you are
le, spend time cuddling skin-to-skin whenever possible, carry
r in a sling and consider having her in bed with you at night. If
u enjoy routine, don't impose this until after you've had your
by at home with you for several weeks. Initially you need time
d commitment to connect with one another's rhythms and
come intimate. Touching with massage now and swimming
er will reinforce her security and continue to help her
velopment. Complementary therapies such as cranial
teopathy can also be very effective in soothing your baby's
ergy. As for knowing who you are, there is no doubt that your
by will recognise your voice, which she heard daily from the
th week in your womb, and feel a strong attraction to your
miliarity. She may grow to love the embrace of a nurse, but
nnot confuse a nurse with her mother.

y baby loves it when my husband tickles and jiggles him, yet he hates
when I do. Does he like his daddy more?
ke adults, babies have their own style when they strike up a
lationship, and this style will differ with each person. There's no
mpetition from your baby – he goes with each moment and
presses his emotions freely, and will enjoy some things with you
d some with his daddy. Each of you will relate to your baby in a
ique way: he responds to you, you respond to him, you make
le another feel good and sometimes you clash. Conflict happens
tween the best of friends, and it is part of the closest
other–baby partnership without affecting the love involved. No
oubt there will also be times when your baby reaches out to you,
king to be taken away from his daddy's arms. Remember, you
nnot take control of the way your baby responds to other people
give him love, welcome, acceptance and encouragement, and the
st is up to him.

y baby's 11 weeks old and rarely drinks a whole bottle without a break.
he losing his appetite?
ur baby isn't losing his appetite, he's gaining interest in the
orld around him, and gaining control of his body so that he can
llow what interests him with his eyes, his head and, to some
tent, his hands. This is exciting for him, he loves gathering
formation and he takes every chance he gets. Go with your baby,
d respond to his added interest. Chat to him and talk to him
out the things he sees, tell him what the noises are that distract
m. You might want to limit distractions at a few of his daytime
eds to encourage him to eat enough. If you're worried that his
eight or his intake has dropped significantly, though, do talk to
ur GP or health visitor.

y baby is 10 weeks old and barely lifts up his head when he's lying on
s tummy. Is he a slow developer?
u needn't worry about your baby's neck control. Let him spend
gular time on his tummy and wait another month to see how his
rength improves, and then reconsider your concerns in the light
his overall development. If you are still worried consult your
P, health visitor or paediatrician.

Every baby passes the same milestones on the developmental
ad, but no two do it at exactly the same rate. Yours may not yet
ld his head up, but might have smiled 2 weeks before your
ighbour's baby. His hands may reach for what he can see by

10 weeks, or by 13. Don't expect too much – next week will be
very different. If you are always looking for the next stage of
development, or encouraging him to go one step further than he is
capable of, you will miss the magic of the moment. Helping him
to do what he is already trying to do and delighting in each small
achievement will bring the biggest rewards for you both.

Could having a night-light on harm the way my baby's eyes develop?
Short-sightedness, or myopia, the inability to focus on distant
objects, is caused by excessive growth of the eyeball, which grows
particularly quickly before the age of 2 years, and some scientists
believe that light at night may stimulate growth. There are many
factors that contribute to a person's eyesight, including genetic
inheritance and the amount of close work done in childhood
(which may include TV watching).

Sleeping without artificial lighting may help your child to
cope with the dark in the long term. If your baby doesn't like the
dark it is best to turn the light off gradually, perhaps using a
dimmer switch or leaving the hall light on and gradually closing
the door.

Is a baby intercom really necessary?
While being able to hear your baby when you're watching
television or enjoying a noisy party can bring peace of mind,
having an intercom while you are trying to sleep is not always a
blessing. Often parents become 'addicted' to listening to their
baby breathing and babies who are naturally restless in sleep get
woken frequently because they are disturbed as soon as they
make even the slightest noise. Your baby will surface from sleep
more than 20 times a night, and sometimes might sniffle, mumble
or give a little cry before settling down once again. If you can hear
his cry without help from an electronic microphone you may get a
better night's sleep without the intercom switched on, knowing
that you will wake when you are really needed. Having an
intercom does not reduce the incidence of sudden infant death
syndrome (SIDS) (p.510).

I am trying to do the best for my baby and following all the latest advice
on development. How do I know I am doing the right thing?
Knowing about baby development, good stimulation and the
latest methods of care will help you look after your baby well. But
women have been having babies and babies have been thriving
for as long as humans have walked the earth, and long before
psychotherapists and neuro-scientists analysed development. So
while it's fascinating to learn more about how and why babies do
what they do, it's important to remember that you and your baby
will work together best on an instinctive and emotional level.
The media, including the Internet, is full of information. Some is
useful and well informed, some is useless and ill-informed.
Gather as much information as you can deal with, and try and
discuss with other informed individuals before drawing
conclusions as to what is right or wrong for your baby and you.
There is no such thing as a perfect parent or a perfect baby, and
getting it right often is fine. Babies don't need perfect parents –
they need normal parents who teach them about the ups and
downs of life and how to recover from them. Don't forget that the
best part of having a baby and the fondest memories come from
the times you have fun together. Babies learn best when they are
having fun. Enjoy, relax and interact with your baby – you are
both naturally inclined to do this well.

Your developing baby: months 4, 5 & 6

From 3 months onwards, your baby is on a fast ride of exploration and discovery: he's finding out just how much his body can do, he learns that he can control his hands and he can reach things by rolling or from a propped sitting position. Along with these leaps in bodily control come exciting advances in communication. All this helps him become more sociable with anyone who's attentive, and every game he plays, every conversation he has or listens to, lets his brain register and store an increasing amount of information as he forms a complex map of his world.

Your laughing baby

By the time your baby is 3 months old he will be smiling broadly, at you, at his toys and at your friends, and laughing openly, revealing a developing sense of humour. He has his own special language of gurgles and burbles, and by the end of the sixth month he might be a real chatterbox at times.

His laughter and language help him engage others in conversation and play. By the end of 6 months your baby might be sitting up, and may even pull himself up to stand. He'll probably be experimenting with food, and might even be able to move from one end of the room to the other, either by bottom-shuffling or belly crawling.

You will know your baby well now, and be quicker to trust your instincts. You'll probably notice when he's tired, in pain or discomfort, know when he's hungry, and be quick to diagnose boredom. He knows you better too and, knowing that you understand him, will begin to use you as his interpreter as he communicates with other people. As he learns through play, you are still his most important companion, teacher and comforter, and he is still a great teacher for you. His trust of other people is a reflection of the good foundation you give him and is a great asset while he is learning so much.

Your baby's social life

Although your baby knows that he is physically separate from you, he has no concept that you and he have independent minds (or, indeed, any mind at all). His short-term memory is only 3–5 seconds at 6 months, so although he may cry for a toy that's taken from him, if he's given a replacement or loses sight of it, he'll quickly shift his attention to something new. The same happens when people leave: a short feeling of loss soon disappears and your baby will calm down if he's with someone who makes him feel secure, loved and entertained.

Behind his short-term memory are longer memories that help him recognise people and things. While he may not miss you, when you return he'll recognise your face and instantly expect the other things that make up 'you' – smiles, a certain voice and a comforting smell. He won't

remember what he was doing 10 minutes ago, but much of his world will now be familiar. This familiarity breeds trust, and he may often turn to his parents and adult carers to check their reaction when he meets something or someone new, or if he is trying to solve a problem ('How do I get to that toy I can see?'). By the sixth month your baby may already have a number of different signs to greet different people: for example, when he sees you he may put his arms out as if to say, 'There you are, here I am, let's have a cuddle.'

Communication

Although many of your baby's movements are still unconscious, he is increasingly using his body purposefully. He reaches up to your face and grips your nose between his tiny fingers through curiosity and when

---

Self-awareness games

- As he develops relationships, your baby will enjoy games that are specific to each person and may love games involving waiting, such as 'incy wincy spider' with tickles starting at the toes and ending on his chin. This is a great time to do peek-a-boo by hiding your face behind your hands. At 4 months if you peek through the gaps in your fingers you'll see a total lack of expectation on his face, as if he has no idea where you are, followed by a peal of laughter as you reappear. By 6 months he'll have learnt the rules of the game and giggle as he waits for your face to appear.
- You will repeatedly do what he finds funny because it makes you both feel good. It doesn't matter if you jump up and down, sing funny songs, sit in front of him wrinkling your nose or gently tickle him: the fun games will spice up and strengthen your relationship. He learns from everything: 'If Dad can dance like that, can I? How does he get his feet off the floor? He moves but he's always the same daddy. Where did that tongue come from? Have I got one? If I stick it out, will he laugh? I like that tickle – I'll ask for another one by smiling; I know that will make him do it again.'

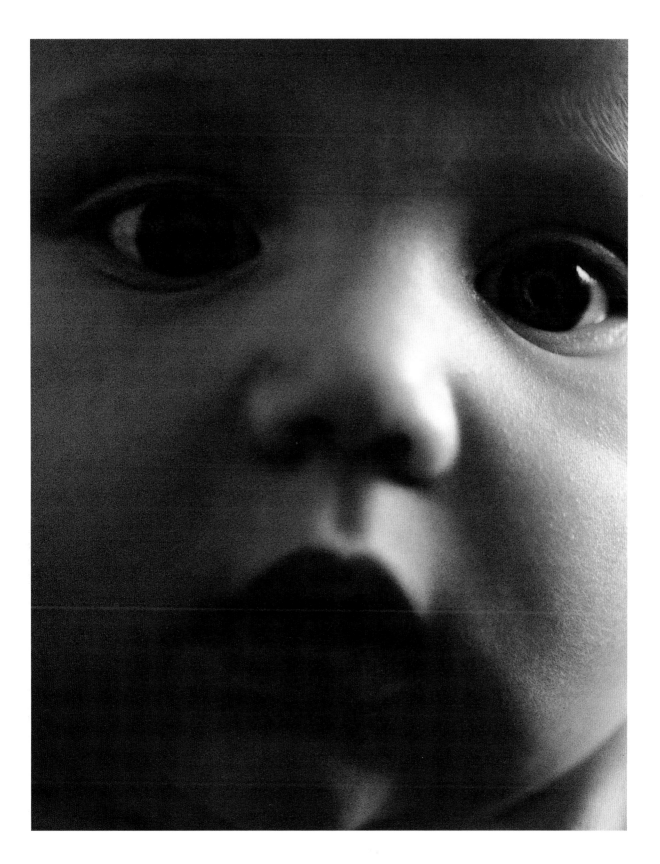

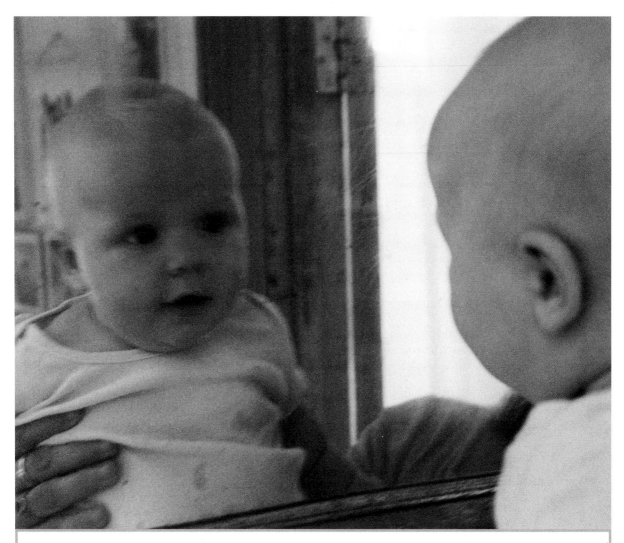

Visual games

- Let your baby play the mirroring game as much as you and he want to: hold him in front of you and move your mouth or blink, wrinkle your nose or shake your head. He'll probably laugh at you (who wouldn't?) but if he's in the mood he'll copy you as well, and if this makes you laugh he'll enjoy it and try again. He's having fun while learning about controlling his face. You may enjoy holding him in front of a mirror (or use tin foil pressed nice and flat). One day he will break into a grin and ripple with laughter – he sees an instant response to his smile and begins a conversation with 'another' baby.
- Give your baby a selection of colourful and noisy toys and mobiles and let him study them for as long as he likes. You can help him develop his arms and keep the games engaging by putting visually exciting toys within his reach. See what he does if you cover a toy with an upturned bucket. He won't search for it, but will turn his attention to something else. By 6 months if he is sitting on your lap and drops his toy on to the floor and it rolls out of sight, he may look where he expected it to fall, but search no further. It's not because his vision isn't developed but because he has little concept that the toy continues to exist when he can't see it. If he is interested in something you do not want him to have, removing it from his sight will take it out of his mind. If you give him something else at the same time there will be less fuss at the loss of the original object.
- When your baby is sitting sturdily on your lap, books become excellent playthings. Use books made from cardboard or cloth. If you read or talk while he looks at the pictures, and choose books that have textures or pop-up sections, he'll be even more drawn in to this intriguing world.
- Don't forget that he also gets a chance to develop his long-range vision each time you go out, so draw his attention to things that are on the other side of the road, at the top of a tree or across the garden.

he sees a bottle in your hand, he may open and close his mouth with expectation or wave his arms up and down. When he's hungry but doesn't see a bottle, he may use similar signals to let you know what he wants.

You can follow his eyes as he looks at a toy and pass it to him; from 4 or 5 months he can follow your gaze to something and take an interest in it. He can grip your shoulder or arm while you hold him, to reciprocate your loving touch, and can reach towards your plate to let you know he's interested in trying your food.

Most of the time he communicates so well and so clearly that you respond without needing to think about his messages. You imitate him automatically and he copies you. This is crucial: what he learns through imitation teaches him what he isn't genetically predisposed to learn – the nuances, attitudes and body language of his social world. By 6 months, he will have learnt a great deal about his culture. And he's learning how to be an active part of it: how his body language develops now provides the basis for making signals that may he may begin to use from 7 or 9 months.

He opens conversations with eye contact and body movements. Vocally, his outbursts of crying will probably be shorter and more widely spaced. He is learning to make sounds, control them, link them and thread them together with musical intonation. Every bit of practice he gets will help him understand you, and by the end of the sixth month he may exhibit patterns of sounds that reflect your own way of talking.

His voice box descends at around 4 months, allowing him to make guttural noises that are between vowels and consonants ('marginal babbling'). What he understands far exceeds what he can convey. Experiments have shown that at 6 months most babies show surprise if a sentence is spoken with stresses in the wrong place (for example, 'THIS appLE is rEd', instead of normal emphasis). Your

baby can tell the difference between questions and statements, and can tell what some words refer to by following your eyes or your movements. By the end of his sixth month, he will probably recognise his name and is linking the shape of your mouth with the sounds that he hears; he's building a mouth-to-sound map and can use this to try out his own sounds.

Vision
Your baby is better at concentrating on the details in faces and objects that are close to him, and can focus to at least 5 m (5 yd). His vision has become binocular; that is, the images from both eyes are merged to give a three-dimensional impression. This is why he can judge speed, depth and direction with uncanny accuracy: he is now able to predict the direction familiar objects will follow and can track something whizzing past (his sister on her tricycle, perhaps). As his hands become more co-ordinated he learns about and tests the objects in his world.

In the fifth month, your baby begins to use his eyes more expressively. An inviting glance may tell you he's ready for a game; a single look could tell you he's about to break into a cry. He watches you keenly, and learns a lot by your facial expressions. He may very well show surprise if you greet him with a blank face rather than a broad smile. When he's convinced that his hands are a part of him, he'll be so enraptured by them he'll spend minutes at a time gazing at the way they fan out and interlock.

By 6 months, your baby's vision is around 20/200 (10% of an adult's). He can see things that fall within his field of vision well, but is not adapt at perceiving distance and depth. The more he studies things and the more contact he has with what he can see (your face, his toys, the armchair, the saucepan, the phone), the more easily he remembers things. Each time he sees something familiar he assesses its texture and heaviness, and recalls information his brain has already stored – whether and how it moves, the sound it makes, how it smells and how it feels in his mouth. By the end of the sixth month he will have no trouble recognising you if you have been away for up to 2 weeks.

Hearing
In these months your baby's ability to locate sounds improves. Already able to locate noises made in front and to the side, he will soon begin to look towards noises made above him and below his face and by 6 months he may locate noises made behind him, though his response won't be as quick as yours for around a year. As he gets better at using his hands he'll test anything for noises, and delight in any sound he can, from rambling baby-speak to the repetitive clonk of his heels banging on the floor. A lot of the energy your baby puts in to hearing at the moment relates to his language learning and it is significant that he

---

Communicating games
• Let your baby have his say and then reply, and wait for him to speak again. If he's not trying out his vocal repertoire on you or when he's on his own, plan some sessions when there is no other noise (radio and television off and other children quietly occupied) and play the mirroring game: make some simple noises with your face close to his and give him spaces to fill. If he responds with a smile or a look in his eyes rather than cooing, accept it and continue the conversation; his language entails many strands of expression. Talking to people and taking turns is the best way for him to learn now. When he knows that you've heard him, and taken an interest, he'll feel good. He'll also like watching you talk to friends or even on the phone, and may enjoy hearing you sing.

understands so much more than he can vocalise. Your baby expects people to talk when they open their mouths – mouth at him like a goldfish and he'll wait for a sound, and may be puzzled if none comes.

Smell and taste

Your baby uses his sense of smell unintentionally yet all the time, and it is still one of the sharpest senses. Taste is also extremely significant – as he puts anything and everything into his mouth he learns about texture and size and tastes a whole range of flavours with his lips and tongue. It's an important part of learning and helps his brain make associations between how an object looks, feels, tastes and smells; this 'cross-modal' matching enables him to understand and predict properties of things he can only see

or hear. If he has played with balls often, licked, bashed and rolled them, he may expect all balls to roll. When you choose to offer solids (any time from 16 weeks onwards), a whole new world of taste and texture opens up and he can learn more about the food he has previously only seen and smelled.

Body development

Your baby's strength and co-ordination increase daily. When he first rolls from his tummy on to his back, which may happen by the fifth month, he links movements in his lower back, legs, arms, shoulders and neck, and makes them happen in the right order. Meanwhile he becomes more flexible and starts using his hands to explore his feet as he lies down; by around 5 months, he'll get his toes into his mouth. By then he'll already be using his feet together with his hands to hold toys, a trick that he'll abandon by 7 months.

Your baby is also keen to become upright, and will welcome help. From around 4 months he may love being held and bounced in a standing position and will bear his weight for a few moments before his knees give way and he falls with a soft nappy-plop on to your lap. Learning to sit will also take up a lot of time. At 4 months he begins to support more of his weight if you prop him in a sitting position and might jig up and down and move him back away from the cushion, even though if he stretches too far he'll keel over. By 5 months he'll probably be able to maintain his balance for a moment if you place him in a sitting position without support and by 6 months he may stay upright (perhaps with a few wobbles) for as long as 30 seconds, perhaps using his arms to support his weight.

How your baby uses his arms and hands

Muscle control progresses from your baby's shoulders to his fingertips, so at 3 months, though his swiping may be quite accurate, his hands won't be ready to take hold of what he's aiming for. By around 4 months he may begin to use both hands when he reaches for something and he'll often kick or push with his legs as he tries to propel his arms forward. As he gets more balanced he will often have his hands open, ready to grasp as he reaches for something.

At first his grasp is unrefined: he uses his thumb as one of his fingers and holds things low in his hand so they protrude out of the bottom, and finds it difficult to test them further through sucking. But he won't give up trying. He may try to grip a flower on a flat rug or a face in a picture book, and will only ever catch a swinging object by chance. Over time, he'll learn that some things can be picked up and some can't, and hand control will increase. He may pass an object from one hand to the other and will begin to use his thumb in opposition to his fingers. By around 6 months he may reach and grasp with only one hand, without losing his balance.

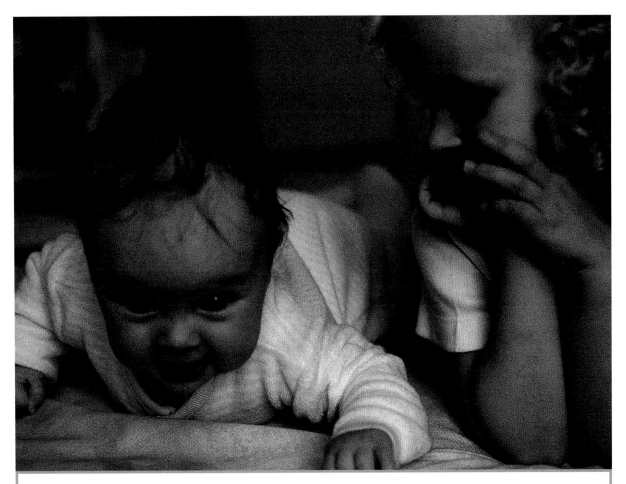

Developmental games

- Your baby may enjoy sitting in his baby chair. Yet when he starts straining to sit up, the chair becomes a hazard because he may topple forwards, and he'll develop better strength from sitting on a flat surface. So instead of sitting him in his baby chair hold him on your lap or prop him up on the floor with cushions around him, and arrange interesting toys within his reach. But don't leave him sitting for too long – lying down still offers the best support for his growing spine.
- When he's lying on his back, tempt him to kick against your hands or face, and give a little resistance; this helps him build strength.
- Give him plenty of time on his front too, and if he's reluctant to lift his head off the floor, lie next to him and talk – the temptation to see what you are doing will give him the impetus to look up, and he'll build strength.
- If your baby has an older brother or sister, his or her input might be very helpful and fun to watch – siblings can demand response and often love repeating games over and over again.
- Your baby may love to pat an open book, or grab his favourite toy, and will still try to bring everything to his mouth. His hands are the tools he needs to satisfy his curiosity and the more practice he has at reaching, opening, closing and grabbing, the more he will learn.
- Your baby will show delight every time he feels he has made an achievement – imagine being able to see something for 5 whole months and finally being able to reach out, grasp it and explore it at will.
- While he lies on his back, pass him toys that he can grip easily, and let him wave them around and feel their weight and texture.
- When he's on his tummy or side or sitting, place a range of toys within easy reach. If he falls while he's trying to reach something, he'll try again and again until he succeeds. After a few attempts, make it easier so he can definitely reach his goal – otherwise he may try, try, try and never succeed, and end up tired and grumpy.
- In his pram or pushchair your baby may love hitting and grabbing a string of toys hanging across the seat, and while he's in your arms, your face, lips, hair, buttons or necklace will be perfect playthings. He will be increasingly curious about the way you look and behave, and what it is that is so similar about the two of you.

How your baby sleeps: months 4, 5 & 6

At 3 months your baby is making a transition from her newborn stage. At 6 months she is well down the road towards independence. There will be a huge difference between her sleeping habits at the beginning and the end of these 3 months. She may already sleep through the night as she travels through her fourth month, or not until the sixth month or later. Her sleep affects yours; while parents do get used to broken nights, none complain of the pleasure of a good long sleep.

Sleeping soundly

If your baby gets guidance and support, she's likely to sleep through the night sooner rather than later. Not every parent yearns for this, however. Some are very relaxed about sleeping patterns and are happy to respond to their baby, whatever she needs, knowing that babyhood is a very short time and the closeness and support it involves do fade. Generally this is easier if there are no problems, but the range, as ever, is wide. Some adults are lucky and have a baby that sleeps through, some still consider themselves lucky to be breathing in their baby's scent after a feed in bed, whatever the time is.

At 3 months, the average time spent sleeping is between 13 and 15 hours, with roughly 5 of these hours during the day, and most babies continue to wake once or twice a night. If you enter the fourth month and still haven't had a full night's sleep, you're not alone. Have faith: as your baby grows, gets more active, eats more and sleeps less during the day, a full night's sleep will come. Some babies give up night waking of their own accord, and others need encouragement. Now is a good time to approach the issue.

Waking at night

Getting your baby to sleep is the first challenge. To begin with, use a bedtime routine that includes darkening the room and reducing noise levels to relax your baby and give a cue for sleep. You may want to introduce a soothing tape or a mobile above the cot to lull her and help her feel secure. As she gets older she may become attached to a particular toy or 'cuddly' and settle better with this in bed, but don't give her anything too big that could act as an insulator and contribute to dangerous overheating. Your baby may suck her fingers or thumbs, or relax with a dummy. If your baby continues to complain, follow the advice for settling her given on p.205.

The second and greater challenge is reducing night waking. This may be due to a number of causes:
- The most likely cause is hunger. If your baby is not hungry she may drift back to sleep after a short suck, having satisfied her thirst or need for comfort.
- She might be uncomfortable, perhaps with a full nappy.

- Her clothing may be too tight.
- She may be too hot or too cold. Check her temperature by feeling her tummy.
- She may find the room too light or too dark.
- If you suspect she is ill stay with her and seek a medical opinion as soon as possible.

A significant cause of night waking is often behaviour during the day.
- If your baby has recently begun eating solid food, feelings of digestion may unsettle her and she'll benefit from a regular eating pattern, with no solid food for at least 1 hour before bed. Check that she is still getting adequate calories and enough milk; you will be reassured if she is gaining weight.
- Look at the pattern of daytime sleep and try to limit this to 5 hours at most, with no sleep for 3 hours before 'bedtime'.
- Your baby needs exercise and fresh air. She will probably get enough exercise in the course of a normal day but not if she has been confined, for instance, in the car. She may enjoy being played with, swimming or a massage. If the weather has been dismal and you've been inside all day, open windows or take a quick walk in the rain.
- Your baby's bed may be uncomfortable – try changing the sheets, using natural fibres or warming the sheets and blankets before bedtime. Is there a toy or cot bumper that could get in the way? Is she getting too cold or hot? Adjust the bedding according to temperature and use a sleeping bag if she's happy with this.
- If your baby is waking herself up with a cough, try using some eucalyptus oil or a plug-in vaporiser to help keep her airways clear.

Breaking the habit of waking at night

If your baby wakes at almost the same time each night but falls asleep as soon as you cuddle her or let her suck, she is probably waking through habit. One day you may feel that the time is right to try and stop her waking – you'll need to put in some concerted effort if you want to break this habit. Stick with it, and you will almost certainly get results. One or more of the following suggestions may suit you.

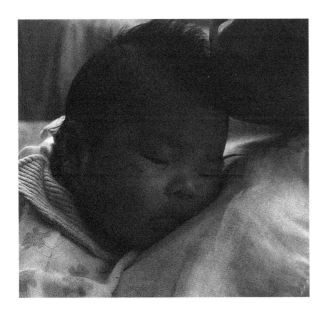

- Each time your baby wakes, start off by doing as little as possible. Stroke her head and back and tuck her in. Give her a dummy if she uses one. Talk to her to reassure her.
- This may help or she may wake up again. Try the same thing again.
- If she does not go back to sleep, she may need her nappy changing. Try to do this without turning the lights on, or entertaining her, but don't do it if it isn't necessary.
- If she wakes again, offer some water. The water has two functions. It tells your baby that night is not for eating, but she can have water if she is thirsty. Tell her this with a firm but gentle tone.
- Repeat the above activities whenever your baby wakes. Remember that the night is supposed to be boring, so don't do anything that is likely to make her excited.
- If she's still unhappy, give her some milk for the first nights, but not as much as she usually eats so she doesn't stock up on calories at night. If she usually feeds from both breasts, or 175 ml (5 fl oz) from a bottle, give one breast, or 100 ml (3 fl oz). Cut down gradually over the first week. If you are sharing your bed you can still reduce the feeds, and she may settle back to sleep quicker than she would in her own cot.
- You may decide that the only option is to see if she will fall asleep after a little crying. Only you can decide whether to wait for 1 minute, 5 minutes or 15 before going to her. Remember that you are not disciplining but training her to fall asleep without help. As she surfaces from deep sleep and glimpses a world where she can't see your face, she may cry out for reassurance. If you can gradually lengthen the time between her first whimper and your appearance at her bedside, you may be surprised that she can actually go back to sleep without a reassuring cuddle.

Remember that sometimes your baby will need to eat during the night: illness or growth spurts could make her extra hungry. And if her cry stirs something near to panic in you, go to her immediately. Whether it's a bad dream, a sore tummy, an unexpected vomit, a painful gum or fear of being alone, she'll feel soothed and protected when you're with her.

Most importantly, don't be hard on yourself. If you can't bear to leave her to cry, don't feel that anyone is telling you that you must, or that you are wrong. You will hear a variety of opinions from friends or relatives and from your health visitor. It is best to try to follow your intuition, remembering there is no single 'correct way' for all families.

Daytime sleep

As your baby gets older you may gradually extend the time between day time naps. If she tends to sleep for one long stretch, let her sleep as she needs, but not beyond 4pm if you want her to go to bed by 7 or 8pm. For her other naps during the day wake her gently after around 45 minutes when she surfaces from deep slumber, and encourage her to eat or play, depending on your schedule. To make her naps worthwhile try not to let her sleep with an empty tummy or a full nappy or just before you're due to go out. The better she sleeps, the more likely she is to fit into a regular pattern that will help you organise her days as well as her nights.

If your baby simply doesn't need to nap during the day it's still good to have a quiet time, perhaps after lunch, when you read a book, massage her or take her for a walk. Without a rest she may feel strung out at the end of the day and this can lead to unsettled sleep.

How can I make my baby's transition from her Moses basket to her cot easy? She seems so cosy in her basket now, even though she's almost too big for it.

Your delicate, tiny little newborn has grown. She's no longer resting in her basket like a single pea in a big pod; instead she's bashing the sides, even in her sleep. She needs to move to a larger space, and this will probably help her sleep better. You can help her take the move in her stride with a few simple steps:

- Let her play in her cot during the day so it becomes familiar.
- Place her Moses basket inside her cot and let her have a few daytime naps there before putting her there for the night.
- When she's too big for the basket, make up the cot with blankets that smell familiar, and line it with some pictures or fabric that were part of her basket. The familiarity will reassure her.

When your baby cries: months 4, 5 & 6

As the second 3-month period begins, your baby will be settled and, probably, crying less than he did as a newborn. Now his crying develops as he masters many other ways to make himself understood and he may often flit between babbling and crying as he tries to get his message across. And, as you settle into parenthood, you may be clearer about what your baby means when he cries, and though he will still throw you from time to time, you'll have more faith that you can give him the right response. There may, however, be days when crying persists or you find it harder than usual to cope.

What your baby is telling you

By now you may have a clear idea of your baby's character: he may be placid and quiet, demanding and vocal, or have a time of day when he simply needs to cry and wants you to hold him. Against this background his cries may be easier to decipher and placate. Yet he has changed from a newborn or fledgling to curious explorer and chatterbox. With wider spaces between feeds and longer sleep, he has longer wakeful periods and his range of needs has extended.

Many of the things that might have made your baby cry in the first 3 months may still cause him to cry now. You may be quick to recognise a trigger and expert at offering the right comfort, but the checklist on this page may still be very helpful. A marked difference is that he will love – and expect – interactive play and may complain if he's not getting enough attention or is not being acknowledged and made part of your conversations. He can object more if an interesting object is denied him – you'll know that it's dangerous, while he has no idea. If you remove it from sight he will soon forget about it. His transition to solid eater may also influence his crying – he might have discomfort from digestion or cry out to you when he is hungry, or eager, for food, or surprised by an unexpected flavour.

Crying and sleep

At night, or at bedtime, your baby could begin to fight his sleep, probably because he wants to stay with you and continue to learn, explore and play. With a relaxed bedtime routine you can calm his body and mind and settle him. He might settle well to a bedtime story, starting a habit that continues throughout childhood. When your baby surfaces from deep sleep at night he may be better at calming himself – indeed, many babies make less night-time fuss after the third month. If you are trying to reduce your baby's habit of waking (p.238), however, you will be in for some persistent and insistent wails in the short term.

Crying from illness

If your baby's cry suggests illness or pain, call a doctor if you're at all worried. He might be uncomfortable from colic (p.431), although this commonly passes by the end of the third month. The other common cause to watch for is teething (p.541), which may give intermittent pain or discomfort over a number of days. If your baby is unwell, give him love and comfort and help him fall asleep or eat when he wants so he can recuperate. Relax all your routines. He'll need your support and may want to share your bed, your armchair, your bath – put everything else on hold.

Why does your baby cry?

Communication
- Crying is still a central part of your baby's communication.
- Sometimes he still needs comfort and space simply to let it all out.

Hunger and digestion
- You may know your baby's 'I am hungry' cry by now, and be familiar with his feeding pattern.
- He may cry from digestive discomfort, particularly as his body adapts to eating solid food.

What's happening
- Your baby may become more clingy in his sixth month, and be a little nervous on meeting new people or visiting new places. This is normal.
- He may be quicker to complain if he feels bored, wants company or interaction, or is frustrated when he can't do what he wants to.
- He may cry if he wants more physical stimulation.
- He may cry if he wants peace and quiet.

Illness
- Persistent crying or unusually insistent crying may signal illness.
- If you are at all concerned, contact your health visitor or doctor.

Crying and emotions

Of course crying is still a vital part of your baby's communication. He may by now have a particular tone of wail to express frustration, for instance. Often, a short-lived cry is not a sign of being upset but may instead be the outward sign of the way he feels inside. He could be frustrated because he cannot reach his toy or upset because you are not paying attention to him while you talk on the phone – and express these feelings quickly and loudly. This kind of crying often stops when the problem disappears (you pass the toy to him or finish your phone call) and does not indicate that your baby is spoilt. It is an entirely natural way for him to express himself at this age.

Crying and the family atmosphere

Your baby's crying pattern, and the urgency and persistence of his cries, will also reflect the atmosphere at home and at his place of care, if he goes away from home while you work. This may not be easy to spot, as you may not notice the atmosphere in the same way as your baby does. Sometimes it is helpful to try to consider things from his perspective. He may feel anxious, unsure or left out if you have been rushing around or if you have been upset and arguing and feel unenthusiastic at the moment. He may feel vulnerable if there is conflict among the adults in his life or in a care situation if he does not feel secure with his carers. His personality may clash with another child's.

At home, if the atmosphere is strained or things don't feel quite right, making space for quality time with your baby may soon help. If you build quality time into each day, when he feels that he has your full attention, he may feel more settled. If you think that the care situation may not suit your baby, try to arrange some time off work so you can spend time with him. It may be possible to spend time observing him when he cannot see you, or you could ask his carers to keep notes of his actions and behaviour patterns during the day. You may need to consider changing his carers.

Crying and comfort

When your baby cries, it is your instinct to imagine what might be wrong and try to fix it. It is also your instinct to act appropriately, most, if not all, of the time. So if your baby is hungry and you offer him milk or food, you will have solved the problem. If he is bored and you begin to play with him, his frustration will disappear. If he is uncomfortable or in pain, you may help. If he is upset or scared, and needs the security and reassurance of your embrace, this too is easy to give. Nature plays its cards well, because your response serves not merely to reduce crying – it also gives your baby what he needs for normal development: your attention and interaction make him feel heard and wanted, adding to his sense of self-esteem; your embrace and caresses stimulate his skin, give him pleasure

and increase his sense of bodily awareness; and your encouragement and love are important for his ongoing emotional development.

Your responses, well-rehearsed in the first 3 months after birth, may now be automatic. To anyone else, your baby's crying may sound unfathomable, but to you it is a straightforward method of communication. That you can respond appropriately is a sign that the dance of communication between you is flowing well. When he or you is out of step – either he won't stop crying, you can't cope or you feel an unusual sense of panic – this is an indication that you need further support or even medical opinion. This is nature playing its cards right, once again.

If your baby cries a lot

Although it's reasonably safe to say that most babies cry less as they get older, this is not always the case. If your baby cries more now than he did in the first 3 months, or has always cried a lot, you will probably be exhausted. You may be worried there is something seriously wrong with your baby. As you try to find possible causes, see if there are triggers for his outbursts – a time of day, a thing, a person, a place or a position he doesn't like it. Make some notes and take your baby to see the doctor, or ask your health visitor to come to your house. Both of you need support through this difficult time.

Some babies have more than the usual dose of excess energy and cry less if they are stimulated sufficiently. Some are simply 'needy' babies and cry quickly if they are left or feel at all unhappy. Some babies don't like sudden changes and if something is different – perhaps you've gone to work, introduced a new carer or redecorated your baby's room – give extra-special comfort and attention and see if things improve. If you have excluded illnesses you might consider a complementary therapy such as homeopathy, massage or cranial osteopathy, with guidance from a practitioner qualified to care for babies. In the sixth month many babies begin to cry more than before. Often this is a sign they are feeling anxious about being left alone – confusion and insecurity are quite normal as your baby begins to work out that he is separate from you (p.262).

Still crying?

If you have tried everything, excluded illness and still he cries:
- Put your baby down, walk out of the room, shut the door and take a short break.
- Give him to someone else, for a few hours if possible – perhaps he or she could take him for a walk.
- Use any time away from your baby to look after yourself.
- Go out with your baby and visit other parents if possible.
- Phone a friend or relative, your Health Visitor, GP or the CRY-SIS help line.

Your baby's evolving diet: months 4, 5 & 6

In the second 3 months your baby will have new hunger feelings. Now that she's so physically active, she'll get hungrier and will drink more, and from her perch on your lap she can watch closely as you eat. One day you may be surprised as her little hand reaches towards your food. She's ready for a taste. By the end of her sixth month she will probably be enjoying meals with you in addition to regular milk feeds. Her exploration of the world of food is just beginning and promises to be fun, and messy, for both of you.

Milk

In these 3 months it's vital that your baby continues to drink formula or breast milk as the largest part of her daily diet. It gives her superb nutrition with a full quota of vitamins and minerals and the contact at feeding time helps her feel loved and protected. Breast milk continues to provide antibodies and essential nutrients and is still the best source of milk. Some mother and baby partnerships give up the breast in the first month, others in the fifth month and others not until much later. If you want to switch from breast to bottle, or supplement some breastfeeds with a bottle, turn to p.195 for guidance. If you're already bottle feeding, stick to the formula that your baby is used to. Before 6 months her system is not mature enough to cope with 'follow-on' milk.

Scheduling milk feeds

During this period you may be keen to help your baby drop or reduce night feeds. Her intake of milk and feeding schedule during the day have a direct bearing on her sleep at night. If you are still feeding her once or twice between 8pm and 6 or 7am, the month before you introduce solids is a perfect time to build a milk schedule. If you know roughly when your baby will be hungry you could find the transition to solids at meal times simpler.

- View your baby's day with a beginning (morning) and an end (last feed and sleep), and give her regular feeds.
- A typical day's feeding schedule could be: a feed at 6 or 6.30am, a 'breakfast' at 9am, 'lunch' at noon or 1pm, afternoon feed around 3 or 4pm, and 'dinner' around 6 or 7pm. Around 3 hours between milk feeds is average, but the range is wide.
- As your baby gets more active and hungrier, give her more milk at each sitting rather than introduce another mealtime.
- If your baby eats well at each feeding time (from both breasts or around 175 ml/6 fl oz of formula, although this can vary widely according to individual babies) she should have eaten enough to see her through the night. If you are happy that she has, but she still wakes, you may want to help her sleep through by attending to the other causes of waking (p.238).

Weaning on to solid food

Opinion regarding the best time to start a baby on solid food has changed over the last 50 years, and across the world there are different philosophies about the benefits of adding solid food to a milk diet. The current recommendation is that weaning should not begin until 16 weeks after birth or after the expected due date if your baby was premature. By this time your baby's digestive system will have matured enough to break down food. Some babies are reluctant and stick to their milk diet for longer. It may take your baby up to the end of her sixth month to get used to eating food. Even if she doesn't eat much, her experiments with food help her learn and help her body adapt. Take it easy and support her as you go into this together.

Giving your baby non-milk food before she is ready may bring on colicky symptoms, or worsen existing problems or lead to constipation or (less commonly) diarrhoea. If your baby has a tendency to food intolerance (p.391), it may be activated by early solid feeding. It takes time for every baby to develop the enzymes to cope with non-milk food and to build up the immune system.

Your baby's first tastes of solids

Weaning your baby does not mean an overnight change from a milk-drinking baby to a three-meals-a-day girl. Solids supplement but do not replace milk feeds and progress is best made gently in response to your baby's signals. During the day if she shows curiosity and is reaching out for your food or mouthing like a goldfish as she sees you eating, you can assume she's ready to try some. Offer something smooth with a gentle flavour, cooled to room temperature: soup or very sloppy mashed potato would be better than olive paste or gravy. As she takes her first tastes she'll rely on you for moral and physical support. Hold her on your lap and give her food with your finger. She may suck thoughtfully, feel the texture with her tongue and then squeeze out a mush through pursed lips. If so, she's made the perfect start – she needs to acquaint herself with food before she begins to swallow it. It's a new concept and she'll take time to get used to it.

After she has had her first taste, your baby might open wide and ask for more or sit back and close her mouth. At your next meal she may show interest again, or may not ask for another taste until tomorrow or the day after. Offer your baby food when she's alert and content and let her set the pace. What's important is that she should feel supported and learns to associate eating with fun and socialising. Smile, encourage her and praise her – to her, it's another game of discovery.

When to give spoon feeds

When you and your baby have completed the 'trial' stage and you're ready to move on to regular meals, you can introduce a soft plastic spoon and give her her own specially prepared food. It is best to sterilise all the spoons and bowls that she uses (p.201).

Begin with baby rice mixed with her usual milk: this won't taste very different from milk but will feel different. Give one spoonful a day, and guide it gently into her open mouth: you'll find it easier if you keep the spoon above her tongue. She may even need two or three mouthfuls to eat this amount. If she spits out what you give her but seems happy, she's learning; if she cries or turns her head away from the spoon, she doesn't like either the taste or the experience. Rather than trying to force the food on her, stop the meal then and there and try again later. If she eats

eagerly and enthusiastically tries to catch the spoon each time it approaches, give her a spoon to play with while you feed her with another.

Begin with the solid at lunchtime following half her usual milk feed; if she has difficulty digesting she should settle down before bedtime. If she doesn't enjoy it, try moving her 'meal' to another time of day. Whenever you feed her, don't offer the spoon when she is howling with hunger, and until she's over 6 months always begin her meal with milk.

If your baby drinks from a bottle, break half-way through and introduce the solid part of the meal and then offer her milk again. If she's breastfeeding, give her one breast, then her solid and then as much as she will take from the second breast. If your baby seems happy after between 4 and 7 days of having one spoonful a day, introduce another, and then continue to build up gradually. Always end the day with a milk feed, last thing before she settles down for the night.

What can you feed your baby?

Research over the last 10 years has given valuable insight into healthy diets for babies. What has become clear is that excessive salt can be harmful, as can excessive sugar, so don't add any extra to food you cook: the natural levels are quite high enough. Specially prepared baby rice or cereal is

---

A rough guide to mealtimes

These meals are in addition to your baby's usual milk feeds.

Day/week	Time of day and food	Notes
Days 1–4	**Late morning/midday:** 1 tsp baby rice or cereal mixed with bottle or breast milk.	Give half of milk feed first, then the solid, then finish with milk.
Days 4–7	**Late morning/midday:** 1 tsp baby rice or cereal mixed with bottle or breast milk. **In the evening, at least 1 hour before bed:** 1 tsp puréed pear.	Stagger with milk feed, as before.
Week 2	**Lunchtime:** 1–2 tsp puréed vegetable (e.g. carrot). **In the evening, at least 1 hour before bed:** 2 tsp puréed vegetable and baby rice followed by 1 tsp puréed fruit.	Stagger with milk feed, as before.
Weeks 3–4 (up to 5 months)	**Lunchtime:** Vegetable or fruit purée. **In the evening, at least 1 hour before bed:** Baby rice mixed with puréed vegetables, with fruit to follow if your baby wishes.	Gradually increase quantities and vary types of vegetables and fruit, introducing something new every 3 or 4 days.
Weeks 5–8 (months 5–6)	**Breakfast (after a milk feed):** Introduce some baby cereal with fruit purée. **Lunch:** Give potato or rice with vegetables. **Evening meal:** Sweet vegetable (carrot, swede or cauliflower) and 1–2 tsp of cereal, plus fruit to finish.	Give your baby as much as she is happy to take – she is unlikely to overeat and will vomit up any excess. It's better to have food left over than a hungry baby.

a great food to start with, mixed with a little breast or bottle milk, and an easily digestible fruit is puréed pear. After a few days you can introduce a finely mashed or puréed vegetable such as carrot or sweet potato (yam). Unless you have a history of allergies (p.391) or are concerned about some of your baby's symptoms, there's no need to introduce foods with a space of 3 days in between, as was thought until recently. Yet you do need to keep an eye on the way your baby copes with different foods. Some foods, like banana, may reduce her number of motions while others, perhaps summer fruits, may increase them. If your baby seems uncomfortable or has an unexplained rash, think over her diet in the last 24 hours and exclude anything suspicious. Re-introduce it in a few weeks and watch her reaction.

If you are eating something suitable and share it with your baby, you'll know just what she's getting, and will make the first steps towards family meals. Although most babies love sweet food they are not as partial to it as toddlers seem to be. Give your baby lots of vegetables, with fruit purées as a second choice, and avoid sweets and biscuits at all costs; they will not give her the calories that she needs and can cause decay in her developing teeth.

Ready-made baby food

Baby food in jars and powder is processed with a sensitive digestive system in mind. The recipes and flavours are chosen by a taste panel of adults, and based on years of experience and feedback. Each 'meal' follows strict national weaning directives, which limit the content of salt, sugar and additives, and is prepared under the strictest code of

---

Can I start my baby on solids before she's 16 weeks old? Could this help her sleep longer at night?

If you are keen to introduce your baby to solids before she is 16 weeks old, you need to consider her individual needs. Usually babies who are bigger than average and weigh more than 7.3 kg (16 lb) by 12 weeks can cope with solids because their digestive system may be mature enough, but the response may be less favourable from a small 12-week-old or younger baby; this includes a baby born prematurely who hasn't reached 16 weeks following her expected due date.

If you want to give her solids in order to get a good night's sleep, think again. If you try to give her solids before she's ready, whether you offer potato, custard or baby rice, she'll feel pressurised and sense your frustration if she refuses to eat. If you persist, an unhappy relationship with food may continue into toddler years and beyond, making mealtimes a struggle for the whole family. There are other ways to help her sleep better: be patient, ensure she gets enough milk, and work on her sleeping pattern, day and night (p.236).

Sample day for a 6-month-old baby

This plan allows for five breastfeeds or five bottles of 250 ml (8 fl oz), giving a total milk intake of around 1125 ml (38 fl oz) a day. Remember that all babies are different so timings and milk intake may vary. Your baby is likely to settle well if there is a daily structure that helps her eat and sleep well, feel full and have stable energy levels.

7/8am	**Breast or bottle in bed in the morning:** This may be combined with a solid breakfast. If she has woken early (6am) and had milk already, give breakfast and a milk feed at around 9am.
Around 10am	**Mid-morning milk feed:** Some babies like this unless breakfast was late. As solids increase, this feed will drop.
12/1.30pm	**Lunch:** Milk plus solid food
Around 3pm	**Afternoon milk feed:** Most babies enjoy this.
5/6pm	**Tea/dinner:** Solid food and small drink; give water if your baby is happy to let go of milk.
Bedtime	**Breast or bottle before bed.**

If you are concerned about your baby's eating habits, consult your doctor or health visitor and monitor her weight

---

hygiene and sterility. They are made with the expectation that should a baby be fed pre-packed food exclusively, she would get all the nutrition, vitamins and minerals she requires. Even so, some processed meals can have unusually high quantities of sugar (check the ingredients) and shouldn't be given on a regular basis; pure fruit purées have a high level of sucrose.

Keep jars and packets for outings, or those days when you're just too busy or exhausted to prepare something yourself, and choose savoury dishes over sweets, every time. If you only use half a jar keep the remainder in the fridge and then throw it away if your baby doesn't eat it within 24 hours.

Wherever possible, buy organic. This applies to the vegetables and fruits that you mash as well as eat raw. Your baby's tender new system is very susceptible to the harmful effects of excessive pesticide residues and other artificial chemicals that are found in conventionally produced food. If you choose not to buy organic produce, at least always wash fruit and vegetables and peel them if possible. It is worth giving your baby the best start in life by shielding her from chemicals, even if the risks from ingesting them are still unclear.

Foods to try and to avoid

Start with plain fruit and vegetables and after a few weeks introduce a twist. Boil up potatoes with onion or parsley, mix swede with carrots or yams with broccoli. You could mix pear with puréed apple or banana with kiwi fruit, and when you give rice or cereal blend it with a fruit or vegetable. Try unusual combinations too, such as avocado and banana: it's amazing what your baby may like.

Remember that your baby gets the lion's share of nutrients from her milk, either breast or formula, so keep it up.

Foods to try

- In the first 2 months, stick to vegetables, fruits and 'first' baby foods.
- Sweet vegetables such as carrot and yam (sweet potato) are good to start with, followed by potato, plantain, courgette and broccoli. Steam them to keep the goodness in, then mash. Purée hard fruits, such as apples, and finely mash pears, bananas, peaches, nectarines, etc.
- There is a vast range of first baby foods on the market. The most important thing to remember is to follow the instructions on the packet about mixing, storing, and age category. To boost their nutritional value, mix the baby foods with breast or formula milk.

Foods to avoid between 4 and 6 months

- Unmodified cow's milk.
- Dairy products such as yoghurt and cheese.
- Hard un-puréed food.
- Small items, such as grapes or raisins, which can be inhaled.
- Wheat-based foods such as wheat cereals or bread, including toast sticks.
- Meat and fish.
- Egg whites.
- Protein-rich beans, which are hard to digest.
- Citrus fruits.
- Strong spices.
- Foods with added sugar or salt.
- Processed snacks such as crisps, biscuits, chocolates, packet potato mashes.
- Peanuts and peanut oils.

Juice and water

Once your baby is eating one or more meals a day, you can begin to introduce cooled, boiled water in addition to but not instead of milk. Cups vary greatly in the size and shape: the best are soft plastic and have handles, and many are designed to be drip-free and balanced to avoid tipping. Some babies find it easier to drink from the rim of a cup than from a spout. You can add some juice from 5 months onwards, but dilute it by adding seven parts of water to one part of juice. If your baby likes water don't introduce

sweet juices – the longer she goes without something that has the potential to harm her developing teeth, the better. Adding juice to every water drink will lead to your baby having a 'sweet tooth' and wanting sugary foods later on and can increase to boost their nutritional value tendency to obesity (p.565).

Preparing and storing food in your home

In the days before food processors, mothers would chew food until it was the right consistency and then give it to their baby. Powdered baby rice and cereal reaches the right consistency when mixed with milk (formula or expressed breast milk) and it's simple to mash food with a fork or in a food processor after it has been cooked. Towards the end of the fifth month or when your baby is competent at swallowing her food, you can start to mash more coarsely. She may enjoy the texture.

Some people always set aside a few spoonfuls of their own food. This isn't always convenient, though, and is not appropriate if the meal is curry or steak. Another option is to purée vegetables and fruit and store small pieces in an ice-cube tray in the freezer, taking out the blocks you require each mealtime. They will keep for up to a month. Alternatively, cook enough in the morning for lunch and dinner, and store it in an airtight container in the fridge. Bring it out 20 minutes before feeding time so that it's not too cold or add a little hot boiled water to bring it to room temperature.

Using a high chair

Initially it's nice for your baby to sit on your lap and taste food from your plate. But as soon as she's holding up her head and seems happy about experimenting with food, you can put her in a high chair. If it is well padded and fitted with a safety harness, she should be comfortable, even if she can't quite sit without support. If she's not happy, place her in her baby chair or car seat for meals until she's stronger and more confident.

Letting your baby explore

Tasting new flavours is just one way to explore food – touching, squeezing, smelling, licking and patting are just as important as your baby figures out the business of eating. As soon as you like and she is comfortable sitting in her high chair, give her the chance to take control and let her play. Give her different textures to explore: mashed potato or banana are great for squelching while large slices of apple or pear are good for biting on. A piece of plastic or newspaper beneath her chair will catch the drops. If it's a warm day, you could undress her: skin is much easier to wash than clothes. Otherwise use a plastic or cloth bib – one with arms will give maximum protection for her clothes. Stay with her and join in, and give her a clean and a cuddle when she has had enough.

The learning curve: months 4, 5 & 6

After 12 weeks with a baby many parents feel a marked change that's comparable to the 12-week milestone of pregnancy. You will now be looking back on the newborn stage and can congratulate yourself for having learnt a great deal, and coped well. The second 3 months are typically easier; there aren't so many new things to deal with and the mother's body has healed, or is well on the road to recovery.

What's special

The waves that came with the storm of change have subsided. Yet the ripples still remain and you may still be tired if your baby is not sleeping through the night. Many parents find their energy is spent simply getting everything done, which may be a greater challenge if you have returned to work. But if your baby begins to sleep better, this will make a difference to your energy levels and your outlook on life.

Mum's body

Within 3 months of the birth your uterus will have returned to the size it was before you conceived, although your cervix will have altered in shape from circular to oblong. The ligaments in your spine and pelvis will no longer be softened and your vagina will be back to the pre-pregnant state unless there was stretching or tearing during the birth. Doing pelvic floor exercises will help your muscles to tone and improve urinary control. The curves in your spine will be back to normal function unless your pelvic joints twisted during birth.

On the outside of your body, your skin continues to shrink, and the final state of stretchmarks or loose skin will be evident later. The same applies to the veins in your legs. If you are feeding, your breasts will still be large but probably not as big as they were 3 months ago and your periods might not return for up to 6 months. Until menstruation returns, your ovarian hormone levels, including oestrogen, will be low and your vaginal lining may be sensitive during sex.

Your feelings

You may feel a mixture of sadness as you bid farewell to the newborn phase and enthusiasm as you watch your baby's exciting and rapid development. You could still feel emotionally turbulent, particularly if the hormonal effects of breastfeeding continue or if you are not sleeping well. Although this stage is usually easier than the first, it may lack the magic that goes with new life and some parents do feel a bit melancholy as the reality of parenting hits home. The postnatal blues may hit you now. Fortunately, babies usually bring their parents round with huge smiles, surprising rolls and gurgles and loving touch. Many parents feel this is the happiest time of their lives and the pride and joy they feel in themselves and in their baby are much greater than they hoped for. The same applies to many grandparents.

Your relationships

You and your partner may now have more time and energy and continue to build an even stronger partnership. If you have been feeling distanced or upset with one another, it's important now to spend time together, build bridges and gently go through any issues that cause conflict or confrontation. You will both have learnt a great deal and as your relationship strengthens, your roles and expectations may change to fit the reality of parenting.

Time is a great healer, but be wary that a baby may also be a great excuse for spending time apart and skirting difficult discussions about issues that may have been present before pregnancy. If a mother focuses on her baby and neglects her partner, this may be a decisive time for each family member. It is important to give your relationship attention now because time passes rapidly and this is a formative stage for your family, just as it is for your baby. Love, support, acceptance and communication are crucial ingredients in the bonds that keep you together as parents and as friends (p.285).

Outside your partnership, new friendships may spring up through parenting networks. If things feel easier now, you might be able to get out a lot more and enjoy a more varied social life.

If you feel isolated it can be hard to muster the confidence to build friendships with other mothers. Parents are often surprised that depression may hit 3–6 months or more after the birth, and this has a knock-on effect on social confidence. Feeling loved and valued will help you out of isolation – you may try baby groups or lift the phone to find a listening ear or professional advice.

Making time to enjoy

At home you may find a routine has slotted into place so it is easier to enjoy time with each member of your family, and your baby has a framework. Outside the home, work may begin to feature more strongly or you may find time for leisure or to enrol in a class, visit friends more often or go out as a couple. You may wish to take an objective look at your life, consider some of the following questions and use them in conjunction with the Wheel for Living (p.58) as a way of keeping things in balance.

- How is our new family getting on?
- How much quality time do we spend together?
- How are we dealing with parenthood?
- How do we need to be supported?
- What is our family structure like? Does it suit Mum, Dad and baby? Could it do with any changes?

Baby groups

Some mothers don't make it to baby groups until after the third month when their baby is easier to handle, tiredness has passed or they have plucked up the courage to go along and meet new people. The range appropriate for you now that your baby is older may have grown considerably – for example, music workshops with nursery rhymes and gentle dances, swimming classes, baby massage for mums and tots where your babies play together while you natter over a cup of tea. You may still be in touch with women or couples whom you met in pregnancy, and there may be groups that you can attend with other parents while your baby is cared for in a crèche – these commonly offer the best chance for honest advice and moral support.

Dynamic boundaries

You will now be able to see more clearly whether the boundaries that have fallen into place suit you, your partner and your baby. If you are discovering differences in your approaches, or are trying to break away from the ideas you inherited from your own family, you will be on a learning curve of trial and error. You have a firm basis from the first 3 months upon which to reassess boundaries defining your time and space, and you may need to make many adjustments because your baby's needs have changed. If there are some boundaries you and your partner disagree about – for example, feeding – you may find the advice in the partnerships chapter helpful as you discuss the conflict in question (p.290).

Your body image

You may now be completely in tune with your baby, and with yourself as a mother, and feel fine. If your weight is not falling, however, you may be upset. Given your other commitments, eating well may be a low priority but simple changes help enormously. How you get on with your partner and whether you have resumed a sexual relationship will also affect your body image. So will the time you devote to yourself – mothers of young babies so often put themselves last on the list of priorities and if you have not found time to wash your hair, you are unlikely to feel positive. Raising your self-image is possible with a combination of belief in yourself and creating time and support. Mixing the ingredients is the challenge and, with support and planning, you may soon find a balance.

Eating

The adrenalin of the first trimester has passed and you may have space to think more clearly about your family's eating habits. If you ate a lot soon after birth, perhaps because you were often hungry while breastfeeding, your urge to graze may settle down. But if you are still eating too much, or reaching out for high-sugar, high-salt snacks, a committed exercise programme will help you get back on track. Have another look at your multivitamin and mineral supplementation as well.

It is surprising that if you become aware of how and what you are eating, it may be relatively easy to make simple changes with a big effect on your body and your energy. Eating slow-burning foods every 3 hours can make a big difference to your desire to eat. If you are not eating well because you don't have time to get to the shops or cook nutritious meals, ask for help with one or both of these chores.

Exercise and rest

If you have been exercising regularly since birth, you will probably feel pretty fit now, though your body will not have regained full fitness. It is safe to continue with a programme that includes aerobic and strengthening exercises.

Walking, swimming and running are excellent aerobic activities. Yet you might lack the inclination to exercise. Often this is because of the time it takes, and even in the home it is hard to do a floor routine if you are distracted by such things as the phone, the washing-up, your baby, etc. It might be easier to commit to exercising if you have a club, gym or postnatal exercise group in your area, particularly if there are crèche facilities. If you can get out into the fresh air with your baby as often as possible, you will both feel the benefits.

Yoga is active relaxation as you stretch your body and if it is combined with attention to your breathing it is meditative as well (p.346). It is easy to do simple stretches as you play with your baby on the floor at home and there may be a class in your area that welcomes babies. You may find that yoga helps you to feel calm and sleep well.

Exercise for your baby includes playing at home, massage, swimming and baby gymnastics – a simple programme of stretches. Babies thrive on being stimulated and their bodies love being used. Massage and other complementary therapies may help you both feel calm and balanced.

Dad's issues

After the first few months you may be settling into family life happily and learning a lot about your baby and brimming with pride and love. Fathers often begin to enjoy their baby a lot more when there is head control and less crying, and revel in physical play.

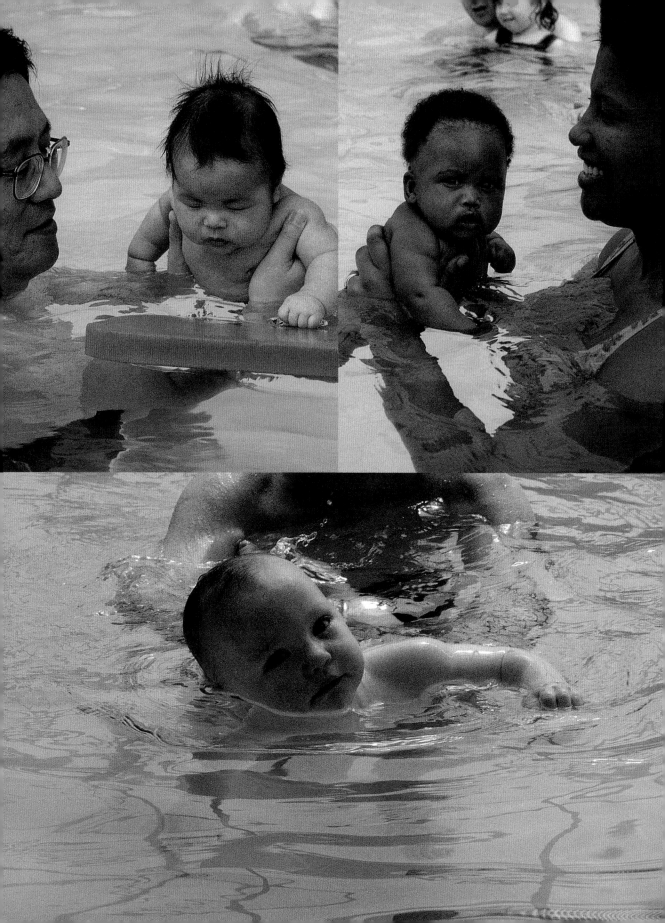

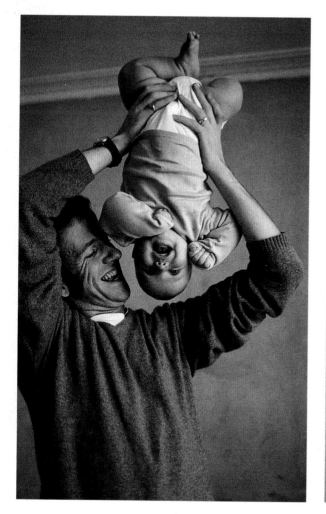
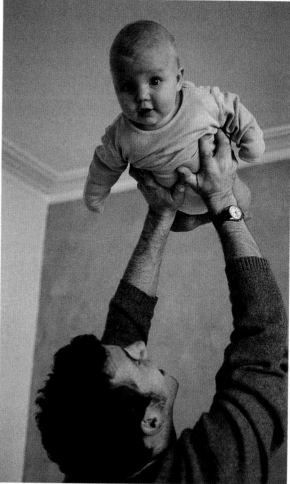

If you share babycare you will know what it's like to be with a baby for hours or days on end and meet his demands while managing other aspects of life. Because your attention is so constantly focused on your baby, you might feel somewhat different from people without babies and it will help if you can arrange regular spaces for socialising with your friends. If you work long hours you may miss being with your partner and baby, and be surprised at your baby's recently mastered activities and his changing preferences. Ask for an update from your partner each day.

Sometimes the second 3 months after your baby has been born feel like something of an anticlimax for a father. There is no longer any waiting as there was in pregnancy, no new baby or recovering mother to care for, and life may be very busy and frequently restricted. Men who become primary carers may feel this especially strongly. In addition, some men feel shut out of their partner's world if her attention is always on their baby, and miss being listened to. If you are feeling down it is important to make

time for yourself and possibly confide in someone: postnatal depression is a common problem for men (p.299) as well as women.

Sex and intimacy

A healed body and some predictability about your baby's sleeping and waking patterns might give space for relaxing into sex once again. If menstruation has begun, your libido may increase. Many couples enjoy their sex life at this stage and this can really boost the relationship. Some, however, don't feel that sex is a priority, and this is more likely if you are tired, fully breastfeeding or if one or both of you feels down and has a low body image.

Arranging time to be together without distractions may be easier now that your baby is likely to be more settled, and a night away could keep the flame of intimacy glowing. This 3-month period is a common time for men to feel lonely and isolated and to grow apart from their partner. Being aware of this could encourage you both to maintain your intimacy.

Medical care for your baby

In this period, standard checks are not commonplace. You will, however, be welcome to attend your local baby clinic to monitor your baby's development.

Physical development

Weight, height and head circumference can be measured and plotted in your child development record. If your baby's weight appears to be dropping or rising excessively, your health visitor will discuss it and give advice about maintaining sufficient calorie intake (p.565).

Vaccination

If you began a course at 8 weeks (p.554), this will continue: usual programmes include vaccination against diphtheria, tetanus, whooping cough, meningococcus C, haemophilus influenzae Type B (Hib) , and polio virus.

Hearing

By now you will know that your baby can hear you, and that he listens as well. At 3 months he will only be able to turn to sounds made at the level of his ear. By 6 months he will be able to pinpoint your voice with great accuracy.

If you have any concerns, your health visitor will check hearing using a test that's standard at 7 months, with a similar follow-up if problems are indicated (p.452).

Vision

Your baby can be expected to see well, to fix on your face when you are close and to follow your movements around the room. As with hearing, if you are concerned your health visitor may offer the check that is usually done at 7 months. If you are worried that your baby has a squint (p.465) there is a simple test: one eye is covered and your baby is encouraged to look with the uncovered eye at a bright object. The covered eye is then uncovered and its movement observed. If it moves to locate the object then a squint will be suspected and your baby will be referred to a specialist.

Teething

Long before the first tooth breaks through your baby's tiny gums, he begins 'teething'. The pain this brings varies from hardly noticeable to extreme, and may occur between the fourth and sixth month, earlier, or not until the 12th month – every baby is different. The signs of teething are:

- Your baby may cry, dribble excessively, gnaw on his fists or fingers or toys, make pained shapes with his mouth and have red, flushed cheeks.
- When he is eating he may cry because it hurts to suck.
- He may develop a slight cough or cold, or diarrhoea, or hit or rub his ears, which may ache.
- Nappy rash is often associated with teething.
- There may be fever.

It is important to note that your baby may coincidentally develop any of these symptoms of common illnesses and you may need an opinion from a doctor.

Usual remedies for teething include ice cubes, rubber teething rings, some of which can be cooled, carrot sticks for nibbling, teething gels and homeopathic remedies. There is detailed advice on p.541.

Work and finance

If you are returning to work, the guidelines for taking it easy and sharing the load outlined on p.322 will help you settle in. Many mothers find it exciting and energising to be back in the adult world. Many are also surprised at the strength of their maternal feelings and the change that having a baby has brought to their outlook – you may miss your baby more than you expected and at work find yourself more understanding, better at prioritising or very sensitive. You may also need time to harness your energy and get used to concentrating again. Fathers can have similar feelings.

You may work in shifts with your partner so that one of you is always with your baby or you may need extra childcare. Budgeting for this can be difficult – once your costs have been taken into account, you might earn very little. This is reality for many parents.

If you enjoy your work, you may not worry too much about the finances – indeed, you may qualify for some governmental help with childcare or rent. If you do not enjoy your job, it may create more stress and separate you from your baby for very little reward. The 'Catch-22' – needing to work and the cost of having your child cared for – is often unavoidable. You may decide to look for new work that could suit you better – perhaps a job-share, working from home, or training to do work that can involve your baby. The Wheel for Living (p.58) may reveal some possibilities for you.

Going away from home

Travelling with your baby will now be easier, at least before he is crawling. One thing that may have changed is your routine, and if you are worried about upsetting this you'll need to travel during sleeping times, stop for regular meals and re-create bedtime at your destination, wherever possible. Your baby may really enjoy being in a new place and meeting new people.

Some hotels and holiday companies run crèches for babies of 3 months and up, and you may be able to take a real break from parenting for a few hours a day. If your baby does not enjoy the change or becomes very clingy, you will need to devote time to him.

Common concerns

Extended information on these concerns, and a range of other postnatal health issues, are covered in the A–Z Health Guide.

My baby, who is 5 months, is very attached to a little white blanket and likes to hold and suck it while he sleeps. But it's getting dirty. Should I wash it?

Many babies become attached to a comfort or security object – this is a normal thing to do. It may be a dummy, a toy, a blanket or an item of clothing. There's nothing wrong with your baby's need for comfort: sniffing and sucking his blanket reassures him and helps him feel secure. And he likes it because of the way it feels, smells and tastes. If you think it needs washing, you can do this without depriving him of these sensual familiarities. Cut a section off the blanket, or cut it in half, and wash one section. When it's clean, give this to him during the day, and give the worn section at night. In a few days the new piece will have the same comforting smell and he can hold it to his face and sleep easy while you wash the first. In the long run, having two comfort blankets is very worthwhile: once your baby gets mobile and starts to drag it around the house or drop it over the side of the cot, you'll be thankful that there's a replacement at hand.

My 5-month-old baby tries to grab everything that comes within her reach. Yesterday she grabbed a leaf off a tree. What plants and trees should I keep out of her reach?

Despite the fact that we are all aware that there are many poisonous and unpleasant plants around, and babies spend a considerable amount of time exploring and eating the natural world around them, few if any children ever come to serious harm as a result. The worst you are likely to see is some unpleasant vomiting or diarrhoea, with occasional abdominal pain. For over 20 years, no child has died in the UK from eating native plants or leaves. You may feel more confident if you read a plant encyclopaedia to discover which plants in your house, garden and park may cause illness. By far the most dangerous substances are in the kitchen and bathroom cupboards (p.388). Every year hundreds of children are harmed, some fatally, by commonly available but highly toxic household chemicals or medicines, and water – in the bath, a bucket or a pond – is also dangerous.

We love sleeping with our 5-month-old baby but miss our private space. Is it time to put her in her own bed, or in her own room?

If you are feeling deprived of intimacy in bed, then you have a strong reason for making some changes. Talk it through as a couple and, if you both agree, help your baby make a gradual shift to her own sleeping space. Introduce her to her cot, and use a blanket that smells of you. Let her sleep there for daytime naps over several days and then put her there at bedtime. If she usually falls asleep with you beside her, she'll probably object and you'll need to withdraw gradually (p.236). She's not only used to feeling and smelling you, though: by now she'll be used to the noises you make in your sleep. If she moves to her own room where she can't sense you at all, she may be unhappy. Begin by keeping her cot in your room and, when you feel ready, introduce her to her own room. If you make the change this month you'll avoid the risks of your baby wriggling or crawling out of your bed once she is able to. In a

few months, when she is likely to be anxious about being left, she could find it harder to adjust.

My 13-week-old baby has begun to roll over, but when he gets on to his back he cries because he can't get on to his tummy again. How can I help him?

Rolling from the back on to the tummy is a skill that's rarely mastered before 7 months – it usually follows rolling from tummy to back by 16–20 weeks. Your baby will try and try again and this is just what will help him build strength and control. He needs to develop 'neck righting' so that his shoulder follows his head as he turns. You can help him by letting him continue this often frustrating experiment, laying him on his tummy regularly so he can strengthen his shoulders, neck and arms and trying massage and light stretches (p.368) to encourage flexibility and co-ordination. Remember that he may take you by surprise: never leave him where he may roll himself into danger. He is likely to roll that little bit further when you least expect it.

My baby doesn't seem to turn to me when I call her, but she did at 4 months. Why has she stopped responding?

The usual reason for this kind of behaviour is that your baby is just too interested in the world around her, and you are now familiar and can be ignored. In fact, her brain is inclined to ignore familiar 'background' noises and sights so that it can learn about new ones. If she continues to ignore you and you are worried, ask your health visitor or GP to arrange an appropriate hearing test (p.268). If there is a problem, it's best to find it early because early treatment can be very effective. The most common cause is glue ear, which is thick mucus in the middle ear cavity and affects up to 30% of babies under 12 months for up to a third of the year, usually in the winter months, and usually clears up of its own accord (p.454). Less commonly, some babies are born with normal hearing but lose it after a serious illness such as meningitis or measles. If there is an inherited cause of hearing loss it may be progressive (up to 50% are). This means that a baby with normal hearing at 3 months may have reduced hearing by 6 months or later. Usually there are clues in family history.

My baby is 5 1/2 months and is refusing his meals. Is he fussy?

Babies are like adults: some days they like their food, others they don't feel like eating. They also have their own likes and dislikes. Rejection usually boils down to one of four things: illness (or approaching illness or food sensitivity), sore gums (teething), lack of hunger (too much milk between meals) or not liking the taste. If none of these reasons seems likely, ask yourself whether your baby might be bored. Are you giving him a wide variety? Is eating fun and does he enjoy touching and feeling his food? Is he ready to move on to something with a little more texture?

As for fussiness, if your baby is hungry he will eat; if he doesn't like the food, he will complain. Respect him and offer something else: if he doesn't like parsnip, give him potato; if he doesn't like pear, try peach. You could try a new recipe to include some of the foods you want him to eat. Avoid chocolate desserts or other sugar-laden foods, as this is a quick way to have a fat baby and he'll soon learn that an angry scream and rejected meal leads to sweets, and you might end up encouraging the very fussiness you fear. Remember to persist with healthy foods at mealtimes. Your attitude about eating will have a very powerful influence on your baby, and the habits he establishes will probably determine his habits for life. If you are having battles between your anxiety about his wellbeing and his strong will, it might mirror your relationship in general – food and eating can be emotive issues. You may wish to discuss your feelings with people you trust.

My 6-month-old seems frightened of all men except her dad. Why?
A loud 'No!' or shaking head, a sharp cry or turning away in defiance or aversion are not uncommon and may stem from the desire to be independent. Sometimes it is only seen in association with certain things, for instance people with glasses, men with beards. Usually this is because a single episode, perhaps when someone came to the door, was connected with an unpleasant feeling – maybe your baby was crying and was reprimanded and told to be quiet. Now she may associate men with an unpleasant feeling. Your baby's aversion may contribute to feeding, sleeping or behavioural difficulties, and the best thing to do is gently to introduce her to men to break the negative association. If you're worried about her behaviour you may need support from your health visitor or GP or advice from a child psychologist.

Does my baby need to take a vitamin supplement?
There are established guidelines about vitamin supplementation. In the UK it is recommended by the Committee for the Medical Aspects of Food Policy (COMA) and the European Society for Paediatric and Infant Nutrition (ESPGAN) that every baby, whether breast- or formula fed, receives daily vitamin drops containing vitamins A, B, D, E and C, for the first 2 years. While the origins of this advice date back to the 1800s, when many young children had severe rickets due to calcium deficiency, modern nutritional reviews continue to make this recommendation. In reality, probably fewer than 10% receive vitamin supplementation.

Certain babies are at risk from vitamin deficiency; these are the fast-growing premature babies and infants with certain disorders. For example, a baby with cystic fibrosis will need additional fat-soluble vitamins (A, D, E, K). Babies who have been very ill in the newborn period are often given iron or folic acid supplements or are advised to take vitamin drops. Iron deficiency (p.398) is seen very frequently in babies given unmodified cow's milk before the age of 1 year.

This morning my baby had tiny black threads in her poo. Could she have worms? Sometimes she also goes a long time without pooing.
If you have given your baby banana in the last day or two, that might make her faeces look like this. Worms are different and usually appear as fine white threads at the anus and cause an itchy or sore bottom. Many children have worms at some time. They are harmless and are easily banished with one-off treatments available over the counter.

Bananas may be a cause of widely spaced motions. Along with rice, apples and toast, they are common causes of constipation (p.435), defined as fuss and pain when opening the bowels, even if this happens daily. Constipation may also occur if your baby doesn't drink enough. Remember that water is the best fluid. Too many sugary drinks can cause diarrhoea (p.446) and something like apple juice is a binding substance, contributing to constipation. If you are concerned, look at your baby's diet and consult your health visitor.

My baby is 5½months old. He dribbles constantly and has a red patch on his chin. Why does he do this?
Your baby is fulfilling his taste curiosities and developing his appetite now that he is eating solids. As a result his saliva production increases, especially when he is hungry or sees some food. Another reason for excess saliva is that his gums are being stimulated by the developing teeth beneath them.

Keeping fluids in the mouth, and this includes saliva, depends on a complex mixture of reflexes, muscle movements and learnt swallowing, which matures at a variable rate. Many babies find it difficult to control their saliva and as a result they dribble. Most dribbling gets better as the teeth arrive and form a physical barrier, along with the lips and gums. Some children take longer than others to stop the flow, but it is not harmful. Dribble rash, as the red patch under the chin is called, often responds to barrier creams and may need an antiseptic cream if it becomes infected.

My baby has dropped a percentile on the parent-held weight chart – should I worry?
It is unusual for healthy babies to lose weight in the first 12 months after birth after the initial weight loss in the first 10 days. A drop of one percentile is not a cause for concern, but it is unusual for the charted line to cross downwards two or more percentiles. This usually means that calorie input is insufficient (p.563). This is most commonly seen in breastfed babies and among babies whose introduction to solids has been delayed. More rarely, the crossing of two percentiles may be an indication of infection, especially urine infections, or failure to absorb nutrition for some other reason. Introducing more solid food may help, and you should continue to observe the weight gain. If in doubt, ask your health visitor.

Is it safe to use a baby bouncer?
The baby bouncer is harmless unless it is not attached securely, or your baby bounces into a wall or doorframe or is walked into. All the other effects are entertaining and even educational as your baby learns about movement and gets a good view of his world. He may bounce up and down on his tiptoes when in the bouncer, but it is unlikely that there is any untoward effect on his hips, knees or ankles. But use it in moderation – your baby will get bored if he's in it too long. Baby walkers are more concerning as the risk of accidents in them is high, and they should be avoided.

I haven't had a period since the birth 5 months ago. When will they return?
After birth the hormones that control your menstrual cycles are suppressed by your body, which releases prolactin, the breast-feeding hormone. If you feed frequently your periods may only return when you wean, and it may be more than a year. In some women, though, menstruation begins within the first 6 months. Even if you bottle feed it is not unusual to wait 4–6 months but remember that you could conceive before.

I had a caesarean section. When can I start exercising?
With modern surgery, wound healing is rapid and by 3 months your scar should be healing well. If you have had any discomfort, this should now have passed. However, the tissues need a few more months to mould and blend into your body. By the fourth month you will be able to do all the normal daily activities and exercise normally. It is best to do stomach and lower back exercises, gradually allowing time for the muscles to strengthen and the sheath that surrounds them to heal, and it may take 6 months before you can do a full stomach routine (p.362). Yoga stretches are useful to help the healing process and reduce muscle tightness and pain (p.354).

My skin is still greasy as it was in pregnancy, though it never was before. Will it get better?
The hormonal changes of pregnancy have passed and the effect on your skin should be over. It might be that your diet is contributing to greasiness – fried and fatty foods, milk and dairy products, chocolate and wheat are common culprits. Try to make a change in one area, see how it goes and then go on to the next. At the same time you could increase fibre-rich and raw foods and supplement with multivitamins and minerals and essential fatty acids. Use soaps that reduce greasiness but are not harsh on you skin.

I am feeling low. I thought postnatal depression happened in the first month. What can I do to feel better?
Unfortunately, depression can strike at any time and it frequently happens when the excitement of the birth is over and you have time to think about how your life has changed. There may be obvious factors such as a difficult birth, feeling lonely or isolated or difficulties in your relationship, and deeper issues that go back to your own childhood could be coming to the surface now and contributing to your sadness. Practical matters like sleeping, rest, exercise and eating will have a considerable influence on your emotions. This is a long list of possible issues for you to deal with. It is best to start small and make changes you can stick to that may help you feel better – these could include some time away from your baby, more time out of the house, adjustments to your diet, practical help so you can sleep and someone to talk to. If the black feelings persist you may need the support of your health visitor, GP or specialist (p.462).

I switched to formula milk 3 weeks ago and my baby has had a rash ever since. Could she have eczema?
Most formula milks are based on cow's milk, and cow's milk is a trigger for eczema in babies who are genetically determined to develop the condition at some time. Yet other triggers also include immunisations, teething and viral infections, and it is not easy to ascertain whether your baby is allergic to the milk. There are many other rashes in babies that you may confuse for eczema (p.530). Visit your doctor or health visitor, who can base her response on visual evidence.

I feel upset with myself because I think I am not being a good father to my daughter. What can I do?
These feelings are very common and most people go through doubt about their ability to parent well. If you create good quality time (p.296) to spend with your daughter, you may enjoy yourself and feel really good, and as you get to know her better you can relax more.

Your worries may be unfounded but it is important to take a look at the reasons for being upset and see what you can do to improve your enjoyment of fatherhood. If you are a high-achiever and find babycare difficult, it may be frustrating when you do not know all the answers. Underlying tension may rise if you feel excluded from your relationship with your partner. It could help to recall your own childhood – if you felt insecure or unhappy you may project these feelings on to your child or imagine she sees you as you saw your own father. It is a good opportunity to look back and perhaps talk to your parents about what you were like as a baby. If you feel supported, you may feel loved and let go of any expectations you have of your baby. Feelings of doubt, expectation and uncertainty are covered in Emotions and feelings (p.300).

I have an itchy bottom. Could I have piles?
Your bottom may be itchy from piles (p.523) although they usually cause pain and bright blood in the stools. You may have a vaginal infection of candida (p.423), which may cause intense itching and redness on your labia and on the perineum between the vagina and the anus. Skin conditions such as eczema may begin at this time but the itch is usually not confined to the anal area. Another possible cause of itching is tiny white pinworms. It is best to consult your GP to be examined, establish a diagnosis and begin treatment.

If we smoke outside the house could the smoke on our clothes and breath harm our baby?
If you always smoke outside then your baby is not exposed to passive smoking unless you are breastfeeding where some of the small molecules from the cigarettes pass into the milk. It is only too easy to 'forget' and have a cigarette in the house and passive smoking has a major health effect on your baby. The more he inhales, the worse the effect. This may be a good time to kick the cigarette habit for ever.

How much alcohol can I drink while I'm breastfeeding my 5-month-old baby?
There was a time when breastfeeding women were advised to drink Guinness beer to increase milk flow. It's now known that alcohol does depress the release of oxytocin, one of the hormones that are essential for breastfeeding. Although there is no watertight evidence to suggest that a little alcohol can be harmful or even beneficial, your baby may be intolerant to alcohol. It is best to limit yourself to the occasional drink.

Is it too early to give my baby a cup?
Cups aren't usually functional before a baby can hold objects steadily in both hands. If your baby can do this, then go ahead, and choose a variety that drips as little as possible. If she is still using one hand, she's likely to bash the cup and get the contents all over herself, the floor and you. It may not be until around 8 months that she gets the hang of it. If you have finished breastfeeding and are thinking of introducing a cup for milk feeds, don't. Give your baby the pleasure of sucking from a bottle and the close contact that comes with this. Sucking helps the mouth mature and contact is crucial for her security and development.

Your developing baby: months 7, 8 & 9

By the end of the ninth month you and your baby are as far away from birth as you were at the moment of conception. There's a poignant symmetry. When you discovered you were pregnant you began to share your life and your body with your baby. She was entirely dependent upon you and became more and more active and explorative as her birth approached. As a newborn she relied on you for everything. Now she is more lively – very possibly mobile – and delightfully interactive. She has carved a niche for herself in your family and is beginning to realise she is unique. Wobbly, noisy, demonstrative and ever more curious, your baby is getting ready to move from the formative primal period and into the fascinating world of a toddler.

Changing from 'Us' into 'I'

Some time around the sixth month your baby may get extremely upset when she can't see you and cry as if her world has been overturned. Her behaviour is what sets this stage apart from others of her early life – she is beginning to miss you when you're away. Having believed you and she were one, she is now faced with the realisation that you can both exist separately. At times she may feel very alone.

This 'separation anxiety' or 'individuation' is entirely normal. It is a result of her experiences, the trust she has built with close family and carers and her love of social contact. It's also down to the sophisticated workings of her brain: the area controlling spatial awareness is maturing and her short-term memory lengthening. All of a sudden she grasps the fact that things can exist even when out of sight – a concept known as 'object permanence' (p.30). When her parents leave, her crying outbursts will be most unyielding and distraught, and these difficult partings may continue for months. She may also cry bitterly when she is separated from a carer or a brother or sister.

Different babies respond in different ways to this feeling of separation. Your baby doesn't have the capability to philosophise but is faced with a very disturbing thought, perhaps something like, 'Where can Mummy be if she's not with me? Who am I without her?' 'Who is here to protect me, to play with me, to smile at me if Daddy's not here?' She can only learn about being both separate *and* secure through experience while you are the one who leaves her and returns with a warm welcome. She also learns about the difference between herself and others by exploring – something she can now do more easily if she is crawling. She wants to discover new things and she wants to be with you. She can have both as you hold her in your arms, introduce her to new things and new people, and give her time and space to be separate when she's in the mood.

Giving your baby support

Your baby needs to feel emotionally supported and physically close to her parents and most trusted carers. You may need to devote more time to her; again, this ensures that she gets the attention she needs in a period when her emotional development is rapid and may be overwhelming. Take her with you when you move from room to room in the house, and play lots of games involving disappearing and reappearing: hide behind a door and jump out; crouch behind a chair and peep your head over the top, then the side, then the other side; let your baby pull a cloth that's obscuring your face and cover her eyes briefly with your hands. You'll be helping her understand disappearance through fun and games. You can't always avoid upset, though: when you leave her with someone else, even if it's her favourite grandmother, she may be 'clingy' and reach out for you.

You may be able to organise your days so she is with one of her parents or a carer most of the time. Gradually she learns about self-reliance, trusting others, and the fact that you will return. It's a hard lesson, so take it gently. While she is coming to terms with separation, starting a new nursery or crèche will be difficult. If your work commitments mean you have to use childcare, see if you can take time off to spend with your baby in her new environment and reassure her as she gets to know her new carers in the first of many lessons in independence.

Developing play

When she is sitting, crawling or pulling herself up to stand, your baby's extra control and confidence makes for play that gets ever more exciting and amusing. She is likely to get more enjoyment – and learn more – from games that involve movement, change, disappearance and interaction. She'll throw things on the floor from her high chair, look excitedly at them and expect you to bring them back to her. She's investigating space, working out the difference between *here* and *there* and getting an invigorating sense of control: 'I drop this, I look at it, you pass it back!'

If your baby is absorbed in something, let her continue and try not to suggest how she handles it or offer any distraction – she learns well through doing the same thing again and again, and when she is left to do things entirely at her pace she learns about individuality and is free to conduct her own experiments. When she feels like interacting or wants help, your baby will love the company and fun this brings.

Communication

By 6 months, and certainly by 9, you'll be something of an expert when it comes to deciphering your baby's gurgles, squeals, yells and grumbles. Some noises will be general chit-chat, some requests, some will be observations and comments, and others will be made for the sheer pleasure of making sounds.

Between 6 and 9 months she will make huge advances in communication. Your baby uses eye contact and stretches her arm towards things or holds them out to you as a way of sharing what she has discovered. Her increased bodily awareness is significant because although she's getting better at controlling, refining and joining noises, she won't be able to 'talk' in your language for a few months yet. With her body, though, she may be able to communicate very clearly.

Making signs

Some babies grasp basic signing from 6 months, others don't show interest until 10 or 11 months or later. But your baby will make signs whether you teach her or not, and it's great if you can tune into them. It's more pleasant for you to understand something simple like 'no' than it is for your baby to have to cry as a way of making the same communication.

It is a natural evolution of the mirroring dance between every parent and baby that helps you understand one another and promotes socialisation. The timespan from your baby seeing a sign and making it may be more than a month or two, but it is worth remembering that she always

understands more than she can communicate, and indeed there may be times when she might be one quick step ahead of you.

You can expand the vocabulary of signing by introducing gestures and by watching and learning those that your baby uses regularly. If you see your baby making a sign or mimicking your own gestures, make a big deal about it to let her know you have understood. There are suggestions in the box below.

Making words

As your baby gets more talkative, she'll have more conversations that wander between her and someone else and fewer that have a fixed end point (cry–feed). At around 7 months she'll begin stringing noises together in what's known as 'canonical babbling' (bab ab ada da da ga ga ga) because she's finding it easier to change the shape of her mouth and throat and move from consonant to vowel, and back again. By around 8 months she may even say 'Mama' or 'Dada' as she experiments with sounds – these 'm' and 'd' consonants are easy for her.

By the age of 9 months your baby's brain will have developed enormously and the connections between the neurones are responding to her experience by developing pathways known as hard wiring. She will understand many of the words you use every day – her name, your name and a string of other words, such as bottle, bo-bo, teddy, yum-yums, mummy, daddy, granny, kitty-cat, ball, car, more, etc. And the way she is putting sounds together begins to reflect your speech patterns (a French baby sounds French, an American baby sounds American). Many babies grow up in an environment where two or more languages are spoken, and they learn to speak both equally well. Gradually you will find that your baby's babbling becomes more and more refined until one day she utters her first proper word.

Communicating games

- Your baby can now sign keenly and will definitely respond to your signs. At first movements of the head and mouth will be the easiest way to sign. Shake and nod your head for 'no ' and 'yes', open your mouth for 'more' or make kissing motions for 'kiss'. Try tilting your head to one side while she watches, and see what she does. Tilt it to the other side and wait . . . she may also copy simple hand movements or introduce her own, perhaps putting her hands in the air when her dinner is finished.
- As long as you understand one another, it doesn't matter what the sign is. At first, accompany signs with words and repeat them slowly and gently. Build up gradually. You could use a thumb in the mouth for 'bottle', or stroke your eyes for 'sleep'.
- You can introduce signs for naming objects as well and she may

appreciate being able to talk about them even if she doesn't make use of them – this can help an early love of books. Body parts are easy – point to each part and name it, and make a game of it. A hat can be signed with a pat of the head, a bird with flapping arms and a cat with a stroking gesture.

- Your baby may seem a long way away from the newborn you spoke to slowly and melodically, but still benefits from 'Motherese' speech (p.179) and from clues you give with your body and eyes. Give her every chance to absorb language: keep conversations going, repeat, take turns, leave spaces and ask questions: 'Do you like that? Do you? Shall I do it again?', 'Where is your ball? Oh, is this your ball? Shall I give this ball to you? Here it is, here is your ball.' Use her name often: 'Does Jenny like that?'

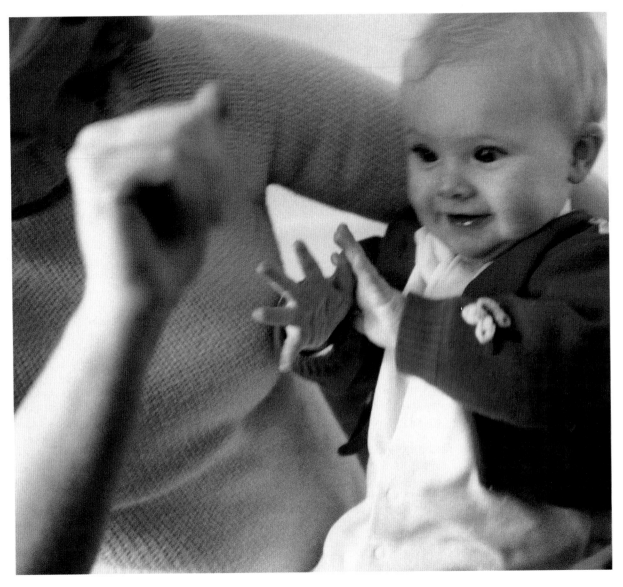

Vision and hearing

By the age of 9 months the average baby can see, in focus, for about 25 m (28 yd). Your baby's hearing ability has also progressed considerably, not such that she can hear any more than she could before, but such that she can judge where the noise is coming from and also sense the distance it travels.

By 7 months each time your baby looks at something she analyses it in many different ways. It has been found that most babies of this age prefer to attend to detail, taking the outline or overall shape of something for granted and focusing on patterns or details such as size, texture and solidity, and any protruding or coloured bits that will move or make a noise when pressed. Give your baby a toy that has opening doors, squeaking buttons or

pop-up elements, and she will soon find them, even if you don't show her where they are. This is because, from their appearance, she expects them to behave in a different way from the solid body of the toy.

Towards the age of 9 months, your baby begins to develop the apparent ability to see through things. She's no more superhuman than you are, but she is testing her suspicion that things can exist when she can't see them – another example of object permanence.

If you hide a toy under a blanket she will lift the blanket to find it, rather than look at you as if to say, 'Where is it?' as she might have done just a month or two before. She may even start her own peek-a-boo games, although her attempts to pull a jumper or cloth over her face may be more amusing than effective: her head is still disproportionately big, so when she raises her arms her hands only just meet above it.

By the end of the ninth month, if she drops a ball she'll look along the route she expects it to take. This is an important step in understanding how things behave when she can't see them: she can make predictions and remember things that have happened in the past. The world is a little less like a magic show, and although it will take many years for her to imagine fully what goes on when she's not around, she's certainly well set on the right road of discovery.

Body development

Between 6 and 9 months the most astounding change, in addition to leaps in communication, is your baby's increasing mobility, agility and control. With repeated practice, she has strengthened her muscles and bones and her brain has formed enough connections to permit co-ordination and balance. The age at which babies achieve the different stages of mobility and dexterity varies enormously.

Using arms and hands

Practice, practice and more practice has strengthened your baby's arm muscles and improved co-ordination many times over. Inside her brain connections have formed that allow her to judge her place in space, as well as distance,

movement, texture and size, with increasing accuracy. Following the pattern of muscle control from the head downwards and from the chest out, your baby's manual control has now progressed from her shoulders all the way to her fingertips. And that's not all: she can also hold out her hand or position all her fingers so that she's ready to grab something, having worked out how big and how heavy it is likely to be.

By 9 months, she'll be able to catch a swinging light cord in the bathroom if you hold her high enough, or stop a ball rolling slowly in front of her. Of course, she won't be successful every time she tries this trick, but even a few successes spur her on to try again and each one helps her brain link the information she receives through her eyes, hands and ears. It may seem easy to you, but she needs to judge space and speed, decide which hand to use, decide when to reach out, when to close her fingers and how to use her thumb.

Once your baby is sitting unsupported she can use both hands without falling over. Her hands will more often be open than closed and soon she'll try to bash two objects together. It sounds simple, but it isn't – she needs to use each hand differently, at the same time. It's comparable to a novice piano player trying to use his hands in syncopation and play ragtime. When your baby succeeds, she can make lots of new discoveries: a wooden spoon and a pan make a loud noise, her teddy and the pan together don't make a noise but feel quite different. She learns about impact, compressibility and stability: how things affect one another, what fits inside what, what things balance on one another. When she hits your cheek with a spoon it's not because she wants to hurt you, it's to see what happens. This may be a part of her greeting to you.

Your baby's hand–eye co-ordination will be more advanced than her dexterity because controlling her fingers relies on a part of the brain that develops more slowly, and building fine motor skills is a longer process. The more she manipulates objects of varying shapes, weights and sizes, the more she'll build her motor and mental skills. Experience is important to further these skills and you can help her in her task by encouraging her to play with a range of objects.

By 9 months your baby will probably have enough manual control to enjoy playing with blocks or tubs that can be made into towers or put inside one another. She may also be able to put simple shapes into the right holes (square, circle, triangle) if she is a patient type who likes to learn by a process of trial and error.

By the end of her ninth month she may start to point to things with one tiny index finger. This is a wonderful discovery that can lead to many forceful games of, 'Show me', 'Take me there', 'Bring me back', 'Let me feel that' and will allow her to poke you, often quite unexpectedly, in the mouth, nose or eye.

Rolling

By 6 months, your baby may have begun to roll over. Rolling over from front to back is generally easier: she may first do this unintentionally, having raised herself up on her hands and tipped the balance slightly too far. She'll try again and again to repeat this surprising feat. Rolling from back to front requires much more planning and is seldom achieved before 7 months: first your baby has to rock and lift all her body weight on to one side, then arch her upper body, head and neck, move each leg slightly differently and push her trunk to follow her legs. She needs to develop 'neck righting' so that her shoulder follows her head as she turns.

Sitting

Your baby may have already made some progress towards sitting with confidence by the time she reaches her 6-month birthday. Building on strength in her head, neck and shoulders, she'll be increasingly able to support herself for longer. First she may sit unaided for around 30 seconds before toppling over, but she'll want to try again and again.

The greatest challenge to the fledgling sitter is getting balanced. Sitting depends on sideways protective movements – as she wobbles to left or right, the corresponding arm comes out to prop her up. Falling is common, at least until these protective reflexes are established. Even a few millimetres off-centre can make her topple backwards or take her forwards until her nose presses the floor between her knees. It is wonderful to watch her rapidly master this intricate balancing act and increasing co-ordination that leads to reliable sitting. It won't be long before she can put her weight on one or two hands and lift her buttocks slightly, beginning a 'bottom-shuffle' that can get her from one place to another.

Crawling

Your baby may be adept at moving around with a combination of rolling, bottom-shuffling and belly wriggling weeks or months before she even thinks about crawling. In fact, some babies are so good at one or all of these that they don't bother to crawl: around 15% skip it altogether. Yet crawling is the most practical way to combine balance and speed without making the leap to walking. Most babies who are going to crawl begin by 9 months, with a few holding back for a further month or two. Some babies begin their crawling adventure by going backwards.

At first, your baby will limber up for the full crawling position by pushing herself up with her hands while she is in a tummy-down position on the floor. Sometimes she may find herself on hands and knees if she leans forward from a sitting position on to her hands and finds that her waist tilts, her bottom goes in the air and there's space under her tummy. She may then begin to rock backwards

and forwards, or put pressure on her legs so that her bottom goes even higher and she gets into the hands-and-feet position for what is known as bear- or spider-walking.

Crawling can be fast and accurate, and equally it can lead to crashes and bangs when concentration slips. It follows a universal method similar to that used by most four-legged animals – alternation between the two pairs of diagonal limbs. First one pair moves (left hand, right knee) and then the next (right hand, left knee), which gives optimal balance and uses energy most efficiently.

Inside the brain, activity relating to crawling is at first intense while movement, planning, visual assessment and balance skills are co-ordinated. After sufficient practice the brain has hard-wired connections and your baby doesn't need to think about how to crawl – instead she can focus on her objective, move fast and turn corners with precision.

Standing up

With legs only a third of her body length (as opposed to the half they'll account for in a few years' time), your baby faces a big challenge when it comes to standing up. And it doesn't stop there: it's just as hard to get back down to a sitting position. She has a strong forward 'parachute' reflex to extend both arms equally if she falls forward, although most often she'll fall flat on her nappy-padded bottom. Your baby may begin to stand by pulling herself up, on your legs, your hands, a chair or a sofa, look delighted, and then look puzzled at the thought of getting down again.

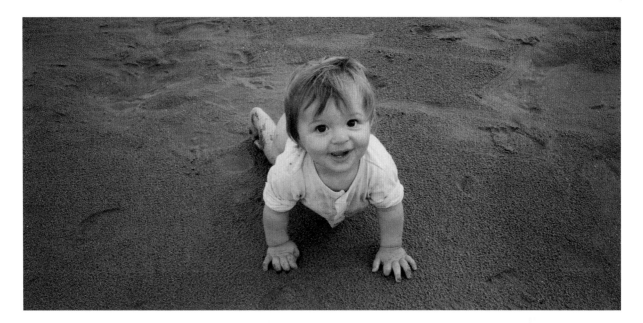

Once she's able to stand, your baby will probably do it frequently. She's powerfully driven to get upright, and a few months of practice gradually build up her muscles and hone her sense of balance. In time, she will stand without support and this gives her the confidence to move in an upright position .

Cruising

The intermediate stage between standing and walking is known as cruising – holding on to a piece of furniture or another person with one or both hands and moving sideways. It's almost an upright version of crawling, because your baby will rely on her hands as much as her feet. Some babies cruise very soon after learning to stand, others may wait weeks before making the progression – 1 in 4 babies do it from 9 months onwards. A minority, especially the bottom-shufflers, never try it, but move straight on to walking.

Cruising presents challenges that need some working out. Whatever your baby uses as a prop – a chair, a wall, a person or even a well-sized and very patient dog – will eventually come to an end (or want to be elsewhere). Looking at the space between chair and table, your baby learns a lot about distance and how this relates to her own size, and about balance. She'll either cling on and cry out for help or resort to her usual method of self-propulsion, plopping down on to her bottom or hands and knees and bridging the gap before lifting herself up once again.

Walking

The problem with crawling or cruising is that your baby cannot use her hands – she may be able to carry one toy, but not two, and will feel limited in what she can do. And if she wants to point to something or wave at you, she has to stop moving to keep her balance. Walking, however, frees up the hands and it is the most energy-efficient way to move. Moreover, it's just what Mummy and Daddy do. A small minority of babies (around 3%) walk before or by the age of 9 months: more wait until their 12th or 13th month. Some don't take the plunge until they are 18 months or older: all these are normal.

The lifting and placing of feet that you take for granted is very difficult to master: one foot needs to be raised and moved forward while the other pushes down and takes all the body weight and keeps balance, then the first foot comes back down, takes over the balancing role, and the next is lifted.

If your baby is ready for help, let her fingers grip your fingers at her waist or shoulder level, and go at her own pace. Don't hold her by the wrists with her hands above her head or actively pull her along: this may be uncomfortable and can interfere with her sense of balance, which she has to learn to keep. Practising with you will help but doing it on her own is quite a different matter. She will start with one step and might go sideways before managing to propel herself forwards. Later she will get half-way through the second step before wobbling and sitting down in a hurry.

Her progress will depend on her own tenacity and daring – some babies are fearless and seem unruffled by bangs, bumps and failures, while others are more wary of danger. You'll never forget the first time your baby takes some steps unaided, and she'll notice your pride and happiness: there's nothing quite like the sense of achievement and freedom that radiates from a baby's face in the early stages of walking.

How your baby sleeps: months 7, 8 & 9

Between 7 and 9 months of age, while every baby has different tendencies, a total of 15 hours sleep in every 24-hour period suits most well. Ideally, this is made up of 12 hours at night – a blessing for parents if this is in one stretch – and two or three naps during the day. The challenge for you is to encourage your baby into a pattern that suits your lifestyle, and help him to stick to it. Sleep during the day can ensure that he has plenty of energy to play and exercise and that he eats well. It also gives him peace to relax and absorb everything he's learning and helps him sleep well at night. And if your baby sleeps well at night, so will you.

Difficulties with sleep

By 7 months your baby will have lost the knack of falling asleep when the need takes him (although a few remain adept at nodding off in company for the rest of their lives!). If you have already been working on a bedtime routine (p.205), he may respond to this well and settle comfortably, knowing that a good peaceful sleep lies ahead. If he begins to object to being put to bed, or you are beginning to set a bedtime and are finding it difficult, there may be a number of reasons that you might like to consider. And if night waking is problematic, there are many possible solutions.

Getting to sleep

Almost all babies, at least on some occasions, object to being put to bed. It may help if you take him to each member of the family and say 'goodnight', or, if no one is with you, say 'goodnight' to some toys, some pictures, the kitchen – anything with the word *goodnight* in front of it. Often the complaining lasts only a minute or two: you may be able to settle your baby, tuck him in, say 'goodnight' and leave the room, then stand outside the door while his wail fades to a whimper, and his whimper dissolves into quiet sobs and finally the deep breathing of sleep.

If you find it hard to step outside and let your baby calm himself down, you could spend a few minutes putting some clothes away in his room or tidying some toys. In this short space of time he may settle, awake but happy, knowing that he's not alone. If he's tired, it could help him relax and he might take to comforting himself, perhaps by sucking his thumb, holding a blanket or snuggling into his teddy – security objects are normal and very important for some babies and can give comfort in the middle of the night.

Waking during the night

Babies who have slept well from a young age usually continue to do so. Infrequent night waking is often due to illness, discomfort, overheating or coldness, vivid dreams or hunger during a growth spurt, or an unfamiliar environment. Unless your baby is ill or has persistent teething discomfort, he's not likely to wake again or on following nights.

If your baby wakes once, twice or even several times almost every night, there will be some reason. It may take observation and a process of deduction before you find the cause, but the detective work will be worth the effort. The reasons that applied to your baby earlier (p.236) continue to apply. What might be new are your baby's fear of solitude and his anxiety about being separate from you. It is hard to reduce his need for company but you can make steps during the day to help him feel contented, loved and secure. Give him plenty of quality time and a lovely long bedtime routine where he really feels your attention. It might help to include the parent who is normally absent during the day.

Persistent night waking is draining on parents and may be unsettling for a baby. If you are happy to give your baby a quick cuddle or snuggle up in bed with him, and don't mind this habit persisting, then you need do nothing beyond waiting for him to change his own pattern. If you want to eliminate night waking, you'll need to be patient and follow the advice for breaking the habit that applied in months 4–6. Some parents start well but give in soon, giving a cuddle or deciding to read a story or sing a song by the cot – some babies respond better to this more gentle approach.

Your baby in your bed

If your baby sleeps in bed with you, at some point between 7 and 9 months safety becomes an issue. If he rolls out of bed or slides down he will almost certainly cry out and need settling; in addition, when you put him to bed, you or another adult will need to stay with him while he falls asleep, and this may eat into your own time considerably.

You may overcome the risk of him coming to harm by using a futon close to the ground next to your bed or put a soft rug around the bed and install a gate to keep him away from dangerous stairs. There are cots designed to fit

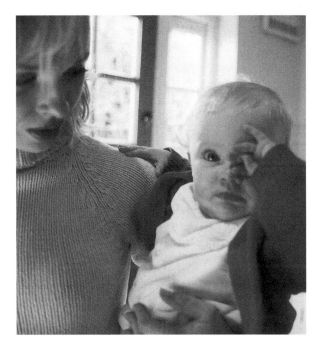

alongside an adult bed. In the morning your baby will probably wake, sit up and begin chatting away and poking you in the face with an enthusiastic greeting.

Sleeping during the day

It does not follow that a baby who doesn't sleep during the day sleeps longer at night. In fact, missing out rest during the day can make for a cranky baby who's demanding and may sleep less soundly at night. Up to the age of 9 months all babies benefit from at least some daytime rest. The average total daytime sleep is 3 hours.

Your baby may be happier if he is guided into a routine. The usual times for naps are mid-morning and early afternoon. Set nap times may put some restrictions on your movements and activities, and although you may be able to combine a rest period with a walk in the pushchair or drive in the car, structured days don't suit every parent. Often it is a toss-up between organised sleep and a spontaneous, routine-free life. If you take a relaxed approach, do still keep an eye on how long he sleeps for: wake him gently if he has more than a total of 3 hours at any one stretch, and try to keep him awake for the 3 hours before bedtime.

If your baby is really energetic and simply will not sleep during the day, give him two quiet periods of at least 20 minutes, one in the morning and one in the afternoon: tidy away toys, put on some relaxing music, give him a massage or take him for a walk. He needs this time to relax, otherwise his excessive energy may wind him up like a tightly coiled spring and make it difficult to let go of the daytime world and fall asleep at night.

Early mornings

A major part of the whole sleeping equation is what happens each morning, and many babies wake up, joyous and excitable, long before their parents want to. The average time is 7am. Some babies sleep later, but it's very common for wake-up time to get earlier. For some families 6.30am may seem reasonable but if this creeps to 6 or 5.30am the whole day is affected.

Changing an early-waking habit is not easy. Often babies continue to wake early well into their second year. The first thing is to attend to the daytime routine: reduce the length and number of daytime naps if he's sleeping excessively, encourage him to eat heartily (try new recipes or textures of food) and keep him exercising and getting fresh air on a regular basis.

The second thing to attend to is tackling the early-morning waking itself. Check that the curtains keep the room dark and that your baby will have nothing to suggest that it's daytime when he wakes. You could introduce a light with a timer-switch that gives a sign for morning. Set it to come on at his usual time of waking (say 6.20am) for 2 or 3 days and draw his attention to it: 'Look, the light is on and it's time to get up.' Then set it to come on 5 or 10 minutes later for the next 2 days and gradually move the intervals forward to an acceptable time. Your baby may associate the light with waking up and if he surfaces from sleep before the signal for morning is clear, he could drop off or wait.

Lastly, put some toys in or near your baby's cot where he can reach them – he may amuse himself for a while when he wakes up in the morning. If he takes a liking to a certain toy during the day, place it in his cot when you go to sleep so he finds it on waking – giving him something unexpected is a good way to keep him occupied for longer than he might otherwise be. If he wakes at 5.30 or 6am crying with hunger, you may want to bring him into your bed for a breastfeed and dose off together. If he is drinking bottles and can hold one himself, you could leave a bottle of water where he can reach it (not juice, which is harmful for his teeth). He may drink happily in his cot while you get another reprieve.

Blissful sleep

By the end of his ninth month your baby may love sleeping, and happily wave 'goodnight' as he is carried to his cot. Like adults, babies and children relax completely in deep sleep, and it is important for their emotional and physical health.

As your baby accepts it as part of each 24-hour period, you will be able to enjoy your sleep more, and the hours you have to yourself at the end of the day. Mothers and fathers who resolve a sleeping problem often experience huge positive changes to their energy as their fatigue disappears and they feel a new lease of life.

When your baby cries: months 7, 8 & 9

Your baby has come a long way since the uncertain weeks of newborn life. By 7 months she will feel secure in the family she has come to know. By 9 months she may be communicating with gurgles and body language and cry less often to get your attention. She won't, however, stop crying altogether.

What your baby is telling you

What may have been a great challenge in the newborn stage is now second nature: you've most definitely graduated into the 'experienced parent' class. You'll recognise the troubled, surrendering cry of tiredness or the urgent demand for food, symptoms of overheating or coldness, signs of illness or the grimace of a mouth sore from teething. Yet your baby's cries will now express her emotions in a different way and she is becoming more curious, more expectant and more aware of her ability to control things.

Some babies do cry more than others and every baby flits between seeming content and seeming upset. There are some babies who will launch into a cry over what to you may seem trifling, and stop after less than a minute, and some who rarely cry but, when they do, howl as if the world is coming to an end. And then there are all the babies in between.

Solitude and novelty

Much of your baby's crying at this stage is caused by anxiety about being separate from you (p.254). Her cry on your return ensures that she gets the reassuring embrace she needs. She may cry when you leave her and then cry again when she sees you once more. In the long term, though, rest assured that she will get used to hearing the words 'bye, bye' and seeing a wave of the hand or being kissed goodbye, and understand that things, and people, can come and go.

Every day your baby can hold a thought for a little bit longer and form more lasting memories. Her experience expands but sometimes things don't go quite as she expected, or something is so new that she can't find a place for it in her framework of reference. At times like this she may want you beside her. On some days she may appear to be bold and fearless, and on others rely on your moral and physical support.

Beginning to show frustration

As your baby approaches the age of 9 months, she may begin to show frustration with bursts of hot tears streaming down a red and angry face. Some babies shout rather than cry while others collapse ruefully in a whimpering heap. Usually the reason is a physical difficulty or not feeling understood. Imagine wanting to go through the stair gate and being completely unable to; knowing that the red peg fits in the hole but being unable to match the two; wanting a drink but not being able to make anyone understand that you are thirsty.

Frustration comes with a lack of desired results and your baby will have many of these for many years ahead. As she angrily tries to fit pegs in holes, she's learning, and the relief that comes with success will make up for the frustration tenfold. You may be able to help by guiding her or setting things up but not by actually fitting the pegs for her. There's a fine line between helping and interfering with your baby's development, and only you will be able to judge this, taking into account your baby's determination and current ability.

Sometimes it may feel as if your baby is very frustrated or angry with you. Few parents forget the first time their baby hits them full in the face. Unfortunately, it happens to most. Psychologists believe that it is healthy and normal for a baby to express herself forcefully. Your baby is too young to set out to hurt you deliberately, yet, like the rest of her species, has a tendency to take her anger out on the person she loves the most.

In her eyes you are a constant and essential part of her life. But if you decide that her playtime is over and it's time for a bath before going to bed, she will not necessarily agree: if she points to the pepperpot and wants to shake and suck it, and you refuse, why shouldn't she let you know that she's angry?

Each time your baby's irritation will be momentary. If her crying turns into howls of rage, by the time she calms down in your embrace she will have forgotten that she was ever angry with you in the first place. She will still be attracted by the pepperpot, however, so keep it out of sight, and out of mind.

Being fearful

Some babies show particular fears. If your baby cries each time she sees a dog then you can accept that she is afraid of dogs, even though you may not know the reason. Some of her fears will not be rational – she may hate the pink bouncy ball, but love the large heavy blue ball. The first snowfall may set her off in floods of tears and only an hour or a day later be welcomed with whoops of delight and a passion to touch the cold white flakes that tickle the end of her nose.

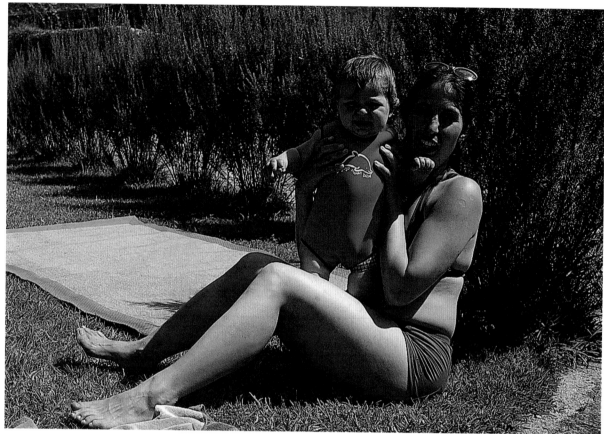

By the age of 9 months your baby may show his grumpy face more often in advance of, or instead of, crying. His communication has become more varied since his first months out of the womb, when he may have launched into a cry the instant he felt like complaining.

If the snow makes her cry, give her protection while she looks. When she's calmer, introduce her to a flake or watch from the window. This is more helpful than being plonked bottom-first in the very stuff that terrifies her, or being cosseted and kept away until the thaw.

If you force your child to face what frightens her, you could shatter her trust in you; if you protect her from everything she fears, you could nurture timidity. This delicate balance is something that most parents achieve by following their natural instinct to guide and protect their child at the same time.

What crying means for you

With months of practice behind you, you will probably not jump to attention the moment your baby begins to cry. Many parents are more relaxed by now and, without ignoring the cry completely, can approach it without a sense of urgency.

Of course, when a cry signals distress, danger or pain, you'll know. And there may be days, or weeks, when your baby seems to cry more than usual or you are less able to put up with it. If the crying persists and makes you upset, it is important to get help. You may have cried a lot when you were a child and your baby's distress may be very disturbing.

What crying means for your baby

As a general rule, it does no harm if your baby cries for between 30 seconds and 3 minutes before she is picked up or given what she is asking for. This applies particularly at night when she surfaces from sleep because she may drop off again if left undisturbed. A little undisturbed crying from time to time, even from the most temperamental of children, can be an important step on the ladder of learning about give and take.

The most important thing about your baby's cry is that it gets you to respond, just as it did when she was born. For many months yet she will need you to be there for her and every time you soothe her your bond through touch grows. Even when she becomes a toddler and beyond, she may continue to value your embrace above any other form of comfort you can give.

Your baby's evolving diet: months 7, 8 & 9

Eating progress is remarkable in these 3 months when your baby may grow from a gummy, mush-eating baby to a toothed, balanced sitter who can feed himself. By the age of 9 months he'll be able to handle more coarsely mashed solids and nibble on a range of finger foods, and may hold his own cup. Some babies love mealtimes and rarely turn down anything offered to them, while some need gentle coaxing to try new flavours and textures. Babies have an instinctive reaction to test novel foods gradually, possibly stemming from their distant ancestors' need to check for safety.

What your baby needs

By 7 months, your baby's diet will feature many more solids. Each day, he needs roughly 80 kcals per kilo of body weight, although from day to day his appetite may vary. He gets around half of the calories he needs from his breast or formula milk, and half from solids. As well as calories, he requires vitamins and minerals, protein and a small amount of fibre. He also needs plenty of iron. Breast milk and formula milk offer all these constituents, and as solids feature more and more, they need to provide goodness too.

If you aim for a low-fat diet yourself, remember that your baby has different requirements: fat is crucial for his growth and development, and his diet needs to contain it. Foods such as cheese, yoghurt and eggs are as important as vegetables and fruits. Meeting his requirements involves giving the right kind of meals, spacing his feeds appropriately, introducing new tastes and textures, going at his pace and making mealtimes enjoyable.

Foods you can introduce

From 6 months it is safe to introduce some of the things that were excluded earlier, and this will make meals more exciting. You can begin to mash instead of liquidise and, little by little, introduce grated food or easy finger food so he can enjoy feeding himself: the best time to do this is when he has his first teeth.

Fruits: Introduce a wider range, including kiwi fruit, pineapple and citrus fruits, many of which are best mixed with plain yoghurt or porridge. He may enjoy chewing on dried fruits such as apricots or apple rings.

Vegetables: Now it's time to introduce some of the more strongly flavoured vegetables such as parsnip and peppers. Green leafy vegetables (spinach, seaweed, cabbage, etc.) are great sources of iron and other minerals and their strong flavours can be toned down by mixing with a cheese or creamy sauce or a blander vegetable such as potato. Steam your vegetables and give them as finger foods when they're cool: carrot sticks, baby sweetcorn, thin beans, swede, broccoli florets, etc. Buy organic where possible and leave the skins on when cooking, for they contain a lot of the vitamin and mineral goodness.

Dairy products: It is not appropriate to give your baby cow's milk or made-up skimmed milk powder in his bottles until he is 12 months old. Use breast or formula milk in cooking as well. You can introduce hard cheese such as Cheddar, Edam or Lancashire, but don't give soft or blue cheeses such as Brie or Stilton. When he's eating finger foods you could give a slice of cheese or make cheese sticks.

Fat: Fat is an excellent source of energy for a baby and should not be cut out: it is also crucial for the development of the nervous system throughout the body and brain. Your baby will get fat in his breast or formula milk. He can get more from egg yolks (scrambled are good), cheese and in yoghurts – natural is best, mixed with fruit (flavoured varieties are often loaded with sugar).

Fish: Fish is an excellent source of protein and can be mixed with things such as tomatoes, orange juice or cheese. Begin with white fish, such as haddock or cod, when your baby is about 7 months old, making sure that the fish is fully de-boned and thoroughly cooked. Don't use smoked or tinned fish such as tuna or salmon, which may be very salty.

Meat: From 6 months your baby's digestive system is able to cope with meat, an excellent source of iron and zinc, but it needs to be introduced gradually. Start with chicken, finely puréed, and move on to puréed or minced red meat from around 8 months. If your baby has strong front teeth he may enjoy nibbling at chicken strips. When you cook chicken you can use the stock to mix with vegetables. Don't give sausages or other meat-mix food whose exact contents are not clear.

Pulses and grains: Your baby can digest lentils and a range of beans from the age of 6 months. These will be more palatable as part of a soup or stew and should not be given more than twice a week because they can cause a build-up of wind. Chickpeas have a lovely nutty flavour and are full of goodness but should be drained and washed if they have been soaked in a saline solution in a tin.

Tofu, quorn and other vegetarian sources of protein: Vegetarian sources of protein are satisfactory for a baby's needs, providing they form part of a balanced diet. One thing to be careful of is salt content. If in doubt ask at the store or call the manufacturer's help line.

Gluten and wheat: It is best to limit foods high in wheat and gluten before the first year, but you can begin to introduce it gradually if there's no history of allergies in your family. Bread and toast sticks are fine. You can also use cereals such as porridge with warm milk, which is a good supply of slow-burning carbohydrate. If you give your baby rusks, check the ingredients because some are high in sugar.

Pasta: Pasta is a good source of carbohydrate and is quick to cook and to chew. Tiny 'baby' shapes are available but there's nothing wrong with giving your baby what you eat, providing it is finely chopped and hasn't been cooked with salt. Pasta is generally made from durum wheat, a good source of gluten. If your baby is sensitive to gluten, use egg or rice pasta.

Rice: You can use flaked rice in both sweet and savoury dishes. Unless you have a food processor to break up rice pieces, save whole rice until the end of the first year.

Foods to avoid
- Peanuts and peanut oils.
- Sesame seeds.
- Salt.
- Too much sugar.
- Egg white.
- Oily fish.
- High-fibre foods such as bran or granary bread, which fill your baby up without giving enough calories.

Cooking for your baby
As you expand your baby's repertoire, follow the same guidelines for safety and cleanliness outlined for the early stages of weaning (p.242) and put some aside when you cook so you always have something reserved in the fridge or freezer. You can transfer frozen blocks from ice-cube trays into freezer bags marked with the date – don't keep anything for longer than a month. Fish doesn't always freeze well when it's cooked but can be frozen uncooked, and most banana dishes are disastrous if frozen. You'll learn a lot through your own trial and error. If you're not a keen cook or seldom have the time, a recipe book and some practice could set you and your family on an enjoyable road to tasty meals, while reassuring you that your baby is eating healthily.

Balanced meals
Balancing your baby's diet is important and can make a difference to his moods and sleeping pattern. The same general rules that apply to adults (p.332) also apply to babies: give a good meal every 3 to 4 hours and avoid eating in between these times. This helps to keep energy levels stable and allows the acidity levels in the mouth to

Pre-processed foods for the older baby
Powdered baby foods contain a full quota of vitamins and minerals and will be more nourishing for your baby than a corner of your sandwich. Jarred 'wet' foods can also be full of goodness but they are more likely to contain non-essential extras. Look out for anything that contains lots of sugar (these are called by several names including maltose, glucose, dextrose, lactose and fructose).

If the list of ingredients is very long, there may be a high number of additives, among them thickeners (e.g. starch, gelatine, xanthum or carob gum) and improvers (e.g. emulsifiers, caseinate, demineralised whey, hydrogenated vegetable fat). Although these are probably not harmful, it's preferable to choose a food with a short list of ingredients so you know the meal is balanced.

settle, protecting developing teeth and gums. Between 6 and 9 months you may give your baby three meals – breakfast, lunch and tea. Each needs to contain good servings of carbohydrate (pasta, flaked rice, potatoes are the main sources). A particularly hungry baby may enjoy a snack after tea.

For breakfast, give fruit and baby cereal mixed with milk or yoghurt, so that he gets adequate vitamins and a lasting supply of energy from the cereal.

Introduce protein at lunchtime – beans, pulses, cheese, meat or fish – because it can take time to digest, and combine it with a fruity pudding and a drink of diluted orange juice. The vitamin C in fruit will help absorption of iron (cow's milk can reduce iron absorption considerably).

For the evening meal give vegetable purées or finger foods, pasta with vegetable sauce or soup, and a yoghurt or piece of fruit as a pudding. By 8 or 9 months you can introduce protein-rich foods for dinner.

Think about portions: it's better to leave a little than to finish and still be hungry.

When I give my baby anything with lumps in, he coughs and seems to choke. Why?
Many babies are very sensitive to lumps in their food, even very small ones. As soon as they feel one they gag and cough, and seem to be choking. For most babies this soon passes with experience but for some the stage persists. Try going back to purées and give finger foods, like bread or apple. A very small number of normal babies remain sensitive to lumps, and the help of a speech therapist is needed to desensitise them. This occurs more often in children who have been born prematurely or have had other difficulties in the newborn period. If milk feeding has been traumatic then these sensitivities to lumpy foods are more frequent.

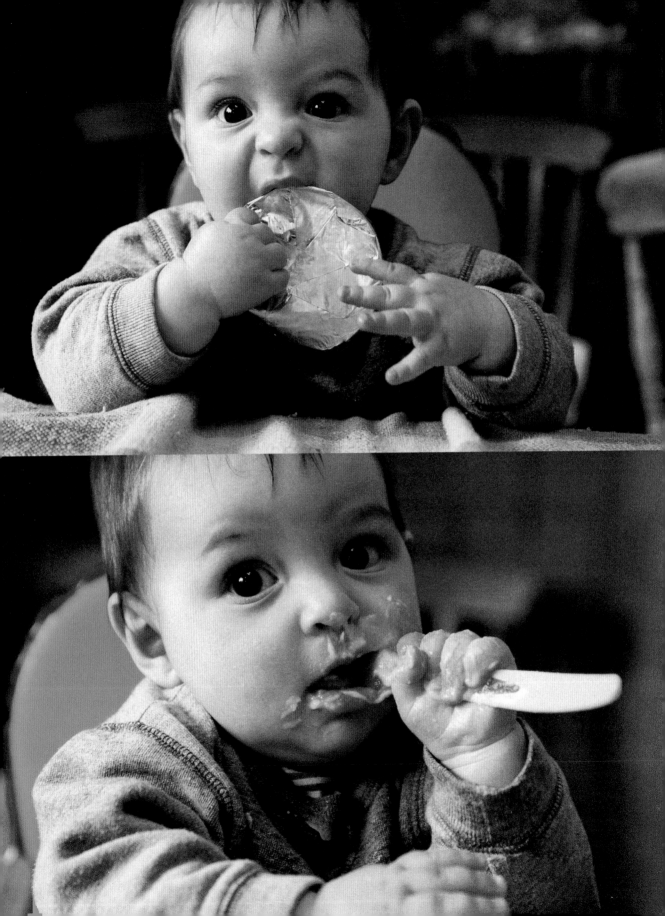

Milk

Your baby needs to consume at least 600 ml (20 fl oz) of milk a day. You may give some of this as part of his cooked meals – for example, 30 or 60 ml (1 or 2 fl oz) in a cheese or creamy vegetable or pasta sauce – but most will come from your breast or a bottle.

Between 6 and 9 months most babies have three or four milk feeds a day, usually at breakfast, mid-afternoon and bedtime, and an optional extra mid-morning. Except for the possible exception of breakfast, it's best to keep milk and solid feeds separate, using a cup for water or dilute juice at mealtimes. Keep the number of feeds constant: if your baby goes through a growth spurt or goes off his food when he is teething, increase the amount of milk at each feed.

The final milk feed before bed is the most leisurely and your baby can drink as much as he wants. It's much better for him to have too much than too little milk, and far better for him to go to bed without any lingering hunger. If he's still hungry after a large bottle or two breasts, look back over what he has eaten during the day: you may need to increase the size of his meals.

Water, juice and other drinks

When he regularly has three meals a day, your baby is ready to drink water or juice with each meal. Use cooled, boiled water or natural juices without added sugar and heavily diluted with water. Keep his juice away until he has eaten his main course or until he asks for a drink: if you give him the drink first he may gulp it down and feel full. Don't give your baby aerated or fizzy drinks because the air will make him burp and may make him uncomfortable.

If your baby is thirsty between meals and you don't want to give him a full milk feed, offer him water instead of any other liquid. Juice between meals can be a potent cause of tooth decay.

Snacks

With a structured day incorporating three rounded meals and a number of milk feeds between, your baby probably won't be hungry for anything in between. However, all babies are different. Some prefer a snack to a morning or afternoon milk feed, and some do not always have the appetite for a full meal.

Keep snacks nutritious. Instead of giving a biscuit or piece of chocolate, offer a rice cake, sugar-free rusk, cheese straw or slice of fruit or vegetable. You can also give snacks that are small portions of what you would otherwise give as a main meal.

When your baby feeds himself

As hand control gets better, your baby will become curious and want to feed himself. He won't be fully successful until he's a few months older but will enjoy trying. To avoid

Sample day for a 7–9-month-old baby

6/7am	**Milk feed:** Two breasts or 150–250 ml (5–8 fl oz).
8am	**Breakfast:** Baby cereal mixed with milk and mashed banana or another fruit purée.
11am	**Milk feed or snack:** One breast or 150 ml (5 fl oz) or: dried apricot with toast or sugar free rusk, or steamed vegetables.
12/1pm	**Lunch:** e.g. Chicken purée or lentil stew with vegetables, fruit purée and juice; or cauliflower cheese, pears and flaked rice, juice.
3/4pm	**Milk feed:** Two breasts or 150–250 ml (5–8 fl oz).
5.30/6pm	**Dinner:** Vegetable pasta, fruit jelly and water to drink; or spinach with potatoes, rusk and juice; or soup and bread, yoghurt and juice.
7.30pm	**Bedtime milk:** Two breasts or 150–250 ml (5–8 fl oz).

Calculate the size of milk feeds so that your baby gets 600 ml (20 fl oz) a day (or as nearly as possible). If you give a morning feed (11am) make the afternoon feed smaller.

angry objections, give him one spoon to hold, and use another to feed him. Every now and then, load his spoon with food and help him guide it to his mouth. If he grabs your spoon as well, so that he is holding one in each hand, get yourself yet another spoon rather than take the second one away from him. It's best to continue the feeding while he experiments.

If your baby makes feeding time difficult by constantly reaching out for the food to play with it, take the bowl and hold it under the table or elsewhere out of his sight. In his seventh and eighth month he won't be able to figure out where it has gone, and you may be able to distract his attention while getting a spoonful of food into his mouth every few minutes.

Around 8 or 9 months your baby's short-term memory will have developed sufficiently to allow him to carry on looking for his food if you take it away, but he is old enough to understand and respond to a firm 'no'. So if you don't want him making a mess, tell him firmly and calmly and keep it away from him. He may get the message but remember that touching and feeling everything – including food – is a normal part of his development. Remember, too, that your baby will eat what he needs and will make signs when he has had enough.

The learning curve: months 7, 8 & 9

The seventh to ninth months for your baby are quite distinct. She will probably become a mobile and very active participator in your family, with a growing command of language and communication through signing. As your baby makes her most significant change – the realisation that she is separate from you – there may be a new feeling of increased personal space and a different dynamic to your family.

What's special

There's often a sense that life now seems 'normal' as the whole family eats at similar times, the mother's body feels fully recovered and you all begin to sleep better. You could feel that you're moving on: caring for a baby is now second nature and you may find it easier to devote more energy to other areas of your life, particularly to your partnership.

Many fathers now become more confident with their babies when they seem less fragile, communicate more openly and move around. This can bring a sense of fun and confidence to the family, and may be particularly important if the mother is returning to work. In some families there may be the thought or reality of a new pregnancy.

A time for reflection

The passing of the ninth month is not always a joyous time, however, particularly if there are ongoing health problems or relationship difficulties. If you have been unhappy, moving on may be a relief. If you still feel down it is very important to get support – your feelings cannot be explained by hormones alone and there will be other aspects of your situation or issues from your earlier life that may contribute to current problems. With attention, love and encouragement you may be able to work through these. In a number of cases, depression is due to biochemical factors and medical treatment is a useful option (p.462).

Medical care for your baby

The 7-month developmental check

In most areas a 7-month check is standard. At any time you can visit your health visitor for monitoring and assessment, and should contact your doctor if you are worried about illness.

Growth and development

Your baby will be checked for normal development with a standard checklist about her ability to be sociable, whether she is familiar with her family, how she sleeps and eats and whether there is anything that worries you in her nappies.

- Weight and height and head circumference are measured and plotted on the development record. Your baby's head shape will be checked and her spine assessed for straightness.
- Boy's testes are inspected to ensure they are descended.
- Gross-motor development is monitored – this allows your baby to roll over.
- Her fine-motor co-ordination is checked – this allows her to reach out for and grasp objects.
- Language development is noted, with the expectation that your baby can babble using vowel sounds.

Hearing

Testing a baby's hearing is a skilled task. Currently, methods are rudimentary and done by distracting your baby. The health visitor will make sounds, usually using a sound box or warbler, and another person sits in front of your baby, keeping her visually occupied. At the moment a sound is made, the distracter looks for a response. Many babies don't score highly in this test because there are so many things in the average surgery or clinic that may distract. If your baby fails to respond this does not necessarily mean there is a problem. It just means that at the time of testing a positive response could not be obtained. She will be tested again after a few weeks. If she fails to respond again, she may be referred to a professional for the next level of hearing test.

The majority of babies will be tested by the distraction method. Electronic methods of testing using a mini-EEG (evoked auditory potentials that measure the electrical activity of the cochlear) are being introduced and there are proposals to test every newborn electronically within the first few days. The main reason is that earlier identification of hearing loss allows intervention and planning of treatment, as well as any special communication education that may be required. In addition, early use of amplification or hearing aids may prevent subsequent hearing loss and help speech development.

Vision

Most of the testing at this age involves the health visitor's observation of your baby during the visit. She will also ask you about her visual behaviour with questions about how she fixes on your face, follows you around the room, seems aware of the world around her and reaches for small objects. Only if your answers give cause for concern will further visual testing be advised.

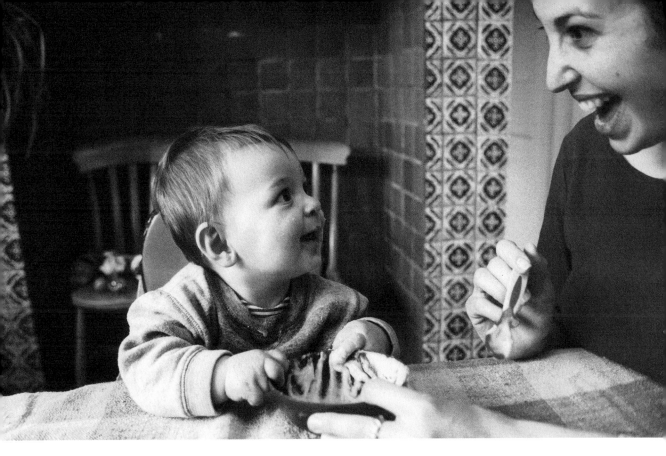

Dynamic boundaries

Once your baby begins to move around and her play area and your personal space overlap, you will need to reconsider physical boundaries. You may be making the first amendments to your furniture arrangements to keep things safe, and this will determine the layout of your house for roughly 2 years, if not longer, as you keep precious objects well out of your baby's reach and automatically place cups of tea and water high up. Parental reflexes like this last until your child(ren) become less curious or clumsy.

You might also want to make areas of your home off limits to your baby, and use a gate to enforce the restriction. Your baby will know exactly what the gate is for, and through human nature will, of course, find what's on the other side extremely interesting.

Personal space is much more than physical space. An important aspect is that you have space to do something for yourself, and this may be easier now. If your baby has a settled sleeping pattern there will be peaceful evenings and nights and more time for intimacy with your partner. You may feel greater freedom to find space for yourself outside the home and go out and socialise more often, with or without your baby.

Feeling ready for taking time out and reclaiming adult hours in the day is one thing. For it to happen you'll need support, and because your baby may be going through a phase of separation anxiety you'll probably be concerned that babysitters are people she knows and trusts. The Wheel for Living (p.58) might help you create space and enrol a selection of carers.

Where are you now?

Looking back over the 9 months since birth, you may be amazed by the challenges and changes you have been through, the way your child has developed, and the things you have achieved separately and together. If you and your partner were to draw a graph of your emotions, it would no doubt look just like a roller coaster, with a range of highs and lows.

As your baby begins to crawl with confidence or even take her first wobbly steps, the end of the primal period may bring joy as things just keep getting better, or it may be an anticlimax for you – the fantasy of pregnancy, birth and babyhood fades, your baby begins to challenge you because she now knows she is separate, and a new reality sets in. As your baby becomes more independent, other aspects of your life come back into focus. The 'you' that existed before birth reasserts itself alongside your parenting role as you marry the old and the new. As you have learnt to care for your baby and make time for your own needs and those of your partner, so you have assimilated one of life's valuable lessons – everybody thrives on time, attention and love.

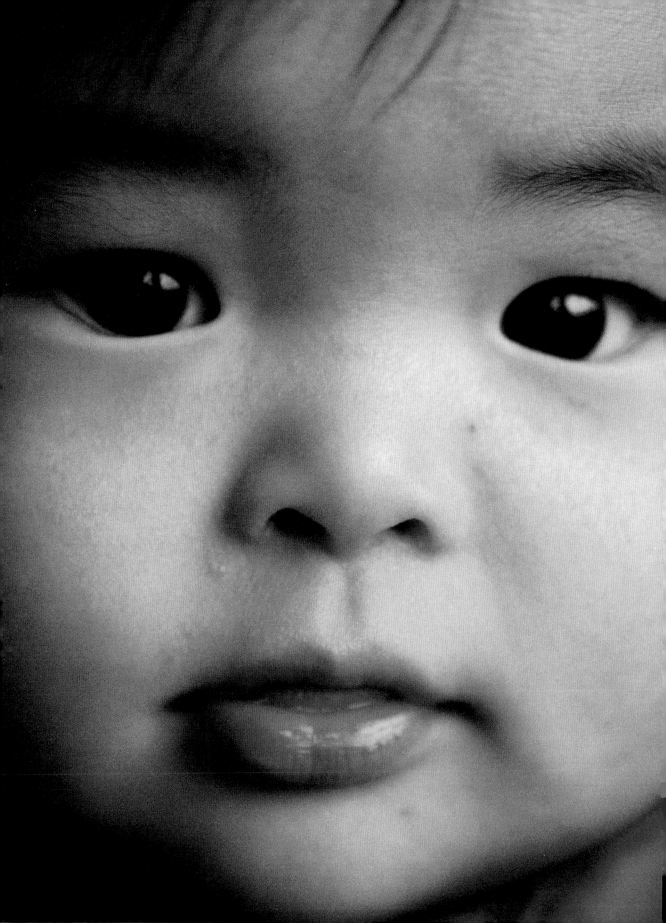

Common concerns

Extended information on these concerns, and a range of other postnatal health issues, are covered in the A–Z Health Guide.

How can I look after my baby's teeth?
Even before they have broken through the gums, your baby's teeth and gums are vulnerable. You can help to prevent decay by limiting sugar-containing foods and avoiding prolonged use of a bottle for comfort, particularly when filled with juice, diluted squash or carbonated drinks. If you give your baby syrupy medicines when she is ill, use sugar-free varieties. When your baby's first tooth appears, begin to clean it. Some parents use a flannel cloth, moistened gauze or clean handkerchief wrapped around a finger but you can use a special baby toothbrush and paste – your dentist can advise you about the appropriate fluoride content. Brushing twice a day helps to prevent the bacterial build-up that leads to decay and is particularly important in the evening.

Now my baby seems very robust. He loves it when I throw him up in the air and catch him above my head, bounce him on my lap or fly him round and round in my arms. My wife cringes each time I do it, but he can take it, can't he?
Most certainly he can. Providing you don't drop him or suddenly jerk him, this is ideal play for developing lightning reflexes and an acute sense of self in space. Many babies seem to love the terrifying feeling of momentary weightlessness as they shoot upwards, then plunge downwards on a parent-driven roller coaster. So, mind the low ceilings and light fittings and slippery hands, and indulge him in boisterous play! One interesting sociological observation is that female babies are less likely to receive this kind of physical play, and this may be an explanation of their slight delay in motor skills and perception of self in space – they tend to lag behind boys and catch up around the age of 2 or 3 years.

My baby seems to prefer to use her left arm and leg. Does this mean she is left-handed?
The average baby will use each side evenly up to about 18 months of age. Some babies show a preference for one side and then the other but can use each side equally well. A persistent over-reliance on one side should be investigated. If the opposite side is stimulated there will be a response, suggesting that the baby is unaware of the underused side. If this is the case, a physiotherapist will suggest ways to stimulate the less-preferred side and will supervise and reassess your baby at intervals.

I have a close relative who has a child with a disorder of communication (autistic spectrum disorder). What can I do to reassure myself that my child is not similarly affected?
Babies communicate subtly from birth and continue to do so with zest and increasing clarity in their early months – communication skills are evident long before spoken language begins. When a child has a communication difficulty, there may be clues very early on. How your child relates to you visually, through play and touch and with her own code of signs, can give clues to you and your health visitor or specialist. The earlier a potential problem is recognised within the first year, the sooner extra attention and therapy can begin.

Clues that are often recognised in retrospect (p.402) include late appearance of babbling, lack of visual interest, unusually settled behaviour, unusually unsettled behaviour and especially disturbed sleep with no recognisable day–night pattern by 9–12 months.

Are baby walkers dangerous? And can they interfere with learning to walk or crawl?
Being in a baby walker can give the baby who can't yet crawl an exhilarating sense of independence and fun, and manoeuvrability far beyond her natural capabilities. In a family where there are other children it can bring the younger baby into the others' world. It can also give adults time and space to get on with their own chores because the baby in a walker may entertain herself for longer, and come to Mummy and Daddy when she wants company rather than sit and cry for attention.

Despite these apparent advantages many health professionals warn against baby walkers. There is a safety risk. Baby walkers can tip up, either of their own accord or when a wheel gets snagged or tips over a ledge, and this could result in a nasty injury, probably to the face or head. Although the height of the seat is adjustable, your baby may use her toes and the balls of her feet to propel herself, and this does not encourage the natural development of the feet to be flat, which they must be for standing and walking. Your baby may not be spurred on to crawl and explore with her head at ground level.

Can my baby have too many toys?
You might see joy and entertainment in every one of 50 or more toys, but your baby may find it much easier to concentrate and experiment if her choice is narrow. Concentration skills are extremely important for learning, listening and socialising and right now she is ready to learn a lot through exploring and examining her world closely. You may want to filter out things your baby ignores, sticking to those she loves and any that exercise her potential to move, grab, sort and position.

My baby gets really angry when I take something from him – I often do this if he has something that might bring him harm, like a pen. He screams and I feel he's doing it to provoke me. Can he be naughty at 8 months? How can I give him a sense of discipline?
Your baby cannot be naughty. He doesn't have the reasoning capability to annoy you on purpose and cannot know when something is not safe. At 8 months he can't be self-disciplined – he is driven to discover as much as he can and acts immediately to follow his desire and express emotions. And at this stage he may be very clingy to certain things and people and easily get angry at any kind of separation.

Every family has a different approach to discipline, and this is usually established on the basis of each parent's background. But until your baby is at least 18 months old he cannot learn by correction or reasoning. Discipline through seclusion, physical hitting or any other form of punishment is inappropriate (p.279) and could be very damaging for his self-esteem, his confidence and his sense of trust. Give him safe things to use: a wide, plastic spoon rather than a narrow and hard metal spoon, for instance. If you want him to try hand

and vision skills, give a thick non-toxic crayon to scribble with. Make your home child-friendly, keep harmful or precious things out of sight and do what you can to give your baby more 'yes' than 'no', more 'well done' than 'bad boy'. When he does something unsafe, remove him from the situation. Some difficult behaviour (such as biting) may fade if it is ignored.

Your whole family needs to be aware of the boundaries between what is and isn't acceptable. Remember that you are all role models and your baby will copy what you do rather than what you say: if you regularly shout or become short-tempered, he may also do this, and if you are regularly calm he may be more inclined to follow your example.

My baby is playing up at mealtimes and sleeping badly. Is this because we went on holiday?
It is common for babies to have a settling-in period after a break and you will need to guide her gently back to her old ways. Your baby may actually miss her holiday location and the social activities there. You may have relaxed too and she'll have picked up on this. Now she needs to settle down to normal everyday life, just as you do.

Next time you make a break, if you have a routine at home, try to continue it as much as possible while you're away, but remain flexible, particularly at bedtime or during the night when your baby may need you with her. On arrival, introduce her to the room where she's sleeping and explore the whole house with her to reduce her fear of the unknown. If you can, do this well before bedtime so she can get used to the different smells and sounds, lights and shadows. If you're using a travel cot let her sit or crawl on the floor as you get things ready, and use the sheets from her bed for a familiar smell. When you return home, spend time with her in her bedroom as she adapts to the change.

Every night my baby throws off his blankets. I wake him when I tuck him in but I know that he'll wake cold later if I don't. What can I do?
It's very common for babies to kick off their covers. It's also very common for parents to wake their babies in an effort to make them more comfortable. He may be perfectly happy as he is. If he hasn't woken up, are you sure that he will later? Is your instinct to cover him and keep him warm based on your own experience? A good way around the problem may be to use a warm all-in-one sleepsuit or a baby sleeping bag. If your baby is just beginning to stand, however, choose the sleepsuit instead of the bag, which may make him fall if he tries to stand up in the morning. Be sure that you are not overheating him.

It's hard leaving my baby at a crèche. Is it best to leave quietly when she cries?
It is not a good idea to sneak out when your baby is not looking. At the moment she is facing the confusing realisation that she is separate from you and is very sensitive to being left. Repeatedly leaving when you think she won't notice may, in the long term, undermine her sense of trust. She may cling more fiercely to you, actively keeping you by her side. Or she may withdraw and become quiet, unsure whether your love and commitment are constant. Even if she is crying, talk to her and say goodbye, tell her that you love her, and go. This may be heart-wrenching for you. Ask the carer how long your baby cries and how she is settling and stand outside the door if you

want to reassure yourself. If you're worried that she is unhappy with the carer, there is an important practical issue that needs to be addressed immediately (p.324).

My baby cries in relation to feeding, sometimes before, sometimes just after – could she be allergic to the milk?
If your baby is crying more than usual, her milk feed may be the cause, although there are a few other physical problems, other than colic (p.431) and teething, that might not be apparent. One is acid reflux (p.561), which gets worse with hunger and just before feeding when digestive juices are stimulated. Most commonly, intolerance is to cow's milk protein. If crying continues with most feeds, then your doctor may advise trying a cow's milk- or lactose-free diet. If your baby draws up her knees while crying, shows signs of constipation or there is blood in the motions, your doctor may want to check for a bowel disorder (p.408). Hernias, more common in boys, may cause crying, but these are usually obvious as swellings in the groin.

How do I know if my baby is eating enough?
If your baby seems healthy and happy and is reliably putting on weight, then he is probably fine. It is completely normal for his appetite to vary because his nutritional demands will change from day to day and he may not feel like eating if he is teething, feverish or under the weather. The only way you will really know if he is eating enough is by regularly monitoring his weight and growth, on a weekly basis if you are really concerned, although fortnightly or monthly is usually sufficient. Weight gain should be steady and follow a growth line or centile on the chart (p.565).

Appetite and hunger vary enormously from baby to baby and eating patterns and behaviour at mealtimes are some of the most frequently encountered problems in childhood. They can cause parental and professional anxiety but rarely lead to genuine disease. The main nutrition problem is overeating, leading to obesity, which is generally ignored as it is still thought to be reassuring to see a fat or chubby baby. If your baby is not gaining sufficient weight, your doctor will look at possible causes of failure to thrive (p.563).

My 7-month-old baby has four teeth and bites me. Should I wean her from breastfeeding?
Many mothers who breastfeed for this long encounter the problem of biting. If she bites, take her off the breast by slipping your finger into her mouth to break the suction, say 'no' firmly and end the feed. Your baby is capable of making the connection between biting and being denied a feed if it's repeated a few times. When you feed, make sure that the two of you are undisturbed, just in case your baby thinks that a quick nip will get your attention. She might be less likely to bite if you keep eye contact as she sucks. And if she has recently got her teeth she may think that biting is good fun – persuade her otherwise and don't encourage her to bite your nose or your fingers as a game.

If you want to stop breastfeeding this could be a good time to make the transition. Start by substituting your breast with a bottle of formula or expressed breast milk (p.195). If she doesn't take to the bottle it may help to get another adult, who doesn't smell of milk, to feed her for the first few days.

My baby is always demanding attention and I can never do anything for myself. How can I get her to amuse herself?

Some parents feel that a baby's need for attention is constant. This isn't far from the truth: you cannot do something that requires your baby to be silent, like prepare a work document or have a long lazy phone call. Yet you can help her feel heard and entertained without your being constantly pulled. When you are busy, encourage her to play in your space but not with you. Have a cosy corner in all the rooms you use frequently and choose toys that she likes to puzzle over. Talk to her every few minutes, making eye contact and maybe giving her a light touch. Hold your attention on her for long enough for her to respond, and then return to what you are doing. Most babies learn to recognise that everyone needs their own space.

Your baby also needs your full attention from time to time. Twenty minutes two or three times a day may make a huge difference to her behaviour at other times. While you are focused on her, leave the washing-up, turn off the television, forget the problem at work and ignore the phone. Let her lead the play. She might choose to crawl all over you, explore your face, throw a ball to you, lie back and be tickled or be carried and shown things on high shelves, touch the curtains or feel movement as you dance with her. One period of quality time may be in the evening when you wind down with a story or song and help her relax with a soothing massage.

I'm worried that my baby is not digesting properly because peas, sweetcorn and raisins come through his system looking just the same as when they went in.

The appearance of undigested peas, carrots, tomato skins and other fibrous materials is quite normal. These take longer to digest fully and for some babies there is a short time from eating to evacuation, leaving insufficient time to digest. Be reassured that all the essential elements have been absorbed, and there is no danger of poor nutrition. If this persists into toddler years the condition is called toddler diarrhoea. Right now, purée his food to help his digestion and use fewer offending foods.

My baby seems to eat earth and all sorts of revolting creatures from the garden – is this dangerous?

In common with most young animals your baby's sense of adventure drives her to experiment with all her senses, and taste is no exception. You can rest assured that a few mouthfuls of garden soil will do no harm, unless there has been recent use of pesticide, and a few insects or even earthworms do not cause a problem. In general, it is very rare indeed for babies to develop any illness from the small amounts of soil they eat, although there are some bacteria and other organisms in soil that are potentially harmful. These are related to animal faeces, which you will be able to see and avoid. Do limit the amount of soil eaten.

Is thumb sucking bad for my baby's teeth?

This comfort behaviour is quite normal. Over half of all babies suck on thumbs or fingers, and 95% have finished this habit by age 6 years. The babies most likely to persist with this behaviour are those for whom thumb sucking is part of the ritual of getting off to sleep. Years of observation have led to the conclusion that thumb sucking does no harm, is usually a comfort behaviour, does not mean your child is disturbed and insecure and doesn't harm teeth or thumbs. If you don't find the sucking acceptable it is worth looking at your own reasons – it is best to allow your baby the comfort she seeks.

My baby wants to be put down all the time. Doesn't he like me?

Some babies become impossibly wriggly and fiercely independent once they realise they can move about. This is part of development and, on the one hand, you will be freed up and no longer have to carry him wherever you go. On the other hand, you may miss the closeness. Some mothers who might have lacked physical contact or close and trusting relationships in their own family become quite addicted to their own baby's nearness.

Your presence is still important, for reassurance and companionship, for an embrace when your baby cries, for guidance in games and to make sure that everything is safe – explorative babies are often not far from trouble. You are probably your baby's most valued friend and his trust in you may be the basis of his growing self-confidence. His wriggly phase may pass soon, or persist for a few months. If you want to keep up the bond of touch you could try massage (he may wriggle through that as well), swimming and baby gymnastics. If your baby is bad-tempered and all touching aggravates him, ask your doctor to check his health and development.

My wife seems to be so clingy to our baby that I don't get as much time as I'd like with him. What can I do?

It seems that you need to organise time with your baby. At first this could coincide with your wife spending time out of the house doing something she enjoys. You will also need to tell your wife that you would like to have more contact and time with your baby – try not to blame her or draw attention to her clinginess and take time to listen to her view. There are tips on p.290 that may help. If you ask your wife to guide you through some of the basic skills, she may feel better about letting her baby out of her embrace.

It could take your baby time to get used to being with you, particularly if he is always with his mum, but he'll gradually relax if you are together regularly and you will develop your own special relationship. You have discovered that boundaries defining time, space and the way each of you feels are central to family life. These work best when they are dynamic, and are looked at more closely in Families (p.276).

Playtime, safety and tidiness are becoming difficult now that my baby is crawling. Is a playpen a good or a bad thing?

Playpens can be a boon for parents, keeping baby and mess confined to one place, and a great thing for the babies who love to explore their toys and amuse themselves. But many babies who hate being confined will need just as much stimulation in the playpen as they did out of it. Also a favourite game is to throw all the toys out and then cry to get them back. Usually babies who are introduced to the pen before they crawl object less but this isn't always the case. In the playpen your baby may actually be deprived of the attention and interaction that is crucial for developing physical and social skills. It is better to get a stair gate to block off doorways, alter your perception of 'tidiness' and make an area of your home into a play space. Join in and enjoy playtime while it lasts.

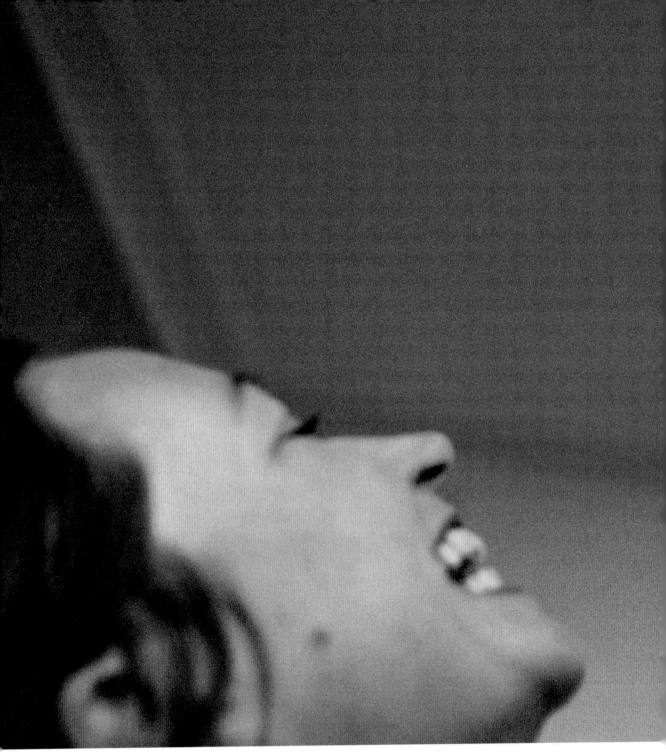

part iv **the journey into parenthood**

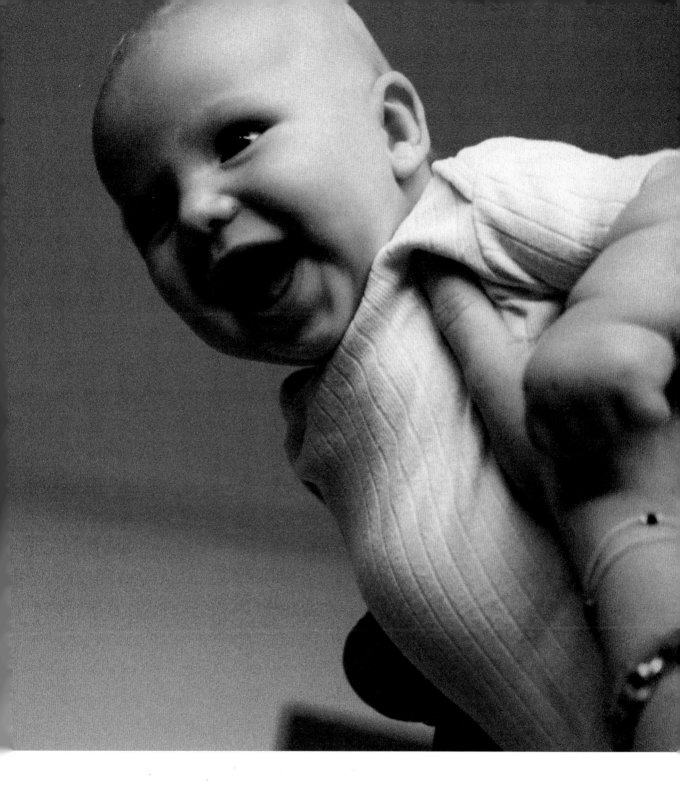

Families

Everyone is a member of a family, whether it is small, large, divided or extended. Whatever your background, your family relationships will be among the most influential of your life. Of course you will also be influenced by your financial, educational, religious and ethnic background, by your friends, colleagues at work, and by the media. But the values and opinions you have inherited from your parents and from the way you interacted with your siblings are part of you and will affect your approach to your new family. Your children will in turn inherit values from you because they are branches of the same family tree.

Family culture

Every family has a culture that shapes the way its members behave towards each other and towards people outside the family. Some families, for instance, are very emotionally expressive while others are private; some value manners highly, others have a free-for-all attitude; some argue openly; some are quick to criticise. Together every mother and father, even when they have separated, evolve a family culture that is distinctive and has rules and expectations. The most powerful ones are often unwritten.

Recalling your experience of how your mother and father behaved towards one another and the way they shared the responsibilities may be very revealing. You may believe that some of your family values are good or you may not wish to follow in your family's footsteps. The same applies to your partner. A lot becomes clearer when you have your first baby and your family cultures will be tested for compatibility. Whether you embrace or reject your parents' ways, they will be your strongest role models. Some couples are lucky and their expectations about roles and behaviours dovetail neatly, some find differences and for many these may be considerable.

Your new family

In your family you, your partner and your baby all have your own needs and make your own contributions. The family is a dynamic unit and it has needs and exerts as much influence as any of the individual members. The balance shifts: one day your baby may determine which choices are made, on another your health may dictate decisions, and on another your home may take priority. The challenge is how to adapt to your situation. This is often easier if you have been raised in a family that tended to negotiate and find the middle ground.

As you get a feel for the way your new family is evolving, it might be interesting to assess it against the background of your individual family experiences. You can apply the questions below to your new family and to your experience with your own parents and siblings. If you are nervous about doing this as a couple, you will still gain from doing it alone. If you do exchange views, you may more easily understand one another's reasoning, and predict some of the potential upsets that lie ahead of you. It's good to talk as much about your differences as your similarities. At times you may feel that one of you does not measure up to certain standards, wherever they come from. If you both believe your opinions are right, it helps to agree to let go of blame and anger, and simply lay your cards on the table. Remember, every partnership faces upset and disagreement at some point (p.287).

- Think about your family as if it were a single person with a developed personality. Is the personality: Generous? Ambitious? Happy-go-lucky? Uptight? Happy? Depressed? What other personality traits could you apply? How is this different from your partner's family?
- Consider the way your family resolves conflict – by discussion, by shouting, by pressure, by silence or by asking someone outside the family to help?
- Imagine your family as a team. Does it work well as a collective unit or is it segmented? How does it organise itself to succeed? How does it encourage individual team members to do their best? What does it do when one of the team members is not pulling his or her weight?

Dynamic boundaries

Everyone has boundaries without consciously thinking about them, based on what was learnt from parents, friends or teachers. There are boundaries that define three main areas of your life: time, space and feelings.

- A 'time' boundary might apply to bedtime or how long it is acceptable to let your baby cry before picking him up. You may have a very clear boundary that says, 'I am committed to meeting my friends every Tuesday night', or set times around the way you share childcare with your partner or another carer. One of you may function on approximate time – 'I will get there when I can' – whereas the other prefers to be meticulously punctual.

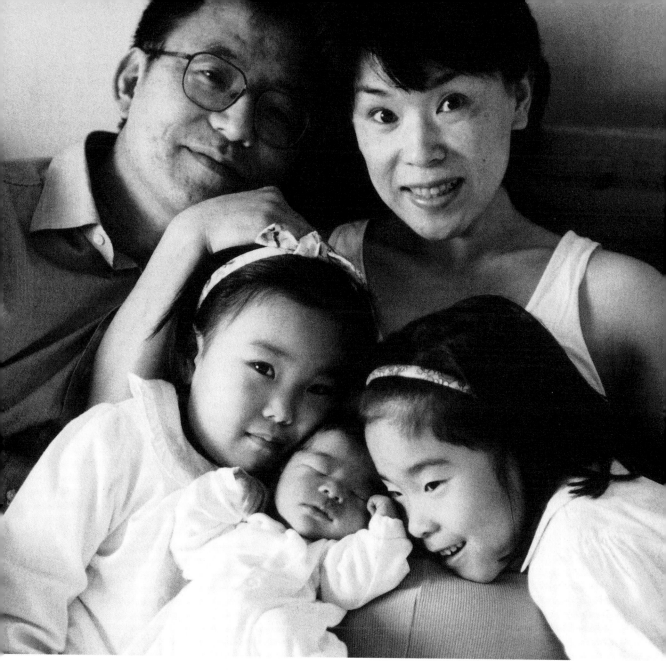

- There are also 'space' boundaries; some families have just one room for the baby and all his paraphernalia, some have a separate adult room, others allow a free cross-over throughout the house.
- When it comes to 'feelings', boundaries are more difficult to identify. You can start by asking yourself what level of expression is acceptable in front of your partner and in front of your baby when you are angry, upset or jealous, or joyous and excited. Do you think it is OK to cry in front of other people or to jump for joy? Do you prefer discussion or argument when your views clash with someone else's?

When boundaries are made clear and agreed upon, they contribute to a secure base from which love and individuality can thrive. Some boundaries will simply appear without discussion. Others may need to be thoughtfully set to strike a balance. Acknowledging your boundaries with your partner is always interesting, even though you may be unsure in some areas.

Defining your view may be embarrassing, difficult or it may spark an argument; doing so may be one of the most challenging aspects of the way your new family evolves. In many families, boundaries are not defined or spelled out in words. Where boundaries are static ('I refuse to talk about that; my baby will *never* sleep in my bed') they act as barriers and become obstacles. It may take a lot of motivation to recognise and alter patterns but the effort is worthwhile if you get used to a way of talking that allows you to discuss your views without conflict, and where the issue is important to negotiate in order to go forward.

Dynamic boundaries for your baby

In pregnancy the amniotic fluid and the womb acted as a physical boundary and your baby felt 'held' emotionally. After birth, if your child continues to feel 'held', it allows him to experiment and confidently express himself from a secure place. He may get this feeling from a structured day, from your ever-welcoming arms or from the way you communicate with him. Gradually he will push the frontiers of his development and the boundaries will alter. Life evolves and boundaries need to be constantly reset. What is appropriate for a 3-week-old is inappropriate for a 4-month-old baby, and when your baby is unwell the usual framework of the day will change.

Your baby will have a strong voice and there may be conflict as well as harmony between your personalities. At any one time, there is always a balance to be struck between the needs of each of you as individuals and the needs of your family. With boundaries in place, quality

---

My baby is 4 weeks old and loves to fall asleep on my chest and I really enjoy the feeling. My mum says that we will spoil our baby.

In the early days your baby may need to be held physically but as time goes on he will change. Hold him when you think he needs to be held and put him down to sleep when he drops off. Initially you may put him down in your bed and later you may move him. This is gradually imposing a boundary and listening to your needs and your baby's needs: you will be building a framework with gentle guidance rather than confrontation. As you do, remember that you and your mother are different and it's your choice for your family.

You may worry that once a pattern is learnt it will be impossible to alter it. One of the features of the human brain is plasticity and the ability to learn; this applies very much to your baby, whose experience of the world is rapidly evolving. Guiding your baby gradually is not a way of spoiling him, even if it takes him weeks to get used to his own sleeping space. In fact, it is a way of teaching him that things change and people adapt. If, however, you suddenly decide to put him in his own room, alone, he will probably object. Some parents may interpret this crying as the mark of a 'spoilt' baby, others call it being honest and self-expressive. Take things step by step. For your baby the feeling of being loved and emotionally 'held' is the most important aspect of his life.

time comes more easily because you can block out other things and feel committed to being fully 'present' for the other person.

Part of the parenting package is to take the lead. Surprisingly, often it is adults who rebel against their own disciplined upbringing who find this difficult. Babies have an inherent drive to fit into the family culture so they need boundaries and it is the parents who set the balance. The ideal environment supports as well as teaches your baby, where there is space for him to be heard, and to adapt. It also supports and teaches you and provides a place for you to feel heard and understood.

You may be determined to do the opposite of what your parents did as you aim to give your child 'better' experiences. The intention is admirable but there may be a catch. As with conformity, when you rebel you continue to define your life in terms of other people's values and expectations.

Rigidity (strong discipline) and a lack of boundaries (very little discipline) may be seen as two sides of the same coin: if a boundary is too tight there is no room to move, yet if a boundary is too loose the space can leave a child without orientation. The ideal balance lies between the two where the parents listen to their baby and set dynamic boundaries. The parents do not negate their own needs, nor ignore their baby's needs. This is a state of symbiosis and because things alter from day to day, the boundaries can change accordingly. Being in a state of harmony is fleeting for most parents. You may be surprised by how variable each day can be in the months after your baby's birth. Altering patterns that are deeply embedded in your past takes a long time, so start small, set little, achievable goals and see how it goes. The more secure you feel about your role in the way your new family evolves, the less you will be inclined to behave as you think you 'should' because other people expect things of you.

Honesty and love

The basis for creating boundaries that cause the minimum of friction for everyone are honesty and love. If you are honest, others may find it easier to respect your boundaries even when they do not agree, and you may find it easier to respect theirs. Love and honesty make it easier to acknowledge that there are different views and none is the absolute truth.

Your confidence will improve with time. What happens now continues as an ongoing process, and if you remain aware and honest, you will evolve throughout your life. When you are offered advice, see if you can take a step back from your preconceptions and expectations, and listen openly with a good heart. Then consider what has been said and decide whether you will act upon the advice. It takes courage to do what you feel is correct, particularly when you choose not to follow the advice of your parents

Smacking and hitting

The subject of hitting as a quick way of reprimanding a baby or child continues to fuel discussion and debate. Some parents were physically punished as children, both at home and at school. Many say that this 'did no harm' but an increasing number are admitting that, on the contrary, being hit has had a lasting, negative impact.

Receiving a smack, whether it be on the bottom, the hand, the cheek or the leg, is confusing for a child. Even if the lightest tap does not physically hurt, children say that it hurts inside, and some may feel pain and confusion – is being hit by the people who love you an expression of love? If parents tell their child not to hurt people (e.g. by biting, which may happen in the first year), what message do they give by hitting? Babies will always learn by what they see and experience, not by what they are told. A lot of research evidence, and common sense, suggests that children who are hit learn to become hitters themselves.

What hitting can do

There is nothing to prove that *not* hitting can do a child harm. The arguments against hitting, however, are numerous. Here are some:

- A baby is a person and deserves the same respect as an adult. Physical punishment undermines a child's self-esteem.
- A young baby cannot be purposefully naughty, so reprimand is inappropriate. A baby usually cries excessively or lashes out angrily when he wants something that is a basic need – food, contact, love or comfort.
- Hitting is painful and makes a child afraid. Fear is not the same as respect and when a relationship is based on fear there is little room for honesty.
- A child is fragile. Hitting can hurt and may cause serious damage. The line between slapping and 'abuse' is very fine.
- Hurting someone does not solve a problem. It causes emotions to be buried deep and issues of conflict rumble on. It may teach a child that it is not right to have certain emotions, nor to have an opinion that differs from his parents'.
- When an adult hits a child, the child receives the message that hitting is right, and that it is OK for a stronger, larger person to hurt someone smaller. It sends a message that bullying works.
- When a parent hits, he or she continues a cycle of violence.

If you feel out of control

All parents sometimes feel out of control, and angry. Sometimes hitting happens because a parent doesn't know what else to do. If you are angry with yourself, your child or something else, and are driven to smack your child, try the following:

- Begin to slow your breath and breathe deeply, focusing on the out-breath. Count to ten.
- Do not shout at your child. Shouting can create fear, just as hitting can.
- If you are really tense, take yourself away to another room for a few minutes. Make sure your child is safe.
- Call a friend on the phone if you want to let it all out.

- Try things that you know will calm you, perhaps yoga. Possibly phone a friend. If you're still mad, take it out on a cushion.
- Come back to your child and explain how you are feeling and why you became angry or afraid. Apologise if it feels appropriate. It may seem strange to do this to a tiny baby but it is good for you and your baby will understand your tone of voice.
- Make time to look at your feelings – why did you feel the urge to hit? What could hitting do for your child?
- If you are concerned about your feelings, there are many people you can turn to for help, including your friends or family, your health visitor and a number of children's charities.

Discipline

In the long term, discipline without violence is more effective. You will find your own way that suits your family boundaries, and may use some of the following tips.

- Try to be honest and set clear limits for behaviour according to your child's age and your ideas. Make sure that everyone who cares for your child knows what these are.
- Set limits to your own behaviour (e.g. settling disputes with your partner) and try to give your child good examples.
- Listen to your child and acknowledge he has his point of view.
- Tell him that you love him.
- Praise his good behaviour.
- Give him quality time when he knows that he has your attention. If one parent is more often absent than the other, perhaps because of work, it is really important that he or she creates this quality time. Listening is the key.
- Do what you can to help your child avoid getting into danger or encountering a situation that often makes him angry.
- Explain why you are doing things and why you are setting limits – even for a tiny baby it is a good habit to start early. He will understand that you are treating him with respect and this will probably be reciprocated in years to come.

The law

Attitudes to the use of physical punishment are, of course, highly individual. When faced with legality, politicians may struggle with the contest between appeasing the adult-voting population while sticking by cultural and religious traditions, and making the right choice for children. The legal aspect is important because when a law is introduced it begins a process of change. Most often, this change gives priority to human rights.

In many European countries hitting at school and at home, by parents or childminders, has been made illegal – a criminal offence. But this is not the case everywhere. Persistent lobbying from parents and children's charities is slowly pushing countries to outlaw physical punishment for young children and clarify the legal distinctions between discipline and abuse. In the UK, Scotland is leading the way as it joins this trend of change. Only time will tell whether the English and North American governments will come into line with Europe.

or someone you admire. It takes even more courage to admit that someone else is correct and alter your thinking accordingly.

As the dance with your baby evolves, boundaries are dynamic and alter. The rules (boundaries) in a dance create a flow and allow for self-expression and fun as you follow the rhythm together, and get better and better at avoiding treading on one another's toes.

Healthy and unhealthy families

There is no such thing as a perfect family. Every family has its own sense of humour and irony, its own good and bad days, its ghosts and demons. Family therapists attempt to define the 'healthy' family but there is general acknowledgement that 5% or fewer actually meet a full list of attributes. The ideas below of healthy and unhealthy families are loosely based on the insights of John Cleese and Robin Skynner (*Life and How to Survive It*). They represent two stereotypes that almost certainly cannot exist in real life. Reading through them, however, may help you to focus on the many ways a family works. Everyone will identify with some aspects in both the 'healthy' and the 'dysfunctional' family. The downside of reading the following lists is that you may feel upset or pessimistic about your life; but it could stimulate you to initiate change in your new family.

The 'functional' family

Mr and Mrs 'Healthy' and the 'Healthy' children (Very, Happily and Absolutely) show the following attitudes and behaviours:

Attitude to life: They tend to accept people for who they are and not what they do. They accept life for what it is.

Response to change: The family is not ruffled by change: its members enjoy immense emotional support from each other and from the family's common value system, which encourages rest and play. They have the confidence that they will be supported emotionally in the decisions they make. Sometimes they draw on moral values based on spiritual beliefs.

Attitude to success and failure: Each family member has learnt to accept that success and failure are part of life, and each one is relative. They feel supported in difficulty and praised for their achievements, and consequently feel very confident to exploit their potential.

Respect for individuality: The family members are capable of great intimacy and affection but they have confidence to cope well on their own and explore their own lives. There is no guilt that makes them cling to loved ones.

Discipline: There are clear boundaries, Mum and Dad are agreed on the principles and are prepared to lay down the law if they have to. Manipulation does not work because the boundaries are clearly defined and consistency leads to self-discipline.

Openness in communication: The children know that all feelings they experience are acceptable and not forbidden. Sexuality, anger and envy are all regarded as a normal part of human experience. This leads to a sense of freedom, lots of fun and high spirits. The children are able to be honest and don't feel ashamed or lie, and learn to be open and respect other points of view.

Conflict resolution: Everyone can be honest, openly disagree and vocalise their opinion. There's no need to guess at what each other thinks and people are asked how they feel. Communication is easy, though it may be noisy.

Blame: When powerful emotions such as anger or envy arise each person can see what is his or her responsibility and own it. The children are encouraged to acknowledge their anger and feelings, knowing they are loved and not rejected. When they were babies they were treated like this, and were able to take responsibility for their own feelings from an early age. They tend to have a well-defined set of values and are more likely to achieve goals because they are objective.

The 'dysfunctional' family

The following list gives an indication of the way a 'dysfunctional family' behaves.

Attitude to life: The members of the family don't feel emotionally supported and are not clear about a common set of values. When confused they are often angry towards one another or the family in general. Love manifests itself as demanding, possessive and jealous and the family members cling to one another for fear of abandonment.

Response to change: Change is often feared because the individual members have not been encouraged to recognise and trust their own strengths and potentials.

Attitude to success and failure: The parents are rarely quick to praise their children and make a habit of criticising them and emphasising what they've done wrong. The children expect the worst of themselves. One child is often praised more than the others. The children may grow up to believe that they are incapable of being successful.

Respect for individuality: Mr and Mrs Dysfunction are possessive and don't recognise that each of the family members has a separate identity. Often they pry into private affairs, and the way the family interacts shows there's confusion about where one person ends and where another starts. The feeling that each member of the family should behave in a certain (family) way blurs the distinction made between their individual and their collective identity.

Discipline: In the dysfunctional family there is often a lot of jockeying for control and some members of the family feel oppressed. Often the parents give out very different messages indeed, and the children learn to manipulate and set one parent against the other. There may be violence in the family.

Openness in communication: The parents try not to be emotional, and do not encourage emotional expression. The children habitually conceal their real emotions.

Conflict resolution: Unclear boundaries, discussion with feelings of blame and disapproval instead of honest admission make conflict resolution rare. Conflicts are either shouted out and end in an angry exit, or are quietened by one family member taking on responsibility for something that wasn't actually his or her fault. The underlying problem does not disappear, and anger and misunderstanding increase.

Blame: The family atmosphere encourages its members to take on other people's feelings and soak up their problems. The individuals get into the habit of projecting feelings on to others instead of feeling them themselves. They blame the family, and grow up to project blame on to others.

Finding a balance

Looking at your own past you will see some things that a psychologist would deem 'healthy' and some 'dysfunctional'. It is useful to take an objective look at your background, particularly your early years, because it can help you fathom why you feel and do some things the way you do. This process can offer relief from guilt, anger or self-blame. Acknowledging your past experience is seldom easy and works best when you feel supported by honesty, love and commitment. As you relate your past to your present, you may be inspired to work at your positive, healthy tendencies and to avoid awkward, repetitive patterns. Every family requires effort and hard work to pull through difficulties and enjoy good times, and every family has a 'history'. Accepting this history, however different it may be for you and your partner, and working with it, is a great way to express your love for one another.

As your baby forms his first emotional experiences, he also forms a set of expectations. If he sees you together regularly and feels that you are happy, he will think this is normal. If he sees one of you during the day and another at night, this will be normal. Equally, if he feels tension and hears arguments, this will be normal for him. Your baby uses your relationship with each other, and with the rest of your family and community, to form an understanding of the way culture works and human beings interact.

Your parents and you

As you become a mother or father, your position in your family hierarchy shifts, so while you are still your parents' child, your relationship with them changes. Adapting and entering an adult-to-adult relationship is part of your own journey of growing up and your mother or father may become a close, or closer, friend and your relationship might be more smooth, loving and easy than it was. You may also begin to appreciate how much your parents did for you over the years.

This is not the case for every new parent, however, and sometimes the reverse can be true: some people dread the involvement ('interference') of their parents. Your mother or father may try to control you and want more than ever to treat you as 'their baby' and resist the reality of you growing up and doing things your way. Allowing your own parents to express themselves without feeling that they are interfering requires patience. If you feel smothered or dominated, albeit in a caring way, you will need to establish your limits and be firm about your decisions. You may need courage to insist, preferably in a kind and loving way, that your choices are acknowledged and respected. Sometimes it's hard to know whether the stand you take is based on true conviction or the need to exert your individuality. Time will help you to differentiate, and you may need to change your opinion later rather than clinging doggedly to a certain point of view.

Even in the sunniest of parent–child relationships there may be differences of opinion. Grandparents – most often it's grandmothers – can have difficulty settling in to an advisory role, particularly if this is the first grandchild. The line between advice and criticism can be thin, and your parents may find it hard to be sensitive and sit back as you find your feet.

A mother's mother

When a mother watches her own daughter becoming a mother the mixture of pride, love, sadness and anxiety may be confusing. For the two women involved there may be a great deal of communication that is never expressed through words, but is based on an understanding that both have gone through a pregnancy and birth, known what it is to create and meet new life, and felt a mother's love. Often this is strong in the hours and days after birth, and it continues to grow. Many mother–daughter relationships thrive on this shared experience of maternal energy. When there is conflict or confusion about the practical approaches to parenting it may help to acknowledge the bond between you. The details of parental care are much less important and less powerful than the love each of you feels for one another and for the baby.

When your relationship is difficult

Problems in parent–child relationships are responsible for many emotional struggles that adults face. Difficulties in getting on with your parents may affect your self-esteem and the relationships you form. At some point, working through the feelings may help you heal parts of yourself and move forward. While you are setting out as a parent, you are in a very good position to take a really close look and consider the impact your relationship with your parents has on your current attitudes and dreams.

If you feel that childhood issues may be important or obstacles exist between you and your parents, you may

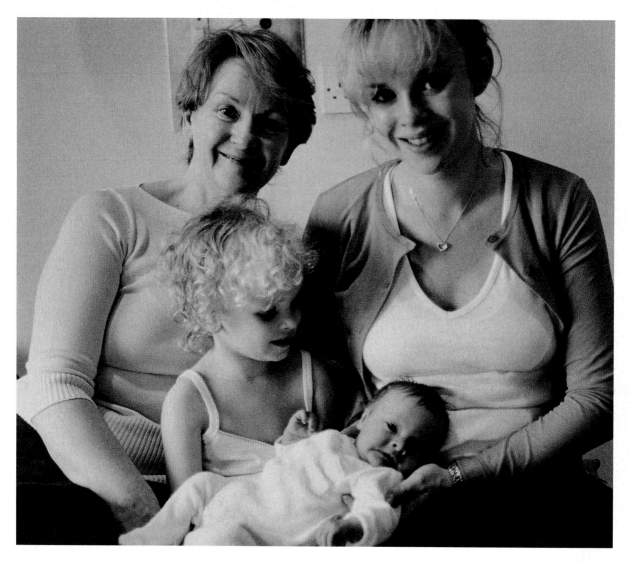

identify with one or more of the thoughts listed below. Some are quite common, some are very unusual and most are seldom admitted openly.

- 'My parents still treat me as if I am a child and I make decisions based upon whether they would approve.'
- 'I'm sure that what I do is never good enough for them.'
- 'I remember that I was often criticised.'
- 'My dad sometimes hit me, and I remember being bullied at school. I find it hard to trust people and can't stand arguments.'
- 'My relationship with my dad is over – he abused me and I'm so angry.'
- 'My mother was always out and I had to take care of myself.'
- 'I spent my childhood looking after my sick mother.'
- 'My mother had an alcohol problem and we could never rely on her to be there for my sister and me.'

Problems relating to parent–child relationships are among the most difficult to resolve. If you do identify with any, some of the advice in this book may inspire you to seek emotional and practical support, lift your self-esteem and improve your relationship. As you work through the issues, you may begin to feel better about yourself and have fewer worries about how you are parenting.

Grandparents

There's a very special bond between children and their grandparents, who hold promise and mystery, hide a wealth of surprises in their pockets, offer warm embraces and allow secret treats. Even tiny babies recognise the unique quality of a grandparent's love. How your parents bond with your baby depends on your baby and them and on your own relationship with them. Your baby will sense whether you trust, love or resent them. If there are issues

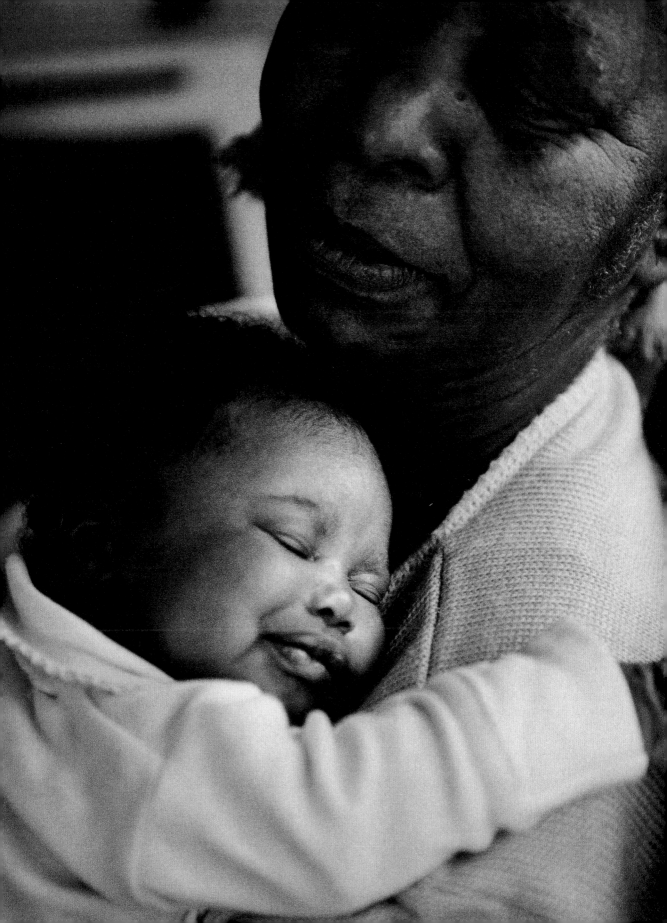

In-laws

Parents are parents and in-laws are in-laws. However much you like or love your partner's parents, there will always be a sense of difference – their cultural background and family views are bound to be different from yours. There may be problems if you always believe your parents' advice is best, or your in-laws are too interfering – it is equally difficult if you favour your in-laws' views over your own family's. Any conflict may impinge on your relationship with your partner, and it often helps to discuss your feelings about your respective parents and their role in your new family.

Conflict between a new father and his partner's mother is common, even though they may become closer in time. Initially he may be protective and resent her intrusion. If his mother-in-law feels displaced she may react by being distant or critical or voice her point of view even more strongly. The mother-in-law issue can become a major source of strife, particularly if the new mother feels torn and hurt when two people she loves are fighting. Listening and acknowledging everyone's thoughts (p.290) is a good starting point.

If a dad and his father-in-law find a deeper level of bonding, the mum can become jealous, or she may get on better with her dad as well as her father-in-law as a result. The way every relationship develops is just one part of the process of growing up and growing into parenthood and your extended family.

---

between you, try to resolve them and explain to your baby in a gentle tone that your upset is your problem and not his, and encourage him to enjoy his grandparents.

Grandmothers are often expected to have a confident and experienced hand when it comes to babycare. But fashions have altered and your mother may feel out of her depth. Grandfathers in the current generation, on the other hand, are more often viewed as gentle, protective figures who are not expected to be involved in the same, hands-on way. If the grandfather was an absent father himself, he may need considerable time to connect with his grandchild, rediscover the parts of himself that can relate to babies and children and strengthen his relationship with his own son or daughter.

However your parents begin on the road of grandparenthood, they will need space to develop their own special relationship with your child. It may be years, or even decades, since they cradled a baby, and many aspects of babycare will be new to them. Thoughts about children and birth have changed and your parents are on a learning curve. It will take time for you all to experiment and find the best way forward.

If your parents don't want to get close to your baby, it is better, in the short term, to accept the situation and focus on building your own new family. Your baby's personality and the passing of time may alter their relationship.

How do they see it?

The birth of a grandchild often heralds a new lease of life for grandparents and a huge amount of joy as the family gets bigger. This transition is another stage in growing up. For your parents, being with your baby – their own flesh and blood – will conjure up memories of holding you in their arms, and may bring their own inner child to the surface again. They are likely to be proud of you and full of love, but their own anxieties may also surface.

Grandparents have the privilege of being able to indulge in their grandchildren without being burdened by 24-hour responsibility. While enjoying this, they may also feel melancholy. Some are sad to see their own children grow away and make a fresh start. If their advice or help is rejected, grandparents feel sore, and they may react strongly to modern childcare practices. Most are loaded with the gift of patience, however, having parented their own children, and know that time smoothes things out, teaches lessons and heals wounds.

Your parents may feel guilt, rather than pride, at the way they raised you or the distance they feel from you now. If this is the case they may find it difficult to relax with you, and, like you, will benefit from enjoying the present while thinking over the past. In time they may find it easier to let go of their uncomfortable feelings, enjoy the way your new family is evolving, and feel better about themselves. How you welcome them and communicate with them may help this transition – you may find the advice on p.290 helps you and your parents feel comfortable with your relationship and reach a position of mutual respect. It may also help to build loving bonds between your baby and his wider family.

I simply cannot stop my mum from giving my 7-month-old sweets. Why won't she listen to me?
Parents want the best for their children, and so do grandparents. Often, however, grandparents take great pleasure in the smile that lights up their grandchildren's eyes when they produce a surprise, and the gleeful welcome they receive on visits. Giving treats is a way of expressing love and revelling in joy and fun. If your mother's visits are far apart then it is best to let her indulge her own and your child's enjoyment. Your child may remember her kindness and unconditional love with great affection. Your baby will easily recognise that you and your mother have different views and your mother's behaviour will not undermine your authority with your baby. If your mother gives sweets frequently, much more often than you would like, then it is a good idea to sit down and explain your reservations, and suggest some limits – perhaps sweets on a certain day or at a certain time after a meal. You may then find it easy to enjoy the smiles and warmth.

Partnership

The partnership between parents provides the foundation for the family to live and love together. Your relationship will change considerably: some things will be positive and strengthening, bringing joy, support and security, and some will test your commitment to one another.

What about sex?

Sex brings the two of you together in a way that needs no words and gives you the chance to lose the rest of the world as you express yourselves purely for one another. It can bring incredible relief from stress as well as intense enjoyment, and this may be particularly heightened for the woman if physical changes brought by childbearing help her experience multiple orgasms.

For some couples sex in pregnancy and after childbirth is better than ever before, but as parents most couples make love less than they used to. The issue of sexual comfort and libido at each stage of the primal period is explored in Parts II and III. Here, it's interesting to see what a wide range of views there are:

She thinks . . .
- I never had such good orgasms.
- I can really feel my vagina and the sensitivity is amazing.
- I love not worrying about contraception.
- I love my body and enjoy being touched.
- I'd love to have sex but he doesn't seem to fancy me any more.
- I'm embarrassed that when we do have sex I can't feel it in my vagina like I used to.
- I feel fat and unattractive.
- Nature is telling me that I don't feel sexy.
- I just can't connect with that part of me.
- My vagina is sore and I need time to recover.
- There are so many demands on me – every minute is taken up feeding and caring for my baby and family; another demand is too much.
- I need time to get to know my baby.
- My breasts are for feeding, not sex.
- I'd rather have oral sex but he doesn't like it.

He thinks. . .
- I don't want to intrude on our growing baby.
- I'm afraid I will hurt the baby in the womb.
- I really like her as she is now, and find our love making is getting even better.
- Sex is fun now that we have conceived.
- I love feeling her softness and warmth.
- I'm too anxious about the labour and birth.
- I feel fantastic after we've made love, and really miss it now that she's not interested.
- I can't get turned on by her now that she's a mother – her body is for our baby, not for me.
- She loves the baby more than she loves me.
- How can we get intimate with our baby in our bed?
- I have been patient and supportive during pregnancy, and think it's time my needs were addressed.
- She went through a lot in labour, and I don't want to hurt her.
- She does not understand that men have a physical need to make love.
- She acts like her mother – how can I possibly make love to my mother-in-law?

Intimacy

Maintaining intimacy is part of sustaining your relationship, and there are many ways to do this. Not all are sexual but being physically close can keep the flame of romance burning. The bond of intimacy is strengthened with trust and understanding, and communicating openly with one another. Intimate actions, such as lying in one another's arms watching telly, massaging each other or holding hands as you walk, can be more powerful than communication with words. Many couples find that pregnancy brings them closer as they share their hopes and their love. This feeling sometimes reduces after the birth when there are new demands and the baby's personality affects the dynamics of a relationship.

Sex and intimacy during pregnancy

No woman feels the same every day for the 9 months of pregnancy, and men feel differently too. In early pregnancy nausea and tiredness and fear of hurting the baby are likely to interfere with sex-drive. In late pregnancy the pressure of the growing abdomen and increased tiredness can have a similar effect. Commonly, sex is most frequent in the middle trimester but all variations are possible. Some women feel sexually charged and bring a new fire into their relationship, and some feel that they want to abandon sex altogether.

But it does take two to tango. Men are often put off by their partner's physical changes, images of childbirth and the idea of having sex with a 'mother'. The reverse also applies: some men become passionate about their partner as they watch her change, see her breasts grow and her hips fill out, and feel more intimate than ever before.

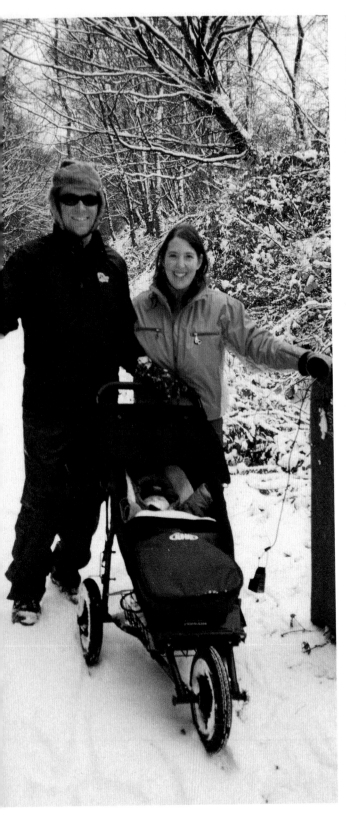

You may both feel strange about having sex with your baby so close but your baby, in fact, benefits from the 'feel good' hormones rushing around the woman's turned-on body. For a baby these are just movements and noise and she does not interpret these as right or wrong. It is safe to make love provided there is no vaginal bleeding (p.406), or a history of miscarriage, and in late pregnancy unless your baby's membranes have ruptured. It is also safe to experience orgasm and there is no risk of initiating premature labour.

Increasingly in pregnancy, you will need to explore different positions and this could bring novelty and extra enjoyment. Penetration from behind might be comfortable, or you could sit or kneel or use a chair to make access easier. Your genitals may be more sensitive, making external stimulation more enjoyable, and it's quite common for women to experience multiple orgasms.

Occasionally penetration might be uncomfortable, and you may prefer oral sex. The taste and consistency of vaginal fluid can also change, however; some men do not like it, some really enjoy the female ejaculation. If you're shy about expressing pleasure with moans or sighs, try to let rip. This is a wonderful opportunity to let go of vocal inhibitions and is excellent practice for being vocally expressive during labour.

Sex after birth

Some couples resume sex very soon after childbirth but most take weeks or months. You will both almost certainly be tired, and will need to rest and sleep when you can. Women need time to recover from birth, and few feel happy to make love before bleeding and postnatal pain have passed. Men can also take a long time to believe that their touch won't hurt.

If you feel as if you've lost sight of your sexual drive, don't worry. In the early days you will be directing most of your energy into nurturing and getting to know your baby. Women who breastfeed are often less sensitive to their partner's touch, and this is due to the hormonal changes and low oestrogen levels that can also reduce vaginal lubrication; libido may fall for 6 months or more. Many couples find the idea of being close again quite daunting, a little like losing virginity.

Resuming full sexual intercourse after childbirth needs to be gradual; penetration must be unhurried with particular care near the perineum and the vaginal entrance. As the outer third of the vagina is the most sensitive, shallow thrusts can be more arousing and comfortable than deeper ones. With the woman on top she can control the amount of pressure.

Vaginal dryness caused by hormonal changes is very common and can be painful and off-putting, but lubricating with natural oils (such as almond or grapeseed) or KY jelly helps and could become part of foreplay.

Intercourse actually helps to stretch and heal vaginal tissues, and can be a great way of strengthening pelvic floor muscles.

It can help to be aware of things that are likely to put you off. First, it will be your baby, whether she is sleeping in your room or elsewhere, because you will probably be subconsciously listening out for her. You may not feel comfortable having sex with your baby in the same room. Another interference is the leakage of breast milk: this is very common as soon as the woman gets turned on and may be contained in a bra with breast pads, or with a towel. Some men find the milk erotic, but it can also dampen sex-drive.

Some couples feel empowered by their experiences of pregnancy and birth and become more open and even daring about voicing their sexual preferences. Discussions between the two of you might bring great results. If sexual intimacy means a lot to you, it is worth creating time by cutting down on other commitments. For some couples, particularly for the man, making love infrequently can be a major cause of upset.

The two of you

Your relationship will change when pregnancy is confirmed. Optimism and closeness may increase, you may need to work through some differences or take time to come to terms with the pregnancy. For pregnancy to bring hope to a fragile relationship, you need to commit to one another in a new way.

It's usual for new parents to be completely absorbed by their baby after birth in a period of euphoria and celebration. Yet in the early days you may seldom have time together, and it's quite common to lose sight, temporarily, of your connection. If one or both of you needs reassurance, it will help to create space and time so you can be friends and lovers as well as parents. The advent of parenthood could be like a new beginning for your relationship, a chance to rekindle the flame of romance and reinforce a foundation of trust and respect.

Love

Love is expressed in many ways – through consideration, physical closeness, sexual intimacy, small gestures and conversation as well as through anger, sulking or jealousy. Love is beyond words and moods, and actions can communicate more powerfully than talking. Often love is expressed in a way that has been conditioned through childhood (p.276). You may discover new strengths that you never before suspected as well as areas of weakness that could do with some loving attention. At its strongest love is unconditional, asks no rewards and has no limits. You may experience unconditional love for the first time when your baby is born and find this love so inspiring that your partnership blossoms.

Sometimes love may be confused with control: 'If you love me you'll stay in with me', 'If you love me you'll do this with me.' The more you give your partner freedom, time, support and space to enjoy life, develop and grow, the more your relationship will benefit. Of course, this freedom needs to operate on both sides. It may be worth talking about how you both organise time and space so that each of you feels supported. We look at this in the Wheel for Living (p.58).

Working with your differences

It is exciting to leap into the unknown together. Most couples start out with fantasies about parenthood. It is likely that your expectations of family life will be different in at least some areas; perhaps you have different views of the role of a mother and father, of the behaviour expected of a baby, of routine, feeding or sleeping patterns.

You may find that being different can lend strength to your relationship if you encourage both of your positive sides; but differences can also weaken your bond. If you find you have unresolved differences, you will need patience and time to find a compromise. Emotional tension

In the 4 months since our baby was born I feel we have drifted apart. We don't talk about ourselves any more. I would love to get our partnership back in balance.
Having a baby does hugely reduce time for parents to be alone together. Even lying awake in bed in the morning may be rare. Sometimes it takes planning and effort to remember to do things for – and with – one another that will help spice up, and cement, your relationship.

- During the early months, particularly if sexual intimacy is reduced, thoughtful gestures and enjoyable activities are great ingredients for a healthy relationship. Cooking a meal, shopping or arranging a babysitter and a night out may make your partner feel loved and wanted, and there are many ways of enjoying time together with your baby.
- You could turn a day that might have been spent in front of the television into a more exciting adventure where you show your baby the delights of a park or zoo, or wander round an exhibition together. While your baby is small, take advantage . . . you can go to cafés and restaurants together without having to chase around after her.
- The concept of quality time (p.55) applies as much to each other as it does to your baby. Creating space is the best medicine for a healthy or ailing relationship.
- When you do have time together you will probably find that you begin to open up to one another. You could start by following one person's choice one week, and the other's the next.

and friction are energy-consuming and draining and affect the ease and enjoyment of parenthood. Love can alternate with dislike, tenderness with anger, and trust with fear, and sometimes both of you may feel completely overwhelmed and need support.

Almost all couples experience difficulties, and while these may be minor, breakdown is common after childbirth, and sometimes in pregnancy. The signs include feelings of distance, silences, increased arguments, dissatisfaction and lack of sex without any willingness to talk it over. Usually the catalysts are reduced time together and lack of communication. Other reasons include a mother being so involved with her baby that her partner feels left out, or a father spending time away from home because he is unsure how to parent.

Often a couple is completely surprised by the differences that appear between them when they are faced with family issues. It is not unusual for the mother and father unwittingly to behave like their own parents and for each to assume that their way is 'right'. In these cases, arguments inevitably arise.

Communication

Communication lies at the heart of every relationship, yet just a small proportion of it is spoken – most takes place through body language and tone of voice. If you feel close to someone, you 'mirror' him or her by sitting or standing in a similar way and having eye-to-eye contact. You find that small gestures of acknowledgement or tenderness go a long way towards maintaining a good flow of communication and body language reaches its height during love making.

In every relationship and in every family, from time to time communication breaks down. Relationships can be restored most easily when the breakdown is acknowledged and someone sets things in motion in an attempt to correct it. In the primal period your relationship becomes extra-vulnerable.

Research studies have shown that by 9 months after the birth a quarter of couples feel their relationship has improved, for another quarter it is about the same and half find that they are not getting on as well. Take heart that conflict and discomfort stimulate change, and it will take time for the 'old' to be discarded and the 'new' to be established. Try to take a step back, think over your feelings, and then create space for communication with your partner: make time to be together undisturbed and re-introduce activities into your lives that may have taken a back seat for a few months. Breakdown is not always final: it can provide the basis for a breakthrough. The new relationship can arise like a phoenix, reborn from the ashes of the old.

It may take time and patience for both of you to feel that your needs are being met and that you have been

Keeping intimate without sex

Time together is the most important thing for your partnership, and can be fruitful in many ways. If you feel that your time together is insufficient, try out some of the following ideas or develop some of your own.

- If you are out with friends you may both catch the 'buzz' of fun and social excitement, and when you are with your baby a cuddle or kiss between you is easy and effective.
- You can create a wonderful atmosphere to talk and laugh at home with a few candles, some music and delicious food (it can be very sensuous to feed each other).
- A gentle massage at the end of the day will almost certainly bring relaxation. Touching one another's bodies in a loving but non-sexual way is very intimate and trusting, and can reinforce the bond you feel as friends, particularly when neither of you feels the pressure to perform.
- You may like the idea of having a luxurious bubble bath or shower together. Undress each other slowly, keep the lights low, and afterwards dry each other before moving to the bedroom for a massage.
- If you both lead busy lives, book time together in your diaries and make a commitment to keeping the appointment even if you feel embarrassed at using a diary to meet one another. This is particularly important if either of you feels upset or lonely. Even half an hour works well and could create space for you to discuss what you both feel about your sex life or bring up any other issues that are making you tense. The active listening techniques that are described overleaf are very useful.
- Could you find time and someone to care for your baby so that you could go somewhere? A night away in a hotel would let you dine together, fall asleep together and wake up together without interruption from your baby.
- When you're separated by work or other commitments you could reinforce your intimacy with messages by phone, text, email or pager.

heard and understood. It can be reassuring to remember that all partnerships need to be worked at, and every couple has its good and its bad times; ultimately, it is the work that you put in, and the compromises you reach, that keep you together.

Resolving anger and conflict safely

Anger is an integral part of any relationship. If your partner has made you angry, ask yourself what he or she was trying to do or say, and why you reacted as you did. Acknowledging feelings and difficulties is not easy. The thing about anger is that until you can accept it, it controls you. It is sometimes used as a way of avoiding change. When you're angry you often lay blame on others, although you may actually be angry with yourself for the way you are acting. Anger may mask feelings of not being acknowledged or loved. If you have looked forward to being a parent you might be thinking, 'Why is it so hard? It's just not fair.'

The most constructive way to deal with anger is to accept that you have a choice, let go and find love inside, and use active listening (overleaf) to 'hear' yourself and your partner. Some cultures or families openly express anger, while others suppress it – you and your partner might benefit from acknowledging one another's backgrounds and talking about the many ways of expressing feelings. You could turn the energy outwards and release anger without hurting others, perhaps by exercising vigorously or sitting in the car and screaming and swearing at the top of your voice. You might need to express your anger in private several times before you can let go of it.

In times of conflict, a safe physical and emotional place is needed. Try not to address important issues when your baby is crying, you're cooking dinner or you have only 5 minutes to spare. Choose instead a long car journey or a relaxed meal with soft music. You may need a third person to act as a guardian angel or a counsellor to help you see one another's points of view.

Where conflict cannot be resolved, communicating is still important, because even if a family separates, the link with your child and your partner will continue. You might find it helpful to refer to the list below as well as to the Wheel for Living (p.58).

- Spend quality time together at or away from your home – book it if you have busy diaries.
- Take things day by day and make space in which to relax so that you can reduce your feelings of being overwhelmed.
- Remind yourself that it is normal to feel different after the birth of a baby.
- Try not to make rash decisions – time can heal.
- Talk about the support available and see who could help with childcare to give you some space.
- Find a postnatal group in your area. There are groups for mothers, fathers and couples.
- You may consider seeking out the help of a support counsellor to improve your communication skills as a couple.
- Express yourself honestly but gently. If you are honest with yourself, you will find it easier to be honest with your partner.
- Above all listen, and then listen, and then listen again until you 'feel' what is the best thing to do.

Breaking up

From a child's point of view, it is likely that two parents, and a secure and loving relationship between them, are better than one. Sometimes, however, there is simply no way to live together when love has disappeared and/or irreconcilable differences emerge. In reality, partnerships are not always 'for life'.

If you are facing this dilemma you may become angry and blame your partner for all that is happening between you. But it will be better if you can try to let go of blame, be objective about the relationship and take as many practical steps as possible to help the transition. Each day rests in the context of a longer period of time that can bring opportunities, closeness and healing.

In many ways divorce can be more upsetting for men, who often lose touch with their children and shoulder a considerable financial responsibility. This can bring even greater anger and blame. Only a tiny percentage of men gain full custody. Using time well – making it quality time rather than quantity time – is particularly important when it is so scarce, as is being honest with your baby and doing the best you can to leave aside negative feelings when the two of you are together.

The mother is usually left with the main responsibility for the baby and she will need considerable support from her family or friends, perhaps in addition to financial and practical support from the social services. The confusion of being pregnant, giving birth, becoming a mother and losing a partner is likely to be huge, even in cases where the partner was often absent anyway. A break-up in the first year following the birth of a baby will raise sadness and questions as well as the conflict between being positive about a new baby and negative about a lost partnership. It may take many years and a great deal of support to come to terms with this.

If you have split up from your partner you will know that no one takes such a decision lightly. You may wonder if being alone will actually improve your parenting skills and your relationship with your child. This can be true: for many, parenting alone (p.307) is an empowering experience and, in the long term, the relationship with the child may be stronger for both parents. In spite of the pain of separation and fear of taking such a big step into unknown territory, each member of the family may be happier in the long run.

Sticking together

Making a commitment to stay with another person for life may be an adult's greatest challenge. 'For life' is a very long time, and individuals and relationships change a great deal. Often these changes are greatest in the early years of parenthood. If you have the friendship and bonds that help you to stay together, you are in a win-win situation and have much to offer each other, and the rest of your family, for years to come. Riding the hardest patches together can build unparalleled strength into your relationship and forge a firm basis of love and support for you, the parents, and for your children.

The power of communicating

Active listening

Sometimes just being listened to can be wonderful. Often a conversation takes place where one person talks much more than the other, and the process of listening can be more powerful than the process of expressing. When you are tuned into a person's words and body language, you may perceive what isn't being said – 'read between the lines'. In addition, when you concentrate on listening you have the space to view your own reactions with a degree of objectivity. As you spend more and more time with your baby you will get lots of practice at listening, because you need to learn to interpret her language.

Many people, particularly those who felt they were never listened to as children, find it difficult to 'listen' and this is particularly true if they disagree with what is being discussed. Initially you will need to make a conscious effort to 'listen' to your partner honestly and 'hear' the words that are said and the meaning behind them. If you take time now to try, you will be surprised how powerful and rewarding listening and being listened to can be for both of you as individuals and for your partnership. Listening actively is a powerful way to reach a compromise or a new solution. One possible outcome is that you may have a change of opinion, and disagreement may become agreement.

To actively listen to your partner:
- Create a quiet time and focus on he/she is saying.
- If you are distracted by thoughts, be aware of them, and let them go and listen to your partner again. If you become angry acknowledge it to yourself and then come back to actively listening. This is particularly difficult if you feel that you are correct.
- Appreciate that your partner's view may be different from yours but it is valid. There is always more than one way to solve a problem. This process may be very difficult at first if you are convinced that you are right and he/she is wrong but it becomes easier with practice.
- If each of you has a turn to listen and be listened to once or twice a week, you will be amazed how many of the disagreements disappear. This is particularly the case if you are able to express your own values thoughtfully and acknowledge your differences without blaming one another. Just a few minutes talking together in this way may be enough – it is the quality of the time spent together that is important.
- Try not to react immediately to what is said, rather let it settle and come back to the subject later. Treat problem solving as a joint effort and let go of believing that there is only one correct solution (yours).
- Where your conversation brings up several issues, you may need to agree to talk about each one individually when you next create time.
- Compromise will be easier in some areas than in others. Begin with the minor issues and approach larger problems when you have practised this way of conversing. Remember that some issues that seem large are actually made up of several smaller points – agreement and compromise may be reached in stages.

The YES strategy

Everyone knows what it means to be disappointed, angry or upset. You probably hear a voice in your head blaming yourself or someone else for a situation that is causing you to be unhappy. All parents – both mothers and fathers – have moments or prolonged periods of feeling upset. When either of you is feeling bad, you probably expect the other, and your baby, to behave differently. Inevitably the expectation causes the whole mood of the family to change and as a result your feelings may intensify further.

The YES strategy is designed to help you to communicate honestly and sensitively with one another, after thinking through the reasons for your feelings. You are then in more of a position to create positive change – the third step of the YES system. It is best to use this approach with the active listening techniques outlined to the left as your foundation and anchor.

Y   **What do you yearn for?**

E   **What do you expect?**

S   **What could you say?**

Y – What do you yearn for?

When you feel unhappy, first find a calm space. Try to get to the root of your unease: what is it that is making you unhappy or frustrated? You will yearn for something that you do not have, or a state of affairs that is not happening. 'I wish I was not feeling as tired', 'I yearn for more time to go out', 'I wish my partner did not have to work so hard', 'I wish I had more money', 'I wish . . .'.

E – What do you expect?

If you are angry it is helpful to look at what you expect yourself and the other person to do. When you look at your expectations (p.304), you may decide that they are fair, and you are ready to and want to express them. Or you may realise that they are not justified – you may have expected something of someone else that is not appropriate, or not realised clearly the role you play. When you have reviewed your expectations, you will be able to look again at what you yearn for. Is it still the same thing? Have its limits changed?

In some cases, simple changes in the way you feel or behave may change the way you communicate. For instance, if you realise that your expectations of the other person were unfair, you may let go of them, apologise and the problem dissolves.

S – What could you say?

In many instances you will need to say something to begin a process of change. After what may have been a complex process of looking at your frustration, the words that trigger a way out may be very simple. If you speak honestly and sensitively it may provide a basis for negotiating a change and lead to incredibly powerful results, whereas if you have an aggressive or hostile, blaming tone, then you and the other person may become entrenched and locked in negative, opposing positions.

Sarah's dilemma

'My partner works late and when he comes home he expects dinner to be ready and the house cleaned. He appears to be insensitive to what the baby and I need. I feel tired, resentful and unsupported, and upset that we're not getting on well.'

Y – What I yearn for

'I want to feel loved and supported and I yearn for my partner to have a more equal role in looking after our child. I had an idea that being a family would mean spending lots of time hanging out together to enjoy our baby, yet we rarely do this. At the weekend he is often out of the house. I want us to be a close family and I would also love to have time for myself.'

E – What I expect

'I expect my partner to be here for me and for my baby. I expect him to leave work behind, be more of a hands-on father and think about his priorities regarding work and family.'

S – What I want to say

'I would like to talk with you about how I am feeling. I think we could share the responsibility for looking after ourselves and our baby in a way that allows for each of us to feel relaxed, and gives us time as a couple. I miss the closeness we used to feel, and instead of adding to our relationship it seems that having a baby has put a distance between us. I'm aware that it's still early days, but I'm sure there's something we could do. Could you think about readjusting your work hours so we could have more time together?'

His response might be: 'I am pulled between work and home, and I think we need more money at the moment. When I get home I often feel tired and I can imagine how you must feel after feeding three times in the night and spending all day with our baby. I am unsure how I can help and get nervous when she cries. I also feel that you disapprove of how I deal with her. Let's try to talk when we are both relaxed and she's asleep.'

She says: 'It feels good that we can talk. I feel we are closer again. I thought of a way to get some help with the house chores – Mum has offered to shop for me and cook a meal once a week. This will give me time to get out and I look forward to a bit of exercise. I understand how important your job is to you but I really want us to use the non-work time well.'

He replies: 'Everyone says that this is a time of high stress for families, and I now know it's true. Thanks for being supportive right now. You have reassured me that it does not matter if we each do things in a different way with our baby and I feel less nervous. I shall talk to my boss and see whether I can start and end early on one day a week. It will be a relief for me to let go of the work issues on my way home and try to make our time together good quality and loving.'

She says: 'I realised that my mum always said that my dad was not there for her when we were growing up. A lot of my disappointment in recent weeks may stem from feeling that you and I are going in the same direction as my parents. It feels really good to be able to talk like this without becoming angry, and know that we don't have to be like my parents.'

He says: 'I'm pleased that we can talk about all this too. We're both feeling less stressed, just by talking. Let's organise some time together this weekend. Let's get our favourite food, a good video and some great music and have a night in. There's plenty of time to ourselves once our baby is asleep.'

Mike's concern

'I am really upset that my wife hasn't touched me in a sexual way for 4 months. Whenever I try she turns over and says she doesn't feel like it. I'm afraid we won't get our sex life back.'

Y – What I yearn for

'I want our sex life to resume.'

E – What I expect

'I expect her to respond to me and for us to be making love as we used to.'

S – What I want to say

'I am upset that we have not touched one another or kissed and cuddled for over 4 months. I know that after having a baby your hormones have changed and that you are physically tired. I would like you to know that I feel left out and lonely and miss the closeness that I know we both used to enjoy.'

Her response might be: 'I agree that our love life has been neglected and it makes me sad too. Sometimes it seems that you are not taking my feelings into account. Please remember I love you but my breastfeeding hormones have decreased my desire and mothering is a full-time job – I don't have much spare energy. It could help if we created time for us to be together even if we are at home, and maybe we could start gently, perhaps with a massage or a bath. If I have a chance to rest during the day I will feel less tired and possibly I will feel more giving physically. Can we arrange some extra help?'

His response might be: 'Is it possible to share childcare with Lucy next door on one or two mornings so you could rest or get to the gym? When we are at home together I am happy to help. You know that I am happy to spend time together without needing to always have full sex. I already feel better knowing we are communicating.'

Your dissatisfaction

Sharing your dissatisfaction can resolve it and make space for new possibilities to appear. There are usually a number of different ways of resolving a disagreement and this two-way process will work best if you are both willing to express yourselves, consider one another's opinions, try things on one another's terms as well as on your own, and make concessions. Begin with things that may be remedied with simple commitments and move gradually on to the more confronting issues that need longer discussion and ongoing changes. As time passes you will each have a chance to reflect and review the way changes have worked – this can be an effective way to avoid falling back into old patterns where you both feel 'right' and think the other is 'wrong'. Looking at how you are doing, and continuing to express yourselves gently but openly, is a powerful way to weather the changes of parenthood and a tool that will be profoundly useful in many other areas of your life.

Fatherhood

Being a father is one of the most wonderful things a man can experience. It is one of life's greatest transitions and can bring an unimaginable amount of joy, delight, wonder and love. It can coax the playful boy in you as well as the protective man, the trusty supporter and the feisty lover, the poet and the pioneering prince. As you share time with your children you will learn and grow through your interaction with them.

Men and a changing society

Social, medical and political changes over the last few generations have affected men in ways that have changed the face of fatherhood dramatically. At the same time, the 21st century is heralding a new willingness among men to talk about the way they feel and what they want out of life.

In many modern families men are drawn into the day-to-day aspects of family life, perhaps unlike their own fathers. Their participation in pregnancy and birth has also increased and it's the majority who see their child being born. This significant involvement in the early days has, in many cases, had a really positive effect: many men bond with their babies early on. Hands-on contact helps men to understand their babies and makes a close relationship more likely over the years.

While this sets the scene for a father and baby to have a more open and emotionally expressive relationship, it often brings confusion in another area. As the parenting roles begin to overlap, the traditional functions a man once held – most notably bringing in the money and imposing discipline – are no longer his alone. On a different but equally important note, physical exclusion is becoming more common as the numbers of separations increase and more fathers are separated from their growing children, apart from an occasional visit. Balancing the financial, social and emotional impact of these changes poses one of the major challenges of this century.

A father's value

In the 21st century, men are still asking the questions about their role and value that have been asked for generations. Is it strong for a man to cry? Can a man protect his wife and children? Can a man still enjoy football matches and nights out if he's a dad? If women talk about using sperm banks to get pregnant, has a father any value at all? As separation becomes more commonplace, do children need their fathers? The answer to all of these is 'yes'. A father brings an energy to parenting that is born of his personality and his masculinity, and children benefit from the balance between male and female parents as they grow. A father is the other half of the equation and babies can tell the difference between Mum and Dad.

Because of the prevalence of Freudian views, for many years 'parenting' meant 'mothering' and there were few studies on the importance of fathers. Most literature concerning babies focused on the needs of the mother and on the effect of mothering on the subsequent emotional development of the baby. Newer studies have shown that

---

I'm so worried for the baby's health, but at the same time I know I shouldn't be neurotic. What if the baby is deformed or has mental problems? What if the birth goes badly? There are so many tests available, should Chloë be having them all? Paranoia! And worst of all, I don't want to show these fears to her because I feel my responsibility is to provide support and stability. I don't want to freak her out because I imagine this will, in turn, freak the baby out.

You are not alone in having so many worries about your baby. Almost every father before you has had them – that's millions of men. It's only natural. As you look at your concerns, try tackling them from two angles: first find out about your baby, and second look into your feelings and how your own life experience may affect how easily you become anxious. Remember, too, that being a supporter is as important as being supported, and this goes for both of you: if you show your fears to Chloë she may reassure you that she and your baby are fine and offer you the best support you could wish for.

If voicing your concerns to Chloë isn't a good idea, try talking to someone who is a father. Your anxiety may be realistic if you or your family have had significant medical problems in the past. If you are feeling excessively anxious you may choose to see your GP or obstetrician for advice and help, or visit a complementary therapist whose treatment may help you to shift emotional blocks. No one can tell you that everything will definitely be all right, but if the antenatal visits and the tests are normal, it almost certainly will be. Go to a scan appointment and see your little baby kicking and punching in the womb.

Finally, if Chloë worries, her feelings will not harm your baby – women cannot turn off their emotions for 9 months, and babies in the womb feel a while range of emotions. Anxiety is just one of many.

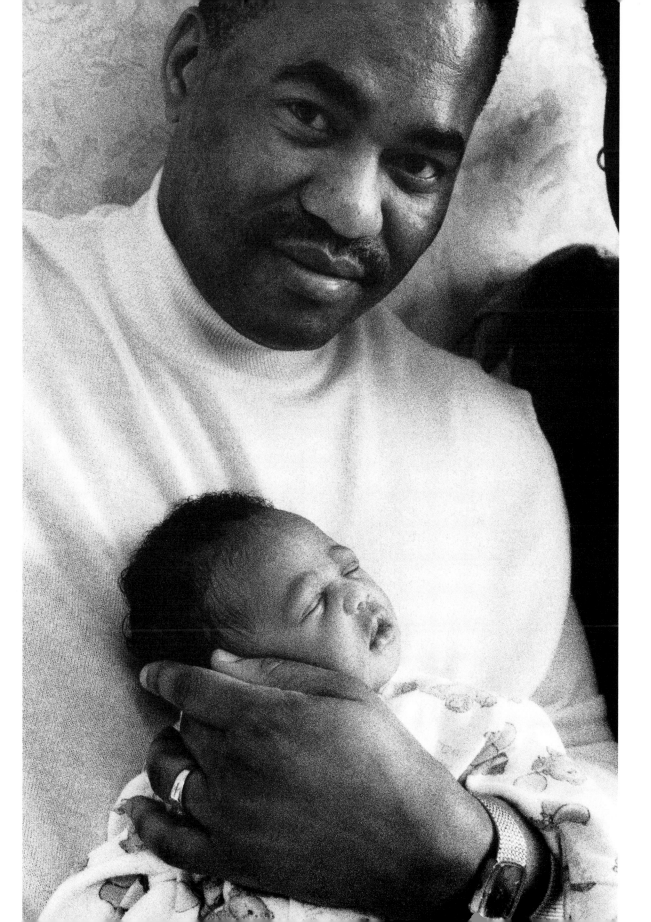

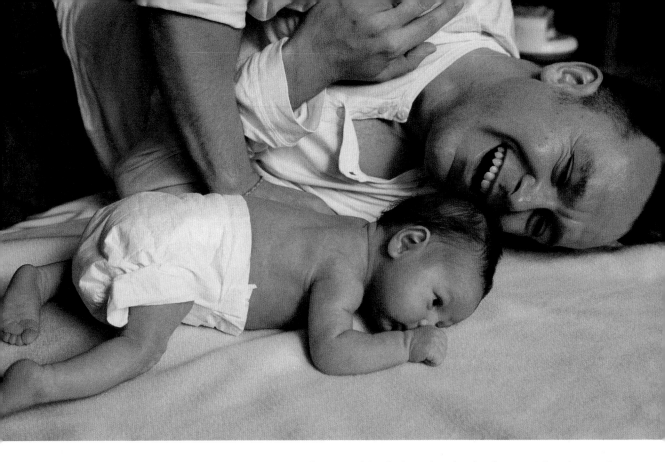

from the baby's and the child's point of view it is equally important to have a man in the home.

Many people of the current parenting generation – men and women alike – mourn the distance that frequently exists between them and their fathers. This in itself illustrates how important a close relationship is. Ask yourself what you think the value of a father is. It may help you to recognise the unconscious drive to copy your own father, and be there for your family on your own terms.

Pregnancy and birth

For 9 months, like your partner, you may hardly ever be able to get the pregnancy, your baby and the idea of the future out of your mind. You will not have the hormonal or physical changes but you'll have strong emotions and a string of questions about your own aspirations and your attitude. There is a section for you in each pregnancy trimester where you will also find tips on work, time management, emotions and health.

Tuning into your baby

Your baby can hear your voice from Week 15 of pregnancy and even at this early stage can accept you as part of his world. When your baby is bigger you will be able to feel him move if you place your hand on your partner's abdomen. Your baby will feel the pressure and this will soothe and stimulate him. Your baby also receives the effect of the 'feel-good' endorphin hormones he releases when he's happy. If you have fun regularly, by the time your baby is born he will already associate your voice, singing or playing with pleasant feelings.

Not all men find it easy to accept their baby, or bond with him, before the birth. In this they are not so different from women. You will not be alone in feeling excited, anxious and confused all at once. You may be able to connect with your baby during pregnancy or you may be the kind of person who needs to feel his baby in his arms before he can really believe it.

What you can do for yourself

Many men find it difficult to look at their own needs and desires, often because their energies are directed towards supporting their partner and their work. They may even be ambivalent about having a baby.

The most powerful way to prepare yourself for being a parent is to look after yourself. Caring for yourself entails caring for your physical health and for inner, emotional needs that influence every aspect of your life. You and your partner will be your baby's world and the whole family will benefit if you provide a strong foundation. If there are difficulties in your partnership, follow the advice on p.287 and aim to work through certain issues before birth.

If you are anxious about the birth and what comes after, do what you can to find out about labour and birth and talk to your doctor or midwife. If you learn about basic care or spend time with friends who have new babies, your confidence may be greater. Seeing things from a baby's viewpoint is fascinating and if you're confident, you are more likely to spend and enjoy time with your own baby.

Caring for your partner

Pregnancy hormones and a constantly changing body make most women feel emotional in pregnancy. You may be surprised to find that aspects of her personality that have previously been hidden surface at this sensitive time. Your partner, whether needy or fiercely independent, may value love and companionship, and simply being there can make her feel good. She may want your input to make decisions about antenatal testing, choices in labour and care after birth (for example, inoculations) and one of the best things you can do for her is to find out the facts about her pregnancy and the birth ahead. She'll also be touched if you can come to ultrasound scan appointments and share the excitement of seeing your baby on screen. If she is finding it difficult to accept motherhood, she will find things easier if you are by her side supporting her. It's quite common for women to get upset about other people always paying attention to the baby and she may love some focus on her.

Many couples really enjoy making love during pregnancy but if you find her changing body off-putting or if she feels out of touch with her libido, be there for her in other ways. Sex and intimacy are explored in each pregnancy trimester in the relevant chapters.

Finally, don't forget that the best way to care for your partner is to be yourself. If you continue to enjoy activities that fulfil you, you'll have positive energy to offer. Have fun, take a holiday together, do the overtime you need and, of course, reserve some loving and undisturbed time with your partner – this will be at a premium once there's another person in your family.

What you can do at the birth

The birth is the major event – the end of pregnancy and 9 months of waiting, and the beginning of a new life and a new relationship. Your physical involvement may be intense and hands on, or more relaxed; you might choose not to be present. During labour and birth your partner will benefit from your love, encouragement, patience and support. You will benefit from feeling relaxed and keeping up your own energy levels. Your role has been taken into account throughout Part II where you can find out about support in early and advanced labour, positions for birth, possible intervention, relaxation techniques, pain relief and the feelings that may arise in you when you see your partner in pain.

Once your baby has been born, you are there to welcome him with your familiar voice and a loving embrace, to look into his eyes and touch his soft skin. You may hold him for many minutes if your partner is tired or needs medical attention. From the moment the two of you meet, you mirror one another and begin a lasting relationship.

Settling into fatherhood

Some men feel that they are fathers before the birth, but most don't really feel the reality until they hold their baby in their arms. It's amazing how much you learn as you go along.

After birth, most couples feel the division into Mum and Dad. Often Mum does the bulk of the babycare, which includes regular feeding day and night. A father's role will include financial support, arranging visitors, cooking and domestic chores and general support. Some men are around all the time in the early days and become the primary carers, others make it home for bathtime and a goodnight kiss and only get chunks of time with their babies at weekends.

There is no 'right' situation. What matters most is not the quantity of time you spend but the quality – if your baby feels that you're connecting with him, his psychological health is bound to be better and the relationship between you will flourish. Think of the first few months as an introduction. You would get to know an adult through spending time with him or her, and the same

---

I desperately wanted a boy, and now I have a daughter. One part of me loves her like nothing else on earth and one side of me is disappointed. Might this affect our relationship?
Some men, some families and some cultures prefer their first child to be a boy, a son and heir and someone who will continue the family name. Many women wish for a girl. It may be that we identify with our respective sexes more easily, and before the arrival of the first baby many parents wonder how they might deal with seeing and cleaning the genitals of the opposite sex. Some worry about not understanding their child as they grow up, particularly in adolescence. Child sexual abuse is a spectre that hovers over us and may cause anxiety about experiencing uncomfortable feelings. It is actually quite natural to be embarrassed if your first child is a girl and you may at first feel strange changing her nappy or bathing with her and having skin-to-skin contact, particularly if you have not grown up with sisters. But after a few weeks the embarrassment subsides and you will accept your child for who she is rather than for what she is. If this does not happen and you still find it hard to come to terms with the sex of your baby, it will be interfering with your love for her and you may need support to explore your feelings.

applies to your new baby. In the first months the pace is slow as you get to know one another. This may be the easiest thing you have ever done, yet if you are ambivalent about being a father, it could take a long time to settle into your new role.

Bonding

Bonding is a term for love and acceptance that can begin in pregnancy but is often strongest after birth. In some families the father bonds faster than the mother, although it is usually easier for women; there is a natural hormonal mechanism to enhance the connection. There are a number of ways to encourage your feelings of bonding (p.302). Touch is a powerful and intimate communicator and spending time holding your baby, whether he's awake or asleep, can help you sense him and connect with him.

The early days

The first week of being a father could be compared to a whirlwind. Most men feel euphoric after the birth and float around on cloud nine even if they've been awake for 40 hours. Then the realisation dawns: this baby is for life. Along with him comes love and joy and limitless exciting possibilities – in addition come responsibility, restriction on personal freedom, sleepless nights and anxieties.

Learning how to satisfy a new baby is a huge challenge for both you and your partner, and days and

---

I love my wife and baby daughter dearly, but it feels as if they have a really close relationship and neither of them needs me anymore.

The 'mother cat with her kitten' instinct sometimes surfaces in a new mother. If your partner is like this, it may be hard for you to take an active part in babycare – she may not give you time to calm your crying baby, or she may not trust you to do things in the correct way.

Men also play roles. The 'upset little boy' sometimes emerges, and a man expects to be mothered by his partner, but feels shunned when there's a new baby. These jealous feelings often arise from the maze of childhood experiences.

The first months are for 'trying on' the roles of parents and juggling your family's needs. Your partner's hormones focus her on your baby. Try not to take this personally – nature has ensured that she concentrates on nourishing and protecting your baby. If you feel left out, instead of stepping back and feeling upset, step forward and see how you can make yourself part of the process. You will both be more relaxed when you trust one another with your baby and some couples take a few weeks to do this. If you can sit down and talk about the way you're feeling, you may more easily plan your time so that none of you feels left out (p.58).

nights may be turned inside out as you settle into a pattern. If you have the time to be with your family, you can snuggle up with them in bed and enter into the new-baby world where adult time is put on hold and the baby takes centre stage. Your baby will sleep between 16 and 20 hours in each 24-hour period. If he prefers to sleep in company, you can take turns to hold him. It can be magical to gaze into your own baby's face and watch his mouth twitching or his eyelids flickering as he dreams on your chest.

You won't regret it if you make time to enjoy these early days. They pass very quickly and set the scene for the relationship between you and your baby that continues for the rest of your lives. You might be surprised just how equal the parts are: you mirror your baby as he puckers his lips and stares at you, and he mirrors you. If you are anxious and restless, he may be unsettled, or his calming influence may relax you. You may be able to calm your baby when his mummy cannot. And don't forget that all parents – men and women – make many mistakes as they learn: many babies have survived perfectly after wearing a nappy back to front.

What your baby needs

Initially there is a never-ending round of feeding and changing and sleeping with virtually no distinction between day and night. You may help with all these areas, or your partner may take on the main caring role. Many babies actually have their nappies changed exclusively by their fathers in the early days because their mothers need to recover.

Aside from the practical aspects of care, your baby's main needs are to feel warm and fed and cuddled and to be surrounded by loving faces – he'll love to watch and interact with people. He'll know you; by the end of the first week he'll know your smell and will differentiate between the way you and his mother hold him.

Like every other newborn baby, yours will express himself and within days you may begin to get a sense of his personality – easy-going, extra demanding, cuddly, anxious, relaxed; and you may recognise different levels of cries. As your baby grows and becomes more physically interactive, he'll love to be stimulated and entertained. He'll begin smiling at around 6 or 8 weeks and by 12 weeks will be chuckling. Physical play is a great way to entertain him, and he'll always love watching your face. You'll find guidance on play and development in Part III.

You will benefit enormously from spending time with your baby, who has a lot to give and can lift your spirits. And the early days set a precedent for the future: the more you put in, the more you get back.

What your partner needs

Your partner needs to have someone to share her joy and love her precious baby. She also needs help so she can give her best to your new baby. She needs to sleep as much as she can between feeds, eat well and will experience intense mood swings. It can be very hard for a man to fulfil this supportive role, particularly if his partner cries a lot or if he feels excluded when all her attention is focused on the baby and on sleeping.

As the days become weeks you might be back at work and the tiredness of broken nights can build up. The first 3 months are often the toughest and you both need support and rest. You could help your partner to regain other areas of her life. This may involve making the space for her to exercise or arranging to have friends around and joining her and your baby on days out or evening visits.

One of the greatest demands on you will be to be patient and tolerant. Schedules are not always met if your baby needs a feed or a nappy change and your partner may seem distant and forgetful for months. You may also have the responsibility for the household. It can be tough to let her focus on mothering while you cope with everything else, but the balance will redress itself as time passes. Try to avoid being over-critical: err on the side of encouragement and praise, and voice any advice gently because she is likely to be very sensitive. Evenings may be difficult if your baby cries a lot and both of you are tired. It is a common upset among fathers that after a tiring day they look forward to coming home but their arrival coincides with their baby's crying time and their partner is fraught. You may discover that your partnership has 'flash points' that recur at similar times of day and it helps to anticipate the feeling of upset so you can be gentle with one another.

What you need

After the birth you need time to recover and time to meet, get to know and enjoy your new baby. Get as much help as you can, from friends and family or from a paid help if you can afford one. What you need is time to yourself as well as time with your family (p.51). Remember that time for yourself does not equal time at work, even when you find work extremely fulfilling. See if you can fit exercise into your week and, if you have a heavy work schedule, sleep in a room away from your partner and baby before busy days. You may also find it helpful to talk to other fathers who can empathise with your position. Many men feel isolated and having support prevents this.

When you feel upset or confronted, the advice in the chapter on partnership about communicating (p.290) may help you to avoid staying angry and blaming your partner or your colleagues for your mood. Try to keep love uppermost and take practical steps to alter problematic situations. After the birth you may be short of sleep and reducing your emotional stress will improve your energy.

Though it's hard to admit, you may resent the intrusion of your baby into your previously predictable life and feel jealous that your partner has been taken over.

A family man?
The experience of feeling present varies from family to family. Some men enjoy being hands on but others prefer to show their love by caring for organisation and finances. In one family, coming home at 8pm is considered late whereas in another it is fine. For a baby 1 hour is a long time, a day is a very long time and a year inconceivable, but for an adult, time frames are longer. Your family will define its own boundaries.

'Couvade' refers to the custom in some parts of the world whereby a father takes on the mother's physical or emotional symptoms. A man might gain weight, feel nauseous or injure himself around the time of birth, and after birth behave in a childish way. If you have identified intensely with the pregnancy you may have very strong opinions about birth and parenting. This works well if you and your partner are in agreement. If your views are different, it is essential to remember that it is your partner's labour and your baby's birth, and after birth your baby's personality and preferences need to be taken into account as your family becomes established.

I've no idea what it's like to be a father, or even if I'm ready. Do I have to change? Will I be forced into a life of nine-to-five and middle management? Will I have to sacrifice my personal dream of becoming a novelist?
This bundle of questions shows that you're anxious and need to make changes. You're not alone. You are thinking about who you are, what you have to give up, whether you need to fit a stereotype and how you can provide financially for your family. It's not easy.

Some of your questions will be answered over time as you see how life evolves, and some will disappear as you simply get on with it. In one sense you're in a position with little prospect of escape but in another sense it promises incredible opportunity for personal growth and happiness. Sometimes the most feared, unpredictable challenges in life teach us the most.

Middle management is only one among a vast range of choices; you may elect to take the risk of being an entrepreneur with greater responsibility and potentially greater rewards. If you feel your needs and aspirations are being dwarfed, there are many things you can do.

As you ask yourself whether you are ready to be a father, it might be helpful to forget about the practical aspects of fathering, and look at its essence instead. Are you ready to love and provide for your baby? As a father you may find that since your baby's arrival you have a stronger purpose in life, a new zest and a clearer sense of direction. You could relish bringing up your child, and will certainly learn a lot from him. Be yourself. Don't give up your dreams.

Some men also feel criticised by in-laws and many feel inadequate if their partner takes on all the babycare. These feelings are very common and normal. If you do feel upset or angry it may help to talk to someone – a trusted friend, a work colleague, or a midwife or your GP. You'll meet plenty of other men who feel as you do, and others whose brimming enthusiasm can be very infectious and healing. Many men simply need to have feelings acknowledged. Remember that many men also suffer from pre- and postnatal depression (p.462) and you may need help.

The later months

After the first 3 or 4 months have passed, things get easier. Your baby will begin to reach for things; he'll sit and then crawl, and soon will be standing up while he babbles. Play becomes more exciting as your baby gets more interactive. He will probably sleep for longer at night and your energy levels will rise. You'll also be more relaxed once you know that you do have the basic skills needed to be a father and you may feel freer to take time out and plan for the future.

The later months can be confusing for mothers who are going back to work. Sometimes this period is very stressful and your partnership needs a great deal of support. A lot of strains may be financial. The blues – for you and for your partner – often hit after 4 months and many people do not expect this.

I was keen on becoming a father during the pregnancy, but now my baby is here I feel differently. He seems to do nothing but cry, sleep and eat. It seems that there is nothing for me in a family. I'm not made to be a dad.

It can be very hard to admit that you are not feeling good about being a dad. Your feelings are common and it can help to share them. At some point it is important to let your partner know how you feel. She will see how you act and sense your unease, and the atmosphere could become very difficult if your thoughts aren't out in the open. She might be supportive and help practically so that you can spend time with your baby and get to know him.

As you think over this, ask: What is it that you don't like or are uncomfortable with? This could be a question that is a catalyst for action and change – use it together with the Wheel for Living (p.58) or for looking at a way out of your dissatisfaction (p.290).

Many partnerships break up within the first 5 years of having a baby (the figure in Britain is around 1 in 4) and in 90% of these the father becomes the absent parent. If you are not comfortable with your young baby, you may still have time with your partner and keep the flame alive. You may have a wonderful time with your baby later when he is a toddler or pre-schooler. These early days are just a tiny part of your baby's life and it is best to look at the bigger picture before stepping back.

When your baby settles into sleeping and eating patterns it might be a good time to take another look at the family boundaries. From around 6 months on, differences in family values concerning discipline frequently upset parents. If your own family was structured along paternal lines where your father's view ruled the roost, you may expect this to continue, although your partner may not agree. Differences, and bridging them, are discussed in Families (p.276).

Many men put work priorities on the back burner to start with. Once things settle down you may find more energy to review your work and ensure you are performing well. It may be easier now to leave work concerns at work, and home concerns at home, perhaps using the commuting time to make a separation so you can focus on each area as well as possible and avoid the flash points that often occur when you get home.

Your transition into fatherhood

Bowled over by the pride of having powerful sperm and, later, the amazement of holding your own baby in your arms, you may slip into fatherhood as if it's the best thing you've ever done. It can make you feel fulfilled, empowered, protective and full of hope. While these feelings can continue for months or years, your adaptation to fathering can be emotionally demanding. There may be a strong link between what you feel now and your early life, in particular what you felt towards your father.

Your self-esteem and your father

Becoming a father can send your self-esteem rocketing through the roof. Having a baby has been the catalyst for countless men to pursue long-held ambitions and mend ailing relationships, and is often one of life's most positive turning points.

There are some issues that apply more to men than to women. Self-esteem for many men is generated through achievement at work. Some struggle in the transition to parenthood because they have been taught to turn their caring energy away from their most intimate relationships and into work and altruistic endeavour.

When there is mutual respect and love, some men get tremendous joy and enthusiasm from their relationship with their own fathers. Moving into parenthood can reinforce this. For others, however, the gap between generations may result in a gap of understanding, or a confusion about how best to act. It is common to unconsciously act like your father, reflecting characteristics that you like and some you do not. It may be helpful to remember that you live in a difficult time, a different political and financial world, have different friends and unique dreams and ambitions.

If you do not want to be like your father (and around 1 in 3 men do not), you may feel driven to do better than he did. If you feel self-doubt or inner criticism, this may stem from a subconscious search for your father's approval, even when you accept that different values are normal. Your new role as a father is in the context of you, your partner and your baby. You may consider talking openly and listening actively (p.290) to your father to find out how he feels and you may discover that he admires you for being the person that you are, and living life in the way you have chosen.

Some men feel very distanced from pregnancy and mothering and keep themselves away from home and family. Some fear that being a father distracts from a successful career. Yet studies have shown that there is no conflict between career achievement and fatherhood: men who spend time with their families and have good relationships with their children perform better as managers, community leaders and role models, and usually have more fulfilling marriages. Often difficulty in feeling close reflects experience in childhood and it may take intense commitment on your part to alter old patterns. There are possibilities for creating regular quality family time when you communicate well with your partner and you have support.

Fathers who are primary carers

Most commonly, men who stay at home feel a conflict between their hunter-gathering and caring sides. It is unusual for men to have been brought up by their fathers, and the idea of being the main carer, which involves keeping up with washing, cleaning, ironing and cooking, can seem foreign and demeaning. Some men who stay at home love this side of life and get a kick from supporting their successful partner. It's just as common, though, for them to get frustrated with day-to-day drudgery and to feel resentful.

As a primary carer it is important to arrange your days and weeks so there are activities to get you and your baby out of the house. You may take on a part-time job. Even if you don't mix work with childcare, it is vital that you make time to do things for yourself as well as with your partner. The reversal of roles that sees Mum earning and out of the house for hours or days at a time suits some couples well although sometimes it may bring conflict. It is reasonable for each of you to have time for yourself outside of work or childcare. The way you do this will reflect your family structure.

Although your partner has fewer hours with her baby, she may find it hard to step back from a position of 'knowing best' – the maternal instinct is very strong. If your partner offers her view when you feel it's inappropriate, or even criticises the way you care for your baby, it is important to make time to talk. Both of you will have strong feelings about these matters and it is helpful to share these.

Your partnership

The months of pregnancy that lead up to the birth of your baby can be a warm, nurturing time for you as a couple, particularly if you spend regular, quality time together. Yet you will find conflict as well as support in your relationship as parents. The chapter on Partnership (p.285) examines this closely, touching on issues of communication, sex, intimacy, upsets and breakdown.

In the early days of parenting, which are recognised as among life's more stressful times, sometimes a man finds comfort and closeness in another relationship, in part because he can feel comforted and listened to without the distraction of a baby. Communicating with your partner is the best way to prevent this occurring. By making her aware of your needs and being aware of hers you can take an active role in the family, and rekindle the flame of romance if it has died down. Expectations need to be discussed, tried and established; couples who do this often find that disagreements can be reduced.

Depression and conflict

Antenatal and postnatal depression in men are not formally recognised as medical conditions. Parenting, however, can bring men down, and depression, whether or not it reaches the clinical stage, is common (p.462). Reasons are various: some men have too many work commitments, some feel excluded, some feel angry and find responsibility overwhelming. It can be difficult to imagine that the short months of baby-centred life will pass very soon.

If you feel down and the feeling continues, turn to p.459. Seek support, whether it is from your partner, your best friend, your father or a counsellor. Feeling low is not a crime, yet men are much more reluctant than women to reach out and confide in others. Depression has negative effects on the whole family and for some men feelings of upset or anger are turned outwards through violence. If you have feelings of rage that are difficult to control, it is best to seek help or professional counselling in resolving the underlying conflict so that you can feel more at peace and avoid harming your family. To prevent the problem spiralling out of control, the ideal is to seek support as soon as signs appear.

Growing up, moving on

When you become a father it can feel as if you've crossed a bridge. You know, and feel, a lot of things you never did before. At the same time, you are probably feeling a slight panic as you look back at the place you left behind. Some old friendships will fall by the wayside but others persist and flourish. You will also find you make new long-term friendships through the network that springs up around your child. As your baby passes out of his primal period at 9 months, you too will complete a rite of passage. The lessons you have learnt will arm you for the years ahead.

Emotions and feelings

Being a parent is a true adventure. As you sail through smooth times, you'll feel as if you're floating down a river on a warm sunny day, unable to wipe the smile from your face. And as you struggle through harder times, it's as if you're climbing a mountain, physically and emotionally exhausted, yet you find relief and reward at the top.

What's happening to your life?

When you become a parent, you can expect your outlook on life and your priorities to alter. For both parents it's perfectly normal to find that rational activity diminishes and emotive thoughts predominate, and you may find that you feel more closely in touch with your emotions. After the birth, emotions often intensify and even become overwhelming but this intensity usually softens as the months pass.

When emotional pressure or confusion arises, it can be exhausting and may have knock-on effects. It is reassuring to know that psychologists classify pregnancy, giving up work, financial pressures and moving house as among the most stressful life events. Two or more of these are likely to occur around the time your baby is born. As part of your preparation for parenthood, you may want to talk to your partner and close friends about the strains that await you. As a human, you can't help how you feel, but you can attempt to put things into perspective and take control of choices and decisions – this challenge becomes more pressing, and more exciting, as the next generation arrives and waits to be guided.

Over the 18-month period from conception until your baby crawls, parts of your emotional view of life will change for ever. Being aware of these changes as they occur is the most positive step that you can take towards getting pleasure out of your family life, and it will help you to offer your baby a loving environment in which to grow.

Gains and losses

Parenthood brings many gems and it also entails changes. The balance between gains and losses shifts from day to day. Some of the wonderful gains include watching your baby smile, hearing her laugh, feeding and cuddling her, loving and feeling her love, and other relationships may blossom as if infected by this new life. But some days or weeks are difficult, and apart from your baby other areas of life can present challenges.

During pregnancy the presence of a baby in the womb can make a woman feel loved and cared for, complete and happy. After the birth, despite all the love and hope the new baby brings, it is common to sense loss. This loss is related to you; you and your baby were one and you may feel that an integral part of yourself has gone. You may feel both physically and emotionally empty and the hormonal changes following the birth enhance this perception.

Men often feel loss as well, particularly those who enjoy sharing and feeling mothered by their partner and have to give this up when their baby needs so much attention. This feeling of personal loss could be vocalised simply as 'I've lost part of me' and you may be surprised at the intensity of your feelings. The feelings of grief and sadness pass with time but, while they are there, the person may show them by being irritable or upset and difficult to get on with. Anger is a common way to show loss and it is part of accepting the situation for what it is and moving on. Emotionally it can be confusing to have the gift of a new baby as well as feeling that you have lost something important. You may also feel guilty about feeling upset when you 'should' be happy.

Lost independence

It is common for women and men to be taken aback by the level of commitment that being a parent demands. As you take on your responsibility you will sacrifice the independence you had. Parents who find this easy often create a social support network and are energetic and keen to make new opportunities. For those who mourn lost independence, being a parent gets in the way of living a rich and fulfilling life. As you would expect, most parents alternate between these two stereotypes.

What do you feel?

Many books, and certainly most people, talk about the positive emotions connected with being pregnant and becoming a parent – pride, love, fulfilment, bliss, contentment, harmony. But in reality these are only part of the picture: while positive feelings exist they are rarely exclusive. Upsetting emotions are part of the deal.

It is often extremely hard to look some of your more painful feelings in the face. Some are more unsettling than others: one may linger for decades, another may be resolved in minutes. As an initial step it is helpful to be honest with yourself about how you are feeling, and let your baby know. The tendency to smile and say everything is OK when it is not sends a strong message to your child

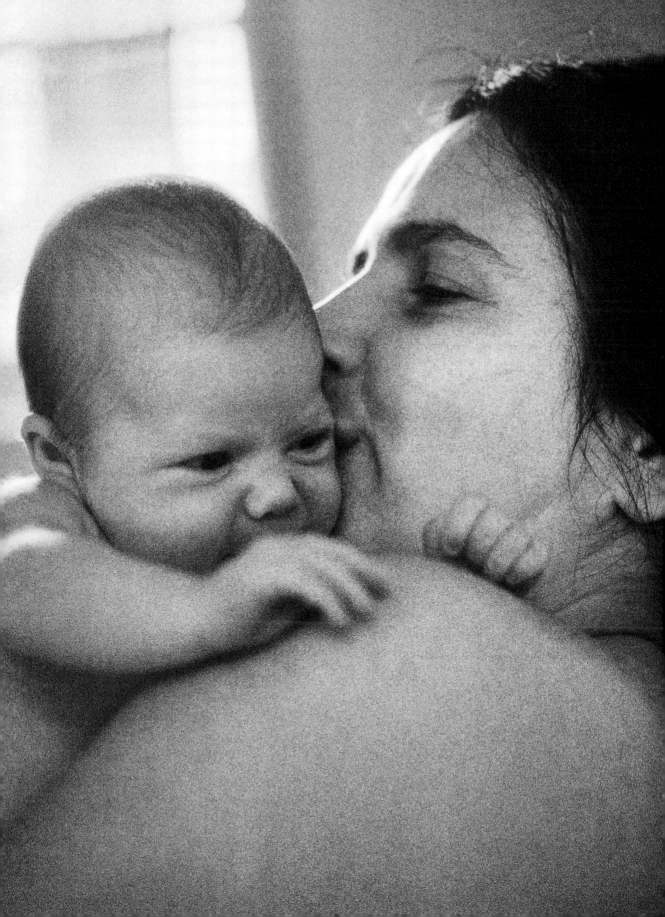

that it is wrong to feel unhappy: there is nothing wrong with feeling unhappy, which is quite simply a part of life. You could tell your baby, 'I am feeling really angry right now, and I still love you,' and then let your anger out elsewhere. You can start doing this before birth; when you are upset, try telling your baby that it is not about her, it is not her fault and you love her. Admitting emotional feelings and identifying what they are related to is a very positive way of living.

Negative emotions may not be more common than the positive but may be more difficult to deal with, and they may become more problematic when they are denied. In almost every case, a difficult emotion arises because of something that is happening in the present but has roots in the past. Recognising the link is often the first step towards finding an alternative way to approach a situation. You may find it difficult as you experience negative emotions or discover parts of yourself that you do not like. It is tempting to want to throw these away. But because they will always be a part of you, the challenge is to live with them and get to know them, in the hope they won't get you down so often.

Being loved

A common concern that many parents have is whether their baby likes them, particularly when there is a lot of crying, or when she is older and asserts her desire to be independent. You don't need to do anything special to make your baby love you – she has a basic drive to be emotionally attached to you from before the birth, and will love and trust you for who you are. Her demands are intense and ongoing – she needs love, food, warmth and touch – and the rewards she gives are huge. As she grows, the physical distance between you may increase but her eagerness to explore life reflects the background of love and trust you have shown her.

Bonding

Many men and women find the deep love for their babies among life's most rewarding experiences. Every adult has an inherent reflex to connect with babies; this is part of your natural urge to protect. And while you may smile at someone else's baby, when you hold your own this protective instinct is many, many times stronger and is coloured by a love unlike any you have felt before.

Bonding seems to imply that you and your baby become gelled by an unmovable love and commitment. Rather, it is about how quickly or deeply you fall in love and how this love flows. It defines your reaction to a new life stage, your degree of confidence or fear and all your feelings about your baby. It is also affected by instincts that have been moulded by your life experience.

There is a wide variation in how mothers and fathers 'bond' with their baby. Some do so from conception or before it, some at birth. Some parents feel distanced from the experience of birth (especially if it was difficult) and from their baby for some days or weeks following labour. A tiny proportion of parents are unable to welcome and bond with their child. Falling in love after birth is not only down to you – your baby has her own character and expressions and her feelings affect how you feel. The mothers and fathers who bond quickly are often those who have created the time and space to welcome and focus on their babies.

Your self-esteem

Your own self-esteem arises from your 'inner child' and reflects your life experiences. It is coloured by the way you have been praised, encouraged and reprimanded in your life. If you have been shown love and respect and urged to believe in yourself, you will probably have a high level of self-esteem. If you have not been commended for your achievements, or you have felt disrespected or abused, it will be low.

My baby is now 2 weeks old and I don't feel as if I've bonded. I thought it would happen automatically but I don't feel the magic. What's happening?
What you are feeling is not uncommon. You may be recovering physically from the birth and having a baby can be a huge shock. You may find it hard to connect with your baby until you see some smiles and feel some feedback for all the effort you are putting in. Your baby's 'language' is easier to read as the weeks pass.

If you still feel unconnected with your baby in a few weeks' time, you might find some or all of the following advice helpful.
• Try to make quality time for you and your baby and tune into her special ways of communicating. It may help if someone takes over babycare for part of the day.
• How are you and your partner (if you are together) adapting to being a family? If your partnership feels neglected or intruded upon you might have problems accepting and loving your baby.
• You might find bonding difficult because of something that happened in your own childhood, perhaps if you felt your parents or carers were distant or aggressive.
• Some parents find it difficult to bond because they lose sight of their own identity. If you feel out of touch with yourself, make time just for you (p.51). It is tough in the early days of sleep deprivation but you can start off gradually and build up.
• There are a number of parent and baby groups or clinics that provide good environments for discussing difficulties such as yours. You might be surprised how easy you find it to open up when you meet other parents who share your feelings.

Wherever you start from, your self-esteem may soar and plummet during the primal period. So many things affect it – love, smiles, laughter, tiredness, pain, a crying baby, irregular meals, a restricted social life or feelings of exclusion are just some factors. And self-esteem can fall away without familiar props such as work. Being a parent is a new role and a great challenge. You are everything to your baby and may never be valued by anyone as much as you are by your own children.

It can be difficult to imagine that there will be time to put balance back into your life and enjoy non-baby activities. There are tips on making this possible with the Wheel for Living (p.58). Many parents feel a drop in self-esteem; for some it returns after a few weeks, for some it takes a few months, and others don't feel they have it back completely until their children are at school.

Being jealous

Jealousy is a common human emotion shared by many fathers who so often feel excluded in the early days of family life and it also affects a number of women. Some people are more prone to it than others. You may be jealous of the relationship your partner has with your baby, or jealous of the freedom that others have, or of other people's relationships or financial circumstances. Jealousy often goes hand-in-hand with low self-confidence or can be compounded if you feel undeserving because of your own family background. Having a baby opens the doors to a new and powerful love whose underlying power is acceptance.

The best way to reduce jealousy is to make time for you to be with your baby and, when the early days of intensive babycare have passed, to aim for time when you and your partner can be alone together. If you share your feelings with your partner, your love may flourish. It is often healing to talk to your parents and siblings about how they felt when you were a child and you may identify some feelings that have been with you for many years. When you hold your baby and feel good, you may be able to let go of being jealous. The focused love for your baby is enriching, and you could apply this feeling of plenty to your other relationships. Remember that you can also direct love to yourself.

The blues

For many parents having a baby is the most wonderful thing in the world, but it is true that most go through at least some periods when life isn't so rosy. Positive feelings may be mixed with, or even overwhelmed by, anger, guilt, frustration and unhappiness. This is quite natural. Sadness marks the end of one life stage (independence/childhood) and the beginning of another (parenthood). Though natural, being sad is not always accepted – a whole industry exists to try to stop or hide it with anti-depression pills and a range of distractions. Yet feeling down is often a trigger for tackling personal issues and you may find that once you have passed through the blues you continue with renewed strength and enthusiasm.

The blues in pregnancy

Pregnancy, and thoughts of the future, can be very daunting, and getting the blues before birth is common. Antenatal depression is becoming more widely recognised and recent studies have shown that it is almost as common for women to feel depressed in the last trimester of pregnancy as it is after the birth. Women have to deal with a changing body, hormonal fluctuations, tiredness, apprehension about labour and thoughts of the future while getting on with everyday life. Men can also be overwhelmed – watching the baby grow, accommodating

I am 7 months pregnant and I'm hardly interested in my job – most of my attention is focused on my baby, the birth and the future. In fact, I feel like a bit of an airhead when other people start talking about politics or even prices of food. It's as if nothing matters but my baby, and my brain automatically switches off. Is this normal?
Retreating into yourself and focusing on your baby are entirely natural at this time. Hormonal influences definitely contribute to the feelings but men also have similar experiences.

According to the Taoist tradition, everybody has both yin ('dark') and yang ('bright') aspects to their personality and the balance between them may change from hour to hour. Yin is feminine and maternal, creative, dark, emotional and instinctive. Its energy is said to fluctuate, much like the phases of the moon. Yang is masculine and paternal, light, steadfast and rational, protective and supportive. Its energy is likened to the sun's.

Almost all women feel that during pregnancy their instinctive, feminine (yin) energy has more influence and the rational male (yang) energy recedes. Rational decision-making, memory and mathematical ability diminish and motherly feelings predominate. Sometimes the yang aspect remains uppermost and there may be conflict between work and mothering. Men often experience the emergence of their yin during the primal period, and some relish this as emotions surface and love emerges.

Another influence attributed to yin is a resurfacing of childhood memories and experiences stored in the unconscious mind. The yang influence is believed to balance this by giving a logical context for dreams and emotions and making it possible to apply these to new situations such as birth and parenthood. If you embrace the mothering – or fathering – instinct, you will nurture yourself and your baby. The Taoists see this as flowing with, rather than against, the stream of nature.

mood swings or tiredness, fearing what the birth may bring for mother and baby, worrying about money or about the health of the growing baby. In addition, both partners may be upset about losing independence. Becoming the focus of medical attention and being asked how you feel and what your plans are can bring pressure to perform. For some expectant parents this triggers anxieties that have lain deep beneath the surface for many years.

Dealing with sadness and anxiety during pregnancy can be healing and can clear away the blues in time for the birth, however. Often, coming to terms with difficulties in pregnancy can prevent postnatal depression, which is a very real problem and affects roughly 15% of women. The advice given on p.459 for dealing with 'blue' feelings applies in pregnancy and beyond.

Feeling down after your baby is born

Almost every mother feels down at some point. The 'third-day blues' with weepiness may occur on any day and are very common after birth. They usually pass. It's also common to feel down if you are tired or feel isolated, and the first months with a baby may be interspersed with low periods. For some women, however, unhappiness may persist for many weeks or begin 2, 3 or even 6 months after birth when the enormity of change and the reality of life with a small baby really hit home. Most get over it, but some, often those who lack support, do develop postnatal depression (p.462).

Fathers can be as ecstatic and euphoric as mothers when their baby is born, and can also feel a slump or let-down a few days, weeks or months later. There is an incredible build-up of tension in the run-up to birth, and men use a lot of energy tuning into their partner, supporting her, fitting work in and just keeping going in the face of such anticipation.

A feeling of anticlimax can bring confusion or even guilt, and many men feel abandoned or excluded: having cared so closely for their partners they feel unsure of how to help with babycare. Ways of avoiding some of the more common pitfalls of fatherhood are explored on p.292. Things don't always get easier quickly, particularly if work commitments are intense and sleep is broken. Feeling down can lead to a vicious cycle where self-esteem falls, exercise is neglected, and the outlook seems cloudy – in short, depression sets in.

I didn't plan to get pregnant and I'm finding it really hard. I hate to admit it – in fact, it makes me feel really guilty – but I often resent my baby. How can I get out of these uncomfortable feelings?

If you chat with other mothers you will find that they sometimes resent their own situation; knowing that what you're going through is normal may reduce your guilt. Some adults who easily feel guilty were brought up where guilt and blame were part of the family culture. Guilt is often associated with not doing something you feel you should do. 'Should' is the key word and it usually arises from your expectation of how you or someone else 'should' behave.

Acknowledging resentment or a feeling that you are trapped or controlled by outside forces is a positive thing – perhaps a good goal is not to get rid of your uncomfortable feelings but to notice them and then take steps to improve the situation.

It's also good to remember that quality time with your baby is more beneficial for both of you than the actual number of hours. Forcing yourself to spend time with your baby when you resent doing so is counter-productive; the message will be negative to your baby who is acutely sensitive to your energy levels and emotion, and your resentment will affect the whole family. You may find it helpful to talk to people you trust and create time for you away from babycare, perhaps with the use of the Wheel for Living (p.58). You might choose to use this time to work through your feelings, or to do something completely different so that you feel you have had a break.

Can you be the perfect parent?

The desire to give your baby the best is universal and every parent goes about this in a different way. It is commendable to aim for high standards but it is important to remember that there is no such thing as a perfect parent – just as there is no such thing as a perfect baby. Parenting, like anything else you do in life, is a task that cannot be mastered in an instant: you bring your talents, instincts and skills and in some areas you may benefit from support and guidance, learning as you go along.

Remember that there is no 'right' or 'wrong' way to parent – no rules are written in stone and different cultures around the world have different ways of doing things. Below are a few guidelines that may help you to offer your baby the best you can in the context of your own particular lifestyle, without imposing rigid or restricting goals on your family.

- Love is the key. Let your baby feel loved, wanted, welcomed and adored for who she is rather than what she does. This is infinitely more important than whether your routine is rigid or flexible. Babies love to feel 'held' emotionally and physically.
- You will develop a partnership with your baby that lasts for life, and if you listen and adapt to her needs and encourage her to adapt to yours, the relationship will be more powerful and comfortable. She has an inherent drive to communicate and rely on you. You will learn her language and fine-tune your senses to both her obvious and her more subtle signals. She will appreciate being loved for who she is rather than for how she behaves.

- Getting it right as often as possible is most definitely good enough. You will learn from your successes and your mistakes and so will your baby. You are both on a learning curve. Let yourself have ups and downs, do well and not so well, and give your baby space to have good and bad times, be quiet and noisy and have happy and sad moments.
- Conflict between your values around parenting and those of your partner, family or peer group may upset or discourage you. See if you can acknowledge areas where opinions differ as the first step. Actively listening to each other (p.290) is a good way to start. The concept of dynamic boundaries allows all of you to adapt as life ebbs and flows.
- Many parents feel torn between the needs of their baby and other aspects of their lives. You may need or want to return to work very soon, which brings an inevitable conflict along with feelings of guilt about your child spending time with a carer, or sadness at missing the first smile, first step or first word. In reality, being a parent encompasses caring for your baby and caring for yourself, and both areas need attention. Consciously weighing up the gains and losses of a decision that you need to make may help you feel satisfied with the final choice. Once you have arrived at a decision, be honest with your baby; even if she cannot understand your

words, she will sense the feelings you express, and you may feel relieved about being open.

What do you expect of yourself?

Expectations will unquestionably reflect your own understanding of 'achievement' and 'failure' and this has an effect on how well you think you're doing as a parent. Sometimes your expectations are appropriate and offer helpful guidelines, but at other times they are a product of your background and family influence, and do not actually suit you or your baby.

You can get an idea of what your expectations are by completing the following sentences. You could apply them to a topic that is playing on your mind at the moment. It is also useful to look at the expectations you have of your partner and, indeed, of your own parents.
- A good mother never . . .
- A good father never . . .
- My mother would . . .
- Fathers nowadays . . .
- Mothers I admire do . . .
- My father thought that fathers ought to . . .
- My generation believe that a baby is . . .
- I believe that . . .

As you fill in the answers, the emerging picture contains the view you have inherited from your family (not necessarily only your parents, but possibly grandparents and siblings, too) as well as what your heart tells you. In some instances the two may be the same, and in others there may be opposition. You may doubt your heart if your inner critic is loud – an internal voice that says, 'I am not good enough, they will not approve.' This little voice has been with you for many years and, while it has a positive role to remind you of certain principles, it may interfere with your happiness.

What do you expect of your baby?

Do you have thoughts such as, 'Babies should sleep through the night from 6 weeks,' or, 'Babies should have at least one tooth by the age of 5 months'? How many times do you find yourself saying or thinking in terms of, 'Babies do', 'Babies should', 'They always do'? Try turning the words around: 'My baby does x, y and z and that is fine even though my sister's baby does a, b and c,' or 'This is the way my baby behaves in this situation.' Try to hold on to the knowledge that every baby behaves differently, and that when a baby is young the perceived need to be first belongs only to the parent.

Children can tell from a very young age if they meet, surpass or fall short of their parents' expectations by the encouragement they receive and the energy of pride or disappointment conveyed in tone of voice and body language. You may know that this is true from your own

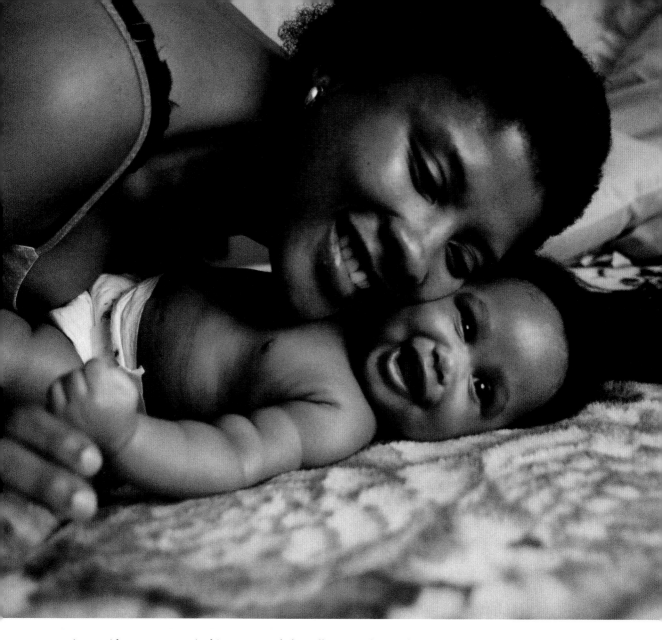

experience with your parents. At this stage your baby will feel good if she knows that she is loved for who she is and not what she does and this includes crying as well as smiling, demands for cuddles as well as sociability, anger as well as joy. If you find it difficult to relate in this way to your baby who is not yet talking, remember that she understands an incredible amount before she utters her first words and the first 9 months are among the most emotionally formative of her life.

Your baby does not think like a mini adult and often when you think you know how she is feeling the truth is quite different. You know how you would feel or react, and simply assume the same will be true for her. Over time it will be easier to distinguish between your separate feelings. You will find it easier to relate to your baby if you can let go of preconceived ideas and expectations and live with her in what is naturally happening from day to day and week to week.

Loving and learning

Your baby, and the relationship between you, will always contribute to your general sense of wellbeing. Sometimes she will be the cause of difficult emotions, sometimes she will be your healer as she replaces sorrow with joy, and sometimes she will be a valued listener as you pour your heart out. You, your baby, your partnership and your family continually affect one another. Perhaps the most important lesson your baby will teach you is how to love freely and accept people for who they are, and enjoy being loved and accepted in return.

Parenting alone

When one parent has responsibility, some things will be harder to cope with and some things will be easier. Being alone inevitably demands a different approach to family arrangements. This chapter is not a 'how to do it' guide, but, combined with the information given in the rest of the book, aims to encourage those who parent alone to enjoy their family. As the 21st century began, there were three times as many single parents as in 1970. Today many children are, at some stage, cared for by one parent and 'lone parenting' is seen as part of the life cycle of a family. Nine out of ten single parents are women.

Being a single parent

Some women choose to parent alone, some become single mothers because of a break-up during pregnancy and some split up from their partner after the birth. In fewer cases a father is left with the main responsibility of rearing a baby. And for some men and women being a single parent is not a choice but follows the tragic death of one partner.

Stigma

In western society today there appears to be increasing freedom to pick and choose how to live, yet there is also a complex array of moral judgements. For single parents the pressure of being judged is often intense. Parenting alone is frequently regarded with suspicion, as if someone somewhere along the line has done something wrong, renounced responsibility, or is otherwise regarded with pity or as unable to be a 'good' parent if he or she leaves. These assumptions are widely held, even by health professionals. Without realising it, people can act inappropriately. This is much more likely where the single parent is a man.

Two parents who are in a stable relationship can offer each other support and give their baby a stimulating and secure environment; two parents who have a volatile relationship, however, may create an unstable environment. There is also a common experience where one parent (usually the father) works such long hours that the mother is effectively left to parent alone. Single parenting is not necessarily more difficult, or even that different, from what some people consider to be the norm, yet in many circles it carries a stigma. Families have many permutations – mixed couples, lesbian couples, primary carers (both male and female) and single parents. All have a unique set of difficulties and advantages and none fit into a prescriptive way of living.

How much reproach you encounter as a single parent will depend on your circumstances, where you live, the culture you live in, and the personal experiences of friends and family. You may find that you are particularly vulnerable to social criticism about financial independence. This can hurt when you know that you are doing the best

you can and giving the best you know how to give to your baby; it's also saddening to think that people can be so quick to disapprove and don't see all that you have achieved. Yet it is heartening to know that you are one of many in a similar situation and there is plenty of support available in your community.

Pregnancy and birth without a partner

Pregnancy is an emotive time when love and support are both invaluable. If you are living alone you will appreciate a group of friends or family with whom you can share your excitement and joy. Some mothers whose relationship has broken up need additional emotional support. If you can, make new connections and friendships, which will be valuable after the birth, particularly with people who live locally. You could get advice and contacts from your midwife or health visitor and follow the general advice for caring for yourself throughout pregnancy given earlier in this book (p.51). You might need to make some difficult decisions, perhaps about where to live, and seeing these through as far as possible in pregnancy will help you to settle in to parenting.

Being with your new baby

All new mothers, whether with or without a partner, have to absorb a huge amount of information and are flooded with emotions. Life with a new baby is magical, but can be tough. You may feel strong, proud and happy, and blessed by the wonderful baby in your life. You might also feel overwhelmed or very alone as you deal with all your new feelings and challenges without the company of your baby's father. You may be able to draw a lot of strength from your own tiny bundle, but you will find practical support invaluable so that you can find your feet as a parent and care for yourself and your baby in the best possible way.

Support from your community

With the sole responsibility for one or more children, staying healthy and financially afloat, nurturing self-esteem and making crucial parenting choices may be the most challenging things you will ever do. Without a live-in partner, even one who is only around at the end of the day or weekends, there is no one to offload problems on to, to help you soothe your baby at night or give you time for yourself. It may be hard to keep up the enthusiasm but being alone usually stimulates action.

A common experience for many single parents is the lack of a community and the sense of isolation. If you have separated from your partner and encountered disapproval or ostracism from your parents or in-laws, loneliness may be intense. You may feel deep inside some sense of failure if you think that your parents and friends disapprove of your relationship not working out, even if you feel better off without your partner.

You need as much care and attention as your baby does. It is often most difficult to reach out for support when you feel low, and if your situation follows a painful breakdown in family relationships, you will need to look outside your family. It will take time to nurse your feelings and rebuild a network of friends and supporters.

Every process begins with a small step. Your health visitor or GP will have valuable experience from helping many other parents in your situation, and will be able to offer a listening ear and practical advice and contacts. There are many options for single parents, which include help in the home, crèches and groups where you can take your baby and meet other parents. It can take courage to make use of these resources, and it may take time to re-establish your confidence if your self-esteem has taken a knock. If you feel a lack of confidence, you might find it useful to refer to the Wheel for Living (p.58) to learn about turning problems into possibilities.

Time

A lot of stress can be avoided if arrangements and schedules are regular and reliable, and this will also create the space for quality time, both for yourself and for your baby. Although you will have personal preferences, boundaries that define sleeping and eating (p.276) will help you have time to yourself as well as time with your baby. With a structure you will find it easier to delegate by letting those who share your childcare know about the boundaries your baby is used to. One of the hardest jobs is maintaining consistency and balancing the time that your child spends with you, with the other parent and with other carers.

Support from the 'absent' parent

Many separations can be bitter and sad affairs resulting in temporary and sometimes permanent loss of communication between parents and, more tragically, between the child and a parent. If you are still in touch with the other parent (whether your relationship is close or distant), you will be able to share some emotional responsibility for your child. Whatever your arrangement,

you are linked in a unique way. In the long term, you could find that communication between you is more important than financial support.

If you have recently separated from your partner, you may experience the extremely common scenario where feelings of anger, abandonment and loss are played out between the two of you. In the process of separation parents often blame one another for what has happened. Actively listening and acknowledging one another's point of view are particularly valuable and may reduce the time you spend in conflict. These are covered along with upsets, honest communication and separation in the Partnership chapter (p.285).

If you can reach an agreement for your ex-partner and child to have regular time together this will help them foster a close and healthy relationship. You may struggle to agree on this and, like many people going through the separation, could benefit from the objective support offered by professional mediation. Where an amicable arrangement is reached, you may share joy in your child's development and support one another when your child goes through difficult periods.

Some mums or dads do not have contact with the other parent, whether this is through choice, death or traumatic separation. Around a third of lone parents experience violence in their relationship, and are concerned about their child having contact with the other parent. There are support groups offering help and encouragement. When the second parent is completely absent, the balance may be redressed by forming strong relationships with others who take an active interest in your child's life. Babies are quick to place trust in loving carers and are experts at striking up friendships, but they also notice if familiar people disappear from their lives.

As a single parent you are faced with the challenge of continuing to live your own life and form your own close relationships, and remaining honest and consistent for your baby, who may show jealousy when he feels your

I am the third generation in my family who has had a baby as a single parent. I am very well supported by my mother and grandmother and we have a close and warm relationship and live near one another. What shall I do to help my baby?
It is best to encourage the close relationship, support and consistency from your family and friends, and the work you put in to maintaining your relationships will bring benefits for both you and your baby. If you have the support of your mother and grandmother, you may draw some useful lessons from their experiences as single mothers. If your baby's father is around it may be good to encourage him to retain a relationship with your baby. The main thing is for your baby to feel loved and wanted by the people around him.

energy directed towards someone else. It will help to communicate clearly with your baby, and even if he is very young he will feel you are committed to him. This is good preparation if you then welcome a new partner into your life, whether or not he or she stays indefinitely.

How might your baby feel?

When two adults are around regularly, working as a team, a baby feels two different energies and quickly learns to distinguish between them, and to act differently with them. Being on your own with your baby can put extra pressure on your relationship, particularly if you need relief and have none immediately to hand. Your child may be more frequently exposed to all your moods if there is no one to bail you out at short notice. Yet exposure to a wide range of human emotions contributes to a child's healthy development. Even from an early age your baby can learn that it is normal for all people to be quiet or sad, irritable or tired, as well as to be happy, and to accept his own and others' mood swings.

A baby or small child can't know, in the same sense that an adult knows, what is happening if the relationship between his parents is breaking down. But a tiny baby can sense tension and feel loss. If you have separated after the birth, your baby may be confused or upset, and his automatic reaction will be to look to you for love, honesty and support. He will feel more secure when you set clear boundaries, giving him a sense of containment within which he can express his feelings.

When you are going through your own grief or anger it will be hard to remain consistent for your baby, and you will both benefit from support and time out from one another. When you are with him, let him know you are upset but emphasise that you love him and it is not his fault. He will sense your meaning. When he expresses distress or anger it may be heartbreaking for you, but his feelings may not be related to your break-up. Because he is so young, however, he will flit between emotions much more rapidly than you do and may quickly change and show excitement, happiness and joy. Your baby's zest for life may spur you on.

Finances and work

Balancing finances may be particularly difficult when you are on your own: many single parents choose parenting over work and need to become experts at living economically. In terms of statistics, single parents are worse off financially than pensioners and poverty is the biggest challenge they face. Lack of finance for childcare is a major factor inhibiting a return to work and difficulties are often exacerbated when maintenance payments are not met.

Some people are naturally good at being frugal, others are not, and many lone parents find themselves with financial commitments, such as house ownership. In some cases these can be maintained and in some there has to be a change in lifestyle, which may entail moving to a new neighbourhood. Such decisions are difficult and may be traumatic.

Decisions regarding work may be particularly tough. The broad issues for parents are covered in the chapter on Work and finance (p.320). If you are single before your baby is born, talk to the decision makers at work as soon as you can. There may be a way for you to stay on at work. If a compromise at your present workplace cannot be reached, take time to think about some new occupation to balance your role as a parent. Information is available through your local social security office, and ask your health visitor for details of childcare and support schemes.

There are no rules about how to negotiate this complex area and each decision will be unique. It will help to acknowledge that your arrangements, once established, will need to be reassessed at regular intervals. Many single mothers get very little or no financial help from ex-partners; sometimes this is in return for an amicable relationship and trouble-free childcare arrangements. While having sole financial responsibility can be very difficult, some find the independence empowering.

Moving forward

A journey that begins in partnership, involves separation and then living as a single parent, is often a long and difficult one. At first the outlook may appear to be bleak and the pain and anxiety may be intense. In the long term, however, you may feel much happier, stronger and more confident as an individual and as a parent. With a focus on your personal strengths, your support network and your baby, there will almost certainly be possibilities that can improve your situation, even though you cannot step back in time. The Wheel for Living (p.58) offers a worthwhile guide, however you feel. The most helpful strategies for coping and enjoying life as a lone parent are to listen to yourself and to your child, trust and respect your own instincts and seek and accept the support that will help you do this.

There is no easy way to adapt to unexpected separation or to parenting alone. Yet life goes on and you and your baby will move forward and build a life together. Ultimately, the relationship between you is the most important thing in both your lives, and this can thrive whatever people in the street say or do. As it develops there will be a new richness to your life. Now, and as your baby grows, you will need hands-on help and emotional support so that you can do the best for yourself and for your baby, and this may bring blossoming relationships and unforeseen possibilities. As your confidence grows you may find that fewer people show disapproval or suspicion. Many people will, in fact, draw hope and strength from your example.

Having a second baby

The addition of a second baby to your family can bring a wonderful sense of fullness and growth, and yet more wonder at how amazing babies – and parents – can be. Along with the excitement you may also be apprehensive. This is entirely normal, and is a good trigger for finding possibilities and support to create the time and space each member of your family needs. Some changes to your lifestyle may be inspired by experience with your first baby, but many things will be different this time around.

Pregnancy number two

A common complaint from women who are pregnant for the second time is that they do not have time to rest or pamper themselves as they did during their first pregnancy, and find coping with a baby inside and a baby outside extremely demanding. The key is to focus on quality of time rather than quantity and to broaden your network of friends, family and helpers who can babysit so you can take time out. The same time restraints apply to fathers. Where there was space to indulge in the first pregnancy, when the second comes a father often spends more time with his first child than he does relaxing with his partner and the baby inside her. For both parents the second pregnancy may seem to pass much more quickly.

For a woman physical strength depends on fitness and diet. Even if you have less time to exercise alone you can incorporate your first child into some simple activities: walking with a pushchair or as your child rides his tricycle, yoga or antenatal stretches in your bedroom or classes for mums and tots are all possibilities. If you lead a busy life you may need consciously to pay more attention to when and what you eat and take supplements to replace the vitamins and minerals used up as you care for both your children as well as yourself.

Every pregnancy is different. You might accommodate this pregnancy with ease and cope with symptoms more easily than you did first time round: discomfort and nausea are usually not as bad. Your abdomen is likely to enlarge sooner and expand more, so by 3 months you could look like you did at 5 or 6 months last time. If you had varicose veins and haemorrhoids, they may flare up again. The changes in your skin and hair tend to be similar to last time. If you experienced urinary incontinence or vaginal prolapse after your first pregnancy, this may increase during this one but is likely to decrease after the birth.

It's also common for the pelvic joints to cause more discomfort, having already expanded and settled before, and this can lead to pain in your back or pelvis (p.519). You'll need to pay attention to your posture, particularly when you lift and carry your older child, and ensure you exercise and rest adequately. You may need to get advice from your doctor or osteopath about alleviating pain.

Is there a perfect age gap?

If you look around, you'll notice that brothers and sisters survive, and thrive, on all kinds of age differences. There is no perfect age gap, and each scenario brings blessings as well as challenges. Each of your children, however many months or years between them, has his or her own strong character and will react to the environment you create and the love and acceptance you show.

Some people find that a small gap – that is, having two below the age of 2 years – means that the children have similar interests and make great companions for one another. In the early days, however, both will be in nappies and require close attention throughout the day and possibly at night too. Other people find it easier to wait until child number one has passed through the terrible twos, left nappies behind or begun pre-school before they bring the next on to the scene.

Involving your older child during pregnancy

Children, however young, are very perceptive. They pick up on moods and get the gist of a conversation by listening to tones of voice. When you choose to tell your first child about your pregnancy, whether he is 1, 2, 3 or 6, he will react. He may be excited, angry, confused, or all three, with behaviour to match. He might also find it difficult to understand that he will be waiting a considerable time to meet the new arrival. You may prefer to leave it until the fifth month when he can feel kicks inside your tummy.

When you tell your child about your pregnancy, try to involve him every time you talk about it: 'You are going to have a very special friend who will be your brother or sister,' or, 'Mummy has a baby in her tummy who can't wait to meet you.' This will be accepted with more enthusiasm than, 'Mummy and Daddy are having another baby.' If you know that you are having a boy or a girl you can explain things even more clearly, and if you have a name in mind, your unborn child can become a named member of your family even before birth. To your older child, 'Can you feel Matthew's foot kicking my tummy?' will feel more real than, 'The baby's kicking.' If you're talking with adult friends in the presence of your child, use terms like 'Sam's new sister' in place of 'my baby'.

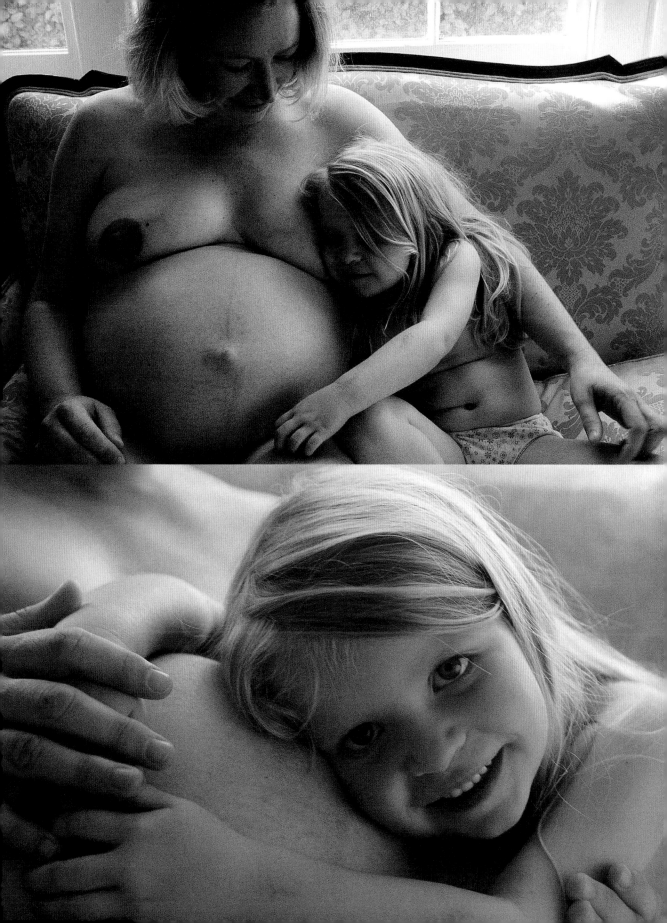

It is common for an older child to demand more attention from his parents. Some demands may be disruptive, such as bed-wetting, tantrums, clinginess or aggression. This is where quality time becomes important in order to let your child feel special, using love and attention and gentle encouragement as he builds his sense of individuality. Often fathers devote an increasing amount of time to the first child.

If your older child is passing through his 'terrible twos' (which can happen any time between 13 months and 3 years), he will be finding out what is and isn't acceptable and who is boss. Testing and pushing boundaries is an essential stage in growing up. You might enjoy dancing with his fiery, defiant side as well as the gentle angel in him and letting him know that you love him for who he is, not only when he's a 'good' boy. Sometimes, of course, going with troublesome behaviour may not be appropriate, and where you draw this line will depend on your family boundaries. The concepts of naughtiness and discipline could be debated for ever and you and your partner must decide what is acceptable. Now could be a good time to reassess boundaries (p.276) in the light of impending change, and to ensure your child receives the same messages about what is acceptable from each of his carers. You might get tips and support at a parenting class or advice from other second- or third-time mothers. And don't forget, your health visitor may be an excellent support and source of further contacts.

Older children often feel valued and respected if they go into a more 'grown-up' environment, and it may be appropriate to begin at a playgroup or enrol your child at a nursery where you leave him for an hour or even a day. It can also help enormously to introduce a routine if you don't already have one. A reliable framework helps most children feel secure, particularly while things around them are changing. And for you, predictable mealtimes and a set bedtime may help.

Approaching the birth

As your due date gets nearer, you'll need to organise support so you know your first child will be cared for while you are in labour, even if this is in the middle of the night. If you are giving birth in hospital you may be away from home for anything between 24 hours and 4 days, or longer if you or your baby need special care. Your child will miss you and may need extra reassurance while you're away. If he is cared for by a familiar person whom he loves, the transition will be easier.

Your eldest child may be very excited about meeting the new baby and show his eagerness to be involved. Ask him if there's anything he would like to give his little brother or sister. You could also buy or make something as a present from the new baby, and give it to your eldest when they meet for the first time.

Second birth

Many women look forward to having an easier time than they had before, and most men feel much more comfortable about being present for the labour. If you had a good experience first time round, you may be eager to repeat it, and the chances are you will. If you had a difficult experience you may be able to take steps to reduce the chances of complications arising again as you care for yourself in pregnancy. The majority of second labours are shorter and easier than the first.

It is a good idea to create a birth plan based on your past experience. This will open the way for you to talk

---

My second baby is due in just under 8 weeks. One part of me is very excited, but another is nervous. I'm afraid that I will lose the very special relationship with my daughter; I'm unsure about labour and I wonder if I can get through caring for a newborn again.

Your concerns are completely normal. Every parent has worries, usually centred on time, money and space, and many wonder how they can possibly love anyone else as much as they love their first baby. Love is infinite and actually thrives when it is extended and shared. Many parents feel love for their first child even more deeply when a second arrives. As for time, you know that the early days are intense and can plan in advance to get through this, perhaps with extra help. And with parenting practice already under your belt you will not stumble over nappy changes, bathtimes or general babycare.

Here are some worries that mothers and fathers commonly feel. Many disappear when the new baby arrives, although some are best worked through before birth and some concern areas that need extra effort after the birth. You can use the Wheel for Living (p.58) to tackle any issues that concern you.

- What if the labour is as difficult as last time?
- My first was not the sex I preferred. How will I feel if it happens again?
- Will I cope if depression strikes again?
- I am nervous that my partner and I will lose touch.
- I dread the thought of our sex life being put on hold again.
- I can't believe we will be lucky again and our second baby will be as wonderful as the first.
- What if there is something wrong with my baby?
- How can I possibly cope with months of broken sleep, piles of washing and a screaming baby?
- We can't afford two. I'm fed up of working really hard and living hand to mouth.
- Last time my productivity at work decreased a lot. I am afraid I will lose my job if it happens again.
- I barely have enough time to enjoy one child, let alone two.

about your first baby's birth and is particularly important if you had a problematic time and suffered from post-traumatic stress (p.461), a well-recognised phenomenon. Your partner may feel less nervous about the labour being difficult if he also has a chance to talk through his fears and suggest some things that may help you both. You can be guided by a midwife, obstetrician or family therapist. The memory will always be there but the emotional effect and fear can virtually disappear: you will then be able to put the past in the past, enjoy the pregnancy and look forward to a different birth.

The physiology of giving birth a second time

In your second and subsequent pregnancies your baby's head is likely to engage later because there is more room in your abdomen and uterus, but it is less likely that you will give birth more than 10 days after your due date. Your second labour is also likely to be shorter. The cervix usually dilates with fewer contractions and the ligaments and muscles of the pelvis and the vagina open more easily. If your second baby is much bigger than the first, or in an awkward position, labour may be longer, but this is unusual.

Your contractions may be more efficient and more painful. If you have given birth vaginally before, the final phase as your baby's head emerges should be faster and you will stretch more easily; any tears you get are likely to be smaller and heal more quickly. In the hours and days after birth, particularly when you breastfeed, afterpains, or uterine contractions, are strong: they are felt more strongly after each birth.

Recovering after giving birth

If your second birth is easier than your first, particularly if you do not need intervention or stitches, you will be surprised at how good you feel. In the first 24 hours after birth it's still important that you rest, hold your new baby and get feeding off to a good start. If you are in hospital for several days, it may be one of the few chances you have to be really close without interruption from your other child. Your partner, if he is at home caring for your older child, may take longer than you to replenish his energy and catch up on sleep.

After second and subsequent births, pelvic and abdominal muscles and stretched skin can take a little longer to recover. Second-time mums very often find their body heals well after birth, but tiredness can persist and it's hard to stock up on energy while coping with the 24-hour demands of a newborn. Plan in advance to eat well and gather help for the first few weeks so you do not feel overwhelmed.

Begin pelvic floor exercises as soon as you can, particularly if you have previously experienced vaginal prolapse or urinary incontinence. Your vaginal tissues and pelvic floor muscles will recover as fast or faster than last time and if you have had an incontinence problem it will not be greater second time around. If you have previously experienced postnatal depression then you could consider taking stock during pregnancy of any underlying causes that are still present and discussing them with your doctor, midwife or counsellor. If depression may have been brought on by hormonal changes, using progesterone after the birth may be effective (p.459).

Family life with more children

There's a marked difference between welcoming your first child into your home and welcoming your second. The concerns are not whether you will drop the baby but how you can meet two children's needs as well as your own. Your first child's presence, his behaviour and the way he treats your baby will have a huge influence on how you settle in.

You may settle down for a relaxing feed only to be disturbed by your toddler, or be playing with your toddler and interrupted by your baby's cry. This is the fun, and the challenge, of having a larger family, and your time management skills will be put to the test. On some days you will think that two children amount to more than twice one. On others having two may be as easy, or easier, than having one.

Parents are often amazed at how different their two children can be, in looks as well as in temperament, and

---

I needed forceps for my first baby. What are the chances that I will need intervention again?
The partnership between you and your second baby is different from the first, and you cannot predict how your birth will progress. It is reassuring to know that a forceps or ventouse is more common with first babies. Unless your second baby is much bigger or awkwardly positioned, you are unlikely to require this level of intervention because your muscles and tissues will open more easily. Based on statistics, it is safe to say that your second birth will be easier and achievable without forceps. It is also true that most women who had a caesarean in labour the first time round are able to give birth to their second child vaginally if the indication for the original caesarean is no longer present.

Although you are unlikely to need forceps you may wish to make a birth plan that includes the possibility of intervention. Remember that, in addition to giving birth before, keeping fit and nourishing yourself well during pregnancy and adopting an upright posture and moving your body freely in labour make a normal birth more likely. If your first baby was very large, avoiding fast-burning sugary drinks and foods during this pregnancy may help to reduce your baby's weight (p.332).

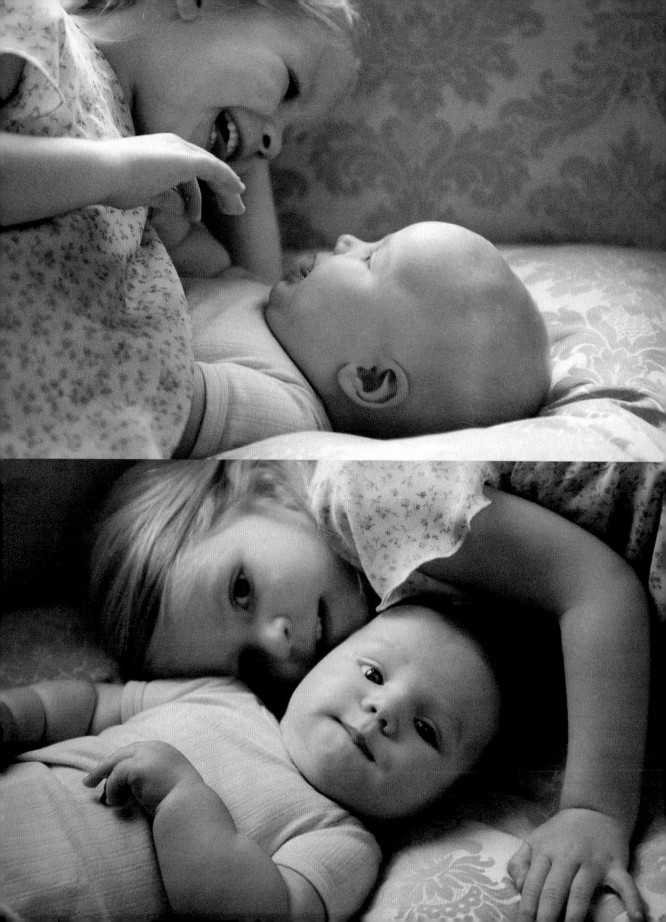

notice it from the first moments after birth or even during pregnancy. This difference is a wonderful bonus and can work to everyone's benefit. The key to adapting is to take each day as it comes, honour your new child's individuality and guide your first child carefully.

As your baby gets older she will compete more actively for your attention. As a parent of two, you will become an expert at doing two things at once and juggling your children's needs, and perhaps something of a diplomat as you explain and bargain for a balance. The most important thing is to remember that each child is an individual and give them space to be themselves. Comments such as 'Why can't you be quiet like your sister?' or 'He was never as messy as you' can undermine self-esteem. It is tempting to think back and compare what your first child did but it is healthy to recognise and encourage differences and enjoy the richness this contributes to your family.

Your new baby

Your baby will be welcomed by proud parents, and by an excitable (or moody) brother or sister. In the early days, the new baby needs time and love to come to terms with the transition from womb to room and learn to trust her family and carers. She will love to watch all of your faces and hear you talk and sing as she forms her new relationships. The relationship she forms with your other child is as important as those she forms with her parents and will be completely different.

You may find you are less anxious about your baby when she cries because you know more about babies' communication. A second child often learns quickly that her needs do not always come first and as a result is often more patient than the first. Repeatedly putting your new baby's needs second, however, can have detrimental effects. However young, if your new baby feels that her cry always goes unheard, she may have a sense that she does not deserve attention.

Some parents who feel they could have done better with their first child try to compensate by doing things differently. In some instances this is appropriate but doing some things in the same way may be also be OK. If you have regrets related to your older child, they may influence you in the way you behave with your new baby. Ask yourself what your expectations are and remember that your enlarging family has new dynamics. The surest way to discover what suits you all now is to be open, listen to everybody's needs and learn by trial and error.

Your older child

Common reactions from young children to new siblings are wonder, love and tenderness. You can encourage these by letting your older child touch and stroke his sibling, watch feeding times, help with baths and nappy changes and choose clothes for the baby to wear. Tell him that the baby enjoys watching him and loves to be with him. If he's old enough, he can carry things for you or tidy up, or he might use a doll or other toy and imitate you. When you feel confident, step to one side and leave your two children together: they have a special relationship and this can thrive without interruptions. When you're all together ask him what he thinks the baby wants. This nurtures his self-esteem and he may spot things you haven't thought about: young children can tune into one another and he may know whether your baby is asking for a cuddle or a feed.

This romantic picture of child with baby is only part of the reality, however. An older child often shows anger and jealousy, and begins to crave attention. It's common for an older toddler to revert to nappies, become more dependent on a dummy or comfort object, wake more often at night, play up at mealtimes or want to share your bed. Often an older child's call for attention, whether he's asking for a drink or falling over, coincides with the time you are most busy with the baby.

If you sense that your older child is jealous, don't worry; it is very common. In his eyes he is being forced to share his favourite people with someone else, and he wasn't even asked. On top of that, he'll sense that he's supposed to like this new person, and may also feel that she has taken his place as favourite. He might express his jealousy through tantrums or through nastiness, perhaps by shouting at or hitting the baby, waking her up, poking her or giving her things she's not allowed, like chocolate or toast. In many families, sibling rivalry and jealousy can continue for decades.

Attention-seeking behaviour, often misdiagnosed as naughtiness, does pass, although it often reappears when the younger baby sits, crawls, stands and walks, and again when she learns to talk with confidence. You could make a game – play at putting a nappy on your older child or feeding him, for instance. He may enjoy hearing stories about himself as a baby, and laugh when he realises he also used to put his food in his hair. Sometimes you'll need to be calm but firm if he demands attention at inappropriate times. Explain gently and make sure he gets a good dose of quality time with you each day. You could build this into a routine that involves someone else caring for your baby.

Sometimes children ask if their new brother or sister can go away, if they can have a new mummy and daddy or if they can go and live with their grandparents. This can be very upsetting. But these reactions are normal, healthy and infinitely preferable to your toddler suppressing his feelings. Try to deal with these outbursts calmly.

Try not to ask your first child to grow up, stop crying or stop asking for cuddles: if you do, the opposite is likely to happen. Many parents learn to make their arms big enough to cuddle two at a time. This can begin a long tradition of sharing that creates strong family bonds.

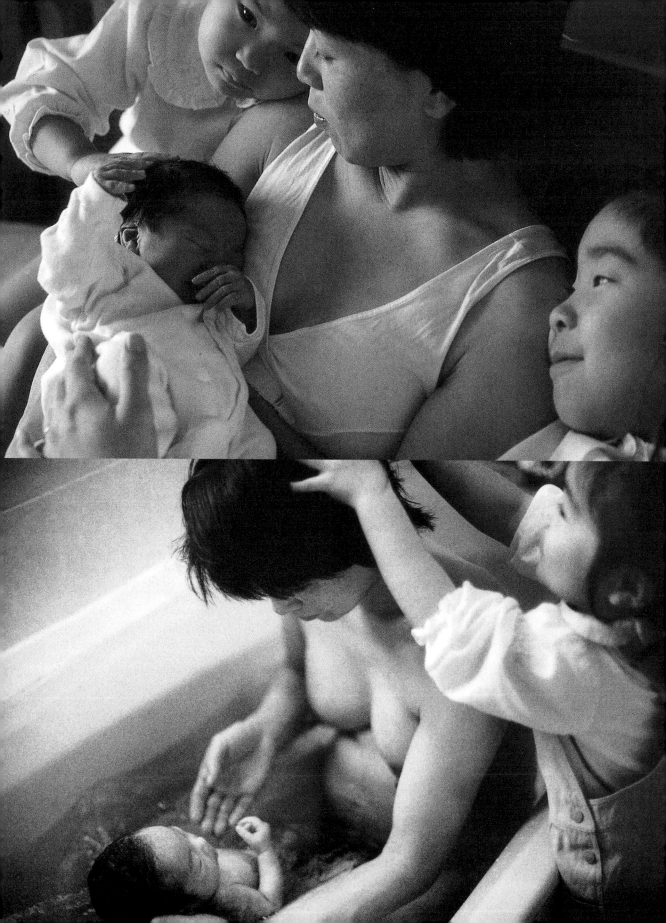

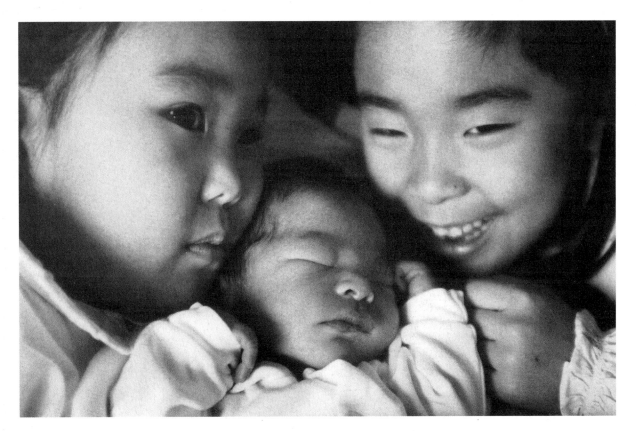

Sibling love, sibling rivalry

Many parents worry whether their children will love one another and sometimes this reflects their own experience with their siblings. You cannot force your children to become friends. Although most children get on well, all have squabbles and some have conflicting characters that may be a recipe for discontent. You can encourage their relationship but you will also need to step back and let them find their own ground and this process can begin early. Right now, you can do your best to help them both feel valued. Standing by and watching, though sometimes it can be hard not to intervene, allows you to see your children's personalities blossom and gives them the space to form the ground rules for their own relationship.

An older child plays a powerful role in your baby's early learning experience. Whatever examples he sets, or games he plays, he is an important teacher and, for the younger baby, there is nothing but benefit from this guidance. An older child is frequently more direct and expressive than parents tend to be, carries few expectations and will accept things at face value, and is usually much less protective. This is great for a developing baby, who naturally strives to copy and keep up with her older sibling and there is often a sense of deep companionship between the two children. They can live in their own world and entertain one another in a way only children can, and may develop their own language or understanding of one another – sometimes your older child may interpret your baby's cry for you. Their mutual entertainment will certainly include arguments or conflict, particularly as your younger child becomes more mobile and expressive. This is part of the interaction between all siblings, and is essential practical experience that gives valuable lessons about sharing, expressing opinions and being part of a group, about being upset, expressing it, and learning to move on.

More babies for the grandparents

When a second, or indeed a third or fourth child joins your family there will be yet another shift in the relationship that your parents have with you, and with your children. The arrival of your first child may bring anxiety from your mother and father as they are unsure how you will cope through pregnancy, how the birth will go and how your partnership will travel through the tests of parenthood. When another baby is on its way, they usually have less pressing concerns if they know that you have already managed one pregnancy, one birth and one newborn.

If your parents feel more confident about your ability to care for and enjoy your new baby, they may have more energy to focus on you and the children. At first this may be extra-special attention for your older child while you wait for birth. Indeed, many grandparents are 'on call' to step in and help when labour begins, and this role often entails many months spent with the older child, when a relationship blossoms. And when the new baby is home they may have time to give hands-on help as you feed and care for your newborn and they entertain your older child.

Feeding with two

Your older child will be eating solids whereas your newborn will need frequent feeding and attention as she gets settled. Older children often get more clingy to their bottle, want to be spoon-fed when they are capable of feeding themselves or get jealous of the new baby each time she is being held. Try giving your older child a bottle or a light snack when you feed your baby, and arrange your house to make this practical. If it's not the right time for your older child to eat, the three of you may be able to snuggle up together while you feed your baby and read a story to him. Alternatively, he may play happily while you're feeding your baby and is more likely to do this if you let him know that you are watching him and enjoying it. You won't be able to lose yourself in your baby at each feed, but you can still relish the quieter feeds late at night.

If you are breastfeeding two children, always give priority to the youngest, who needs the calories and nutrients. Your older child may enjoy the sucking and closeness, but doesn't need the nutritional boost. He might grow out of breastfeeding of his own accord. You could make a cup of juice or bottle of milk seem more attractive – buy a cup together that's decorated with his favourite storybook or television characters.

Sleeping with two

In an ideal situation your older child will already be sleeping soundly through the night by the time number two comes along, whatever his age. In many families,

though, the older child still wakes regularly. On top of this, it's quite a common reaction for the older one to begin to kick up a fuss at bedtime and wake more frequently as a cry for attention. These difficulties usually recede but can be trying, particularly if the baby cries a lot in the evening.

Try as far as possible to stick to any routine you have already set for your older child, but in the early days allow him to have extra cuddles or go beyond bedtime so that he feels special. If he has no bedtime routine put your energies into settling your baby and let him help. Dealing with bedtimes will be easier if you have some support. It is useful for one adult to read to the older child while the other feeds and settles the baby.

Moving on

Almost all parents find the newborn period the most trying. Though a second baby is often less demanding than the first, adjusting to the change is a challenge. You may feel torn if both children want all of you all of the time, and you may feel very tired, but there are many rewards and most come from watching your children interact. Your older child will surprise you with his perception, entertaining suggestions and amusing offers of help and your younger child may surprise you with her wit and an amazing capacity to learn that flourishes when there's another little person to copy.

The family unit will have changed considerably, and will change again if you have more children. The requirements from you, including time, love, responsibility and patience, increase with each child but with each new addition there is potential for countless rewards. With each baby you learn, and your parenting skills will get better and better. If you remember to include you and your partnership in the family equation, you will sail through the years with a growing team of loving supporters.

I'm worried that my baby will wake her brother if I let her cry for longer than a second at night. I want them to share a room soon, but will this ever be possible?
A baby's cry is programmed to wake people up. But, surprisingly, all but the one who's doing the feeding can sleep through a certain level of wailing. The chances are you will get to your baby quickly and this is easier if she is in your room. Initially, if your toddler wakes he may need a quick cuddle before he drifts off. He might want to come into your bed. Within a week, however, he'll be used to the change and may ignore the crying. If he isn't woken, which is likely, there will be few problems with sharing. If he always wakes, you could wait until your baby wakes less, before moving her into his room. Your children will probably enjoy sharing. Across the world and for countless generations brothers and sisters, and even whole families, have slept in the same room and managed fine.

If I had my child to raise over again
If I had my child to raise over again
I'd build self esteem, and the house later.
I'd finger paint more and point the finger less.
I would do less correcting and more connecting.
I'd take my eyes off my watch, and watch more with my eyes.
I would care to know less and know to care more.
I'd take more hikes and fly more kites.
I'd stop playing serious, and seriously play.
I would run through more fields and gaze at more stars.
I'd do more hugging, and less tugging.
I'd see oak trees in the acorn more often.
I'd model less about the love of power, and more about the power of love.
Anon

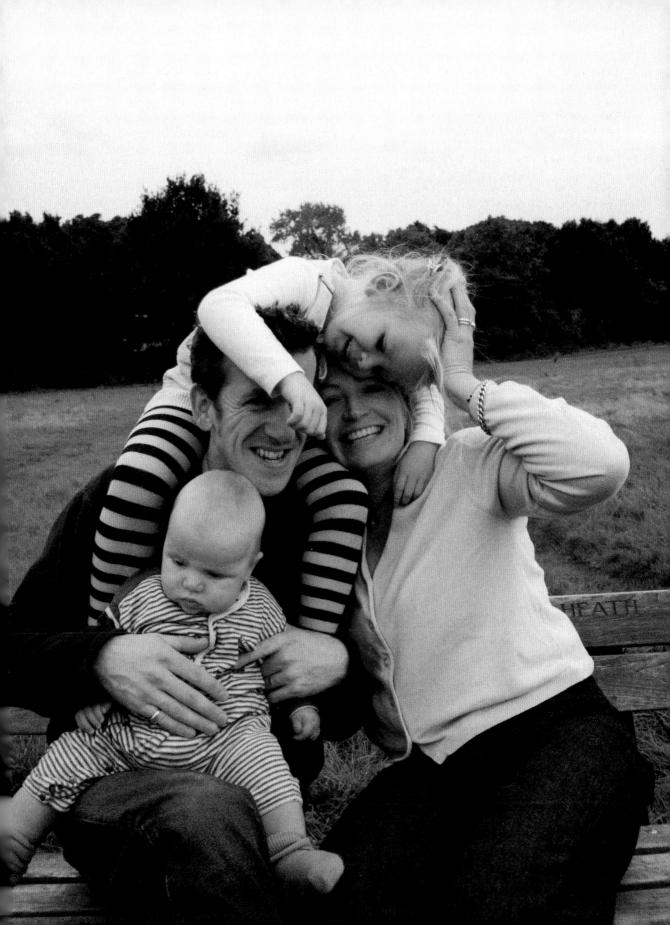

Work and finance

Having a family requires financial commitment, and increasingly mothers work as well as or instead of fathers. For many parents juggling work and home and budgeting for a family is a tough challenge. As you make choices about what to do and how to mix family and career, you may need to make compromises.

Time and money

Forward planning is almost essential as you decide how much time to take off and when to return, if at all. As you plan, it will help to make the most of your rights and find out what you are entitled to. Managing your time to make space for different aspects of life is a skill you'll build on as a parent, whether or not you work. The Wheel for Living (p.58) suggests ways to assess your situation and find the support to help you achieve your goals.

The costs of parenting

Most expectant parents have concerns about finances and almost all find their income drops significantly just at the time their expenses are growing. If you or your partner want to reduce your hours or leave work, you will lose all or part of one salary. If you both intend to go on working, you will almost certainly need to pay for childcare. The range of expense related to your baby varies. The changes you decide to make may be as minimal as cutting down on non-essential luxuries or as huge as moving house. It might help to look at the areas where costs can be involved and see which apply to you:

- Midwife and other birth supporters: NHS, family and friends, or hired support?
- Maternity clothes and baby clothes and equipment: handed down from family and friends, received as gifts, second-hand or new?
- Nappies: disposable or washable?
- Milk: breastfeeding is free; the cost of formula milk can be reduced if you receive financial support or if your baby needs it for health reasons.
- Where you live: will you stay put without making changes, redecorate, put in heating, buy a washing machine, build a nursery, move house?
- How you travel: will you keep your current car, remain without a car or buy a new one?
- Childcare: will you have help or use a crèche?
- Family food: will you make changes, e.g. to buy organic?

Work and pregnancy

Work and pregnancy are compatible. Although pregnancy may bring symptoms that affect your working life, such as tiredness, backache, nausea or reduced concentration, equally it can enhance your abilities, making you more focused, determined and better at prioritising. As your pregnancy advances, a few changes may help. Chiefly, these will revolve around safety but they may also include altering your posture, changing the way you apportion time and incorporate rest, adjusting your role and delegating as your maternity leave approaches.

Employers who help staff to balance work and family commitments generally have employees who are much more likely to return to work after maternity leave. Some employers continue to see pregnant women as a burden, however, and can be inflexible. If you have problems, remember you do have rights: do some research through your local DHSS office and check company policies.

If you are self-employed you may have greater flexibility to fit work in around drowsiness, antenatal appointments or relaxation. In addition, you may be more anxious about taking a break, maintaining your client base and planning for the months beyond birth. It will help to let your clients know about your future availability.

I have worked in increasingly senior roles for my company for 8 years and always felt I had a strong professional image. Now that it's obvious I'm pregnant, I feel that several of my colleagues don't take me seriously any more.
Pregnancy is one of those things that gets tongues wagging and brews up excitement, and your colleagues would not be human if they didn't show some interest. It does not follow that your colleagues respect you any less. In fact, many of them may enjoy the opportunity to talk with you on a more personal level.

The novelty of your pregnancy may soon wear off and you may notice that as the months go by they will be focused on ensuring that the business functions when you are not there. If you continue to perform well in your job you may win even more respect. You can assert yourself honestly by drawing clear boundaries around the tasks you wish to delegate, and delegating ahead of time.

It might help to think about the role work plays in your life. If you have been career-orientated, you may be more unsettled by your pregnancy than you care to admit. You may fear that you will miss colleagues who have become close friends and feel lonely because you will lose their emotional support. Think about seeing your work friends socially and look forward to forging some great friendships outside your work community.

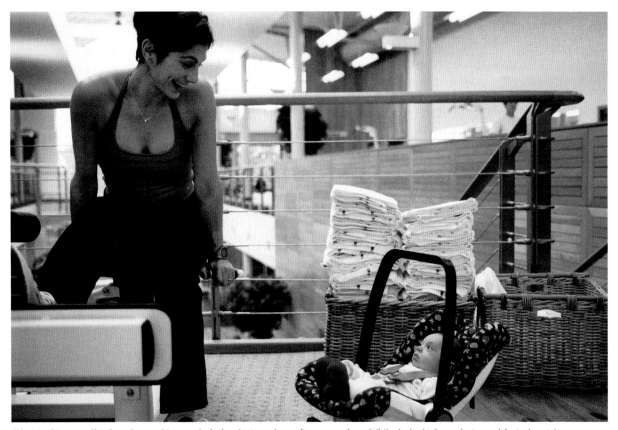

Jake joins his mum, Shirel, as she gets things ready for her day's work as a fitness consultant. While she leads classes, he is cared for in the crèche.

Comfort and safety at work

Whatever your job it's important to consider your baby and your body and not to exceed your limits: eat well and often, rest intermittently, pee whenever you need to, sit, stand and lift comfortably and eat well to keep up your energy. Sitting down all day isn't good for circulation or energy levels, so if you're an office worker stand up, stretch and walk around every hour or so and make use of any space that's available for you to relax (even for 5 minutes) and perhaps do some simple antenatal exercises.

Where work involves standing for lengthy periods, you may become uncomfortable and it may aggravate backache, varicose veins or any giddiness. Although your baby is at little risk, it is best to sit down while working or change your role; if this isn't possible you may need to stop work early. If you feel fit enough to continue as before, you still need to take account of your pregnancy. As your ligaments soften, you will be less capable of bearing heavy weights safely, and doing so may lead to strain or injury. Studies suggest that if you have discomfort or pain, you should not remain past Week 20 in a job that involves heavy lifting, pulling, pushing, bending or climbing. Heavy manual labour may predispose to premature birth.

More subtle risks during pregnancy include chemicals and other toxins and you need to take every measure possible to limit your exposure to dangerous substances (p.388). Subtler still are the stresses you may put upon yourself if you take on too much. It might be possible to split your workload between workplace and home or switch to part-time work or job-sharing.

While you are pregnant you might feel stressed more easily. Signs range from persistent anxiety to insomnia, from stomach pains to runs of Braxton-Hicks contractions. In a large company it is the human resources manager's task to evaluate stress at work. Dealing with stress is an integral part of a complete programme of self-care, and reducing your workload is an important element that it is better not to ignore.

When to leave work

Many women thrive at work during pregnancy and enjoy working until the last minute. If work is not a priority or a financial necessity, you can leave without sacrificing your maternity pay, on the date confirmed by your employer. This is commonly 11 weeks before the baby is due. In early pregnancy it can be hard to imagine what you may

The earth-mother type may have unlimited time with her children to enjoy every moment of their amazing growth. The downside may be that by staying with them continually she unwittingly smothers their independence and sacrifices her own. The Superwoman who continues her career has less time with her children but may feel more fulfilled on a personal level; if she has delegated to good carers and spends real quality time with her family when she is at home she may achieve a balance. There's another stereotype of the successful couple in an egalitarian marriage where both parents work and share domestic chores equally, although in reality maintaining an equilibrium may not always be simple.

As role models, the earth mother radiates altruism and commitment; Supermum demonstrates success and independence. The egalitarian parents exhibit teamwork and good communication. All three can offer love and consistency.

There is no 'better' way to do things, and no ideal that suits everyone. As you look at other people you only see a fraction of their life; you need to do what suits you financially, emotionally and your family. The key factors are to give your baby quality time when he can feel loved and valued and to be true to your heart as you aim for your own contentment.

What's best for you?

The days of career-long, full-time, office-based employment with one company are gone. With this change the communal voice of working parents has grown and inspired innovative developments, from job-sharing to work-based crèches, and a range of legislations to ease the conflict between work and family. Many new mothers plan to return to work then reverse the decision. There are also many women who, during pregnancy, can imagine nothing better than being a stay-at-home mum and then after a few months yearn to go back to work.

Whatever decision you make there will be pros and cons. If you return to work, you may never have felt so busy, and if you become more tired as a result it will be even more important to build exercise and relaxation time into your weekly schedule and focus on a healthy diet. You may also find that becoming a parent gives you a powerful impetus to take a new or unexpected direction.

Your decision about working after your baby's birth will be based on at least five criteria whose order of priority will depend on your own circumstances: your income requirement; your baby's personality and how this fits your image of your family; your wish to work for personal fulfilment; appropriate, affordable childcare; and flexibility in the workplace.

feel like at Week 30, 36 or 38, and it is quite common for women to anticipate working longer than they actually do. If you feel great and want to stay on at work, do give yourself space and time to wind down and prepare your mind and home for your baby's arrival.

Your body image at work

If you dress yourself up and look good, you'll probably feel good (p.54). As a result, you may feel more confident, even if you are suffering lapses of concentration. You may need to invest in a pair of shoes that will accommodate and support slightly swollen feet. And underneath your skirt or trousers you could wear support tights – they are no longer ribbed and do help prevent varicose veins.

Work and motherhood

Your own ideal mix between work and home might be easy to realise. Alternatively, there may be a period of adjustment as you discover what suits your family. Until you are a parent, you may never appreciate just how much of a full-time job parenting is and how challenging it can be to combine it with paid employment. With each passing generation the goals and rules of the working world change. You may be doing something your parents would never have dreamed of doing or you may be following closely in their footsteps. Their reaction to your decisions may be central to the way you value yourself, and how you choose to work.

Back to work

Once you settle back into working you may find that you have new confidence and a clearer direction. Knowing that you need to leave on the dot can focus your mind on the tasks to be completed. On the other hand, working again may be very hard, particularly if you don't want to be there and the demands placed on you are intense.

Looking after yourself and using the support of your community can help you integrate the workplace and home, and discover alternative possibilities. You will need time to find the right balance, and you will need to re-adjust on an ongoing basis as your baby grows. When you return to work, whether it is earlier or later than you originally planned, be gentle on yourself:

- Before beginning, try an interim period where you gradually have more time away from your baby to ready you both for the separation.
- You may need to phone home frequently at the beginning and express milk if you are breastfeeding.
- Allow yourself time to adapt. The first few days away from your child and back at work are the most difficult.
- If you feel guilty, explain to your baby why you are working – he will sense your honesty even if he cannot speak, and talking will help you see things clearly.
- Be firm about your limits from day one. Both you and your colleagues need to adjust to the idea that your working hours are less flexible, particularly if your baby is ill or needs your attention.

- If your company doesn't make allowances for the responsibility of a new baby, you may have to sell them the idea that a committed mother can also be a committed employee.
- Use the support of your colleagues and delegate so that teamwork brings results effectively.
- If things prove very difficult, it may be best for you to take a break, even if this means making financial compromises. Deciding that work and a baby are not a viable combination can be a courageous choice.

Working from home

Successful home working demands self-discipline and a suitable working space, and both may take time to build. Generations of women have boosted their family income by working from home in the hours that their babies sleep. For many, however, these are the hours that offer time to rest, finish household chores, eat and share time and conversation with other adults. If you need to dedicate hours – or days – on end, you won't be able to get by without childcare. If you try to work intensively and care for your baby, you may not give your optimum performance, your baby may feel sidelined and become more insistent and demanding, and you may be exhausted and feel there is no time to relax.

If your child is being cared for at home, you need to allow her carer to organise the day, while you forsake your mothering role, as much as possible. Drawing boundaries around your space is as important as being strict about your time. It's also crucial that these boundaries can be flexible when the need arises.

Work and play

Having a family and a job may be like having two full-time jobs; having both may also be like having the best of both worlds, and when the two are balanced this can happen. Yet life is capricious, and perhaps never more so than when children are involved.

Some days and weeks may flow beautifully smoothly. There will also be times when life with work and a family feels almost impossibly full, and when the unexpected, such as illness, crops up, you'll need help to stay afloat and avoid feeling overwhelmed.

The golden rule is: 'Don't try and do it all yourself.' At work and at home, you have a pool of supporters who can share your load, take difficult tasks off your hands or free up your time so you can channel your energy elsewhere, whether into a work project, a day with your baby, or a weekend away with your partner where neither work nor baby infringe.

Childcare

Finding childcare that is right for you and for your baby may take you into a maze of choices, waiting lists, contracts and compromises. As you explore the field and find out what's available and affordable, you may also feel a tug as you begin to share the care of your baby. Where childcare suits you both, the tug is replaced by a feeling of trust and sharing, and relief that you can have time to yourself without worrying. When childcare isn't suitable, you or your partner and your baby may get frustrated and upset.

Your priorities

You are delegating your parental responsibility to another person. This is not always easy, but because you have a duty to your baby to ensure that she is safe, happy and well looked after, and to yourself to keep your anxiety to a minimum, there are a number of practical considerations that you cannot ignore. Wherever your child is cared for, your views need to be clearly laid down, preferably in writing, so there is no room for uncertainty or misunderstanding. You also need to show the carer respect and part of this is giving clear and honest guidelines about your expectations, while acknowledging and fitting in with his or her expectations. Remember that a carer's qualifications are important, but your intuition and impression of whether he or she loves babies is more important. It is also essential to take regular stock of the arrangements and assess how well they are working for your baby, for you and for the carer.

Interviewing a potential carer

Most carers are women. When you interview a prospective carer you'll form a strong impression of her character. You will sense whether or not you're likely to get on in a working partnership and how she gets on with your baby. Armed with a list of questions, you'll be sure you won't miss out anything important. The points to the right might help you and could be used to form a contract if you need to draw one up.

Setting ground rules

An integral part of entrusting your child to someone else's care is that you trust the carer and the two of you respect one another's views when it comes to bringing up children. Once you have chosen a carer, it's up to you to set the ground rules and be clear about what you expect.

Basic boundaries concern issues such as feeding, sleeping and toys to play with, activities such as swimming or going to baby groups, and being outdoors each day, and so on. The best way to set ground rules and to stick by them is to have them written down so you can both refer to them. Try to be as clear as possible about your wishes, your baby's routine and the days and times you require care, but

---

Interview discussion points

The carer's background

- Ask about her feelings about the needs of tiny babies and her experience with them.
- Ask about her qualifications.
- Ask why she left her last job (if applicable).
- Have a look at references and follow them up.
- Ensure that she has first aid qualifications.
- Find out if she has a driving licence and whether she has a car of her own.
- Does she have any allergies (for instance to your pets) or dietary needs that may affect her work?
- IAsk if she smokes or drinks alcohol during the day.

The carer's approach

- Discuss her ideas about being there for your baby. Does she enjoying playing with and entertaining children, can she sing or play an instrument, is she happy to go swimming with your baby?
- If you're leaving your baby away from home, find out about sleeping arrangements and spaces for play.
- Ask about any other children in her care – how many and what ages.
- Discuss her approach to food and breastfeeding and what kind of food she considers 'healthy'.
- Ask her about safety, how she minimises risks and what she would do in an emergency.
- Find out how she perceives discipline for babies and young children.
- Discuss training in sleeping and toilet training.
- You may want to ask about the way she remembers her own childhood, as this will affect her approach to children now.

Finances and conditions

- Discuss pay, holidays, overtime and sickness.
- Find out if she has insurance or arrangements for paying tax.
- What are the limits on the time she can work for you?
- Discuss what might be an acceptable period of notice if either of you want to terminate the arrangement.

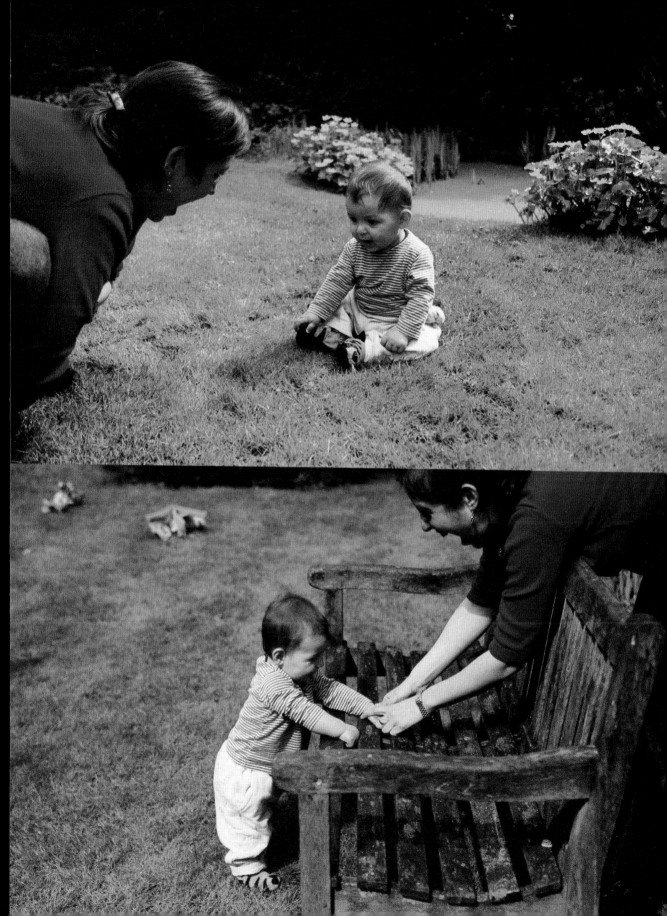

avoid being dictatorial. Establishing a few guidelines will allow your carer to be spontaneous and loving with your baby within a comfortable framework, and this will help them develop a good relationship.

- Discuss important issues such as smoking, food, sleeping times, etc.
- Give clear instructions on contacting you and your partner, with back-up contacts, e.g. grandparents, friends, neighbours, doctor.
- Make a list of things to do if your baby's unwell or there's an emergency.
- Provide a book for the carer to make a record of each day.
- Make a list of what to do if domestic emergencies arise, e.g. plumbing, electricity, car breakdown.
- Be clear about the carer's duties and whether these include housework.
- Be clear about hours of work and holiday times.
- Arrange a date when you can go over the arrangements together and assess how they are working.

Your options

Your choice about childcare will hang on the following issues: whether you want care in your own home or away from home, from birth or later. You'll get details of childminders, maternity nurses, nannies, nurseries and crèches from your local health visitor or Children's Information Service, or from advertisements in local and national publications, and they may indicate how far in advance you need to book.

A maternity nurse: A maternity nurse is a qualified nurse specially trained to care for newborn babies. She will take over the care of your baby when you want, and bring her to you for breastfeeding. Maternity nurses aim to get a baby into a routine and sleeping well through the night from an early age, and offer postnatal support to mothers. Your maternity nurse will be on duty 24 hours a day and will be a major part of your baby's life for the few weeks she stays. Focusing on a routine so early does not suit all parents or babies.

Mother's helps and doulas: A mother's help can be a great support around the home, doing a variety of domestic duties to leave you free to rest and care for your baby. If she's a mum herself, she may also offer pearls of wisdom that help you care for and bond with your new baby. A mother's help may be a regular part of your life for years.

A doula fulfils a similar role with a greater emphasis on babycare and feeding, and some doulas begin to help women before and during birth (p.76). The main qualification is to be friendly and caring, offering emotional support and practical help and advice wherever she can. Doulas are still rare in the UK; they're more common in the US. They tend to stay for a few weeks or longer if the parents have the funds.

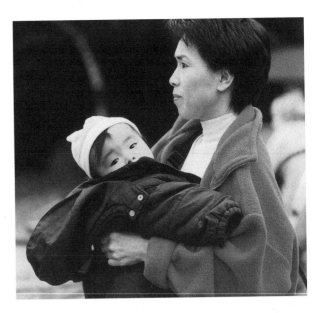

A nanny: Nannies will care for your baby in your home and may live with you or come to your house for agreed hours. Nannies vary widely in the qualifications they hold, the amounts they charge, the services they offer and the treatment they expect. You could explore the possibility of sharing a nanny with another family to reduce costs.

An au pair: Au pairs are young people who come to the UK to stay with a family and help with childcare while getting a taste of another culture and learning English.

If your baby does not adapt well

- Look at how you feel. Are you ready to separate from your baby?
- Consider whether the environment suits your baby's personality. For example, an extrovert child may thrive in a crèche, while an introvert may prefer personal care.
- Have courage to give yourself, your child and the carer time to adapt, and be committed to change if it becomes necessary.
- Look at the possibility that your baby is being mistreated. Trust your intuition and ask other parents about their children's behaviour. Be observant and notice any cuts, scratches and bruises.

If you're concerned that your baby cries excessively when you leave, or she seems despondent or unhappy when you return, talk to her carer. This may be a signal of approaching illness and your carer may have noticed it too. Alternatively, your baby may not be happy with the current arrangement, perhaps because she doesn't get on well with the carer, or because she misses you; some babies are more dependent on their mums than others and take a long time to settle. If you feel that the arrangement is not right, you will need to try alternatives.

Their working conditions are regulated and they expect a minimum weekly payment as well as accommodation, meals and involvement in family life. What your au pair does in her spare time is up to her.

Because they are young and may be away from home for the first time many au pairs need emotional support, and this may involve a considerable amount of mothering from you. Your au pair won't necessarily be trained in childcare. It's common for au pairs to move on after around a year.

A childminder: A childminder uses her own home as a mini crèche. Childminders usually have their own children, many are flexible regarding hours and most are significantly less expensive than nannies. They are self-employed and are not obliged to have any childcare qualifications but they are expected to have a good understanding of child development and experience of caring for children. Every childminder is required by law to register with the local authority and must attend a pre-registration course run by the local Social Services department. Disadvantages may be the absence of care through school holidays or cancellation at short notice if there's a contagious illness in the house.

A nursery or crèche: In a nursery or crèche your baby will be cared for along with a group of other children and babies by a team of qualified nursery nurses and people undergoing training. The great bonus is the social interaction and the resources and space that are seldom available at a childminder's or in your own home. One of the greatest disadvantages is the high rate of infection from common childhood illnesses.

Quality of care and resources can vary widely, as can price, and popular nurseries can have long waiting lists. A good guide of standard is the frequency of staff turnover. Most nurseries offer a degree of flexibility concerning hours. Some don't take children below the age of 2 years.

All nurseries must be registered with the local authority and are thoroughly inspected each year to ensure that they are providing a safe, happy environment for young children.

A grandparent or other relative: There's a very special bond between many children and their grandparents. Grandparents have often grown in patience with the passing years and take unrestrained pleasure in playing with their grandchildren.

If one of your parents has offered to look after your baby, and you get on well together and share similar values, it may be a perfect arrangement whether or not you give payment. However, some people find it hard to be completely straight about expressing their preferences to their own parents and using them for regular care is not a suitable option.

If childcare seems unaffordable, visit your local Social Service office or ask at a Citizens' Advice Bureau about your entitlement to financial assistance. You may be able to get costs partly or fully covered.

If you are a single parent, you may be able to get some assistance while you train or look for work. Your baby may also be eligible for a place in a community nursery operated and subsidised by your local authority.

About 1 in 10 employers offer assistance with childcare through an allowance or voucher scheme or with subsidies.

Your baby's happiness

When you have chosen someone to care for your baby, it is time to settle in. If the care is from birth, you will all be together. If it is care to cover you while you work, spend time with your baby at the nursery or with the carer – if possible, do this on several days for increasing amounts of time. You and your baby can get used to the new environment and begin to form a relationship with the carer. While you're there, your child will sense your feelings about the arrangement and will feel a positive atmosphere if you and the carer get on well and trust one another. Everyone has heard about carers who injure children. Although these are rare, it may take many weeks before you are sure your child is in safe and loving hands. If you have doubts it is best to follow your intuition.

When you feel ready, leave your baby for a few minutes and you can then leave her for longer and longer. Tell her that you are going and you are coming back: even if she doesn't understand your words, she'll understand your tone of voice. If your workplace and carer are flexible, you may be able to build up the hours you spend apart over a week or two.

Your baby may cry when you leave, and her crying may be particularly distraught if she is going through a period of separation anxiety, usually after 6–8 months (p.254). It may take her time to calm down: wait outside the door if you need reassurance before turning your mind to work. If she does not cry, try not to take it personally: it is an excellent sign that she feels loved and secure. Most babies adapt well to change and enjoy going to a nursery or spending time with a childminder or nanny.

Handing your baby over to someone else can be heart wrenching and it's common to have anxieties: 'Will she be happy?', 'Will she miss me?', 'Will she be angry with me?', 'Will she love the carer more than she loves me?' Rest assured that babies are never confused about who their parents are. Your baby has the capability to receive love from both you and her carer. Although it may be hard at first, it helps to welcome and encourage the carer's love because if there is fondness between them you'll find it easier to trust that everything is going well. The carer will become an important person in your child's life and may have many positive influences. You too may form a lasting friendship with her and, in turn, with her children.

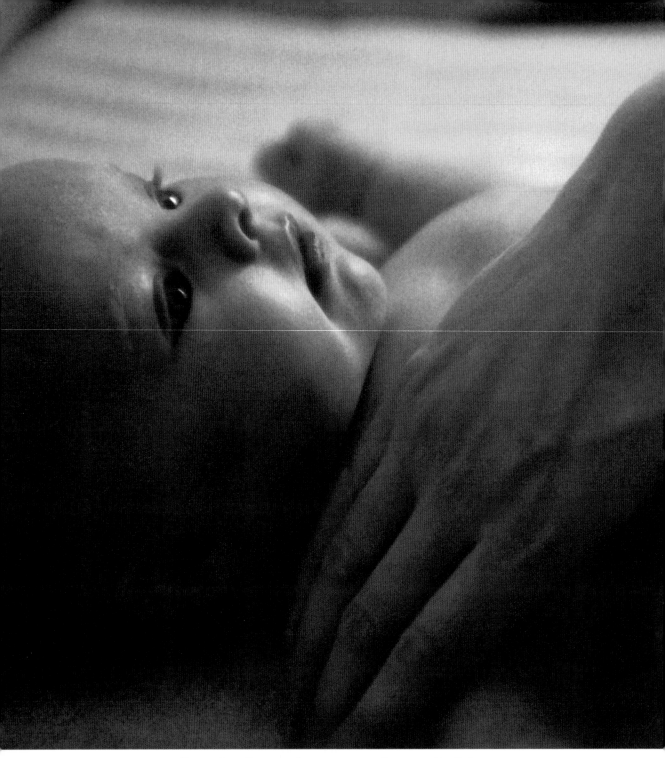

part v mind, body and spirit

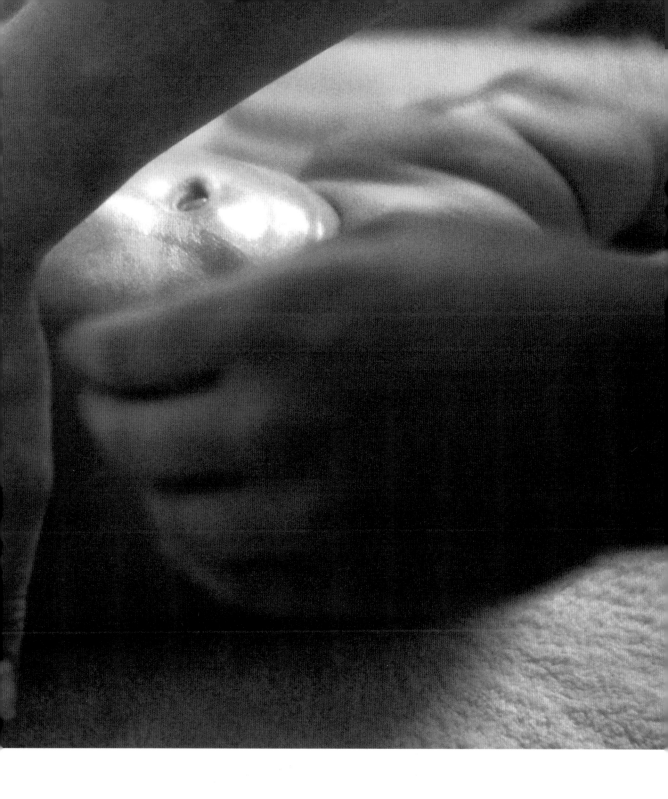

Integrated, holistic care

Over the centuries there have been many approaches to health care. Not every approach suits every person, and using a mixture of options available from different disciplines, both conventional medicine and complementary therapies, often brings the best results. The past decade has seen the number of people who use complementary therapies rise exponentially.

The holistic approach

Medical care during pregnancy in the 21st century offers modern obstetric and paediatric practice and high-technology interventions alongside traditional midwifery skills. In addition, there is a range of therapies that complement conventional medical care. An increasing number of people rely on these and they can be combined with conventional modern practices, often to great effect. This holistic approach considers physical, emotional and spiritual issues against a background of lifestyle: what your work involves, how stressed you feel, how you sleep, how you exercise, what kind of diet you have and how you react to day-to-day situations in your family. One of the most significant factors is emotional health – what you love, what you fear and any underlying emotional issues that may manifest with physical symptoms.

When you visit a complementary therapist he or she will gradually build up a picture of who you are and where you are in your life in order to advise the most appropriate treatment. Complementary medicine can be a catalyst for you to look at your own lifestyle, expectations, emotions and residual anxieties, and begin a process of healing from within, aided by the therapist's guidance and treatment.

Complementary therapies are based on nature and rest on centuries of experience and, as with conventional medicine, practitioners must go through training in order to qualify. As the use of these therapies becomes more widespread, they are more thoroughly researched and monitored. It is difficult to evaluate their effect in the same way as conventional medical treatments and there is still a lack of information about the pros and cons of different techniques. There are, however, an increasing number of studies comparing the two and in many countries regulatory bodies are being set up to improve training and standards. The overall aim of continuing research and regulation is to improve safety and success rates.

Integrated care

The term 'integrated care' implies the free use of both conventional and complementary techniques. The treatment chosen will depend on your symptoms at any one time. The same mother or baby, for instance, may use homeopathy one day and require an epidural anaesthetic in labour the following day.

During pregnancy, complementary therapies may be your primary resource. You may use them as you prepare for birth and as pain relief in labour, knowing that modern obstetrics can act as a safety net if the need arises. A number of midwives have complementary skills, bringing to the labour ward and postnatally techniques from disciplines such as homeopathy, aromatherapy, acupuncture and massage.

The disciplines used most commonly during labour, birth preparation, postnatal healing and baby health care are covered in subsequent chapters in this part of the book. In such a short space only brief details can be given, however, and there will undoubtedly be unanswered questions, but what is contained in this book may give you the interest and inspiration to investigate further for yourself. You may also be interested in emotional support offered by counselling and psychotherapy. This is discussed on p.459 of the A–Z Health Guide.

Making your choice

Integrated health care is not new. The term 'holistic' is a modern one, but the integrated approach has been used for thousands of years. We all eat, exercise and breathe, and how we approach even these apparently simple parts of our normal daily lives plays a role in our attitude to health. The purpose of this part of the book is to stimulate interest in several areas of alternative health care, suggesting possibilities that may help you improve your health, enjoy

---

The benefits of complementary therapies

Used alone or when integrated with modern obstetric and paediatric practice, complementary therapies:

- Can improve breathing, circulation, heart function and sleep patterns and treat many diseases.
- Can improve emotional health, positivity and energy.
- Can aid relaxation without resource to addictive drugs.
- Can be very useful as part of babycare.
- Can become a welcome part of daily life.

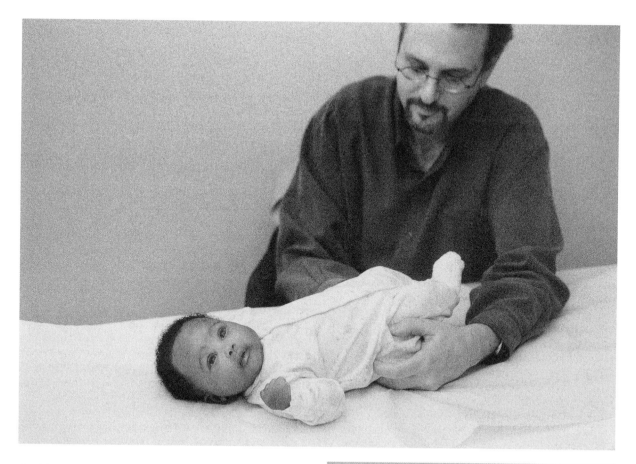

Cranial osteopathy after birth is a powerful way to calm a baby and relieve any tension that may have built up while in the womb or during birth .

your pregnancy more, and improve your family's health.

You will undoubtedly find a diverse approach to complementary therapies among the many people involved in health care. Some doctors and nurses are open-minded about combining alternative practices with conventional medicine; some know little about them and choose not to become involved; some are cynical and may discourage their use. As with any choices for labour, for nutrition or for general health, your most powerful tool is knowledge – so find out what you can and then you can make your own decisions.

An appealing concept is the use of complementary techniques against the background and safety net of modern obstetric care. The clinical examination, tests and ultrasound scans provide an increasingly sophisticated background in which more problems are discovered and understood. Complementary care may be used as the primary method for affecting a cure for a condition, or alternatively it may be used in a supportive role to ameliorate symptoms and relieve distress.

Seeking help from conventional medicine

Alternative therapies must be augmented by conventional drug therapy when there is an emergency or when the condition being treated does not respond. It is best to consult a medical practitioner in the following situations:

- If symptoms do not respond to the measures you have tried.
- If symptoms become worse.
- If there is a persistent high fever that reaches or climbs above 38°C (100.4°F) or if there are acute indications of infection such as fever, pain, pus formation.
- If there are signs of drowsiness, disorientation, confusion or a sudden loss of vision or there is loss of consciousness or fitting.
- If there is a severe headache with neck stiffness and sensitivity to light.
- If there is severe or persistent pain or crying.
- If there is severe loss of fluids and dehydration as a result of vomiting and/or diarrhoea.
- If there are respiratory and breathing difficulties.
- If there are signs of a severe allergic reaction.
- If there is excessive bleeding.

Eating and weight

'Prepare yourself for a major life change and start eating to live rather than living to eat. You'll be amazed at the difference.' Dr Marilyn Glenville is a nutritional therapist, psychologist and author; her approach to nutrition forms the basis of this chapter.

Eating well

Optimal nutrition is one of the cornerstones of health. 'You are what you eat' remains as true today as it was a thousand years ago. Nutrition includes everything you eat, drink, smoke and inhale; all the elements that your body absorbs, uses, stores and excretes. It is surprising how your nutrition – what, when and how you eat – affects everything about you from minute to minute: your weight, susceptibility to illness, appearance, energy levels and sleep, and your moods, feelings and relationships.

Many women are naturally inclined to take a fresh look at food when they become pregnant. This life-changing event may be an opportunity to introduce new eating habits that will benefit you as well as your family. And when you do eat well in pregnancy, and beyond, you give your baby a nutritional start that will influence the way she eats for the rest of her life.

Good nutrition is not dieting – it is about moderation and balance, enjoying food and maintaining good health and fitness. Before pregnancy, nutrition is an important factor in your own wellbeing and influences the conditions you will provide for your unborn baby. When you are pregnant, a balanced diet ensures you meet you baby's needs while nourishing your own body and strengthening it for the demands of birth and breastfeeding. If you choose to breastfeed, everything you eat will be present in your milk and you will remain your baby's sole source of nourishment until you introduce other food.

This chapter looks at what's in food, what's good and not so good, how food is related to emotions and how

healthy, fun eating can be achieved. It has to contain a lot of details, so it's a long chapter – skip the bits you already know about and use the new information to make good nutrition a part of your life.

Weight and pregnancy

One of the most common concerns among pregnant women is weight gain. It is an important issue and it is best to discuss your own weight at your antenatal visits, watch your progress and have a target gain.

Ideally, weight gain begins with the first missed period and continues until the birth – precisely how much you gain depends on your physiology, your baby and your eating habits. More significant than the gain during pregnancy, however, is your weight before conception. If you are underweight or poorly nourished this can be harmful. The classic example is the famine in Holland during the Second World War: babies born to mothers who were malnourished before conception were subject to more miscarriages, low-birth weight and prematurity than those whose mothers lacked food in pregnancy but were not underweight to start with.

Too much or too little?

It was once thought that weight gain should be limited to 6.8 kg (15 lb) but this is insufficient. Recommendations endorsed by the American College of Obstetricians and Gynaecologists are based on pre-pregnancy body mass index (BMI). BMI is a formula identifying the percentage of body tissue that is actually fat. It is preferable to measuring only weight because it takes height into account. Taking your weight in kg and dividing it by the square of your height in metres gives your BMI. BMI charts are available in most clinics.

Women who gain less than 6 kg (13 lb) during pregnancy run the risk of having a baby who is premature or underweight. In rare cases low weight gain is linked with maternal illness in pregnancy that interferes with proper nutrition. Other cases may stem from a fear of gaining weight or other eating disorders (p.455) such as anorexia or bulimia. Women with these problems may be helped with sensitivity during pregnancy.

Many women do gain more weight then necessary. Though overweight women stand a greater chance of having a larger-than-average-sized baby, the mother's

---

Recommended weight gain

Weight	BMI: gain recommended
Underweight	Below 19.8 BMI: 12.7–18.2 kg (28–40 lb)
Normal weight	19.8–26 BMI: 11.4–16.0 kg (25–35½ lb)
Overweight	26–29 BM: 6.8–9.1 kg (15–20 lb)
Obese	30–40 BMI: 6.8 kg (15 lb)

Pregnant with twins: Target weight gain 15.9–20.5 kg (35–45 lb). Women who are 1.6 m (5 ft 2 in) or smaller should gain at the lower end of the recommended range.

How your body gains weight in pregnancy

Breasts	450 g–1.3 kg	(1–3 lb)
Placenta	675 g	(1½ lb)
Amniotic fluid	900 g	(2 lb)
Uterus	900 g–1.6 kg	(2–3½ lb)
Maternal fluid/blood	2.9 kg	(6½ lb)
Foetus	3.1–3.8 kg	(7–8½ lb)
Maternal fat stores	3.6–4.5 kg	(8–10 lb)
Total	12.5–15.8 kg	(27½–35 lb)

weight gain and that of her infant do not always correlate. What is vitally important is the quality of the food that contributes to the weight gain as well as the quantity. Excessive weight gain may, however, spark a weight problem following pregnancy, which could need a lot of attention and loving care to overcome; this is the most common time for a weight problem to begin and excess weight gain may give rise to postnatal depression. Excess gain is most often down to the consumption of fast-burning sugars in the form of colas and fruit juices, sweets and chocolate, biscuits and white bread and cakes. It is easy to consume 'empty calories' – foods that are empty of goodness, but full of calories.

Weight gain in each trimester
These are guidelines and there is a lot of individual variation: do not be too rigid.
In the first trimester (Weeks 1–13): The ideal weight gain is 1.4–1.8 kg (3–4 lb). Fortunately, nature protects babies of mothers who feel too sick to eat well during the first 3 months: a baby does not need many calories at this stage and the reserve of vitamins, minerals, essential fatty acids and proteins built up by the mother before pregnancy will be sufficient. Not gaining or even losing weight in the early weeks isn't likely to cause problems.
In the second trimester (Weeks 14–26): The ideal gain is 225–450 g (½–1 lb) per week. This amounts to a total of 3–6 kg (6½–13 lb). It is often the easiest time to eat well.
In the third trimester (Weeks 27–birth): A similar gain should continue until the end of the eighth month. In the final month, weight gain may slow down, so the gain for the whole trimester is between 3.6 and 4.5 kg (8 and 10 lb). During the last months of gestation calcium is laid down in bones and the iron store is built to get your baby through the first few months of life when iron intake will be low. Eye, brain and nerve development are being completed, and important components of essential fats are necessary. Especially good are the oils from fish and linseed. Your baby is putting on weight at the rate of up to 50 g (2 oz) per day during the ninth month, so you need to eat sufficient

proteins and calories. The third trimester is definitely not the time to go on a weight-loss diet, neither is it a time to binge and gain excessive weight.

Monitoring your weight
It is best to keep weight gain as steady as possible – your baby requires a daily supply of nutrients throughout the pregnancy. There will be fluctuations, but with good antenatal care your doctor or midwife will help you to keep on track. As a general rule, try to weigh yourself no more than once a week.

If you recognise that you are out of your target range, it is time to take stock and get advice. For example, a rapid weight gain of more than 1 kg (2 lb) per week could signify the onset of pre-eclampsia (p.410). However, it is more likely to signify excess calorie intake in the form of sugar, fruit juices or refined foods. You may say, 'To hell with it' and use pregnancy as an excuse for letting go. However, it is better for you to acknowledge the reality and get back to eating well.

Weight after pregnancy
Within a month of birth most women lose around two-thirds of the weight they have gained. The rest – or most of it – falls away over the following many months unless your diet contains an excess of fatty and sugary foods. While you're breastfeeding a sharp fall in weight could affect your milk supply, so it's important not to try to lose it too quickly. Whatever your body shape or your tendency to gain or lose weight, it's more important to attend to nutrition than to the figures on the scales.

Eating well
The fundamental point about eating well is that it involves enjoying food and allowing abundance. Eating well really can mean eating regularly, consuming delicious food and ignoring calorie quotas when the food you choose to eat is nutritious. Dieting and counting calories, on the other hand, involves guilt about eating 'too much' and a feeling of being denied great taste experiences and the fun of sociable mealtimes.

As you introduce new approaches to eating, it is good to remember that it may take months or years before it becomes second nature. Even so, as you commit to each small change, it will improve the way you feel, physically and emotionally. It is also helpful to remember that every person – and every family – has individual nutritional needs, requires a unique number of calories and enjoys differently sized and spaced meals.

The hormonal changes of pregnancy and breastfeeding may alter your appetite and you may be surprised that food you always enjoyed tastes awful or that you are driven to eat unusual combinations (p.455). Reduced physical activity, sleep deprivation, leaving work, financial strain and many other things will also have an effect on how you eat. Yet eating well may make it easier for you to deal with potentially stressful events.

What about calorie counting?
Throughout pregnancy and breastfeeding you need 200–300 extra calories each day – that's the equivalent of an extra 250 ml (8 fl oz) glass of milk and a sandwich made from one slice of bread spread with margarine, and filled with approximately 25 g (1 oz) of meat or cheese. When you are breastfeeding you need the same as during pregnancy. If you follow the advice in this book about a healthy balance, however, you'll no longer need to count calories. Instead, you can know that you are eating well and that your body will tell you when you are hungry and when you have eaten enough. You could find it much easier than you expected. When you have experienced a feeling of balance without excessive hunger or peaks and troughs of energy, even for a day, you may choose to continue along the same lines. Of course, it's not always easy to stick to resolutions or overcome cravings, and even the most dedicated plans may fall away amid the hormonal swings of the primal period. What's important, and healthy, though, is a good nutritional foundation. Deviations or binges now and then are not harmful as long as you come back on track.

Dieting
Dieting is a short-term plan to lose weight whereas altering eating patterns is a long-term strategy. Most people in the west do eat more than they need, and there is a tendency to reduce intake drastically in order to lose weight. Very often the dieting cycle alternates between eating too much, eating less and losing weight, and then eating more and gaining again.

Eating less than your body needs sends it into 'famine' mode: it slows down the rate at which energy is used and encourages your body to store as much as it can. In other words, your body does what it can to avoid burning calories. When you diet you may feel colder than usual, and tire easily, because your body is not freeing up energy. When you return to your normal intake of food because your body is in the habit of using as little energy as possible, it continues to store, rather than burn, calories, and you will put on weight rapidly.

What you feel about eating
Food is an emotive issue. Eating too much, too little or inappropriately is often due to underlying feelings, even though the link may be unconscious. Often feelings originate from your youth. For instance, you may reach for food to comfort yourself, as if you are having a biscuit to take away the pain of a nasty fall or enjoying something sweet when you're in a boring or unpleasant situation.

If you find you sometimes turn to food when you are feeling low or anxious, now is as good a time to begin to make practical changes. If you have a balanced diet this reduces the low points and anxiety during the day, and this will help you to deal with your feelings without reflecting them in the way you eat.

When you are pregnant you will have to live with a gain in weight and your body image will shift. You may also have dietary likes and dislikes that you never had before. Some women find pregnancy easy and enjoyable. Others find it a challenge and feelings range from being angry about becoming heavier, to using pregnancy as an excuse to eat more.

You may know what your physical and emotional triggers are in relation to food. If you do, you are lucky. If you suspect there are issues affecting the way you eat, the following points may be helpful.

Triggers for eating
There is a hunger centre in your brain that tells you when you need food. There is also a reflex in your unconscious mind that has been built up over your lifetime and brings on the urge to eat in response to a particular situation. Often its strongest foundation is in childhood and teenage years, although pregnancy can be the start of new appetites. You may find it useful to keep a diary of the feelings or day-to-day situations that encourage you to eat when you are not actually hungry.

Feelings: Does the way you eat, what you eat and when you eat reflect how you are feeling from hour to hour, and from day to day? Being aware of how your feelings influence your appetite can be very powerful. You may not always find it easy to be objective in pregnancy or when your baby is young, when the range and strength of your feelings may be intense. You could take time each day to look back over what, and when, you have eaten – feeding your baby last thing at night may be a good opportunity for this.

If you notice a link between your feelings and your diet over time you may find it easy to be objective and take the choice about whether to follow your usual pattern or break out of it. Small decisions made once or twice a day have a greater effect than big decisions taken every few months.

Habits and environment: Everyone has habits. You may feel hungry each time you pass the cupboard where the biscuits are stored. You may find that when you relax and watch television you reach for a sweet or a snack, or when you go for a long drive you stock up on nibbles.

Make a note of your habits: this simple awareness may bring change without the need for big resolutions. Something as straightforward as not having colas, sweets, biscuits and chocolates in your home may make a big difference. It will mean that you have to go out to buy

The building blocks of food

One way of looking at nutritional balance is to use the illustration of a pyramid. This looks at food in terms of its basic components. For optimal nutrition the greatest part of a diet should be made up of complex carbohydrates and vegetables and some fruit. Protein-rich foods are essential, but are needed in much smaller quantities. Fats are needed in yet smaller quantities and are best consumed in unsaturated form (p.337). Of course, each food has several properties – for instance, a potato is a complex carbohydrate that also contains minerals and proteins, red meat is protein-rich with fat and also a good source of iron, beans contain protein and complex carbohydrates and minerals. You can choose the best food in each group for your own diet and budget: for instance, you can eat pulses instead of meat and fish.

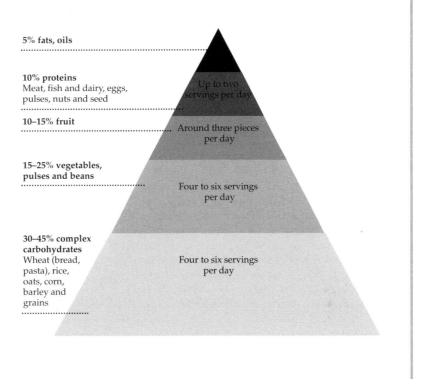

5% fats, oils

10% proteins
Meat, fish and dairy, eggs, pulses, nuts and seed

10–15% fruit

15–25% vegetables, pulses and beans

30–45% complex carbohydrates
Wheat (bread, pasta), rice, oats, corn, barley and grains

Up to two servings per day

Around three pieces per day

Four to six servings per day

Four to six servings per day

---

chocolate when you crave it, and it also reduces the likelihood of bingeing. Consider clearing your house of these foods. You will miss them at first but later you may be relieved that the temptation isn't there.

How to avoid picking

Provided your general nutrition is good and you eat regularly spaced meals, the following tips may help you cut down on excessive snacks or sweets:

Exercise: Exercise makes you high. It releases feel-good hormones called endorphins and it mobilises sugar from you body stores so you get a natural sugar boost. It also stimulates your metabolism to work for hours after you have finished and suppresses your appetite for a while, providing you haven't exercised on an empty stomach.

Distract yourself: You may be surprised at how cravings subside if you do not satisfy them. If you feel the urge to pick, do something else or have a slow-burning snack instead of a sugar or chocolate fix.

Don't deny yourself: Against a foundation of good nutrition you can afford to eat the extra things you like and enjoy them. If you have a chocolate fix and then eat less 'good' food at the next meal, your calorie intake will not shoot up. This is provided the binges are occasional. If you follow the recommendations in this chapter, your cravings

will decrease and you will really enjoy a treat every now and then. You will need less willpower and a single indulgence will not spark a week of overindulgence.

Getting a balance

Good nutrition is balance in the way you shop, cook and eat. Once you have a grasp of what's in food, for instance the nutritional value of an orange compared to pasta, you can look at how often you eat. Some foods keep you going for longer, others satisfy you in the short term. Some have a high calorie content, others are low in calories. The right mix for you will be meals and snacks eaten in moderation that keep your energy levels stable without piling on extra calories. Some people find this a difficult balancing act.

Balance in cooking, balance in eating

The process of breaking down food for digestion begins in cooking, and it is ideal for cooked food to make up around 70% of what you eat. How you cook is important: over-cooking depletes nutritional value, and deep frying increases fat content. The remaining 30% is best eaten raw and this applies to many vegetables and fruits. The breaking-down process continues as you chew so it's best to take your time and eat at leisure whenever possible. This increases the chances of having a relaxed, sociable meal, and if you take time to rest afterwards your digestion works more efficiently than it would if you began moving as soon as you finished.

Sugar highs, sugar lows (hypoglycaemia)

Every food contains sugar in some form, as sucrose, glucose, lactose or dextrose. The body breaks down food and uses the sugar component for energy. When you eat, your blood sugar level rises as the glucose enters your bloodstream. This lifts your energy. Anything that isn't used by your muscles for energy is stored in fat deposits or as glycogen in the liver so it is available at a later time.

Some foods are more easily broken down than others, which means that the sugar energy they provide does not last so long. An example would be to compare a spoonful of pure glucose with a bowl of lentils that contains the same amount of glucose combined with fibre, protein and other components. If you were to eat the sugar, you would experience an energy rise and feel good. The sugar is so easily accessible, however, that your body would use (or store) it quickly. Your blood sugar would rise rapidly, and after around an hour it would fall again and you would

feel hungry. If you were to eat the bowl of lentils, it may take up to 15 minutes longer to feel the initial energy rise. But because your body needs to work harder to break down the lentils and extract sugar, the sugar would remain in your bloodstream for longer. Your blood sugar level would not fall sufficiently to make you feel hungry for 3 hours – three times as long as the spoonful of sugar.

It may seem strange to compare pure sugar with lentils. Yet a lot of convenience food – chocolate bars, sweet pastries, cakes, biscuits and even white bread, and drinks such as colas and fruit juice, sweet tea and hot chocolate contain a vast amount of sugar. Consuming these brings about a pattern of short-term satisfaction followed by renewed hunger. And when blood sugar rises rapidly and then plunges, emotions and energy levels do the same: when your blood sugar is high you feel energetic, enthusiastic and positive; when it plummets you are hypoglycaemic and feel tired, irritable, anxious and unable to concentrate.

Hypoglycaemia is another word for 'low blood sugar'. Your body reacts to this by releasing adrenalin, which works to stabilise blood sugar levels but it is also a stress

---

The glycaemic index of common foods

Keep foods with a score of over 70 to a minimum. These are 'fast burners'. When you eat a number of foods in a meal, you can work out the glycaemic score by totalling all the figures and calculating an average. Protein foods such as milk, meat, fish and cheese do not cause the same fluctuations in blood glucose as carbohydrates, so are not listed on this index.

Food	GI score	Food	GI score	Food	GI score
Sugars		**Grains and cereals**		**Pulses**	
Glucose	100	French baguette	95	Baked beans	48
Honey	87	White rice	72	Butter beans	36
Sucrose (sugar)	89	Bagel	72	Chick peas	36
		White bread	70	Blackeye beans	33
Fruit		White spaghetti	70	Haricot beans	31
Orange juice	86	Ryvita	69	Kidney beans	29
Apple juice	80	Brown rice	66	Lentils	29
Watermelon	72	Muesli	66	Soya beans	15
Pineapple	66	Pastry dough	59		
Melon	65	Basmati rice	58	**Vegetables**	
Raisins	64	Porridge oats	49	Potato (boiled)	70
Banana	62	Wholegrain wheat bread	46	Beetroot (cooked)	64
Kiwi fruit	52	Wholemeal spaghetti	42	Sweetcorn	59
Grapes	46	Wholegrain rye bread	41	Sweet potatoes	54
Orange	40	Barley	26	Peas	51
Apple	39			Carrots	49
Plum	39				
Pear	38				
Grapefruit	25				
Cherries	25				

---

hormone that fuels tension. Hypoglycaemia thus brings with it some of the following: irritability and anxiety, increased aggression or tearfulness, exhaustion, nightmares, headaches and hunger pangs. Eating sugary foods puts you on a roller coaster with energy and emotions rising and falling every 1 or 2 hours. If your blood sugar rises and falls like this while you are pregnant or breastfeeding, your baby will be subject to the same highs and lows. If her sugar levels are elevated for prolonged periods each day while she is still in the womb, she may grow excessively large.

To know whether what you are eating provides a rapid or prolonged release of sugar, refer to the hypoglycaemic index opposite. Pure glucose (sugar) has the fastest release and is given an index of 100. Everything else is measured against this score. Going back to the lentils, a score of 29 means that the body's blood sugar level remains stable for just over three times as long as it would with pure sugar. If the lentils were sent to a factory to have the sugar extracted and you ate that sugar, the exact amount of sugar from the lentils would go through your body three times faster than it would as part of a lentil and you would not have eaten the fibre and minerals.

Carbohydrates
Carbohydrate is another word for sugar. The body breaks down carbohydrates to release glucose, which gives energy for body cells to function. Some carbohydrates have a fast-burning effect and others have a slow-burning effect.

Slow-burning complex carbohydrates
These have a low score in the glycaemic index. They are found in plants, wholegrains (such as oats, whole wheat and brown rice, millet, barley and corn), beans and pulses, whole vegetables and nuts and seeds. Because they must be broken down by digestion, they provide energy for long periods, giving a smoother feeling of wellbeing, and protect against hypoglycaemia. They are the foundation of a good daily diet, the basis of the food pyramid.

Fast-burning simple carbohydrates
These have a high score in the glycaemic index. They are found in soft drinks, colas, fruit juices, sweets, chocolate, white flour, biscuits, cakes and other foods containing refined sugar. They contribute to hypoglycaemia and are the most common cause of excessive weight gain, because the sugar not used as energy is stored as fat. Generally, they should be kept to a minimum. However, a fast-burning carbohydrate can be useful when you are being physically energetic and will use up the energy, instead of storing it. To make it easier to eat slow-burning foods you may need to exclude fast-burners from your home. If you have a sugar craving, eating at 3- or 4-hourly intervals and taking vitamins and minerals regularly may help.

Calories
Calorie is the term used to describe the energy-producing property of food. Everyone needs calories, and there are no foods without calories. In excess they contribute to weight gain; when you don't get enough they contribute to weight loss. If you are concerned about calories, it is useful to use the food pyramid and look at the glycaemic index (opposite). The relation between the index and calorie counting is that a food with a high glycaemic score will be broken down quickly and the calories it contains will be stored if they are not used in this time. Yet a portion of food with a low glycaemic score, containing a similar number of calories will provide energy for longer, and the calories will be used rather than stored.

Calories are highest in fatty foods, which are essential to health but are only needed in minimal quantities (5% of your diet). Don't forget that sweet drinks, even so-called 'healthy' fruit juices, are loaded with sugar, and are a potent cause of weight gain. The food industry has promoted fruit juice as healthy but if you drink more than one glass per day you will gain weight because the sugar content of two to four oranges is concentrated in the juice, and there may be added sugar. If you do drink fruit juice, dilute it with at least three times as much water. Aside from the occasional exception, it is best to drink water and choose from herbal or fruit teas – a selection of teas and their benefits is explored on p.344.

Proteins
Proteins consist of amino acids and are essential for the function of every cell in your body. You could not survive without them. There are eight essential amino acids that you cannot make in your body so you have to eat them. Proteins are present in many foods, but the concentration is highest in meat, fish, eggs, many vegetables, beans and pulses, nuts, cereals and grains. Soya beans (tofu) contain the full complement of amino acids essential to build proteins. Vegetarians can get all the protein they need from plant sources. During the ninth month of pregnancy, your baby is putting on weight at the rate of up to 50 g (2 oz) per day, so sufficient protein and calorie intake is important.

Fats
Despite media fascination with fat-free foods, the truth is that in moderation fat is good for you and essential fatty acids are crucial for health. Fat keeps you warm, insulates nerve cells and is a component of every cell in your body. What matters is the distinction between saturated and unsaturated fat.

Unsaturated fats
These provide essential fatty acids to allow the enzyme systems in the body cells to function optimally. Unsaturated fats are oils and do not coagulate. There are

two main types, both important to normal health; the Omega 3 oils are derived from vegetable sources (nuts, seeds) and the Omega 6 oils are from oily fish and linseeds and dark green vegetables. Linseeds are obtainable as seeds to be added to food or as purified oil. The purest 'cold-pressed' unsaturated vegetable oils, squeezed out during pressing without heating, come from sources including sesame and sunflower seeds, corn, walnuts and olives. Olive oil is best for cooking because when heated it does not form carcinogenic free radicals (see box, opposite).

To get sufficient essential fatty acids, have a handful of nuts or seeds or a salad dressing made with a cold-pressed oil each day, or try three meals a week of oily fish (mackerel, sardines or salmon). An alternative is to take an essential fatty acid supplement.

Saturated fat

This is not necessary in a nutritious diet, and in large quantities can cause harm. Not easily digestible, this form of fat tends to increase the risk of heart attacks. Saturated fats are usually derived from animal products such as butter, lard and red meat. Deep-fried food and fatty meat is best avoided. Saturated fat is also found in hydrogenated margarine as trans-fat, an artificially modified and plastic-like fat, which does not occur naturally in such high levels. Your body is put under undue stress if you ask it to perform the very difficult task of eliminating or digesting unnatural trans-fats.

Fibre or roughage

Fibre, also known as roughage, aids digestion and promotes intestinal movement. It also helps to balance blood sugar levels, removes toxins from your body and reduces the risk of bowel disorders, cancer and heart disease. By increasing the feeling of fullness, fibrous food will reduce your desire to eat excessively. You'll get roughage from your diet if you eat complex carbohydrates that also contain fibre: these include grains, brown rice, wheat, oats and millet, skins and pulp of fruit, vegetables and salads and nuts and seeds. Linseeds added to cereal or salads add roughage, help prevent constipation and also contain essential fatty acids. Bran is a good source of roughage when eaten in its natural form but note that wheat bran contains phytates, which reduce the absorption of iron, zinc, calcium and magnesium, so choose oat bran instead. A rapid increase in the bran content of your diet may actually increase constipation, so raise your intake gradually.

Vitamins

Vitamins A, B, C, D, E and K act in conjunction with minerals and enzymes to help the body's metabolic system work as efficiently as possible. The human body cannot function without them. They occur naturally in many

The no-fat–high-fibre health trap

Twenty-first century western ideas present fat as bad, but you need the essential fatty acids. There is a whole range of products labelled 'fat-free' or 'low-fat'. Many of these contain unnatural trans-fatty acids or other chemicals that the body finds very difficult to process. It is best to avoid these and choose unprocessed foods containing fat that is good for you – this is, fat in its unsaturated form (see left).

It is very important to remember that your nutritional needs are not the same as your baby's. When you wean your baby on to solid food, it would be a mistake to give her 'fat-free' foods, skimmed or semi-skimmed milk or margarine instead of unprocessed butter or pure olive oil. Your baby needs lots of calories and fat and cannot easily cope with processed foods and chemicals that don't occur naturally. Unlike you, she needs full-cream milk.

The same caution should be taken as you choose bread and flour: it is OK for you to eat high-fibre food, but if you give these to your baby she will feel full before she has eaten enough to get the nutrients essential for her growth and she may develop diarrhoea.

vegetables and fruits, particularly in the skins and in green leafy vegetables. It is safer to eat the skins of organic fruits and vegetables as these do not contain pesticides. It is possible, however, to destroy or reduce the vitamin content of vegetables by overcooking, so steam or stir-fry instead of boiling, or eat raw. Vitamin deficiencies or excesses may be harmful to you and to your growing baby – this is particularly true of folic acid and vitamin A respectively during pregnancy.

Vitamin A, also called retinol

Essential for the skin and mucus membranes, it is present in vegetables, dairy (overleaf) and liver. Avoid liver, paté and liver oil in pregnancy because of high concentrations of vitamin A, and if you take vitamin supplements ensure they contain less than 10,000 IU of retinol. Excess may affect foetal brain and eye development.

Vitamin B

The B vitamins affect the nervous system, mucus membranes, digestion, oxidation, cholesterol levels, fluid retention and blood cell formation. Vegetables, fruit, pulses, nuts and seeds, eggs, poultry, fish and milk all contain elements of the vitamin B complex.

Folic acid

This is a B vitamin that assists a growing baby's neurological development in the womb and reduces the chance of spina bifida (p.538). Fresh or steamed vegetables such as broccoli, sprouts, asparagus and spinach are a rich source of folic acid, as is fortified wholemeal bread. The recommended dose of 0.4 mg (400 mcg) per day is particularly important during the first 12 weeks of pregnancy and before conception. Regardless of diet, all women are advised to take folic acid supplements daily during this time.

Vitamin C

This helps oxidation and prevents infection, is an anti-pollutant, boosts connective tissue, reduces cancer risk and is important in iron absorption. It is present in all raw fruits and vegetables. Excess vitamin C may be harmful: the maximum safe dose is 1000–1500 mg daily.

Vitamin D

Necessary for calcium absorption and skeletal development, it is an important factor in guarding against osteoporosis. It is made in the skin by exposure to the sun, and is found in liver, dairy products and eggs and it may be added to bread during baking.

Vitamin E

This assists normal blood clotting, tissue healing and skin oxygenation. It is found in wholegrains, dairy products, soya beans and many seeds.

Vitamin K

Essential for normal blood clotting, vitamin K is made by bacteria in the bowel. However, newborn babies do not have bacteria for a few days so currently vitamin K is given at birth (p.226).

Minerals

Minerals are essential to wellbeing. Each one performs a specific task, maintaining your health while supporting the development of your baby.

Iron

In combination with other minerals and vitamins, iron is instrumental in maintaining sufficient haemoglobin levels to allow the blood to carry oxygen around the body. Low iron levels are common during pregnancy because the baby absorbs large amounts of iron to form muscles and blood, so it's important to increase your intake of iron-rich foods such as meat, seaweed, green leafy vegetables, spinach and cabbage, raw vegetables and salad, beans, pulses, tofu, millet and lentils.

If you take iron supplements, it is best to take them an hour before a meal and decrease Indian tea, which prevents iron absorption. Iron supplements are widely available from chemists or health food shops if you need a boost. During the last months of gestation your baby's iron store increases to get her through the first few months of life when her iron intake will be low.

Antioxidants and free radicals

Antioxidants are the subject of intensive research and they are thought to protect the body from the effects of substances known as 'free radicals'. These are chemically unstable atoms produced by oxygen metabolism in living cells that can cause cell damage and are linked to health problems including heart disease. They speed up the ageing process by destroying healthy cells and they may also attack the DNA in the nucleus of a cell, causing cell mutation and cancer.

Pollution, cigarette smoking, fried or barbecued food and UV rays from the sun can trigger free radicals but there is protection in the form of antioxidants, which occur naturally in food, especially in fruits and vegetables when eaten raw. Vitamins A, C and E, plus the minerals selenium and zinc are all antioxidants and are contained in many different foods. These include orange and yellow fruits and vegetables, green leafy vegetables, nuts and seeds, vegetable oils and oily fish.

Calcium

Intake of calcium is vital during pregnancy because your baby needs calcium to form strong bones. It is present in meat, many vegetables, nuts, seeds, beans, pulses, seaweed and dairy products. Routine calcium supplementation is not essential and women who do not eat dairy products can obtain calcium from vegetable sources. Food additives and processing, sweet fizzy drinks (which contain phosphates), sparkling water and bran wheat or oats interfere with calcium absorption.

Magnesium

This is an essential mineral acting with calcium in your baby's bone formation and replacing your spinal bone mineral density after birth. This mineral is also used by other tissues and cells in the body. Magnesium is found in sprouted seeds, leafy vegetables, seaweed, nuts, avocado, dates and apricots.

Zinc, selenium, manganese

Together with other 'trace minerals', these are extremely important in foetal development since they are integral to the make-up of every cell. Zinc plays a vital role in cell division, and zinc deficiency can block folic acid absorption. Zinc is in pumpkin seeds, wholewheat, rye, oats, almonds and peas. Selenium is an antioxidant (see box above) and helps in normal function of the chromosomes. Selenium is found in tuna, sesame seeds, avocados and grains. Manganese helps activate enzyme systems and is particularly important for bone development, thyroid hormone and sex hormone production, as well as helping to protect tissues against free radicals. Nuts, brown rice, wholegrain bread, pulses and cereals are good sources.

Foods that nourish

You can be sure that your nutrition will be well balanced if you eat a varied mixture of foods, expecially whole foods. Divided into food categories, the following text shows how to get the best from your diet.

Grains

Grains are a great source of slow-burning carbohydrates and roughage.

- Upping your intake of grains is an easy way to radically improve your nutrition – oats, wheat and brown rice, millet and barley.
- Choose wholemeal bread without added sugar or flour improvers and a sugar-free muesli.
- Soak muesli for 10 minutes to 12 hours: this helps to break down phytates that can block uptake of minerals from food.

What to avoid

- Because grains are small they easily absorb pesticides, so try to buy organic.
- If you are sensitive or intolerant to wheat (p.391) you may need to substitute bread made from other grains.

Vegetables

Eat vegetables for vitamins, fibre and minerals, antioxidants and phyto-chemicals that offer protection against diseases and boost the body's healing capacity. Vegetables high in vitamin A are fine to eat in pregnancy. The risk of excessive intake applies to animal foods, where vitamin A is in the form of retinol.

- Eat raw vegetables as well as cooked for maximum goodness. Boiling removes the minerals and vitamins but this does not happen if you steam them or stir-fry in a little light oil.
- There is a huge range. Some more unusual vegetables include kelp or seaweed (wakimi, nori and arami), a rich source of iron and minerals.
- Organic vegetables are safer to eat because they are free of pesticides, and better for you because the soil is likely to contain more minerals.
- You can eat the skins too, which hold much of the goodness.

Pulses – beans, peas and lentils

These are good sources of vitamins (particularly the B group), minerals and protein. Soya beans also contain all the amino acids essential for a normal diet.

- Great for soups, stews, curries and pastes.
- When they are allowed to sprout, beans are easier to digest and contain more minerals. They keep for a few days in the fridge and are a delicious, crunchy addition to salads and sandwiches.
- Buy soya beans in bean form, tofu or as soya milk.

What to avoid

- Cut down if you feel bloated or have flatulence.
- Look out for added salt in tinned beans and soak and boil all dried beans as the pack instructs.

Fruit

Eat fruit for their vitamin (mainly vitamin C), roughage and mineral content.

- Eating a whole fruit (with skin or pith) gives energy for 1–2 hours longer than a fruit juice.
- If you find it hard to eat enough fruit, build it into your meals: chop a pear into breakfast cereal, add berries to yoghurt or chop an apple or pineapple into salad.

What to avoid

- Eat fruit daily but stick to three pieces on average as more may cause weight gain.
- Hard fruits like apples and pears contain less sugar than soft fruits like grapes or plums; dried fruits are very sugary.
- Bananas are fast-burners and best consumed infrequently.
- Beware of fruit juices; they are deceptively high in sugar content.

Meat

Meat is high in protein and calcium and a range of vitamins and minerals, yet high in fat. So it is best to consume meat in moderation, to make up no more than 10% of your daily intake.

- Poultry is less fatty than red meat, which is filled with saturated fats that can be harmful for the heart.

What to avoid

- In pregnancy, avoid all uncooked meat (e.g. paté) to prevent toxoplasmosis and other infections and if you reheat cold meat, do it thoroughly.
- Avoid liver and liver products that contain more vitamin A than recommended.
- Non-organic meats may contain added antibiotics and hormones.

Fish

Fish is packed with vitamins, minerals, protein and essential fatty acids, including omega 3 fatty acids, recommended for pregnancy and essential for your baby's development.

- Oily fish (sardine, mackerel, tuna and salmon, trout and herring) are excellent sources of essential fatty acids and vitamin D – aim for three sea fish meals a week.
- White fish (cod, whiting, haddock, etc.) is a rich source of vitamin B12 and protein.
- Grill or bake fish with very little oil – if you deep-fry, you'll lose much of the goodness.

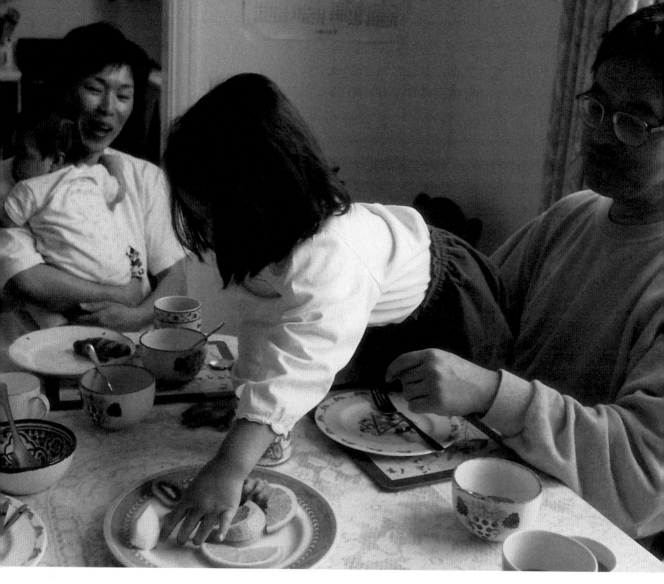

- Tinned fish contains minerals and vitamins but processing removes most of the omega 3 fatty acids, so essential for a heathy pregnancy.

What to avoid
- Don't take fish liver oils because they contain vitamin A in levels not recommended in pregnancy.
- Farmed salmon is not as nutritious as wild salmon and may contain high levels of mercury, as may swordfish, shark or fresh tuna.
- Fresh-water fish is more likely to contain pesticides.
- Avoid raw fish – it may carry infection.
- Choose tinned fish soaked in brine rather than oil to keep calories down.

Dairy products
Dairy products are a good source of protein, vitamins (mainly B), minerals and calcium, but they are high in calories and saturated animal fats. They are great for children, who need fat and calcium for growth, but adults need them only in moderation.
- Yoghurt is the easiest dairy product to digest. Choose live, 'bio-' or pro-biotic yoghurt, which contains natural inhabitants of the gut (lactobacillus acidophilus and bifida bacteria) to improve digestion and increase resistance to infection.
- If you are on antibiotics, bio-yoghurt helps to replace lost bacterial flora in your gut.
- If you want to cut back or avoid dairy products altogether, substitute calcium intake with nuts, seeds, pulses, cereals, leafy vegetables, beans and soya milk, tofu, fish and meat.
- A carefully planned dairy-free diet can provide enough nutrients to nourish your baby and sufficient calcium to replace any bone-mineral loss that occurs during pregnancy.

What to avoid
- Switch to semi-skimmed or skimmed milk, which contains all the mineral goodness but less fat.
- While you are pregnant avoid unpasteurised milk and soft and blue-veined cheese, which can contain harmful listeria bacteria unless fully pasteurised.
- Fruit yoghurts often contain a lot of added sugar, so it is preferable to add your own fruit to plain pro-biotic yoghurt.

Eggs
Eat eggs for protein, minerals and vitamins, especially vitamin B12.
- Eggs are an easy fast food as long as they are fresh and well cooked. Scramble, boil or poach them.

What to avoid
- Fried eggs pile on the calories – cut down.
- Avoid mousses or mayonnaises or dishes made with raw eggs (risk of salmonella infection), especially when pregnant.

Nuts and seeds
Nuts and seeds are available in many different forms and are excellent sources of essential fatty acids, protein, calcium and slow-burning carbohydrates.
- They make good snacks and add flavour to salads and stir-fries.
- Nut spreads are nutritious.

What to avoid
- Avoid fried or heavily salted nuts.
- Peanuts in your baby's diet are best avoided as a precaution against nut allergy, and if you have allergic tendencies, avoid them while you are pregnant and if you are breastfeeding.

Foods that do not nourish
It is best to keep your consumption of processed foods to a minimum. In most cases this is simply because they have little nutritional value or an excess of fat, salt or sugar. While you are pregnant, particularly during the first trimester, you may need to avoid foods that carry a risk of infection or disease. The principle for risky as well as non-nutritional foods is 'prevention is better than cure'. Don't worry if you have already slipped up because the effects depend on how much you have consumed and over what time period.

Processed food
Processed food may contain additives, emulsifiers, gelatines, stabilisers, food colourings and flavourings, some of them listed as E numbers. They are chemically based and may have negative long-term effects on health.

- Some processed food is made with the minimum of additives and may contain nutrients you wouldn't otherwise get from your diet, e.g. nut spreads. Check the labels closely.

What to avoid
- Steer clear of heavily processed foods whenever you can. You may need to dramatically rethink your basic food stocks, change your shopping habits and shift to fresh produce.

Sugar
Sugar is a good source of quick energy but too much may lead to weight gain and tooth decay, and causes peaks and troughs of energy. Sugar does not contain vitamins, minerals or fibre.
- Provided your diet is balanced and nutritious, it's fine to eat sugary foods in moderation.

What to avoid
- Cut down or avoid sweets, chocolates, biscuits and highly sugared, processed foods.
- Cut out colas and sweetened soft drinks and fruit juices as these are a potent cause of weight gain as well as poor dental health.
- Try to shift gradually to slower-burning carbohydrates so you don't need to boost your energy with sugar.
- Artificial sweeteners may be harmful to your health in the long term – they certainly do not contain any goodness.

Salt
Salt helps to maintain fluid balance, regulate blood pressure and supports the nervous system. Too much salt is harmful – it promotes fluid retention and raises blood pressure and may cause your body to excrete an excessive amount of calcium.
- You only need 1 level teaspoon of salt a day, and much of this comes from fresh produce. When a dish really needs salt, use sea salt, which contains a variety of minerals but has not been treated with chemicals that make it flow easily.
- You could substitute herbs or spices for salt in your cooking to add new flavours – try lemon juice, garlic or pepper.

What to avoid
- Try to avoid processed foods and salty snacks like crisps, and adding salt to your meals. Over the years this can lead to a preference for salty flavours and it may subsequently take you months to change your taste and avoid craving it.
- Your baby cannot process sodium so never add salt to her meals.

Wonder foods

Many plants that are used in every-day cooking also have healing and strengthening properties and are commonly used as herbal medicines. Each of the foods listed below has particular benefits, and can become part of an extensive and imaginative diet.

Alfalfa sprouts: High in calcium and vitamin K, which increases blood clotting and therefore reduces the likelihood of heavy bleeding; they help lower blood cholesterol.
Almonds: Rich in protein and minerals.
Apricots: Extremely rich source of iron. When dried, use the dark or Hunza apricots.
Artichoke (globe): Helps to support and improve liver function and thus the function of the whole digestive system; improves bowel function and helps to reduce nausea.
Asparagus: High in folic acid, vitamin C and potassium. It is a natural diuretic and also supports liver and bowel function.

Barley: Rich in protein, vitamins and minerals. It also helps to reduce cholesterol and is a very nourishing source of food. Barley water is famously good for urinary infections.

Cane molasses: Extremely rich in iron (take a dessertspoonful daily).
Carrots: Rich in a wide range of vitamins (A, B and C) and minerals; they aid poor digestion.
Celery: Rich in minerals; supports kidney function and is generally cleansing; well established reputation for use in arthritis and rheumatism.
Chickweed: Chopped fine and used in salads, it is highly nutritious; try cooking it with spinach and/or combine into a soup. It has traditional use for soothing rheumatism.
Chicory: A bitter form of lettuce that stimulates liver function.
Coriander: A highly nutritious herb, rich in iron, which can be used extensively in salads and cooking. Increases lactation; used in cooking, the seeds aid digestion.
Cranberry: The juice reduces urinary infections.

Dandelion: The leaves are generally cleansing and nutritious; they contain substantial amounts of potassium and are a bitter tonic for the kidneys; helpful for joint and skin problems. Chop finely and add to salads or blanch and eat as a vegetable.
Dill: Aids milk production and digestion and relieves flatulence. Relieves cramps and colic in babies.

Echinacea herb: Available in tonic and teas, this is a powerful boost for the immune system in adults (but not suitable for your baby).
Endive: Another bitter form of lettuce, which stimulates liver and digestive function.

Fennel: Highly effective in increasing milk supply after birth and as

a digestive aid; eases flatulence and colic in babies (may be safely given as weak infusion). Also relieves water retention and bloating.
Fig syrup: Very effective in relieving constipation.

Garlic: Good for just about everything. Daily use strengthens the immune system and reduces vulnerability to infection, lowers cholesterol, improves circulation and helps to reduce high blood pressure. Wild garlic (ramsons) may be picked in the spring/summer and chopped finely into salads or soups.
Ginger: Helps to warm and increase the circulation; is a digestive aid used to relieve nausea.

Horseradish: Heats the body, so use for fevers, rheumatic conditions and increasing circulation. Stimulates digestion while calming stomach cramps and wind.

Mints: All the mints can be used in salads and cooking to improve digestion and ease indigestion cramps.

Nettles: Contain large amounts of iron, vitamin C and other minerals and vitamins. They increase lactation and tone and strengthen the whole body. Commonly taken as tea or soup.
Nuts and seeds: A rich source of protein, essential fats and minerals. Consider using almonds, cashews, brazils and hazel nuts and sesame, pumpkin and sunflower seeds regularly. Avoid peanuts.

Oats: Especially good for nourishing the nervous system, to relieve exhaustion, stress and anxiety and help restore vitality. Eaten as porridge, muesli and oatcakes.
Onions and chives: Stimulate digestion and increase absorption of food; prevent growth of harmful bacteria in the digestive and urinary systems.

Parsley: Rich in iron and other nutrients; strengthens metabolic functions and relieves water retention.

Seaweed: Rich in minerals and iron; strengthens metabolic functions. Add seaweed to salads, soups, stir-fries and stews.
Sesame seeds: Worth a special mention because they are especially rich in calcium and therefore a good alternative source of calcium when avoiding dairy produce. Sprinkle on salads and food or eat in form of tahini or hummus.
Spinach: Rich in iron, potassium, calcium, vitamin C and other nutrients, it is good for building and restoring body strength.

Thyme: Will improve sluggish digestion and soothe abdominal cramps.

Watercress: Very high mineral and vitamin content and is generally cleansing.

Drinks

Most people are under-hydrated most of the time, which produces the negative effects of dry skin and a sluggish digestion. The best way to provide adequate fluid for your body is to drink water, the most powerful drink at your disposal. Your body is made up of approximately 70% water, which is needed for every process from digestion and absorption to circulation and excretion. If you choose to breastfeed you'll need to drink more than usual and may find that sipping water as you feed your baby helps your milk to flow. Throughout the primal period (and the rest of your life, ideally) the optimum intake of water is between 1.5 and 2 litres (2½ and 3½ pints) daily. It is best to drink earlier in the day to avoid disturbing your sleep at night.

The cheapest and easiest way to get hold of pure water for drinking and cooking is to use a filter to purify tap water. If you are drinking bottled water, choose glass bottles – there is a risk that xenostrogens (foreign oestrogens) may be absorbed from plastic containers. These can affect hormone levels in men, women and children and may be linked to breast cancer. Water that is labelled 'sparkling water' does not necessarily come from a pure or spring source, and may simply have carbon dioxide added to it – it is not as good for you as simple tap water.

- Spring water: water that may have been taken from one or more sources and has undergone a range of treatments, such as filtration and blending.
- Natural mineral water: water bottled in its natural state (without treatment). It has come from an officially registered source and conforms to standards of purity. It will carry details of its source and a mineral analysis on the label.
- Naturally sparkling water: water that comes from an underground source with enough natural carbon dioxide to make it bubbly.
- Sparkling water: water with carbon dioxide added to it during bottling. Sweet fizzy drinks also contain carbon dioxide.

Tea and coffee

These drinks contain a number of toxins including caffeine, which draws water from the body, exacerbates concentration problems and mood swings, hinders iron absorption and can cause anxiety, insomnia, indigestion and even a rise in blood pressure.

Avoid tea and coffee in excess and do all you can to phase out regular use. Caffeine crosses the placenta and travels in breast milk and the effects your baby experiences are likely to mirror your own.

Instead, use herbal and naturally caffeine-free alternatives, as suggested in the box on this page. If you usually have a heavy caffeine intake, cutting down or quitting may not be easy and you may have intense withdrawal symptoms, so plan a gradual reduction. While

Herbal teas and fruit drinks

Water is the first and best drink. You can jazz it up with a slice of lime or have it hot with lemon for a revitalising drink that's also good for digestion.

Tea and coffee contain a number of substances that are of no benefit, affect absorption of vitamins and minerals and contain stimulants that give a short-lived energy rush. Indian tea reduces the absorption of iron and other minerals. As alternatives you could try any number of herbal teas, many of which also act as general tonics. Try one herb at a time and judge how you respond, and when you have got used to the taste and effects of each herb you could use two or three in combination.

You can buy herbal tea bags in a variety of mixtures. If you are familiar with herbs you could prepare your own.

- **Camomile tea** helps relaxation and can diminish morning sickness. Try drinking a mug before bed or when feeling anxious.
- **Caro/vanoh/bambu** are instant caffeine-free coffee substitutes.
- **Fennel tea** helps aids digestion, reduces water retention and bloating and encourages milk production after birth.
- **Ginger tea** is one of the most effective ways to prevent and alleviate nausea.
- **Lime flower, lemon balm, and camomile or St John's wort** may have a calming effect as an infusion ilf you're feeling emotionally turbulent.
- **Marigold tonic** is useful for boosting your immune system, as is echinacea.
- **Nettle tea** helps the absorption of iron and is a good tonic for the kidneys.
- **Peppermint tea** aids digestion and relieves heartburn, wind and nausea, so it's an ideal drink after food. Herbs with similar effects include lemon balm, spearmint and catnip.
- **Raspberry tea** strengthens the womb and may assist contractions, so try drinking a few cups each day from the Week 34 of your pregnancy. Red clover and Lady's Mantle have similar properties and all three encourage hormonal balance.
- **Rooibos (red bush) tea** from South Africa is caffeine-free.
- **Freshly squeezed juice** – fruit or vegetable – diluted with water makes a long drink. But beware of the high sugar content of fruit juices; they are a common cause of excess weight gain. Fruit teas including apple, lemon and orange contain much less sugar than fruit juices.
- **Fruit milk shake** made by blending skimmed milk with peach or berries and a few ice cubes is delicious; although the fruit adds calories so limit to once or twice a week as a treat.

you are doing this, keep your energy levels high with regular meals, a balance of exercise and sleep and a vitamin and mineral supplements.

Vitamin and mineral supplements

A balanced, varied diet, with nutritious meals at regular intervals could supply all the vitamins and minerals that you and your baby require during pregnancy and beyond. But no diet is ideal – like everyone else you may have days when you skip meals or eat badly and even with a balanced organic diet there may be nutrition deficiencies. The mineral content of fruit and vegetables is dependent on the quality of soil in which they grow: many are deficient because soil is poor, has been chemically treated or is over-farmed.

So however dedicated you are to eating well, it's sensible to take a daily supplement. There is a lot of research information to suggest that pregnancies where the parents are well nourished have a lower rate of miscarriage, birth abnormalities and low birth weight. After birth, supplementation helps to replace what your body has lost and helps it to provide for breastfeeding. Beware of the temptation to treat supplements as a substitute for good food: they work best and are most efficiently absorbed when taken in conjunction with a healthy diet.

Vitamin and mineral supplementation needs to be considered in relation to the way different supplements combine if they are to work optimally. Minerals like zinc, iron or calcium don't work effectively unless they are taken as part of a wider vitamin and mineral programme. If you take iron on its own, it will reduce zinc absorption. It is best to take supplements with food, which aids their absorption. Iron, zinc and calcium, however, are best taken at least an hour before other minerals, unless they are part of a multi-mineral pill.

Iron will be best absorbed if you take it on an empty stomach with diluted fruit juice or vitamin C, followed by food an hour later. Indian tea blocks its uptake so avoid it for an hour before and after taking iron. Try drinking nettle tea instead, which can improve mineral absorption and contains iron.

Choosing your supplements

Choose your supplements carefully – not all are equally effective. For example, many iron supplements are difficult to absorb and can cause digestive problems, especially constipation. Iron EAP is an organic iron compound that is suited to women who develop digestive problems with iron supplementation. You may find that a tonic containing iron and other vitamins and minerals is better for you: choose one with high absorbability, and minimal or no yeast, sugar, talc, lactose, preservatives or colours.

Recommendations are given above for vitamin and mineral supplementation during pregnancy and the postnatal period. If you are in any doubt about a suitable mix of supplements, talk to your family doctor or midwife, or consult a qualified nutritional therapist.

Vitamin and mineral supplements

Minimum supplementation for pregnancy and after birth
This will cover all the important vitamins and minerals you and your baby need during the primal period. The amounts, including folic acid and vitamin A, are safe:
• Multivitamin and mineral designed for pregnancy: 1 daily, with breakfast.

Moderate supplementation for pregnancy and after birth
This will cover diets that may not contain sufficient essential fatty acids or vitamin C. The fatty acid and vitamin content suggested is safe during pregnancy:
• Multivitamin and mineral designed for pregnancy: 1 daily, with breakfast.
• *Essential fatty acid: 1 at breakfast, 1 at dinner.
• *Vitamin C (500 mg): 1 daily, before a meal.

Maximum supplementation for pregnancy and after birth
This is necessary if your iron level is low or you have anaemia:
• Multivitamin and mineral designed for pregnancy: 1 daily, with breakfast.
• *Essential fatty acid: 1 at breakfast, 1 at dinner.
• *Vitamin C (500 mg) plus **Iron EAP: 1 daily, an hour before lunch or dinner.

*Avoid essential fatty acids (EFA) and vitamin C if you are taking aspirin or heparin.
**Don't take Iron EAP if you have a history of epilepsy.

Making good nutrition easy

Eating well becomes most enjoyable when it is easy, and over time you will develop ways to cut corners and learn about cooking nutritious food in a matter of minutes. For time-saving techniques you might keep olive oil-based dressing in the fridge; cook large quantities of certain dishes and freeze some ready meals, buy washed salads or have dry-roasted seeds in a jar for sprinkling on your lunch. There are many possible routes to fun and easy eating that don't involve 'fast food' or unhealthy snacks such as crisps and biscuits. You may find it useful to keep lists of the food you want to concentrate on, of recipes for snacks or full-blown feasts, or of herbs and spices that carry medicinal qualities. This way you have a constant visual reminder of the benefits of eating well.

If your attempts to eat well leave you feeling stressed remind yourself to make changes gradually and enjoy all that's good for you. It's worth remembering that eating is not simply a way of giving your body fuel – it's an opportunity to indulge your senses and join with friends and family and socialise. Before and after birth your baby will pick up on the feel-good vibes that flow through your body when you're eating well and enjoying company.

Yoga, breathing and posture

'Yoga is an ideal form of exercise and relaxation during pregnancy. Just as pregnancy is a bridge into parenthood, yoga illuminates a path from the hectic, outward-focused life most of us lead, to a calmer, more peaceful and centred existence, from where we can welcome the birth of our children.' Jill Benjoya Miller, active birth and yoga teacher.

Yoga as balance

Yoga, a practice begun in India thousands of years ago, means 'yoking' or union, and refers to the link between mind and body. The aim of yoga practice is to restore the balance between the two and bring a feeling of peace. Yoga is active relaxation – by stretching and toning your body you will improve your energy and relieve stress. It is safe and beneficial to practise during pregnancy and after birth, providing you work within your own personal limits and do not stretch excessively. Yoga postures developed at a time when people walked everywhere and they were basically fit. Lifestyle is different now, and yoga practice is most effective when done in conjunction with a basic exercise programme that tones the body.

As a discipline, the fundamental purpose of yoga is to achieve comfortable, balanced posture with full, free movement of the diaphragm and lungs. This harmony of body and breath allows you to let go of conscious effort and focus energy on meditation. A vast collection of postures, movements and breathing exercises has been devised and practised over thousands of years to loosen and balance the body, improve circulation and breathing and heighten awareness. Yoga does not have to be followed by meditation or visualisation, although you may choose to combine them. Each time you practise, you stretch, strengthen and balance different parts of your body, boosting overall wellbeing, strength and vitality, and easing physical or psychological ills. Many of the postures look simple but when undertaken with an awareness of the sensations inside your body, the lengthening of your spine and the movement of your breath, they are dynamic and your body becomes simultaneously relaxed and energised.

The guidance in this chapter has been derived from Hatha yoga in a style pioneered by Vanda Scaravelli, an innovative yoga teacher from Italy. Many of the postures have been adapted to suit the changing body throughout pregnancy and after birth, and to help you prepare for labour. For the majority of women who try it, yoga is the perfect way to enhance the enjoyment of pregnancy and relieve common discomforts such as back and pelvic pain, heartburn and exhaustion. After birth yoga is an ideal exercise to begin with when your body is recovering.

One of the greatest benefits of a yoga class is the nourishing effect of sharing with an experienced coach and with other women, some of whom already have children. Breathing and 'opening' together, partner work and massage bring unity and trust and promote honest and open communication that can begin with shared thoughts and grow into long-term friendships.

Yoga with a baby

It becomes harder to make time for quiet yoga practice once your baby is born, or during a subsequent pregnancy when you already have children. Your baby may be happy to lie down and watch and you can hold him during some postures. If you have a toddler he may enjoy imitating your movements and playing around you. You will be distracted but you can still benefit from a few minutes of stretching and relaxing. For more focused practice, use the time when your baby (or children) are asleep or enrol someone to care for them or take them out for a walk while you have 30 minutes to yourself or attend a local class.

Breathing (Pranayama)

Every living creature breathes without conscious effort. From the moment of birth your body is engaged in the continuous and imperative task of inhalation and exhalation, bringing oxygen and energy to every cell in the body, and releasing carbon dioxide. When you are pregnant, this process becomes even more dynamic as you breathe for both yourself and your baby. To achieve stillness, yoga practitioners have used 'Pranayama' meditation for centuries. Breathing awareness is an integral part of yoga postures but a separate time devoted to breathing is a powerful way to connect with 'prana', your life force. Your breath is always there and can become an effective tool to centre and calm you.

The mechanism of the breath

Breathing is not just about oxygen. As you exhale, your diaphragm contracts and curves up against your lungs to push air out. This creates a vacuum in your upper body so air is drawn into your lungs in an involuntary in-breath. As your lungs expand again, your diaphragm presses against your underlying organs (stomach, liver, kidneys, intestines and reproductive organs), creating a massage-like movement through the upper body. This stimulates energy flow and healthy function of all the vital systems.

- *Gentle yoga done with awareness will cause no harm to your baby or your pregnancy and will not bring on premature birth.*
- *Stop any exercise and seek immediate medical care if you have vaginal bleeding.*
- *If you feel dizzy or light-headed in any position, and particularly while standing, lie down on your left side and rest until it passes.*
- *If you experience heartburn, avoid all the forward-leaning positions on pp.350-6.*
- *If you have circulatory problems such as varicose veins or piles, avoid positions that put pressure on the pelvic region (squatting, forward bends). These can be alleviated with daily pelvic floor exercises done in the all-fours or knee-chest position – p.352.*
- *If you experience pelvic pain either in the back or front, avoid open-legged positions. Instead, kneel on or between your feet, sit with legs crossed or straight out.*
- *Use cushions to make yourself comfortable and ease pressure on joints (for example under your bottom while kneeling or under your thighs in tailor sitting).*
- *Whenever your spine feels tired or aches, sit with your lower back flush against the wall.*
- *If you have been advised to rest in bed, you can still do many of the upper-body and leg stretches, which can help maintain your energy and sense of wellbeing.*

Most people, unknowingly, take quick shallow breaths into the upper chest. This is exacerbated in stressful or rushed situations, and when you feel down. The result is that the lungs do not take in enough oxygen and the diaphragm does not massage or stimulate the internal organs and muscles as it might. Damage to the body from insufficient breathing can range from lethargy to digestive disorders. Simple breathing exercises, including regular deep breathing, are very powerful.

Breathing exercises

The following exercises are useful to develop awareness of your breath, and to become comfortable with full, healthy breathing. They can also help you to slow down, soothe anxiety and relax physically. You can do them in any comfortable sitting position, or lying on your back in early pregnancy or postnatally. When you become familiar with the exercises you will feel more confident to rely on your breath in labour (p.152). You may also enjoy combining breathing awareness with visualisation or meditation (p.370).

Getting comfortable

Lie down or sit, making sure your back is well supported with cushions or against a wall. Start each session with the natural breathing exercise and then choose one or two of the other exercises described below. You can do the exercises alone or as part of a longer yoga practice. It may suit you to record the instructions on an audiotape, speaking slowly in a soft voice.

Natural breathing

- Close your eyes. Allow your body to settle and all of your muscles to relax. Take your time. Focus your attention on the flow of your breath and try to let go of all other thoughts. Do not change your breathing pattern in any way; simply observe your natural rhythm and the movement within your body as you inhale and exhale.
- Place you hands on your lower belly or focus on this area. Now follow your breath as it enters and leaves your body and feel the movement of your lower belly rising towards your hands as you breathe in, and moving away as you breathe out. Feel your lungs filling with air each time you inhale, and feel them emptying as you exhale. Notice that this is a natural, automatic process. Feel the wave of breath rising and falling along your spine. Lengthen your spine. Your lungs and rib cage should expand without effort or strain as your breath naturally deepens.
- At the end of the out-breath, there is a brief moment of stillness until the next breath follows. At the end of the in-breath, there is another still point before the out breath begins.
- At the end of each exhalation, try to release a bit more breath, and then a bit more. Gradually you will breathe more fully, with comfort and ease. You may be surprised how revitalising it feels just to breathe healthily, taking in new energy with each breath and expelling all the waste products your body does not need.
- Continue to breathe in an easy, gentle rhythm for a few minutes.

Following each breath and becoming fully focused on its journey quieten the mind and connect you with your source of vital energy. When your body and mind are so still, you heighten your awareness of internal activity and may feel the beating of your heart and the flow of vital energy. Over time you will become familiar and comfortable with your natural breathing. Your body will automatically breathe more fully and you will instinctively use breathing to relax and re-energise yourself.

It may take years to learn to sustain your concentration. If your thoughts intrude, simply try to observe them and let them go without following them and return to concentrating on your breathing. Try not to be despondent if you lose concentration – everyone does at one time or another. Instead, learn to persevere and enjoy relaxing into the stillness of this time-honoured form of meditation.

Counting while breathing

This exercise is easy to do anywhere in order to slow down or calm yourself.

- Inhale to a slow count of four or five, letting your lungs expand gradually to their fullest capacity.
- Pause for a short moment at the top of the breath, staying relaxed throughout your body, then exhale to the same count or just exhale slowly. Repeat several times.

Deep breathing

You may like to use this exercise to ease yourself into your yoga session, or at the end as you relax. It can also be helpful for insomnia.

- Take slow, deep breaths. Empty your lungs completely with the out-breath, pause, and then fill up the entire space when you breathe in. As you inhale, silently tell yourself, 'I'm breathing in one.' On the exhalation, tell yourself, 'I'm breathing out one.'
- With the next breath, tell yourself, 'I'm breathing in two. I'm breathing out two,' and so on, counting up to between five and ten breaths.

Interrupted breath/interval breathing

This exercise is good if you feel short of breath or anxious as it expands your lungs and restores full breathing.

- Begin to inhale slowly, then pause for a moment, without tensing any part of your body. Inhale a bit more, and then pause again. Inhale fully to the top of your breath and pause.
- Release the breath in one long continuous exhalation down the spine.
- After three cycles pausing on the in-breath, pause instead on the out-breath for three cycles.

If you find it helpful, imagine filling a glass with water, one-third at a time, until it is entirely full.

Breathing with sound

Releasing sound with your breath is a natural way to let go of tension and pain. You will instinctively make noise during labour, and it is good to get used to the sound of your voice now so that you don't hold back during contractions.

- Kneel comfortably, perhaps with your buttocks resting on a pile of cushions or a low stool. Relax your shoulders and let your arms hang loosely. As you inhale, slowly raise your arms above your head. Lower your arms as you exhale and make a long, deep 'ooohh' sound. Repeat four times.
- Stretch your arms out to each side at shoulder height. Open your hands. Breathe in fully. Exhale with a deep 'aaawww' sound and bend your elbows, bringing your hands in to cover your heart. Breathe in and open your arms. Repeat four times.

Mumbling breath

This exercise can help you to focus or balance your energy and get used to the sound of your voice as practice for labour.

- Relax your facial muscles, particularly around your jaw, tongue and lips.
- Part your lips very slightly and inhale deeply through your nose.
- As you exhale, let the breath escape your lips very softly and make a light mumbling sound.

Over time mumbling breath should feel more and more like a vibration working its way down your vocal cords and spine. A sensation of warmth and calm may gradually build inside you.

Breathing during labour

You can also practise breathing for labour and birth, as described on p.152. To practise, take a position that feels comfortable – hands and knees may suit you, the upright kneeling position on p.352 or standing – and imagine a contraction rising, peaking and then passing away over a period of roughly 60 seconds.

- Breathe in deeply and slowly at the beginning of the contraction and feel as if you are breathing out the pain with the out-breath. You can move or rock as you breathe.
- Moaning or sighing with the out-breath may further help you – bring the sound up from deep within your pelvis.
- Continue breathing calmly while the 'contraction' lasts and then relax, returning to your natural rhythm of breathing.

Posture

Posture affects the entire body: the way it feels and the way it functions. Good posture helps to improve muscle tone, strength and energy levels. It also improves the circulation of blood and lymph fluids, affecting the way nutrients are fed to every cell and toxins are released. Good posture also enables full, easy breathing, enhancing the supply of oxygen and the release of carbon dioxide for yourself and, when pregnant, for your baby. Once you learn and practice good postural habits, they come automatically and will improve your health for life.

Pregnancy is a wonderful time to improve your posture, as you become naturally more aware of your body and physical sensations. As your pregnancy progresses, it becomes essential to adjust the way you sit, stand and move to alleviate the normal physical pressures of carrying a baby. Correct posture ensures your skeleton evenly supports your weight and takes the strain off your back and pelvic joints. After the birth, for several months or more, your spine, ligaments and muscles are vulnerable while your body returns to its non-pregnant state.

Good posture in practice

Attention to your posture will protect your body in pregnancy and postnatally as you lift, carry and feed your increasingly heavy baby. Think about your back and bend your knees before you pick up your baby and don't lift heavy weights. Make sure your lower back is in a neutral position (neither arched, nor flexed) by centring your weight and lengthening your spine.

Imagine a tree. Its roots extend deep into the soil from ground level, giving support, while above the solid tree trunk and branches grow upwards and blossom. From the pelvis, your legs and feet extend down and gravity holds you to the earth. With this secure foundation, your spine can elongate, enabling you to stand upright and move your upper body freely.

Basic standing is an excellent position for good posture (illustrated and described on p.353). As you get comfortable standing in this balanced position, you will have a strong sense of gravity holding you while your upper body feels light and free. Try walking and turning, carrying and resting again. Wherever you are, standing or walking, brushing your teeth, doing dishes, waiting in a queue or talking on the telephone, try to come back to your central position: feet parallel, weight balanced and spine lengthened. You will feel relaxed and natural in this posture and notice the effects throughout your body.

Getting ready to practise yoga

Whether you are going to practise for 10 minutes or an hour, it is important to be in a quiet, comfortable place where you can relax. Choose a time of day when you generally feel well and unhurried and your home is peaceful.

Have some cushions within reach and a soft belt or tie. You can practise on the carpet or use a yoga mat, which makes practice safer and easier. You'll need a clear wall to sit against. Wear soft, loose clothing.

It is best to eat 1 or 2 hours before a practice, and avoid heavy foods. If you are hungry and want to start, have a light snack or a glass of milk or juice. In this way your body's energy can be focused on your breathing and movements instead of on digestion.

Yoga is an individual experience and relates to how you feel, physically or emotionally, on any given day. Take time before you start in order to focus on yourself. As you practise, try to keep your attention on your body and breath, feeling and respecting the sensations. If a certain posture or breathing exercise does not feel good one day, allow yourself to modify or skip it.

Most importantly, let your breath guide you through each pose. Inhale and exhale in a natural, gentle rhythm. Never hold your breath, as your muscles need oxygen to work and the constant flow of the breath keeps your body relaxed. Take your time, even if you only have a short while to practise a few poses. Move into and out of each pose slowly, holding the position only as long as you can keep it soft and fluid with your breath, and without straining. Try to keep the muscles of your face and neck and the rest of the body free from tension. Rest between poses. It is ideal to start and finish each yoga session with a few minutes of relaxation, sitting or lying in a comfortable position and breathing easily.

Antenatal yoga sequence

As you practise yoga, listen to your body and keep within your limits of comfort. Choose a space where you feel comfortable and won't be distracted and take a few minutes to become aware of your breath and the way your body is feeling. Acknowledge your thoughts, any concerns or excitement that distract you, and try to let them go – they can wait as you refresh your body and mind.

Neck release (quieten your mind)

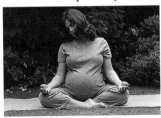

Sit comfortably with your ankles crossed, or kneel. Relax your shoulders and feel your lower body (pelvis and legs), releasing towards the floor. Let your head fall forwards. Breathe softly and enjoy the stretch at the back of your neck. Slowly roll your head to one shoulder, then back and around. Pause wherever your neck feels tight or tender, breathing and releasing tension with the exhalation. Keep your jaw, shoulders and knees soft. Circle your head several times, alternating directions.

Quiet sitting (turning inward)

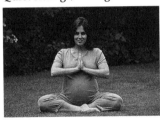

Sit comfortably with your ankles crossed. Sit just on the edge of a firm cushion (or yoga block) to support your spine. Centre your head, then drop your chin slightly to lengthen and open out the back of your neck. Bring your hands together in front of your chest. Relax your shoulders. You may wish to close your eyes. Let your breath flow naturally and become aware of its movement along your spine. With each breath, the sacrum and tailbone release downwards and your spine lengthens up from the waist.

Note: If your back aches, try sitting against a wall. The back of your pelvis and lower spine should be flush against the wall. If your legs or ankles are stiff, place a firm cushion under each thigh for support. If you have pain in the front and centre of your pelvis, avoid open-legged positions. Instead, sit with your legs outstretched and knees together, or kneel.

Easy sitting eagle arms (shoulder and upper spine release)

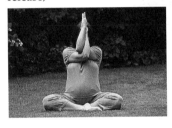

Sit comfortably. Feel your sitting bones rooted to the earth as your sacrum and tailbone release down into gravity. Stretch your arms out at shoulder height, opening your chest and lengthening your spine. Cross your right arm over the left in front of your chest, resting the right elbow inside the left one. Wrap your forearms round, bringing the fingertips of your left (bottom) hand against the right palm. Raise your elbows slightly, softening your shoulders, then lower your chin to open the back of your neck. Feel each breath expanding the back of your lungs and spreading behind your shoulder blades. With each exhalation, release tension from your upper spine and shoulders. Hold for several breaths, then unwind and shake your arms. Repeat with the left arm on top.

Kneeling with cow arms (shoulder and upper arm release, opening the chest)

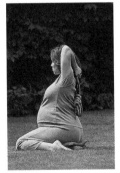

Kneel with a few cushions between your heels and bottom to reduce the pressure through your legs. Let your breath flow softly, deep into your lungs, and feel your lower body releasing down while your spine grows. Holding a belt or cloth tie in your left hand, raise that arm over your head and drop your hand (with the belt) behind your neck. Stretch out your right arm, then bring it behind your back and take hold of the hanging belt, as high up as possible, or hold your fingertips if you can reach. Tip your head forwards away from your arm. Stretch up through your top elbow, opening your chest. Gradually work through the tension in the shoulders and upper arms and let your spine elongate. Hold for a few breaths, then repeat on the right.

Note: If you have circulatory problems, such as varicose veins, piles or cramping, or stiff knees or ankles, it is best to sit on a low stool or a big bolster cushion and then place your knees down on the floor. For slight discomfort in the ankles, try kneeling with a small cushion under the front of your feet until they become more supple.

Tailor sitting (nourishing the pelvis)

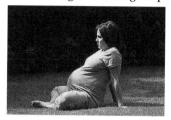

Sit on the edge of a cushion. Bring together the soles of your feet and draw them in, letting your knees drop towards the ground. Place a cushion under each thigh to allow your hips and inner thighs to stretch gradually with support. Rest your hands on your knees. Take several gentle, flowing breaths and have a sense of gravity drawing your knees downwards with each exhalation. Do not bounce. Place your hands on the floor behind you and lean back, keeping your spine straight (not arched or sagging). Release your head comfortably forwards. Take long, full breaths, imagining the inhalation entering your feet and travelling through your legs and pelvis, enriching your womb and expanding in your chest, then rising to the crown of your head. The inhalation nourishes you and your baby and moves vital energy through your body. Imagine the long exhalation moving down from head to feet, carrying away your fatigue, anxiety and tension and leaving you feeling light and fresh.

Note: This position enhances circulation to the pelvic region, and can improve varicose veins and piles and increase hip flexibility. Avoid it if you have pain in the front of the pelvis. If you have pain in the back of the pelvis ease the position by placing your feet further out in front of you.

Legs outstretched (lengthening the spine)

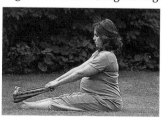

Sit on the edge of a cushion with your legs outstretched and feet together. Wrap a soft belt around the balls of your feet. Keep your shoulders and elbows soft as you hold the belt. Lengthen your spine. You should not be leaning back or pulling on the belt. Extend your heels to feel a pleasant stretch along the back of your legs. Relax your knees and the front of your thighs. Imagine the S-shaped curve of your spine, from the tailbone up to the top of your neck. Feel your breath rolling up and down, softly touching each vertebra. Breathe for a few minutes in this position, with great awareness of the movement of your breath. As you become comfortable sitting and breathing in this position, your spine will feel invigorated and strong.

Reaching up with legs apart

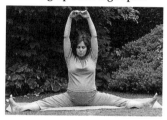

Spread your legs as wide as you comfortably can and pivot on to the front of your sitting bones, with your spine straight and tall. Extend your heels and soften your knees, enjoying the stretch at the back of your legs. Touch the floor with your fingertips, shoulders relaxed and chest open. With a long, slow exhalation, raise your arms. As you breathe, focus on opening. Create lightness through your upper body, making room for your abdomen and for the expansion of your lungs. This is especially helpful later in pregnancy when your breath may feel shallow or constricted.

Side stretch with legs apart

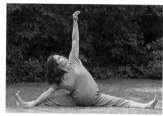

Sitting with legs apart, rest your right hand on your right knee. Inhale, stretching up the left arm and let your right hand slide along the leg. Look up to your left hand. Take the breath into your fingertips and as you exhale release your sitting bones into gravity. Keep your top shoulder back so your chest is open. Hold the position for 4 breaths. Release and repeat on the other side.

Seated twist (spinal rotation)

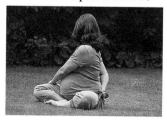

Sit comfortably on the edge of a cushion, with your ankles crossed. Wrap a soft belt around your left knee and hold the ends of the belt in your left hand, behind your back. Stretch your right arm behind your back and take the belt in your right hand. Let your empty left hand rest on your knee. Breathe evenly, relaxing your shoulders and growing through your spine. Have a sense of gravity holding your pelvis. On an exhalation, slowly turn towards the right, letting the movement begin at the base and travel up the spine and through the neck, until finally you gaze over your right shoulder. Let your breath flow up and down your spine, keeping the posture soft and fluid. Turn back to the centre slowly. Repeat on the right.

Note: This position nourishes and invigorates the spine. It is important to turn slowly, and move with awareness to your breath.

Cat arch (spinal release)

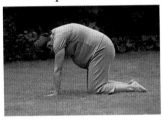

Come on to your hands and knees, with your hands directly under your shoulders and your knees parted. Keep your spine long and straight. Inhale gently and relax. As you exhale, drop your head, tuck your pelvis under, and arch your spine as if you are pushing away from the ground, like a cat when it stretches. Breathe evenly, lengthening from your tailbone to the top of your neck. Sense the release of compression from between the vertebrae. Hold the position through a few breaths, or stretch on each exhalation and release on each inhalation, as it feels comfortable. Try to keep your abdomen and thighs relaxed. This stretch, done several times throughout the day, offers wonderful relief for backache.

Note: This may aggravate heartburn. An alternative is to kneel in front of a wall and extend your arms up the wall, dropping your pelvis and stretching up through your spine and shoulders.

Upright kneeling (labour practice)

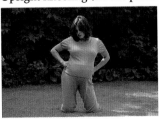

Kneel upright with a cushion under each knee. You can lean on to a low table or the seat of a chair if this is more comfortable. Relax your head, neck and shoulders. Gently close your eyes, letting go of conscious thought and turning inwards to feel the sensations inside your body. Take long full breaths, in through your nose and out through your mouth. Roll and sway your pelvis, moving freely and without inhibition. Let your breath flow softly and continuously. Surrender control. Just breathe and move with the feelings.

Pelvic floor exercises

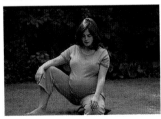

Choose a comfortable position, half kneeling or half squatting, as pictured, and use a cushion if you like, or on your elbows and knees (knee-chest position). Take a few easy breaths to relax your entire body, including your jaw, hands, abdomen and thighs. Close your eyes and visualise your pelvic floor muscles. Let your breath flow easily. As you exhale, squeeze all around the vagina and back passage, lift deep into the pelvis and hold for 2 seconds. Release slowly, with control, and completely soften around the perineum and sphincter muscle. Repeat these quick lifts 15 times. Then do each lift in three stages, pausing at intervals and squeezing deep inside the pelvis. Release and soften in one long, slow motion. Repeat 10 times. Finally isolate your sphincter muscle (anus) and do 10 quick lifts.

The strength and tone of the pelvic floor muscles – developed through squeezing and lifting – help to support the heavy pregnant uterus. During birth, good muscle tone aids the necessary rotation of the baby so he can move smoothly through the birth canal. By consciously releasing and softening the pelvic floor you are conditioning your body to open more easily during birth. Pelvic floor exercise also increases circulation to the entire pelvic region and can relieve symptoms of piles and varicose veins (pp.523 and 559). After birth do at least 50 daily, working up to 100, until you can do them easily. Then repeat several times a week, throughout life, to maintain pelvic/genital health.

Deep squatting (increasing flexibility in the pelvis)

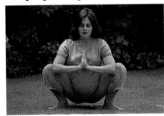

Stand with your feet slightly apart and your toes pointing out. Exhale and bend your knees, lowering your pelvis, until you are squatting. Keep your knees and ankles open and strong, taking care they do not collapse inwards. Place cushions or a rolled yoga mat under your heels if you need support, or try squatting with the back of your pelvis touching a wall. Soften your pelvic floor. Feel the increased space in your pelvis and visualise your baby, head down, descending towards the birth canal. Hold the position through five easy breaths, letting the exhalation flow down and out through your centre. To move out of the squat, place your hands on the floor and kneel forwards.

Note: Deep squatting should be avoided during the last 6 weeks of pregnancy if your baby is breech or if you have varicose veins, haemorrhoids, pain in the back or front pelvic joints or lower back pain. Instead, sit on a stool with your knees no higher than your pelvis and your back flush against a wall.

Mountain pose (basic standing posture)

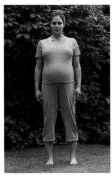

Stand comfortably with your feet a hip-width apart. Turn out your heels so the outer edges of your feet are parallel. Sense your sacrum and tailbone releasing, as if you have a heavy tail hanging down, but do not tuck under your pelvis. This helps to undo compression of the pelvic joints and lower spine. Soften your kneecaps and thighs, relax your shoulders down and back, and let your arms hang at your sides. Do not arch your back. Feel your head at the centre of the top of your spine, with your chin very slightly down to lengthen the back of your neck. Breathe gently. When you exhale, let your heels drop down and the soles of your feet spread. You will feel a release at the back of your waist, knees and neck, which allows the spine to grow. As your spine realigns itself, the connecting muscles become balanced – uneven tension is released and your lungs can expand easily.

Note: It may not be comfortable to stand for a long time during pregnancy. Do what feels comfortable and do not strain yourself. If you feel dizzy or faint, lie down immediately on your left side until it passes. For minor discomfort, try swaying gently for just a short time while you stand. If you have high or low blood pressure, stand for short periods and only while you are completely comfortable.

Triangle with raised arms (pregnant warrior)

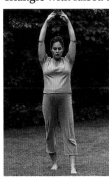

From the basic standing position, have a keen sense of your weight, evenly balanced and dropping through your heels. Shift your weight over your right foot and take a small step forwards and slightly out with your left foot. Your legs form a triangle. Let most of your weight drop through your right leg and into that heel, anchoring the back foot to the floor. Quieten your feet. Breathe and relax through your upper body. With a soft, slow exhalation, float your arms up until they stretch above your head. From the waist down your body is strong and sturdy. From the waist up it is light and free to grow. Keep breathing and opening while the posture feels dynamic. Rest, then repeat with the left foot at the back.

Standing forward bend (elongating the spine)

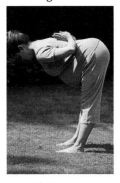

Stand with your feet slightly wider apart than your hips, heels turned out. Feel your weight dropping through your heels. Bring your palms together behind your pelvis, then raise your fingertips to the middle of your back. (If this is uncomfortable or you are arching your lower spine, hold one wrist in the other hand behind your pelvis.) Release your sacrum and grow with your breath. On an exhalation, slowly bend forwards from the hips. Keep your chest open, shoulders back and spine long. Relax your head. Breathe, dropping your heels and lengthening your spine. Move out of the posture by bending your knees, tucking under your pelvis and rolling up through your spine.

Note: Do not hold the posture long if you have high or low blood pressure.

Stork pose (full body stretch)

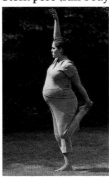

Stand arm's width from a wall to your right side. Touch the wall for balance if you need to. Focus ahead. From the Mountain pose, shift your weight over your right foot. Bend your left knee, taking hold of your left foot behind you to stretch the front thigh. Once you are steady, slowly extend the right arm over your head. Let your sacrum slide down and lengthen the lower spine. As you breathe, drop the right foot into the floor and stretch up into your fingertips. Enjoy growing and opening with your breath. Turn and repeat on the left.

Deep relaxation

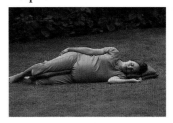

Lie on your left side with cushions between your knees to balance your pelvis and avoid strain. Stretch your right arm up, then extend it along your right side and rest your hand on your hip. Let go of the weight of your body, allowing the earth to cradle you. Try to relax deep within your body, letting go of busy thoughts. Be soothed by the gentle rhythm of your breath. Let it warm and massage the tender places in your body, and release fatigue and tension with the exhalation.

Postnatal yoga sequence

Basic lying position (deep abdominal breathing)

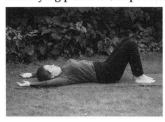

Lie on your back with knees bent and parted. Position your feet a hip-width apart, heels turned out, comfortably close to your bottom. Your arms can be at your sides or outstretched behind your head. Centre your head, then lengthen the back of your neck by tucking in your chin slightly. Inhale deeply, feeling your abdomen expand. Exhale slowly, releasing your lower spine to the ground and pulling in your abdominal muscles. Feel your spine lengthening towards your tailbone. Rest for a moment at the end of the exhalation before the new breath begins. Breathe deeply for a few minutes to begin to tone your abdominal muscles and to relax.

Raised arms and legs (relaxation into gravity)

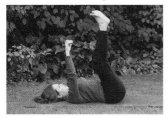

From the basic lying position, raise your arms and legs into the air. Soften your elbows and knees and feel your arms sinking into your shoulder sockets and your legs dropping into your hips. Breathe naturally, and on the exhalation be aware of the pull of gravity on your spine and limbs. Enjoy being held by gravity.

Crossed arms (upper spine release)

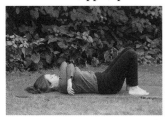

From the basic lying position, stretch your arms out to the side and breathe, feeling your lungs and rib cage expand. Then hug your chest, feeling your shoulder blades spread and your upper spine release. Relax your hands and lengthen the back of your neck. Take the breath into the back of your lungs. On the exhalation, concentrate on letting go of tension along your spine. After several breaths, stretch your arms out to the sides, letting your chest expand, then cross them the other way and repeat.

Supine charioteer (long leg stretch)

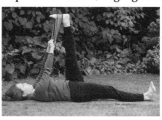

From the basic lying position, draw your left knee into your chest. Wrap a belt around the ball of your left foot, then stretch that foot into the air, straightening your leg. Soften your elbows and shoulders so as not to create upper body tension. If your lower back is strong, stretch your right leg along the floor, otherwise keep the knee bent to protect your lower spine. Extend both heels. Breathe into the soles of your feet and the backs of your knees as you lengthen both legs. For a longer stretch, hold the belt in your left hand and lengthen the right arm along the ground behind your head. Stretch all along your right side from foot to fingertips.

Bridge posture/pelvic tilt (strengthening the lower spine)

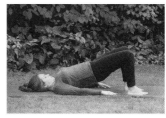

Start in the basic lying position with your arms along your sides, palms down. As you breathe quietly, feel the soles of your feet dropping into the floor, as if you are sending down roots. On an exhalation, draw in your navel, pressing your lower spine into the ground and tilting your pelvis. Using the strength in your thighs, lift your pelvis a few centimetres off the floor. Keep your pelvis tilted and your spine lengthening as you breathe into your spine and lift. To release, slowly roll your spine on to the floor from your shoulders down to your tailbone. Rest, then repeat.

Little boat (lower spine release)

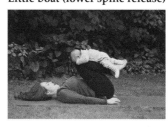

Lying on your back, draw your knees into your chest, one at a time. You can rest your hands softly on your knees. Slowly roll your knees as if you are drawing circles. Enjoy the massage of your spine and the back of your pelvis against the ground. As you exhale try to let go of tension and fatigue. Do this whenever your back feels tired or sore. This is also a good way to rest in between postures.

Spinal rotation (nourishing the spine)

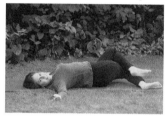

Lying on your back, stretch your arms out just below shoulder height and relax your shoulders. Cross your left leg over your right. Just after birth and whenever your back feels weak, do not cross your legs, but hold a small cushion between your knees. You can also use cushions on both sides of your knees. As you exhale, slowly roll your knees over to the left until they rest on the ground or a cushion. Look to the right. Send the breath down your spine, nourishing the places where you feel the rotation and opening of the vertebrae. Try to lengthen along your right side, from shoulder to hip. Turn your head back to centre, then follow with your knees. Rest and breathe. Repeat to the other side.

Yogic sit-ups (strengthening the abdomen and spine)

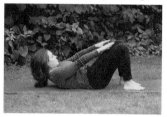

Lie on your back with knees bent and feet parallel. Tuck in your chin slightly. Rest your hands below your navel. Take several long, full breaths, releasing your lower spine down and feeling the movement of your abdominal muscles. On an exhalation, pull in your navel, press your lower spine into the ground and slowly slide your hands up your thighs to your knees, lifting your upper spine, shoulders and head off the ground. Inhale, holding the position. Keep your neck and shoulders soft. Exhale and roll down slowly. Rest and repeat.

Sleeping or supine tailor pose (relaxation)

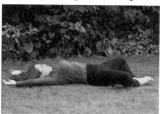

Lie on your back with knees bent, knees and feet together. Just after birth and whenever your back feels weak, place a large cushion beside each hip. Gently part your knees and lower them to the ground or cushions, keeping together the soles of your feet. Let your lower spine rest on the ground – if you feel it arching, concentrate on releasing down. Extend your arms behind your head. Bend your elbows enough to let your shoulder blades rest comfortably on the ground. Breathe gently and relax.

Extended cat arch (dynamic leg and spine stretch)

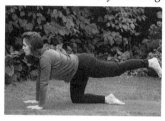

Come on to your hands and knees, with your weight evenly balanced. Raise your head just halfway, so as not to arch your spine. Breathe and lengthen your spine from the top of your neck to your tailbone. On an exhalation, draw your left knee into your chest, drop your head and pull in your abdominal muscles. As you inhale, lift your head and stretch your left leg, extending your heel. Lengthen your spine instead of arching. You will feel increasing strength through your abdomen, back and leg, and a stretch at the front of your hip. Repeat a few times, then switch sides.

All-fours warrior (strengthening through balance)

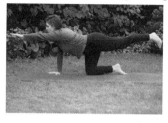

Come on to all fours, hands in line with your shoulders and knees directly under your hips. Focus your gaze ahead. When you feel steady, stretch your left leg back, toes on the ground. Slowly lift that leg, then lift and stretch your left arm in front of you. Lengthen your spine. You may wobble slightly – breathe and quieten your right hand and foot on the ground. Hold for a few seconds. Repeat on the right. Balancing postures create a sense of inner calm and strength. When you achieve balance you may experience great freedom and release through your body. The more you practise, the longer you will be able to hold the position. If this isn't comfortable, begin by stretching the opposite leg and hand.

Dog posture (opening the back of the neck, waist and knees)

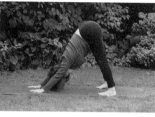

Come on to hands and knees, with your toes tucked under. Breathe easily, releasing your palms into the ground. On an exhalation, slowly lift your pelvis and stretch your legs, dropping your heels. Tuck in your head and extend your pelvis. With easily flowing breath, stretch from the palm of your right hand to the heel of your left foot, then left hand to right foot. Then lengthen from your hands back into your pelvis, and from your pelvis down into your heels. Come down on to all fours and relax in child's pose (next).

Child's pose (resting the spine)

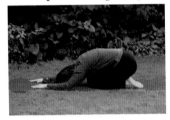

Kneel with your knees and feet together. Place your hands on the floor and walk them forwards until your upper body rests over your legs. Part your knees if your breasts are uncomfortable. Keep your bottom in contact with your heels. Breathe and relax your spine. You can stretch your arms out to release your shoulders, or reach around to your feet and drop your shoulders to release through your upper spine. Lean over a beanbag or pile of cushions if this pulls uncomfortably on your spine.

Cow sitting (balancing the pelvis)

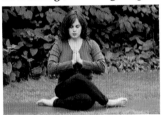

Starting on all-fours, cross your left knee behind the right. Spread your feet wide and ease yourself back to sit between your feet. Place a small cushion under your left hip. Massage into your lower spine and sacro-iliac joints, then shake your arms and hands to release tension. Bring the backs of your hands lightly together in front of your breastbone. Lengthen the back of your neck. Breathe quietly, dropping your knees and shoulders and growing through your spine, as long as the position is comfortable. Stretch out your legs and roll your feet. Repeat, crossing your right knee behind the left.

Dynamic standing stretch

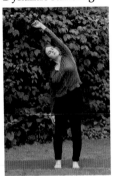

Stand with your feet parallel, hip-width apart. Inhale and raise your left arm, dropping down through your left foot. Reach and extend your arm over your head, letting your right arm slide down your leg. Breathe deeply, lengthening along your left side. Feel the release of tension through your hip, rib cage and shoulder. Gently drop your arm across your front. Stretch four times on the left, stretching straight up on the inhalation and reaching over on the exhalation. Keep the movement flowing with your breath, then hold the last reach through a few easy breaths. Switch sides.

Forward bend (chest expander)

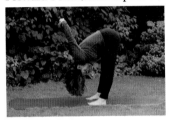

Stand comfortably, with your feet a hip-width apart and parallel. Lace your fingers behind your pelvis. Relax your neck and shoulders. On an exhalation, drop your heels into the ground and slowly bend forwards, keeping your spine straight and long, lifting your sitting bones. Take your time, breathing and enjoying the stretch through your spine and legs. Eventually, raise your arms to release tension from your shoulders and open out your chest. To come up, lower your arms, bend your knees, tuck your pelvis under and slowly roll up though your spine.

Tree posture (balancing, strengthening and growing)

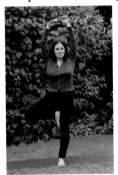

Stand with a wall to your left side. Touch the wall for balance as needed. Focus your gaze ahead. Place your feet apart parallel, your heels beneath your hips. Feel your pelvis centred and your weight evenly balanced. Relax your shoulders. Shift your weight over your left foot, then lift your right foot and place it against your left thigh. Press foot and thigh together and lengthen up from your waist. As you breathe, have a sense of strength through your foundation leg (like a tree trunk) and lightness in your spine and chest. Extend your arms over your head (if unsteady, place your palms together in front of your chest). Turn and repeat on the other side. If this isn't comfortable begin by placing your right foot on your left foot.

Corpse pose (relaxation)

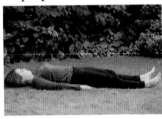

Lie on your back with your legs outstretched and arms slightly away from your sides. Soften your shoulders, hips and knees. Empty your limbs, hands and feet of any stiffness. Close your eyes and breathe in a natural rhythm. Feel the ground along the back of your body. As you exhale, release your spine down, letting any tension, fatigue or tenderness flow into the earth. With each exhalation try to become a little lighter, and let gravity hold you. Inhale energy.

Exercise

'If I can pass on a few tips and perhaps inspire a few women to get active I would feel I had really achieved something. I understand how hard it is to start a programme after a baby, but I would definitely encourage a woman to try. It is one of the best ways to feel better about yourself. When Robbie was born I would often be in my pyjamas at 5pm and I would forget to eat or even have a cup of tea all day. I wish I had known 5 years ago what I know now. But that's experience, isn't it?' Shirel Stemmons, fitness consultant

Why exercise?

The main reason for exercising is to get enjoyment from it. If you do, then other effects will follow – fitness, acceptable weight, heightened energy, buoyant body image, lower stress levels, peaceful sleep, healthy immune system and a glowing smile. You'll also want to continue. The human body is designed to be moved, stretched and challenged and will not work optimally without exercise. Being active and becoming fit will give you a stronger, more youthful and athletic body; neglecting exercise will make you feel lethargic and may contribute to feelings of depression.

Pregnancy and childbirth are physiological upheavals and being a parent is a demanding job. Being committed to a balanced exercise programme will strengthen, stretch, revitalise and relax your body and it will give you a sense of wellbeing. Hand-in-hand with a nutritious diet, it forms the core of your physical health.

Balanced exercise

A balanced exercise programme combines strength training (building muscle strength) and aerobic conditioning (continuous motion, such as walking or swimming).

Strength training increases muscle mass and physical strength through exercises and working with weights. It also encourages your bones to lay down calcium: this increases bone density and helps to fend off osteoporosis in later years. Because muscle is metabolically active, it burns calories even when your body is at rest. The more muscle you have, the higher your resting metabolic rate becomes, and you use more calories while resting.

Aerobic exercise involves continuous training where your body keeps moving and your heart rate stays in an appropriate range for a specific length of time. This raises your metabolic rate (thus burning calories), trains your heart to work more efficiently and tones your muscles.

For best results, exercise regularly. If you stop, the benefits quickly reverse. Set yourself realistic goals that suit your stage of pregnancy or body after birth, and begin with achievable targets. There is no recommended training zone for pregnant women: each person's targets depends on her level of fitness and stage of pregnancy and any symptoms she is experiencing, such as breathlessness or nausea.

Taking care

When you exercise, especially when you are pregnant, it is important to listen to your body. Trust your instincts and do what feels good, and always seek advice from a professional trainer and from your doctor to ensure you have no pre-existing conditions or conditions related to your pregnancy that affect the way you should exercise. You have limitations, and it's best to acknowledge them. Remember that:

- Every pregnancy is different and one woman's experience will be different from another's, and you may feel able to do less or more during different pregnancies.
- You are not in competition with anyone, least of all your past performance.
- Exercise should be balanced with rest and fuelled with a nutritional diet – without these your body will be under strain. Remember too that it's important to warm up and wind down with gentle stretches when you do exercise – you can also use the stretches outlined in the Yoga chapter (p.350).

Ten reasons why exercise is great

1. Increases muscle control and body awareness. As your shape and posture improve, so will your self-image.
2. Increases energy levels, leading to a positive state of mind. Endorphin hormones rise when you exercise, making you feel good and reducing feelings of anxiety.
3. Increases aerobic capacity, building stamina for the demands of labour.
4. Helps your body adjust to the growth of pregnancy, giving better balance and making it easier to bear the extra weight.
5. Strengthens the back and abdominal muscles, improving posture and movement, and reducing aches and pains.
6. Improves muscle tone, supporting the joints through pregnancy.
7. Helps to regulate weight and prevent excessive gain.
8. Speeds recovery after birth.
9. Improves your strength and energy as a new mother.
10. Is good for your baby.

Exercising in pregnancy

As your baby grows, your body will adapt to the increasing load and become more efficient. Pregnancy is a perfect time to exercise. Your body will respond, even though you may not notice improvements as much as you would have before you became pregnant. Your baby will also benefit from your healthy cardiovascular system and your 'feel-good' hormones.

If you are used to working out regularly, you will need to adjust your programme as pregnancy progresses. For instance, you may ordinarily do a step routine on a 20-cm (8-in) platform; by Week 25 a 10-cm (4-in) platform may suffice and still give a good aerobic workout.

If you have never exercised before or have exercised only infrequently, if you begin now your body will adapt to a training regime quickly and easily, whatever level you choose. Take guidance, start gradually and increase time and intensity as you get fitter. It's important not to push yourself, so stay within your comfort zone. Try out a few options because some will suit you better than others. For instance, you may like the motivation of a class environment or prefer to exercise alone. You will need to adjust your routine as your pregnancy progresses.

Strength conditioning in pregnancy

Strength conditioning is the fastest and most effective way to tone and shape your body and builds up the stamina and strength you'll need in labour. If going to the gym is not an option for you, don't worry. You can buy a set of dumb-bells consisting of 1 kg, 2 kg and 3 kg (2, 4½ and 6½ lb) weights. Weights like these do not take up much space and you can use them in your own time, starting with the lightest and building up as you get stronger. You only need to find 20 minutes three to four times a week.

In-studio weight-training programmes are held at most gyms. Unless there is a special class for pregnant women, now is not a good time to join. If you already participate and are familiar with the exercises then it may be possible to continue, but because the instructor will be teaching a group of people, he or she will not be able to give you much individual attention. It's important to get medical clearance from the doctor during each trimester. You will have to modify the programme in the last 6–8 weeks and you may wish to stop this type of training altogether, settling for a gentler programme instead.

The goal of weight training is to maintain joint stability and improve posture with appropriate weights, not to make great advances. It will be impossible to make big strength gains because pregnancy hormones soften joints, which may be damaged if you exceed your limits.

Aerobic conditioning in pregnancy

As part of a balanced programme you'll need to do 20–30 minutes of aerobic exercise three to four times a week.

Choose something that you enjoy, that is appropriate to your fitness level and that you can continue without a break. You should feel physically pushed, but not out of breath. As your pregnancy progresses you may need to reduce intensity or the time you spend exercising.

Step and low impact aerobics: These are safe and effective forms of exercise if you enjoy exercising in a class. Remember to work at your own pace and avoid moves that may affect your balance.

Walking: Walking is a simple and relaxing way to exercise that costs nothing and gives you the added benefit of being outside in the fresh air. Anyone can walk her way to fitness. All you will need is a pair of supportive, well-fitting athletic shoes and a place to walk.

• The pace is in your control. It can be gentle, moderate or at race speed if you are already fit.

• You can walk for 2 hours or 30 minutes. If you walk at a mild pace, you will need to walk for longer to achieve the same training benefits resulting from a short walk at a quick pace.

• Take comfortable strides and let your arms swing naturally. You can create a faster swing by bending them at the elbow, which will make your legs move faster too.

• Push off each step with the toes of the rear foot, allow the ankle full range of motion and land heel first.

• Be aware of your posture. Walk from the waist and keep your tummy tight to prevent your back from arching.

Swimming: Doing aerobic exercise in water makes you feel light because your weight is supported. Most leisure centres and health clubs have aqua aerobic classes for pregnant women. If you can, go swimming regularly and gradually increase the duration or the number of lengths you do. Providing you are disciplined about maintaining a good rhythm and do not take frequent breaks, you will get an excellent aerobic workout. The only downside is that, because your weight is borne by the water instead of by your bones, it does not increase bone density, so swimming should be part of a wider programme.

Cycling: In early to mid-pregnancy, cycling is a good form of aerobic exercise, with the main danger coming from falling off. In late pregnancy, the discomfort of sitting on the saddle may make cycling impossible, although you may not choose to try because your large uterus could alter technique and make your legs turn out at the hip, putting pressure on your joints, particularly at the knees. In the gym the upright rather than recumbent bikes will be more comfortable. The position used and the intensity of 'spinning' classes are not appropriate for pregnancy.

Exercising after birth

After the birth take your time returning to exercise. You may not feel like doing anything strenuous for 6–12 weeks but begin light exercise within 2 weeks. Start with a gentle activity like walking and build up slowly. Pregnancy

Guidelines for safe exercise in pregnancy

- Get your doctor or midwife to confirm that what you're doing is safe during each trimester.
- Exercise regularly and within your natural limits.
- Avoid going to the point of exhaustion. Lower the intensity if necessary and be able to talk during the workout.
- Only 10% of women maintain their pre-pregnancy fitness level. Don't aim to gain.
- Avoid rapid twists, jumps, high impact and rapid shifts in direction. Find your balance, then move.
- Avoid exercises that take any joint to the maximum point of resistance. You will feel more flexible but don't push it – you may over stretch. Be careful not to sway or arch.
- When you stand up, keep your body in good alignment and use the strength of your muscles equally.
- Pay close attention to how you feel. Ask yourself: 'Am I too hot?', 'Am I working too hard?' Ensure that you do not overheat.
- Drink plenty of water before, during and after exercise.
- Warm up before and stretch after exercise.

- Wear comfortable, loose-fitting cotton clothes. Outside, wear layers that you can remove as you get hotter. Inside, make sure the room is well ventilated.
- If you have pain, bleeding or contractions see your doctor as soon as possible. If you experience severe breathlessness, palpitations or faintness during exercise stop immediately.

First trimester (Weeks 0–13)
- Most exercises are safe providing you don't feel nauseous or tired.
- Don't over-exert yourself while your body is changing and your baby's organs are developing.
- Avoid the step machine, which may overstretch ligaments attaching the uterus.
- Begin pelvic floor exercises (p.98). This will help prevent prolapse in the postnatal period.
- If you suffer from intense sickness, dizziness, palpitations, and even fainting you may need to stop or reduce the amount of exercise you do until it wears off (normally Weeks 12–15).

hormones can stay in your system for 5 months or more, particularly if you are breastfeeding, so your joints may still be unstable. If you want to return to strength training, start with low weights.

If you cannot find the enthusiasm or the time, rest assured that many women feel the same. It can be very hard to fit exercise around life with a baby, but it is not impossible. With support from people who can care for your baby while you take 20–30 minutes, three times a week, exercise can be part of your life. The Wheel for Living (p.58) may help you take practical steps to make this a reality.

If you want to begin a new exercise programme, your body will respond well because it is receptive to cardio-vascular training after having a baby. Your heart and lungs have already undergone a training regime through pregnancy because they had to pump an increased amount of blood and circulate more oxygen than before.

Try not to set yourself impossible goals – it will take time to regain your pre-pregnancy shape and longer if you want to improve it. Your joints and ligaments will be soft so allow at least 6 and preferably 12 weeks before you are back to intense activity. Try not to judge your progress by your weight – now is certainly not the time to cut down on calories and if you are building up your muscles you may gain because muscle weighs more than fat. Instead, try to judge your wellbeing by the way you look and feel and use exercise as part of a wider programme of caring for yourself (p.51). If you are breastfeeding, you may find that you lose weight gradually, or continue to carry a couple of extra pounds of fat so that your body can produce enough milk for your baby.

The first few days
After a couple of days of complete rest, you can start to do some gentle walking. Being active within your comfort zone will help your recovery, stimulate your circulation, reduce build-up of fluid and any stiffness you feel. It will also encourage your digestive system to return to normal.

The first 6 weeks
You can start doing pelvic floor (p.98) and certain abdominal exercises (start with belly breathing, overleaf) as soon as you feel able to. These help realign your pelvic joints after birth, help your pelvic floor and abdominal muscles return to pre-pregnancy function, provide support to reduce lower back pain and increase urinary control. Improved muscle control of the pelvic floor also heightens sexual pleasure.

Walking is the perfect way to begin getting back into shape after childbirth. You can start slowly, build up gradually and move on to more intense forms of aerobic exercise when you are ready. You won't need a babysitter or a crèche, you can walk alone or with a friend and with a sling or big-wheeled stroller you can walk on rough ground. Babies enjoy being outside and the motion of mum's body or the stroller is usually very restful. You can also join swimming classes when you feel ready, and take your baby with you as soon as you can (p.219).

After 6 weeks
Increase the duration of your walks and start some strength training, so you get a balanced combination of aerobic conditioning and strength training. This is the best way to reduce excess fat and build a strong, fit, lean body.

Antenatal exercises

Abdominal/waist
Belly breathing

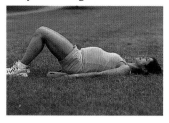

Lie on your back with your knees bent and feet flat on the ground. Raise your head and shoulders up on a couple of pillows. Inhale and inflate the abdominal area making your belly bigger. Then exhale and compress, pulling your navel in towards your spine. Think of flattening rather than shortening the abdominal muscles. During the first two trimesters you can add a forward curl by reaching up your thighs as you exhale and compress, then release back as you inhale. Repeat 8–12 times. Ensure you maintain neutral alignment throughout. If you start to feel uncomfortable or breathless, roll on to your side. Later in pregnancy or from the time you can no longer lie on your back comfortably, perform this exercise on all fours or sitting.

On all fours

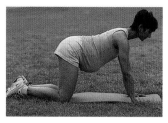

Kneel on all fours and start with your spine in neutral alignment so your back is not excessively flexed or extended. Keeping your back in this position, inhale and inflate the abdominal area, then exhale and contract. Compress and pull in your tummy. Imagine that you are pulling your belly button up towards your spine without arching. Release and inhale, performing each stage slowly, then repeat 8–12 times. Maintain neutral alignment throughout. This is an extremely effective exercise during pregnancy as the weight of the baby plus gravity provides your muscles with excellent resistance.

Sitting

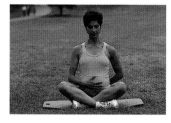

Sit upright with your spine in neutral. If you feel you need support, sit with your back against a wall. Inhale and expand your belly; exhale and compress, contracting your abdominal muscles. Perform this slowly and with control. Repeat 8–12 times.

Legs
Squats B

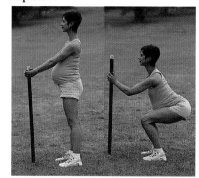

Stand with your legs a shoulder-width apart and your knees and toes parallel. Squat down until your thighs are parallel with the floor. Your knees should only cover the knots of your shoelaces, not your toes. Think of sitting back over your heals, flexing at the hips rather than the waist. As you push up bear your weight on your heals and contract the back of your legs as you extend your hips. Check your spine remains in neutral alignment. Keep your head and chest high and your eyes on the 'horizon'. This exercise should be a low, controlled movement. Repeat 16–32 times or until your muscles feel tired. If you feel unstable, use a chair for support.

Side-lying abduction

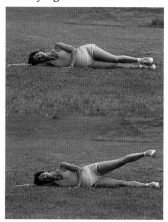

Lie on your side with your bottom leg bent and your top leg extended. Keeping your hips with the top hip directly over the lower, lift the top leg to about 30 degrees then return to your starting position. Don't make the lift too high because if your hips move out of alignment you will not be working the muscle effectively. Repeat 16 times on each side.

Warming-up

Before exercising, warm up for 5–10 minutes. You need to raise the core temperature of your body. The best way to do this is to move the muscles you will be working and increase your pulse rate. Your body will then be prepared for the extra demands of exercise. A good way to warm up is by walking outside or on a treadmill. Follow or combine this with large upper body movements, such as arm swings and circles to loosen up the joints and get the blood flowing.

Chest
Standing press-up

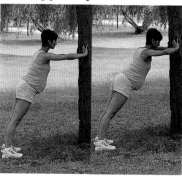

Stand at arms-length from a wall with your feet a hip-width apart and your heels on the ground. Place your hands on the wall slightly wider than a shoulder-width apart. Bend your elbows and lower your body towards the wall keeping your elbows over your wrist and your body in a straight line (make sure your hips remain in alignment and avoid arching the lower back). Push back slowly, returning to your starting position. You can make the exercise harder by increasing the incline and thereby increasing resistance from gravity. Repeat 8–16 times.

Back
Seated row

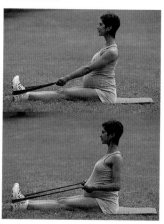

Sit upright on the floor with your shoulders pressed down and back in neutral alignment. Loop an exercise band/tube around your feet and hold it with your palms facing inwards and your arms extended. Squeeze together your shoulder blades and pull back your elbows until your hands are at the side of your rib cage. Return to the starting position with control. Repeat the seated row 8–16 times.

> ### Posture
> Don't forget to check your posture. Poor posture will pull your body out of alignment and put additional strain on your back. Due to the increasing weight of the uterus, your body is pulled forward and you tend to lean back to compensate. This causes increased curvature of the lower back and backache. Once you have warmed up, listen to your body, begin your routine gently and build up slowly. Do each exercise in a controlled manner so you get maximum benefit. It is quality, not quantity that counts.

Reverse flye

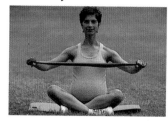

Sit upright in neutral alignment with your legs crossed. Hold the band/tube in front of you at chest level. Your hands should be a shoulder-width apart. Pull together your shoulder blades and as you do so, let your arms follow without extending the elbows. Focus on the muscles between your shoulder blades. Imagine there is a penny between your shoulder blades and you are trying to squeeze it. Return to the starting position and do two sets of 8 repeats.

Arms
Shoulder press

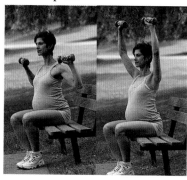

Sit upright on a chair with your knees bent and feet flat on the floor. Hold a dumb-bell in each hand at shoulder level with your palms facing away from you and your elbows tucked into your sides. Extend your arms overhead so your hands move towards each other slightly and avoid locking out your elbows. Bend your elbows and return to the starting position, keeping your elbows close to your sides. Do two sets of 8–12 repeats.

Biceps curl

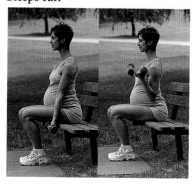

Stand with your feet a shoulder-width apart or sit upright in a chair. With your arms extended at your sides, hold a dumb-bell in each hand, palms facing towards your knees. Slowly curl the arms towards the shoulder, rotating the forearms so your palms face your shoulders at the top. Slowly return to the starting position, keeping your elbows tight to your waist throughout. Do two sets of 8–12 repeats.

Triceps kickback

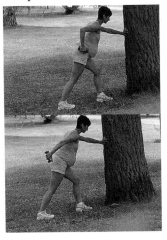

Stand with one leg behind. Lean forwards slightly with one hand on the front bent leg. Hold a dumb-bell in the other hand (the same side as the extended leg) and bend the elbow so it is lifted at shoulder level and your hand is on your hip, palm facing in. From here extend your elbow, keeping the arm close to your body and the shoulder lifted. Return to the starting position. The elbow and shoulder should be in a fixed position throughout.

Postnatal exercises

Abdominals
Standing vacuum

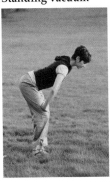

Bend your knees slightly and place a hand on each knee for support. Inhale and fill your lungs and abdominal area, then exhale and suck in your stomach so it is concave. Ensure your back remains in neutral alignment throughout. Be particularly careful you don't flex your spine as you exhale and pull in. Repeat up to 10 times.

Basic crunch

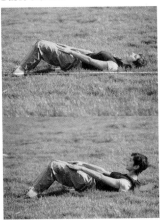

Lie on your back with your knees bent at a 45-degree angle. You should feel comfortable, but you should also feel you need to pull in your abs slightly to maintain neutral alignment. Inhale and inflate the abdominal area, then exhale and compress, reaching up your hands towards your knees as you do so. Keep your tummy tight as you curl up. Inhale and uncurl, returning to the floor. Repeat 8–32 times. Avoid using your neck and shoulders to perform the curl instead of your abdominal muscles. Try to focus on contracting the abdominal muscles before you start to curl and keep them tight until you return to the floor.

Plank

This is an excellent exercise for stabilising your torso muscles. Start this exercise at Level 1 at 6–8 weeks after childbirth then progress to Levels 2 and 3 as you build up strength and confidence. If you have had a caesarean section, wait until 2–3 months after your baby is born, starting with Level 1.

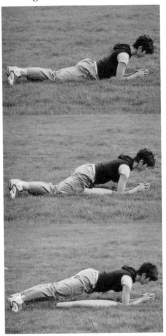

Level 1: Lie on your stomach, upon your elbows, with your hands together. Contract your abdominals, pulling your tummy in until you create a vacuum.

Level 2: Lift your hips off the floor to your knees.

Level 3: Extend your knees into a full plank position. At each stage check your spine is in neutral alignment and you are not pushing your hips up to the ceiling or sinking in the spine. Hold the position for 10–30 seconds.

Legs
Squats
See Antenatal exercises (p.360).

Lunges

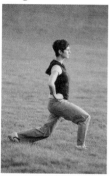

Use the same starting position as for squats. Standing, step forward with one leg, lowering your back knee towards the floor. Keep your front knee over your ankle and both knees at a 90-degree angle at the base of the lunge. Keep your hips in alignment under your shoulders and your tummy tight throughout. Squeeze your buttock muscles and pull the lunging leg back in to standing position. Repeat 8–12 times on each leg. As your strength increases you can hold dumb-bells for extra resistance.

Adductor lifts (inner thigh) and abductor lifts (outer thigh)

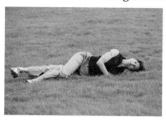

Lie on your side with your body in a straight line. Place one arm under your head for support, the other in front to help you to stabilise. Keep your bottom leg extended and your top leg over in front. Lift and lower your bottom leg, keeping it extended. Focus on contracting your inner thigh muscle, which should be facing up to the ceiling. Make sure your hips remain one on top of the other. You can do this exercise while pregnant, resting the front leg on a cushion. Repeat 8–16 times for each leg.

Chest
Press-ups

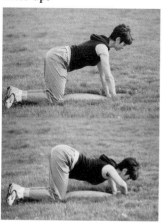

This is a variation of the standing press-ups in the Exercises for Pregnancy section. Kneel on your hands and knees with your knees under your hips. Keep your hands slightly wider apart than your shoulders with your fingers facing forwards. Keeping your head in line with your spine and your elbows over your wrists, bend your elbows and lower your chest to the floor. Keep your abdominal muscles tight so your back doesn't arch as you go down and keep your weight forwards as you come up, rather than pulling back. As you get stronger, you can increase the intensity of the exercise by moving your knees further back to create a longer lever. Be sure you can perform the exercise with good form and your abdominal muscles are strong enough to support neutral alignment. Repeat 8–16 times.

Back
Seated row
See Antenatal exercises (p.361).

Reverse flye
See Antenatal exercises (p.361).

Arms
Shoulder press
See Antenatal exercises (p.361).

Biceps curl
See Antenatal exercises (p.361).

Triceps dip

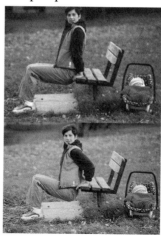

Sit on the edge of a sturdy chair or low bench. Place your hands on the edge of the bench, a shoulder-width apart, with your fingers pointing towards you. Bend your elbows and lower your body to the floor until your elbows are bent at a 90-degree angle. Make sure your bottom stays close to the bench. Straighten your elbows and return to the starting position.

Repeat 8–16 times. You can make this exercise easier by sitting on the floor so your body moves backwards as you bend your elbows, or harder by extending your legs in the bench position.

Stretches

Stretch the appropriate muscle group after each exercise (e.g. follow squats with quad and hamstring stretches) or do a sequence of stretches after you finish exercising in an order that feels comfortable. Stretching during pregnancy is important but be careful not to over-extend. The effects of relaxin will make you feel more flexible, but pushing too far can cause joint instability. Stretching after exercise will reduce the risk of injury, cramp and muscle soreness.

Back

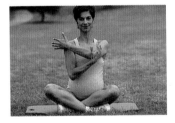

Shoulder

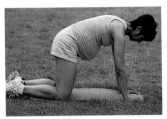

Upper back

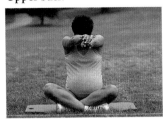

Calf (seated)

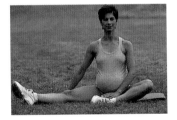

Side stretch

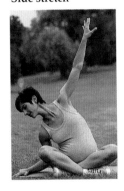

Chest

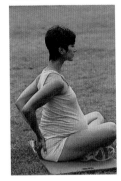

Triceps

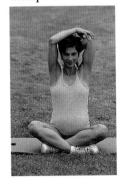

Biceps

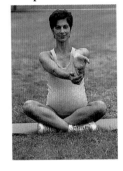

Neck

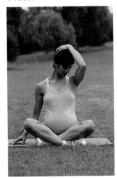

Calf (standing)

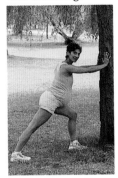

Quads

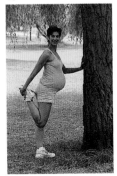

Hamstring

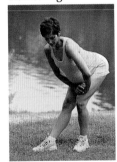

Massage

'Western society has become so impersonal and desensitised to the value of loving touch that from the very first moments of birth many mothers are discouraged from expressing this, by having their babies routinely removed. Disempower any other mammal after such a momentous event, deny her the opportunity to feed or feel her offspring, and the mother will almost certainly reject her newborn or change her mode of behaviour towards it . . . Fulfilling the tactile needs of the baby is the first step towards maintaining the concepts instilled in the womb of a benevolent and caring world.' Peter Walker, baby massage therapist.

The power of touch

Massage has been used since ancient times across the globe to enhance wellbeing and heal the body, ease pregnancy and labour, assist recovery after the birth, and to stimulate and soothe babies. Throughout the east, where mother and child are traditionally given a daily massage, the practice is an essential skill. In many parts of the world babies are massaged until they are a few years old.

Touching and being touched is non-verbal and universal among all mammals. Massage converts this basic instinct into a skill that brings pleasure to both the giver and the receiver. Western parents may not be used to massaging one another. Beginning in pregnancy, it may become a new habit that has great benefit for the family.

In western society massage is now recognised as a complementary form of treatment. There are many types of massage available from a variety of health-care professionals (including Swedish massage, Shiatsu, sports and deep-tissue) but you don't need extensive training to receive its benefits. Couples can massage each other and it is a great way for parents to communicate with their child.

How massage works

The skin and brain develop from the same area in the foetus, and every touch on the skin initiates a mental response. It is obvious that internal feelings and health directly affect the skin; for example, exhaustion leads to dark areas under the eyes, and flushing of the skin reflects moods. Likewise, sensations on the skin can affect moods. Massage stimulates the acupressure points situated along the meridian lines of the body to balance the body's energy, and this also affects the function of all the internal organs. In an experiment in the 1950s, babies were fed but not touched: sensory deprivation caused failure to gain weight, poor muscular co-ordination and apathy. Holding, cuddling and touch are essential for infants to thrive.

It brings emotional pleasure: Being lovingly touched is an expression of affection. The language of touch, ranging from gentle stroking with the pressure of a butterfly to powerful pressure into the deep tissue, has considerable healing power and is a fundamental part of communication with a baby. Developing this in partnership with your child is one of the gifts of becoming a parent.

It relaxes: The parasympathetic nervous system is activated and the endorphin 'love' hormones released. This brings the body back into balance by reducing the metabolic rate, blood pressure, anxiety and improving circulation and sleep.

It promotes growth and development: Stimulation of the tactile nerve endings in the skin provides information about the outside world and helps the brain organise its circuitry. Touch is known as the 'mother sense' and is highly developed in the newborn, whose skin area is relatively large and very sensitive. During massage muscular co-ordination is encouraged and growth hormones flowing from the pituitary gland increase. Premature infants who are touched gain more weight.

It stimulates the skin and boosts the immune system: Massage helps to keep the pores open for the skin to eliminate toxins and the therapeutic effects of oils are absorbed through the skin. It also assists the flow of the lymphatic system that transports immune cells through the body and removes waste products.

It promotes optimum muscular and joint activity: As a muscle contracts, metabolic waste is 'milked' into the venous and lymphatic systems ready for excretion. Over-use does not allow sufficient relaxation time, so waste products are formed faster than they can be eliminated, while under-activity does not provide an opportunity for the muscles to be sufficiently milked. Massage can assist this milking process, reducing the stiffness and soreness that occurs after activity. Together with gentle joint movements it can also help maintain joint mobility.

It reduces pain perception: massage stimulates the brain's release of endorphin 'feel-good' hormones that also act as pain suppressors, and occupies sensory pathways to the brain, 'gating' out some of the pain signals. It also lowers levels of stress hormones and it is very useful in labour.

It aids digestion: Relaxation through massage can help digestion (chronic stress is known to disrupt it). Abdominal massage can aid the elimination process in the large and small intestines. It also influences intestinal functions by stimulating the vagus nerve to facilitate food absorption in newborn and premature babies. Abdominal pain, colic, constipation and indigestion can be reduced by regular massage of the abdomen and the back and babies are particularly responsive.

Massage for mothers

Massage during pregnancy promotes relaxation, helps tone your skin and can relieve nausea, heartburn and headaches. If your partner massages you, he'll feel close to his growing baby, particularly when he concentrates on the abdomen.

Massaging the head, neck and shoulders, all common sites of emotional tension, can bring a sense of relief to the whole body. Massaging the feet and calf muscles is soothing and, along with the postural muscles – back, legs and buttocks – can relieve general fatigue. Massaging your abdomen and breasts with oil rich in vitamin E may minimise stretchmarks. Towards the end of the pregnancy perineal massage will help prepare your vagina for stretching at birth (p.98). When it comes to labour, massage can help enormously by relieving pain of contractions and of pressure on the joints in your pelvis and aiding relaxation. During the birth a skilled midwife can massage your perineum and vaginal entrance to encourage the area to stretch and open.

After birth, being massaged is soothing and you will feel cared for when you are spending most of your time caring for your baby. You could also treat yourself to a session with an aromatherapist. Massaging the calves, thighs and buttocks and the spine, neck and shoulders relieves tired muscles and joints and can help you regain shape and improve posture. The whole body routine is not needed every time – even a simple foot massage can be really relaxing – and one area, such as the lower back or shoulders, may need more attention than another.

Massaging your baby

In the womb your baby is massaged by contractions that reach their height during labour and birth, stimulating his nervous system and awakening his survival mechanisms. After the birth this stimulation continues when he is caressed and held by loving hands, held and cuddled at the breast, preferably with skin-to-skin contact. A mother's touch is instinctive: as you stroke your baby with tenderness, you are massaging intuitively. Fathers are usually just as sensitive. Regular massage brings peaceful togetherness, increases your confidence in handling your baby and allows you to share in your baby's innate and beautiful energy.

When to massage

Periods of massage create space for relaxation and balance in your day. At first your newborn baby may enjoy massage for only a few minutes. In time you will be able to lengthen the sessions. You can start with a single session, perhaps when your baby is alert in the morning, or as part of a bedtime routine, and progress to up to five short sessions every day if you enjoy it and have time.

Good times for massage are at bathtime, when the water will increase relaxation; an hour or two before your baby's usual crying time (often in the evening), or before his usual sleeping time. When your baby is lying or sitting quietly, start by massaging his feet or hands or stroking his face or his body through his clothes. Choose times when you are feeling relaxed and unhurried and your baby is calm but alert.

How to massage

Massage for a baby involves very gentle touching and stroking. It is most effective when your baby is naked, but some very young babies don't like this. Progressing from instinctive touch to massage is a pleasure and a natural transition demanding only sensitivity and love. It is best to begin at birth and gradually increase the frequency as your skill improves and your baby's attention span increases. Your baby will learn to trust your hands and you will learn to feel instinctively when something is wrong, and naturally smooth out tensions in his body.

Choose pure oil such as grapeseed, sweet almond or sunflower oil. If you want to add some essential oil, always do a skin test on your baby first by applying it and leaving for 30 minutes, then checking for an adverse reaction. You could use one of the following, putting 5 drops in 100 ml (3 fl oz) of carrier oil or lotion:

- **Camomile:** noted for its calming effects, good for calming digestion and inducing sleep.
- **Frankincense:** relaxing, and encourages steady breathing.
- **Lavender:** clears nostrils and airways, so good when your baby has the sniffles, and also good after immunisations.
- **Myrrh:** another aid for breathing and to encourage the elimination of mucus.
- **Rose:** for dry skin, though it is expensive.
- **Teatree:** an antiseptic healer, which is good for minor skin infections (e.g. nappy rash) if your doctor has consented.

You may also enjoy burning some essential oil such as lavender or camomile to relax you both, and play some soothing music. Find a warm place where you will not be disturbed – it may be your bedroom or the mat in your bathroom – and take the telephone off the hook and switch off your mobile. Take a few minutes to ease the tension

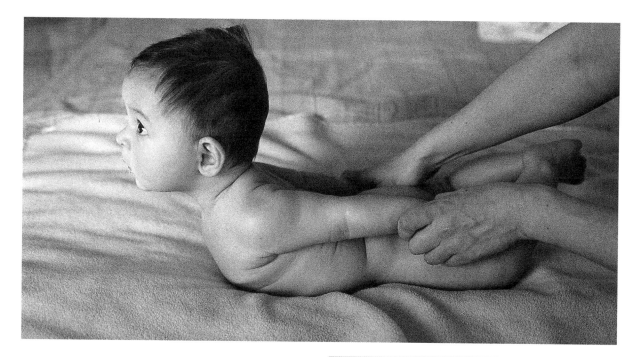

from your face, neck, shoulders, arms and hands and focus on calming your breathing with the emphasis on the outward breath.

Remove jewellery from your fingers to avoid rubbing your baby's skin, check for torn nails and make sure your hands are warm. When you feel ready ask your baby, in your own way, if he would like a massage.

Newborn massage

A good way to introduce massage is to lie on your side facing your baby and, with a well-oiled hand, stroke his upper back in a clockwise circular motion for about a minute. Then massage his hips and the base of his spine for another minute. Now lie on your back and lift your baby on to your abdomen (preferably skin-to-skin) and stroke hand-over-hand down his back on both sides of the spine for a minute or two.

Massage as your baby grows

The basic massage routine will suit you both for months and years to come. As your baby grows, the keys are to take his mood into account, and adjust your technique and the amount of support you give as he grows. For instance, at 6 weeks you may hold him under his arms in a standing position, while at 7 months a light support around the hips will suffice. When you feel ready – from 3 months onwards – you can make massage more dynamic and move into 'baby gymnastics', helping your baby to bend, flex, strengthen and move in a balanced way. If you have a baby massage or exercise class near you, you will be able to learn a number of postures together.

Points to remember
- Always keep your hands well oiled.
- Repeat each stroke several times.
- Never force your baby's limbs into positions.
- Stop if your baby cries and give him what he wants. Sometimes stopping and resting your hands on your baby will give enough reassurance to allow the massage to continue, sometimes he'll want a short feed, sometimes it's best to stop altogether.
- Always keep your baby warm. When it's cold, you may need to massage through clothes and without oil.
- Be aware of your own positions and ensure your back is comfortably positioned.
- Relax and enjoy this time with your baby.
- Don't wake your baby for a massage.

Do not massage:
- If your baby has an elevated temperature or is otherwise unwell.
- If your baby has any cuts or skin disorders, such as eczema.
- At all in the 48 hours following immunisation.
- Around the injection site for a week following immunisation.
- If your baby has had surgery or has any fractured bones.

Conditions that respond well to skilled massage include colic, reflux, constipation and digestive difficulties, sleep disorders and excessive crying, muscle tension and irritability. It is always advisable to have your baby examined if he is unwell.

Baby massage

When your baby is about a few weeks old or when he is ready, he will happily lie in front of you on his back on a towel and you can introduce this simple routine. Repeat each movement several times.

Legs

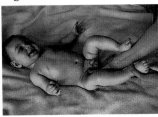

- With well-oiled hands, take your baby's leg and give it a gentle shake. Pull his leg, hand-over-hand, through your palms from thigh to foot. Repeat several times. Hold the ankle with your inside hand and, using the outside hand, massage up the front and down the back of the thigh.
- Let your hands slip down to your baby's knee and gently pull the calf and foot hand-over-hand through your palms, feeling your baby's feet and toes as they slip through your palms.
- Stroke the top of his foot to extend the toes and then gently pull the toes one by one through your thumb and forefinger.
- Gently trace your thumbs up the sole of the foot, from heel to toes – being aware that you may touch the kidney acupuncture point and, therefore, stimulate urination.
- Remembering to keep checking that your hands are well oiled, now repeat, several times, the first stroke of hand-over-hand from thigh to foot. Give the leg a gentle shake and repeat all these movements on the other leg. The massaged leg often feels lighter than the un-massaged one. Never massage one leg and leave the other leg, even if you cannot devote as much time to the latter.
- Having massaged both legs, gently bicycle them, holding the ankles. Keeping your baby's knees together, bend them into the abdomen and straighten them out again. Repeat three or four times (good for releasing wind).
- Tap your baby's feet alternately on the floor.
- To finish the legs, still using plenty of oil, pull your hands down both sides of the body from under the arms, then over the chest, hips and legs.

Abdomen

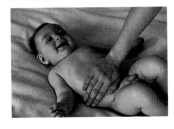

- This is a sensitive area where massage can help with colic and can be generally comforting but some babies find it uncomfortable. Start by moving your fingertips of one hand in a clockwise circle and then, after a few circles, use the relaxed weight of your whole hand, make further clockwise circles moving across the abdomen from left to right.
- Cup your other hand and place it horizontally across your baby's abdomen and then gently push in sideways between your baby's hip and lowest rib. Pull back gently using the pads of your fingers.

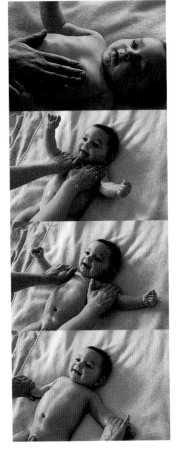

- Massage, hand-over-hand, from between the hip and lower ribs on the left side to the belly button and repeat on the right side.

Chest and arms

- Place your hands on your baby's chest and massage upwards and outwards over the shoulders and then back to the centre of the chest.
- Next, place your hands on your baby's chest and massage upwards and outwards over the shoulders and then bring your baby's hands down by his sides.
- Now place your hands on your baby's chest and massage upwards and outwards over his shoulders and draw his arms out horizontally through your palms, feeling his hands and fingers. Do not force any movements – if your baby is reluctant to open his arms, try clapping his hands together and then open them, little by little.
- Stroke down his whole body from the front of the shoulders to the legs.

Head

- Give your baby's head a gentle 'shampoo', being careful not to get oil into his eyes.
- Then, using your forefingers and thumbs, work your way down the ears. Head massage is very powerful so spend a minute or two on this area.
- Gently stroke from the bridge of the nose over the cheeks on each side.

Back

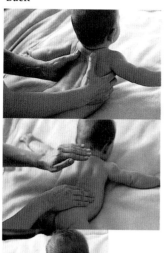

- Pick up your baby and give him a cuddle and then place him on his tummy. If he dislikes this position, try laying him across your knees
- Stroke down your baby's back to the base, with the palms of your hands on either side of the spine.
- Now cup your hands and pat your baby firmly but gently from the back of the chest and shoulders down to the base of the spine.
- Massage the base of the spine and the buttocks in a circular, clockwise motion, with relaxed hands.

Finishing

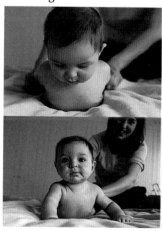

- To finish, trace your hands from the top of the rear of your baby's head and down the back and legs to the toes.
- Then tell him how much he is growing and how well he is doing. Cuddle him in a warm towel. By now, he will probably be ready for a good feed, followed by a sleep.

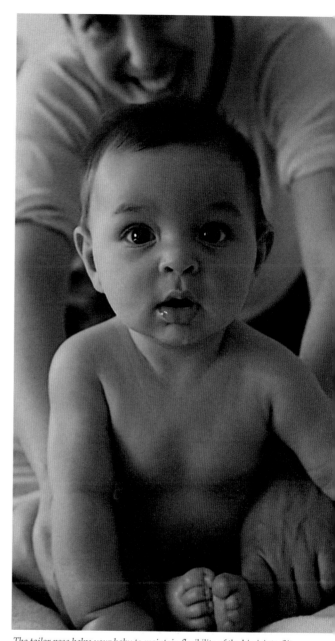

The tailor pose helps your baby to maintain flexibility of the hip joints. Sit with him in front of you or on your lap, and place the soles of his feet together. When you are confident that he can sit sturdily, and you and he enjoy massage together, you can take this a step further in more active baby gymnastics and move into swinging tailor pose. Start with your baby on your lap, and your hands coming beneath his arms to hold his lower legs. Your forearms make a harness and you can swing him gently, just above your lap, backwards and forwards. This is a fun exercise that you can continue until age 2 or 3 years, and encourages your baby to sit upright on the backs of his legs, leaving his spine completely free.

Meditation, hypnosis and visualisation

'True meditation does not begin and does not end. In fact, the true art of meditation is to always meditate. There is no place to arrive, there is nothing to do. Meditation is to simply stay at home as being.' Papaji (Sri H.W.L. Poonja).

The peaceful mind

If you measure the brain waves of a baby who is awake and quiet, they will be identical to those of an adult in deep meditation – babies can naturally enter a peaceful meditative space. Every adult naturally enters a similar state for short periods of time and may not recognise it. Many parents slip into a meditative state as they become absorbed in their baby's consciousness and mirror what she is doing. Being peaceful in this way helps the body and the mind to relax. As you do this, the benefits to your body and mind are many: your heart rate and blood pressure fall, your circulation flows and you breathe more deeply, promoting health. Furthermore, the levels of stress hormones fall, physical and emotional tension is released, and with relaxation comes revitalisation.

Many people find that a short session of meditation or visualisation – as little as 10 minutes – is as refreshing as an hour of sleep. Visualisations are active imaginings, a part of everybody's dreams and wishes. Against a background of feeling relaxed it is encouraging and exciting to practise specific visualisations to prepare for birth and for welcoming your baby.

Being meditative is to be peacefully still and fully in the present, in touch with oneself and free to love and be loved; not worrying about what has happened in the past or what will happen in the future. Everyone naturally experiences moments of stillness and meditation from time to time. The power gained from 'doing nothing' but being fully in the present is amazing. Feeding or sitting calmly with your baby gives you opportunities to connect with her and join in and be still. You may also choose to breathe consciously, watch your thoughts or do a visualisation and feel the joy.

Meditation

Some people attempt to remain aware of their thoughts and feelings throughout the day. To do this consistently requires attention, perseverance and years of practice. Others need to schedule a time when there won't be distractions and set aside a quiet place where they are able to be comfortable, with cushions, soft lighting and perhaps some soothing essential oils scenting the air. With guidance you could follow the meditation of your choice or practise on your own. The example given here is to give an idea to inspire you.

'The ocean and the waves'

Waves arise from the ocean and return to it. Thoughts and feelings arise and fall like waves in your mind; some may come and go quickly while others surface repeatedly for months or years. Sometimes your thought waves may be whipped up by hurricane winds and you flounder, overwhelmed by the activity in your mind. At other times you may be as still and unruffled as the sea in moonlight on a hot summer night.

Although some thoughts that arise may be unsettling, making the choice to experience them can be liberating. The secure and calm nature of your inner 'self' is always there and when you remain quiet and aware of your thoughts, you can return to this peaceful, unsullied place.

Begin by consciously observing your thoughts. Acknowledge each one, observe it, and you will find that it falls away of its own accord, back into the ocean from whence it came, unless you become involved. Some people find it difficult to reach a state of 'no thought' and if you do, it may only last for a very short time. During this you will feel blissfully calm, happy and connected, with a peaceful and harmonious energy. By practising this awareness of thoughts, calm periods will increase and you will be less anxious. You can be aware of your thoughts as you go about the routine of your daily life and you can cultivate this state by setting aside time to be still.

Visualisation and self-hypnosis

Taking time to relax through visualisation is rewarding, it recharges your batteries and expands your mind. You can perform a visualisation at any time of day, for example when you're feeding your baby or having a bath. If you want to make it more formal, set aside some time when interruptions will be rare. Watch thoughts arise and intrude on your visualisation, but let them fall and then re-focus. The visualisations here are for you to play with and use whenever you wish – their power will surprise you.

When you spend time doing a visualisation, you often slip into a state of self-hypnosis. Hypnosis is, in fact, a natural state of mind and the human brain drifts in and out of hypnosis spontaneously. It derives from the Greek word *hupnos*, which means 'sleep' but hypnosis is closer to an altered state of mental awareness when the brain waves flow as 'alpha' waves as they do when in a state of meditation, or in babies who are calm and awake. The hypnotic state of mind can be used to create a state of relaxation and calmness and to inspire confidence.

Everyone knows in theory and many people have discovered through their own experience that the mind can have a significant influence over the body. For instance, a fear of birthing can be transformed into eager anticipation of the joy of birth using self-hypnosis for positive thinking. Likewise, labour can be visualised and experienced as segments of contractions that can be managed easily. For some people previous traumatic memories may need to be worked through and healed, and hypnosis and visualisation can help this.

Hypnosis in practice

Entering hypnosis is easy if you know how. To be guided into hypnosis you can talk silently to yourself or ask someone to talk to you in a flowing and gentle rhythm, as if there is no punctuation and no break between sentences. You can learn this method if there is a class near you. Your birth partner can then 'talk' you into a calm and focused state for birth.

Signs of successful hypnosis include a reluctance to let your eyelids open and increased moistness within your eyelids. You may also notice a feeling of tingling in your hands and feet as the muscles relax and the blood vessels dilate, increasing blood circulation. Hypnosis has the benefits of stabilising blood pressure, slowing your heart rate, and helping you to feel calm.

The simplest method for achieving hypnosis is to (spoken in hypnotic language): stare at an imaginary spot directly overhead on the ceiling without moving your chin; keep your gaze focused on that same spot until you begin to feel your eyelids becoming heavier and you will notice that your eyelids want to close; take three deep breaths into the lowest part of your abdomen and with every deep breath allow all the muscles in your neck and shoulders to relax more deeply; and then allow the relaxation to flow downwards towards your lower back and feel the muscles of your buttocks and thighs and legs relax all the way down to your feet until you are relaxed all over.

Visualisation in practice

Under the influence of focused hypnotic visualisations, some of the changes that happen on the day of labour can be encouraged to occur more easily, and discomfort may be reduced. Looking into your body and imagining your ligaments, muscles and tissues gently stretching and opening may encourage your baby's smooth descent (as guided on p.128). This may be part of your antenatal preparations for labour (p.102).

After the birth it is vital for you to have lots of good quality rest. Visualisation and self hypnosis may help you to slip away into your own inner realm where you enter a safe and quiet space. This is a sanctuary for deep rest and recuperation: you can go there by closing your eyes and saying, 'I am going to my safe place now.' Over time, this will become a trigger that helps you leave daily demands to one side and enter your well-deserved space of relaxation and peace.

Once you have taken yourself away, you can do 'brushing down' and scan your body with your inner eye as you visualise all your muscles getting firmer and stronger. You may want to gently ask your body to heal and replenish itself, and might enjoy several short visualisations, perhaps while you feed your baby. Some women find it useful to visualise milk flowing during a feed. Before sleeping, or after a night feed, visualise all the muscles in your body relaxing very deeply so that when you wake up in the morning you will fell comfortable all over, especially in your neck and back.

Being in nature – a revitalising visualisation

Imagine yourself on a warm summer day walking through a meadow. You can hear the sound of a river. You lie on soft, green grass and look up at leaves moving in the breeze.
Let yourself relax and watch wisps of cloud moving across the blue sky . . .
Feel your body sinking into the softness of the grass and hear the sound of birds and wind-rustled leaves . . .
Feel that you are warm and comfortable as you become one with nature . . .
You are in harmony.

Relaxing in water (good for the bath)

Imagine yourself walking along the beach on a warm day. There is a lagoon where the water is almost completely still. Watch the gentle waves and look at the ocean ahead of you . . .
As you walk into the ocean you feel the water lapping at your ankles, knees, thighs, pelvis and abdomen and then you chest. Stand like this for a while as you feel the weightlessness of the water beginning to take over . . .
You are now floating weightlessly as the water supports you and your breath softly rises and falls . . .
As the water takes your weight and the sun warms your body, you feel yourself blending with the warmth and comfort of the water. You are connected with the timelessness of the ocean . . .
When you are ready, you float gently back to the shore.

'Brushing down'

This is a powerful way to relax and to focus on your baby.

Sit or lie comfortably and relax. As you breathe, gently focus your attention at the top of your head.

Now move your attention gently and slowly towards your left ear and focus on the shape of your ear and on the warmth and the sensations of your skin.

'You are your baby'

Lie in a relaxed position (possibly on your side). Breathe slowly and gently, focusing on inhaling energy with the in-breaths and slowly exhaling any anxiety or tension with the out-breaths. Allow your body to feel very heavy as if you are growing roots reaching down, down deep into the 'mother' earth . . . At the same time allow yourself to be very light, like a feather drifting in the air currents, weightless, floating without gravity . . . As you breathe you can go deeper and deeper into relaxation and rest.

Now focus on your pelvic area, your womb and on the new life growing within you . . . Imagine how it is to be your baby, secure, completely naked and surrounded by water at the perfect unchanging temperature . . . enclosed in a warm darkness, feeling safe and open to every subtle experience . . . Imagine the pulsing at your navel of your umbilical cord coiled around you and connected to your placenta, which is warm with the energy of constant unconditional nurturing . . . Perhaps you cuddle up to your placenta, your 'twin' . . . Maybe you play with your cord or you play with your fingers and toes . . . or you suck on your thumb, twist and turn. Listen to the sounds around you, two hearts (yours and your mother's) beating as one but at different rhythms . . . the constant swooshing sound of your placenta . . . the sound of your mother's voice, her digestive processes . . . a symphony of nature . . . and also the familiar voice of your father . . . You and your mother are as one, there is no separateness . . . Her feelings are your feelings but not defined by concepts or judgements . . . Just an experiencing of what is . . .

Water is your element . . . if you are still very small you have an ocean in which to swim and dive and kick and play . . . if you are approaching birth you will feel the silky lining that is your 'bag of waters' and smoothly massages you as you move . . . And then you sleep, dreaming of . . .

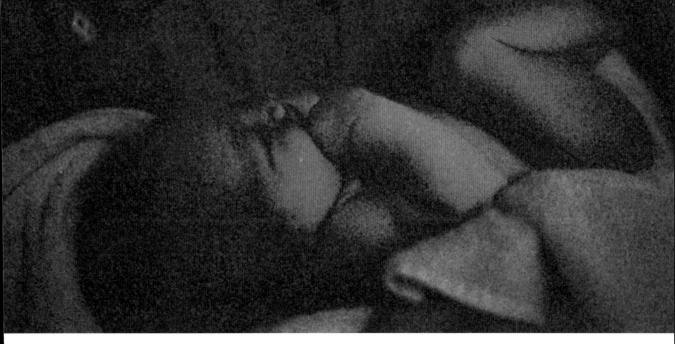

Continue through your body, covering your ears, face, head, throat, shoulders, arms, hands, fingers, chest, lungs, spine, abdomen, pelvis, legs, feet and toes.

As you 'brush down' the body, feel the energy warming and relaxing you. Feel the connection between the top of your head and the end of your toes and fingers. If you encounter areas of tension, stay with them and let them relax.

Sometimes it helps to imagine a spot of light, soft and beautiful, moving slowly over, into and through your body, or a warm feeling of energy focused on and moving through you.

You will be distracted by thoughts. When you notice them, do not fight them. Simply acknowledge each thought, watch it and refocus on your body. The visualisation becomes easier with practice, your level of relaxation will increase and you will be able to stay with the visualisation for longer.

When you have 'brushed down' your body, focus on your baby and do the same thing.

Meditation in daily life

Meditation and visualisation may already be part of your life, or become an enjoyable activity during or after pregnancy when you are naturally more inclined to focus inwardly and relax. Once you have felt the benefits you will find it easier to take yourself into a peaceful space,

'To be free from thoughts is itself meditation.
You begin by letting thoughts flow and watching them.
The very observation slows down the mind till it stops altogether.
Once the mind is quiet, keep it quiet.
Don't get bored with peace, be in it, and go deeper in it.
Watch your thoughts and watch yourself watching your thoughts.
The state of freedom from all thoughts will happen suddenly
And by the bliss of it you will recognise it.'
Sri Nisargadatta Maharaj, 1973

follow your breathing, relax your body and re-centre yourself. In the years ahead the ability to step out of the busy-ness of daily life, even if only for a couple of minutes, will be a true asset. It may also improve your sleep. If you feel overwhelmed, sit down and take yourself into this still space, let go of all the demands momentarily, and recharge. This is a gift to yourself, and to those around you because you will radiate a sense of peace and stillness and stress levels may seldom spiral out of control. Looking at and accepting your thoughts and watching them rise and fall is a powerful way to feel at one with your life. Remember that you can take your lead from your baby, who naturally lives in the moment, and will often enter a peaceful, meditative state.

Homeopathy

'Homeopathy can safely ease you through the transitions of pregnancy, labour and parenting, bringing physical and emotional balance. It is also a wonderful support for babies. It is a privilege to watch its magic in action.' Felicity Fine, homeopath.

Gentle healing and support

The gentle, non-invasive, healing approach offered by homeopathy suits many pregnant women and newborn babies. It was founded 200 years ago by Dr Samuel Hahnemann, a German physician. The underlying principle of homeopathy is that 'like cures like' (omnio-pathos means 'same-suffering'). The substances are specially diluted and prepared to promote a curative response by stimulating the body's natural healing forces. In pregnancy, and in babyhood, the body is very receptive and has strong vital energy that quickly responds to the homeopathic 'prompt' as natural healing takes place. Homeopathy is completely safe when used appropriately and can encourage health and balance, increase vitality and offer support at many different levels.

Homeopathy is based on an holistic understanding of health. It takes a wide view of illness and its causes and the ways in which people express their illnesses. Each time a homeopath assesses a patient, emotional, mental and physical conditions are taken into account. The remedies are made to suit an individual symptom picture and each remedy has a 'personality' that matches the symptoms.

A remedy may be taken as a 'once-off' for specific acute situations or prescribed 'constitutionally' to treat deep-seated issues over time. In many cases, homeopathy can be used on its own but it is also effective if used in combination with a number of other methods of treatment, such as conventional ('allopathic') medical care, Yoga or exercise, massage, aromatherapy or cranial osteopathy.

Remedies – origin and potency

Homeopathic remedies are mostly derived from plant, mineral or animal sources diluted and succussed (mixed according to homeopathic principles) with a mixture of distilled water and alcohol. The process that results in the final tablet defines a remedy's potency. The potency of a remedy is really the energy at which it resonates, and the aim of prescribing is to match the potency to the energy of the disease and to the energy of the individual. As a remedy is produced, potency is determined by its dilution and succussion, e.g. 1:9 or 1:99. Unlike conventional medicine, where a low dilution gives a high potency, in homeopathy, potency increases as dilution increases.

Remedies are prepared according to a variety of scales, most commonly the decimal (x) and the centesimal (c) scales. In the decimal scale, a remedy is diluted and succussed in a proportion of 1:9 drops of water and alcohol. In the centesimal scale, a remedy is diluted and succussed in a proportion of 1:99 drops of alcohol and water. The figure of potency denotes how many times a substance has been diluted and succussed and the letter indicates which scale has been used.

Low potencies, e.g. 6x or 6c, are usually most suitable for treating localised symptoms over a short period. Medium potency, e.g. 30c, is often used as first line treatment for an acute case, or for an ongoing problem. This is the usual dose for home prescribing and the one that is most widely available in chemists. Higher doses, e.g. 200c, are more powerful and often work quickly to aid emotional balance. This is the usual potency for use in labour as the intensity of the situation warrants using a higher potency (p.162). When you are given advice by your homeopath, she will prescribe a remedy in a potency that suits your symptoms and personality. If she recommends a higher potency, she may mix this for you.

Finding the remedy for you and your baby

The approach of homeopathy is to treat you as a unique individual rather than tackle a disease. If you visit a homeopath she will form a picture of your personality, your physical and emotional symptoms, your personal and medical history and your lifestyle. As your symptom picture changes, so too will the remedy that suits you. The key to sound homeopathic prescribing is to match remedies to symptoms and choose the correct potency to match the complaint. Each remedy will be administered at an appropriate potency for your circumstances.

Prescribing for babies involves a different level of perception and awareness because babies cannot verbalise how they feel. Having said this, babies often present very clear and uncomplicated remedy pictures that can easily be prescribed for. The most important symptoms are those that differ from the baby's usual state. For example, if your baby is usually very alert and active and becomes floppy, or a typically thirsty baby refuses to drink anything.

How to take remedies and what to avoid

Remedies usually come as small tablets, occasionally as powders, or as liquids. Creams, ointments, lotions and tinctures are also available for external use. Tablets should

Taking an acute case

When prescribing a remedy each homeopath takes a personal approach. But the following framework may be generally applied.

1 What is the chief complaint?

2 Time and onset
- When and how did the symptoms start?
- Was the onset fast or slow?

3 Aetiology – studying possible causes
- Is there a known cause?

4 Pain/sensation
- Is there pain?
- What kind of pain? For instance, is it sharp, dull, throbbing?
- Is it constant, spasmodic, irregular, changeable?
- What sensations are there?
- Does touch or stimuli affect the complaint?

5 Location/extension?
- Are there any symptoms associated with the main complaint?
- Does the pain, for example, extend somewhere else?
- Does motion, position or pressure affect the complaint?

6 Modalities
- Does anything make the patient feel better or worse?

7 General states – how do these differ from normal?
- Temperature – feverish/chilly?
- Perspiration?
- Sleep?
- Thirst?
- Desires/aversions?

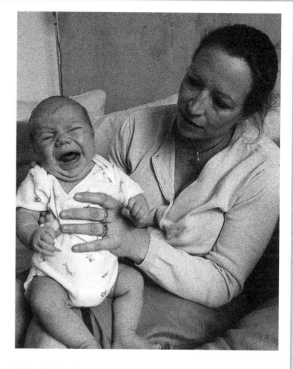

8 Mood – how does this differ from normal?
- Bad-tempered/irritable?
- Clingy?
- Anxious/agitated?
- Lethargic?
- Compliant?

9 Peculiar symptoms
- Anything that is out of the ordinary?

be taken in a clean mouth and no other substance should be put in the mouth for at least 20 minutes either side of taking the remedy (not even toothpaste and cigarettes). The effects can be reduced with coffee, peppermint, menthol, eucalyptus and camphor, which are best cut out of the diet completely while treatment continues.

When administering remedies to babies, it is often easier to use soft tablets, which dissolve quickly in the mouth. Hard tablets can be crushed and the resulting powder can be placed in the corner of the mouth or diluted with a little boiled cooled water on a teaspoon.

Using homeopathy at home
The best introduction to homeopathy is a consultation with a homeopath. After a number of visits you may feel ready to buy a home-remedy kit and use this in conjunction with advice from your homeopath. Many pharmacies and health food shops have a basic stock of remedies, and there are special kits for labour and birth and kits for first aid. Over time, you will become more familiar with the remedies that suit your family's symptoms and personalities. Your homeopath may recommend a book to help you match symptoms and remedies.

Safety
It is safe to use homeopathic remedies provided the symptoms do not indicate an underlying acute or serious medical condition that requires urgent medical diagnosis or treatment. Throughout the A–Z Health Guide you will find advice for self prescribing. If you are in doubt, consult your midwife or doctor and use homeopathy in conjunction with allopathic medicines and treatment. Remember to take care: like any medicine, homeopathy is most safely used with the advice of a qualified practitioner.

Osteopathy

'Imagine the structure of the body as an intelligent web where everything is connected. Besides voluntary motion there is a dynamic orchestra of tidal rhythms, helping the body's physiology to balance, nurture and heal itself. This is the world of osteopathy.' Lynn Haller, osteopath.

The value of alignment

Osteopathic treatment realigns the body's structure, gives it balance and assists the natural process of self-healing. It can be an immensely powerful way of reducing areas of tension and can also release the emotional stress that underlies a physical complaint. The discipline was founded in 1874 by Dr Still. Cerebrospinal fluid bathes the brain and spinal cord. It causes the bones in the skull and the spine to make tiny movements as the fluid ebbs and flows from the head to the pelvis, 10–15 times each minute. This is called the cranio-sacral rhythm. A cranio-sacral osteopath senses this rhythm by using her hands and can gently locate and release areas of tension, rebalancing the body's energy. Osteopaths are trained to assess the severity of a strain pattern in the body and to identify how long it has been there: some long-standing tension patterns arise from very early life (such as a forceps birth) or have been forgotten (perhaps an accident in childhood).

Performing cranial-sacral osteopathy does not involve 'manipulation'. The osteopath gently holds the client's head or back and follows and guides the flow of the cranial rhythm. It is a non-invasive practice that's extremely safe for adults and babies and can have far reaching effects, particularly for newborns. Structural osteopathy (as opposed to cranial-sacral osteopathy) involves manipulating the bones to correct the alignment of the bones and the joints.

Treatment for conditions related to birth is most effective, both for mothers and babies, soon after delivery while the body tissues are still soft and malleable and before any pattern of strain has become established. Babies respond more rapidly because their tissues are less rigid, and they usually improve within five or six treatments.

In adults treatment may be needed over a number of months to release patterns that have been present for years as the body slowly adapts and deep tension is encouraged to rise to the surface. The cranio-sacral osteopath is treating symptoms such as pain, but the main aim is to release the underlying cause of tension because this will have a positive long-term effect on health.

Osteopathy in pregnancy and beyond

In pregnancy osteopathy can balance your body, maximise energy and assuage nervous tension and may release long-term strains, relieve nausea and sickness, backache, pelvic and pubic pain and headaches. If your ligaments cause discomfort while they are softened, you may feel better after repeated osteopathic treatments. Once tension in your pelvis is released your baby is encouraged to engage her head in your pelvis and also take an 'optimal position' for birth (p.120).

If you have had a difficult birth, a caesarean, stitches or an epidural, cranial-sacral osteopathy may greatly relieve the associated postnatal pain. The physical and emotional experience of even the gentlest birth can result in strain. Where you are sore, your muscles react by becoming tense to protect the area; osteopathy can release this tension pattern and alleviate the underlying cause, such as twisted joints or stretched tissues.

If you suffer from insomnia or anxiety and feel low and tearful, the calming effect of osteopathy can reduce adrenalin levels, promote relaxation and peaceful sleep and lift your energy – all qualities that help to prevent postnatal blues, encourage successful and enjoyable breastfeeding and enhance recovery after birth.

Osteopathy for babies

Every baby is subjected to significant forces in the womb that reach a peak during labour and birth. Even in the gentlest birth a baby's body may show strain as a result of position in the womb or the journey through the birth canal. Stress patterns may also relate to tension picked up in pregnancy. The head, whose soft bones overlap as it moulds to fit the shape of the birth canal, has a remarkable ability to absorb strain. After birth the shape gradually changes as the moulding releases but areas of tension may persist. Some babies cope well with the changes and are content and happy, but others may react by being unsettled or crying excessively – for them osteopathy provides a very gentle method of relief.

Osteopathy is often the chosen treatment for relieving strains following forceps or ventouse delivery, malposition of the head in labour or a prolonged labour, and may be valuable for a baby who experiences breathing difficulties or requires resuscitation at birth.

Osteopathy can also address feeding difficulties, colic and excess wind, irritability or the need to be constantly carried and rocked to sleep. For the older baby it can treat sleep and digestive problems. The A–Z Health Guide indicates where osteopathy may be useful.

Acupuncture

'Chinese medicine offers a rich store of wisdom and health care for women and babies, and has been used for over 2 millennia to support families during pregnancy, birth and the postnatal period.' Wainwright and Meredith Churchill, Traditional Chinese Medical practitioners.

Acupuncture and qi

Acupuncture is a branch of traditional Chinese medicine based on the concept of *qi* (pronounced chi), which is sometimes translated as 'vital energy'. Every part of the body is associated with a certain type of *qi* that has a specific quality and function, and each internal organ generates or affects various types of *qi*. In health, the body is balanced as the different types of *qi* interact harmoniously, giving physical, psychological and spiritual wellbeing. In illness some types of *qi* may be deficient or excessive, and the resultant imbalance leads to symptoms, which might be physical – from feeling generally unhealthy to having indigestion or a medically diagnosed illness – psychological or spiritual. Diagnosis determines the underlying state and balance of the *qi*, and treatment adjusts it, restoring health.

Acupuncture treatment involves stimulating minute points on the body surface where *qi* is concentrated. There are approximately 350 classically recognised acupuncture points, and another several thousand 'extra' points. Most of the main points occur along meridians – recognised *qi* pathways that travel up or down the body. The internal organs are represented at different acupuncture points and one organ may have many points.

When you visit an acupuncturist he will take a case history and then feel the pulses at your wrists and inspect your tongue. This diagnostic practice indicates how your body is out of balance. For long-term health problems a rule of thumb (of course there are many exceptions) is that it takes 1 month of treatment for each year of imbalance.

Scientific research into acupuncture

There has been a significant amount of research into the mechanisms of acupuncture, which was first recorded in a detailed written treatise, *The Yellow Emperor's Classic on Internal Medicine,* around 220 BC. Despite clear physiological effects there is no single scientific insight to explain all the results. Acupuncture works, at least in part, via the central nervous system and affects the function of the brain. For instance, it can stimulate the brain's production of endorphins, which may explain some of its analgesic effects (useful in labour). Acupuncture increases the rate of wound healing by 50%: light pressure applied on the skin around the wound stimulates chemicals that promote healing.

Applying acupuncture

Using needles: The most frequent application uses one or more very fine needles lightly applied to acupuncture points. Many people find this painless, or only slightly uncomfortable momentarily, and often feel harmonised and relaxed. The needles may be taken out immediately, or left in, usually no longer than about 20 minutes. Pre-sterilised disposable needles are used to prevent transfer of infection.

Moxibustion: A herb, traditionally *Artemisia vulgaris,* commonly known as 'moxa', is burned and used to warm a specific acupuncture point or a whole area of the body. Moxa placed on an acupuncture point on the little toe from about Week 33 of pregnancy is traditionally used to turn a breech baby.

Moxibustion is also used for women who feel the cold unduly, who in Chinese medical terms would be diagnosed as having a deficiency of yang energy.

Massage and acupressure: Acupressure is the technique of massaging acupuncture points. This is not as powerful as using needles or moxa but nevertheless can be very effective and is often recommended for people who do not need strong stimulation, or fear needles. It can be very useful for treating babies.

Acupressure also underpins massage therapy, which has many forms: one treatment in Chinese medicine is called *tuina,* while *shiatsu* is a Japanese form of massage using acupuncture theory.

Reflexology

The practice of reflexology originates from Chinese acupuncture philosophy and also has roots in American Red Indian and Inca traditions. It uses the principle of acupressure on the soles of the feet, where acupuncture points relate to the entire body. Gentle pressure on particular points on the soles of your feet can bring about relaxation, assist rebalancing when you are not in optimum health, relieve physical symptoms of illness and relieve pain during pregnancy and labour.

Once you have picked up the basics of reflexology, perhaps from a reflexology practitioner, a simple foot massage can be easy to do on yourself or on someone else, and may have a beneficial impact on your health. Reflexology can be very powerful in labour and many midwives now incorporate it into their practice.

Aromatherapy

'I cannot imagine a better use for aromatherapy than in pregnancy and in childbirth, and for mother and baby after birth. Its holistic, calming and healing qualities have a profoundly therapeutic effect on mothers, babies and midwives.' Anita O'Neill, midwife and aromatherapist.

The power of plants

For thousands of years herbs and plants have been used to balance the diet. They are also used as medicines, in many different ways across the globe, and their essential oils are used in aromatherapy. Plants support and nourish your entire system. They can be used to trigger healing, strengthen organs, generate feelings of calmness and relaxation or enhance self-esteem and re-establish emotional balance.

Aromatherapy is based on the use of essential oils extracted from plants. Each oil carries with it the life force of the plant and its smell stimulates one of the most powerful and instinctual senses. When applied to the skin, the constituents of the essential oil are absorbed directly into the body.

The effects of different oils range from relief of mild health complaints and aches and pains to relaxing or revitalising the mind and body. Throughout the A–Z Health Guide their use has been indicated where relevant so that you can choose the oil that suits you.

Provided they are not contra-indicated for use in pregnancy or while breastfeeding, oils can be used simply and safely, and many women find them helpful during labour and birth and for relaxing in pregnancy and the postnatal period. When used appropriately, oils can also relax your baby. You may wish to visit an aromatherapist for a relaxing massage and find out which oils best suit you. Alternatively, you can use them in your own home: always ensure that you follow instructions, because excessive doses may be harmful.

How to use aromatherapy oils

- To bring the scent of an essential oil into a room, put several drops in water in an oil burner or vaporiser, or put them on to a tissue or into a bowl of water placed over a radiator.
- For soothing yourself, put a couple of drops on cotton wool, and place this in your pillowcase or your shirt pocket.
- For many complaints oils are most effective if mixed with a nourishing carrier oil (almond, grapeseed or wheatgerm, for instance) and massaged into the skin. When you are pregnant, use 20 drops per 100 ml (3 fl oz) of carrier oil: you can prepare some oils in advance for use in labour (p.162).
- When you are not pregnant, use 40 drops in 100 ml (3 fl oz) of carrier oil. For babies use 5–10 drops in 100 ml (3 fl oz) of oil or lotion.
- In your bath, use 4–6 drops of oil, preferably mixed into a tablespoon of carrier oil, which nourishes the skin. In a baby's bath only use 1–2 drops. Add the oils to the warm full bath when you have turned the taps off as agitation of the water destroys the oils. Stay in the bath for 5–15 minutes and relax. You can use single oils or blend two or three oils which enhance each other's properties; don't use more than four oils at a time.
- For long standing pain (or early labour pains) you can use a hot compress. Fill a basin with water as hot as your hand can bear and add 4–5 drops of oil. Fold a clean absorbent cloth and dip it into the water to pick up essential oil from the surface. Wring out surplus water, cover the cloth with plastic and place it on the painful area. Replace it with a fresh one when it has cooled to blood heat. Hot compresses are especially good for backache and other muscular pains.
- Cold compresses are good for headache, acute breast engorgement, mastitis and sprains. They are made in the same way as hot compresses, with water as cold as you can get it. Add ice before use.

Using oils safely

- Do not use any oils until you are 13 weeks pregnant unless you have been advised to do so by a qualified aromatherapist or midwife.
- Avoid bay, basil, clary sage, comfrey, fennel, hyssop, juniper, marjoram, melissa, myrrh, rosemary, thyme and sage during pregnancy.
- Always follow the instructions provided with oils and, wherever possible, seek advice from a qualified aromatherapist.
- Never add more oil than the stated dose.
- Never take oils internally.
- If you have a history of miscarriage, avoid camomile and lavender for the first 16 weeks.
- Don't apply oils to your breast while you are breastfeeding as they are absorbed through the skin and can pass to your baby in breast milk.

Herbal medicine

'For thousands of years, herbs and plants have been used as an integral aspect of a balanced diet and as medicine. Used correctly, they can alleviate physical, mental and emotional suffering, and support and nourish the body, and treat acute and chronic health problems.' Delphine Sayre, medicinal herbalist.

Ancient plant lore

Across the world people have used local plants to treat their ailments and to support them, in pregnancy and birth and at other times of health and sickness. There are many different disciplines and as world-wide communication improves, more varieties become available. Some treatments are available in tablet form, others come as tinctures or teas, syrups, lotions or extracts. Although most substances used are from plants, Chinese herbal medicine sometimes uses minerals or animal products. It has a long history, and was already advanced thousands of years ago. For instance, a text written around AD 750 describes diabetes and recommends that pig's pancreas be used to treat the problem, pre-dating by 1200 years western medicine's use of insulin derived from the same source.

It is relatively simple to make your own infusions (teas from leaves) or decoctions (teas from roots and bark) if you have guidance. However, herbs can be very powerful and although many have great value in pregnancy, many are not advised for use (see box). If you decide to use herbal medicines, it is best to visit a qualified practitioner.

How do herbal medicines work?

By using plants in their raw and complete form, a complex fusion of chemicals – a combination of minute amounts of plant constituents – can be introduced into the body in a gentle and natural way. Plants have a natural balance and energy and when prescribing, the constitution of the plant and the person are considered equally and their 'temperaments' matched.

The most straightforward way to harness the power of herbs is to use them in cooking and make them a part of your diet. 'Wonder' foods, from onions and garlic to almonds and watercress, are listed on p.343 and there are tips for what to eat if you are unwell throughout the A–Z Health Guide.

Using herbs safely

Herbalists stress the importance of using the whole plant as other compounds present in the plant counteract any toxic constituents. Side effects from herbs are rare and only likely when large doses are consumed. Nevertheless, natural does not necessarily mean safe and particular care should be taken during pregnancy. You should always seek the guidance and expert knowledge of a medical herbalist for conditions that would normally warrant a medical opinion.

- As a general maxim, avoid herbal medicines during the first trimester unless you have been advised to continue treatment. Teas for nausea, constipation and lethargy are safe.
- Highly concentrated extracts should be avoided throughout pregnancy because the danger of side effects is considerably higher than in preparations that contain the whole plant. Use infusions (teas) or decoctions, not tinctures, which need to be provided, with advice, by a herbalist.
- When in doubt, or if worrying symptoms persist, seek the help of an appropriately qualified herbalist or ask your GP's opinion.
- From conception to the cessation of breastfeeding ensure you only use herbs that are safe. It is always best to avoid herbs known to have a stimulating, or irritating, effect on the body. Self-medication with herbs from the following list drawn from herbs in common use is not advised.

Herbs to avoid

Aloes (*Aloe vera*) (External application of the gel is unlikely to cause problems)
Barberry (*Berberis vulgaris*)
Blue cohosh (*Caulophyllum thalictroides*)
Cascara sagrada (*Rhamnus purshiana*)
Castor oil (*Ricinus communis*)
Celery seed (*Apium graveolens*) *
Golden seal (*Hydrastis canadensis*)
Juniper (*Juniperus communis*)
Parsley (*Petroselinum crispum*) *
Pokeroot (*Phytolacca americana*)
Rue (*Ruta graveolens*)
Sage (*Salvia officinalis*) *
Senna (*Cassia angustifolia*)
Southernwood (*Artemisia abrotanum*)
Tansy (*Tanacetum vulgare*)
Thuja (*Thuja occidentalis*)
Wormwood (*Artemisia absinthium*)
* These herbs are unlikely to cause harm when used as food in cooking.
Pennyroyal (*Mentha pulegium*) can be used in small doses to help contractions during labour, expel the afterbirth and reduce fever linked with mastitis. It should **never** be used in pregnancy.

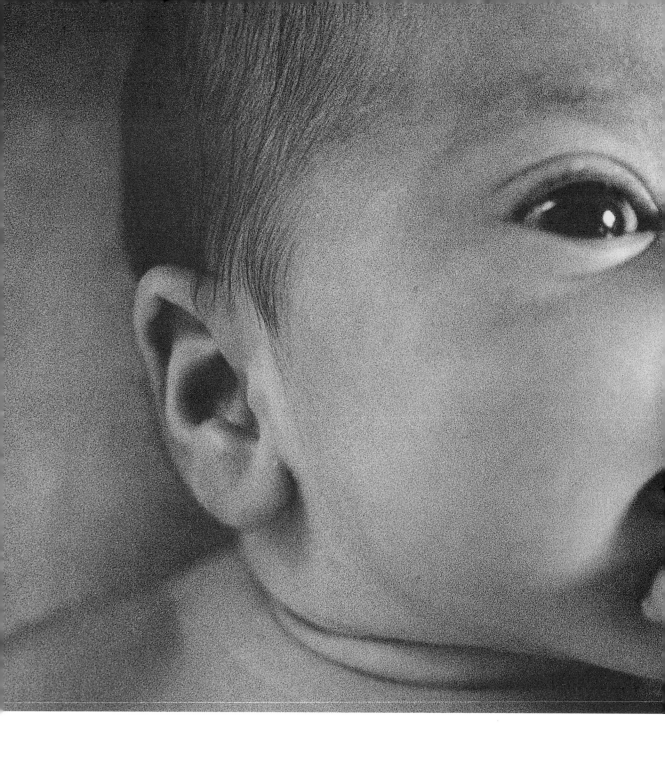

part vi a-z

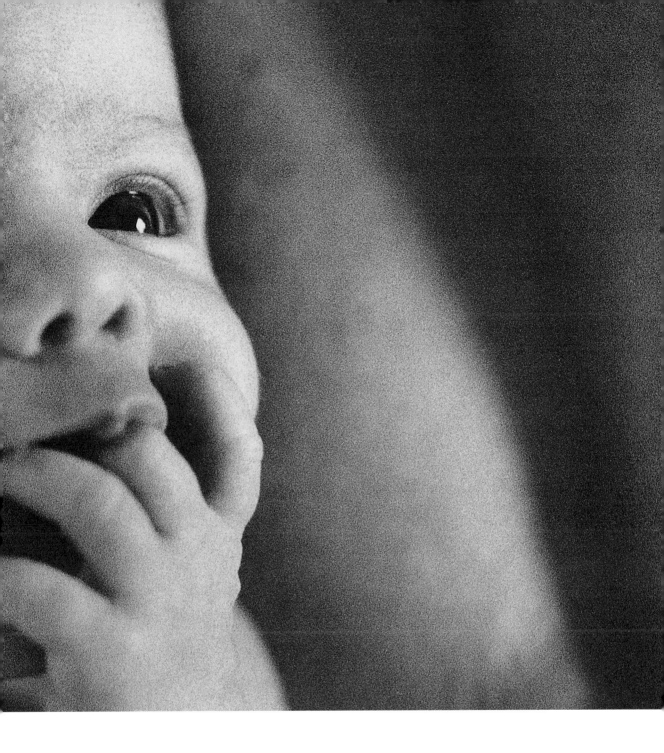

How to use the A–Z Health Guide

This A–Z Health Guide is designed for easy use to help and empower you to make an informed decision if you are concerned about any aspect of your or your baby's health. Early diagnosis and treatment usually help to bring results and improve the outlook. The integrated approach examines the nature of a condition and possible medical or complementary care, beginning with self-help where appropriate, and outlines further treatment or procedures that may be advised by your midwife, doctor or complementary practitioner.

In some instances, direct or even urgent medical action may be essential. In others, complementary care is sufficient and you may find a persistent complaint becomes a thing of the past when you make simple changes to your lifestyle. This guide encourages an integrated approach to prevent difficulties and to enhance recovery. An essential part of using it is to follow your hunches and not to hesitate to seek help.

Use the A–Z Health Guide by looking up a symptom (e.g. bleeding), or a condition (e.g diabetes), or a subject (e.g. drugs). There are cross-references to related subjects within each entry. Those referring to other entries are indicated in small capitals (e.g. VACCINATIONS). Page numbers refer either to items within entries or to Parts I–V of the book. There are some important subjects (e.g. labour) that are covered earlier in the book as well as in the guide and you may find the index helpful to access answers for a particular question.

In each of the entries we indicate whether symptoms suggest that a condition is minor or needs emergency medical treatment. If it is an emergency, call an ambulance. If you do not think it is an emergency but are at all concerned, contact your midwife, doctor or the relevant specialist in your local hospital, or your complementary therapist to discuss the best course of action. Most often, an ailment is minor but when there is something seriously wrong, diagnosis and treatment are best. Try to write down your concerns, so that even if your baby is crying you will remember the important questions. Sickness makes everyone anxious, and you may be tense and distressed. Broadly speaking, the following symptoms warrant immediate medical attention:

Mother:
- Bleeding.
- Breathlessness.
- Severe or increasing abdominal pain.
- Persistent headache or convulsion.
- Reduced foetal movement in late pregnancy.

Baby:
- Fever: temperature above 38°C (100.4°F) alone or with rash or stiff neck.
- Temperature below 35.5°C (95.9°F).
- Convulsion and/or difficulty breathing.
- Persistent diarrhoea and/or vomiting.
- Refusal to feed for more than two feeds.
- Behaviour changes: excessive crying, lethargy, pale appearance, vacant look.

Use the A–Z Health Guide as a source of information and advice in conjunction with the support of your friends, family and medical community.

If there is cause for concern

During and after pregnancy you and your baby will be examined frequently. The aim of medical care is to prevent problems and in most instances monitoring is done as a precaution. If, however, there is a serious problem, you will naturally be concerned.

Receiving news

Everybody varies in the way they react to bad news. Some people feel out of control, some feel angry, some feel numb and others are calm. There is often disbelief. You may need to express your feelings and want reassurance and information. Most hospitals have a supportive team for parents but sometimes information is not easy to come by. You will need time to assimilate the information and it is usually best to talk about the issue again after you have thought it through. It might be easier if you make notes and take another adult with you to get the facts straight.

It is often hard to keep track of all the facts, particularly when you are anxious, but do try to make sure you understand the issues involved. Don't be afraid to ask again and again until you understand difficult medical terms. You might need to ask the doctors if they can say things in a different way. It is important to express your feelings and concerns – your carers are trained to help if you feel upset or disappointed.

What's next? Adapting to the reality

In the main, doctors are progressively more up front and honest, but sometimes they don't know exactly what is wrong and need time to make diagnoses and predictions. This is difficult when you want to know the facts immediately. Feeling well informed is important, but unfortunately this does not always mean knowing the complete answer. If you worry that information is being withheld you can contact the director of the obstetric or paediatric service to ask them about your concerns. You may be given a number of opinions about causes and treatments and it may be up to you to make choices about further tests or treatment.

Planning for the future: orientation

You will need to consider the problem, treatment and outlook, and think about ways to feel supported and cope with practical matters with the help of your family, friends and medical team. Some health issues require careful forward planning. Many parents faced with difficulties feel more positive and hopeful once they are able to make plans. Emotional advice (p.459), perhaps combined with counselling and complementary therapies or help from local or national organisations, may be useful for you and for other members of your family to help you move on.

The rest of your family

You may find it difficult to share bad news with other people who might also be deeply affected, such as grandparents and siblings. It is usually best for the news to come from you because this minimises the likelihood of misinformation and unnecessary anxiety. Even the honesty of a 3-year-old can be healing and your family may be very supportive to one another.

Accidents & First Aid

Children do have accidents. Their curiosity and spirit of adventure are healthy. Whatever your baby's reaction, your care will make her happier as she recovers. If she has a serious accident it will be distressing for everyone. It is your role to make her comfortable, remove any danger, and seek appropriate medical care, even though you may be in shock and upset. If an accident is serious don't hesitate to call another adult for help.

This guide gives basic tips. It is also worth familiarising yourself with baby First Aid in theory and in practice at a local clinic. The suggestions for homeopathic First Aid apply equally to adults and babies.

Is it an emergency?

Many minor injuries can be handled at home. If you are ever unsure about whether an injury needs emergency care, treat it as an emergency. Call 999 or NHS Direct or your local GP. The following situations require emergency attention:

- Trouble breathing – shortness of breath, inability to feed or speak.
- Blue or purple colour to lips, skin, or nail beds.
- Chest or stomach pain or pressure.
- Sudden dizziness, weakness, or change in vision.
- Change in conscious level, e.g. loss of consciousness, confusion, or trouble waking.
- First seizures – a fit or convulsion of any type.
- Animal, snake or human bites.
- Pain or loss of use of a limb, which might indicate broken bones.
- Bleeding that does not stop with direct pressure.
- Burns or scalds above the size of your baby's palm or any burn or scald to the face.
- Puncture wounds to the skin at any site, due to sticks or sharp points.
- Head, neck, back or eye injuries.
- Signs of allergic reaction such as hives, swelling of the face, lips, eyes or tongue, fainting, trouble breathing or swallowing, or wheezing.
- Swallowed drugs or household cleaners.

If you do provide First Aid treatment for your baby, call your GP to see if any follow-up care is needed.

Broken bones and fractures

It is very unusual for small babies to break a bone. If it happens, it may be immediately obvious, or only brought to light when your baby is less settled than usual – there may not even be bruising or swelling. If your baby stops using a limb or seems in pain when a limb is moved, take her to the nearest emergency medical service. An x-ray is the only sure way to diagnose a fracture.

- A broken bone will usually be set in a cast – roughly 3 weeks for an arm bone and 6 weeks for a leg bone. If the bone needs to be straightened, your baby will be given an anaesthetic.
- Once the cast is in place the fracture is unlikely to give much

---

The ABC of resuscitation

If your baby stops breathing or is unconscious and cannot be roused:

- Call for help – quick call to neighbour, friend or relative, even a passer-by.
- Stimulate your baby by very gently shaking her.

If there is no response, act quickly and as calmly as you can:

A – Airway: Ensure the airway is clear. Lie your baby along your forearm with her head supported on your hand and lower than her chest. Give five firm slaps on back to dislodge any foreign object.

B – Breathing: Check for breathing movement of the chest. If there is none:

- Position head to 'sniffing the morning air position' – chin lifted and head tilted back slightly.
- Give five rescue breaths: put your mouth over your baby's mouth and nose and blow just hard enough to make her chest move, as though she is taking a deep breath for herself. Take a breath for yourself between breaths.

C – Check pulse: You can feel your baby's pulse at her neck or groin, or where her heart is beating on her chest. If above 60/min, give regular mouth to nose and mouth respiration at a rate of 20 breaths per minute, about double your own rate. If below 60/min, start chest compressions to boost the heart and to maintain blood supply to the brain. Continue chest compressions until the heart rate (pulse) is above 60 and remains above 60 for 1 minute. If in doubt continue chest compressions.

- Use two fingers and place them in the centre of your baby's chest, roughly two finger-widths below her nipples and press hard enough to depress the breast bone 1-2 cm (1/2-3/4 in).
- Aim for five chest compressions to one mouth to nose and mouth breath. That's 100 compressions to 20 resuscitation breaths per minute.
- After 1 minute check again – **A**irway, **B**reathing, **C**irculation – and call for help.
- Repeat the cycle until help arrives.

If your child starts breathing again:

- Turn her on her side so secretions can run out of the mouth.
- Keep watching her breathing rate to make sure it continues.
- Check her pulse every minute to make sure it stays above 80/min.

Keep checking these until help arrives, and be prepared to restart the ABC if her breathing rate or heart rate falls.

---

pain, but if your baby seems uncomfortable, infant paracetamol will help. If she has a large fracture, your doctor may suggest other painkilling medications.

- Modern casts are lightweight. To bathe your baby, wrap the cast in a plastic bag and seal it with tape. Keep the limb out of the water if at all possible.
- Homeopathy: Give *Aconite* (30c) as soon as you can, to treat shock. Give *Arnica* (30c) for shock and pain relief and to begin the healing of muscles and tissues – 1 dose every 15 minutes for an hour, then 3–4 times a day for a week. When the fracture has been set, give *Ledum* (30c) 3 times a day for 4

days in conjunction with *Arnica*. After the initial pain and swelling have reduced, *Symphytum* (6c) speeds the bone-healing process – from 1 week after the accident, use 3 times a day for 2 weeks, then twice a day for 2 weeks. If the fracture has not healed after using *Symphytum*, use *Calc Phos* (6x) twice a day for 2–3 weeks. If the ribs are broken, use *Bryonia* (30c) twice a day for 2 weeks.

Bumps and bruises

Your baby will almost certainly get bumps and bruises. If she tumbles, give loving care. She may let you rub the area lightly – this increases circulation and begins the healing process.
- Witch hazel solution is good to use in the first instance to reduce bruising.
- Homeopathy: *Arnica* is the no. 1 remedy following an injury or accident, for trauma and bruising and is effective nine times out of ten. Use 30c every 15 minutes for 4 doses and then 3–4 times a day for 3 days. If the skin is not broken, apply *Arnica* cream twice a day for a few days. Use *Ruta* (30c) 3 times a day for 3–4 days when an area thinly covered by skin is bruised (e.g. elbow, shin), or bruising follows a fracture, dislocation or sprain and *Arnica* does not help; *Ledum* if arnica does not help and the bruise feels cold to the touch. Use in the 30c potency, 3 times a day for 3–4 days.

Burns and scalds

Burns and scalds are the most common cause of serious injury in babies, caused by hot liquids, flames or hot ashes, electricity, friction, chemicals or even radiation. The most common cause is spilt tea or coffee.

In a superficial burn the skin may appear red or form a blister filled with fluid. It usually recovers well without scarring. A deeper burn or scald causes the skin to come away. Recovery may be prolonged and there will be scarring. Occasionally skin grafting is necessary. Very deep burns result in blackening of the skin. Inhalation of hot liquids or gasses can cause damage to the airway – seek expert help immediately.

If your baby is scalded the immediate treatment is:
- Remove her from the source of the heat.
- Remove clothing if necessary (clothes hold hot water on to the skin).
- Pour cold water over the injured area.
- Keep the skin area exposed, allowing it to cool.
- A loose covering can be applied, cling film is ideal, especially if you are moving your baby to hospital – do not apply greasy dressings.
- If the burn is smaller than the palm of your baby's hand, use a proprietary burn cream. If it is bigger, seek help and do not apply cream.
- Infant paracetamol is ideal as a pain reliever. Use the dose recommended on the bottle.
- Seek help.

Homeopathy

Give *Arnica* (30c) for the shock every 15 minutes until the situation is under control; *Combudoron* burn ointment (available from most chemists) for minor burns or scalds; *Urtica Urens* tincture 10 drops to 250 ml (½ pint) water for minor burns, scalds without blistering or with minimal blistering where there is stinging, soreness and redness, scalds from boiling water; *Cantharis* (30c) alongside medical treatment 4 times a day for a week if the burn is severe and very painful; *Causticum* (6c) 3 times a day for up to 2 weeks for burns to the tongue or burns that look healed but still hurt. After initial healing, use *Calendula* cream twice a day for up to 4 weeks – it soothes and can help minimise scarring.

Sunburn

Even very short exposure to strong sun can cause redness and blistering of a baby's sensitive skin. Prevention is the best thing. If there is burning:
- Infant paracetamol or ibuprofen can help relieve pain.
- After-sun lotion or simple emollients such as E45 stop the burned skin from drying up.
- A weak hydrocortisone steroid cream (0.5–1%) available over the counter will reduce the discomfort of mild sunburn where the skin is red but not blistered.
- *Calendula* cream can be soothing.
- *Combudoron* cream, also used for scalds, is effective.
- Homeopathic *Belladonna* (30c) 3 times a day for 2 days can relieve the burn.

Cat scratches

Cats usually avoid babies but babies are curious and can provoke them. Apart from the discomfort from a scratch – worst if on the face or eyes – there is the risk of an infection called cat scratch, which is usually only contracted from kittens. After being scratched, redness spreads up the arm or leg, and then settles down. Later the glands in the groin or armpit on the affected side flare up.
- Simple antibiotic treatment settles the condition over a 2–3 week period.
- Homeopathy: Use *Calendula* tincture – 10 drops in 250 ml (½ pint) water – to bathe and clean the scratch, and apply *Calendula* cream to soothe and promote healing.

Choking

If your baby chokes on something, she will struggle for breath, may become red in the face, cough, grasp her neck and seem terrified. You will need to act quickly. The cause is likely to be food or a toy stuck in the airway.
- Call for help.
- Check your baby's airway and give her five back slaps (as in ABC, p.383).
- Check if the airway is clear and she is breathing.
- If not, turn her over to face you.
- Place the heel of your hand on the lower part of her chest and give five firm thrusts.
- Check her airway is clear and she is breathing.
- If not – give five rescue breaths (ABC).
- Start chest compressions if the heart rate has slowed to less than 80/minute, or has stopped.
- Keep repeating this cycle until help arrives or your baby improves.

Cuts, lacerations and abrasions

Cuts among babies are unusual, although broken glass on the

ground or a sharp knife left in reach might cut fingers, and stumbles, particularly on to open doors or table corners, can cause nasty head cuts. In babies cuts bleed easily.

For minor cuts:
- Wash the affected part.
- Apply firm pressure and the bleeding will usually come under control in 3–5 minutes.
- When bleeding has stopped do not disturb the injury, as this will often start the bleeding again. Apply a firm dressing if possible, or a plaster.
- If the cut continues to bleed, keep the pressure on and ask for help from your doctor.
- Homeopathy: *Calendula* cream is good – you can also bathe the graze or cut with 10 drops of *Calendula* or *Hypercal* tincture dissolved in 250 ml (½ pint) cooled boiled water to guard against infection and promote healing. For a deeper cut, give *Hypericum* (30c) 3 times a day for 3–4 days.

For deep cuts:
- Act quickly.
- If your baby has lost consciousness or appears to be in shock, ask someone to call the emergency services while you begin First Aid.
- Lie your child down with her feet elevated about 15 cm (6 in). This increases blood flow to the brain and reduces the risk of shock. If possible, elevate the site of bleeding as well; that helps reduce blood flow.
- Use a sterile bandage or cloth to apply firm pressure with your hand directly to the wound. If nothing else is available, use the palm of your hand (after washing your hands, if possible). Maintain steady pressure until the bleeding stops. If an artery has been cut, it will take at least 10 minutes of constant pressure. If blood soaks through the bandage you're using, don't remove it; instead, add another layer on top and exert finger pressure. Try to keep calm and calm your baby (anxiety will pump more blood to the site).
- Once the bleeding stops, leave the bandage or cloth in place. If more blood seeps through, apply another bandage or cloth on top. To maintain pressure keep pressing with your finger and wrap cling film or tape tightly around the bandages and the injured area.
- If your child is awake and alert, take her to casualty immediately and if she is woozy or unconscious, call for an ambulance.

Dog bites
Dog bites are common and usually no more than a playful nip. Severe dog bites can cause serious injury, including fractures and deep cuts, and wound infection.
- Clean the bite with water, and apply a dressing to stop bleeding.
- Seek expert help from your GP or casualty department. Professional care is essential because the risk of infection is high.
- Homeopathy: Give *Ledum* (30c) hourly for 2 hours followed by *Hypericum* (30c) hourly for the next 2 hours. *Hypericum* tincture – 10 drops in 250 ml (½ pint) water – can also be used to bathe and clean the bite.

Drowning and near-drowning
A young baby can drown in very little water. Many children do survive drowning without brain damage, especially if they are very cold because this slows down the body's system so that it can operate without oxygen for longer. But prevention is certainly better than cure – do not leave your baby unattended in or near water.

If you find your baby face down in water, not breathing, lifeless and perhaps blue and cold:
- Call for help.
- Shake her gently and see if she responds.
- If no response, give five rescue breaths (as in ABC, p.383).
- Check for breathing or response.
- If no response, continue to give rescue breaths and chest compression.
- Call for help.
- Continue until help arrives.

Ears
Never poke anything into the ear. Treat bleeding from the ear as from the nose (p.387).

If a foreign object is pushed into the ear canal, do not try to remove it, as it will be pushed in further. Take your baby to the local casualty department, or to your GP, who will arrange for an ear, nose and throat specialist to remove the foreign body (p.453).
Homeopathy: Seek medical help and en route administer 1 dose of *Silica* (30c), which will facilitate the removal of the object. After it has been removed, give 1 dose of *Hypericum* (30c). *Arnica* (30c) 3 times a day for the next 2 days will help reduce any swelling.

Eyes and eyelids
The eyes are very well protected behind the bony ridges of the eye socket and serious eye injuries are very uncommon. If your baby does injure her eye, take her to your GP or nearest casualty department – it is important to be careful.
- If you can see something in your baby's eye, such as an insect, eyelash or piece of grit, use a clean cloth or tightly rolled piece of cotton wool and gently encourage it to come out. You can also try using plain tap water to flush it out. If she is crying, it may come out of its own accord.
- If you cannot get to the foreign object, don't poke and prod, go to hospital.
- If her eye appears swollen and you are unaware of any accident, she may have an EYE INFECTION or be displaying an ALLERGY OR INTOLERANCE.

Homeopathy
Any eye injury needs medical attention. If a small foreign body is stuck, give *Aconite* (30c) for shock and fear and then *Hypericum* (30c) hourly for 4–5 hours, which reduces pain and sensitivity. Once the foreign body is out, bathe the closed eye with a mixture of 8 drops *Euphrasia* tincture to 250 ml (½ pint) boiled cooled water every 3 hours until there is relief. Never use undiluted tincture. Hold your baby in front of you so she is facing you, soak cotton wool in the diluted solution and gently squeeze it over the eye area. You can also give *Euphrasia* (30c) 4 times a day until the eye settles.

For a black eye, give *Arnica* (30c) or *Arnica* cream (do not use on broken skin) immediately and then hourly for 3–4 hours. If bruising is painful and soothed by cool compresses, give *Ledum* (30c) 2-hourly for 8 hours then 3 times a day for 2–3 days.

For a minor cut to the eye area use *Calendula* (30c) 4 times a day for a few days and *Calendula* cream rubbed lightly around (but not on) the cut. You can combine this with *Hypercal* tincture – 10 drops to 250 ml (½ pint) water – and bathe the area 4 times a day.

Falling downstairs

If you fall down the stairs holding your baby or your baby falls down without you:

- Check airway, breathing and circulation (ABC, p.383).
- If your baby is unconscious, call for help.
- If your baby is awake, make sure she is using all limbs fully and equally. Check for bumps and bruises. Notify your doctor or go to casualty if you are concerned.

Hands, fingers, feet and toes

Small babies love to put fingers where they don't belong, and as a result often get minor cuts and grazes (p.384). Sometimes a finger or toe may be caught in a door, and as a result a nail or tip will be crushed or torn.

- Wash the affected part and look at the damage. Even small cuts will bleed heavily. Apply firm pressure to stop the bleeding.
- If the nail has been torn, it will probably need removal at the nearest casualty department. Once removed, future growth depends on how much damage there has been to the base of the nail.
- If the end of a finger or toe tip been crushed, the bony tip may be exposed. A few stitches are needed to close the cut, and the digit will heal well.
- If the tip has been amputated, find it, place it back on the finger or toe and go to the nearest casualty department. It may be sewn back on. These kinds of injuries have good rates of recovery.
- Babies can get thread wrapped around a toe or finger, and if this is not noticed for a few days the digit can turn black. If possible unwind the thread, but it may be buried in the swollen skin. Go to the nearest casualty department.
- Homeopathy: *Arnica* (30c) every 15 minutes for the 1st hour treats the shock and *Hypericum* (30c) given hourly for 4 hours following works on alleviating pain and repairing nerve endings. Bathing affected part with *Hyperical* tincture – 10 drops to 250 ml (1/2 pint) water – will also promote healing as it acts as an antiseptic.

Head injuries

Most children who injure their heads suffer no ill effects. Even a skull fracture is not always a bad thing, as it indicates that most of the force of the injury was taken by bone rather than brain. The most severe injuries are those associated with rapid acceleration then deceleration – for example, falling from a low height on to a hard (or even a soft) surface, or receiving a kick to the head from an animal (especially horses).

A common cause of serious brain injury is shaking. Because the head of a baby is heavy and the neck muscles are weak, even two or three shakes of a baby under 12 months of age can lead to brain damage caused by bleeding into the brain (p.407).

- If after a head injury, however trivial, your baby behaves in any way differently from normal, consult your doctor. While most children survive injury with no harm, symptoms may be delayed for a few hours, so watch your baby closely.
- Seek medical attention if your baby is conscious but drowsy, pale and listless, vomiting, crying incessantly or is abnormally quiet and unresponsive.
- While you are travelling to hospital or waiting for your doctor to arrive, *Arnica* (30c) is an effective initial treatment.

Insect bites and stings

Insect bites and stings are a common problem for babies, particularly in the summer and in temperate regions. The best treatment is prevention.

The most common biting insects are mosquitoes and midges whose bites usually cause intense itchiness and a raised spot, often with a dark centre. After a few hours the skin may become hot and swollen (due to histamine) and redness may spread around the site of the bite. Very often there is a crop of bites within a small area. The spots can become fluid-filled blisters. Symptoms usually disappear within 48 hours but you can treat the bite with proprietary creams and/or with oral antihistamines available over the counter (e.g. Piriton), particularly if the swelling is significant: 2.5 ml (½ tsp) of Piriton syrup or 0.5–1% hydrocortisone cream is quite OK for babies. If the bite(s) become infected, antibiotics are usually effective within a few days.

If your baby is stung by a wasp or bee, keep a close eye on her. These stings, although rarely, can cause a serious allergic reaction known as anaphylactic shock: swelling of the face or mouth, noisy or difficult breathing or difficulty swallowing (p.417), which needs emergency medical attention.

- Bee stings are often left in the skin. The chemicals in the sting can be neutralised with an ammonia pen, available from all chemists, and you can pull the sting out with tweezers.
- For a bee sting you can dab a diluted mixture of bicarbonate of soda and water on the site; vinegar soothes wasp stings.

Homeopathy

Use *Aconite* (30c) immediately if your baby is in shock. Then give the most appropriate remedy (30c) every 15 minutes for the 1st hour, reducing to 1 dose every 2 hours for the next 8 hours. Use *Apis* for ant, bee or wasp stings leaving hot, puffy, red skin and burning, prickling or stinging pain; *Hypericum* if pain is shooting upwards from the site, and the skin feels tender, numb, tingly and hot; *Ledum* if the skin is punctured, becomes puffy and swollen yet feels cold, and is soothed by cold compresses; *Rhus Tox* if the sting comes from a plant and scratching makes it worse, or it is worse at night or from warm bathing; *Urtica Urens* for itchy, blotchy skin, like a nettle rash that feels better for rubbing. You can bathe the irritated skin in a tincture of *Hypercal* or *Urtica* – 10 drops to 250 ml (½ pint) water. If you have *Pyretheum* spray in your First Aid kit, use it 2-hourly for the first 8 hours.

Mouth and nose injuries

The soft tissues of the face are so well supplied with blood that any injury to the mouth or nose tends to bleed a lot. The bleeding will probably stop in a few minutes.

- If the nose is cut and bleeding, don't squeeze it – it will be bruised. Apply gentle pressure to obvious bleeding areas on the skin. Only if there is a constant flow of blood from inside try to apply a gentle squeeze, but this may be painful.
- Lips and tongue bleed easily, and the volume appears greater because it's mixed with saliva.
- Recovery from a mouth injury can take time, particularly if there is bruising or if mouth ulcers develop. Avoid acid drinks and foods for the first few days.
- Homeopathy: Give *Arnica* (30c) every 15 minutes for the 1st hour to treat shock and to curb the bleeding, then *Hypericum* (30c) hourly for the next 3 hours. You could also bathe the area in a solution of *Hyperical* tincture – 10 drops to 250 ml (½ pint) water.

Swallowing objects and liquids

If you think your child has swallowed a medicine, tablet or dangerous fluid:

- Clear chewed tablets/liquid from the mouth.
- If your child is drowsy, do not make her sick. Never give salt water.
- If she has drunk a toxic liquid (household cleaner), do not make her sick; she will probably vomit anyway.
- Call an ambulance.
- If she is choking, take the appropriate action immediately, and then call an ambulance.
- Look around on the floor for tablets that have been dropped rather than swallowed, or check for spilt liquid.
- What quantity was originally in the pack/bottle? Take any remaining medicines and containers with you, especially of household cleansers, when you go for medical help.

If your baby needs surgery: homeopathic tips

- *Aconite*: Very useful for fear. Use 1 dose (30c) just before surgery.
- *Arnica* (30c): Excellent for dealing with shock and trauma, and to help the healing of inflammation and bruising that are inevitable with surgery.
- *Hypericum* (30c): The arnica of the nerves. It is especially useful for surgery involving nerve tissue with or without stitching, particularly to feet, hands, eyes, head or teeth.
- *Calendula* (30c): Speeds up post-operative healing of wounds and scars. Also available in cream form.

After surgery, these three remedies can be given 4 times a day for 3 days and then 3 times a day for 4 days.

- *Phosphorus* (30c): Helps your baby to deal with a general anaesthetic. Give 2-hourly for the first 6 hours after surgery.
- *Staphysagria* (30c): Heals lacerations and helps with the trauma of an invasive procedure, for instance if a catheter is used. If your baby seems jumpy, give this in addition to the top three, 4 times a day for 2 days.

First Aid kit for your baby and family

Your baby's 'normal' body temperature is individual to her. Take a measurement when she is well so you know what is normal. As a general guide, consider a temperature of 38°C (100.4°F) to be a fever. Accompanying symptoms, such as seeming unwell or too warm, having sweaty skin or being unusually out of sorts are also important. If you are worried, follow your instinct. Feeling your baby's forehead is not an accurate measure of temperature – use a thermometer to be sure. Your paediatrician may refer to the following figures:

	Normal	Fever
In the mouth	37°C (98.6°F)	37.5°C (99.5°F)
In the armpit	36.4°C (97.6°F)	37°C (98.6°F)
Rectal	37.6°C (99.6°F)	38°C (100.4°F)

Keep a First Aid kit easily accessible and replace anything you use as soon as possible. Specifically for your baby this should contain:

- List of useful telephone numbers.
- Loving Care and Patience.
- Thermometer (range from simple strip for placing on the forehead to electronic – simple is usually adequate).
- Tweezers for splinters and stings.
- Infant paracetamol suspension (one brand is Calpol) or Junior Disprin for bringing down temperature and relieving minor pains. Use dosage as instructed, according to your baby's age. The dose of paracetamol recommended for babies is 2.5 ml (½ tsp) no more frequently than 4-hour intervals.
- Paracetamol suppositories are useful for older babies (above 3 months) who have a fever illness with vomiting. Use a dose of 125 mg for a 3-month-old.
- Ibuprofen/Junifen for night use and those more severe pains not helped by paracetamol. This is stronger than infant paracetamol suspension and only needs to be given 8-hourly.
- Teething gel or homeopathic teething granules.
- Rehydration sachets (e.g. Dioralyte), to use if your baby has diarrhoea or vomiting.
- Barrier cream for severe nappy rash.
- Antiseptic cream (suitable for your baby's age group).
- Small sticking plasters.
- Small roll of adhesive tape to stick down dressings for scalds and burns.
- Antihistamine syrup – Piriton.
- Cotton-wool balls – for cleaning skin, but not for a dressing as they stick to the damaged skin surface.
- Homeopathic remedies: You can buy First Aid kits that will suit your whole family and your homeopath can prescribe anything that suits your particular needs. Useful applications include *Calendula* and *Combudoron* for burns, Bach Flower rescue cream, *Arnica* cream, *Hypercal* tincture for cuts and grazes and *Pyretheum* spray for bites and stings. *Aconite* (30c), which is best given straight away for shock, is also handy for parents as it reduces panic and fear.

Safety

Keeping safe in pregnancy

During pregnancy most women are aware of potential hazards and avoid activities that carry risks. Recreational DRUGS, SMOKING and ALCOHOL are covered separately and there is guidance on eating in Eating and weight (p.332). If you've already done some of the things that are better avoided, don't worry – the risks are small and you can now carry on safely.

Sport and exercise

Exercise is very good for you, but keep within safety limits (p.357), take care not to overheat, and make it fun. Exercise on a regular basis is better than widely spaced spurts. Always ask a professional teacher if you are unsure of safety.

In general, don't start a new exercise in pregnancy without guidance, and avoid climbing, horse riding, scuba diving, squash, step classes, water skiing, sky sports and anything that is fast or involves impact or sudden twists or turns. If you're already a jogger, do no more than 2 miles a day. If you're not a jogger, don't start now. In mid- to late pregnancy fast walking is safer than jogging. If you are a competent skier it is safe in early pregnancy to cross-country ski below 2000 m (6500 ft); downhill skiing and high-altitude skiing are out.

Sex

If you have had a history of MISCARRIAGE or BLEEDING DURING PREGNANCY, it is wise to abstain from sex for the first 14 weeks. Otherwise, making love is safe and the penis cannot damage your baby. There is no risk if you use condoms and spermicide. In late pregnancy sex is safe unless you have a history of PREMATURE BIRTH or your waters have broken.

As long as you are comfortable, the following are safe: oral sex, anal penetration, masturbation, vibrators (but not deep penetration) and lubricators, including natural oils and KY jelly. Vaginal douches may not be safe.

Leisure and day-to-day activities

Bleaching facial and body hair and electrolysis: Both are safe, though avoid the nipple area if you are breastfeeding.
Body piercing: Don't have a new piercing in pregnancy. If your labia are pierced, it is better to remove the rings for birth.
Depilatories: It may be preferable to shave or wax during pregnancy.
Electric blankets: Turn off an electric blanket before getting into bed to avoid overheating. It emits an electro-magnetic field, though levels are considered to be safe.
Gardening: Wear gloves to avoid TOXOPLASMOSIS from the soil, keep your posture in mind to avoid strains. Delegate jobs involving lifting and climbing.
Hair colouring and perms: There is no conclusive evidence that chemicals involved in dyeing are unsafe, nor that they are safe. You absorb hair-colouring agents through your scalp, not through each hair shaft, so streaking or highlighting may be better. Always wear plastic gloves when dyeing. Henna is a semi-permanent vegetable dye considered to be very safe. Perming may not work well in pregnancy, and the chemicals may not be safe; to achieve curls use rags or plaiting instead.
Heaters in the house: These might carry a risk of carbon monoxide poisoning. Arrange inspection of any gas stoves, heaters, fireplaces or wood-burning stoves in your home.
House cleaning: Wear gloves and avoid direct contact with products that have strong fumes and warning labels. Keep windows open for ventilation. Look into alternative products (such as vinegar for cleaning windows).
Loud music, rock concerts: Your baby is cushioned and will be fine. Even so, don't stand too close to the speakers and if you feel your own ears hurting, move.
Massages: For safety, check the oils are safe for use in pregnancy (p.378).
Painting and decorating: Avoid contact with oil-based paint, polyurethane floor finishes, spray paints, turpentine, white spirit and liquid paint removers. Water-based paints are a safer choice. Good ventilation is a must. Take care if you are removing or sanding old paint (pre-1970), which may contain lead, a toxic chemical, and avoid electrical work.
Pets: If you have cats, be very hygienic when dealing with their faeces because of the risk of TOXOPLASMOSIS infection.
Saunas and jacuzzis: Raising your core temperature significantly has the potential to cause birth defects, especially in the 1st trimester. Using the facilities for very short periods may be safe but avoidance is best.
Tattoos: Existing tattoos are no problem. New tattoos are best not done in pregnancy.

Chemicals and work hazards

A drug or chemical that is known to carry a high risk of causing birth defects is known as a teratogen. The link is a difficult one to ascertain, and although some chemicals and drugs have been proved dangerous, not every drug has been tested. Moreover, the risk of harming a baby's development in the womb is often associated with a combination of environmental factors or some genetic factors. It is estimated that of the 2–3% of babies born with birth defects, fewer than 10% of cases can be linked with exposure to teratogens.

Most chemicals are present in extremely low doses and pose very little threat to you or your developing baby. The risk depends on the level and frequency of exposure, the stage of pregnancy and your genetic make-up. It inevitably rises if you are exposed to a dangerous chemical on a daily basis and do not take adequate precautions Take steps to avoid exposure to: the dry cleaning chemical tetrachloroethylene, Ethylene glycol ethers, Insecticides, lead, mercury (most commonly found in contaminated fish), aromatic hydrocarbons, phenols, xylene and vinyl chloride (used in laboratories, art work and ceramics), radiation (e.g. x-rays and gamma rays) and infections (e.g. if you work in health care).

If your line of work involves exposure to potentially dangerous chemicals, your employer is obliged to tell you if any may be harmful in pregnancy. You are entitled to ask to move to a safer position, as you are if physical demands may endanger you or your baby.

Pharmaceutical drugs

In general it is preferable to avoid taking medication in pregnancy. Yet if you are unwell it is important to treat the cause and reduce symptoms. You may be able to do this without medication. Sometimes the risks associated with taking a drug (e.g. for epilepsy) may be lower than the potential risks of not taking it. If you require medication you need to consult your doctor who will recommend a safe dose or an alternative. Over-the-counter drugs are usually labelled clearly if they are contraindicated in pregnancy, but to be safe it is always best to consult a doctor. Research into the effects of drug use in pregnancy is limited, for obvious reasons.

Your baby is particularly vulnerable between Days 17 and 57 of pregnancy while crucial organ development is taking place. If you take a drug that affects your baby, there is a chance of a birth defect. Before Day 17 the effect may be total (causing MISCARRIAGE) or absent. After this date, if a drug has an effect it is more likely to interfere with growth of the organs (leading to INTRAUTERINE GROWTH RESTRICTION), although the brain and nervous system can also be affected.

This list gives guidelines; your doctor will give you details. There are details for specific health conditions within the A–Z Health Guide.

Anti-anxiety drugs and antidepressants: These can carry implications for a growing baby and can be passed on in breast milk. There is a detailed list on p.460.

Antibiotics: Penicillins such as amoxicillin, erythromycin and a number of other antibiotics appear to be safe. Your doctor will advise you depending on the treatment you require. There are antibiotics that are contraindicated in pregnancy including tetracyclines (affect bone and teeth), streptomycin (affects hearing) and trimethoprim (affects cell development). Chloramphenicol can cause a serious illness in the newborn. There are usually alternatives available from your doctor.

Anticancer drugs: The cells in a growing baby's tissues multiply rapidly and are very vulnerable to anticancer drugs. It is preferable to consult a doctor before conception.

Anti-clotting drugs: Heparin is the safest option, taken under supervision (p.409). Warfarin may cause birth defects but low-dose aspirin is safe in pregnancy.

Anticonvulsant drugs: Some drugs to reduce FITS may cause an increased risk of congenital abnormality (7%). It is preferable to use single medications rather than a combination. The drugs may reduce a baby's blood-clotting ability and this is minimised with injection of vitamin K at birth.

Aspirin: Nonsteroidal anti-inflammatory drugs (NSAIDs), such as aspirin and ibuprofen, are best avoided, particularly in the last 4 weeks. If you need to take aspirin for an underlying medical condition, your doctor will advise you. Low-dose treatment is unlikely to have a significant effect on your baby. Taking large doses during pregnancy may delay labour and may also cause early closing of the ductus arteriosus in the HEART, overloading the baby's circulatory system. These drugs in large doses could cause BLEEDING problems in the mother or the newborn around the time of birth and contribute to JAUNDICE in the newborn. Aspirin intake during a viral infection has been associated with Reye's syndrome in babies, a rare condition that causes brain and liver damage and death and it is best avoided during breastfeeding.

Painkillers: It is safe to use paracetamol in low doses to control temperature symptoms or as pain relief. If you require a stronger painkiller, morphine and codeine are the options. It is best to avoid a large dose of codeine before delivery.

Sex hormones: Used to treat hormone disorders, excessive body hair and endometriosis, these can affect a baby's genital organs. The contraceptive pill has not been shown to affect foetal development if it is taken in pregnancy.

Skin treatments: Of the retinoid type, these can cause birth defects and it is best to stop use for up to 1 year before conception. It is best to consult your doctor.

Steroids: Taking corticosteroids (e.g. for ASTHMA or irritable bowel syndrome, p.448) carries a small risk to a baby but this is often smaller than the risk of complications if drug use is stopped. The exposure is minimised when steroids are taken as inhalations or enemas and the doses are kept low.

Vaccines: Except under special circumstances, vaccines made with a live virus aren't given to women who are or might be pregnant (p.546).

Safety for your baby

Even before you bring your baby home it is a good idea to try to anticipate the everyday dangers that you might encounter. Most childhood accidents happen in the home. It is the easiest place to guard against accidents, yet also the easiest place to overlook dangers. It is not always possible, but try to keep one step ahead of your baby, because she may do something you don't expect (like roll for the first time while you are not watching).

Surfaces and falling
- Never leave your baby on a surface other than the floor when you leave the room or even turn your head. Babies can fall from beds, sofas, etc., very quickly.
- Always strap your baby into her car seat before lifting it.
- Never leave the seat on a raised surface with your baby in it.
- Always strap your baby into her chair, pram or pushchair.

Bathroom
- Never place your baby in a baby bath resting on a raised surface.
- Never leave your baby unattended in the bath or bathroom.
- Always run the hot tap last, and watch your child when it is running and once she is in the bath.
- Support your baby in the bath.
- Place a towel on the floor and lift your baby out before you step out of the water, to avoid slipping.
- Wash the bath thoroughly after using essential oils.
- Keep all your toiletries and medicines well out of reach.

Kitchen
- Your baby may pull a jug, cup of tea or a plate of hot food off the table. More babies get burned by cups of tea and coffee than by anything else.
- Turn all pot handles away from the edge of the cooker, and use the rings furthest from you as often as possible.
- Keep sharp knives out of your baby's reach.

Food
- Avoid the risk of choking – never prop up your baby's bottle.
- Help toddlers to understand that babies only eat milk so they shouldn't offer food, however friendly they are trying to be.

- When your baby is weaned always stay with her at meal times. Don't give small morsels or peanuts as they can obstruct breathing if inhaled and, if sharing your food, be aware of risks (e.g. fish bones and unevenly distributed heat).

Bedroom
- Don't use too much bedding and avoid cot bumpers and a gathering of soft toys, which could increase the risk of overheating (p.214).
- Don't put pillows around a bed. Although they may reduce injury if she falls, your baby can suffocate in them.
- Keep your baby's cot away from shelves because she may reach up and pull things on to herself.

In the car
- Always use a car seat for your baby and fix it where it is safe with the correct seatbelt and away from fitted airbags. Upgrade the car seat to suit your baby as she grows.
- Use sunshades to prevent overheating. Never leave your child alone in a parked car.
- Use child locks.
- Never start the engine before your baby is fully strapped in.

Outside
- Watch what your baby picks up, or where she puts her hands – they will almost certainly go into her mouth.
- Always strap your baby into her pushchair or pram. Don't ignore the middle strap in a pushchair. Always use the breaks when you are not moving.
- Don't use a pushchair on an escalator. Take your baby out and hold her, or use a lift.

Sun safety
Your baby's skin is very sensitive:
- Keep your baby out of direct sunlight if possible.
- Keep her legs and arms covered in loose clothes and encourage her to wear a sun hat.
- Use an umbrella for shade in the buggy or pram.
- Always apply a high-factor sun cream (25 or higher), especially if at the seaside or by a swimming pool.

Pets
- Family pets may get jealous – watch their behaviour and don't leave them alone with your baby. Even familiar dogs may bite.
- Don't let your dogs lick your baby's bottles.
- If you arrange your space so your baby is never physically lower than your dog, she will remain the boss.
- Prepare your pets, especially cats; if they sleep in your bedroom move them to another room for sleeping a few weeks before the birth.
- When your baby has arrived, where necessary use a cat net over doors and a stair gate to keep your dog out of a room. Also use a net over the pram when your baby is sleeping in it.
- Try to keep your pets' routine as normal as possible, as this can reduce jealous reactions.
- Be careful with other people's pets, they may be curious.

Poisonous substances
Most cases of poisoning in children are with household cleaners, unused tablets (commonly iron tablets and painkillers among new mums), and tablets stolen from grandparents.
- Keep detergents, shampoos, medicines, fertilisers and other poisonous substances out of your baby's sight and reach.
- Medicines may be locked in a cupboard for extra safety.
- Throw away tablets and medicines that are not being used.

Safety for your mobile baby
Be accident aware – judge everything from your developing baby's point of view.

Inside
- Once your baby is sitting, a lightweight rocking seat is no longer appropriate – she has the strength to tip it over.
- Don't leave pens, sharp or small objects within reach – they may be swallowed or cause choking.
- Guard the top and bottom of stairs with a stairgate as soon as your baby is mobile. A baby who can crawl can climb stairs but not descend safely and younger babies can roll.
- Use a fireguard around any fire, radiator or hot-water pipe that may scald.
- Cover electric sockets – blank plugs can be obtained from chemists and baby stores. If possible use safety plugs, which are fused, and a trip switch to prevent electrocution.
- Keep all electric wires out of your baby's reach – she will be tempted to play with them.
- Avoid free-standing shelves. If you keep them, fix to the wall and ensure they do not wobble, causing objects to fall.
- Use a guard on your cooker.
- Remove unsteady stools or tables until she is much older.
- Use cupboard locks.
- Avoid standing lamps.
- Use window locks if you have low windows.
- Use non-slip socks or soft shoes for your baby so she doesn't slip when pulling herself to standing.
- Don't leave your baby unattended in a baby bouncer or walker. When your baby is cruising, keep obstacles that may trip her up out of the way.
- When grandparents visit ensure their handbags are closed – they can be a source of colourful but dangerous tablets.
- At other people's houses watch out for drapes over tables that your baby will love to pull, perhaps bringing down hot cups of tea or coffee. When visiting friends who don't have small children, be baby aware – it's amazing what you do automatically in your own home to protect your baby.
- Don't give your baby toys with small parts, which carry the risk of choking.

Outside
- Be careful of open water, including ponds, buckets and water butts.
- In playgrounds, stay with your baby at all times.
- If you cycle, use a child seat once your baby is big enough to fit in safely and wear a protective helmet. Buggies that attach to the back of a bike with a body harness are safer.
- In public sandpits and parks watch for animal faeces and broken glass or plastic.

The A–Z Health Guide

ABDOMINAL PAIN
See PAIN, IN THE ABDOMEN

ABUSE
See BATTERING & ABUSE: MOTHER; CHILD PROTECTION & ABUSE

ACNE
See SKIN, RASHES, IRRITATION & SPOTS: BABY; SKIN, RASHES & IRRITATION: MOTHER

ALCOHOL

See also DRUGS, RECREATIONAL

Alcohol – in beer, wine and spirits – is a central nervous system depressant that affects nearly every organ in the body. Drinking, especially heavy drinking over a period of time, can contribute to a number of serious problems, including muscle, brain and heart disease, malnutrition, digestive and liver problems, and can significantly affect the developing system of an unborn baby. Whenever you consume alcohol, so does your baby, in pregnancy and after birth if you are breastfeeding, although the levels are lower in milk.

The World Health Organisation suggests that no alcohol at all during pregnancy is the safest approach. Bingeing probably has a more intense effect than the same amount of alcohol taken over a few days, although a single binge on one occasion is highly unlikely to affect a baby.

What happens
Inside the womb a baby's liver has a very low capacity for breaking down alcohol and eliminating toxins. Alcohol interferes with the ability to obtain sufficient oxygen and nourishment for normal cell development. At any stage in pregnancy a baby receiving more alcohol than he can cope with may develop problems: severity increases with the amount consumed and it is probably more intense in early pregnancy. Problems may relate to physical development or to mental acuity and could persist to school age and beyond. When a newborn shows symptoms of excessive alcohol intake, he is said to have foetal alcohol syndrome.

Action plan
If you are a light, recreational drinker, as soon as you know you are pregnant, cut down or stop altogether. It is up to you to set your boundaries and to stick within them. If you drink regularly and find it hard to give up, you may be addicted. The guidance for quitting drugs on p.451 also applies to alcohol. Mothers battling with an addiction often have a number of practical and emotional difficulties, and giving up can be a long and difficult journey.

Foetal alcohol syndrome
See also Neonatal abstinence syndrome (p.451)

When a mother consumes alcohol excessively, and for a prolonged period of time during pregnancy, her baby's cell development is affected to a degree reflecting the amount consumed, and the duration of consumption. Babies who appear to be affected are said to have foetal alcohol syndrome (FAS) or, with less severe consequences, foetal alcohol effect (FAE). At least 1:750 babies are born with FAS each year in the UK, although the true number may be higher and FAS may be the leading cause of learning difficulties later in life. It is an entirely preventable cause of birth defects.

FAS refers to a collection of mental and physical birth defects that can include developmental delay, learning difficulties, impaired growth, abnormal functioning of the central nervous system, physical abnormalities of the face and behavioural difficulties when older. The facial features are relatively easy to recognise, and include a HEAD with a small circumference (**microcephaly**), low-set ears, thin upper lip, small chin, short upturned nose and smaller-than-usual eye openings. FAE gives a less severe set of the same symptoms and there is no way of reversing the damage. Babies born with FAE may also suffer from neonatral abstinence syndrome (p.451) after the birth and symptoms may persist for months.

ALLERGIES & INTOLERANCES

The word 'allergy' is derived from the Greek words *allos* (different) and *ergos* (action). An allergy is an abnormal reaction or increased sensitivity of the body's immune system to certain substances or 'allergens'. An allergic individual produces symptoms when exposed to substances that are harmless to non-allergic people.

The frequency of allergies and allergic disorders has increased over the last 60 years. More adults are discovering intolerances or allergies in themselves and their children as there are more chemicals in the food we eat, the air we breathe and the substances we put on our skin. Also, more people are aware of the origin of the symptoms. Sensitivities now affect between around 1:3 people by adulthood. On some occasions parents incorrectly suspect allergies in their children because many common illnesses in young babies have symptoms that are similar to those connected with allergies or intolerances.

The difference between an allergy and an intolerance
The distinction between an allergy and an intolerance is medical. Although the symptoms may be similar, the body's reaction is different: an allergy involves an immune reaction with the production of antibodies, while an intolerance is a reaction that does not involve the immune system. Intolerance appears to be more common than allergy, particularly where food is the cause. Treat by avoiding the trigger, e.g. wheat.

What happens: allergic mother or baby

The body's immune system is a highly efficient defence mechanism that gives protection against foreign materials, such as bacteria and viruses, by producing antibodies. These protective antibodies, called immunoglobulins, help destroy a foreign particle by attaching to its surface, thereby making it easier for other immune cells to destroy it.

The allergic person develops a specific type of antibody called immunoglobulin E, or IgE, in response to a foreign substance such as pollen. The substance evoking a reaction combines with IgE, irritates the body's cells and leads to the release of chemicals, including histamine, that cause inflammation in parts of the body where they affect the mucus glands. If the glands in the respiratory tract are affected, there may be excess coughing (asthma) or a runny nose (hay fever); if the glands in the gut respond, DIARRHOEA or CONSTIPATION may result. Other organs can be involved, from the SKIN, with a rash, to the nervous system, bringing on symptoms that include irritability, migraine, depression or insomnia.

When allergens are eaten, inhaled or absorbed from the skin or injected, they may gain access to the bloodstream and travel around the body: this explains how symptoms can occur in different areas and a single allergen can affect multiple organs. For example, a food allergen may cause digestive problems, asthma and tiredness; latex on the skin may cause hay fever and intestinal symptoms.

The immune system remembers allergens and becomes 'sensitised' so that on subsequent exposures there is a rapid antibody response, giving a reaction. Most allergies cause mildly uncomfortable reactions that may become tiresome to deal with. Some cause more acute symptoms requiring urgent attention and may even be life threatening. The symptoms can impact upon the entire family, particularly when an allergic baby has COLIC or cries excessively.

Symptoms

Allergies and intolerances usually become evident by about 6 months, often in response to weaning food. But extremely sensitive babies may have a reaction in the first days or weeks, or some people believe from Week 22 of pregnancy, and some sensitivities do not become apparent until adulthood. While children usually 'grow out' of an intolerance by the age of 3 years, many intolerances and allergies may continue for life and an allergy can begin at any time, including old age.

Some symptoms appear a few minutes after contact with or ingestion of a trigger. Others appear within a few hours and sometimes, often where diarrhoea or constipation are involved, may not appear for 2–3 days. Symptoms may affect:

- The digestive system (bowel): abdominal pain and bloating, COLIC and irritable bowel syndrome (p.448), diarrhoea or constipation, nausea and VOMITING and INDIGESTION.
- The SKIN: rashes (blotchy, itchy, raised and red) and eczema.
- The lungs (chest), nose and ears and eyes: COUGH, allergic ASTHMA or bronchitis, a runny nose and sore eyes.
- The brain and nervous system: hyperactivity, irritability or TIREDNESS, LOW ENERGY & INSOMNIA.
- Headache (p.521) and migraine, lethargy, anxiety (p.461) and depression (p.462).
- An emergency with anaphylactic shock (above right) may

If you or your baby has a severe allergy that may bring on anaphylactic shock

Anaphylaxis is a rare but acute allergic reaction that affects the whole body and requires immediate medical attention. Common triggers are peanuts and insect stings. Symptoms include anxiety, itching of the skin, headache, nausea and vomiting, sneezing and coughing, abdominal cramps, hives and swelling of tissues such as lips and joints, diarrhoea, shortness of breath and wheezing, low blood pressure, convulsions and loss of consciousness. If you or your baby are allergic to this degree, you need to carry an epinephrine (adrenalin) syringe, known as an epi-pen, and wear some form of medical information bracelet. A quick, decisive epinephrine injection can be a life-saver. There are 3 recognised levels of allergic reaction, and 3 levels of response:

Level 1
Skin and mucous membrane reactions – usually mild. Skin rash appears, lips tingle and eyelids may swell.
- Treatment for all age groups: antihistamine by mouth, e.g. Piriton.

Level 2
A wheeze and cough in addition to level 1 symptoms. No colour changes nor reduction in consciousness.
- Treatment: as above, with the addition of 10 puffs of salbutamol (Ventolin) via a spacer device, which can be repeated every 10 minutes.
- Begin taking prescription oral steroids and continue for 3 days.
- Call your doctor or the NHS Direct service.

Level 3
As above but with life-threatening wheeze and colour change due to lack of oxygen. This is true anaphylaxis.
- Treatment: as above, with addition of epi-pen adrenalin injection (epinephrine).
- The emergency medical team will give oxygen and intravenous steroids and immediate transfer to hospital.

---

cause fainting and collapse and facial swelling, particularly around the eyes and mouth (not itchy). If the swelling occurs in the throat, there may be difficulty breathing and swallowing. Anaphylactic shock may be fatal.

Possible causes of allergy or intolerance

Although some people develop allergic reactions when there is no history of it in the family, many inherit the tendency. An adult may carry the genes responsible for an allergic reaction without having any apparent signs of allergy. Similarly, a baby may inherit the genes but it may be years before the allergy appears, if indeed it appears at all. And allergies do not always present themselves similarly – if your mother has hay fever, you may have asthma, and your child may come up in a violent rash when eating a particular food. The range of triggers is almost limitless, as each person's system is different. Possible causes can be divided into four broad groups.
Contact: Allergic contact dermatitis is an inflammation of the skin caused by a local allergic reaction. Examples include latex,

dyes and chemicals, perhaps in washing powders, metals in jewellery, and cosmetics. Some allergens are transported by the bloodstream and react in the skin with eczema (p.530).

Eating: Food is a common cause of allergic-type reactions and it is perhaps not surprising that reported cases are on the rise given the widespread use of chemicals and modifiers and genetically modified plants. Many people are intolerant of components such as monosodium glutamate (MSG), and sulphites, used to enhance crispness and prevent the growth of mould, and additives and preservatives, which often give rise to rashes. Naturally occurring histamine (e.g. in tuna) commonly leads to diarrhoea or wheezing, and nuts are also significant – in the UK around 1:100 people has a nut allergy and this may cause serious or fatal reactions.

Inhalation: Potential allergens include pollen, dust mites, flakes of dead skin and hair, and industrial by-products. Usual symptoms are allergic rhinitis, asthma, and conjunctivitis, although some people may experience a reaction in a different area of the body. Children below the age of 9 months are seldom sensitive to inhaled allergens.

Injection: The most severe reactions can occur when allergens are injected into the body. Commonly this is through an insect bite or sting but some people react to medications (e.g. penicillin). Allergic reactions to vaccines are extremely rare.

Sensitivity to cow's milk

Cow's milk is one of the most common food allergens among babies. This may be because it is usually the first foreign substance encountered or because it is a powerful allergen. Cow's milk allergy affects about around 5% or more of babies and adults. As many if not more have a milk intolerance that is not always a true allergy. These babies can tolerate moderate amounts of cow's milk. Symptoms of cow's milk allergies are up to seven times more common in babies who are fed formula rather than breast milk.

Sensitivity to cow's milk protein: In some babies, the immune system produces IgE-antibodies against milk protein: this is a true cow's milk allergy. Reactions not involving the immune system are cow's milk intolerance.

The two main components in milk that trigger allergies are casein and whey. An individual may be allergic to either or both. Casein is the curd that forms when milk is left to sour and whey is the watery liquid that remains. Casein is the most significant allergen in cheese. When milk is heated it may alter the whey proteins, so a whey-sensitive adult may be able to tolerate evaporated, boiled or sterilised milk and milk powder. These milk-substitutes are not suitable for babies. Most babies do not encounter these proteins until they are given formula milk or dairy products. For a tiny number of very sensitive babies, however, milk protein in breast milk from a mother who has consumed dairy products can cause allergic symptoms.

Of people allergic to cow's milk 50% develop an allergy to other food proteins (e.g. egg, soya, peanut) and fewer than 50% can tolerate the proteins in goat's and sheep's milk. There is also a tendency to develop allergy to air-borne allergens before puberty, and asthma or eczema on the skin.

Lactose and sucrose intolerance: Lactose is a sugar (carbohydrate) found in all milks. Usually, an enzyme called lactase in the bowel breaks it down and allows it to be absorbed. If this enzyme is absent or reduced, then large amounts of lactose remain in the bowel. Diarrhoea and frothy stools are characteristic signs of lactose intolerance. Breast milk encourages the activity of lactase. If a baby does not have sufficient lactase, he may react to the lactose in breast milk and will need to be fed with a specialised milk formula. Adults have relatively little lactase in their bowel so that if they drink too much milk they may react in the same or a similar way, revealing an intolerance. This is more common among people of Asian or African heritage.

Sucrose occurs naturally in many foods, including fruit, and processed food and drinks that claim to be 'sugar free' or 'reduced sugar'. Intolerance occurs due to the deficiency of the digestive enzyme sucrase in the small bowel. Sucrase or lactase enzyme deficiency may be a genetic disorder, but it may also develop as a complication of gastroenteritis (p.446), and is temporary.

Coeliac disease

Coeliac disease (gluten intolerance) is a disorder in which ingesting gluten leads to the formation of antibodies, which cause damage to the lining of the small intestine. This results in malabsorption of nutrients and vitamins. Gluten is one of the proteins found in many of the cereal grains – mainly wheat, rye and barley. It is very useful to help the grains to stick together when making bread. Rice, maize, sorghum and millet do not contain gluten. The intolerance may be inherited and is more common in Mediterranean families, where wheat originated, and in people of Celtic origin. More than 5% of the population of Europe, at least 1 million people, has an intolerance to gluten and there are 10 times as many 'carriers' who are at risk of becoming intolerant.

A baby with coeliac disease is likely to show symptoms 6–24 months after the introduction of gluten-containing foods, although if the intolerance is mild, symptoms may not develop until adulthood and are likely to be minimal. This is why the introduction of large quantities of gluten-containing food is best delayed until 12 months or later. The baby is likely to have frequent bowel movements producing bulky, putty-coloured stools with an offensive smell. Left untreated, protein and fat malnutrition is intensified by inadequate absorption of vitamins and trace minerals. In severe cases insufficient absorption of nutrients may lead to low WEIGHT gain, muscle wasting, distended abdomen, ANAEMIA, listlessness, irritability and immature bone development.

In adults coeliac disease may cause a few or many of a variety of symptoms, which include abdominal pain (p.518); constipation or diarrhoea and FLATULENCE; ongoing tiredness; weakness; dizziness; headaches (p.521); numbness and tingling; flu-like symptoms; irritability; muscle and joint pains; asthma and sinusitis; and greater susceptibility to other intolerances and allergies. It may resemble symptoms associated with chronic CANDIDA (thrush). If you have had persistent problems that have not been diagnosed, you may have a mild gluten sensitivity that is worth investigating.

Gluten intolerance can be diagnosed after excluding gluten from the diet, a blood test for antibodies directed to the three proteins in gluten and, in selected cases, possibly a biopsy of the wall of the small intestine. True coeliacs need to stay on a gluten-free diet for life with advice from a dietician.

Diagnosing an allergy or intolerance

Finding the trigger and excluding it can make a huge difference to your life, and if your baby is allergic the change from a whiny, aggressive, rash-prone, doesn't-know-what-he-wants, non-sleeper to a pleasant, clear-skinned, easy-going child who sleeps well may be extraordinary.

For both you and your baby observation linking symptoms with what has been eaten, drunk or inhaled, is the first step. Avoiding the possible cause is a way to implement your own test system. If symptoms improve, this is a good sign. There may be a few days between exposure and an allergic reaction. With an intolerance, the symptoms may get worse before they get better: you may have to wait a week until they diminish. When you resume contact or reintroduce the food, if the symptoms return a diagnosis of allergy or intolerance can be made. Some doctors prefer you to note this pattern several times before making a firm diagnosis since symptoms such as diarrhoea or rash often come and go, particularly in babies.

Clinical tests support or supplement observation. Lactose intolerance, for instance, is diagnosed through detecting excessive sugar in a baby's stool (there is more sugar because it has passed through the bowel without being digested). Yet even in a specialist allergy clinic a long process of trial and error may ensue before a cause is identified. Skin tests are difficult and seldom performed in children under the age of 9 months; in adults the results are not always accurate. Blood tests are becoming increasingly sophisticated in pinpointing the presence of antibodies that react against known allergic triggers, although they are more commonly used for adults and older children than babies and need to be combined with avoidance of suspected triggers for a true diagnosis. There may be antibodies in your blood but these may be dormant and not causing the symptoms you are experiencing.

Kinesiology, which remains a controversial method that has nonetheless been used for years, involves dissolving a suspected trigger in water while you hold the vial and testing muscle power for a reaction. It can be used on babies.

Allergy & motherhood

Some women enter pregnancy with a known allergy. If avoidance of a trigger is difficult, you may be concerned about using medicines. In general, babies are very hardy and take it in their stride. Keep the doses as low as possible.

- Inhaled steroids and bronchodilators (for asthma) are considered safe in pregnancy and during breastfeeding. Steroids used on the skin for eczema are safe – there is very little absorption. The same is true for steroid enemas used to treat colitis. Doses are kept as low as possible and avoided if possible in the 1st trimester.
- Antihistamines have been used for decades to treat pregnancy nausea and to date they have not been shown to harm a developing foetus. Once again the doses are kept as low as possible in the 1st trimester. After birth your breastfed baby may be sleepy or irritable but relatively small amounts filter through, so the effect will be slight.
- Complementary therapies such as homeopathy,

acupuncture or herbal medicine can often be used in conjunction with conventional medication, and may help to reduce the dosage.

Action plan

If you take medicines to treat your allergic reaction, check with your doctor to ensure they are safe for use in pregnancy. The next step is to keep your life free of the allergen, as far as possible, and take steps to reduce your baby's chance of developing allergic symptoms.

Diet and lifestyle

- If you need to avoid certain foods, ensure you obtain adequate vitamins, minerals and nutrients from other food sources. Take advice from a dietician or nutritionist.
- If you suspect an allergy or intolerance in pregnancy you can try to diagnose it through observation or clinical tests (left). After pregnancy it may disappear. If you were reacting to a food, you may feel better if you continue to restrict consumption of it.

Homeopathy

Homeopathy has a lot to offer but it is inappropriate to self-prescribe. Treatment involves careful case management by a qualified homeopath, who may work alongside doctors, nutritionists and allergists.

Protecting your baby in the womb and after birth

The most proactive approach you can take in pregnancy to help your baby develop a healthy immune system and delay or avoid the onset of allergies is to look after yourself, eat a balanced diet, avoid family allergens and stop smoking. After birth, the best thing to do is breastfeed. This is particularly significant if your baby is born prematurely or there is a family history of allergy. If there is no history, there is no need to avoid things in pregnancy simply because they are potential allergens, with the possible exception of peanuts.

- Breastfeeding has a protective effect. It coats the insides of the intestines and impedes leakage of foreign substances from the gut. It also reduces your baby's exposure to potential allergens, such as the protein in cow's milk.
- Breastfeeding for longer than 1 month without other milk supplements offers significant protection against food allergy at 3 years of age, and also against asthma until 17 years of age. Six months of breastfeeding may prevent eczema during the first 3 years and reduce the chances of allergies developing in adolescence.
- If you have a family history of food allergy it is best to avoid the foods in pregnancy and while breastfeeding delay weaning until 6 months and avoid introducing those foods until 1 year. If your baby was born prematurely, apply these time scales after his expected date of delivery. This can reduce the chances of an allergy developing, and if the allergy does occur may reduce the severity of symptoms.

Allergy & babies

In the first 6 months a baby's immune system develops in response to the substances he breathes, touches and ingests. Gradually his system produces the range of immunoglobulin antibodies that protect against harmful substances. In an allergic baby, allergies such as eczema are often apparent by 6 months, but some develop later and inhaled allergens seldom cause hay fever or asthma under 9 months. In a baby below the age of 6 months the most common intolerance or allergy is to cow's milk.

Action plan

If you suspect your baby has an allergy, visit your doctor. There is no cure for allergies. The best treatment is to avoid the allergen(s). If it is not possible, for instance with persistent hay fever, do what you can to make your child comfortable. Make sure that everyone who cares for him is aware of the allergy, knows how to avoid it and what to do if symptoms arise. This also applies to drugs he may be given on prescription.

- If the allergic reaction is severe – breathing difficulties, fainting, listlessness, swollen throat, unconsciousness – call an ambulance. You may need to resuscitate (p.383).
- If the reaction is less severe, but you are very worried, for instance your baby is crying uncontrollably and seems to be in great pain or has excessive vomiting and diarrhoea, call your doctor immediately.

Diet

- If you are breastfeeding make a note of your baby's symptoms and behaviour. The usual symptoms are of the bowel, chest or skin. If your baby is very sensitive you will need to exclude the allergen and continue to breastfeed under supervision from a paediatrician.
- If your baby is allergic or intolerant to a component of cow's milk, your doctor may recommend a milk substitute, perhaps a soya or hypo-allergenic formula. You may be able to get this on prescription. If your baby reacts to the alternative formula, your doctor will prescribe a specialised milk. If you are no longer breastfeeding or have introduced solid food into his diet, you will need advice from a paediatric nutritionist or dietician who will provide milk-free recipes to ensure a nutritionally adequate diet including sources of minerals and vitamins.
- If your baby displays an allergy to another food, it is best to avoid it. You could reintroduce it again in 3 or 4 months and watch for reaction, as some allergies and many intolerances do pass. Because an intolerance may be caused by a chemical component related to a certain food, you could try organic produce. It is important, however, to avoid potentially dangerous allergens: do not give your baby anything with peanuts in because he may be susceptible to peanut allergy. If you have older children it is important they understand about the allergy and do not share inappropriate food.
- Reintroducing a food is the only way to discover if an allergy has passed. If your baby's allergic reaction is severe, it is best to do this under specialist medical supervision. You may be advised to wait until your child is 3 years old.

Environment and lifestyle

If your child is allergic to something in the atmosphere, for example pollen or animal dander, you will need to do all you can to reduce the triggers.

- Smoking is significant – never smoke near your baby and keep time he spends in a smoky atmosphere to a minimum.
- If the cause is house dust or mites, take steps to reduce them. This may involve using a special vacuum cleaner, cleaning curtains and furniture coverings regularly, keeping soft toys and clothes in drawers, avoiding feather pillows and quilts, replacing carpets with wood-type flooring or improving ventilation. Avoid blown-air heating. If your child is sensitive to pollen you may need air conditioning to keep the house cool instead of opening windows.
- With a pet allergy it might be possible to reduce or stop contact or to keep the pet clean and well brushed. Sometimes the only option is to find another home for the pet – this is often the case with cats whose saliva, which causes the allergy, dries to a fine dust and gets everywhere.
- If your baby is sensitive to something else (e.g. a metal, fabric or chemical used in washing) you may need to buy hypo-allergenic products. These are produced without the use of substances that cause allergic or intolerant reactions in a significant number of people. Even so, hypo-allergenic products still contain chemicals. A baby can still be sensitive to them, although they are less likely to cause allergy.

Medical care

Medical care involves treating the symptoms. It is preferable to avoid the cause. Care may range from making your baby comfortable if he has a persistently runny nose, or using an inhalant if he is wheezing.

- Desensitisation involves multiple injections of the substance known to cause an allergy. These are not easily available in the UK and are commonly reserved for use when there is a severe life-threatening allergic response to wasp and bee stings, although they may occasionally be used in treatment of allergy to house dust or some grass pollens.
- There are other treatments that may desensitise an allergic person, so they can tolerate allergens without symptoms. These are still experimental and consist of placing a dilute solution of the allergenic food under the tongue or developing a homeopathic remedy. As studies progress it will become clear how effective these approaches can be.

AMNIOCENTESIS & CVS

See also CONGENITAL ABNORMALITIES; routine antenatal visit tests (p.78)

If your baby has a high risk of having a genetic or chromosomal abnormality (p.433), or another condition for which the tests are suitable, you may consider amniocentesis or chorionic villous sampling (CVS). In both tests cells originating from the foetus are obtained and analysed in a laboratory. Amniocentesis is also used to treat anaemic babies with a blood transfusion in the womb.

Many parents faced with the option of invasive testing find it difficult to decide (p.81). Invasive testing does carry a small risk of MISCARRIAGE. This is around 0.5% (around 1:200) for amniocentesis after Week 15 and around 1% (around 1:100) for amniocentesis before Week 15 and for CVS. The results will either put your mind at rest, because they will confirm that everything is fine, or, if an abnormality is diagnosed, will help you to make plans for the future. For some conditions, treatment can begin in the womb.

Invasive testing is usually only carried out when a significant risk has been identified of a health condition that may show itself in the structure of the 46 chromosomes or in the genes. The most common chromosome abnormality that may be detected in this way is DOWN'S SYNDROME. There are also many inherited genetic diseases including TAY-SACHS, CYSTIC FIBROSIS and ANAEMIA caused by sickle cell or thalassaemia. Some foetal abnormalities are not related to chromosomal or genetic structure (e.g. SPINA BIFIDA) and a number may be detected by ultrasound scans rather than amniocentesis.

What happens

An amniocentesis allows a sample of amniotic fluid to be collected. The fluid contains cells that have been shed from your developing baby's skin. CVS takes foetal cells from the chorionic villi in the placenta (p.34). The cells are cultured in a laboratory so the chromosomes or the function of the genes can be analysed. An amniocentesis is carried out around Week 15 or 16. It can be done earlier in pregnancy but the risk of miscarriage reduces after Week 15. After amniocentesis, initial results using a DNA probe test are available in 3 days but harvesting to confirm these results takes 14 days. CVS can be done between Weeks 11 and 14, and gives results within 3–4 days but there is a slight increased risk of miscarriage.

Amniocentesis and CVS are done in the ultrasound scan room by an obstetrician so that during the whole procedure your baby and uterus can be seen clearly on a monitor. This ensures your baby is unlikely to be harmed. The procedure takes a few minutes and you go home within an hour. You may be most anxious before the insertion of the needle rather than during the procedure itself. The feeling of the needle is similar to having a blood test in your arm, but fear of injury to your baby may increase your sensitivity. You will be able to see the image on the screen if you wish to watch. Some women feel no pain; others feel pressure or a needle prick.

During an amniocentesis a fine needle is inserted through your abdominal wall. Using the ultrasound image as a guide, the obstetrician will withdraw 10–20 ml (½–1 tsp) of fluid. The amniotic fluid removed represents 5–10% of the total volume and will be replaced by your baby within 6 hours.

CVS removes a small amount of chorionic villi from the placenta using a needle inserted into the placenta and gentle suction, under ultrasound guidance. Depending on the location of your placenta, your doctor may insert the needle through your abdominal wall or through your cervix. In the transcervical approach, a speculum that is usually used to take a cervical smear is used to view your cervix and the needle is inserted under ultrasound guidance. It may be more uncomfortable than amniocentesis.

If you have rhesus negative blood, you will be given an injection of rhesus factor Anti-Rh D after the procedure. This prevents foetal cells that may be released into your circulation from causing rhesus disease and affecting your baby.

The amniocentesis or CVS sample is sent to a laboratory

where it is divided in two. One half is examined using a DNA probe test. Cells are treated with specific probes, which make the chromosomes visible under a light microscope. Normal cells have two chromosomes in each group. When three chromosomes occur in a group this is known as trisomy. The most common abnormality associated with trisomy is Down's syndrome (trisomy 21).

If the DNA test reveals a trisomy, the results are reliable; false positives do not occur. There is, however, a tiny chance (1:1500) that the initial test result will show a normal chromosome complement although a problem remains undetected (false negative). Because of this, the second half of the sample is incubated and the cells grown over 2 weeks for amniocentesis or 4 days for CVS, then harvested and the chromosomes counted. The result on the incubated cells is totally reliable.

Cordocentesis and foetoscopy

Later in pregnancy a sample of your baby's blood may be taken from the umbilical cord any time after Week 16. This is called a cordocentesis. The advantage is that the cells can be grown more quickly than with amniocentesis but there is a higher miscarriage risk. As more centres offer amniocentesis results in 3 days, this test is used very infrequently. This technique is also used for intrauterine transfusions for anaemia or low platelet levels.

If an ultrasound scan detects a developmental problem that may benefit from surgery in the uterus, a foetoscopy may subsequently be carried out. This is only done in specialist centres and involves inserting a small camera with a light source into the uterus.

Action plan: after the test

After the procedure the needle puncture site seals in a few minutes. You will be asked to stay for 30 minutes and take it easy for the next 24 hours and avoid intense physical activity and sexual intercourse. Though the tests are now used widely, there are still risks involved.

The most significant risk is miscarriage and you will be asked to be aware of any bleeding, cramping or leaking fluid from the vagina. Around 1% of women experience these symptoms and they do not usually result in miscarriage. Bleeding is slightly more common in CVS. Amniotic fluid may run between the amniotic membrane and the wall of the uterus, down to the cervix and emerge from the vagina as a clear urine-coloured discharge. Leakage usually stops within 48 hours as the membrane seals. Continuous prolonged leakage, however, may lead to a miscarriage. If you have these symptoms, call your doctor for advice.

Infection following the procedure is very rare. Harm to the foetus is very unlikely because the obstetrician can see, with the aid of ultrasound, precisely where the needle is. CVS before Week 10 may be associated with a higher incidence of foetal limb abnormalities.

A repeat test is rarely needed, but more common after a CVS (around 1%). If you need a second test this is not because there is something wrong with the pregnancy – the cells may have failed to grow, or results may be unclear and a fresh sample will be needed.

If the test reveals an abnormality

If the test reveals an altered chromosome complement or another genetic abnormality, your obstetrician will discuss the implications. You are likely to feel shocked and may be faced with a very difficult decision. Termination of pregnancy may be an option, particularly if your baby is diagnosed with a severe abnormality. Most parents appreciate genetic counselling (p.434). It often helps to talk to other parents who have had children with similar conditions before making a firm decision about whether to continue with pregnancy, or how to make plans for the future.

AMNIOTIC FLUID EXCESS

An excess of amniotic fluid, **polyhydramnios**, may not lead to any problems if mild. If it is severe with a significant increase in the volume of fluid, the additional pressure may cause BREATHLESSNESS, INDIGESTION & HEARTBURN and abdominal discomfort. More seriously, the pressure from a severe increase may lead to PREMATURE BIRTH. There may be other consequences affecting labour, including malposition where the baby may present as a breech or even as a transverse lie (p.493). If excessive fluid means your baby's head does not engage and the membranes rupture there is a risk of UMBILICAL CORD PROLAPSE.

What happens

In most instances of suspected polyhydramnios, a baby is normal and healthy, and may be quite big, and there no cause for concern. If you have DIABETES and your blood sugar is not well controlled, your baby may urinate excessively leading to the increase in fluid. If you are carrying TWINS the amniotic fluid volume is always high but it may be increased more if the twins are identical. In very rare instances, fluid may accumulate when a baby has difficulty swallowing, either because there is an obstruction in the oesophagus or because of a neurological difficulty, and the amniotic fluid cannot be recycled.

Action plan

An ultrasound scan will spot twins and check your baby's anatomy and swallowing. A glucose tolerance test may be performed to exclude maternal diabetes, particularly if your baby is large. If a cause cannot be found on the scan, your baby is very unlikely to have an abnormality.

- When the amniotic fluid excess is significant you may be encouraged to give up work and rest to reduce the risk of prematurity.
- If you have DIABETES, meticulous control of blood sugar will reduce fluid volume.
- Draining the amniotic fluid by inserting a needle into the uterus is not worthwhile: indeed it may precipitate premature birth.
- When labour begins or if the membranes rupture ,contact your hospital immediately. Approaching and during labour your medical team will watch carefully for umbilical cord prolapse, a very LARGE BABY or a transverse lie or breech

(p.493). If any of these is present you will need a CAESAREAN SECTION.
- After birth a soft tube may be inserted via your baby's mouth into the stomach to check for a blockage of the oesophagus. The long-term outlook is usually good and largely depends on the cause for polyhydramnios and whether birth was premature.

AMNIOTIC FLUID REDUCTION

A reduction in the volume of amniotic fluid is known as **oligohydramnios.** Amniotic fluid volume usually peaks between Weeks 36 and 40 and if your baby is late there may be a natural reduction in the volume, particularly after Week 42. Many normal babies produce low volumes and the baby is healthy. In other instances placental function is reduced and the baby may have INTRAUTERINE GROWTH RESTRICTION (IUGR). In labour, if the fluid volume is low there is a higher risk of umbilical cord compression and this may lead to foetal distress, particularly after the membranes rupture.

What happens

In most instances of suspected oligohydramnios, a baby is healthy. During pregnancy if the reduced fluid is due to insufficient placental function, this may cause slow growth (IUGR) and you and your baby will have to be monitored. Rarely, oligohydramnios occurs if a baby is unable to pass urine because the kidneys have not developed or there is an obstruction to the flow from the bladder. When this is the case, reduced fluid is usually obvious on ultrasound from Week 20.

Action plan

If there is a slight reduction in amniotic fluid and your baby is otherwise healthy, no treatment is needed.

- The natural reduction in the volume of amniotic fluid in late pregnancy may occur earlier and your team will check your baby's health closely using ultrasound scans.
- If there is IUGR and reduced placental function you will need frequent check-ups as for any HIGH-RISK PREGNANCY.
- If your baby has a kidney or bladder problem, treatment will be based upon the individual problem.
- If the reduction is large your doctor may advise labour by induction (p.497) or CAESAREAN SECTION before term, particularly if there is severe IUGR. If the reduction is moderate you may be advised not to go past Week 40 – timing of induction will depend on the fluid volume and the wellbeing of your baby.
- In labour, particularly after the membranes rupture, your baby's heartbeat will be monitored frequently to check for UMBILICAL CORD COMPRESSION and FOETAL DISTRESS.
- After the birth, if there has been significant growth restriction, the paediatric check will pay close attention to your baby's body temperature and blood sugar levels because low levels (p.486) can be dangerous. Your baby's outlook will depend on the cause of the oligohydramnios. Often, IUGR can be corrected with early and good feeding after birth.

ANAEMIA: BABY

See also BLOOD GROUP, ABO INCOMPATABILITY; BLOOD GROUP, RHESUS FACTOR

In the womb, your baby produces his own blood with a special type of foetal haemoglobin, the protein that carries oxygen and gives blood its red colour. Foetal haemoglobin can pick up oxygen and release it throughout the body very efficiently. It is needed because oxygen levels received via the placenta are lower than those obtained when the baby breathes air after birth. After birth haemoglobin changes as the adult type gradually replaces the foetal type. Anaemia occurs when there is an abnormally low level of haemoglobin in the blood.

Prenatal foetal anaemia

Anaemia before birth is rare. The most frequent cause is rhesus disease (p.410). A tiny number of babies have anaemia in the womb due to congenital infection, especially PARVOVIRUS (TOXOPLASMOSIS and CYTOMEGALOVIRUS may also be a cause), or because of the complication of foeto-maternal transfusion (right) or a severe strain of inherited thalassaemia (above right).

Anaemia after birth

Full-term babies are born with a haemoglobin level of 16–20 g/dl (roughly 33% greater than adults) and often look very red at birth. After birth the extra red blood cells break down, giving rise to the yellow pigment, bilirubin, which may cause JAUNDICE. The released iron is stored in the body for later use. By 2–3 months the haemoglobin level is 9–12 g/dl, which is roughly 30% below adult levels and this is normal. Haemoglobin builds up to adult levels over the next 6 months.

In the 1st year, the two most common causes of minor anaemia are inadequate iron intake due to the use of inappropriate milks and excess iron loss. This is usually due to the continuous but small loss of blood from the bowel because of inflammation resulting from cow's milk intolerance (p.393). When the haemoglobin level is 10 g/dl or less, compared to 12 g/dl, a baby may look pale. Treatment is simple – take cow's milk out of the diet and the anaemia gets better. Some babies benefit from iron supplements.

Babies born early are particularly prone to iron-deficiency anaemia because iron stores are laid down in the last 4 weeks of pregnancy. PREMATURE babies may require transfusion for anaemia when there is difficulty breathing or feeding. It is suggested that up to two IQ points can be lost due to early iron-deficiency anaemia. Iron deficiency in babyhood infrequently leads to severe anaemia.

Action plan

If iron-deficiency anaemia is suspected, treatment is generally simple with improvement over a 1–2 month period, after which your baby will look less pale and feel better.

- Replace inappropriate milk with a baby-milk fortified with iron. Follow-on milks, which contain extra iron, can be used after 6 months when iron is better absorbed.
- Remove the food causing an intolerance.
- Iron supplements may also be given.

Sickle cell anaemia and thalassaemia

Sickle cell anaemia and thallassaemia may cause anaemia in the mother (below) but do not generally affect a newborn baby. If mother and father are carriers, an amniocentesis will determine the baby's haemoglobin during pregnancy. If a baby has inherited sickle cell disease, as adult haemoglobin replaces the foetal haemoglobin, abnormal 'sickle' cells build up: by 6 months this brings on symptoms. Rarely, it may lead to a sickle cell 'crisis' where body tissues and internal organs can be damaged through lack of oxygen. Thalassaemia usually follows a similar pattern, affecting a baby as adult haemoglobin replaces foetal haemoglobin. The effect can be minimal, with a haemoglobin reduction to around 10 g/dl at 9 months (the usual level is 12 g/dl). Very rarely there is severe foetal anaemia requiring intrauterine transfusion and blood transfusions may be needed for life. Babies at risk of these causes of anaemia are followed up by specialist paediatricians.

Foeto-maternal transfusion

When your baby's blood circulates through the placenta it does not usually mix directly with your blood, although a small amount can cross into your bloodstream during birth and in pregnancy. In very rare circumstances, with no known cause in pregnancy, a baby may lose a significant amount of blood in this way. Moderate loss usually results in anaemia and if this is ongoing it may lead to INTRAUTERINE GROWTH RESTRICTION and even HEART failure. If the loss involves 30% or more of a baby's blood volume, this is called a foeto-maternal transfusion and there may be FOETAL DISTRESS before or during labour showing a specific alteration in the heart rate that necessitates urgent delivery. If haemoglobin is below 10 g/dl, a blood transfusion may be needed at birth. In very rare cases, foeto-maternal transfusion occurs without warning signs and it is a rare cause of stillbirth (p.509).

ANAEMIA: MOTHER

Your blood can carry oxygen because it contains haemoglobin in the red cells, which consists of a protein with two alpha and two beta chains and iron. It is maintained in sufficient quantities when there is an adequate supply of iron in combination with other minerals and vitamins. Anaemia occurs when there is a fall in the concentration of red blood cells and, with them, haemoglobin. If you are anaemic, you may look pale and feel tired, short of breath or faint. Mild anaemia is not harmful for your baby.

What happens

Before pregnancy, the normal haemoglobin level is over 11 g/dl. In pregnancy the number of red blood cells increases but water in circulation also increases, and there is a natural fall in haemoglobin concentration, usually above 10.5 g/dl. A normal or high haemoglobin level indicates that oxygen supply to your baby is normal, and you have adequate reserves of red blood cells should bleeding complicate the birth. A level below 10.5 g/dl indicates anaemia.

Vitamin and mineral deficiency is by far the most common

cause of anaemia. The most common deficiency is iron but many women with low iron stores are also low in other minerals, mainly zinc, cobalt, selenium and vitamins B12, B6 and folic acid. Sometimes deficiencies in these nutrients can cause anaemia, even where iron levels are normal.

You are more likely to become anaemic if you are carrying TWINS or a very LARGE BABY (they absorb more nutrients from your blood) or if you have had babies in close succession. Some women inherit an anaemic tendency (sickle cell disease and thalassaemia, below). Some people are susceptible to iron and mineral deficiency, perhaps because of poor nutrition before conception, heavy periods, difficulty absorbing nutrients because of a bowel disease or an EATING DISORDER.

After the birth, the amount of water in your circulation diminishes and because extra red blood cells formed during pregnancy the concentration of haemoglobin increases, usually at a rate of 1 g per week for 3–4 weeks. If you have lost a lot of blood in labour, you may become anaemic. Usually this can be simply treated and the level rises over a few weeks.

Action plan

It is routine to check the haemoglobin level in the first 12 weeks of pregnancy and again after Week 30, then on the 3rd or 4th day after birth. If you are anaemic, it is important to raise a low haemoglobin levels because TIREDNESS AND LOW ENERGY may reduce your enjoyment of parenthood and could contribute to depression (p.462), and anaemia may contribute to INTRAUTERINE GROWTH RESTRICTION (IUGR) and breastfeeding difficulties (p.412) with low milk flow. If you are at risk of anaemia from sickle cell or thalassaemia you must have your blood tested because you may need specialist care.

Diet
- Stick to a nutritious diet (p.332) and eat regularly to maintain stable energy levels and nutrient stores. Iron- and mineral-rich foods include meat, seaweeds, green leafy vegetables, raw vegetables and salad, beans and peas, pulses, tofu and soybeans, millet and lentils. Apricots, cane molasses, coriander and parsley are rich iron sources.
- You may need to take iron supplements, together with vitamin and mineral supplements (p.345).

Medical care
- If the haemoglobin level does not rise after supplements, further blood tests can check for rarer causes of anaemia, particularly sickle cell and thalassaemia. If iron and ferritin levels remain low this indicates low iron stores in your body and that you are not taking iron, or you are not absorbing it. If you are not absorbing it a different preparation may be more suitable (e.g. iron EAP, p.345).
- You may need injections of iron to boost the stores.
- For haemoglobin below 8 g/dl after birth you may be offered a BLOOD TRANSFUSION, which will bring the level up immediately. The alternative is to take iron and mineral supplements combined with a good diet, and let your levels rise gradually over a period of days or weeks.

Homeopathy
To aid absorption and assimilation of iron take *Calc Phos* (6x)

and *Ferrum Phos* (6x) daily, morning and night in addition to a nutritious diet.

Sickle cell anaemia & thalassaemia

Sickle cell anaemia and thalassaemia are inherited conditions caused by an abnormality in one of the protein chains (the alpha or beta) that make up the haemoglobin molecule. If you have one of these conditions, you may be a carrier with no or slight symptoms, or have the full condition, causing anaemia.

Beta thalassaemia is an abnormality of the beta haemoglobin chain and is more common among people who live around the Mediterranean Sea and in parts of Africa, the Middle East, India, and Pakistan. Alpha thalassaemia involves the alpha haemoglobin chain and is more usual in Southeast Asia.

Sickle cell disease is an abnormality in the beta chain most common in people whose ancestors come from Africa, Central America (especially Panama), the Caribbean, the Mediterranean and India. With sickle cell disease when red blood cells don't get enough oxygen they become longer and curved, like the blade of a sickle. Sickle cells can get stuck in blood vessels, and can inhibit circulation to some parts of the body. This can damage internal organs and cause pain, particularly if the blocked blood vessels are in the arms, legs, chest or abdomen.

What happens

A carrier has both normal and abnormal haemoglobin, while a person with the full condition only has abnormal haemoglobin and will be anaemic. If you are tested using a technique called electrophoresis and found to have abnormal genes, your partner will also be tested. Severe anaemia due to sickle cell disease may affect the function of the placenta and your baby's growth (p.488). If a baby inherits the condition (a 1:4 chance if both parents are carriers), the anaemia may not manifest for months after birth. If you carry thalassaemia there is a very small risk of your baby being affected in pregnancy (p.398). If you and your partner are carriers, you may request an AMNIOCENTESIS to determine the exact composition of your baby's haemoglobin.

Action plan

The treatment for anaemia due to sickle cell disease or thalassaemia is not the same as treatment for iron-deficiency anaemia. Women with these anaemias may have excess iron in their circulation and it is dangerous to receive more. Treatment is usually needed in specialist units because mothers and babies require monitoring, possibly blood transfusions and treatment for IUGR. During labour and birth it is important to avoid shock or reduced oxygen because this may precipitate a sickle cell crisis and raise the risk of damage to internal organs.

ANXIETY
See EMOTIONS, ANXIETY

ASPHYXIA
See FOETAL DISTRESS & ASPHYXIA

ASTHMA & WHEEZING: BABY

See also ALLERGIES & INTOLERANCES; COUGH & COLD: BABY

There are at least three forms of asthma in babies. Viral-triggered is the most common, then allergy-related asthma and finally asthma due to exposure to tobacco smoke while in the uterus. The common symptom is wheezing, a whistling noise made on breathing out, which is very common, particularly under the age of 2 years, and generally needs no treatment, but it can be worrying for a parent. It is rarely serious and often passes with age as the respiratory system matures.

What happens

Wheezing occurs when the airways have narrowed, either because of mucus blockage or because of inflammation following infection. The respiratory system includes the nose, middle ear, back of the throat (pharynx) and voice box (larynx), the main airway to the lungs (trachea) and the smaller airways in the lung itself. Sensitivity resulting in wheezing and asthma is sometimes referred to as hyperactive or irritable airways. Fortunately, sensitivity decreases with age.

Viral-triggered wheeze

A viral-triggered wheeze is the most common form of childhood asthma, occurring in about 25% of babies and children under 5 years of age at least once, and is three times more common in boys. A virus brings on a cold or cough (usually respiratory syncytial virus), followed by a wheeze. The younger your baby is when he has his first wheezy episode, the more likely he is to grow out of the tendency to wheeze.

Each episode of a viral-triggered wheeze may last for 6–8 weeks, during which time your baby's sleep may be disturbed and his cough may worsen when he is excited or upset. If, just as he is recovering from one period of viral-triggered respiratory sensitivity, he gets another cold, the cycle may repeat. This gives the impression of a respiratory infection lasting all winter. Infection of the airways in the lung, bronchiolitis (p.440), does not cause allergic asthma, but may be associated with the development of a persistent wheeze in early childhood. This effect becomes weaker by the age of 5 years, unless an allergy coexists.

Allergy-associated wheeze

An allergy-associated wheeze is the second most common type. This is a wheeze associated with allergic symptoms and more commonly affects girls. There is also a tendency to wheeze and cough in response to viruses, but because of an allergy there are other symptoms, in particular eczema, and possibly sensitivity to foods. Environmental allergens don't come into play as much until the toddler years. So a baby who lives with a cat won't usually start to have symptoms until he is at least 9 months old. Seasonal allergies such as hay fever sometimes show up in the 1st year.

It is difficult to distinguish an allergy-associated wheeze from a viral-triggered wheeze when there are no other allergic symptoms. Children with an allergy-related wheeze may take longer to grow out of their asthma.

Wheeze resulting from passive smoking

Tobacco smoke affects some babies in pregnancy and after birth by altering their lungs, reducing lung capacity and making them more sensitive to viruses. Babies affected by smoking commonly develop a viral-triggered wheeze. The symptoms improve with age but affected lungs may never achieve optimal function and viruses may later trigger wheezing attacks. As the lungs age, they have less reserve capacity than those of adults not exposed to cigarette smoke before birth.

Action plan

If your baby suffers from a wheezy cough linked with a viral infection, use the comforting suggestions in COUGH & COLD: BABY. Additional care for a wheezy baby includes:
- Avoiding smoking and smoky atmospheres.
- Breastfeeding, to reduce asthma related to allergy.
- Rarely, certain foods (especially eggs, shellfish, cow's milk and nuts) can trigger wheezing if your baby is allergic to them. That is why it is recommended that you wait until a child is at least a year old before you introduce these foods. You may use cow's milk earlier.
- If your baby has eczema and asthma, it is best to avoid contact with pets, especially cats.

ASTHMA: MOTHER

If you are an asthma sufferer you may be concerned that some BREATHLESSNESS, a natural side effect of pregnancy, indicates an attack. If you become anxious, breathlessness may worsen and you may begin to wheeze. Yet severe asthma is rare in pregnancy and labour and for most women (2:3) it actually improves. One reason may be a physiological increase in the production of cortisone. Asthma is often caused by an ALLERGY. It may also be a reaction to a viral chest infection. Very occasionally, asthma occurs for the first time in pregnancy. When this happens, it usually resolves completely after the birth.

What happens

Asthma involves spasm and inflammation of the smooth muscles lining the bronchioles, the small air passages in the lungs. This is called bronchospasm. The passages become narrowed, which makes breathing difficult and may induce wheezing. An asthma attack may last for anything from a few minutes to many days. In pregnancy it will have little effect on your baby, although in very rare circumstances uncontrolled prolonged asthma with reduced blood oxygen can produce complications such as PREMATURE BIRTH or INTRAUTERINE GROWTH RESTRICTION (IUGR).

Action plan

If you are an asthma sufferer the most important thing to do is to prevent attacks where possible. If you are aware of the triggers, avoid them; pregnancy may be an opportunity to reassess your environment. Your asthma will be under good control if you do not have any symptoms, are sleeping well and obtaining your personal best peak expiratory air flow.

Medical care

- If your asthma is mild you will not need medication but there are agents that can be used safely during pregnancy and while breastfeeding. It may be necessary to use steroids if asthma is severe; if the steroids are inhaled very little is absorbed into the bloodstream or passed to your baby.
- Inhaled bronchodilators and inhaled anti-inflammatory steroids do not appear to affect breast milk. Antihistamines, however, can cause sleeplessness and irritability in babies and reduce production of breast milk – so are best avoided.
- If you have a severe attack you will need prompt attention (a bronchodilator and perhaps oxygen) to prevent a fall in your blood oxygen and the potential and dangerous risk of hypoxia (low oxygen) for your baby. Take your usual medication for relief when the first signs appear. If you have an acute attack, call an ambulance.
- In pregnancy, your doctor may want to monitor your lung function by measuring your peak expiratory air flow rate. Your obstetrician may assess your baby by examinations and ultrasound, which can give an early warning of IUGR.
- Some doctors advise physiotherapy to reduce excessive coughing and the strain this puts on the abdominal muscles.
- If asthma symptoms develop while in labour, someone from the medical team will measure peak flow rates. You may be given intravenous fluid as a precaution against dehydration. Pain relief and medication limit the risk of bronchospasm. After birth you may need more medication than in pregnancy.

Lifestyle, diet and exercise

- Aerobic exercise helps by expanding your lungs and draining secretions from the chest and sinuses. Bronchospasm can be avoided or reduced by taking medication before exercise, warming up and cooling down and avoiding exercising in cold air.
- Avoid trigger foods. Focus on foods containing B vitamins (e.g. green leafy vegetables and pulses), magnesium (e.g. fish, sunflower seeds and figs) and antioxidants (e.g. citrus fruits, soya beans, olive oil and apricots).
- Avoid SMOKING and being in smoky atmospheres.
- Do what you can to avoid chest infections, which may spark an attack.
- In the months after birth you may find the normal demands of caring for a baby increase asthma, and attacks may make you more tired than usual.
- Homeopathic remedies may be very useful to treat an attack or to diminish the number of attacks, although home prescribing is not appropriate.

ATTENTION DEFICIT DISORDER (ADD) & AUTISM
See BEHAVIOUR PROBLEMS: BABY

BACKACHE
See PAIN IN THE BACK & PELVIS

BATTERING & ABUSE: MOTHER

It is shocking that battering and abuse against women is most common during pregnancy: around 1:10 women suffer physical, emotional or sexual abuse and most violence takes place in the home. Abuse leading to physical trauma is a more common cause of antenatal complications than vehicle accidents or falls. If you are or have been a victim you may find it difficult to share the truth, even with friends. During pregnancy, however, you have access to a wide network of medical, practical and psychological support. This may be the first chance you have to confide in people who are in a position to listen, offer counselling and help you bring about change.

Many cases of battering in pregnancy follow abuse before conception. Sadly, abuse of a mother is a strong indicator that a baby or child may be abused in the future but taking steps during pregnancy to address the situation could greatly reduce the chance. The ideal is to seek support as soon as signs appear, which can prevent the problem getting out of control. Although separation is sometimes the only way to put an end to aggression, some families do survive the scars of violence.

What happens
Abuse shatters many lives and it can take years to pick up the pieces. It may involve physical, psychological and/or sexual abuse between intimate partners. In pregnancy, physical abuse is often directed towards the abdomen or the breasts. Psychological abuse includes verbal harassment and threats, intimidation and destruction of possessions, and forced isolation. Sexual assault may include rape and mutilation of the breasts and genitals. Sometimes the effect of violence may hinder a baby's growth (p.488), cause PREMATURE BIRTH or LOSS OF A BABY.

Battering is a form of control, where one person maintains dominance over another. It often involves a man abusing his partner although abuse may be present in other relationships (e.g. in a parent–child relationship when the child is grown up). The reasons for abuse cannot easily be simplified. Some people have a personality trait that inclines them towards violence, and some repeat aggressive treatment they received as children. During pregnancy men with a tendency to aggression, jealousy or anger may feel threatened by their unborn child. The baby may be seen as an intrusion or as someone who will take all the mother's love and attention. Often an abusive man becomes a 'different person' when he is violent. An abuser often blames his victim who over time may believe in the illusion that she is at fault. Some battered women deny the truth either because they are afraid of the attacker or feel ashamed, embarrassed or guilty. Many have developed skilful ways to hide the truth believing this protects the relationship and their dependence on their partner.

Abused women are prone to a number of emotional and physical ills and doctors or midwives may sense a problem during antenatal care. Some women delay or miss antenatal visits, perhaps for fear that their physical wellbeing will carry signs of abuse. Battered women are more likely to have pain such as headache (p.521) or chronic pelvic pain (p.519), DIARRHOEA with irritable bowel syndrome, unrelenting

TIREDNESS or significant anxiety (p.461) and depression (p.462). Some women may be afraid of vaginal examinations, a fear that could make the birth experience highly traumatic. Victims of violence are more likely to take addictive DRUGS, which carry their own implications in pregnancy.

Action plan

Effective action that offers comfort, support and practical help, including alternative housing, counselling, therapy and realistic options for the future, can begin once help is sought. The first course of action is to confide in somebody. It is always worth trying a second time if you have previously received a reaction of disbelief or denial. Any counselling will be treated in the strictest confidence. It will focus on your experiences and the impact they have on your life and may address anxiety or depression, which may have been present for years, particularly if you were subjected to violence earlier in life.

Pregnancy and birth

Letting the medical team know about abuse is important. If your fears stop you from attending antenatal appointments, you miss out on care that assures you and your baby are in good health. If you can confide in someone, they may schedule more time for your appointments and take particular care, explaining everything in detail.

During labour if doctors and midwives are aware they may find it easier to support you appropriately. Affected women often react with unusual silence and passivity, incessant screaming or uncontrollable terror, or try to dissociate themselves from the experience as labour pain increases and there are pelvic and genital examinations by one or more people. Understanding and sensitive support, often with epidural anaesthesia, may reduce discomfort and fear.

After birth

Beyond the birth a change in life is the ideal. Many battered women are isolated and appreciate help in seeing ways to make a change. Counselling (p.459) can soon begin to help you acknowledge that you are not alone, nor are you at fault. Practical support and trusted company is also important and many health visitors or local support groups can help to make this a reality. They can also make connections with legal professionals when necessary.

Extra support with childcare may also be an option, and social workers may be involved if CHILD PROTECTION is an issue. A small number of abused women abuse their own children, perhaps because aggression is the only means of control they know. Ongoing support can help a mother form a loving bond with her child and avoid the pitfalls of aggression.

Staying in an abusive relationship

If you remain in an unsafe home, the priority is safety in the event of abuse recurring, particularly if your child is with you. It is a good idea to have to hand a telephone number of someone who can help and/or a police number, identity documents, keys, money and a suitcase with essential items. Social workers or health visitors can help you make a plan and think about the options that you have should you leave your home. They can also help you choose support and therapy

(p.459). On the bright side, in some relationships when abuse is addressed and both partners receive support and therapy, behaviour patterns do change and family life may become loving and rewarding.

Homeopathy

It is best to visit your homeopath for a specific remedy, and to do so regularly if you are receiving therapy, because a number of different emotions may surface. Many people find remedies for depression, grief and anger (p.460) helpful. *Staphysagria* is a powerful remedy for suppressed anger that builds into deep resentment, simmering beneath a façade of pleasantness and compliance before exploding uncontrollably – this is one of the main remedies for long-term abuse.

BEHAVIOUR PROBLEMS: BABY

See also Emotions and feelings (p.300); CRYING

Every normal baby develops motor, visual and auditory skills, in common with every member of the human race. The more variable aspects of behaviour include language and social interaction. Within a given context determined by family, culture and race, if a person – an adult or a baby – does not act as expected, this is considered abnormal. When talking about a baby, behaviour that does not seem 'normal' may be labelled as problematic. In general, a problematic behaviour is one that persists beyond the usual age and stops a baby from interacting normally.

Many factors influence behaviour. Probably the most important is the nurturing environment because a child learns to behave in ways determined by her experience and the response she gets from those around her. If your baby's environment is difficult, she may react with difficult behaviour or behave inconsistently. Yet your baby's personality is well developed at birth and she plays a major role communicating and determining her own way of being.

Parents visit health professionals more often in the first 9 months after birth than at any other time in the next 25 years, and usually discover that a worrying behaviour is perfectly normal and there are simple, practical approaches to change. If you think your baby is behaving unusually, it could help to discuss it with your health visitor or doctor: she will either put your mind at rest or refer you to a specialist if there is cause for concern. Many difficult behaviours fade quickly and some continue beyond the age of 5 years. You may find it useful to take advice about the huge variation in 'normal' early patterns. Sometimes a behaviour only seems strange because it does not quite fit your expectations. On p.305 we explore how powerful expectations can be.

Hair pulling

A baby for whom hair pulling is a problem constantly pulls her hair, breaking it off to leave a bald area or patch of short stubs, and perhaps eating it. This rarely occurs before the age of 6 months and seldom causes health problems, although swallowed hair may become a tight hairball and could cause digestive problems. Cutting the hair is a temporary solution.

Head banging, rolling and rocking

Head banging and body rocking are normal behaviours that can start as early as 4 months or as late as the 2nd year and can last for several months. Some babies bang against the cot headboard, while others are partial to the railings. The rhythmic movements may be a soothing way to fall asleep or distract from other pains, such as TEETHING or EAR INFECTION AND PAIN. It may look painful, but your child won't get hurt banging herself to sleep. Some babies stop if there is a rhythmic ticking metronome or clock in the bedroom. If the sound of your child's head banging bothers you, try moving the cot away from the wall, or make her a bed with a mattress on the floor.

Although head banging in babies and young toddlers is generally not a cause for concern, strong head banging that lasts longer than 10–15 minutes and recurs throughout the night may be a sign of emotional or behavioural problems such as ADD (below, right). If head banging is excessive or begins after 18 months, talk to your paediatrician.

Hitting, biting or punching

As your baby grows older, gets more mobile and sociable, hitting, biting or punching may begin. If there is an aggressive or angry undertone, it may help to remember that anger is part of normal human behaviour. This may be your baby's way of communicating and defending her territory, and she needs to explore the boundaries around her as she learns about independence and tests out her limits. If you are clear about what is and isn't acceptable, in your own and your baby's actions, and express these boundaries in a loving way, you provide support as she discovers how to create limits and how to cope with other people's.

If your baby bites, give a clear, calm and direct vocal expression of dissatisfaction and make eye contact as you show disapproval with your face. Doing this consistently will normally stop the behaviour over a period of time. Laughing and saying 'No' will not, while reacting with a tap or slap is likely to augment, rather than reduce the behaviour. There are many ways to use discipline without aggression (p.279). If you suspect your child is learning about excessive anger from aggressive adults or children around her, you may be able alter the balance in her life.

Genital touching – masturbation

This is common in both boys and girls who may enjoy the feeling of touching their genital areas or the sensation they get by rocking or rubbing against something. This is nothing to worry about and demonstrates the natural urge to explore, discover and experiment.

Thumb sucking

Thumb and finger sucking is extremely common, enjoyed by around 50% of babies. Some babies are seen on ultrasound scans doing this in the womb and may even be born with sucking blisters. Sucking is usually associated with becoming calm, is not harmful and generally subsides of its own accord. It is parents, rather than babies, who have a problem with it (because of the way it looks). Sucking normally stops before the appearance of the second teeth and cannot harm their

alignment before they emerge. It is best not to make your child feel self-conscious. Corrective measures usually backfire: pulling her thumb out of her mouth may make her rebel and suck more forcefully.

Needing a security blanket

From 6 months on, security objects, such as blankets, are used by many toddlers to relieve tension and anxiety. These 'transitional objects' are usually soft, cuddly things, often held close to the nose and mouth. A transitional object serves a mother-like role, providing familiarity and comfort, perhaps when going to sleep or feeling insecure, when angry or unwell. As your baby grows more independent and realises that she is no longer an extension of you, her security object may become extremely important. It allows her to hang on to familiarity without losing the chance to explore and is a positive, not a negative, attachment. Some babies hold one almost constantly and child psychologists and parents alike encourage their use.

Causes of a worrying behaviour

Some babies are more 'difficult' than others and the cause is not always easy to spot.

- It may be a response to the family environment, the way a day is structured, how much and when a baby sleeps, or what and when she eats or by illness.
- Some behaviour is triggered by unsettling change, such as moving bedroom, moving house or going on holiday.
- An unusual behaviour can sometimes be part of your baby's personality. On rare occasions it may indicate an underlying problem and your baby may need a developmental check with your health visitor or doctor.

Parental responsibility

No baby is born to misbehave unless she has a developmental problem where the behaviour is normal for her but not what is expected by others. Understanding how behaviours develop can help you guide your baby, accept her personality and your part in her development. Young babies do not premeditate, they respond to what happens in the moment. The most visible behaviours – feeding, sleeping and communicating – are inextricably linked with other subtle and powerful behaviours – expressing emotions, asking for attention and wanting to try new things. Your child's personality and behaviour can be influenced, but not determined, by you.

As a parent you are your child's chief guide and she mirrors you. Babies do need dynamic boundaries, and so do parents. Creating and modifying them is one of parenthood's challenges (p.276). Your baby also guides you. The balance between who is guiding and who is being led changes daily.

Babies and parents get frustrated, angry, tired and irritable. In discomfort and pain, they can exert large amounts of power. A baby who is unhappy after birth may contribute to her mother's postnatal depression; equally a mother who is depressed may find her baby very demanding. It is a two-way relationship but you as the parent are the principal guide.

Attention deficit disorder (ADD) and autism

ADD and autism (autistic spectrum disorder) are seldom diagnosed within the 1st year but there may be some early symptoms. The symptomatic behaviours are part of every baby's normal development, and on their own do not suggest a problem: only when they are intense or persist for longer than expected might they suggest an underlying behavioural difficulty. As awareness of problems increases, early diagnosis and specialist care and support are becoming more common.

Early signs of severe ADD include irritability, crying inconsolably, screaming, head banging or rocking, fits or temper tantrums, difficulty establishing a routine for sleeping, feeding or playing, difficulty feeding, and COLIC.

Many autistic babies develop normally at first and begin to show symptoms later – some by 9 months and others by 3 years. From birth, suggestive behaviours include arching the back away from an adult to avoid physical contact or failing to anticipate being picked up and going limp. Some autistic babies are passive, others are irritable. By 9 months some persistently fail to point at or look at an object when another person points it out. Slow speech development and the absence of babbling may be attributed to difficulty hearing (p.452), but could be part of an autistic spectrum disorder.

Action plan
If you are worried about your baby's behaviour, you may need the help of your family or your health visitor to get an objective view. If there is emotional stress in your family, it is important to accept your responsibility but it is neither helpful nor realistic to shoulder all the blame. You could also take some of the following steps:

- Make sure your doctor has examined your baby and checked there is no underlying condition causing the problem. Try to treat any pain or discomfort; homeopathy may be helpful.
- Give your baby plenty of love and praise and quality time each day, and make sure there are activities and she is not bored. Ensure she is sleeping and eating as well as she can. Introducing a routine may help.
- Make a fuss of good behaviour – babies love attention. Ignore bad behaviour if it is not harmful – babies are tuned to get attention and often abandon activities that go unrewarded. Try not to be angry if behaviour is difficult; be consistent.
- If the behaviour is harmful (licking outside walls, for instance) gently avoid or remove your baby from the situation when it happens. Provide alternative activities to distract her when she behaves inappropriately.
- Do not force your baby to do something she does not want to do – this can have negative effects on her self-esteem and on your relationship and may reinforce the difficult behaviour you are trying to minimise.
- Sometimes your baby will challenge you as she expresses herself and explores her boundaries. This is an important sign of normal human development. Try not to jump to the conclusion that your baby is difficult.
- Above all, be consistent and be kind. Make sure any carers know the boundaries you have set and that you have also considered their viewpoints (p.324). How a behaviour is approached will influence your baby's sense of value and acceptance, and gentle solutions are usually the best for all concerned and are part of your baby's education.

- If a behavioural difficulty highlights an area of imbalance in your family, it can be a positive trigger for a thoughtful approach to the way relationships and attitudes have formed since birth (see Part IV).
- Seek professional help when you feel the need. Your first point of contact is your health visitor, GP or paediatrician.

BIRTH INJURIES: BABY

With modern obstetric care severe injury, or birth trauma, is extremely rare, affecting 2–7:1000 babies. Minor bruising is the most common injury. If your baby requires medical attention for one injury, she will be checked for others. In most cases treatment is straightforward and recovery is complete within days or weeks. Support and comfort from you, frequent feeding and massage (p.365) may help her relax. Cranial osteopathy (p.376) is a very powerful aid following birth trauma. Some babies are more susceptible:

- PREMATURE babies have more fragile bodies, and may bruise more easily.
- LARGE BABIES are more likely to need forceps or ventouse assistance or have difficulty negotiating the birth canal or shoulder dystocia in labour (p.502). Birth may also be more difficult if there is malpresentation (p.498).
- Babies who go through a prolonged labour may be subjected to excessive force or pressure. This may be caused by a tight fit in your pelvis (p.498).

If your baby is considered to be at risk of injury, your birth team will pay close attention to progress in labour. Using an upright position for birth can reduce the possibility of injury because the birth is more likely to be straightforward. If you need intervention your obstetrician will take care to avoid injury to you and your baby and may decide that a CAESAREAN SECTION is the best option.

Bone injuries
The collarbone (clavicle): The most common bone to fracture, most often when a baby is large and there is difficulty delivering the shoulders (shoulder dystocia). A baby is unlikely to move the arm on the injured side and there may be bruising over the bone. A paediatrician will check for damage to the spine and the nerves associated with the muscles of the arm and hand. The clavicle usually heals after 7–10 days and will do this best if the arm is immobilised by pinning the sleeve to the babygro. You may be able to feel a bump at the site of the fracture; this remodels over a few years.

The upper arm (humerus) and upper leg (femur): More rarely, these bones may be damaged. If your baby does not appear to be moving a limb this may be an early sign, followed by swelling and pain when you move it for her. An x-ray confirms the diagnosis. Fractures are treated by an orthopaedic specialist and a plaster cast may be needed for the humerus but femur fractures can be treated with a weight hung from a bandage wrapped around the leg. The weight (traction) keeps the bones aligned and encourages healing. Very rarely, if there was little trauma during labour, osteogenesis imperfecta (brittle-bone disease) may be considered.

Eye injuries

One or both of the eyes may have a bright red band or red or brown spots on the white area surrounding the iris. This common and harmless subconjunctival haemorrhage results from small blood vessels breaking in the eyes during labour. The blood is absorbed over several weeks.

Injuries to the head & face

See also HEAD & HEAD SHAPES

Soft tissue damage

Some newborns' facial skin appears blue from tiny pinpoint bruises caused by bleeding into the skin as a result of the pressure of birth or if the cord has been tight around the neck. If the bruising affects the eyelids they may swell. These harmless effects improve in a few days.

A few weeks after delivery the appearance of a pea-sized lump, perhaps in the cheek of your baby, is usually due to a small lump of fat that has hardened from its natural liquid state because of pressure during birth. This disappears within a few weeks.

If a foetal scalp electrode has been used for close monitoring, it may leave a small cut or spot that usually heals in a few days. Infection may occur and is easily treated.

Swelling and bruising

Caput succedaneum: Often called 'caput', this is a swelling of the soft tissues of the scalp that protects the underlying bones and the brain during birth. It usually disappears after 36 hours unless there is associated bruising. Babies delivered with the help of ventouse may have more swelling.

Cephalohematoma: An area of bleeding and bruising underneath the lining membrane of one of the cranial bones. It often gives a raised lump on the head several hours after birth. The bruise tends to get bigger over the first weeks and then shrinks as the blood is reabsorbed. It is not drained and a large bruise may take up to 3 months to disappear. If the area of bleeding is very large, an excess of bilirubin, a yellow pigment, may be produced when the red blood cells have broken down, leading to JAUNDICE.

Sub-aponeurotic haematoma: Extremely rare but more serious, with bleeding that crosses over various skull bones and can track down to the face, giving bruising that lasts for weeks. It may follow a difficult ventouse birth and cause a fall in blood pressure and more intense jaundice. It usually disappears completely with time.

Damage with bleeding into the brain

The most common reason for a bleed into the brain (intracranial haemorrhage) is bleeding from fragile blood vessels in the brain of a premature baby if there is a period of low oxygen levels, or even with minor trauma at birth. In a full-term baby bleeding is rare and may be linked with forceps or ventouse assistance or a prolonged labour (p.502) with FOETAL DISTRESS & ASPHYXIA. Sometimes abnormally developed blood vessels may be the cause. The risk of injury to the brain ranges from 1:1000 for a forceps or ventouse delivery (p.496) or caesarean in labour to 1:3000 for non-operative delivery.

A baby who has had a brain injury resulting in bleeding may have anything from the most minimal of symptoms, such as poor feeding and irritability, to major complications such as neonatal FITS. Occasionally the effect of a large bleed may become obvious over a few weeks and the head may visibly enlarge from hydrocephalus (p.476).

If bleeding is suspected your baby may be given an ultrasound scan and a CT or MRI scan. She may also be tested for infectious and chemical disorders as well as BLOOD-CLOTTING abnormalities, and closely monitored. The blood is naturally absorbed over a period of weeks or months and only vary rarely does it need to be removed surgically.

The outlook for babies with haemorrhage is variable and is determined by the size of the bleed, which part of the brain is involved and the underlying cause. While there may be no lasting effect, rarely the injury may lead to learning difficulties or physical disability related to severe cerebral palsy, or unexpected death.

Subdural haemorrhage: Bleeding into the outermost lining membranes due to birth trauma. Significant tears in the membrane may cause blood to collect in the brain stem, an area that controls breathing and consciousness, leading to severe damage.

Sub-arachnoid haemorrhage: Blood may pass into space under the innermost of the lining membranes as a result of foetal distress and low oxygen flow to the brain. The effects and symptoms may be severe.

Intraventricular haemorrhage: Bleeding into the fluid-filled ventricles of the brain. It mainly occurs in premature babies. The bleeding is graded from 1 to 4: effects of the more severe grades may lead to hydrocephalus.

Intraparenchymal haemorrhage: Bleeding into the brain substance due to birth injury, malformed blood vessels, abnormal blood clotting or low oxygen tension. The effects may lead to long-term nerve damage.

Nerve damage

Facial nerve palsy: Thought to be a developmental abnormality where some of the fibres of the nerve associated with the facial muscle of the face are absent, giving a lopsided mouth and stopping one eyelid from closing completely. More rarely it is caused by the facial nerve becoming compressed during a forceps birth. Eye drops stop the affected eye from becoming dry as the nerve recovers naturally. This can take a few days but occasionally takes months. Some babies need to be referred to a plastic surgeon and recovery may not always be complete.

Erb's and Klumpke's palsy: When the nerves supplying the muscles of the arm and shoulder are damaged there may be limited or no movement in the shoulder, arm, wrist or fingers. Depending on which nerves are dysfunctional, this is called Erb's or Klumpke's palsy. Although nerve dysfunction may pre-date birth, the most common cause is delay in delivery of the shoulders (p.502) when traction to assist the birth stretches the nerves in the neck or there is a broken collarbone. Usually complete recovery takes just hours or a few days. Up to 15% of affected babies need physiotherapy and paediatric attention for months. If recovery is incomplete within 1 year, an operation to rejoin the nerves is often successful.

Cerebral palsy (CP)
See also CEREBRAL PALSY

CP is damage to the nervous system, in particular the brain and is usually a non-preventable developmental abnormality. Around 2% of babies with CP may have had a birth injury often related to foetal distress and asphyxia resulting from sub-optimal care during labour. Obstetric and midwifery care is designed to minimise this risk.

BLEEDING, DURING PREGNANCY

See also CERVICAL EROSION & CANCER; ECTOPIC PREGNANCY; PLACENTA PRAEVIA; PLACENTAL ABRUPTION

Vaginal bleeding at any time during pregnancy should always be reported to a doctor or midwife. If bleeding is heavy and there is pain and/or evidence of clots, this is an emergency: see your doctor or go to casualty. Light bleeding not accompanied by other symptoms, although worrying, may not affect your baby. One of the principles of midwifery is to treat bleeding early to reduce complications and improve safety.

Bleeding in early pregnancy

Many normal pregnancies are associated with light bleeding or 'spotting' during the first 12 weeks. Commonly this arises from small blood vessels in the uterus that open as the placenta implants, usually in the first 6 weeks. Implantation bleeding is usually light and does not indicate problems with the baby.

As a sign of a threatened MISCARRIAGE, bleeding often stops and pregnancy continues normally. If a pregnancy is definitely miscarrying, bleeding is profuse, accompanied by pain and the passage of clots and embryonic material. Although rare, an ectopic pregnancy may be associated with bleeding and severe pain. Bleeding may also be due to infection in the VAGINA with no effect on a baby's wellbeing.

Bleeding in mid- and late pregnancy (antepartum haemorrhage)

Light spotting in the second half of pregnancy is usually not a cause for concern. In the last weeks it may be a 'show' (p.121), of blood mixed with mucus, and is a sign of imminent labour: contractions may soon begin. Sometimes it may be connected with a more serious condition that requires close medical care.

- It may be linked with cervical erosion or infection in the vagina (bright red blood). Neither poses a risk to your baby and an infection can be effectively treated.
- Another possible cause is a placenta praevia, or low-lying placenta (painless bleeding, bright red). This potentially dangerous condition may necessitate delivery by CAESAREAN SECTION if the bleeding is heavy.
- Very rarely bleeding can be linked to placental abruption where the placenta separates from the wall of the uterus (usually dark red blood and abdominal pain). A severe abruption is dangerous for you and your baby and an immediate caesarean section may be needed.
- Rarely, bleeding in mid-pregnancy is a sign of miscarriage (heavy loss, often with clots) or premature labour.

Action plan

- If you are passing pieces of solid material, save them for your doctor.
- If the bleeding is excessive you will be examined and given an ultrasound scan to observe the position and function of the placenta and check the wellbeing of your baby. Your baby's heartbeat will also be monitored (CTG).
- Treatment depends on the underlying cause of the bleeding and the urgency of the situation. It may need urgent care or just take it easy.
- Report all bleeding to your doctor or midwife. Heavy bleeding requires emergency attention with intravenous transfusion and possibly early delivery of the baby.

BLEEDING, IN LABOUR & AFTER BIRTH

Bleeding in labour

Labour is commonly accompanied by bright red bleeding in the form of a 'show' (p.121). This bleeding is not usually profuse. If it is, your medical team will assess whether it is arising from a PLACENTA PRAEVIA or PLACENTAL ABRUPTION, where the placenta has separated from the wall of the uterus. If either is occurring, your baby may need to be delivered urgently. Rarely, bleeding may be excessive because of a BLOOD-CLOTTING DISORDER. Most women affected are aware of the disorder but childbirth may be the first time it actually becomes apparent. If there is no obvious cause for bleeding your blood-clotting factors can be checked using a blood test.

On very rare occasions, bleeding comes from a baby's blood vessels. Known as vasa praevia, it occurs when the blood vessels from the umbilical cord track along the membranes and are torn when the membranes rupture. If birth follows rapidly the baby will not lose much blood and may be unaffected, but there may be FOETAL DISTRESS & ASPHYXIA and an urgent delivery. After birth the baby may then need a BLOOD TRANSFUSION.

Early bleeding after birth

The birth of the placenta – the 3rd stage of labour – is always accompanied by bleeding, with a loss that is usually less than 500 ml (1 pint). After birth, the muscle in the wall of the uterus contracts and retracts, compressing the maternal blood vessels that supplied the placenta and slowing the bleeding to a trickle. Natural blood clotting also reduces bleeding from the blood vessels. Excessive bleeding in the 24 hours following birth, known as primary postpartum haemorrhage, occurs in fewer than 10% of deliveries. It is more common after a prolonged labour, with a LARGE BABY or TWINS.

What happens

After your baby is born your midwife checks the flow of blood from your vagina and assesses how well the uterus is contracted. If labour has been long or difficult, your contractions may lack power. Sometimes the uterus cannot contract fully because the placenta has not detached completely from the uterine wall: this is called a retained placenta (right). In some cases this is because the UTERUS is bicornuate (heart-shaped). Bleeding originating from an injury such as a tear or episiotomy (p.494) is usually slight, although it may be profuse and stops after the area has been stitched.

Action plan

If you are bleeding excessively your midwife will want to speed up the birth of the placenta. She may first massage your uterus. If you begin breastfeeding this releases oxytocin from your pituitary gland and boosts contractions.

Medical care

- Contractions can be boosted with an injection of hormones: initially oxytocin (Syntocinon) is administered and this may be followed by ergometrine if contractions are not stimulated sufficiently. Your midwife may pull gently on the cut umbilical cord to speed placental separation. If these hormones do not keep the uterus contracted, prostaglandin can provide a more powerful boost but this is very infrequently needed. Some hospitals routinely administer Syntocinon or ergometrine immediately after the birth to speed the delivery of the placenta (p.138).
- If bleeding is excessive, an intravenous drip can administer oxytocic drugs and keep the uterus contracted and replace lost fluid. Very rarely, a blood transfusion is needed.
- If there is an indication that levels of blood-clotting factors may be low, they will be checked and replaced.
- If the birth of the placenta is delayed, it may have to be removed by the obstetrician. The muscle of the uterus may have clamped down and the placenta is trapped or, occasionally, the placenta is deeply embedded in the wall of the uterus (PLACENTA ACCRETA). The obstetrician uses his hand to separate and remove the placenta from the uterus in the operating theatre, under epidural or general anaesthesia. It is usual to administer antibiotics after surgery to prevent infection. The operation is over soon and you can breastfeed your baby within 2 hours. The milk will contain antibiotics in low doses but your baby is unlikely to be affected. After surgery you may feel your uterus contract strongly and the Syntocinon drip continues, but discomfort and heavy blood flow usually stop within a few hours.

Homeopathy

Homeopathic remedies in high potency (200c) taken after your baby's birth may encourage contractions and thus reduce blood flow, and can be used in conjunction with conventional medical treatment. Reassess the situation after 5–10 minutes. Even if there is a positive reaction, you may need a second dose. If there is no change, try a different remedy.

Caulophyllum after a long, exhausting labour; *Cimicifuga* if contractions are absent, there's excessive fear and you are cold and shaky; *Pulsatilla* if your abdomen feels hot and tender, you are hot, tearful and still in pain – taken at the moment of birth it can be very effective in facilitating the 3rd stage; *Secale* if contractions are strong but ineffectual, you can't tolerate heat and feel distressed (it helps to counteract side effects of oxytocin and ergometrine); *Sepia* if the placenta is slow to descend and you have bearing-down sensations, shooting pains up the rectum and feel emotionally indifferent to your baby. If there are no characteristic symptoms, *Arnica* may help to expel the placenta.

Late bleeding after birth, retained placental tissue

After birth the uterus retracts and sheds its lining together with any remaining fragments of placenta or membrane. This results in bleeding, called lochia, whether birth was vaginal or caesarean, that lasts for 1–8 weeks. Frequent breastfeeding helps the uterus to contract and expel remaining fragments.

If the bleeding has an offensive smell or is very heavy, an infection may be present. To investigate, a vaginal swab can be taken to check for bacteria. If blood loss is still excessive or clots appear after the 5th day, an ultrasound can check for retained tissue. If large placental fragments have been retained, these may need to be removed.

Action plan

If you do lose an excessive amount of blood, you may feel weak, more tired than normal and perhaps light-headed when you stand or walk. Rest and accept extra help at home so you can use your energy to recover and establish breastfeeding. You may have *anaemia* and will need to treat this with good nutrition and appropriate mineral supplementation. If blood loss is heavy, you need to return to hospital for emergency treatment.

Medical care

- Rarely, a blood transfusion is needed if haemoglobin is below 8–9 g/dl.
- If there is retained placental tissue, bleeding will continue. The tissue is visible on an ultrasound scan and needs to be removed with an operative **dilation and curettage (D&C),** up to 4 weeks after birth. Under a short general or epidural anaesthetic the placental fragments are gently scraped from the uterine wall with an instrument called a curette. The procedure lasts 20 minutes and need not interfere with breastfeeding. Within 4 hours bleeding will have reduced. Antibiotics after surgery reduce the risk of infection.

BLEEDING PROBLEMS: BABY

See also ACCIDENTS & FIRST AID; BIRTH INJURIES: BABY

Nothing can be as worrying as seeing a baby bleed. Luckily babies have an efficient blood-clotting mechanism that improves with time and usually prevents any bleeding from becoming severe. Clotting ability is only rarely affected if a baby has an underlying disorder of blood clotting (overleaf) or a disease of the liver. Abnormal blood clotting may cause bleeding from the nose or bowel, or bruising.

Early bleeding after birth

Vitamin K is required by the liver to make factors essential for the blood to clot. Haemorrhagic disease of the newborn arising from a deficiency in vitamin K is a rare disease affecting 1:10,000 babies in the UK. It can cause bleeding from the mouth, nose and gut in the first weeks after birth but can be prevented if additional vitamin K is given in the newborn period (p.226). Without additional vitamin K, the condition carries a high risk of death or handicap if bleeding occurs into the brain. Studies in the UK, the USA, Germany, Switzerland and Sweden have concluded that intramuscular vitamin K prevents haemorrhage completely, and that oral vitamin K offers a significant degree of protection. Vitamin K is not associated with an increase in the risk of childhood cancer.

Your baby may be given an intramuscular injection of vitamin K if she is premature; if you have taken medications that thin the blood in pregnancy (e.g. aspirin, heparin); if she had a traumatic birth with bruising or foetal distress; or if she is ill and vomited the oral vitamin K.

Blood in the stools
Blood in the motions, when it occurs with no other symptoms, is rarely a sign of any serious problem. Seek help early if the bleeding suddenly occurs or your baby appears to be ill and has other symptoms.
- If your baby is breastfed the most likely cause is that you have cracked nipples (p.416). Even without obvious cracks, your baby's suck may be strong enough to cause bleeding. The blood does no harm and you can continue to feed.
- A very common cause in an otherwise well baby is some form of allergic colitis. Common foods that cause this ALLERGY are milk, rice and wheat. The diagnosis is simple to make if the blood clears when a food is excluded: then avoid the food while taking advice from a nutritionist to ensure your baby receives adequate nutrients.
- If blood is bright red and coats the outside of your baby's motion, this could be due to a small tear in the skin of the anus (anal fissure), and is often associated with a large or hard stool. You may not be able to see the tear but there may be a tag of skin. Fissures heal of their own accord if steps are taken to avoid CONSTIPATION.
- Blood mixed with the motion may indicate some infection in the bowel that may also causes DIARRHOEA and tummy ache. Rarely, bloody stools with an ill baby may indicate a serious condition called intussusception (p.437).

Vomiting blood
Even a small amount of blood in the stomach is likely to make your baby sick. The most common source, if your baby appears well apart from the vomit, is if she breastfeeds from cracked nipples. The blood is altered by stomach acid and may appear dark brown. This is harmless, and the best thing to do is to continue feeding and treat your cracked nipples – usually a simple case of attending to latching on.

Some babies with bad reflux associated with VOMITING may occasionally vomit flecks of blood. Although this is usually harmless and needs no specific treatment, let your doctor know. Another, rare, cause is a disorder of clotting. The most common is vitamin K-dependent bleeding (above).

Bleeding from the genitals
It is quite common for newborn girls to have a little bleeding as a result of maternal hormones that circulated during pregnancy: as levels of oestrogen fall after birth, the womb may bleed as the lining is shed. The blood may be pink or red, is usually mixed with mucus and commonly stops after 3 weeks. Any further or persistent bleeding from the vagina needs to be investigated.

Another very common symptom that is alarming yet misleading is pink discoloration on the nappy. This is a harmless deposit of urate crystals from the urine and resolves without the need for treatment.

Bleeding from the nose, ears & skin
Bleeding from the nose is unusual, except when a baby has a cold. If your baby has a bloody discharge from the nose and it lasts longer than a normal cold, something may be stuck up her nose – usually a button or piece of paper that you will be able to see. If removing it is likely to be difficult, take your baby to the local casualty department. She may need an anaesthetic while the object is extracted. Another common cause of nose bleeds is a blow to the nose (p.387).

Bleeding from the ear or, more usually, blood streaks in mucus discharge from the ear usually means that the ear drum has perforated, due to infection in the middle ear (p.453), which weakens the eardrum, and discharges through a small hole that heals. Another cause is a foreign body in the ear canal, or damage to the skin of the ear. Most rarely, bleeding from the ear results from a severe head injury.

Bleeding from the skin usually results from a cut or graze (p.384). A less common cause is a condition called purpura that leads to bleeding into the skin and results in a rash. If the rash does not disappear when a glass is pressed against your baby's skin, and she appears unwell, this may indicate MENINGITIS. Call your doctor. In most cases a meningitis scare is a false alarm, but it is best to be sure.

BLOOD-CLOTTING & BLEEDING DISORDERS
....

See also BLEEDING PROBLEMS: BABY

There is a very complex system that ensures the blood clots when necessary and stays liquid and fluid the rest of the time. Blood clotting requires special cells that make up the blood clot, called platelets, and a sticky protein called fibrin, which mixes with the platelets to make the clot and it then dissolves over time. People bleed and clot all the time. Disorders of clotting include **thrombophilia** with a tendency to clot excessively. This may interfere with the function of the placenta or cause deep vein thrombosis (p.560). Deficient clotting may cause a mother or baby to bleed excessively because the blood cannot clot normally. A bleeding tendency may be inherited or be part of another abnormality affecting mother or baby.

Excess clotting
In a normal pregnancy and after birth a mother's blood has a slightly increased tendency to form clots and there is an increased risk of deep vein thrombosis, particularly after bed rest, caesarean section or long air flights. Women with thrombophilia have a greater than normal tendency for the

blood to clot. It may be inherited (e.g. Factor V [Leiden], protein C and S, and homocysteinaemia) or acquired (e.g. antiphospholipid syndrome associated with lupus, an autoimmune disorder).

What happens

Soon after the embryo attaches to the uterus, the placental cells come into contact with the mother's blood vessels, which are the only source of nourishment. Thrombophilia can cause clotting and reduce blood flow to the embryo, either early or late in pregnancy. In a mild form it may have no effect. Untreated, it may cause: MISCARRIAGE and recurrent foetal loss, pre-eclampsia (p.410), INTRAUTERINE GROWTH RESTRICTION, PLACENTAL ABRUPTION, deep vein thrombosis or, if severe, stillbirth (p.509).

If you or other members of your family have experienced any of these conditions, you may consider a blood test for thrombophilia that includes lupus as treatment greatly reduces the risks to your baby.

Action plan

Medical care
Treatment depends on the type of blood-clotting anomaly. In severe cases when there has been a previous foetal loss, it is best to begin treatment soon after conception. Treatment has transformed the outlook for pregnancies associated with thrombophilia.

- Aspirin tablets can be safely used throughout pregnancy.
- Heparin is more powerful than aspirin for severe thrombophilia. Heparin is administered by injection in doses monitored by your obstetrician. Heparin has the advantage of not crossing the placenta. The disadvantage is that long-term use can lead to bleeding or OSTEOPOROSIS. It is used less commonly than aspirin but it is very effective when used appropriately. Warfarin is not used because of the associated risk of foetal abnormalities.
- If you have thrombophilia, you should not use birth control pills and consider taking aspirin daily and use heparin for surgery, including a CAESAREAN SECTION.

Bleeding disorders

Bleeding disorders may be inherited where the person is born with an abnormally low activity of one of the 12 clotting factors that make up the coagulation system. If the clotting factor is severely reduced, bleeding may occur spontaneously without trauma. A mild inherited deficiency may have a family history or it may surface because of bleeding in adulthood after surgery or childbirth.

A bleeding disorder may be part of another disease process. The most common disorder is following a placental abruption, severe pre-eclampsia or excessive bleeding where the mother's clotting factors have been used up. The deficiency is replaced by a blood transfusion with extra clotting factors until the mother's liver makes the missing factors. After birth, babies, particularly PREMATURE babies, may be deficient in vitamin K and some of the associated clotting factors are low. This deficiency is corrected by giving newborn babies vitamin K (p.226).

Haemophilia

Haemophilia is a deficiency of clotting factor VIII. More than 3000 people in the UK are affected. Haemophilia is usually inherited by male children from their carrier mothers, but every year 60% of newly diagnosed cases have a spontaneous mutation with no family history. Very rarely, females inherit haemophilia.

The problem may not be suspected within the first 6 months but 30% of male haemophiliac babies bleed excessively during CIRCUMCISION. Bruising or bleeding into the joints are the common presentations. Occasionally a baby may bleed from the nose (p.387) or have blood in the stool from the bowel (opposite) or have ANAEMIA. Even more rarely, among 1–2% of haemophiliac babies, there is bleeding into the brain. When your baby is mobile, falls and bumps may lead to profuse or unusual bruising. Unfortunately, this may prompt medical carers to investigate the need for CHILD PROTECTION before a diagnosis is made. It is routine to check a baby's blood-clotting abilities before saying an injury was not accidental.

Action plan

Before the advent of safer blood products in 1985, many haemophiliacs were infected with HIV and HEPATITIS B and C, with catastrophic results. Today safer clotting factor replacement products are available. There are also haemophilia centres for diagnosis and treatment although most patients can be treated at home with the assistance of home-care nurses.

Von Willebrand's disease

Von Willebrand's disease affects 1–3% of the UK population, and passes from parent to child. The blood platelets do not adhere normally and the von Willebrand factor that protects factor VIII, which is essential for blood clotting, is also missing. It rarely causes any problems in newborn infants, but later in life bruising is the most common problem and bleeding can happen after a surgical procedure. With severe forms there may be bleeding from the digestive or urinary tract or from the mouth. Treatment to replace clotting factors is usually less intensive than for haemophilia.

Other clotting factors

There are 12 clotting factors and deficiency and in some families there is an inherited deficiency in one of the factors. The incidence varies in different populations and factors X, XI and XII are found in the UK. The deficiency may be mild without excessive bleeding or it may cause excessive bleeding after birth. If there is a history, family members are usually tested and treated if the excessive bleeding occurs.

Thrombocytopaenia

Thrombocytopaenia involves the absence of platelets from the blood, or a count below normal that results in bleeding into the skin, the mouth, nose and ears. The condition may affect fewer than 1:5000 babies. The usual cause is infection, where platelets are used up more quickly than they can be produced. Sometimes a mother passes an antibody against the platelets to her baby in the womb, and the platelets are destroyed. With treatment the outlook is excellent, providing a baby does not suffer a major bleed (a low risk in cases of thrombocytopaenia).

BLOOD GROUP, ABO INCOMPATIBILITY

ABO incompatibility disease may occur in babies with blood type A, B or AB whose mothers are blood type O. Ordinarily, type O women have antibodies against the blood types A and B but they are too large to pass easily across the placenta into the foetal circulation. However, some foetal red cells often cross into the mother's circulation (p.398). These foetal red cells stimulate the formation of a smaller type of anti-A or anti-B antibody, which can pass into the baby's circulation and cause the destruction of foetal red cells. Destruction of red cells can lead to JAUNDICE after birth, which may need to be treated with phototherapy or even exchange transfusion (p.491). There is no prevention of ABO incompatibility, only treatment of the jaundice in the baby.

BLOOD GROUP, RHESUS FACTOR

The rhesus factor on normal red blood cells has three components, C, D and E. The D is most important. Rhesus carries no implications to general health but may be significant in pregnancy. Roughly 15% of people lack the rhesus factor and are known as rhesus negative (Rh–). If a baby's father is also Rh–, the baby will always be Rh–. But if the father has the rhesus factor and is therefore 'rhesus D positive' (Rh D+) there is a 50% chance that the baby will be positive. If some of the baby's blood enters the mother's bloodstream, the mother's body will react to the baby's apparently foreign (Rh D+) blood cells and produce anti-rhesus antibodies. Foetal cells may enter the mother's circulation in small amounts during pregnancy (p.398) or during AMNIOCENTESIS OR CVS. It is most likely during birth as the placenta separates. Anti-rhesus antibodies may also occur in a Rh– woman after a miscarriage when the baby was Rh D+ or if a Rh– mother receives a BLOOD TRANSFUSION of Rh D+ blood.

If you are Rh– and have rhesus antibodies, they will have no effect on you. But in a subsequent pregnancy, the antibodies may cross the placenta and, if your second baby is Rh D+, they could damage or even destroy her red blood cells, leading to foetal ANAEMIA and severe JAUNDICE after the birth.

Action plan
If you are Rh– incompatibility can easily be prevented if you have an injection of anti-Rh D. The anti-Rh D mops up any foetal red blood cells that may have travelled from your baby into your blood and prevents the development of destructive maternal antibodies.
- During pregnancy the injection is given at Week 28 and 34 and after amniocentesis or CVS or miscarriage.
- After birth the cord blood is tested to establish your baby's blood group and your blood will be checked for foetal red blood cells. If your baby is Rh+ you will be injected with anti-Rh D within 72 hours, which ensures you do not develop antibodies that could affect a future rhesus positive baby.

In the unlikely event that you are Rh– and have developed antibodies before pregnancy, this will be detected in an antenatal blood test. There is a chance your baby may be affected so she will be regularly monitored by ultrasound scan and the concentration of antibodies in your blood will be checked every 4 weeks. If your baby is severely affected, she may need a blood transfusion in the uterus, or, if pregnancy is sufficiently advanced, labour may be induced and your baby will be treated for jaundice or anaemia after birth.

BLOOD PRESSURE, HIGH (PRE-ECLAMPSIA)

Normal blood pressure is less than 140/90 mm of mercury. Raised blood pressure is called hypertension. In pregnancy there is a specific type of hypertension known as pre-eclampsia, **toxaemia** or pregnancy-induced **hypertension**. Although mildly raised blood pressure may not have any effect on you or your baby, severe elevations (below) can have serious results, including eclamptic convulsions (p.471) and reduced blood flow to the placenta with reduced placental function and INTRAUTERINE GROWTH RESTRICTION (IUGR).

Pre-eclampsia occurs in around 5% of first pregnancies and is usually mild. Commonly it does not begin until Week 34 and it almost always resolves after birth. If it is severe it may begin earlier, and sometimes it does not arise until labour, or even until a few days after birth. A woman who has hypertension and then becomes pregnant will have high blood pressure in pregnancy: this is called essential hypertension, is likely to worsen with superimposed pre-eclampsia and needs careful monitoring.

What happens
Because symptoms may not appear in the early stages, blood pressure and urine are tested throughout pregnancy so that treatment can begin early.
- In mild pre-eclampsia, blood pressure rises up to 140/100 and there is slight swelling of the feet or hands and the urine is clear. Women often feel well.
- In severe form, blood pressure may rise above 160/110 and protein in urine indicates an effect on the kidney and on blood vessels throughout the body.
- Other symptoms of severe pre-eclampsia may include headache, dizziness, blurred vision, restlessness and irritability or drowsiness and even FITS (indicating effects on the brain); pain high in the abdomen, and nausea (related to a swollen liver); bruising or bleeding (effects on blood clotting); excess fluid retention with intense puffiness of the limbs or the face, and excess weight gain.
- If pre-eclampsia becomes severe there is an increased risk of bleeding related to PLACENTAL ABRUPTION, which may be dangerous for mother and baby.
- Severe pre-eclampsia becomes eclampsia when fits or convulsions occur. It may lead to coma. This life-threatening condition for mother and baby is unlikely to happen with modern obstetric care, which ensures that treatment begins before eclampsia occurs.

What may cause pre-eclampsia?

The exact cause of pre-eclampsia is unknown. There may be a genetic predisposition and it is likely that the condition is related to the mother's immune system reacting to the placenta or the baby. The reaction leads to a narrowing of the arteries and increases the blood pressure. Researchers believe that pre-eclampsia may be part of a spectrum of disorders that begin in the first few weeks as the placenta implants and invades the arteries in the uterus wall. Incomplete invasion may lead to a number of conditions, including slow growth of the baby (IUGR) with or without pre-eclampsia and pre-eclampsia with normal growth. A diet deficient in nutrition and vitamins and minerals before and during early pregnancy may increase the likelihood of high blood pressure. Hypertension may accompany an existing kidney disorder. It is more likely if you are carrying TWINS.

Action plan

If you have mildly elevated pressure, relax, look after yourself and continue to be monitored. Be aware that excessive weight gain or SWELLING (OEDEMA) may be symptoms of a further rise. If you have protein in your urine or are diagnosed with severe pre-eclampsia, you will need intense monitoring and treatment.

Medical care in pregnancy

- If pre-eclampsia is mild your blood pressure and urine will be checked from once a week to daily, depending on the levels. You may buy a portable machine to check blood pressure at home. If you are nervous of hospitals the level may be falsely high when you are checked by a midwife; this is called the white coat syndrome.
- You will be given blood tests to assess kidney and liver function and blood-clotting ability and urine tests to quantify the amount of protein.
- Your baby's wellbeing will be assessed in line with monitoring for a HIGH-RISK PREGNANCY.
- If pre-eclampsia is severe, you will be admitted to hospital and checks will be frequent.
- If blood pressure remains above 150/100 and particularly if there is protein in your urine or hypertension has been present before pregnancy, anti-hypertensive medication may be needed. The drugs are usually taken as tablets but can be administered by intravenous infusion in hospital. If pre-eclampsia is severe these may be combined with anticonvulsant medication to prevent eclamptic fits. It is preferable to use magnesium sulphate and avoid benzodiazepine (Valium) as an anticonvulsant because it may affect your baby's breathing and alertness for weeks after birth. If anticonvulsant medication is needed for more than a few hours, urgent delivery is usually necessary.

Lifestyle, diet and complementary therapies

In conjunction with medical monitoring these measures may help keep your blood pressure manageable.
- Reduce strenuous activities and cut down on work. If pressure is very high, bed rest may be advised.
- If you have mildly elevated blood pressure, exercise (p.357) and yoga (p.346) within your comfort zone improves

circulation and can stabilise levels.
- Meditation and visualisation (p.370) are also useful.
- Cook with plenty of garlic. It's good for just about everything and can improve circulation and help reduce high blood pressure. Reducing salt is useful to prevent hypertension but does not have a significant effect later.
- Acupuncture and reflexology can help reduce high pressure.
- Homeopathy can have powerful effects but qualified advice must be taken. Remedies for swelling can reduce fluid retention, but do not tackle the underlying cause of hypertension.
- Helpful aromatherapy oils (in the bath or for massage) include orange, petitgrain, tangerine, sandalwood, ylang ylang and bergamot, and low doses of rose and melissa. Take advice from an aromatherapist and consult your doctor before use. From Week 24 lavender can be used.

When early birth is necessary

- You can safely wait for labour to begin spontaneously if hypertension is mild, provided your baby is healthy.
- Where hypertension is significant and your baby is mature, induction (p.497) may be advised.
- If pre-eclampsia is severe and there is IUGR or a risk of eclamptic fits, a PREMATURE BIRTH may be safer. If you have very severe pre-eclampsia or are having eclamptic convulsions, immediate CAESAREAN SECTION is essential.

Treatment during labour

You and your baby will be closely monitored. Notably this involves frequent checks of your blood pressure and urinary protein levels and foetal heart patterns on CTG.
- Epidural anaesthesia (p.159) may reduce high blood pressure and anti-hypertensive drugs may be used.
- If contractions are ineffectual the oxytocin (Syntocinon) used to enhance them needs to be administered with caution because in high doses it may elevate blood pressure. Ergometrine, which is used after the birth to reduce bleeding, must be avoided because it may dangerously raise blood pressure.

After the birth

Blood pressure usually begins to drop within a few hours of birth. Your baby will be examined to check for effects of reduced placental function and IUGR. If she has been born prematurely, care will reflect her needs at birth.
- When pre-eclampsia has been severe, the risk of eclamptic convulsions continues for up to 7 days after the birth, so observation and treatment continue.
- The midwives will monitor your blood pressure postnatally because occasionally pre-eclampsia begins in the first few days after birth.

BLOOD PRESSURE, LOW

Low blood pressure, also called hypotension, is a sign of good health. If you have low blood pressure it may drop lower in pregnancy and return to normal as soon as your baby is born.

The level naturally falls in the middle trimester by 10 mm. If pressure drops significantly, however, it may cause dizziness or faintness. A level below 90/55 mm of mercury is significant, although many fit athletes have levels below this.

Action plan
- If you feel faint, sit down: this helps blood flow back to your heart and if you do faint you will avoid injury.
- Standing or sitting for a long time or getting up suddenly may cause blood to pool in your legs, particularly if you are unfit, have varicose veins (p.559), have consumed ALCOHOL or taken drugs to lower blood pressure or when the temperature is hot. You can prevent fainting by contracting and releasing the muscles in calves, thighs and buttocks for 2–3 seconds, continuing for 1–2 minutes. This pumps blood back to your heart and restores circulation to your brain. Exercise, yoga and massage help to improve circulation.
- For a small percentage of women in mid- to late pregnancy, lying flat on the back means the uterus presses on the arteries and veins at the back of the abdominal cavity and reduces the amount of blood flowing to the heart. You may find it more comfortable to lie on your side.
- A low level of sugar in your blood, also called HYPOGLYCAEMIA, may cause faintness and low blood pressure. This is avoidable with a balanced diet – eat every 3 hours with a balance of slow-burning carbohydrates with vitamins, minerals, roughage and plenty of fluid.
- Rarely, loss of blood from BLEEDING DURING PREGNANCY can reduce blood pressure. This is an emergency that requires urgent intravenous fluid replacement and, possibly, a BLOOD TRANSFUSION.

BLOOD TRANSFUSION

In an emergency if your haemoglobin level falls below 8 g/dl you may need a blood transfusion. Supplies of donor blood from your local service are kept in the hospital. Your blood group is known from antenatal blood tests. A repeat blood sample is taken and the laboratory will cross match it with the donor's blood to ensure the two are compatible. The donor blood is also checked for infections, particularly HEPATITIS and HIV. The possibility of being infected is remote – estimated at less than 1 in a million. The procedure takes about 4 hours but can be speeded up to minutes in an emergency where there is shock. It is given intravenously with a drip and you can sit up in bed during the transfusion. After a transfusion it is best to replace iron stores with supplements.

BREAST & BREASTFEEDING PROBLEMS

See also Positioning and latching on (p.188); WEIGHT, LOW GAIN OR FAILURE TO THRIVE: BABY

During pregnancy, hormonal changes cause your breasts to enlarge. They may feel full, heavy and tender to touch. If your breasts usually become very sensitive before you menstruate, you are more likely to feel tender. Within a day or two of birth your breasts will almost certainly feel uncomfortable as they begin to fill with milk. Swelling may be considerable until your baby establishes feeding. In most cases, discomfort passes within days. Each time your baby feeds, your breast empties, then becomes heavy and full before the next feed. Your milk supply adjusts to your baby's pattern of feeding, and feeding on demand helps your body match your baby's rhythm.

What happens
Pain related to feeding may be due to one of several underlying causes:

Let-down pain: May occur at the beginning of a feed as the small muscles in the wall of each milk duct contract and eject milk towards the nipple. Most women find that after a few days let-down pain diminishes but for a small minority it remains part of breastfeeding. Latching your baby on well increases milk flow and reduces pain. Occasionally this type of pain is due to CANDIDA (thrush) infection in the milk ducts.

Muscle pain: Can stem from the way you hold your baby while feeding or carrying her. You may feel pain in the pectoral muscles on the front of your chest, behind your breast and into your shoulder and perhaps your neck. It may be confused with mastitis but your breast won't be red. Your doctor or midwife can diagnose muscle pain by feeling the tender muscle. For this to improve take care about the way you hold and carry your baby, particularly when feeding.

Breast engorgement (p.414): May occur when your milk comes in or after the 1st week if your breasts produce more milk than your baby drinks, or when you decide to stop breastfeeding and there is a build-up before milk production stops (p.414).

Blocked milk ducts: Cause pain with a hard lump in the breast because of the pressure of the milk and inflammation of the surrounding tissues. If a blockage does not drain it may lead to breast infection, and mastitis may develop – this may need antibiotics and occasionally hospital admission. If the infection worsens an abscess may form.

Cracked nipples (p.416): Can be very painful and may occur if your feeding position is poor and your baby does not latch on properly. They improve with attention to latching on.

A breast lump (p.416): Usually caused by a blocked milk duct or accessory breast tissue and not a cause for concern. Extremely rarely, a single lump may be caused by a tumour so it is important to have single lumps checked by a doctor.

Action plan
When things don't feel right you may worry. Remember that breastfeeding does not always come naturally and it is something you and your baby need to learn. It is common to have initial difficulties, and also common for these to pass with the right approach and lots of support.
- Whatever the underlying cause of discomfort, the treatment almost always begins with attention to position and latching on (p.188). If difficulties begin to resolve, feeding can change from a challenge into a pleasure. Persevere because if your baby does not latch on properly, or you keep feeds short because of pain, she may not receive enough milk.
- Look after yourself: eat well, drink plenty of water – at least

2 litres (4 pints) a day – and get enough rest. Your wellbeing affects your milk, and good nutrition, with supplemental minerals and vitamins, will aid healing and boost your immunity.

- Wear a well-fitting cotton bra.
- Create quality time to feed when both you and your baby are relaxed. Extra company and emotional support from your friends, family and wider network could help you get through the current difficulty.
- Wherever possible, it is important to continue feeding, because this usually helps to treat the problem.
- Your doctor or midwife may be able to put you in touch with a local breastfeeding counsellor. Other sources of information and support include NCT groups and the La Leche League.
- In the short term, you will need to treat the symptoms that relate to your specific difficulty. Treatments are listed under the individual entries that follow.

BREAST, BLOCKED DUCTS, MASTITIS & ABSCESSES

If a milk duct becomes blocked, it swells, forms a lump and your breast may become inflamed. This probably happens because your baby's sucking does not completely drain the milk. If bacteria enter the blocked duct the retained milk will become infected and the lump will be red and very painful – this is mastitis. It can usually be treated and need not interfere with successful breastfeeding. In a tiny percentage of women the infection is severe and may lead to the formation of pus: this is a breast abscess. Mastitis and breast abscesses are the most serious problems related to breastfeeding.

Blocked milk ducts
When a milk duct becomes blocked, the resulting swelling has a sharply defined edge, and may reduce with a light massage. It may also reduce after a feed. Milk can be seen in the swelling with an ultrasound scan.

What happens
Anything that restricts milk flow can cause blocked ducts.
- A milk duct may become blocked if your baby does not latch on well (p.188) and milk does not flow all the way to the nipple. This is the most significant factor.
- If your nipples are painful or cracked, you may avoid draining the sore side or you may have a 'favourite' position that does not allow your baby to drain each segment of your breast equally.
- If there is a build-up of milk in your breasts – perhaps because you are producing an excess of milk in the early days, your baby is sleeping through or you are working – your breast may become engorged. The reservoir of un-drained milk may thicken and block one or more ducts.
- If you are wearing a tight bra or clothing or grasping your breast too tightly while feeding, the duct's opening may constrict.
- Nipple shields can affect the flow of milk.

Mastitis & abscesses
Bacteria are normally present on the skin and if they reach retained milk in a blocked milk duct, mastitis may develop. Rarely, mastitis develops from skin bacteria without blocked ducts. If you have ANAEMIA, experience undue stress or TIREDNESS or are not eating well, your resistance to infection is lowered. Cigarette SMOKING can also lower resistance.

In the early stages, mastitis involves slight swelling and redness, a marginal rise in temperature and may pass without antibiotic treatment. The redness and temperature rise distinguish it from BREAST ENGORGEMENT. If the bacteria cause severe mastitis your breasts will be very red and painful and you may have a high temperature and flu-like symptoms.

An abscess is an area of infected mastitis that has progressed. It is a more severe form of infection and is more destructive: bacteria destroy some of the breast tissue and create fluid (pus) composed of the infected tissue. A breast abscess causes a very high temperature, severe flu-like symptoms and a very red and extremely painful large lump. If you have taken antibiotics, the temperature, pain and redness may be less obvious.

Action plan
If you notice breast lumps, pain and/or redness and particularly if your temperature is high, seek advice from your midwife, breastfeeding counsellor or doctor. In many cases, mastitis can be prevented by early attention to clearing blocked ducts. These and infection are not always preventable but good technique reduces the chances that they will occur. With loving support you may be able to stick with it, continue feeding and get over the infection. If you have had mastitis after your first pregnancy, you will not necessarily get it after a second.

Feeding technique
- Check the way your baby is latching on. This is the most important aspect of treating and preventing infection.
- Do not stop feeding – in fact, feed more frequently if you can. This will help to unblock milk ducts and clear any infective organisms.
- Even with severe mastitis continue to feed – your baby has been exposed to the bacteria causing the infection (usually Staphylococcus aureus) since birth and she will not be harmed. Only if the pain is too intense or the infection does not settle despite treatment may it be necessary to stop breastfeeding.
- Use a different position each time you feed so you drain the affected area.

Breast care
- If you feel lumpy or have tender areas, try gently heating your breast for 10 minutes with a warm compress (not hot) before feeding your baby. This will loosen any dry milk in the ducts. You could try using a small amount of the aromatherapy oils frankincense, geranium or camomile in the compress. Alternatively, take a warm shower or a bath before a feed.
- Massage (p.365) can help milk to flow before a feed or release excess after a feed. Use a natural oil (almond, grapeseed or vitamin E) and mix with the same essential oils

that can be used in a compress. Be gentle so you don't traumatise the breast tissue.

- If your breasts do not empty completely after massage, you could use a breast pump. Try pumping after warming your breasts and after feeding to minimise discomfort and improve efficiency. Do not strain your breasts – once the flow has slowed to a drip, stop pumping as excessive use can exacerbate the problem.

Medical care for mastitis
Continue preventive techniques and follow your doctor's advice to treat mastitis, keeping regular contact. Mastitis may make you feel very unwell but once treatment starts, recovery is usually rapid.

- If mastitis is mild, your white blood cell count is normal (it rises if there is an infection) and your temperature is not very high. Mastitis may respond within 48 hours to anti-inflammatory agents such as aspirin or ibuprofen.
- If mastitis is more severe or you have recurrent mastitis, a fever that is rising and you feel sick or your nipples are cracked, an antibiotic is advisable. It is essential to continue to encourage your breast to empty completely to reduce the risk of an abscess forming. The two most effective classes of antibiotics are cloxacillins and cephalosporins but there are others if you are allergic to these. These antibiotics are safe to take while breastfeeding and it is best to complete the course to reduce the risk of the mastitis returning. If you don't feel better after 2 days on antibiotics, you may need to change. A small amount of the antibiotic appears in your milk but it is very unusual for a baby to be affected by it.
- You may be offered an ultrasound scan, which can detect whether the mastitis is associated with collections of fluid and an abscess.
- CANDIDA (thrush) infection in the milk ducts can lead to breast inflammation and even mastitis. If mastitis does not improve with antibiotics, you may need treatment for candida.

Medical care for an abscess
- An abscess needs to be treated with intensive intravenous antibiotic therapy, possibly in hospital. Your baby is usually welcome to stay and you will be home in a couple of days.
- If the abscess does not respond to antibiotics within 24 hours, the pus will need to be drained. A small collection can be removed in the ultrasound room by using a needle with local anaesthesia, or more usually drainage is in the operating theatre under general anaesthetic. A soft plastic drain is then left in place for a day or two. Early drainage of pus is essential to protect your breast tissue. Although some women elect to continue to feed with both breasts many discontinue breastfeeding after surgery. The operation site is uncomfortable for a few days.

Homeopathy
As a general rule, at the first sign of symptoms take *Belladonna* (30c) once an hour for 3 hours. Then reassess and take the most appropriate remedy (30c) once an hour for 3 hours, then every 2 hours for the next 12 hours. If there is no improvement within 24 hours, seek professional advice. Your homeopath

may advise you to take a high potency (200c) frequently. For an infection or abscess, you will need antibiotic treatment; your homeopath may suggest some remedies to aid recovery.

Belladonna is the first remedy to use when you feel sensitive, don't want to lie down, there is swelling and sudden throbbing pain, with heat and redness around the blocked duct or red streaks running from the nipple to the circumference of the breast, and perhaps a fever; *Bryonia* may help if pain builds up more slowly but you are still sensitive to movement, and your breast feels stony-hard and engorged, you feel dry and dehydrated, irritable and unsociable; *Mercurius* helps if you have flu-like symptoms that are worse at night, you are very thirsty and salivate a lot and the blocked duct forms a distinct, hard lump; *Phytolacca* helps if you have shooting pains radiating from your breasts into your armpits, find it unbearably painful to feed, feel hot and sweaty at night and have swollen glands, your breast is red and needs support; *Pulsatilla* is good if your breasts are swollen, the level of pain varies and you have fever, feel weepy and need consolation – it relieves emotional stress, particularly in the first few days after birth, so that you can focus on the specific breast pain and follow up with another remedy.

BREAST, ENGORGEMENT

Engorgement occurs when breasts become full with milk and swell, becoming heavy and tender to the touch.

What happens
On the 2nd or 3rd day after birth when your breasts begin to produce milk, they may swell to up to three times their normal size. This might be mildly or extremely uncomfortable but it is a good sign that your milk will soon flow freely. The swelling usually calms down within a few days. Engorgement may continue for longer if the milk is not drained completely – this may happen if your baby does not latch on well or does not drink as much as you produce. If your breasts become swollen, your nipples may become flat, making it harder for your baby to latch on. If engorgement continues and the milk is not drained, the milk ducts may become blocked and mastitis may develop. Your breasts may become engorged when you decide to stop breastfeeding and there is a temporary milk build-up.

Action plan
It will be painful to feed your baby but the more milk she drains, the more your swelling will reduce. Pay close attention to your position and how your baby latches on (p.188), and feed her as often as she requests it, or more frequently if she is not a demanding baby. In a few days your breasts will match demand with supply.

Breast care
- A simple remedy for engorged breasts has been used for centuries. Keep a cabbage leaf or a bowl of grated carrot in the fridge. Place one or other between your breast and bra for 10–20 minutes every 4 hours. This can help to draw excess fluid away from your breast and reduce swelling. Do

not keep the cabbage or carrots on the skin for longer as this may crack your nipples.

- Gentle breast massage (p.195) encourages milk to flow to the nipple and drain away.
- Check your breasts after each feed for lumps or tender areas. This will help you prevent further discomfort or mastitis.

Feeding technique

- Successful latching on is the key to successful feeding, and you and your baby may need to work on this for a few days. When you are both comfortable, good positioning will come naturally and this will help prevent future engorgement.
- If your nipples are flatter than usual, place your thumb and forefinger above and below the nipple, and gently press inwards and then together so your nipple protrudes. Once your baby is latched on the pressure from her mouth should keep your nipple erect. Take care your fingers do not obstruct her mouth and her lips cover the areola, not just the nipple. Techniques for inverted nipples (p.417) may help.
- If you have a very sleepy baby, you may need to undress and wake her, particularly if she goes for longer than 5 hours without a feed, so she can drain your milk.
- You could express some milk before a feed to reduce tension and allow your nipple to protrude.

If you have stopped feeding

If your breasts become engorged when you stop feeding, wrap a towel tightly around your chest. This may help to reduce pain because the pressure inhibits milk production. Cabbage leaves or grated carrot reduce engorgement. It is best not to express because this will stimulate more milk production. The discomfort will settle in 48 hours. Some hospitals use a drug, bromocriptine, that reduces prolactin hormone levels, but it may cause nausea and is only useful in the 1st week. When the drug is stopped, breast milk production may recommence.

Homeopathy

Choose a remedy that suits and take it in 30c every 2 hours for 12 hours and then 4 times a day for another 3 days, and then reassess. Use *Calc Carb* if your breasts are swollen but not red, with milk that looks bluish and transparent, you have cold sweats and feel anxious and weak; *Lac Caninum* for swollen, lumpy breasts with pain moving from one side to the other but better for warmth and rest, to regulate milk supply; *Pulsatilla* if your breasts feel stretched, you feel weepy, want company and consolation, feel hot, hate stuffy rooms and are not thirsty.

Aromatherapy

Peppermint and cypress oils are both helpful used on a cold compress placed against your swollen breast(s) for 20 minutes every 4 hours.

BREAST, LOW MILK FLOW

See also WEIGHT, LOW GAIN OR FAILURE TO THRIVE: BABY

All babies are different – some take a big feed quickly, others prefer to take their time, and length of sucking is not an indication of how much milk you are producing. If your baby is happy, passing urine and gaining weight properly then there is no indication you have low milk flow. If your breasts leak or milk sprays out when the let-down reflex is active, you definitely have sufficient.

If your baby does not seem happy or appears hungry after a feed, consider whether she is latching on correctly. Latching on and positioning are the keys to maximising milk flow. There may also be other reasons for your baby's unsettled behaviour: so see your health visitor or doctor if you are concerned. If the growth chart shows that your baby is not gaining weight adequately, the most likely cause is a low milk flow.

Action plan

If your baby is not gaining weight adequately your doctor or health visitor will help you to decide what the cause may be: in most instances the cause is low milk flow, and a low flow is usually due to poor latching on. It is important to have your baby checked closely in case there is an underlying problem.

- Use the checklist on p.188 to determine whether your baby is latching on well and whether your own position might inhibit your milk flow. This is the most important issue to stimulate the let-down reflex and the flow.
- Spend lots of time with your baby – her presence encourages your milk to flow.
- Your baby may need help to burp during or after feeds – some babies retain air and feel full when they are not.
- Feed your baby as often as she wants. You may need to spend time establishing a working partnership so that your body matches supply with demand. Ensure feeds are long enough for her to receive the hind milk (p.187).
- If you are in pain, your physical tension may inhibit the let-down reflex. The pain may also limit feeds: your milk flow will reduce if shorter feeding times or less frequent sucking give your body the message that the demand has fallen. Different positions and treating the cause of pain may make feeding less uncomfortable.
- If your baby is not demanding, you will need to encourage her to feed often. If she tires easily and stops sucking after a few minutes, you will need to feed frequently. You can try to rouse her by undressing her before a feed or lightly blowing on her face if her sucking slows.
- If your baby is frail or PREMATURE or has abnormal development of the tongue and mouth, her sucking reflex may be ineffective. To keep your milk production going you may have to stimulate your breasts using a pump to empty them at the end of each feed.
- Make sure you are exercising and resting enough: being out in the fresh air, moving and doing yoga get your body energised. While you are resting you could follow a visualisation or imagine your milk flowing to your nipples and into your baby's mouth to provide nourishment. Some women find this a powerful way to help milk flow.
- Foods that may encourage milk flow include fennel, dill, coriander and nettles. Fennel and nettles make good tea.
- You may feel upset and question whether you are a 'good enough' mother. This is a normal reaction, but because feeling upset can reduce milk flow it is best to find support as you try some practical measures to improve the situation.

Think about ways to ease your load and consider addressing anything that may lead to depression (p.462).

- If you are working and do not express, your flow is likely to reduce as your breasts are less stimulated and/or because you are not getting enough rest. You may choose to express when you're not at home, supplement feeds with formula, stop breastfeeding or re-evaluate the work–home balance. If you are becoming stressed, you may decide it is better to give your baby the milk she needs with formula feed. This could make both of you happier. You may be able to mix bottle and breast (p.195), or decide to stop breastfeeding.

Homeopathy

To increase your milk supply, try *Urtica Urens* (6c) 4 times a day for 5 days and then reassess. If you are exhausted, *China* (30c), taken morning and night for 1–2 weeks, is a great pick-up remedy. If you think your emotions may be affecting your feeding success, try one of the following (30c) 3 times a day for 3 days and then reassess. Use *Aconite* after a physical shock or fright – the shock may be birth; *Chamomilla* after a bout of anger; *Coffea* if you are over-excited; *Ignatia* after emotional shock or grief.

Aromatherapy

Fennel, jasmine, lemongrass, clary sage or geranium used for a massage or in a compress can stimulate flow. Mix the essential oil with a pure oil (p.378). Take care while you massage your breasts and do so after feeding so the oil will be fully absorbed when your baby next feeds. If it irritates, wash off the oil immediately. Fennel passes through to your milk and can settle your baby's digestion, but should not be used if you are epileptic. Avoid clary sage before sleep, as it causes vivid dreams, and do not use it if you have been drinking alcohol.

BREAST, LUMPS

A breast lump is common during pregnancy and even more frequent during breastfeeding. Your greatest concern may be cancer, but it occurs in just 3:10,000 pregnancies and only 3% of breast cancers are associated with pregnancy or lactation. A painful lump is more likely to be caused by a blocked milk duct. This has a sharply defined edge and is easily diagnosed: either the swelling can be massaged away or an ultrasound scan detects milk inside the lump. Some women have extra accessory breast tissue in their armpit, called the axilla, which swells during pregnancy and breastfeeding. It is normal breast tissue and the swelling diminishes with time, usually within 2 weeks. Ask your doctor to examine lumps and if necessary arrange an ultrasound scan. The ultrasound is identical to the one used to scan your baby and it is safe.

BREAST, NIPPLES, CRACKED

Most women experience tenderness in their nipples at some time during breastfeeding. If your baby does not latch on properly and sucks on the nipple instead of the areola, she will put too much pressure on the nipple. Over time this may lead to cracking, causing sharp, piercing pain during every feed. Cracked nipples are more common in women with a fair or sensitive skin, but seldom occur when latching on and positioning are good.

What happens

Excessive sucking directly on the nipple causes an effect somewhat like a vacuum and draws blood to the nipple. The pressure of sucking and blood beneath the skin can cause small cracks. While you are breastfeeding, your nipple skin is naturally soft but if it remains wet continuously the cracks will not heal well. Infection on the skin, particularly with CANDIDA (thrush), also prevents healing.

Action plan

Cracked nipples usually heal well with care. The cracks will not cause your baby harm, even though some blood may show up in her stools (p.408). Cracked nipples are much more common with a first baby, so don't be put off breastfeeding for your second.

Feeding technique

- Continue feeding. If you reduce feeds because of the pain, your milk may build up, causing BREAST ENGORGEMENT.
- Latching on well (p.188) optimises the flow of milk so feeds may be shorter and more widely spaced, giving your nipples longer to recover between feeds. It will also take the pressure off the skin of the nipple. The soreness at the start of the feed will lessen as your milk flows.
- Alternate breasts and change your baby's position for each feed. This helps to reduce pressure on any one part of the nipple and gives cracks time to heal.
- If your breast still feels full when your baby has finished feeding, express some milk as a precaution against engorgement.

Nipple care

It is important to treat the cracks because they are a route for infection and increase the risk of mastitis.

- Expose your breasts to air for a few minutes between feeds and wear a well-fitting bra of natural cotton fibres. Avoid waterproof breast pads or bras that keep your skin wet. Protect your nipples from being rubbed by your clothing and wash with water only. Your nipple skin is naturally protected and lubricated.
- Massage your nipple skin gently for a few minutes after a feed with a small amount of natural oil, and then expose your nipples to air. A good mix is 90% almond with 10% wheat germ, plus 2–3 drops of calendula tincture in a 60 ml (2 fl oz) bottle. Use a small amount so your nipple does not become too moist. You might prefer calendula or vitamin E cream. Sometimes expressed milk applied to the nipple after a feed and left to dry is very soothing.
- The cold cabbage leaf remedy recommended for breast engorgement is also useful for soothing painful nipples. Do not leave on for longer than 20 minutes or the skin will soften.

- Nipple shields can be helpful but only as a temporary solution until the cracks heal. They are available from chemists or your midwife may supply them.
- If soreness persists or your nipples suddenly become red after months of feeding or antibiotic treatment, you may have candida. Check your baby's tongue and her nappy area for signs. Yeast organisms are sensitive to sunlight, so expose your bra and breasts to the sun and continue nipple care. Thrush can be treated with fungicidal cream or tablets or homeopathy. If it resists standard treatments ask your doctor for a 0.25% solution of gentian violet to apply twice a day for 3 days. It is effective, but messy.

Homeopathy

Take the most indicated remedy (6c) 3–4 times a day for up to 1 week and then reassess. Use *Castor Equi* if your nipples are cracked, sore and extremely sensitive and you cannot bear to have anything near them; *Graphites* if your nipples are cracked and blistered; *Silica* if the cracks bleed and you have burning pains while feeding. You can also use a soothing application of 10 drops *Hypercal* tincture diluted in 250 ml (½ pint) cooled boiled water. Then dry your nipples and apply calendula cream or Bach Flower Rescue Remedy cream.

BREAST, NIPPLES, INVERTED & FLAT

If your nipples are flat or inverted, it may be difficult for your baby to latch on properly. If your breasts are also engorged, your nipples may become flatter. It is very rare for inverted nipples to prevent feeding – begin in pregnancy to help them to evert.

Action plan

You will need to pay extra close attention to your position and how your baby latches on (p.188) and get hands-on help from your midwife or breastfeeding counsellor.
- Hold your breast with your fingers underneath and thumb on top. Press and push back toward your chest and then press your fingers and thumb together lightly to elongate the areola and encourage your nipple to protrude. Gently massaging your areola to draw the nipple out may help – start delicately while your nipple skin gets used to it. You can begin, gently, in pregnancy.
- Breast pump manufacturers sell a small plastic thimble-sized device that fits over the nipple, can be worn under a bra, and has a small suction balloon to draw out the nipple. It needs to be attached for 10 minutes before a feed and can be reused: you need to sterilise it between feeds. You can also use it in pregnancy. Alternatively, try using a breast pump, which may draw out your nipples before feeding.
- Breast shells designed for flat or inverted nipples can be worn for 30 minutes before a feed – they have a rounded dome cover and fit inside your bra. They are plastic with a hole through which the nipple can protrude. You will need to wash the shells between feeds to guard against infection. You can begin to wear these in pregnancy.

BREATH HOLDING

See also BREATHING DIFFICULTIES: BABY

A baby usually holds her breath because she is in pain from reflux (p.561), which can be easily treated. Another cause may be anger or fear. Breath holding is more common after 6 months and 20% of children are affected.

What happens

A breath-holding episode lasts a few seconds but this can feel like a lifetime for an adult who is watching. Your baby will fail to breathe in and her face will go red or blue. She may begin to breathe again normally, or faint: fainting is a safety mechanism that relaxes the body and enables normal breathing to restart. While unconscious, even for a few seconds, she may go stiff and twitch. This is a small FIT, but so short there is no likelihood of brain damage. Your baby will soon be bright and alert, whereas after a more serious fit, she is likely to be sleepy.

Action plan
Medical care
- Ask your doctor if painful reflux may be the cause. This can be treated. He may investigate rare causes, such as an epigastric HERNIA.
- If your baby appears white or pale or holds her breath 5–10 times a day, it is probably a harmless habit, but your doctor needs to exclude fits or a HEART rhythm problem.
- A longer period without breathing could be apnoea (p.418) with a risk of sudden infant death syndrome (p.510) and needs to be investigated.

Coping with, and preventing, breath holding
- Think about possible triggers and avoid where possible. Try to distract your baby during angry crying episodes.
- While your baby holds her breath, remain calm. If you shout or panic, this could increase her tension. Let other carers know what to do.
- If breath holding is identified as attention-seeking behaviour, reassure your baby after each event. You may consider why your baby wants attention and a parenting class or your health visitor may offer advice and support.

Homeopathy

Give the remedy that suits in a soft 30c tablet as soon as possible, and then 5 minutes later. Use *Aconite* if there has been an emotional shock or your baby has been afraid; *Arnica* if there has been injury or physical trauma; *Chamomilla* after a temper tantrum, anger or rage.

BREATHING DIFFICULTIES: BABY

See also BREATH HOLDING; FOETAL DISTRESS & ASPHYXIA

Breathing difficulties in the newborn

Most babies establish regular breathing within a few minutes of birth, during which time there is a back-up supply of oxygen via the umbilical cord. A small percentage – around 2%

– have difficulty breathing. This is known as asphyxia and in rare instances it results in breathing difficulties beyond the first few minutes. A rarer cause of breathing difficulties that gives a baby a blue appearance is a congenital HEART condition.

Asphyxia at birth
Foetal distress in labour may lead to asphyxia at birth. This usually resolves in the first few minutes but a small number of babies require resuscitation and help with breathing and medication, correcting any disturbance in the acid levels of the blood.

Transient tachypnoea of the newborn (TTN)
Rapid breathing and grunting may indicate TTN, which affects up to 5:100 healthy term babies, and is 20 times more common in babies born by CAESAREAN SECTION or induced before term (p.497). In the uterus a baby's lungs contain liquid produced by the cells lining her airway. Ordinarily this fluid is absorbed into the circulation once breathing begins. TTN is caused by a delay in absorption that inhibits airflow into the lungs, and a baby needs to breathe fast to overcome the resistance. This is rarely serious but is a common cause for transfer to a SPECIAL CARE BABY UNIT. The fluid is absorbed into the circulation, usually within a few hours, and the breathing difficulty resolves. A baby may need ventilator support for 1–2 days.

Respiratory distress syndrome (RDS)
During the last 6–10 weeks of pregnancy a baby's lungs produce surfactant, a molecule that lowers the surface tension in the airways and allows the lungs to expand in air. If this surfactant is absent, usually when birth is PREMATURE but occasionally following asphyxia or if a full-term baby's mother has DIABETES, there will be difficulty breathing because the air sacs in the lungs are unable to expand: this is respiratory distress syndrome. RDS requires intensive care that may involve instillation of surfactant into the lungs as part of breathing support. A baby may only require additional oxygen in an incubator, but with severe RDS artificial ventilation is needed. A tube is placed into the windpipe (trachea) and a ventilator blows oxygen into the lungs in a closely monitored procedure. Rarely, if ventilation is needed for more than 28 days, it may lead to a long-term lung disorder and the baby may need oxygen administration at home.

Infection
Among premature babies or babies born after premature rupture of the membranes (p.501) there is a chance that infection from the mother's vagina may travel into the uterus and reach the lungs as the baby performs breathing movements. In the rare case that a baby is infected with the STREP B or CHLAMYDIA bacteria before birth, there is a chance pneumonia (p.441) may develop. This is treated by intensive intravenous antibiotics and breathing support until the infection is cured.

Breathing difficulties in the older baby
Breathing difficulties that may occur later in a baby's life give one of two symptoms – noisy or difficult breathing or cessation of breathing.

Noisy breathing
Noisy breathing, or stridor, is often due to a COUGH resulting from chest infection or ASTHMA. It may also be due to reflux (p.561). In a small number of cases a **laryngomalacia** (floppy larynx) may lead to high-pitched breathing and sometimes grunting, beginning several weeks after birth. It is usually harmless and occurs in about 10% of otherwise healthy children, and passes by 18–24 months of age. The floppiness is caused by an excess flexibility in the cartilage rings, which keep your baby's airway open. In up to 1% of cases it interferes with feeding, leading to failure to thrive (p.563), and less commonly it leads to a breathing difficulty or apnoea (below). Very rarely, noisy breathing reveals a heart condition.

When breathing stops: apnoea and ALTE
If your baby stops breathing – apnoea – you will naturally be concerned and may panic. Apnoea occurs when there is a pause longer than 20 seconds between breaths (irregular breathing alone is quite common between birth and 3 months, but pauses of more than 20 seconds are unusual). Irregular breathing wiht pauses of less than 20 seconds are noticed more during sleep or with a chest infection. It occurs more often among premature babies. In rare cases, apnoea may be a symptom of an underlying cause, such as whooping cough (p.441) or FITS. It may also be confused with breath holding.

If apnoea is prolonged, although terrifying, this will not result in your baby dying. As the oxygen levels in the brain fall she will faint. This will cause her to relax, and her airway will relax too so she can breath normally again. This apparently life-threatening event (ALTE) may be linked with a colour change (to blue, white or perhaps very red in the face) and has previously been called 'near-miss SIDS', but this is not accurate because there is no association with sudden infant death syndrome (p.510). Between 1 and 6% of babies are reported to have ALTE. You need to report such an event.

Action plan
Noisy breathing
You need to seek urgent medical attention if your baby is breathing unusually noisily, coughing or wheezing, seems short of breath and particularly if her skin has a blue tint. There is a small chance your baby may have inhaled a small object and be choking (p.384) or have an infection or ASTHMA.

Your baby may be examined by a doctor listening to her breathing and looking at her larynx. It is likely that the cause is not serious, but your baby may be given further tests:

- A flexible fibre-optic telescope may be placed in the nose or a barium swallow x-ray is used to detect stomach reflux. Reflux on to the vocal cords accounts for about 75% of noisy breathing cases, and can be treated with medication.
- A chest x-ray to inspect her heart and lungs as well as an echocardiogram or ECG heart test or an infection culture test may help. If a fit is suspected, medication can be given.

Apnoea and ALTE
If your baby stops breathing or has difficulties, first assist her breathing using the resuscitation ABC (p.383). Call for help.
- Every baby who has ALTE is investigated fully and admitted to hospital where breathing can be closely

observed. The medical team will want to ensure there is no immediate danger, give your baby essential care, and look for underlying causes.

- She will be monitored for low blood oxygen levels (to avoid reduced oxygen to the brain) and tested for ANAEMIA and infections, including whooping cough. Tests will also check for heart abnormalities and reflux. Your baby will have follow-up assessments and treatment for underlying cause.
- Most babies with ALTE have no breathing difficulties in the future, but you will be advised on action if it happens again. You will be shocked and may be anxious that it will happen again. Your doctor or health visitor can reassure you.

BREATHLESSNESS: MOTHER

See also ASTHMA: MOTHER

Approximately 50% of pregnant women feel breathless before Week 20 and even more by Week 40. Usually this accompanies physical exertion.

What happens
If you are fit and have good cardiac function, the increased demands on your heart may pass unnoticed. Sometimes, if you have ANAEMIA, you may feel breathless. Lying on your back or sitting or standing for a long time may make it worse because this reduces the return of blood to the heart; this might also make your BLOOD PRESSURE fall, giving a feeling of faintness. If you are anxious, you may be unaware that you are taking fast, shallow breaths (hyperventilating).

Breathlessness is usually nothing to worry about, but when it is sudden, severe or prolonged, or happens when you are relaxing, it may indicate anaemia (low red blood-cell count), or, rarely, a HEART or lung problem. It may be due to asthma or a chest infection (p.442), which will also cause coughing. On rare occasions a blood clot from a deep vein thrombosis (p.560) in the leg may travel to the lungs, causing a pulmonary embolus. The sudden onset of breathlessness with no apparent cause may be the first sign of this life-threatening condition, particularly if associated with chest pain and calf pain, although it can occur without pain. It needs urgent treatment.

Action plan
If there is an underlying physical cause for breathlessness, you need to treat it. Otherwise, simple steps may help and when pregnancy is over, breathlessness will no longer be an issue.

Medical care
If breathlessness comes on suddenly or is severe consult your doctor **urgently**. If you have leg or chest pain, call an ambulance.

Diet and lifestyle
- Multivitamin and mineral supplements and good nutrition are generally helpful and help to reduce anaemia.
- A graduated exercise programme will help, provided your heart and lungs are normal. Ask your doctor or a fitness trainer to advise you.

- Try altering posture by lying on your side and avoiding sitting and standing still for prolonged periods. Tightening and releasing your calf and leg muscles or your buttocks 10 or 15 times will help to pump blood to your heart.
- If you are anxious or have persistent emotional problems (p.459), seek support to reduce hyperventilation. Visualisation (p.370) may help you relax and yoga (p.346) 'makes room' for your lungs to expand.

Homeopathy
Take a remedy (30c) 3–4 times a day for up to 1 week and then reassess the situation. Use *Aconite* if breathlessness is accompanied by fear and palpitations, often worse at night; *Arsenicum* if you feel weak yet restless, agitated and worried, are pale and perhaps feel worse around midnight; *Ipecac* when you also feel nauseous, chilly on the outside yet warm inside and worse after eating and at night.

BREECH BIRTH
See LABOUR, BREECH BIRTH

CAESAREAN SECTION

After episiotomy caesarean section is the most common operation performed on women. In the UK over 20% of babies are born by caesarean. Elsewhere the figure can reach 40%.

The need may become apparent during pregnancy (planned caesarean) or in labour (emergency), or it may be your choice (elective). A 'C-section' is a major operation that carries risks of post-operative complications. This book encourages you to be involved actively in your antenatal health and to maintain your energy during labour to increase your chances of delivering vaginally. Many caesareans, however, are necessary and can save the life of mother or baby or significantly reduce trauma that may occur in a vaginal birth: not all caesareans can or should be avoided.

Many women do not expect a caesarean and are upset and shocked by the reality. It is a good idea to discuss it so you and your partner will be better prepared should you need the operation. You might be able to visit the operating theatre and talk to an anaesthetist as well as to your obstetrician and midwife. You could ask about your hospital's rate of caesareans; type of anaesthetic used; whether your partner could stay with you; and postnatal care, including how soon you will be encouraged to feed your baby after birth, pain-relief options and how long you may stay in hospital.

Planned caesarean section
The most common conditions prompting a planned caesarean:
- Your baby is too big to pass through your pelvis (p.493).
- Your baby is small for dates (p.498) or at high risk of FOETAL DISTRESS & ASPHYXIA, and it is safer to be born than to remain in the womb.
- Your baby is in an awkward position (p.493) or is breech (p.492). Or you have triplets, or TWINS where the position of one baby is not optimal.

- Your placenta is low lying (PLACENTA PRAEVIA).
- You have very high BLOOD PRESSURE with severe pre-eclampsia.

Except where it is safer to deliver sooner, the operation is usually set for Weeks 38–39 to ensure that your baby is mature and to reduce the risks associated with PREMATURE BIRTH. If labour begins spontaneously before this date, the operation can be done in early labour. Some women are relieved that a decision has been taken in the interests of safety, others are disappointed, angry or feel they are somehow to blame. These are all natural reactions. It may help to remember that most of the events necessitating a caesarean are not in your control but governed by your baby.

Emergency caesarean section

As an emergency, the decision to operate is often taken quickly and events may seem out of your control. A short explanation of the reasons is usually easy to give, even in an acute emergency, and a longer discussion may be possible. After birth you may need to talk at length with your doctor and/or midwife. While an emergency caesarean may be performed to save you from harm, most often it is essential because your baby will be safer.

An emergency caesarean section may be needed after labour has started:

- When there is slow progress in labour (p.502).
- If your baby moves into an awkward position.
- Where there is foetal distress or abnormal BLEEDING.
- If the UMBILICAL CORD is compressed or prolapsed.
- When forceps or ventouse (p.496) assistance fails.
- With high blood pressure that does not respond to drugs.

Elective caesarean section

Reasons for choosing a caesarean are personal and diverse. The main issue is to avoid labour and vaginal delivery. For some women this may be motivated by a deep-seated fear of pain, perhaps after a previous traumatic labour. Some doubt their physical ability or worry about their baby. Others shy away from vaginal birth because they are scarred by BATTERING OR ABUSE. Knowing there is no need to give birth vaginally may enhance your attitude to pregnancy. If you are afraid of giving birth but not certain that you want a caesarean, your midwife or obstetrician may help you to decide. If you can, talk with other women who have delivered vaginally or by caesarean section.

Most health-care professionals prefer to avoid the operation except where it is needed to deliver a baby safely. This is because it carries higher risks for the mother, is more costly than a vaginal birth and has a longer recovery period. The rights and wrongs are not clear-cut and opinions alter. For some doctors, fear of litigation plays a part: they are rarely sued for performing unnecessary caesareans but are sometimes sued for not doing a caesarean section in time.

Many epidemiologists believe that caesarean section is becoming a preventive plastic surgery operation to maintain sexual attraction as an abdominal scar hidden below the bikini hairline is preferable to a vaginal incision. VAGINAL PROLAPSE and incontinence are less common after a caesarean section, but these by no means follow all vaginal births.

What happens

Your baby is born via your abdomen, usually within 5–10 minutes of the first incision being made. You may hold him while your abdomen is stitched.

Preparation for operation

Standard pre-operative precautions include avoiding food and drink for several hours to minimise any vomiting as a result of anaesthesia. You will be given a tablet or liquid to neutralise your stomach's acid contents. Your abdomen will be shaved at the hairline to pubis level. It is not necessary to remove all the pubic hair.

One dose of the homeopathic remedy *Aconite* (200c) is good if you are afraid or anxious and is useful for your birth partner too. If you are having an epidural, a dose of *Hypericum* (200c) is helpful. If your caesarean is planned, you could have a bath or a massage before going to hospital or in hospital while you wait, scented with oils of neroli (peaceful), jasmine (for confidence) or sandalwood (which sedates).

Into the theatre

You and your partner, if he is with you, will probably feel a mixture of excitement and anxiety. Operating theatres can be daunting. The brightly lit room, sterile equipment and medical staff behind masks and gowns can be unsettling, particularly in an emergency when you are nervous about your baby's safe arrival. You will be escorted to the theatre by a midwife and she will stay with you throughout the operation and talk you through each stage. The anaesthetist will be there on your arrival and will stay by your side until you are on your way back to the postnatal ward.

Once in the theatre you will be asked to sign a consent form. Only if the caesarean section is an acute emergency, which is rare, will your partner be asked to leave. He may be welcomed back when the emergency is under control and the operation is in progress.

Anaesthesia

Most hospitals give an epidural (p.159). If you are already in labour, this offers relief from contractions, and during the operation acts as an anaesthetic so you cannot feel any pain, although you may still feel touch and pressure. It will not send you to sleep, so you can greet your baby at birth, and it can be left in place to give pain relief following the operation. Alternatively, your doctor may choose to administer a spinal anaesthetic (p.160): this takes effect more quickly, and you will be awake. It wears off after 4–6 hours. Usually in an emergency a general anaesthetic is given, although it may also be used if you request it. With a general anaesthetic you would wake up around 30 minutes after the end of the operation and by 60 minutes be ready to hold your baby.

After the anaesthetic has been given, a catheter tube is inserted into your urethra to drain urine from your bladder and reduce the risk of bladder injury during surgery. It is usually pain free. It will remain in place for 12–24 hours following the birth. An intravenous drip is inserted into your arm and will remain until you are drinking normally, usually within 12 hours. The drip is useful should you need extra fluids or medicines.

The operation

In theatre you will not be able to see the operation as your abdomen is screened by drapes. Your partner may choose to watch or to remain close to your face. Your abdominal skin will be disinfected and the obstetrician will make a neat incision along the bikini line in a process that opens the abdomen and gently separates, but does not cut, the abdominal muscles, and exposes the uterus. The incision to open the muscular wall of the uterus is horizontal and in the lower segment of the uterus: this results in a stronger scar that is less likely to break in a subsequent labour. The membranes of the amniotic sac surrounding your baby are then cut and the obstetrician will carefully deliver your baby. Blood loss is kept low, but the average loss is greater than the average lost during vaginal birth.

As your baby is delivered, the anaesthetist may need to push on your abdomen to help the birth – what you feel will probably be within an acceptable comfort zone: if not, the anaesthetist can administer an intravenous sedative. In very rare instances a general anaesthetic may be needed. Sometimes forceps are placed on a baby's head to assist with the delivery. Once your baby has been delivered, the umbilical cord will be clamped and cut and he will be checked quickly by the midwife or paediatrician. If he needs any help with breathing (p.417), oxygen will be given.

Then it will be time for you to hold your baby. If you don't feel up to it, your partner or midwife can hold him. While you are meeting your baby for the first time, the obstetrician delivers the placenta, checks your uterus and begins to stitch the incision. Most hospitals urge mothers to establish contact with their baby as soon as possible and a midwife will probably guide you if you wish to breastfeed. If the operation has come as a surprise, this is a perfect opportunity for focusing on the positive aspects of the birth.

Stitching the uterus and abdominal wall can take up to 30 minutes as there are seven separate layers to be sutured. The time and care is worthwhile, as it guards against scar rupture in future pregnancies. Modern suture material is very strong, and dissolves naturally within 6 weeks, so there is no risk of the wound being disrupted. The only suture you will be able to see is the final line on the skin surface; the stitches here may be of the dissolving type or may need to be removed about 5 days following delivery (a quick and painless procedure).

Common concerns

You may have a number of questions about the risks. It is reassuring to know you are not alone: almost everyone is afraid of surgery. Modern obstetric practice makes operating a much safer procedure than it was in the past. Complications are rare but there are hazards. The recovery period is generally longer than after a vaginal birth.

Risks and concerns for the mother

- Infection of the wound: You will be given antibiotics to guard against this.
- An unsightly scar: The scar will be in your pubic hair and you can wear a bikini later.
- Deep vein thrombosis (p.560): Blood clot and pulmonary embolism (blood clot in the lung) risk is reduced if you wear

elastic stockings and walk around soon. If you have had a blood clot before, you may be given anticoagulant drugs.

- Anaesthetic complications: The safest anaesthetic is an epidural. During a general anaesthetic the main risk is inhalation of acid stomach juices. Restricting food and administering antacids prior to surgery largely prevents this, and you will be closely monitored.
- Excess bleeding: This may occur during the operation if any of the large blood vessels supplying the uterus are severed. Sometimes a BLOOD TRANSFUSION may be needed but severe bleeding is rare.
- Bladder or bowel injury: This is extremely rare. The bladder is gently pushed down before the uterus is opened, and the bowel is also protected.
- Late abdominal adhesions: Adhesions are scar tissue that may involve the bowel, bladder or the uterus and develop in a minority of women. They may cause abdominal pain and occasionally lead to further operations. The wound may also be painful for many weeks after the operation as the muscle layers knit together.
- Effect on breastfeeding: Where there is good support, the rate of breastfeeding is as high as after a vaginal birth. You may want to begin in the operating room.

Risks for the baby

A caesarean section is often done to reduce risks of damage when there may be risk of trauma or foetal distress with a reduced oxygen supply. Some obstetricians believe that hormones released during a vaginal birth may help a baby adapt to breathing in air. Babies born by caesarean are more likely to have BREATHING DIFFICULTIES, but this applies only to a minority, unless the baby is premature. If the caesarean has been carried out under a general anaesthetic, the baby may be sleepy but is likely to recover well within a few hours. PREMATURE BIRTH presents the greatest risk.

Some psychologists believe that a caesarean may affect a baby emotionally and hamper the relationship between mother and baby. These hypotheses are theoretical: babies' brains are able to adapt and those born by caesarean section find little difficulty getting used to life outside the womb. Mother and baby are usually united at delivery and are able to stay together unless the baby requires medical attention. Love hormones (p.37) flow during feeding, and many parents feel strongly bonded with their baby even before the birth.

Action plan for recovery

As with any major operation, you will take time to recover physically. You will also go through the normal after-effects of giving birth vaginally (p.224). Like any new mother, you may experience the blues. The emotional effect of the operation may not be fully apparent for some months. If you feel well supported, getting back to normal will be easier.

Many women are virtually pain-free in a few days because the horizontal stitch line follows the natural 'bikini' line. It is common, however, to feel sore on one or other side of the wound for several weeks. This arises from the stitches at the edge of the incision in the sheath that encloses the muscles of the abdominal wall. Moving and walking realigns the cut sheath and can help to diminish the pain.

Medical care

Pain and discomfort are inevitable and are sharpest over the first few days. Your anaesthetist may leave an epidural in place for up to 24 hours so you can have top-ups, or you may be given pain killing injections and long-acting suppositories. Let the midwives know when you feel uncomfortable so you can be relieved quickly and effectively. As your discomfort reduces you can move on to milder painkillers.

Very rarely, a nerve may be trapped in the suture line, giving ongoing discomfort. Injecting the area with a local anaesthetic solution can numb the nerve. Sometimes, pain in the lower back (p.519) may result from the epidural. Cranial osteopathy (p.376) is useful to alleviate post-operative pain.

Homeopathy and aromatherapy

Post-operatively, these four remedies are invaluable, each taken in 200c potency, 4 times a day for 3 days, then 3 times a day for 4 days. *Arnica* is the main remedy for trauma – it reduces swelling, encourages healing, particularly at the site of the placenta, and controls bleeding. Use *Hypericum* for nerve trauma and after an epidural; *Bellis Perennis* to assist the healing of deep tissue and to help with soreness; *Calendula* to speed up the healing of the scar internally and externally. If you feel emotionally raw, which is often the case if the caesarean was an emergency, take *Staphysagria* (200c) every 2 hours for the 8 hours following delivery. *Hypercal* tincture (10–15 drops in the bath) promotes healing, and if bowel movements are a struggle, take *Nux Vomica* (30c) 3 times a day for 2 days (for other remedies, *see* CONSTIPATION).

Aromatherapy oils in a bath or a massage (perhaps on your feet, hands or face) that can help include neroli, camomile, sandalwood and lavender for relaxation. If you feel angry, guilty or upset, try frankincense, ylang ylang or rose.

Movement and exercise

Within 12 hours the midwives will support you as you sit up, get out of bed and take your first steps. If you feel faint or dizzy, eat something light to boost your blood sugar and get up slowly with help. Be reassured that the sutures are very strong and will not break.

Most women sit unaided within 48 hours. As soon as you feel well enough, walk around. This eases breathing, improves healing and reduces the risk of deep vein thrombosis, provided you also wear elastic stockings until you are completely mobile. You need your energy for feeding so while moving lifts your spirits, doing too much is exhausting.

You can safely begin gentle postnatal yoga stretches (p.354) and pelvic floor exercises (p.98) within 3–4 days but intensive aerobic exercises is best delayed for 10 weeks. You could start walking, swimming or using an exercise cycle within 1–3 weeks, beginning with 5–10 minutes, and gradually increasing to 20–30 minutes over 4 weeks. Take care and you'll have no problems using most gym machines and free weights. Delay abdominal exercises and crunches (p.362) for 6–10 weeks.

Caring for your abdomen, the wound and scar

The dressing on your wound will probably be removed the day after the operation. It's a good idea to take a daily bath or shower as long as you dry the wound well. If your skin becomes red or the wound remains very tender, there may be an infection in the subcutaneous tissues. You will be given antibiotics as a preventative measure but if an infection develops a further course may be needed. Vitamin E oil, antioxidants and vitamin and mineral supplements can promote healing and improve skin condition.

Urine and bowels

The catheter is removed within 24 hours, as soon as you are mobile. You may not have eaten in labour and for 12 or more hours after the operation so your bowels will be relatively empty. When you do begin to eat, bowel movements usually return within 2 or 3 days but constipation is common and the analgesics tend to increase it.

Feeding your baby and day-to-day care

Breastfeeding can be established soon after birth. Your midwife will help you find a comfortable position and your partner or another adult can help you if you still need support once you are home. You may find lying on your side (p.189) easiest at first. In the 1st day or two your partner or a midwife can change your baby's nappy. You will soon be hands-on and provided the changing place is at waist height, this won't put pressure on your wound. Bending down to floor level comfortably will take at least a week or longer.

Your emotions

If you have anticipated a caesarean you will have had a chance to go over your feelings. Even so, you may become weepy and confused as your hormones change, and unexpected feelings may surface. If the operation follows a long labour or has been an emergency, you may feel numb. Some parents ask why the operation was not done sooner; others feel the decision was too quick and a vaginal birth might have been possible.

Initially, most parents feel joy and relief at having a wonderful baby, and for many this remains the dominant feeling. Sometimes, there is disappointment or a feeling of 'if only'. It is often easy to forget that a caesarean is usually performed for reasons dictated by the baby. You may envy mothers who have given birth vaginally. These feelings are natural, but they may take months to surface. As with any aspect of postnatal blues, it is important to give space to your post-caesarean emotions and seek support (p.459).

Your baby

Depending on the reason for the caesarean, your baby will adjust to being born in the same way as he would have had he been born vaginally. If he had difficulty, he may need time to recover, but this process varies – some babies are resilient and some are sensitive. A paediatrician may need to assist if there was considerable foetal distress or if he has been born early, and close care may continue for some time. Babies mirror their parents and if your baby feels welcomed, you will help him to recover. He will appreciate being held and talked to and may be soothed by massage (p.365) or cranial osteopathy (p.376).

Getting back to normal

The physical effects of anaesthetic, surgical incision and discomfort may bring TIREDNESS AND LOW ENERGY and rocky emotions. Try not to expect too much – as each day passes you will feel stronger. Some women recover quickly but others feel exhausted or depressed for weeks or months, which is no different from the recovery times following a vaginal birth.

- Accept practical help, eat well, rest and spend a lot of time with your baby. Remember your multivitamins, minerals and antioxidants to help healing.
- Listen to your body and rest if you feel tired or sore. Keep doing a little more until you are back to your normal self.
- Get out of bed without discomfort by rolling over with your knees together and turning from your shoulder, then swinging your feet on to the floor and sitting up. You need to avoid strenuous activity, including housework and vacuuming, for 6 weeks.
- Check with your doctor when it is safe for you to drive a car, and check cover with your insurance company. It is not necessary to wait for 6 weeks as above.
- You can make love without interfering with healing as soon as you feel comfortable.
- Take care how you lift your baby, your shopping bags and laundry, etc., by bending your knees as you lift.

Future pregnancies

The old saying 'once a caesarean always a caesarean' no longer applies. Women are often afraid to give birth vaginally after a caesarean in case the uterus scar ruptures but rupture is extremely uncommon. Very rarely, for technical reasons, the incision may be in the upper part of the uterus, where it may be weak and a repeat caesarean is usually recommended. If the scar does rupture, it may be dangerous for mother and baby.

- If the reason for your previous caesarean does not arise again, you have a good chance of a vaginal delivery, e.g. if your first baby was breech but the second baby is positioned head down. Between 60 and 80% of women give birth vaginally second time round.
- If your first caesarean was planned, the next labour will be equivalent to a first vaginal birth.
- If you went through labour the first time and your cervix did dilate, even if you did not reach full dilation, the length of the second labour is usually shorter.
- In a subsequent labour it is best to avoid Syntocinon to stimulate the uterus. If labour is progressing smoothly and normally then it is usually safe to continue but if it is prolonged a repeat caesarean is the best option.
- If you have had two or more caesareans, you are likely to have a repeat operation. A vaginal birth may be possible if your obstetrician agrees.

Within a few months your wound will have healed completely, so spacing the next baby depends on personal preferences and your financial and social circumstances.

CANDIDA

Candida is a yeast organism that inhabits the mouth, throat, intestines and genito-urinary tract of most humans. It is one of many 'friendly' organisms kept in balance by a properly functioning immune system. In the vagina it exists in balance with lactobacilli bacteria. If the number of friendly bacteria is decreased, which happens when antibiotics are used, or the immune system is weakened or another condition reduces lactobacilli bacteria (e.g. DIABETES or a diet high in sugar), candida transforms from yeast to a fungal form and starts to invade the body. Pregnancy increases susceptibility because the sugar and acidity balance of the vagina alters. Rarely, candida can be passed from person to person, such as through sexual intercourse or to a baby at birth or when breastfeeding.

What happens

In the yeast state, candida is a non-invasive, sugar-fermenting organism. In fungal state it is invasive and gives a candidiasis infection (thrush). Candidiasis affects a wide variety of organ systems, and is particularly common in warm, moist parts of the body, e.g. the vagina (leading to vaginitis), the mouth (oral thrush), the eyes (conjunctivitis), the nappy area (nappy rash) and the rectum. It can also affect the nipples and breast tissue during breastfeeding. In a person with a compromised immune system the internal organs may be infected and severe illness may result. Nearly 75% of women will have had at least one genital 'yeast infection' in their lifetime.

Oral thrush appears as one or more small white plaques in the mouth and on the tongue, which are sometimes painful. Occasionally candida gives shallow painful ulcers in the mouth or vagina. On the insides of the thighs or under the arms or breasts it can produce painful general redness and white pustules. Infection of the genital area (vulvovaginitis) causes red labia and a white itchy discharge often described as 'cheesy'. One of the main symptoms is intense itchiness and burning in the infected areas.

If your baby gets thrush he may develop white pustules in his mouth, which can make feeding uncomfortable, and may get a nappy rash. If he has oral thrush from birth, there is a high chance that he contracted the infection from your vagina during the birth. He may then pass it to your nipples. You both need to be treated at the same time.

Action plan

Thrush can be very unpleasant, yet it can be easily treated, often with a combination of dietary changes and medication. Treatment to reduce itchiness and consequent rubbing reduces the risk of a secondary infection in broken skin.

Medical care

- Diagnosis can be made with a simple visual examination and confirmed with a swab test. In the case of vaginal or urethral thrush, a laboratory test will rule out a URINARY TRACT INFECTION that may also lead to a burning sensation.
- Ask your partner to be tested since candida can be passed through sexual contact.
- If self-help measures fail, your doctor may prescribe an antifungal pessary to be inserted into the vagina, together with ointment for applying to the vulva. Towards the end of pregnancy, treatment reduces the chance of infection being passed to your baby. Antifungal tablets are not recommended during pregnancy.
- Some strains of fungal infection are resistant to standard drugs. Visit your doctor to receive correct treatment. A swab

test can identify the variant: candida galabrata is more drug-resistant than candida albicans. Gentian violet solution is messy but can cure resistant thrush.

- For oral thrush a mouth rinse with a dilute hydrogen peroxide solution can be effective for adults (beware of burning from concentrated solutions). Oral thrush in a baby may respond quickly to homeopathy or antibiotics.

Lifestyle and diet

- Maintain cleanliness, especially after using the toilet. Always wipe from front to back as organisms from the bowel can be easily transferred to the vagina.
- Candida loves warmth and moisture. Wear loose cotton underwear, which allows air to circulate.
- Reduce scented toiletries, which may irritate. You may be allergic to some.
- Candida thrives on sugar and loves an acidic environment. Reduce sugary foods – including fruit juices and colas – and refined carbohydrates in your diet (p.337). Try to cut out food that is fermented and contains yeast, including bread, wine and beer. Eat whole foods with plenty of immune-boosting, fungi-busting garlic, onions and olive oil. Kale, turnip and cabbage may inhibit fungal growth. Make sure you are getting enough vitamins A, B complex and C as well as the minerals zinc, iron and magnesium.
- You could take pro-biotics in the form of acidophilus and bifidobacteria. These reduce the chances of opportunistic fungi taking hold again, particularly if taking antibiotics is unavoidable. Live yoghurt contains lactobacillus acidophilus cultures and these pro-biotics destroy the fungus and create a natural barrier to infection. Eating 145 ml (5 fl oz) per day can dramatically reduce the chance of a vaginal or bowel thrush infection. Pro-biotic tablets and pessaries with lactobacillus are alternatives.
- Inserting yoghurt into the vagina during pregnancy and straight after birth is not recommended. A month or more after birth you could try inserting a few teaspoons of plain live yoghurt or lactobacillus pessaries before you go to bed until symptoms improve.

Herbal treatments

- Calendula cream or tincture can ease the itching. Echinacea, taken in tea form or as a tincture 2–3 times a day, is good for boosting the immune system of adults but should not be given to a baby. You could also use a dilution of tea tree oil in the bath or, from Week 24, camomile oil.
- After the birth you could insert tea-tree oil pessaries into your vagina: these often work well in combination with pro-biotic pessaries.

Homeopathy

Homeopathic treatment works extremely well for babies. If your baby has candida in the nappy area and the mouth and is being breastfed, it is advisable for both of you to be treated at the same time. Use 30c and give the remedy 2-hourly for 8 hours. Then reassess and give the most suitable remedy 4-hourly for 24 hours, then 3 times a day for a further 2–3 days.

Borax is good if your baby salivates more than usual, his mouth is hot, breastfeeding seems painful, he dislikes downward motion and his nappy area looks red and itchy; *Candida* is made from candida fungus and is very effective; *Natrum Mur* helps oral and rectal thrush, with white patches on the tongue and gums and a persistent desire to feed, serious demeanour and a dislike of fuss or contact; *Merc Sol* is suitable when there is profuse salivation, perhaps smelly breath, the nappy area looks sweaty, moist and yellowish and there are small pimples; *Calc Carb* is indicated when there are white patches on the roof of the mouth, sour possetting, white spots in the nappy area and your baby is lethargic and obstinate. You can also use *Calendula* tincture, 10 drops to 250 ml (½ pint) of water, and bathe your baby with soaked cotton wool at every nappy change. For yourself, use 1 drop of tea tree essential oil and 10 drops of calendula tincture in the bath.

Candidiasis hypersensitivity syndrome

Some health-care professionals acknowledge the existence of candidiasis hypersensitivity syndrome, or chronic candidiasis infection, which is similar in nature to chronic fatigue, and leads to symptoms such as low energy, depression, absent-mindedness, headaches, skin problems and hyperactivity. Some people believe it may also be an underlying cause of persistent constipation, diarrhoea, flatulence, abdominal pain or urinary problems. In some respects, the symptoms resemble complaints that may also be attributed to ALLERGY OR INTOLERANCE. Candidiasis hypersensitivity is not universally accepted.

The basis for the belief is that candida and other related fungi multiply when other friendly bacteria are knocked out. If candida creates yeast and this happens repeatedly, the build-up can weaken the immune system, which may already be weakened if you have been on antibiotics, do not have a nutritious diet, consume high levels of toxins in the form of nicotine, alcohol or drugs, or do not exercise sufficiently. Once the immune system is weakened, you may also be more susceptible to developing adverse reactions to foods and chemicals, and succumb to infections that would normally be easily conquered (e.g. the common cold).

If you believe you have candidiasis hypersensitivity syndrome, it is best to visit a nutritionist, homeopath or other qualified practitioner who will examine your lifestyle, diet and medical history. Holistic attention to lifestyle and diet may increase your general health, immunity and vitality, and may prevent the need for antibiotics in pregnancy and beyond. If it improves your vitality, it is worth it.

CEREBRAL PALSY

Cerebral palsy (CP) is a term used to describe damage to one or more areas of the brain associated with muscle control and body movement that gives rise to a range of abnormalities of movement, muscle tone and posture. About 1:400 children is affected, in some cases only mildly. It is more common in babies born prematurely and in complicated pregnancies, such as those with INTRAUTERINE GROWTH RESTRICTION or infection. The cause is not always clear. Damage usually occurs in the womb long before birth (p.433) but rarely it may occur in labour due to FOETAL DISTRESS & ASPHYXIA. About 6% of babies with CP have had foetal distress during labour or pre-existing difficulties that may have contributed to this distress. In fewer than 2% of babies with CP can the cause be attributed exclusively to asphyxia and sub-optimal care in labour.

What happens

Symptoms of CP depend on the developmental stage of a child because different areas of the brain are brought into use as a child grows. There are three types, depending on the part of the brain affected, and it is common to have a combination of two or more types.

Spastic CP: Causes stiff muscles and a decreased range of movement in the joints. Muscular tightness makes it harder to walk or move. Hemiplegia is where one side of the body is affected; if both legs are affected, the term is diplegia and if both arms and both legs are equally affected, it is quadriplegia. This is the type most usually associated with prematurity.

Athetoid CP: Causes involuntary movements, because the muscles rapidly change from floppy to tense. Speech can be affected because of difficulty controlling the tongue, breath and vocal cords. Hearing difficulties are also common. Athetoid CP can arise as a result of severe foetal distress and asphyxia, and is the type associated with brain damage due to MENINGITIS in the newborn period.

Ataxic CP: Causes poor spatial awareness. Most affected people can walk, but find it hard to balance or judge their position in relation to others. They may also have shaky hand movements and jerky speech. This is the type least likely to be related to factors to do with birth and appears to be a genetically determined CONGENITAL ABNORMALITY.

Associated problems: Other difficulties do not necessarily occur but are more likely with CP. These include: CONSTIPATION, urinary incontinence and SLEEPING DIFFICULTIES, difficulty with speech, chewing and swallowing, epilepsy and visual perception and learning.

Action plan

Diagnosis

It is unusual for CP to be suspected before around 6 months of age, when there is stiffness or failure to reach a milestone, such as head control, rolling or hand control. The only way to detect the condition reliably is by skilled assessment and examination of a baby at 3–6 month intervals from birth to 24 months. Some babies appear stiff from earlier, or show primitive reflexes such as the Moro or stepping reflexes that persist after they would ordinarily pass. A reliable diagnosis can only be made by 12 months. The reason for this apparent late diagnosis is because many parts of the nervous system are developed by this time.

If you worry that your child is not developing as you would expect, you need to arrange to see your doctor or health visitor for a formal developmental assessment.

- You may be referred to a paediatrician and then to a paediatric neurologist (who specialises in brain conditions).
- A full examination of the nervous system looks for abnormality in reflexes and muscle tone and power.
- The doctor may order a series of diagnostic tests that could include: an EEG to record the brain's electrical activity; scans using MRI or positron emission tomography, which can detect the abnormalities in the brain that give rise to the

symptoms; vision and hearing tests; and blood tests to evaluate inherited (genetic) conditions (p.435).

Care

There are no cures for CP, but there are treatments that can minimise the effects and enhance a child's abilities. These may be a mixture of physical therapies, complementary therapies and some drug treatments. Specific treatment for CP will be determined by your child's condition, the type of CP, the tolerance for medications, procedures or therapies and your preference. A multi-disciplinary care team may include: a paediatrician; nurse; social worker; orthopaedic surgeon to treat the muscles and bones; a neurologist; an ophthalmologist to treat eye problems; a dentist, and the rehabilitation team (for physiotherapy, occupational and speech therapy).

- Some children need positioning aids to assist sitting, lying or standing, such as braces or splints.
- Medications may be needed to control fits or improve the tone in the muscles.
- Special social and education care is essential to help a child reach his full potential. Care is usually centred in the home, and supplemented with complementary care from nurses and a rehabilitation team.
- Emotionally and practically, the pressure on parents and any other children is considerable. Many families find the lack of an explanation for CP very difficult to accept. Counselling can be helpful in the short and long term, and practical support allows parents to get some respite.
- Children with more severe forms of the condition often have their needs best met in a special needs educational environment with trained carers.
- Attending group meetings for parents affected by CP could provide a chance to be with people who will encourage you.

CERVICAL EROSION & CANCER

See also BLEEDING, DURING PREGNANCY

During pregnancy the cervix becomes soft and engorged with additional blood vessels. It has an inner lining of delicate mucus-producing cells and as it enlarges the opening may 'pout' and reveal the inner lining. This is known as an erosion, although the cervix is not literally eroded. It affects most women at some time in their life and rarely produces symptoms. Sometimes it produces a clear vaginal discharge. Occasionally erosion leads to bleeding from prominent cervical blood vessels, and this may be stimulated by intercourse, particularly in late pregnancy. The blood is usually bright red and not profuse.

Action plan

If you bleed it is important to report it to your doctor because it may indicate an underlying condition that needs immediate medical attention. When you are seen your cervix may be checked through an internal examination.

If the bleeding is arising from the cervix, you will be advised to refrain from penetrative sex until the bleeding has been absent for at least a week. There is no risk to the pregnancy, nor does the bleeding indicate CERVICAL INCOMPETENCE. If there is an infection it may respond to antibiotics and can be diagnosed on a vaginal swab test.

Cancer of the cervix is extremely rare in pregnancy. When it occurs it may cause intermittent bleeding that continues throughout pregnancy and the changes are visible on an internal check. You may be offered a smear at your first antenatal visit or after delivery to check for pre-cancerous cells.

CERVICAL INCOMPETENCE

The cervix has a valve mechanism that consists of smooth muscle and connective tissue. This keeps it closed during pregnancy although there is room for mucus and fluid to leave the uterus. In the last few weeks it gradually softens so it will open during labour: these changes are called effacement or ripening. Incompetence occurs when the cervix opens early. It happens in around 1% of pregnancies and is believed to be responsible for 25% of 2nd trimester MISCARRIAGES.

What happens
In some women there is no obvious cause. Incompetence may sometimes follow laser treatment or cone biopsy surgery to the cervix for the removal of pre-cancerous cells. It may also result from excessive stretching of the muscle during a termination of pregnancy or a dilation and curettage operation (p.407). Very rarely, it is caused by tearing in a previous vaginal birth. It may be linked with a bicornuate UTERUS.

An incompetent cervix is usually discovered after a miscarriage later than Week 12. A vaginal examination or ultrasound scan in the next pregnancy will show whether the cervix has ripened and dilated early. This process often occurs without pain or vaginal bleeding until the miscarriage begins.

Action plan
When early dilation has been diagnosed, a stitch called a cervical cerclage suture inserted between Weeks 12 and 16 will support the cervix for the remainder of the pregnancy. It is a simple procedure carried out under a light 15-minute general anaesthetic: the stitch around the muscle of the cervix acts like a purse string to hold it closed. After a few days of rest, women usually feel fine and can continue normal activity although it is common to feel menstrual discomfort until the cervix settles into the new shape. You can have sex when the discomfort has stopped.

A vaginal swab will exclude an infection but antibiotics may be needed because the stitch is a foreign substance and organisms may adhere to it. The stitch is left in place until Week 36 when the main risks of early birth are over and it can be removed during a vaginal examination, without an anaesthetic. It is not painful. Usually labour begins 2–4 weeks after removal as the cervix ripens, but it may be sooner.

If labour begins early the stitch needs to be removed by cutting it during a vaginal examination. If you have had a cervical cerclage and have a vaginal discharge with or without blood; leakage of amniotic fluid or contractions of the uterus, go to hospital to ensure you are not in early labour.

CHICKEN POX

Almost all children get chicken pox (**herpes zoster** or **varicella zoster**). Many become infected within 9 months of birth and there are usually no complications. Very few adults get chicken pox, but it presents risks to the unborn babies of the small number of pregnant women who do get it.

What happens
The chicken pox virus is highly infectious and is characterised by an itchy rash that develops into fluid-filled blisters, and a fever that may begin before the rash even appears. The extent of the rash varies. Every part of the body can be involved, including the skin, pain in the stomach if the bowel is involved, joint pain if joints are involved, and headaches if the brain is involved.

Chicken pox is transmitted by droplet spread and symptoms begin to show 10–20 days after this 'incubation period'. Someone with chicken pox is infectious from 48 hours before the blisters appear until they crust over.

Passive immunity (antibodies passed from mother to baby) is effective for about 6 months after birth, but it can be prolonged by the effects of breastfeeding until about 12 months. Some babies under 1 year have a very mild infection with few spots and may have another infection later in childhood.

Action plan
If you have had chicken pox as a child, you need have no concerns if you or your baby are in contact with chicken pox. If you have not had chicken pox, and your baby develops it before he is 21 days old, he needs to be treated for neonatal chicken pox (opposite), which is very rare. After this, if your child develops the infection, the best you can do is to ensure that he is comfortable while the rash is at its worst. Usually this is for 3–5 days.

Medical care
- Try creams, such as calomine, to reduce itching.
- If your baby has a fever, infant paracetamol in doses directed on the bottle will help. This will also reduce headache or joint pains.

General comfort
- Your baby may be very distressed. Do what you can to devote yourself entirely to him.
- He may be more comfortable completely covered up, with socks, mitts and a hat, or he may prefer to be naked. Scratch mitts may reduce scratching, avoiding open sores and infection and, later, scarring.
- Take care of spots in more tender areas – in the nose, eyes, mouth or genitals.
- Some babies like to be bathed in lukewarm water, which takes the edge off the itch.
- Hanging a handful of porridge oats in a pop sock beneath the bath taps as you run the water makes the bath more soothing (almost creamy) and is a tested traditional remedy that works well.

Homeopathy

Before the rash appears and you know he has been in contact with the infection, use *Aconite* if he has a fever and anxiety (probably through the night); *Belladonna* if symptoms appear rapidly, with a very high fever, flushed skin and dilated pupils. Give one of these in 30c, 2–3-hourly for the first 12 hours. Once your baby has a rash, use *Pulsatilla* if he has a low-grade fever, is clingy, weepy and intolerant to heat, has a runny nose and shows no thirst; *Rhus Tox* when the rash is very itchy, making your baby restless, worse at night and if he is worse when cold; *Ant Tart* if the rash looks bluish and is slow to develop into blisters, and is accompanied by a loose rattly cough with lots of phlegm and a coated tongue. Give the most suitable remedy in 30c 4 times a day. You may need to change remedies as the symptoms change. You can also use *Hypercal* tincture in the bath – add 10–15 drops to bath water – or add 10 drops to 250 ml (½ pint) of boiled cooled water and drizzle on to uncomfortable or itchy spots.

Chicken pox in pregnancy

If you have had chicken pox you will be immune and you will give your unborn baby protection. If you have not had the infection as a child there is a small chance that if you catch it when pregnant, your baby may be affected. If you are unsure, a simple blood test can confirm your immune status.

What happens

If you are not immune and come into contact with chicken pox, the infection can produce a severe illness. There is a very small risk (around 2%) of damage to your unborn baby, the most vulnerable time being the first half of pregnancy. Congenital varicella syndrome involves a group of birth defects that can include scars, defects of muscle and bone, malformed and paralysed limbs, a smaller-than-normal head, blindness, fits and mental retardation. If you become infected in the second half of pregnancy, damage to your baby is extremely unlikely. If you develop a rash within 5 days of birth, your child has a 25–50% chance of developing neonatal chicken pox (right).

Action plan

If you are not immune and come into contact with an infected person, you are at risk. Inform your doctor immediately.

- You may be advised to receive varicella zoster immunoglobulin (VZIG) antibody by injection, which helps to prevent chicken pox, or at least lessen its severity. It is not yet known whether VZIG given in pregnancy helps to protect a foetus from infection.
- If you become infected in late pregnancy, delaying the birth for as long as possible reduces the risks to your baby. In the extremely rare event that birth cannot be delayed, your baby will need treatment for neonatal chicken pox.

Shingles in pregnancy

When the chicken pox virus is contracted, it travels from the skin along the nerve paths to the roots of the nerves where it lies dormant. Occasionally, the virus may be reactivated, and travel via the nerve paths to the skin, developing blisters along the way. The illness – shingles – is often very painful. The triggers for reactivation are not known, but contact with chicken pox infection is not a cause. If you have shingles, you can pass the virus for chicken pox to someone who is not yet immune. Your baby is safe because you and therefore your baby already have antibodies to the virus.

Neonatal chicken pox

Babies born to mothers who have chicken pox 5 days or sooner before birth or within 21 days of delivery are at risk of being born with chicken pox or developing severe chicken pox with complications. This 'neonatal chicken pox' is extremely rare as adults only account for 5% of all these infections, and few of these adults are pregnant women. If a baby is at risk, he will be given VZIG antibody by injection at birth, which usually reduces the severity of infection. If necessary, antiviral medicine can help alleviate symptoms.

CHILD PROTECTION & ABUSE

The majority of children are very much wanted and loved. A minority, however, suffer from abuse. The risk of physical abuse to children is highest below the age of 2 years, and even tiny babies may be victims. Emotional abuse, often through neglect, is also significant. Abuse is a very sensitive subject. For everyone involved a great deal of support is needed. Sometimes, if support is available soon enough, abusive behaviour can be avoided and close and loving relationships formed in its place.

Some parents find the job of caring for a child unbearably stressful, particularly if there are other demands, perhaps with finance, housing or relationship or addiction problems. A baby may also be seen as a threat, taking up the lion's share of love or infringing on intimacy – some men feel this strongly when their baby is breastfeeding. A woman can be upset by her baby's dependence on her body. For both parents, having a baby may bring intense emotions (p.300) to the surface and can lead to anxiety and/or depression. In some cases issues that have been hidden emerge, and parents are surprised when they regress into feelings that were part of their infancy. These can be shocking and upsetting if they were forgotten. With support many people who suffered as children can be helped to enjoy parenthood and may find it heals their own traumas.

A parent's emotional state contributes to his or her reaction to the everyday demands of nurturing and caring for a baby. When feelings are powerful or overwhelming a parent may react by neglecting his or her child, or may physically take out anger on him. Unfortunately patterns of behaviour tend to be repeated, sometimes in spite of a conscious desire to change. What has happened in your life before conception exerts a profound influence on your feelings about your baby.

What happens

Abuse may take a number of forms. The risk of abuse rises if there is a stepfather or boyfriend who is not related to the baby. Abuse through neglect rises when the biological father is not around. Father–child bonding is valuable: fathers are five times less likely to abuse if they are included in the early life of their babies in a hands-on way from birth.

Emotional abuse and rejection

It is normal to feel anxious or ambivalent in the face of a huge life change. There are many reasons for a parent to feel reluctant to accept pregnancy and babycare. If there is a strong resistance to the growing baby, parents may reinforce destructive behaviour – continuing to smoke or take drugs, for instance. Domestic violence is very prevalent within such couples. When this happens in pregnancy, the baby is aware of shouting, punches will vibrate into the womb, and he can sense the nervousness and fear the mother feels as her hormones change. In this situation the sense of being unsafe can become part of every day life in the womb (babies have an emotional life and can feel fear). Some unborn babies react by becoming withdrawn (i.e. less active), others have more resilience and others become hyperactive.

From birth babies can sense if they are not wanted. If a baby is ignored or deprived of human contact and stimulation, this is emotional abuse and can be very harmful because human babies need love and stimulation to develop and thrive. In the initial 9 months a baby undergoes a progressive emotional separation process from the mother. Without a feeling of security a baby may become withdrawn, not cope well, or become hyperactive and difficult. Some babies cope by surrounding themselves with an emotionally protective layer almost like a second emotional skin.

Physical abuse

During pregnancy foetal development may be adversely affected by excessive consumption of alcohol, cigarettes or recreational drugs. A baby cannot give informed consent and in some countries this is seen as a form of abuse. Some women succeed in breaking an addiction and some manage to reduce the amount they take but still feel guilty. When use of an addictive drug continues, it is not necessarily because of a lack of concern for the baby. Rather it can be extremely hard to stop, and support is essential. Taking harmful drugs is often founded on a lack of self-respect and a rejection of the baby: in this case emotional therapy may be helpful. Physical abuse may also arise from starvation (anorexia), which deprives a growing baby of essential nutrition. Once again the underlying cause of the EATING DISORDER is the main issue that needs to be addressed, and the effect on the baby is secondary. Excessive and compulsive exercising may also have an adverse effect. During pregnancy a man who abuses his wife is expressing anger at her or at the baby who is intruding into his life.

After birth sometimes abuse takes the form of not feeding or nourishing a baby. Crying is a natural way to express needs yet it may make parents upset and angry. Hitting a baby is inappropriate: violent shaking, usually in an attempt to stop a baby from crying, can cause severe long-term damage, including bleeding in the brain. Babies may also be subjected to sexual abuse.

Effects on a baby

The effect of abuse on an unborn baby is becoming clearer as more is being discovered about foetal development. A baby in the womb has a natural resilience, dreams, has emotions and is born with a perception of life. If a baby is exposed to negative experiences, he may switch off, becoming quiet and withdrawn; he may be hyperactive and find it difficult to relax. If an unloving environment or harmful actions continue after birth, these behaviours are likely to be reinforced and he may have high levels of anxiety, difficulty feeding, COLIC and fail to gain WEIGHT. The effect depends in part upon the baby's personality, and also on what happens with his carers.

If physical or emotional abuse starts after birth, a baby learns rapidly from his experiences, which form a foundation for his outlook on life (p.31). The effects may range from undermining self-esteem and fuelling persistent fear, to physical injury that may lead to brain damage and developmental abnormalities or even death. An abused baby may find it very difficult to form the usual parent–child attachment and to interact with other children and adults. He may smile later than expected, and infrequently. Babies who feel neglected are often slow to reach developmental milestones. They may be slow to develop play skills as well as language and problem-solving abilities and later show inattentiveness or poor concentration; they may act aggressively. Often children of anxious parents are themselves anxious, while children whose mothers have eating disorders may have problems concerning food.

The same mechanism that makes early experiences so important – the plasticity and rapid growth of the brain – can also enable healing and positive experiences to replace feelings of upset and hurt if a situation improves and a baby is given love, support and encouragement.

Action plan

The best cure for abuse is prevention. It is not always possible to alter behaviour patterns, correct rifts in a relationship or change personal circumstances, but taking steps to do so during pregnancy may be very useful. Some parents may hope that things will get better with a baby, but if the situation is already bad it is likely to worsen. Support and therapy can be very worthwhile, and practical help may make a huge difference to the life of a family and the welcome given to the baby. Actively treating anxiety and depression (p.459) may make a significant improvement. Encouraging parents to see their child as an individual who does not plan to be difficult or destructive may be helpful. A doctor, health visitor or a family therapist may be involved in helping with the parent's relationship. After birth they may be part of a wider team that helps family life become settled and gives advice on living with a baby.

It is not always easy to admit to abuse, or to reach out for help. Abuse is often out of control and can be very well hidden. Medical professionals are trained to look for signs of abuse in children and to note signals in a mother's behaviour that may indicate depression or emotional difficulties. There is a child protection team in each county/borough that has a protocol for action should abuse or suspected abuse be reported. If this is the case, usually a meeting is held with the parent or carer.

Parents and grandparents sometimes feel unjustifiably accused but at all times the baby's interests are given priority. If you are in need of help, contact any health-care professional, social worker or a parent help line, as they will be able to direct you to a source of immediate support.

CHLAMYDIA TRACHOMATIS

The bacteria chlamydia trachomatis results in the most common sexually transmitted disease (STD) in the UK and can infect the penis, vagina, cervix and uterus, anus, urethra or eyes. It usually gives no symptoms but it can have serious health consequences, and if infection is present during birth it may affect the baby. Fortunately, treatment is successful.

What happens

In women, the infection usually begins on the cervix. It can spread to the fallopian tubes or ovaries and cause pelvic inflammatory disease and it can scar and block the fallopian tubes. This can increase the chance of an ECTOPIC PREGNANCY, and can lead to infertility. It also may cause premature rupture of the membranes (p.501), leading to PREMATURE BIRTH, and it may be connected with MISCARRIAGE. After birth it can lead to infections of the uterus and pelvis.

Of infected women 85% show no signs. If symptoms are present they begin 5–10 days after infection and may include bleeding or pain, fever, pain on urination or a yellowish vaginal discharge that may have a foul odour. These are like symptoms of GONORRHOEA. Chlamydia can also infect the rectum, giving painful bowel movements. Around 40% of infected men show symptoms, including discharge from the penis, burning while urinating or tender testicles.

Between 20 and 50% of babies born to infected mothers become infected. Chlamydia is the leading cause of neonatal conjunctivitis, which in rare cases may cause blindness, but if chlamydia is identified as the cause, appropriate antibiotic treatment is usually affective. An infected baby may also develop chlamydia pneumonia, perhaps 2–4 months after birth: this usually responds to appropriate antibiotic treatment.

Action plan

In some, but not all, hospitals all women are tested. Treatment is simple and effective.

Medical care

- If you or your partner show symptoms of chlamydia, visit your doctor. Culture tests from the penis, cervix, urethra or anus as well as urine samples give clear information.
- You and your partner need to be treated at the same time with antibiotics. You may be offered azithromycin to be taken in 1 dose, or doxycycline to take for 7 days but these are not given in pregnancy. Instead erythromycin is often prescribed for pregnant women and used to treat babies with eye infections or pneumonia caused by chlamydia.

CHOLESTASIS

Cholestasis is a disease unique to pregnancy where the flow of bile in the mother's liver is reduced. The main symptom is severe itching without a rash, often most intense on the palms of the hands and soles of the feet, usually after Week 30, but sometimes sooner. In Europe cholestasis affects 1% of pregnant women, especially those with twins. With attention to birth timing, cholestasis is unlikely to have any ill effect on your baby and your symptoms will disappear soon after. There is a 60% likelihood of recurrence in subsequent pregnancies.

What happens

The exact mechanism for cholestasis is unclear but it is caused by the hormone oestrogen, produced by the placenta, interfering with the movement of bile salts in the liver in women with a genetic difficulty with bile transport. For them, low levels of bile transport proteins only show in pregnancy or on taking the oestrogen-containing contraceptive pill. Itching may be caused by bile salts being deposited in the skin. In a small number of women the liver is affected causing dark urine and light stools and, rarely, JAUNDICE, which may also be caused by gallstones or HEPATITIS so needs to be investigated.

The itch usually worsens in the 2nd and 3rd trimesters. When the levels of bile salts are more than twice as high as the normal limit there is an increased risk of meconium staining of the amniotic fluid and FOETAL DISTRESS & ASPHYXIA in labour and a doubled risk of PREMATURE BIRTH. Most importantly, the risk of stillbirth (p.509) rises after Week 37. Lower levels of bile also affect the body's ability to absorb vitamin K, responsible for assisting BLOOD CLOTTING, and this may make bleeding after birth in mother and baby more likely. Vitamin K levels return to normal a few days after birth.

Action plan

If you are itching on your hands, feet, limbs and trunk but don't have a rash then your liver function will be tested by analysing a blood sample.

Diagnosis

The main diagnostic test for cholestasis is a rise in bile salt levels in the blood, which may increase before a change in liver function can be detected. You may also have liver function tests to exclude hepatitis and pre-existing liver disease and on a regular basis to monitor the severity of the cholestasis. An ultrasound scan of your liver checks for gallstones, which are rare in pregnancy and usually not treated until after the birth.

Medical care

It may be difficult to treat cholestasis.

- Ursodeoxycholic acid given in tablet form is a bile acid that ameliorates the itch and liver function abnormalities and is safe. Itch symptoms may be relieved in 24–48 hours and although further research is needed, it may improve the outcome for the baby and the only known side effect is mild maternal diarrhoea.
- If cholestasis is severe, you will be given vitamin K weekly, orally, to improve blood clotting, beginning after Week 30. It will also be given to your baby at birth.

Birth

The timing of birth will be decided according to your bile salt levels and liver function tests.

- Birth is usually planned for Week 37–38 if the bile salt levels remain elevated because the risk to your baby of unexpected foetal death rises significantly then and by this time the risks associated with premature birth have passed. In rare and severe cases with deranged liver function and maternal jaundice, birth may be recommended at Week 36.

- Unless there are other indications for a CAESAREAN SECTION, birth is usually stimulated by induction of labour (p.497).

Diet
Attention to your diet, plus supplements to ensure adequate intake of vitamins, minerals and essential fatty acids, helps to reduce the work your liver needs to do.

- Drink a minimum of 3 litres (6 pints) of water a day, stick to a mainly vegetarian diet, reduce dairy products and fried or fatty foods and wheat, and increase wholegrain rice, barley, millet and buckwheat, and vegetables and fruits eaten raw or lightly cooked.
- It may also help to eat more seeds, notably linseed soaked overnight in water and added to food or drunk on its own, and others such as sesame and pumpkin.
- Cholestasis may be associated with a deficiency in the mineral selenium and remedied with supplements.
- Alcohol and saturated fats should certainly be avoided.

Soothing remedies
- Do what you can to relieve the itching – avoid becoming hot; calomine lotion may soothe and a light cream with camomile help. The itch may respond to antihistamines.
- Take time to relax and rest during the day because knowing that your baby may be at risk is likely to make you anxious, and the itch may interfere with sleep.
- Homeopathic liver support remedies such as *Chelidonium* and *Lycopodium* can be useful but need to be prescribed by a qualified homeopath.

After the birth
Provided your baby has been born safely, cholestasis in pregnancy will have no long-term physical effects on either of you. Your baby needs extra vitamin K by injection (p.226). Your symptoms will disappear and you will soon forget the itchiness. Cholestasis does not cause lasting liver damage but your medical team may advise you to be rescanned for gallstones. It is best not to use a pill containing oestrogen as a method of contraception thereafter.

CHORIONIC VILLOUS SAMPLING (CVS)
See AMNIOCENTESIS & CVS

CHROMOSOMAL ABNORMALITIES
See DOWN'S SYNDROME & OTHER CHROMOSOMAL ABNORMALITIES

CIRCUMCISION
....

In the 19th century circumcision was widely advocated as a prevention of excessive masturbation in childhood and there were unfounded theories that it could be beneficial to health.

Today the UK's Royal College of Paediatrics and a similar body in the USA advise against it unless there is a medical need, and recommend that anaesthesia should always be used. World wide approximately 20% of men are circumcised. The main religious groups for whom circumcision remains an important ritual are Jews and Muslims.

The foreskin produces antibodies, antibacterial and antiviral proteins and pheromones, and is designed by nature to be an internal organ like the vagina. Circumcision does not promote hygiene or prevent or reduce the incidence of urinary tract infection, cancer of the penis or the cervix later in life or sexually transmitted diseases. A typical western medical circumcision results in the loss of many of the erogenous sexual nerves and affects sexual pleasure, which is enhanced by the foreskin's gliding action. Under normal conditions a baby's foreskin is attached to the underlying glans of the penis and does not start to retract until 3 years of age at the earliest. Any attempt to retract or remove it causes pain and distress.

Phimosis is a condition in which the foreskin of the penis is abnormally non-retractable. It occurs in fewer than 2% of boys and it can often be treated by the simple application of a steroid cream. If this fails, a circumcision is advised. If, at birth, there is a suggestion of hypospadias (p.523), where the urinary opening is not at the tip of the penis, circumcision needs to be delayed because the skin of the foreskin may be needed for reconstructive surgery.

What happens
If you decide to have your baby boy circumcised, there is no best way. All methods will be painful for him: newborn babies perceive pain as intensely or more intensely than older children and adults. In whatever way circumcision is carried out, almost all babies cry, particularly when being restrained by an adult or on a plastic board with Velcro straps. It is preferable to use a local anaesthetic cream or injection. The anaesthetic numbs the outer skin of the penis but the glans of the penis is not numbed and your baby will feel the foreskin being separated. A sugary or alcohol-based drink may reduce pain perception a little.

Ritual Jewish circumcision is traditionally done at 8 days and does not usually use anaesthetic. It is done by a surgeon or a mohel (Jewish religious officer), who may not necessarily be a doctor. In ritual circumcision the foreskin is separated from the underlying head of the penis then drawn forward. A protective shield is slid across the head before the foreskin is cut off. A similar method is used in some hospitals. Some doctors provoke erections in order to judge the 'cut-off line'.

An alternative method is to use a 'plastibell' device like a plastic bell. After the foreskin is separated, the device is placed over the head of the penis and the foreskin drawn over the bell. A tie is tightened around the base of the bell to cut off the blood supply to the foreskin. After 3–7 days the bell and foreskin drop off, leaving the tissue to heal. The pain caused is probably less severe than the pain of a ritual circumcision but as the bell is in place for a few days, pain may last longer.

Action plan: post-circumcision care
After circumcision by any method there may be 2–3 days of discomfort, usually associated with pain on passing urine.

Frequent breastfeeding and cuddling and regular small doses of infant paracetamol will comfort your baby. If pain continues beyond the 3rd day, get in touch with the mohel or surgeon.

After surgical removal of the foreskin, the penis is wrapped in gauze. It is helpful to keep the gauze moist and to cover the inner surface with Vaseline to prevent it adhering to the underlying wound. The gauze will appear bloody at first, but in most cases the circumcision site heals quickly because there is such a good blood supply to the penis. The gauze can be safely soaked off after 3–4 days. It is safe to bathe your baby 24 hours after the circumcision. No change in the type of nappies or the frequency with which they are changed is necessary, and no other precautions are required.

Following circumcision, the penis may appear swollen for at least 2 weeks. This is not unusual, and is due to the healing process. The pink head of the penis, the glans, will be visible.

Possible complications

The risks associated with circumcision are kept to a minimum by ensuring the procedure is carried out by an experienced person. Infections can be avoided by regularly changing the dressings. Complications with a plastibell are less common. The majority of babies recover from circumcision in a few days and only some show long-term effects.

- If excessive bleeding continues for more than 1 hour after the procedure, let the surgeon know immediately. He may come back or recommend you apply further dressings and check for a bleeding disorder (p.408).
- If bleeding begins after 48 hours, this indicates that the site has become infected. You will see redness and swelling around the line of separation and your baby will be distressed and feverish. This requires treatment with antibiotics.
- If excessive skin has been removed, erections may be painful and the penis may develop a curve, or chordee (p.523), because the tissue on the inner surface of the penis is shorter than the erect length of the penis. This may require extensive surgery.
- Around 1:4 babies have redness and pain for longer than a week, are upset and do not feed or sleep well.
- For a minority of babies, the psychological trauma of a surgical operation without adequate analgesia may have a long-term emotional effect similar to post-traumatic stress (p.462) in an older child.

Homeopathy

Before circumcision parents may be calmer after 1 dose of *Aconite* (200c) 30 minutes before the operation; for the baby a single 30c dose may help. A Bach Flower Rescue Remedy is often helpful; 2–3 drops for the parents and 1 drop for the baby immediately before circumcision.

After circumcision use *Arnica* for trauma and to reduce swelling and inflammation; *Calendula* to heal the wound and *Hypericum* to work on the nerves, each in 30c potency, 3 times a day for 5 days. *Staphysagria* can assist healing and deal with the emotional side of the procedure; use it on the 1st day 3 times at 3-hourly intervals. You can also use 10 drops of *Hypercal* tincture in the bath for 5 days to assist with the healing.

CLEFT LIP & PALATE

See also CONGENITAL ABNORMALITIES

During early pregnancy separate areas of the face develop individually and then join together. If some parts do not join properly the result is a cleft, meaning 'split' or 'separation', that may affect the lip or palate (roof of the mouth). In the UK 1:800 children is born with a cleft of the lip or palate.

What happens

With a cleft lip there is an opening in the upper lip between the mouth and nose. It can range from a slight notch to complete separation in one or both sides of the lip extending up and into the nose. A cleft in the gum may also occur.

A cleft palate can range from a split in the soft palate at the back of the mouth to an almost complete separation between the soft the hard palates at the front. Sometimes a baby with a cleft palate may have a small lower jaw and difficulty with breathing. This condition is called Pierre Robin syndrome.

Babies with a cleft lip alone do not usually have feeding difficulties but a cleft palate may interfere with the creation of a vacuum needed for sucking. The most common associated problems are taking in too much air while feeding, which may lead to painful wind or COLIC, bringing milk up through the nose and low WEIGHT gain. Sometimes, bottle feeding is more successful than breastfeeding. Special bottles and teats are available from the Cleft Lip and Palate Association (CLAPA).

Action plan

A member of the Cleft Team at the hospital usually visits babies with a cleft within 24 hours of diagnosis. A Cleft Team might include a plastic surgeon, paediatrician, dentist, speech specialist, an ear nose throat specialist and a nurse. Fortunately, modern surgery produces excellent cosmetic and functional results.

A cleft lip can be repaired surgically, usually at around 10 weeks after birth. Repairing a cleft palate involves more extensive surgery and is usually done at 9–18 months. Before this, you and your baby may have support to overcome problems with feeding, teething, hearing, speech or psychological development, and care will continue after surgery. Many affected children become self-conscious and love and encouragement from the parents is extremely important for self-esteem. Children with a cleft palate are prone to ear infections and hearing difficulties because the cleft can interfere with the function of the middle ear.

COLIC

See also CONSTIPATION: BABY; CRYING; DIARRHOEA: BABY

Colic is the term applied by generations of parents to the symptoms of inconsolable crying (or even screaming) and apparent severe tummy pain experienced by many babies at some time in the first 6 months after birth. A colicky baby may appear very stressed and agitated, and parents commonly suspect that something is desperately wrong. Usually, it's 'just colic' but it puts pressure on the whole family.

Often an attack begins in late afternoon and continues without a break or in fits and starts through the evening and into the night, but it can appear at any time of day. Colic often peaks in the late evening and may prevent baby and parents from sleeping – a cycle forms because sleep deprivation aggravates the situation.

Most colic starts by 2 months of age, although some quiet babies develop it later, and continues for up to 3 months (hence the term '3-month colic'). By 6 months most colicky babies are more settled. Premature babies may follow the same time scale, with symptoms starting after the baby reaches term. Sometimes constipation or mild diarrhoea, or both, accompany colic, particularly if a baby has a food intolerance (p.391). Constipation or diarrhoea can also give symptoms that may be mistaken for colic but go once the causes have been treated.

What happens

Colic occurs when the muscle wall of the intestine contracts excessively and for prolonged periods. To your baby it may feel like severe discomfort or the pain of trapped wind. You can recognise the signs if usual efforts at comforting fail and the symptoms recur each day or every few days. Babies with colic often draw up their knees or hold their legs straight and rigid, and the abdomen is usually tense and hard. Colicky babies do not sleep during an attack.

A Nobel prize awaits the discoverer of the cause and treatment of colic in babies. Little scientific research exists even to guess at the causes or why some treatments work. If you are breastfeeding, some foods you eat may aggravate your baby, and colic may be brought on if he does not suck long enough to benefit from hind milk or swallows air as he feeds because of a poor latch-on position (p.188). If you are bottle feeding, it may be due to an intolerance to the formula milk, unsuitable teats or incorrect positioning during a feed.

Some people believe that it happens simply because babies need to get used to digesting or that it is an emotional reaction to a stressful birth. Reflux (p.561) and food ALLERGY OR INTOLERANCE can cause discomfort and are commonly mistaken for colic. Very rarely, a bowel disorder, such as HERNIA, may lead to colic, but other symptoms are usually more prominent. If your baby has colic but is otherwise thriving, a serious cause is extremely unlikely.

Action plan

Crying and stress brought on by colic can exacerbate it further, so wherever possible it will help if you can tackle it, first by eliminating the cause (if known), and then by easing your baby's pain when an attack occurs. If your baby has attacks at a certain time of day there are a number of things you can do about 2 hours before to ease, but not necessarily avoid, an attack. Remember that every baby is different and will respond differently. Remedies that one family swears by may not suit another. Don't try every remedy at once – take it step by step.

Before an attack
- A warm bath may help release tension around the abdomen and bowel.
- Gentle massage may help, but perhaps not while your baby

is distressed. Try the abdominal massage on p.368. You can move on to the leg massage, finishing with a cycling motion of the legs, which helps the stomach muscles move and puts gentle pressure on the intestines, encouraging the motion of faeces towards the rectum.
- Try to feed your baby before he gets really hungry. He may need frequent feeds throughout the day.

During an attack
- Try the classic colic-alleviation position with your baby facing outwards with his back or side against your chest, his tummy along your forearm and his head nestling in the crook of your arm. You can try gently patting or massaging his tummy with your free hand. Movement may help him too – in your arms as you walk or a ride in the buggy.
- Distractions and cuddling and your soothing voice may be comforting or a drop of water or cooled mild camomile tea or water with dill may be calming.
- If none of these work, try using gripe water, Infacol or Colic Drops. These are all over-the-counter preparations that are safe and may be effective. At the very worst if they have no effect on the colic, they do no harm.
- Some practitioners do not recommend massage during an attack because the muscles are in spasm, but many parents are certain it helps.
- It is OK if your baby cries during the attack. He may cry without a break or cry off and on as you try a number of different comforting techniques. He will eventually calm down and the crying will cause no physical or psychological damage. Ear plugs may help you cope.

After an attack
- Let your baby rest peacefully. He will be exhausted but he may be hungry and need to feed. Having close body contact with you may reassure him and reduce further attacks.
- If he lies on his side, put him on his right side – when lying on the left side, any air in the stomach tends to pass into the intestines where it may cause discomfort.
- You need to rest as well.

To eliminate attacks
- Take time to feed and check your baby has a good position, eats enough and is winded well. Expressing a little breast milk at the beginning of a feed may reduce air swallowing.
- Changing formula or using different water to make up the milk, or using a different style of bottle or teat may help. A pre-sterilised bag inserted into the bottle contracts as your baby feeds and can minimise air swallowing.
- Your baby may be sensitive or have an allergy or intolerance to his milk or to what you consume that passes into breast milk; try identifying problem foods and discuss them with a nutritionist, midwife or health visitor. Food and drinks that produce lots of gas are orange juice, vegetables, especially onions and cabbage, fruit such as apples and plums, spicy food and products with caffeine. Each baby is different and trial and error is the only way forward. Try to maintain a regular and nourishing diet; if you rush or miss your lunch, resulting breast milk quality may make your baby irritable at around 5pm.

- Cow's milk intolerance is frequently given as the cause. Excluding it from your diet if you are breastfeeding may help. Cow's milk is often tolerated when re-introduced after a 1–2 week exclusion period.
- Cranial osteopathy (p.376) and massage (p.365) are powerful techniques that can release tension in your baby's intestinal wall.
- Body contact and water are relaxing, and can really reduce tension for you and your baby.
- You may have been told that drinking a swig of whiskey before the last feed at night is a good soother but this is not recommended. Alcohol is not good for your baby, and there is a risk of his developing a dependence on its sedative effect. Do not be tempted to use it as a prophylaxis and never give any alcoholic drink, however small, to your baby.

Medical care

If colic is severe, ask your doctor or health visitor for advice and to examine your baby to exclude an underlying bowel or food intolerance problem. There are prescription and over-the-counter treatments, but no single drug therapy has proved to be consistently successful. If your baby is below 6 months old, don't give him anything without consulting your doctor.

- Alcohol used to be part of all colic preparations, but that is no longer the case due to safety. Other active ingredients are usually sugar, which has been shown to have a pain-relieving effect in babies, and drugs that act on the smooth muscle of the bowel, reducing spasm and relieving pain.
- Antacid medications such as Gaviscon or other more potent antacids, such as cimetidine or ranitidine, sometimes help. The doses are prescribed by your doctor.
- Some people try preparations such as Phenergan (in prescribed doses) or gripe water although they are usually no more effective than many of the above suggestions or complementary therapies.

Homeopathy

Finding the right remedy to alleviate colic may be tricky as symptoms are often changeable. Homeopathy is useful in combination with the suggestions above and it is worth persisting. In an acute attack, use 30c every hour for up to 3 hours, then reassess and choose the remedy that best suits the new symptoms. When less acute, give the most indicated remedy (30c) 4 times a day, preferably before a feed for 2–3 days and then reassess.

Use *Chamomilla* if your baby is frantic, irritable, bloated with wind and has a hard abdomen, kicks and draws up his legs, may produce green, watery stools and is only relieved by being carried around or being undressed; *Colocynth* if he is writhing in pain and draws his legs in to his abdomen, is restless, shows sudden signs of pain and seems better if he is leaning against something or his abdomen is massaged; *Dioscorea* when pain is centred around the navel and is better for stretching the legs out and arching the back; *Lycopodium* if pain is worse with any pressure around the abdomen and from 4 to 8pm and perhaps if wind is linked with you eating too much fibre (e.g. wholewheat, cabbage, beans, etc.); *Mag Phos* if pain occurs sporadically with great windiness and reduces with warmth, massage and firm pressure (it acts like an antispasmodic); *Nux Vomica* if you are breastfeeding and have eaten spicy food or drunk a lot of coffee, and your baby is woken by pain and is distressed when straining to pass a stool.

Caring for yourself

At times you will feel down, tired and anxious. Colic can be very stressful and disappointing if things aren't as rosy or easy as you had hoped. The stress and exhaustion may bring difficult emotions (p.300) to the surface. Remember to look after yourself, ask for help, and rest well. Use the Wheel for Living (p.58) to put practical plans into action and seek advice if you might benefit from EMOTIONAL ADVICE AND SUPPORT: existing anxieties or depression can worsen when things are tough.

If you feel at the end of your tether and angry towards your baby, take heart that countless other parents have felt that way. If you feel an urge to hurt your child, it is essential to seek help from your friends, family or your doctor. Many parents feel guilty that they feel anger and need reassurance that it happens very commonly. Whatever you choose to do, the ordeal will come to an end. Only occasionally colic may be a forerunner of irritable bowel syndrome (p.448) if it is caused by a food intolerance. Some parents find that once the colicky attacks have finished, the peace is miraculous. And some worry when their babies are so quiet, not at all like the night terrorists who made them doubt their sanity.

CONGENITAL ABNORMALITIES

Any condition or variation from the normal, however small, is called a congenital – 'born with' – abnormality. These are surprisingly common, occurring in around 1:10 babies, and are usually of no significance. Occasionally they may be more serious. Many of the more major congenital abnormalities can be cured or significantly improved with treatment but some result in disability. Around two-thirds are suspected or diagnosed during pregnancy, and as antenatal screening becomes more sophisticated, the number is increasing. However, even with the most detailed ultrasound scans, blood and other tests, some conditions may not be detected.

What happens

Congenital abnormalities may occur because of:

Chromosomal abnormality: A defect in one of the 46 chromosomes that occurs in every cell of the body. The most widely known is DOWN'S SYNDROME.

Genetic abnormality: The chromosomes look normal but one of the genes present on the 46 chromosomes does not function optimally. Examples include CYSTIC FIBROSIS and TAY-SACHS DISEASE. Chromosomal and gene problems are called genetic abnormalities.

Developmental abnormality: There is abnormal formation of the body during embryonic development. The reason is often not understood because the process from single-cell embryo to multi-billion-cell baby is extremely complex. Examples include SPINA BIFIDA and CLEFT LIP.

The majority of anomalies are not preventable and occur by

chance. If there is a family history of a genetic abnormality, the advice of a genetic counsellor is helpful to assess the risks, provide prenatal diagnosis or early postnatal diagnosis and implement a treatment plan. As molecular biology and pre- and postnatal testing improves, the accuracy of predicting and diagnosing congenital abnormalities will become more reliable. When all the genes of the human genome are mapped, it may be possible to predict before becoming pregnant whether your family is susceptible. In spite of science, the best way to avoid congenital problems is through reducing the risk as far as possible. Some abnormalities are preventable:

Nutrition: The best known prevention is of neural-tube defects (e.g. spina bifida) with nutritional supplements containing folic acid, a B vitamin. It is likely that optimal balance of vitamins and minerals (p.345) will reduce the incidence of other congenital abnormalities.

Medication: There are a number of medications that may cause congenital abnormalities. These include drugs to treat epilepsy, chemotherapy, some acne treatments and warfarin, for thinning the blood. It is best to discuss any medications before conception and to change if necessary.

Street drugs: A number of street or recreational DRUGS may cause congenital abnormalities.

Industrial hazards: Workers in some industries exposed to radiation or chemicals may be at increased risk.

Action plan

If your medical team suspects that your baby has a congenital abnormality, you may initially react with disbelief. The range of emotions that follows may be overwhelming, confusing and difficult to cope with. This is often an anxious and traumatic time for parents, because a problem may be suspected but often a diagnosis cannot be made until further tests have been carried out. Fortunately, in many cases, investigation proves that there is no underlying problem. When this happens, the test result is known as a 'false positive'. Medical research is constantly striving to improve the accuracy of prenatal screening tests to minimise the distress caused by false positive results.

Sometimes the diagnosis is confirmed. Parents are often overpowered by emotions such as hopelessness, guilt, anger, pain and denial. There may be a strong sense of grief and loss but there is often a very strong and overwhelming love for the growing baby. When news of the pregnancy has already been shared and celebrated, it is often very hard to tell your family and friends what has happened. In addition to medical support, emotional support and counselling (p.459) is very helpful. Usually, parents are keen to discover as much as they can about the problem, and for some, full information brings hope and relief if the outlook is not as bad as at first feared. Difficult as it may be in the short term, it helps to ask for and receive honest explanations and answers. If your doctor or midwife doesn't have an answer, this may be because there simply isn't one, or that they do not know but may put you in touch with someone who does. Comprehensive information also makes arrangements for the future more straightforward and this may include termination of pregnancy.

Other parents who have experience of a particular problem are often a superb source of support and frequently offer to share their experience. This can be the best source of support and information although you may prefer not to involve others early on. There are also a number of support groups.

On the bright side, for many abnormalities treatment can begin in the womb and positive plans can be made to ease a condition or correct it completely after birth. On the other hand, anxiety is inevitable, and if the severity of a condition is not clearly known, it is difficult to surmise what might happen in the future. There are some conditions that cannot be treated and some that do not become evident until after birth.

Genetic counselling

Genes (p.14) are what determine how every person functions and their traits, such as blood type, body build and personality. They are all contained in the 46 chromosomes. Genes that are present on the first 22 pairs of chromosomes are said to be autosomal – that means that one gene comes from the mother and the other from the father, and males and females are equally likely to have these genes. The last pair of chromosomes are the sex chromosomes. Here the mix is slightly different: males have one X and one Y chromosome, while females have two X-chromosomes. Therefore women do not have any of the genes present on the Y, and men have only one copy of genes on the X. The basic patterns of inheritance are dominant, recessive and X-linked inheritance.

Genetic testing

Examining genes and the chromosomes to which they are related, or the enzymes that they influence, has become an increasingly accurate way of detecting developmental disorders. With advances in molecular biology and decoding of the human genome, an increasing number of inherited conditions are now detected. Genetic testing is offered to parents who wish to know the likelihood of their baby inheriting a disorder when there is a family history. It is also increasingly offered in standard antenatal screening (p.80).

The main purpose of genetic testing is to establish a diagnosis and enable parents and medical staff to make informed decisions. The ethical and religious debates surrounding genetic testing have been rumbling on for decades and with different guidelines in different countries and in different hospitals within a country the decision about what to do may be difficult.

Diagnostic testing: Used to identify an abnormality or a condition in a person or a family. The information is helpful in determining the course of a disease and treatment. The tests include identifying chromosomes or doing biochemical tests for individual genes. Some are offered in pregnancy.

Predictive genetic testing: Determines the chances that a healthy adult without a family history of a certain disease might develop that disease. This is an expanding field for adult-onset conditions such as some types of cancer and cardiovascular disease. It could be valuable before pregnancy where termination of an affected baby is not an option.

Prenatal studies before implantation: Used following in-vitro fertilisation to diagnose a genetic disease or condition in an embryo before it is implanted into the mother's uterus. One or two cells are removed at the 10-cell stage, about 3 days after fertilisation. This allows diagnosis for conditions where a single-gene abnormality can be detected, such as cystic fibrosis, or sex-linked conditions such as Duchenne muscular dystrophy. Exploration of the cells can also identify some chromosomal conditions and enables unaffected embryos to be implanted. Strict rules govern pre-implantation diagnoses to prevent sexing a baby or breeding a genetically similar child to act as an organ donor – the ethical issues are huge and the debate continues around the world.

Carrier testing: Performed to determine whether an adult carries an altered gene for a particular disease. This indicates the chance that the baby may be affected and follow-up tests during pregnancy can determine whether the baby has inherited the condition. Testing may be based on a family history but they are increasingly offered to all pregnant women. Many conditions are detectable, including cystic fibrosis, certain deficiencies of the immune system, abnormal blood cells (sickle cell disease and thalassaemia, p.398) and disorders of BLOOD CLOTTING (haemophilia).

Testing the foetus and baby

Prenatal diagnosis: Used to detect a genetic disorder in a developing foetus and includes maternal blood screening (p.80), ultrasound, amniocentesis & cvs and umbilical blood sampling. These tests can only be carried out once a pregnancy has reached the end of the 1st trimester. They may not be suitable for couples who would not consider termination of pregnancy. Occasionally a sex chromosome abnormality, such as Turner syndrome, is detected before birth during a test looking for Down's syndrome or another chromosomal disorder. As more couples ask for prenatal chromosome testing this is becoming more common.

Newborn screening: Standard across the UK to check for certain genetic diseases. The tests are usually on blood taken in the heel prick test performed in the 2nd or 3rd week after birth. The blood is tested for a range of conditions, including biochemical disorders such as cystic fibrosis, hypothyroidism (p.543) and phenyl ketonuria, and also sickle cell disease and thalassaemia, which may cause anaemia. With all these disorders, early diagnosis may allow early treatment to begin, leading to a better outcome and fewer complications for a baby and his family.

Genetic specialists

A clinical geneticist is a specialist with up-to-date information on genetic abnormalities. She advises parents and other medical and nursing professionals about tests and about the likely outcome for mother and baby of a particular condition. A genetic counsellor provides emotional and practical support and works very closely with the family to explain the diagnosis and the possible effect of the condition. In many hospitals midwives, obstetricians and paediatricians perform the role of genetic counsellors. A genetic counsellor can help with decisions regarding the organisation and timing of specialised tests. This is important because of the emotional, ethical and personal dimensions to these decisions. She will provide an important communication link between the parents, the clinical and the laboratory teams.

The information a counsellor provides is often invaluable to help parents make decisions: these may involve whether to conceive, whether to use a donor ova or sperm, opting for pre-implantation diagnosis or choosing which tests to have during and after pregnancy. Parents may also be faced with the choice between continuing or terminating pregnancy or looking into the possibility of adoption. The counsellor plays an important role while parents appraise a confusing amount of information and take time to reflect on the choices available.

A genetic counsellor also helps the family manage day-to-day affairs if a baby has a disability, and may be involved in celebrating the life and love of a child despite the health and lifestyle concerns. She also offers bereavement support when a pregnancy ends early or a baby dies and helps the family come to terms with the bereavement process that follows the LOSS OF A BABY. A counsellor recognises that the birth of a child with abnormalities can be like the loss of the expected healthy child and it includes a grief process.

CONSTIPATION: BABY

Constipation occurs when stools become firmer and harder and are not passed regularly enough, and the passing of the motion causes discomfort. There is a wide variation in the frequency of stools among babies. It is normal for a baby to have a bowel movement as often as several times a day or as seldom as once a week if breastfed. In very rare cases, and only if entirely breastfed, there can be up to 2 weeks between bowel movements. Constipation is rarely a problem for an exclusively breastfed baby. The usual time for constipation to become a problem with breastfeeding is when solids are introduced. It is, however, common among bottle-fed babies as formula milk is more difficult to digest. Most bottle-fed babies need to have daily bowel movements to avoid constipation.

If you think that your baby is constipated, look at the possible causes and rest assured that, except in very rare circumstances, it presents no long-term problems.

What happens

If your baby is constipated he may show signs of discomfort, perhaps with bloating in the lower abdomen, and straining to pass a stool. Stools are harder than normal and he may also have COLIC pains caused by the build-up of faeces and gas and the stretching of the intestine walls. He may cry when eating or not want to eat.

Food (milk) passes through the small bowel and on to the large bowel where much of the liquid is absorbed and the stool becomes firmer. It then travels to the rectum, where it is stored, and is expelled by reflex action. If passage through the large bowel is slow or the food contains little liquid, too much water will be drawn out of the stool, which then becomes hard and is difficult to pass. If passing a motion is difficult or painful, your baby may be reluctant and faeces may build up in the bowel. This can happen even when your baby is very young and pain overrides the expulsion reflex.

Causes in a young baby

Solely breastfed babies very rarely get constipation because breast milk is easily digested (p.186). Breastfed babies also have higher levels of a hormone called motilin, which increases the movement of the bowels. Bottle-fed babies suffer from constipation more frequently because formula milk is harder to digest and doesn't contain hormones that assist the digestive system. Stools will be thicker and may have a greenish colour. Unusual causes of newborn constipation, such as disorders of the digestive system (below), often lead to other symptoms such as vomiting and severe abdominal distension.

Causes in an older baby

When you have weaned your baby on to solid food, the frequency of his bowel movements and the consistency and appearance of the stools depends on what he eats and the pattern in the bowel movements will change. Gradually, your baby will develop an awareness of the presence of stools in his rectum and his reflexes diminish, so stools are passed less frequently. If he passes less than one stool every other day and shows disturbed behaviour, such as drawing up the knees, squirming and crying, and these signs persist, then constipation is becoming a problem.

If your baby has an illness and drinks less than usual, his stools will reduce in frequency and will become harder and more difficult to pass. This temporarily leads to constipation, and usually gets better after the illness has passed and eating habits are back to normal. Occasionally, passing hard motions results in cracks (anal fissures) that are painful and constipation becomes more persistent. ALLERGY OR INTOLERANCE to milk and other foods, including coeliac disease, may cause constipation. Behaviour concerning the potty is also significant – although a baby cannot control his bowels before the age of 1 year, if potty use is aggressively encouraged early, babies can become upset and constipated.

Action plan

After birth your midwife will check to ensure your baby is able to pass stools and there is no obstruction. Later, if you are concerned your doctor or health visitor can check whether constipation exists – the accumulation of faeces in the large bowel can be felt by lightly touching your baby's abdomen. Steps to reduce constipation are usually straightforward.

Diet

A good diet can help your baby avoid constipation and enjoy a wide range of food, and sufficient fluid, plus balance and variety when he is weaned, are important preventative measures. If your baby becomes constipated, take a look at how and what he eats.

- You can give your baby extra fluids. If you are breastfeeding, give more feeds. If you are bottle feeding, give extra bottles of cooled, boiled water.
- If your baby drinks formula milk, check you are mixing the powder with enough water (p.201). If necessary, ask your doctor about switching to a different brand.
- If your baby is over 6 weeks old, soak a handful of prunes in boiled water overnight and give the juice to her, either on a spoon or in a bottle.
- Once your baby is weaned, a small increase in fibre will help give the stools bulk and assist their movement through the large bowel. Try porridge and purées made from fruits or

vegetables with skins on. Prune purée is good. Cut down on constipating foods such as rice and bananas and don't be afraid to introduce your baby to a variety of vegetables and fruits (p.264). Be aware of food allergy and intolerance, especially formula milk protein, and later to wheat.

Relieving discomfort

- If your baby is relaxed and enjoys the sensation, massage his abdomen (p.368). You can move on to a leg massage, finishing with a cycling motion, which helps the stomach muscles move and puts gentle pressure on the intestines, encouraging the motion of faeces towards the rectum.
- A warm bath with massage may help release tension around the anus and bowel and encourage a stool to pass.
- When you wash your baby's bottom, apply some nappy cream or Vaseline around the outside of the anus – this will help it stretch as a hard stool passes and may prevent painful cracking.
- Do not put anything inside the anus in an attempt to stimulate a bowel movement – it may cause physical and psychological damage.

Medical care

If the suggestions above are not working, consult a doctor. She may encourage you to pay close attention to your baby's diet and fluid intake. If she believes the condition may respond to treatment she may recommend some of the following, all of which are regularly used in babies of 3 months and above.

- Usual treatments are by mouth. Medicines to soften the motions include lactulose; those that stimulate the bowel to empty, include senokot, syrup of figs or prune juice. Senokot syrup is only available on prescription (granules and tablets are not suitable for children). Usually a combination of softeners and stimulants is required.
- In general the less attention paid to the anus and surrounding area the better. Rarely are suppositories used, although for a very constipated baby there may be no other option, at least at the start of treatment. Very infrequently, enemas may be useful if other treatments are not working.

Homeopathy

The following remedies can be useful when constipation is not an ongoing problem. Give a remedy (30c) 3–4 times a day for 4 days and reassess. For persistent constipation it is best to seek advice on a constitutional remedy.

Use *Alumina* if there is difficulty even though stools are soft, your baby may be lethargic and feels better passing a stool upright; *Bryonia* if he is very thirsty, doesn't pass a stool and has no urge to, and finally produces a hard, dry and dark stool with difficulty; *Nux Vomica* if he is tense and irritable and has a persistent urge to pass a stool but does not produce; *Silica* if stools are partly expelled then slip back again, there is stomach cramping and slow weight gain may be a feature.

Possible associated problems

If your baby appears to be constipated and is not gaining weight or shows any other unusual symptoms such as a distended abdomen or vomiting, seek the advice of a doctor. The bowel may be blocked and obstructed.

Chronic constipation: This gives symptoms lasting for more than 3 months, among older babies, with or without episodes of what is called spurious DIARRHOEA (spurious because the underlying problem is constipation). This problem in infancy and childhood is often reported to doctors. The diarrhoea results because the large bowel does not absorb water from the liquid stools entering from the small bowel. Firm hard motions remain in the large bowel, causing constipation. This may lead to laxity in the large bowel and an inability to empty (megacolon), which needs long-term treatment.

Cystic fibrosis (p.443): This condition is a rare cause of constipation and bowel obstruction in the newborn period due to thick and sticky stools and is called meconium ileus. Usually this can be treated by special enemas to clear out the thick motion but it is a long-term problem for affected children.

Food intolerance and coeliac disease: These more commonly occur in older babies after weaning. In a younger baby, constipation may be one of the symptoms of cow's milk allergy (p.393) and most formula feeds are based on cow's milk.

Hirschprungs disease: This rare condition affects about 1:4500 babies and arises when the nerve supply to the bowel does not develop normally. It is diagnosed by a barium enema x-ray and a biopsy of the bowel. The condition is suspected if a baby fails to have his bowels open within 72 hours of birth, or there is passage of a hard pellet of meconium, called a meconium plug. An operation may be needed to remove the affected piece of bowel. In breastfed infants the motions are very soft and the operation may sometimes be put off for months.

Obstructions: These are rare and are most often diagnosed when there is vomiting (often bile stained) associated with abdominal distension and constipation. The baby may become ill and needs urgent diagnosis and treatment. Some obstructions may be detected during pregnancy ultrasound scans. Obstruction may arise from **intestinal atresia** (narrowing and blockage of the intestine); **intestinal malrotation**, where the bowel twists and surgical treatment relieves the blockage; or **intussusception**, where the bowel folds in on itself and there is also diarrhoea and bleeding. Rarely, the passage of motions is obstructed by an **imperforate anus**, where the rectum and anus are narrowed or not correctly linked to the intestine. This is diagnosed by examining the anus and needs surgical treatment.

Emotions
Constipation can cause parents and babies considerable emotional distress. Social taboos and family cultures may lend meaning to frequency and type of bowel movements and in some families there is regular mention of certain foods or activities that are good for – or bad for – the bowel. Sometimes parents believe that their baby's constipation reflects inadequate parenting skills.

Some people see faeces as dirty, which is not the way a baby sees it, and worry that being constipated retains toxins, although this is contrary to medical view. An unusual focus on bowel activities may affect family balance in the same way as obsession about sleeping or diet. Even small babies may pick up on this. If any of these issues relates to your family, you may benefit from support from your friends and doctor or health visitor.

CONSTIPATION: MOTHER

The range of normal bowel movements among healthy people is between three stools a day to one every 3 days. Constipation may involve passing unusually hard stools or the absence of stools for many days. Some women experience mild constipation when pregnancy hormones and altered eating result in altered bowel activity. This can be addressed with attention to diet and passes after pregnancy. After birth it is normal to wait for as long as 3 days before passing a stool.

What happens
If your diet does not contain enough roughage or fluid, this will affect bowel movement. Inside your bowel, fluid is absorbed from digested food, so it needs sufficient fluid in order to keep it soft enough to pass with ease. Without enough fluid, it becomes hard and difficult to push out. Without roughage, there is insufficient bulk to assist movement in the lower gut.

Some pregnancy hormones relax the smooth muscle in the wall of the intestine, reducing muscle tone and slowing activity throughout the bowel. This may bring on atonic constipation, which can be alleviated with improved muscle tone. The other common type of constipation is spastic constipation, often due to anxiety or linked with excessive SMOKING. The stress hormones may cause the wall of your intestine to be in spasm, which reduces bowel movement, and when stressed you may not eat and drink as usual. It may alternate with DIARRHOEA as part of irritable bowel syndrome (IBS). Occasionally constipation is due to a food ALLERGY OR INTOLERANCE. If you are reluctant to pass stools because of pain or bleeding there is a chance you could have PILES or an anal fissure. If you have been in the habit of using an excessive number of chemical laxatives in the past, particularly if you have had an EATING DISORDER, your colon may rely on the stimulation to contract. On exceptionally rare occasions constipation is caused by obstruction of the bowel.

Action plan
If you feel constipated there are many ways to relieve it and the dietary advice is also preventative – you may decide to make it part of your daily life. In pregnancy, it is preferable to avoid laxative drugs, which stimulate the bowel wall, unless your doctor has prescribed them for you.

Diet
Follow the nutritional advice from p.332 to give your body the fuel, minerals, vitamins and roughage it needs for your digestive system to work well. Introduce changes gradually to avoid bloating and focus on roughage. Some vegetables, nuts, seeds and fruits may be more effective for your bowel activity.

- You might want to note your reactions to what you eat and avoid any foods linked with ALLERGY OR INTOLERANCE. Note that if you are wheat intolerant, extra bran will make the constipation worse. Milk intolerance is common.
- Drink at least 2 litres (4 pints) of water a day to help your bowel movements by keeping stools soft. Try camomile, lemon balm, peppermint and ginger teas, but don't drink

too much after 6 or 7pm to avoid night-time visits to the loo.

- Naturally occurring laxatives encourage the passing of stools. Whole linseeds are safe and effective – 1 tbsp sprinkled into food or added to a glass of warm water once or twice a day should suffice. You could add thyme to your cooking – it is known to improve sluggish digestion.
- The alternative is a bulk laxative, such as lactulose, which works like bran by absorbing water into the stool and increasing the bulk and intestinal movement. It is available without prescription and can be safely taken twice a day.
- It may help to change your iron supplement to an elemental iron preparation (p.345) for easier absorption. Reduce your intake to 1 tablet every 1 or 2 days and take 1 hour before a high-fibre meal with a juice or vitamin C to aid absorption.

Homeopathy

Take a remedy (30c) 4 times a day for 3–4 days and then reassess.

Use *Bryonia* when stools are hard, dry and dark, you feel worse in warm stuffy environments and very thirsty; *Lycopodium* if you feel bloated and flatulent, strain to pass small, hard stools yet feel you have not emptied your bowels, cannot bear tight clothes and may be upset; *Nux Vomica* if you have a persistent urge to pass a stool though none is produced, have fullness in the rectum, feel stressed and have persistent dull headaches; *Sepia* if you have shooting pains up the rectum, pass large, hard stools and feel full and heavy in the abdomen.

Exercise and aromatherapy

For most cases of constipation, exercise (p.357) and yoga (p.346) stretches aid digestion and encourage circulation, stimulating bowel movements. Try walking, swimming or any other activity that is safe during pregnancy. Massage your abdomen in a clock-wise direction. From Week 24 it is safe to use any oil containing lemon and black pepper.

COUGH & COLD: BABY

All children cough. Coughing is a protective reflex designed to stop milk, mucus and other fluids from entering the airway. It is also the mechanism for expelling excess mucus or fluid. A cough is most commonly caused by a viral infection or cold, which a baby gets on average seven times a year. For some children a runny nose lasts all winter, some produce a lot of catarrh and others cough a lot, particularly at night. If your baby shows these symptoms but seems happy, do not worry. Most coughs and colds are self-limiting. Only if your baby appears ill, has BREATHING DIFFICULTIES or a FEVER do you need to call for urgent attention.

What happens

Mucus is produced by cells lining the air passages to protect the airways. Coughing is the reflex to clear the mucus and allow oxygen into the lungs, and may occur if the airways have become irritable following an infection. A dry cough does not produce sputum (spit) but a wet cough does. Green, brown or bloody sputum is usually caused by infection. Continuous coughing often leads to vomiting. When the airways are blocked or inflamed, your baby will breathe more quickly because before 12 months he cannot breathe more deeply.

The majority of infections are viral and usually pass in 3–4 days and fever tends to disappear within 36 hours. Although all babies get viral infections, some are more susceptible than others. The most significant factor that determines this is immune make-up. The antibodies your baby receives from you in pregnancy slowly disappear after 3 months as he replaces them with his own. His immunity is strengthened if you breastfeed because your antibodies pass to him in the milk. Exposure to viruses is also significant – if your baby is cared for in a large group or you have other children, he may have more frequent coughs and colds. Babies born prematurely are generally more prone to infection and being malnourished for reasons such as chronic illness also increases susceptibility.

Bacteria are another cause of respiratory infections and may complicate a viral illness because the irritated airway is less resistant to bacteria. It is not always easy to tell a viral from a bacterial infection. Bacterial infections tend to follow a virus, with persistent fever and listlessness, poor feeding, rapid breathing and a wet- or moist sounding cough. At this stage medical advice and antibiotics are needed.

The key to treating a cough is to treat the cause. These are outlined briefly here and in detail on the following pages.

Common colds: Usually viral and may linger with a cough, runny nose, sniffles or catarrh. After a viral respiratory illness the airways may become irritable. The irritable airways can persist for 8 weeks and your baby may cough, especially at night, when he is laughing or crying or on breathing in cold air. Usually there are no other symptoms but if your baby gets another viral infection the cough or cold will worsen.

Asthma (p.400): Characterised by wheezing and cough. The small airways, the bronchioles, are inflamed and become narrow so there is a wheezing noise as air travels from the lungs. The cough is usually worse at night, it may occur without a preceding cold and it may go on for weeks. The symptoms are usually triggered by a viral infection of the bronchioles but for a few children an ALLERGY can trigger the same symptoms.

Bronchiolitis: A viral illness producing inflammation in the small airways of the lungs giving excess mucus production, generally without a fever. A baby will breathe faster and may stop feeding.

Croup: A viral illness affecting the upper airway and larynx (voice box). It is often preceded by a viral cold and commonly comes on at night with a hoarse, grating sound to breathing and a barking cough – it can be frightening, particularly if your baby has difficulty breathing.

Pneumonia: A relatively rare disease that usually follows a viral infection. An affected baby breathes quickly – more than 50 breaths a minute – looks unwell, seems chilled or shivers and may have blue lips and nails if he is not getting enough oxygen. The space beneath his lower ribs may be drawn in as he breathes and he may cough up blood-tinged sputum. He may indicate pain on the infected side. In bacterial pneumonia a child usually has a very high fever. Pneumonia is a medical emergency.

Reflux (p.561): Coughing can be a symptom, where stomach contents come up the oesophagus and stimulate the cough reflex. Coughs and colds will temporarily worsen the reflux but some coughs are due to reflux alone, so treating reflux may eliminate coughing.

Whooping cough: Can be severe or even fatal and needs immediate medical care. It usually starts with a cold-like illness and prolonged coughing with no rest between each cough. The whoop is the forced breathing in after the coughing bout. The coughing makes a baby go red in the face and often vomit and, if it persists, the baby may go blue (p.441).

Action plan
Prevention
There is no way you can guarantee your baby will not catch a cold, but you may be able to strengthen his immunity so he can recover quickly – as well as breastfeeding, constitutional homeopathic treatment can be very effective. Acupuncture and herbal remedies prescribed by a qualified practitioner can also help. Echinacea is a general tonic used by adults but is not suitable below the age of 3 years.

You may have inherited a number of tips, such as avoiding going out with wet hair and staying out of drafts at night. Many of the ideas that pass down from generation to generation have not been confirmed with scientific information but it doesn't mean they are wrong. Vulnerability to infection is not influenced by cold winds, drafts, too little clothing, going to bed with wet hair or wearing too many clothes, although for a baby who is susceptible these may increase the likelihood. It is true that stuffy rooms and poor air circulation, and, above all, passive smoking do contribute to susceptibility. Cigarette smoke is a very common cause of infant coughing. Environmental pollution may increase coughing.

Calling your doctor
Take your baby to your doctor or nearest casualty department immediately if any of the following occur:
- Rapid, wheezy or laboured breathing, blue lips, grunting while breathing, inability to talk.
- Fever above 39.5°C (103.1°F) over 8 weeks of age or 38°C (100.4°F) below 8 weeks old.
- Coughing to the point of vomiting, inability to sleep due to persistent cough, coughing up blood.
- Excessive sleepiness, refusal to eat or drink, drooling and swallowing with difficulty.

See your doctor if your baby is feverish or stops feeding for more than 24 hours; appears lethargic and more sleepy than usual, or if a cough or wheeze persists for longer than 5 days.

Making your baby comfortable
- Continue feeding. You may need to feed little and often, particularly if your baby has a blocked nose. Feeding has the double benefit of providing nourishment and fluid and comforting your baby.
- He may breathe more easily if you dissolve a drop of eucalyptus/albus oil in some hot water or a vaporiser and place it in the room or beside his cot at night. Before 3 months use vapour rub on his vest rather than on his skin.
- Humidifiers and vaporisers increase the humidity in the air. This may soften the mucus and help clear the cough and is particularly useful if your baby has irritable airways after a viral infection. Cold-mist vaporisers give off cool air and avoid the risk of scalding with hot water.
- To reduce night coughing, prop up the head of your baby's cot at night by 5 cm (2 in). This will help the mucus drain away from the nasal passages. During the day your baby may appreciate being carried upright – a papoose or sling could make this easier.
- Outdoors cold air can trigger coughing if the airways are irritable. This is not harmful but can be upsetting for your baby. Being outside for a while is preferable to being cooped up indoors all day, so wrap him well when you go out.

Medical care
You will almost certainly have to tend to the symptoms of a cough or cold at some time.
- If your baby has a fever or high temperature, give him the treatments described on p.467. Infant paracetamol in the right dosage helps to reduce temperature and relieve pain. Keep your baby cool to help his temperature fall.
- Avoid cough suppressants (cough mixtures are all cough suppressants of some type or other) unless directed by a doctor, or your baby is unable to sleep because of coughing, or is coughing to the point of vomiting. The cough is useful to clear infection.
- Nasal decongestants may help. The best drops are salt water or saline drops, available over the counter or on prescription, which moisten and release mucus blockage and reduce the swelling. Do not make them up yourself as the concentration of salt is crucial. Other decongestant drops may contain medication to shrink the lining of the nasal passages and need to be prescribed; they are only for babies over 6–9 months. They are used for a maximum of 2 days because the swelling may increase if used for longer. If your baby has a blocked nose for months, your doctor or an ear, nose and throat specialist may consider a short course of steroid decongestants.
- The vast majority of coughs and colds are viral and will not respond to antibiotics. However, for the 10% of children whose illness is bacterial, prescribed antibiotics bring rapid improvement. Treatments for individual infections are covered in the following entries.

Massage and aromatherapy
In addition to other treatment you can ease congestion with massage:
- Rest your baby on your thighs, facing you as you sit with your knees raised. Press gently with one finger of each hand and trace the outline of his cheekbones from the top of the nose, down the sides, downwards and outwards to the side of the face. This helps to open the nostrils. Try it on yourself to get the technique right.
- Lie your baby on his back across your knees, with his head and trunk leaning back over the side of your lap. Lightly pat the centre of his chest with cupped hands. You can use a massage oil scented with lavender, myrrh and frankincense.
- After massaging his chest, turn him over so he lies across your lap on his belly, and gently pat his back with your cupped hands. This helps to expel mucus by compressing

the lungs and bronchial tubes. If your baby is very congested, he may vomit.

Aromatherapy oils that can help breathing if inhaled include eucalyptus, pine and lavender. Use a burner and dilute the oil in water (p.378).

Homeopathy

For colds: Over time you will learn which remedies your baby best responds to. Give the remedy (30c) 3–4 times a day for a few days and reassess. If your baby has recurrent colds, constitutional treatment under the care of a fully qualified homeopath would be most beneficial.

The usual remedy for first resort is *Aconite*, for sudden onset, cold after exposure to dry, cold, windy weather, worse at night, lots of sneezing, and perhaps a dry croupy cough, with restlessness and anxiety. Use *Arsenicum* for colds that head straight down to the chest, can be wheezy, with a watery acrid nasal discharge, making your baby thirsty for sips, perhaps accompanying DIARRHOEA; *Kali Bich* for thick, persistent, stringy mucus; *Natrum Mur* for recurrent colds or colds coming on with emotional upset in the family (e.g. bereavement), lots of sneezing in the morning, watery eyes, dry cracked lips, profuse, watery, nasal discharge that becomes thick and white; *Pulsatilla* for sniffles in the newborn accompanied by a lot of crying, and for recurrent colds with thick yellow-green mucus (often from the left nostril) with symptoms worse from lying down, clinginess and whining, and no thirst. For a very snuffly baby you can order a combination remedy to drain the mucus: *Kali Mur*, *Pulsatilla* and *Hydrastis* in a low 6x potency to give 3 times a day for up to 1 week.

For coughs: There are numerous remedies that can be used and there are subtle differences. Give the remedy that suits the symptoms in 30c, 3–4 times a day for 3 days and then reassess. The symptom picture may change several times if this is a lingering cough. If your baby has recurrent coughs, constitutional treatment is preferable as this would address the underlying susceptibility.

Use *Aconite* for a dry, irritating, croupy cough with sudden onset; *Arsenicum* for coughing that's worse around midnight, wheezy with intense restlessness and anxiety, perhaps accompanying diarrhoea, better for sipping at intervals; *Bryonia* for a hard, dry cough that hurts the chest, gives extreme thirst, dry lips and skin and is better for lying still; *Drosera* to help a violent, tickly cough that often comes in bouts ending in retching, choking, even vomiting, and is worse for lying down; *Ferrum Phos* when symptoms aren't intense and a cough follows a cold, is worse after eating and first thing in the morning, dry, hacking and hoarse, and lingers; *Hepar Sulph* for a barking, croupy, croaky cough with lots of mucus and an irritable mood; *Spongia* is good for a barking, croupy cough with hoarseness that may wake your baby in a panic in the earlier part of the night, though your baby won't be irritable – *Spongia* helps to open the bronchioles; *Phosphorus* for a dry, hard, ticklish cough that's worse for lying down but your baby still seems happy; *Pulsatilla* for the cough that is dry at night but productive in the morning with yellowish/greenish mucus, worse from lying down, and there is little thirst but your baby is weepy, clingy and miserable.

Bronchiolitis (RSV)
See also ASTHMA: BABY

Bronchiolitis is a common viral infection that affects over 90% of children by the age of 2 years. It is often caused by the respiratory syncitial virus (RSV), found in the air, but many other viruses cause similar illnesses. Babies are most susceptible in the first 4 weeks after birth. PREMATURE babies or those suffering from congenital HEART disease are more vulnerable.

What happens
Bronchiolitis starts with a cough, initially dry, with a tinny, metallic quality. After 3–4 days, or perhaps as long as a week, the cough becomes wetter, with a runny nose and your baby may go off his feeds. The cough usually brings on wheezing (like asthma) and symptoms tend to worsen for up to 5 days before improving. Usually there is no fever: if your baby gets a temperature after about 4 days, this probably indicates that a bacterium is also present in the bronchioles. The cough may linger for up to 8 weeks, but if your baby is feeding and putting on weight you can rest assured the cough will stop.

Action plan
In addition to the action advised on p.439:
- In general no specific medicines are needed. Your doctor may advise you to give an asthma treatment, such as salbutamol as a syrup. This may help.
- If your baby has a fever (bacterial infection), bronchiolitis will take longer to get better and he may need antibiotics for 5 days or so.
- You may visit your homeopath after a medical diagnosis: before 9 months it is not appropriate to home-prescribe.

Croup
See also BREATHING DIFFICULTIES: BABY

There are few things more frightening than the sound of your baby gasping for air and barking like a seal with a hollow, rasping noise. This is the classical sign of croup, a frightening but rarely serious infection. Croup is a respiratory infection, usually due to a virus, that leads to inflammation of the airways, the trachea, larynx and bronchi. It usually lasts 3–7 days and is generally worse at night. It is common between the ages of 3 months and 3 years, after which time the airways have enlarged, so breathing is less hampered if swelling occurs. If your baby is gasping for air, remember there is a possibility that he could be choking. Check his airway and if you believe he is choking you need to act quickly (p.384).

What happens
Infected by a virus, cells in the voice box and windpipe react by secreting mucus that narrows these air passages. The secretions dry and thicken, making it even more difficult for your baby to breathe.

Action plan
What you can do
- Try not to panic: remaining calm will lessen your child's

anxiety. Hold your baby – if he relaxes he may begin to breathe more easily.

- Take your child to the bathroom and close the door. Turn on the hot water to fill the room with steam. Do not put your child in the shower. Hold him in your arms while you sit on the toilet or a chair, but not on the floor.
- Open the window to let in cool air. This helps to create more steam. Allow at least 15 minutes for the steam to ease the symptoms. If the symptoms continue and this doesn't ease breathing, it is time to seek emergency care.
- If your baby begins to breathe more easily and is ready to go back to sleep, use a vaporiser in his room.
- Crying is a good sign. A crying child is able to breathe.
- A drink of cooled, boiled water may help.
- Feed your baby as usual, or let him suck for comfort.

Calling your doctor and medical care
During a croup attack it is a good idea to keep in touch with your baby's doctor.
Urgent medical attention is necessary if your baby shows the the following warning signs:

- He is struggling to breath in or out and has noisy breathing, even while calm, especially while breathing in.
- If his chest wall is moving unusually, with the front of the chest appearing to cave in towards the backbone while breathing in and there is a crowing noise as air passes through swollen air passages. This often occurs in the middle of the night, when the air is coolest.
- If he is restless, cannot sleep or is too breathless to feed.
- A throat infection known as epiglottitis may give croup-like symptoms, plus drooling and pushing out the lower jaw on breathing. This is very rare, but more dangerous because it may lead to MENINGITIS and needs hospital treatment.

Your doctor may prescribe oral or inhaled steroid medication, which can reduce the severity of symptoms, but your baby may need hospital treatment. Antibiotics are rarely required, but may be given if it is thought there is a bacterial infection.

Homeopathy
If the attack seems mild, try a remedy – if it is severe or you are concerned, get your baby seen by a medical doctor.

Aconite (30c) is usually the best remedy to give when croup begins, and again half an hour later. Then choose a remedy (30c) to give 2-hourly for 3 doses, before reassessing. Use *Aconite* if your baby seems very thirsty and coughs on breathing out, is very frightened and restless and may have a fever; *Hepar Sulph* if he is irritable with a hollow, croupy cough with rattling, thick, persistent mucus that makes him gag, he feels chilly and coughs more in the morning and evening and in the earlier part of the night; *Spongia* if he is terrified with a suffocating, dry, harsh cough that sounds like a saw going through wood, and laboured breathing with gasping.

Pneumonia

Pneumonia is a rare disease. The pneumonias are a group of illnesses involving infection of the lung, either by a virus or a bacterium. Most are viral, need no treatment and pass quickly (10–20:3000 babies). Viral pneumonia is infectious and is occasionally followed by a secondary bacterial infection. Much less common bacterial pneumonias (2:3000) are relatively serious and may be life threatening if untreated. Rarely, bacterial pneumonia is contracted at birth if a mother has CHLAMYDIA. Pneumonia can also be contracted from baby powder – some babies do get hold of it and mistake it for a bottle, gasping a mouthful into their airways. Pneumonia from inhaling powder may be fatal.

What happens
Most pneumonias start after a cold, when instead of recovering a baby gets worse and temperature rises. Newborns whose immune system is not mature are more susceptible, as are disabled children who are always lying horizontally.

Signs of pneumonia
- Your baby's breathing will become faster than 50 breaths a minute and he may grunt. He will look unwell and lethargic.
- He may have a fever. He may also seem chilled or shiver.
- He may have blue lips and nails if he is not getting enough oxygen.
- The space beneath his lower ribs may be drawn in as he breathes.
- He may cough out blood-tinged sputum.
- He may indicate pain on one side of the chest – this is the infected side.

Action plan
If your baby shows any of the above symptoms you must get him seen by a doctor.
- His chest may be inspected through x-ray.
- He will be given antibiotics, which usually bring a marked improvement in 2–3 days.
- He may be admitted to hospital if difficulty with breathing interferes with feeding or he appears to be deprived of oxygen. In hospital he may be given intravenous antibiotics , fed via a tube and given oxygen.

Fortunately, modern antibiotics are extremely effective and complete recovery can be expected in nearly every case within 7–14 days. Unless your baby has other problems, such as heart or lung disease, a further episode of pneumonia is rare.

Wheezing
See ASTHMA: BABY

Whooping cough
Whooping cough (**pertussis**) is a serious bacterial infection associated with severe bouts of distressing coughing and wheezing, and can be life threatening, particularly in babies aged less than 6 months. A baby below 6 months may not cough at all, but may a have episodes of apnoea (p.418), when breathing stops for a few seconds. Whooping cough can persist for months and is exhausting for the whole family.
VACCINATION against whooping cough is routinely offered to all babies in the UK.

What happens
Whooping cough often follows what seems to be a minor cold. It brings on episodes of coughing in runs (paroxysms) lasting

up to 5 minutes with a whoop on breathing in. Your baby will go red in the face and if coughing is severe, oxygen levels may fall and he may faint. Fainting stops the coughing and allows his body to recover. Whooping cough is called the 100-day cough because it may last this long before slowly easing up. If your baby catches a cold in the year after the initial illness, the cough is likely to return, not from re-infection (he has produced antibodies) but because his airways are irritable.

Action plan
Even with antibiotic treatment to attack bacteria the cough may remain, although the risk of infecting other people can be reduced. Often by the time a diagnosis is made the bacteria have been eliminated by the body, and the use of antibiotics makes no difference to the coughing, which comes on because the reflex to cough is quickly triggered when the airways are inflamed and sensitive.

While your baby has the cough, follow the general advice for colds and coughs (p.439). Comfort him and wipe excess mucus from his mouth. If the coughing causes him to retch and vomit, when the coughing fit has passed, offer him another feed. Homeopathy may be helpful but it is essential to see a qualified homeopath. Unfortunately, around eight unimmunised babies die from pertussis every year in the UK.

COUGH & COLD: MOTHER

See also ASTHMA: MOTHER; BREATHLESSNESS: MOTHER

As pregnancy advances and your uterus grows and pushes against your diaphragm and forces the lower ribs forwards, your lung capacity is reduced. For some women it increases BREATHLESSNESS and susceptibility to coughs and colds and chest infections. It can also affect asthma sufferers.

What happens
A chest infection may begin as a common cold, which is usually triggered by a virus. It might linger because you cannot breathe so deeply, particularly in late pregnancy when coughing may be less effective in clearing your chest. Infection may make your airways irritable, so even deep breathing could cause coughing. If you get a chest infection there is no risk to your baby unless you have asthma that becomes very severe.

Action plan
If you catch a cold or have an irritating cough, the priority is to look after yourself.

Medical care
• If the infection is bacterial, antibiotics may clear it. Antibiotics do not treat viral illness and the majority of coughs/colds are viral.
• You can use paracetamol in moderation – up to four 500 mg tablets daily, but preferably fewer. Remember that cold and flu remedy drinks contain paracetamol.
• You can safely take proprietary cough remedies in the second half of pregnancy, in moderation. Codeine linctus is also safe for a cough, in moderation.

• If you have a long-standing cough and irritable airways, your doctor may advise a combination of antibiotics, antispasmodics and inhaled steroids to reduce the cough, clear infection and reduce related asthma. The doses are carefully monitored.
• If you have a persistent cough that does not respond to treatment, a chest x-ray taken while your baby is screened with a lead apron can investigate underlying causes. Tuberculosis may rarely begin in pregnancy.
• For underlying sinusitis, your doctor may prescribe antibiotics. Other treatments include using a hot compress on the site of pain or swelling, steam inhalation, perhaps with eucalyptus oil, and gentle massage over the blocked sinus. A post-nasal drip from inflamed air passages or hay fever may cause a cough from mucus production. It may be viral or related to sensitivity to SMOKING or pollution. It may also be a food ALLERGY OR INTOLERANCE or inhaled molecules. It usually responds to decongestants.

Lifestyle and diet
• Drink plenty of water to keep dehydration at bay and mucus on the move. Keep up daily intake of vitamins and minerals.
• Hot water with a dash of lemon and honey may help: honey soothes the throat, lemon fights infection. Eat garlic and onions, cooked or raw; both are known for decongestant properties. Eat citrus fruits and fresh vegetables.
• When you feel up to it, aerobic exercise encourages deeper breathing and will clear your airways. Walking in the fresh air is particularly useful if your sinuses are blocked and you do not have irritable airways.
• If you smoke try to give up – it predisposes you to infection.
• Inhalation of steam may help to clear your chest: lean over a basin with hot water and drape a towel over your head, or run a hot shower in a small bathroom.
• Some yoga postures (p.346) give the lungs more room to expand, and may relieve discomfort.
• Avoid inhaling or consuming substances that you are allergic to.

Aromatherapy and homeopathy
You can use an oil in conjunction with steam, in your bath or with chest or head massage. Try lemon and, after Week 24, eucalyptus, tea tree, lavender or camomile. Homeopathy can be very effective. The suggestions for your baby's coughs and colds (p.439) also apply to you.

CROUP
See COUGH & COLD: BABY

CRYING

Crying is an integral part of your baby's communication. It is also a normal signal that something is upsetting him and he wants attention or help. At first you may be puzzled or worried by a normal cry, but over time you will get used to your baby's usual cry and your natural instincts will alert you when his cry is unusual or signals the need for urgent attention. Crying can put strain on the whole family and you may all need practical advice, comfort and reassurance. Babies who have a developmental difficulty may not show a recognisable pattern of crying and it may be more difficult to distinguish their normal crying from a cry of pain or illness.

Crying that does not feel 'normal' can indicates COLIC pains, and may come on at roughly the same time each day. This does not normally persist beyond the 3rd or 4th month, but from this time pained crying may be a sign of TEETHING. If your baby is crying and you cannot find a reason, it may signal approaching illness – often a baby cries several hours before showing the first symptoms of a cold, for instance.

It is time to take notice and seek extra support:
- If your baby suddenly cries in an unusual way and sounds distressed or in pain.
- If your baby's crying pattern changes and he cries for long periods.
- If your baby seems listless and does not cry as usual.
- If your baby is colicky and cries at a certain time of day.
- If the crying has no pattern and is excessive and incessant.
- If you are very upset and feel out of control.
- If there are signs of illness or a fever – 38°C (100.4°F) – when you should call your doctor.

There is information on causes of crying and tips for soothing your baby and and yourself at each stage of development on p.208 (0–12 weeks), p.240 (4–6 months) and p.263 (7–9 months).

CYSTIC FIBROSIS

See also CONGENITAL ABNORMALITIES

Cystic fibrosis (CF) is an inherited condition that leads to thickened mucus, which can block the airways and lead to lung infections. It also affects the digestive system. It has a large impact on daily life and can be debilitating. Today, life expectancy is 31 years. About 1:2500 babies born in the UK have the disease. For a baby to be affected, he must inherit a pair of defective copies of the CF gene – one from each parent.

What happens
The defective CF gene causes a protein called the cystic fibrosis transmembrane regulator to function abnormally. The flow of water and salts in and out of the body's cells is altered, creating a thick mucus. In the respiratory system, this blocks the airways and can cause infection and cysts to develop. In the digestive system CF makes it difficult to digest fats, proteins and the fat-soluble vitamins A, D, E and K. Babies with CF usually show bowel and chest symptoms within the 1st year. Some may have an obstructed bowel (p.437) from birth, and a smaller number suffer from recurrent rectal prolapse and CONSTIPATION.

Testing for CF
If a test in pregnancy (p.84) shows that you and your partner are both carriers, you will be offered genetic counselling and an AMNIOCENTESIS OR CVS to analyse your baby's genes. Not

all sufferers are identified in pregnancy but by 2004 all babies in the UK will be tested as part of the heel prick test, which is routine at 5–7 days after birth. Another test is the quick 'sweat' test, which analyses the content of salt in sweat, which is obtained by using a chemical on the baby's skin to make it sweat. The salt content is high in affected children and can be done from the 2nd month.

Action plan
The problems associated with cystic fibrosis can be reduced if the condition is diagnosed early. Caring for a baby with CF involves careful control of diet, including vitamin supplements, physiotherapy to remove sticky mucus, and the regular use of antibiotics to reduce infection in the lungs. A baby with CF is cared for by a medicalteam and usually based at a special centre but the role of parents is important, although their loving commitment can be stressful for them in the face of fear for the baby and concerns for future babies.

It is possible to text for CF in pregnancy (p.443) but at present there is no cure. However, ongoing research brings hope that gene replacement will become a reality. Until then the goals of treatment are to ease the symptoms and slow the progress of the disease.

CYSTITIS
See URINARY TRACT INFECTION: MOTHER

CYTOMEGALOVIRUS (CMV)

Cytomegalovirus (CMV) is a common viral infection in young children and roughly 50% of adults have been infected by age 30. Past infections are insignificant in pregnancy, but rare first time infection in pregnancy carries a small risk to a baby and, very rarely, the effect may be serious.

What happens
CMV usually causes no symptoms but infected adults occasionally develop an influenza-like illness, with a sore throat, fever, aching limbs and fatigue. It is a member of the herpes virus family and can be passed through contact with infected body fluids such as saliva, urine, blood and mucus. It also can be transmitted sexually and from mother to foetus during pregnancy. The infection can be passed to a baby during birth or in breast milk, but in these cases babies rarely develop serious problems from the virus because the mother has protective antibodies.

If you have been infected more than 6 months before conception, the risk of your baby becoming infected is low. If the virus reappears during pregnancy, the antibodies in your circulation will protect your baby. The only risk is if you are infected for the first time in pregnancy – an event affecting fewer than 1% of women: around one-third pass the infection to their babies, and 10–15% of these babies develop a serious illness. Congenital CMV may be obvious at birth but it may not give symptoms for months when it may lead to hearing or vision loss or developmental delay and learning difficulties.

Action plan

The most important thing is to take precautions. Most preventative measures during pregnancy relate to contact with children.

- Wash your hands thoroughly after any contact with the saliva and urine of young children, and carefully dispose of nappies, tissues and other potentially contaminated items.
- Avoid drinking from glasses children have been using – in some day-care centres, as many as 70% of children between the age of 1 and 3 years may be excreting the virus.

Testing for CMV in pregnancy is not routine. If you develop symptoms or request a test, your doctor may recommend two or more blood tests. In newborns CMV can be diagnosed within 3 weeks of birth through tests on blood or body fluids.

- If you are diagnosed with CMV in pregnancy, your baby can be tested for infection using AMNIOCENTESIS. The results are 80% reliable, but if your baby is shown to be infected, there is no way of telling how severe the infection is, or what effects it may have. You may be offered ultrasound scans to look closely at your baby's development. The advice of an specialist obstetrician and a genetic counsellor could help you consider the possibilities.
- At present there is no treatment to halt or reverse the effects of congenital CMV. Doctors are investigating whether a new drug may help: ganciclovir is currently used to treat adults with AIDS (p.485) who have CMV-related eye infections.

DEPRESSION

See EMOTIONS, DEPRESSION

DIABETES

The body's chief source of energy is glucose. The pancreas produces the hormone insulin, which assists the transfer of glucose from the bloodstream into body tissues. Diabetes mellitus is a disorder that inhibits insulin action or production. Pregnancy usually makes diabetes worse. Many women now test and control their blood sugar levels at home. There are three types of diabetes:

Gestational diabetes: Begins in pregnancy and disappears after birth. Women who have had gestational diabetes during one pregnancy are at greater risk of developing it in a subsequent pregnancy. Gestational diabetes is a mild form of Type II and 50% of women who have it develop Type II diabetes within 15 years.

Type II diabetes: 90% of diabetics have Type II or non-insulin dependent diabetes (formerly called adult-onset diabetes). It is often associated with obesity and can be controlled by following a careful diet and exercise programme, or with oral medication. A small number of people with Type II diabetes need insulin.

Type I diabetes: Occurs when the pancreas produces insufficient insulin. It is insulin dependent or juvenile-onset diabetes and the classic symptoms include fatigue, thirst, frequent urination and sudden weight loss. People with Type I diabetes must take insulin daily.

If you have Type I or II diabetes, you need to plan pregnancy carefully. Babies of diabetic mothers are at higher risk of CONGENITAL ABNORMALITIES and pregnancy- and birth-related complications but these risks can be greatly reduced when blood sugars are within normal range: it is best to control them before conception.

What happens

Hormones made by the placenta have a blocking effect on insulin. This is known as insulin resistance and usually begins around Weeks 20–24 and increases until delivery. In gestational diabetes the pancreas does not produce enough additional insulin to overcome the resistance.

Diagnosing gestational diabetes

Any woman might develop gestational diabetes during pregnancy and often there are no symptoms apart from sugar in the urine. Risks rise with obesity, a family history of diabetes or if a previous pregnancy was associated with too much AMNIOTIC FLUID, a LARGE BABY or a stillbirth (p.509). If your urine is shown to contain sugar on more than one occasion, a blood test can confirm diabetes. In some hospitals a blood sugar test is taken 2 hours after a sugar drink to screen for gestational diabetes around Weeks 24–28 because it may not be evident earlier. If the test is positive, a full glucose tolerance test is taken by measuring blood sugar levels on an empty stomach and then 1, 1½, 2 and 2½ hours after taking a glucose drink. If levels are elevated then gestational diabetes is diagnosed and close monitoring and treatment can begin, maximising the chances of the pregnancy continuing without problems.

The complications of gestational diabetes are less severe than with Type I. Women do, however, have a higher chance of contracting CANDIDA (thrush) infection and a URINARY TRACT INFECTION, and these may increase insulin resistance.

Implications for your baby

In pregnancy

The risks to babies of diabetic mothers are only marginally higher than in a non-diabetic pregnancy because it is possible to control blood sugar levels. The lower the levels of blood sugar, the lower the risks of complications. If blood sugar falls too low (hypoglycaemia, p.336) it can make you feel weak, confused, very hungry, shaky or sweaty. It can be dangerous for your baby because glucose is an essential fuel for the brain and for a baby and intense hypoglycaemia can lead to brain damage. Gestational diabetes generally does not cause birth defects, which mostly originate before the Week 13. The main, albeit rare, complications are:

- An excess of amniotic fluid, which may cause PREMATURE BIRTH or encourage your baby to take an awkward position (p.498).
- Excessive foetal growth because if high levels of blood sugar cross the placenta, your baby's endocrine system responds by producing insulin and growth factors that stimulate organ growth and fat deposition. Large babies are more susceptible to BIRTH INJURIES and BREATHING DIFFICULTIES and hypoglycaemia after birth. They may need to be delivered by CAESAREAN SECTION.

• Severe gestational diabetes can rarely lead to stillbirth. When maternal blood sugar is not controlled in Type I diabetes, congenital abnormalities may occur. The incidence is proportional to the severity of the diabetes, the control of blood sugar and if there are vitamin and mineral deficiencies in the mother. Poorly controlled Type I diabetes may also be associated with a higher risk of MISCARRIAGE and stillbirth (p.509) in late pregnancy.

After birth
The level of possible complications after birth relates directly to the extent to which blood sugar was out of control during pregnancy, and many babies of diabetic mothers do not have any difficulties.

• There is a chance that breathing difficulties (respiratory distress, p.418) may develop because the lungs tend to lack surfactant, the substance that allows the air passages to expand at birth.
• If your blood sugar levels have been high during pregnancy, your baby will have produced an excess of insulin to break down glucose. She will not be diabetic but will produce an excess of insulin for 5–10 days after birth. The excess production may lead to very low blood sugar levels. In a mild form this will leave her irritable, with jerky movements and behaving in an unsettled way. A prolonged fall may cause neurological damage because the brain needs sugar to function. The blood calcium and magnesium levels may also fall in the days after birth. Your baby will be monitored and frequent feeding usually prevents these complications.
• Your baby may have high levels of haemoglobin in her blood and has a slightly higher chance of developing neonatal JAUNDICE.
• In the long term a baby of a diabetic mother is at risk of developing Type II diabetes, and of having gestational diabetes in pregnancy.

Action plan
The key to a healthy pregnancy and giving birth to a healthy baby is to maintain blood sugar levels in the normal range.

Medical care
You will need frequent medical checks and help in order to keep blood sugar levels well controlled. If your hospital has the facility, attend a pregnancy diabetic clinic staffed by expert midwives, nutritionists, obstetricians and endocrinologists.

• Your blood may be analysed by looking at levels of glycosylated haemoglobin, a substance that increases if blood sugar levels are high; this gives an indication of the level of glucose in the blood over the previous few weeks.
• If you have a history of Type I diabetes, the team will monitor the retinal blood vessels in your eyes and your kidney function.
• NAUSEA & VOMITING need to be treated to maintain the stability of your blood sugar levels.
• The wellbeing of your baby will be closely monitored as for any HIGH-RISK PREGNANCY.

Monitoring your own blood sugar level and ketones
• You will be shown how to monitor your own blood sugar

levels. These indicate blood sugar control and the need for oral medication or insulin therapy.
• You may also be asked to check your urine for ketones daily, first thing in the morning and if your blood sugar level reads high. Ketones are by-products of the breakdown of fat and may occur as a result of inadequate insulin. When large amounts of ketones are present, they are accompanied by acidosis (p.473), which may harm a foetus over a long time. Acidosis will reduce your energy levels.

Diet
What and how you eat is a crucial aspect of care to reduce the symptoms of diabetes and reduce or exclude complications related to pregnancy. With advice from a nutritionist or a specialist midwife, and using the principles laid out in Eating and weight (p.332), establish and stick to a balanced diet to keep your blood sugar levels normal. Eating small amounts of slow-burning foods every 3–4 hours will help you avoid hypoglycaemia. Plan in advance so you do not skip meals, even if you feel exhausted.

• Use a basis of slow-burning carbohydrates because the sugar release is slow and decreases the need for insulin. Aim to get half your calorie intake from carbohydrates such as wholegrains, wholemeal or granary bread, vegetables, beans and pulses and starchy foods such as potatoes.
• Use the glycaemic index on p.336 to gauge which foods require the least insulin. These are the foods with the lowest glycaemic index score.
• Protein is useful as it acts in the long term to stabilise blood sugar. Have beans, eggs, fish or meat in at least two meals.
• Fibre slows down the release of glucose and helps to keep blood sugar levels from becoming too high. High-fibre foods include brown bread, brown rice, oats, vegetables with skins left on, nuts and seeds.
• Unsaturated fats and essential fatty acids are useful in moderate quantities but it is crucial to keep saturated fats (found in meats, cheese, cream, etc.) to a minimum because a diet high in fat causes insulin to act less efficiently.
• It is extremely important to avoid sugar-based foods and drinks: because your body does not release insulin adequately to respond to sugar intake, these will rapidly raise blood sugar levels. If you have cravings for something sweet, eat a whole fruit: but keep even whole fruits within limits because of their high sucrose content – don't eat more than two or three pieces a day, and space these, eating them after a carbohydrate-based meal where possible. Beware of fruit juice, which has a very high sugar content – avoid it.
• You also need to limit your salt intake: this is important because as a diabetic you are more susceptible to high BLOOD PRESSURE (pre-eclampsia).
• Your blood sugar levels may drop during the night, bringing on hypoglycaemia, which could stimulate your body to produce ketones (above) that are potentially harmful for your baby. A late-night snack providing protein and complex carbohydrates can guard against this, e.g. brown rice and chicken, a small baked potato with a bean salad, or a wholemeal sandwich with poached fish. The starch stabilises blood sugar levels in the early night and the long-acting protein will stabilise them later on.

Weight gain

Weight gain in pregnancy (p.332) is a very important issue. Not gaining enough may result in INTRAUTERINE GROWTH RESTRICTION for your baby with low reserves of energy, while gaining too much gives extra body fat that produces an insulin-resistant effect. Optimal weight gain depends on your weight before pregnancy – your medical team or dietician will recommend a realistic goal. Diabetic women are advised to return to pre-pregnancy weight within 4 months after birth.

Exercise and rest

Muscles use glucose when they are active, thus reducing glucose levels without the need for insulin from the pancreas. Exercise (p.357) may also help to reduce any cravings for sweets. If you are on insulin you will need to take some precautions. Exercise lowers blood sugar levels, as does insulin, and the combination may lead to hypoglycaemia. When you exercise it is important to take sugar with you in case your blood sugar becomes too low. You may be able to avoid this with regular slow-burning meals and small nutritious snacks between meals on the days you exercise. Rest and relaxation are important and help you to plan to cover all your needs, including the control of your blood glucose.

Birth

If your baby is not too large and your diabetes is controlled, you may safely await the onset of labour. If sugar levels are not controlled, it may be best for your baby to be born between Weeks 36 and 40; the exact time will depend on her condition.

During labour it is important to control blood sugar levels by having snacks or using an intravenous drip. If you give birth vaginally your baby will be closely monitored for FOETAL DISTRESS & ASPHYXIA and your doctor will be aware of potential difficulties if she is large. Gestational diabetes alone is not an indication for a caesarean section, but there can be other reasons.

After the birth

Insulin requirements drop rapidly as placental hormones decrease. If you are taking insulin, you will need to decrease the dose. You need to monitor your blood sugar levels, food intake and insulin doses very closely to prevent hypoglycaemia. This is particularly important if you are not eating well while you recover after a caesarean.

If you had gestational diabetes, continue with a nutritious diet and closely spaced meals and take vitamin and mineral supplements. This will keep your energy high, improve the flow of breast milk if you are breastfeeding, and reduce long-term complications. Because of the risk of developing Type II diabetes, have your blood sugar level checked annually.

Your baby after birth

Your baby's breathing will be monitored for a few hours and she will be checked for jaundice in the days that follow. Her blood sugar levels will be monitored for the first few days to check for hypoglycaemia. Feeding her frequently will keep her blood sugar levels normal. Breastfeeding may contribute to your postnatal weight loss, and could reduce your baby's chances of developing diabetes in later life.

DIARRHOEA: BABY

It is quite normal for a baby to pass several stools a day, or just one in several days, and if your baby is breastfed, her stools may be loose. Diarrhoea is a sudden increase in the amount of stools, and looser or more watery stools than usual. The main concern with diarrhoea is that if it persists it may lead to dehydration.

What happens

Most mild episodes of diarrhoea last less than 24 hours and pass without treatment. Mild diarrhoea involves three or four loose but small motions in 24 hours. A child like this who is happy and drinking well is not a concern. Moderate diarrhoea involves five to six medium volume loose stools in 24 hours. Diarrhoea is severe when there are eight or more profuse watery stools that leak out of the nappy and soil the clothes.

Dehydration

Dehydration may accompany diarrhoea. A younger baby will more easily become dehydrated as the other body systems for regulating water in the body, such as the kidneys, are immature. If your baby is also losing fluid from VOMITING, sweating from a FEVER or the room temperature is high, this will increase the risks of dehydration.

Signs of mild dehydration include dry lips, although the inside of the mouth remains moist, and your baby will babble and play for short periods. There will be less urine. With adequate fluid intake and improving diarrhoea, mild dehydration usually passes.

Severe dehydration makes the lips and mouth dry and brings on listlessness and there is no urine for 8 or more hours. Your baby may not produce tears and her skin may appear pale or blotchy. Because your baby feels weak, she may suck feebly or refuse to drink. In addition, the fontanelle on her head may appear slightly sunken. If she is very dehydrated you need to call your doctor immediately – severe cases need hospital treatment. The medical diagnosis for severe dehydration is a loss of 15% of body weight since the illness began. For a very few babies, dehydration may lead to shock and long-term damage if fluid replacement has not been started within 24 hours or the fluid loss is unusually severe.

Causes

Diarrhoea may result from one of a number of causes. When its root is infection, your baby is contagious for a couple of days before the onset of diarrhoea and while diarrhoea persists. The germ can be passed through touch: it is very important to wash your hands before touching food, and before and after changing a nappy. Sometimes diarrhoea is a reaction to antibiotics given for other reasons.

Gastroenteritis and food poisoning

Most cases of diarrhoea result from gastroenteritis, which is caused by a viral infection that affects the lining of the gut and may also cause vomiting. Other symptoms may include a fever or stomach pain. Gastroenteritis may last for a week or longer, and may appear to get better and then flare up again.

If there is blood or mucus in the stools, the infection may stem from bacterial food poisoning. This brings on diarrhoea and often vomiting, together with abdominal cramps, within 1–6 hours of consuming the food. Poisoning is classically caused by a bacterium called Staphylococcus aureus, which contaminates food left at room temperature, particularly dairy and meat products. The symptoms improve within 8–24 hours. In some cases parasites cause the infection, usually from contaminated water. E. coli, a bacterium present in some undercooked meats, can cause bloody diarrhoea and requires immediate treatment, perhaps in hospital, because it may result in a severe illness involving other organ systems, especially the kidneys and liver.

Diet and food intolerance
Diarrhoea can occur if your baby drinks too much fruit juice or has an ALLERGY OR INTOLERANCE. If stools appear to be a strange colour, for instance very red or orange, this may reflect what your baby has eaten (e.g. red cordial, carrots, yams).

Bowel disorders
Stools that look like redcurrant jelly may signify **intussusception**, a condition that may occur from birth onwards where the bowel folds inside itself. This causes an obstruction with diarrhoea (mostly blood and mucus) and acute CONSTIPATION from the blocked bowel, and needs urgent surgical treatment. CYSTIC FIBROSIS is a rare cause of diarrhoea, with sticky stools, and usually has accompanying respiratory symptoms and a failure to gain WEIGHT.

Action plan
If your baby has diarrhoea the most important thing is to avoid dehydration. Your baby's bottom may be sore and she will be more comfortable if you treat the nappy rash (p.531). Remember your hygiene: wash your hands after you have been to the toilet and after each nappy change. Keep your baby's hands clean too.

Medical care
If your baby appears dehydrated, call your doctor. She might need treatment in hospital where she can be given fluids to provide the salt and electrolytes and sugar she has lost. Never administer medicines yourself – they may cause harm.

Give your baby fluids
- If you are breastfeeding, encourage her to feed frequently, and let her suck whenever she shows an interest: the sucking motion is soothing, the milk is good for her and its fluid content hydrates. This may suffice for mild diarrhoea. For moderate diarrhoea you can give your baby a rehydration solution (below) between feeds.
- If you are bottle feeding and your baby is less than 6 months old, stop formula for 24 hours. She still needs fluid, however, so give her cooled, boiled water frequently or preferably use an oral rehydration solution. If vomiting stops, even if diarrhoea persists, re-introduce the milk feed after 24 hours. If she is over 6 months old, 12 hours off the milk feed may be sufficient.
- Rehydration solutions can be bought in chemists. They are powders to be mixed with cooled, boiled water that contain a balanced mixture of electrolytes, which replace those lost in the diarrhoea. If your baby doesn't want to drink, or is vomiting up fluid, frequently offer her sips of the solution – even as little as a teaspoon at a time will help. Do not make your own solution of sugar and salt and do not use a rehydration solution alone for longer than 24 hours without consulting your doctor. If the vomiting has settled, and it usually does within 24 hours, switch back to milk.
- Avoid fruit juices or sugary drinks as their high sugar content can prolong or aggravate diarrhoea and they do not contain the right balance of salts.
- If your baby is still not keeping any fluid down, see your doctor or go to your nearest casualty department urgently. Take your baby's parent health record with you – the doctor can estimate weight loss, and thus the extent of dehydration, by comparing her weight with a recent reading.

Re-introducing solids for your weaned baby
- When your baby feels like eating again and her stools have become semi-solid, begin with easily digestible foods such as *b*ananas, *r*ice cereal, *a*pples and white *t*oast (BRAT diet). Stewed fruits may increase diarrhoea.
- Avoid dairy products (but not breast milk) because while she has diarrhoea she may be susceptible to developing an intolerance to milk. Lactose and sucrose intolerance can occur as a temporary phenomenon after diarrhoea (p.393).
- If she doesn't feel like eating, do not worry, as long as she is drinking well. She is well hydrated if her nappies are regularly wet with urine.

Homeopathy
If your baby's diarrhoea is severe, has lasted for longer than 24 hours or there is any sign of dehydration, consult your doctor. For mild diarrhoea that may be accompanied by vomiting, give the appropriate remedy (30c) hourly for 4 hours, then every 2 hours for 8 hours, and reassess. With improvement, give the remedy 4 times a day for a few days. If symptoms change, use a different remedy.

Use *Arsenicum* when there is chilliness, restlessness, exhaustion and anxiety, vomiting, and if the cause is ice cream or spoiled fruit; *Chamomilla* when diarrhoea accompanies teething, is greenish and your baby is irritable; *Phosphorus* for exhausting diarrhoea that is painless, but profuse, there is an urge to drink but fluid is vomited, or if diarrhoea occurs after a shock and is accompanied by anxiety, although your baby seems good-humoured; *Podophyllum* for explosive stools the consistency of batter (often greenish), accompanied by a lot of wind and COLIC; *Pulsatilla* when stools are changeable and there is vomiting, perhaps after eating rich food, your baby is whiny and clingy, not thirsty; *Sulphur* for watery, frothy diarrhoea, worse on waking, and a red, sore anus.

Recovering from diarrhoea
After a mild bout of diarrhoea it may take your baby 2–3 days to get her energy back, although her stools may continue to be watery for up to 2 weeks as the bowel recovers. Sometimes temporary damage to the lining of the bowel wall results in the loss of the enzyme lactase, essential for digesting lactose in

milk, and a temporary allergy or intolerance that gives rise to watery stools and does pass. For a time, a non-cow's milk formula may be needed – follow your doctor's advice. When your baby recovers, you may return to the usual formula. After a bout of diarrhoea or with prolonged diarrhoea, it is important to have your baby's WEIGHT monitored regularly. If she is not gaining normally, your doctor will advise you how best to treat the underlying cause.

DIARRHOEA: MOTHER

If your stools become loose and watery and you have three or more motions a day, you may have diarrhoea, particularly if they contain mucus or if there is blood. In some pregnancies bowel movements become more frequent because of altered eating and drinking habits or the intestine or colon's reaction to hormonal changes. Diarrhoea is not common in pregnancy. It is a relatively common symptom of pre-labour when hormones released to stimulate the uterus also stimulate the intestinal walls to contract (p.123).

What happens
Diarrhoea is usually due to a viral or bacterial infection (gastroenteritis or food poisoning). In pregnancy it has no effect on your baby. If it continues for more than 3 days, it is worth requesting a stool culture. With a severe infection you may have NAUSEA & VOMITING or a fever.

Diarrhoea may arise from a rapid change in diet: for instance, it takes time for your intestine to adapt to an increase in roughage or to supplements, particularly iron – you can assess this by stopping the supplements and seeing if the diarrhoea lessens and then altering the type of supplement. It may be better to take your supplement before a main meal.

If diarrhoea persists for weeks, it may be due to an ALLERGY OR INTOLERANCE. You may need to watch what you eat and how your body reacts, and then cut down on any suspicious food. On rare occasions diarrhoea is a symptom of bowel disease (below right) that may flare up, or begin for the first time in pregnancy.

Action plan
Diet
- Drink to replace lost fluid and electrolytes. Rehydration powders from pharmacists replace bodily electrolyte reserves faster than water. Electrolyte drinks for runners boost energy rapidly and are available in pharmacies and gyms. Light soups also contain electrolytes. If you cannot stomach these, it is important simply to drink any fluid that appeals but avoid fizzy drinks or sweet cordials.
- After 24 hours if you feel like eating, choose bananas for their high potassium (salt) content, dry white rice and white toast, whose low-fibre carbohydrates won't irritate the bowel. After 48 hours introduce gentle, fat-free foods: soups, boiled potatoes, cooked vegetables and egg. When symptoms subside, gradually return to your normal diet. Leave dairy and milk products until you feel 100% but do try bio-yoghurt to replace normal bowel bacteria.

- If diarrhoea is an ongoing problem it is important to maintain adequate nutrition for you and your baby – you may need supplements so you feel well and avoid the risk of developing iron-deficiency ANAEMIA.

Medical care
- If diarrhoea is severe and you are dehydrated, you need to be examined immediately by your doctor. If you feel dehydrated or blood is in your stools treatment is important.
- If diarrhoea persists, a stool culture can exclude or confirm an infection. Your doctor may also consider inflammatory bowel disease, ulcerative colitis and Crohn's (below).
- Opiate derivatives such as loperamide and diphenoxylate are found in a number of branded treatment drugs and may be prescribed if diarrhoea is severe; although they are not licensed for use in pregnancy your baby is not likely to be affected by them. Codeine phosphate is also an opiate and is safe in pregnancy and can be prescribed by your doctor.
- In late pregnancy, if diarrhoea is present your doctor or midwife may want to examine you; labour may have begun.

Homeopathy
Choose a remedy that suits your symptoms and take it in 30c potency, 4 times a day for a few days unless there is no change within 24 hours, in which case you will need to reassess. If diarrhoea becomes severe, it is best to visit your doctor.

Use *Arsenicum* for diarrhoea accompanied by chilliness, restlessness and anxiety, burning pains in the abdomen and a desire for sips of warm drinks, or when diarrhoea and vomiting follow a meal of spoiled fruit or meat; *Carbo Veg* for diarrhoea with extreme flatulence, abdominal pain and cramping with faintness and breathlessness; *Lycopodium* if you are anxious and your motions are accompanied by lots of wind, or if you have eaten bad shell fish; *Podophyllum* for painless but profuse diarrhoea with sudden motions accompanied by gurgling and rumbling and you feel weak and drained; *Sulphur* for watery, sour-smelling diarrhoea that drives you out of bed in the morning and makes your anus sore, red and burning. When the infection has passed, particularly if you have lost fluids, take *China* (30c) morning and night for 1 week; it acts as a mental and physical pick-up.

Aromatherapy
Essential oil of tangerine used in the bath or for massage may help. From Week 24 of pregnancy you can use camomile oil.

Irritable & inflammatory bowel diseases
Uncommonly, diarrhoea persisting for weeks may be a symptom of **irritable bowel syndrome** (IBS), a condition where the muscle in the wall of the intestine is irritable and contracts frequently, causing abdominal pain and diarrhoea, often associated with bloating and sometimes alternating with CONSTIPATION. The irritability may be sparked by emotional upsets or by food allergy or intolerance. IBS often improves but may worsen in pregnancy. If you are aware of trigger feelings or foods, you will be able to control your symptoms. IBS does not affect your baby and usually predates pregnancy.

Inflammation of the bowel called **Crohn's disease** (small intestine) and **ulcerative colitis** (colon) is uncommon but rarely occurs for the first time during pregnancy. It is characterised by profuse diarrhoea and symptoms similar to IBS, but there may also be mucus and blood in stools, abdominal distension and you may feel very unwell. Women who already have the condition usually find symptoms improve in pregnancy.

Action plan
To make a definitive diagnosis of IBS a bowel x-ray and/or colonoscopy examination (inserting a finger-size camera into the anus to inspect the colon) is needed but these are usually delayed until after birth. The diagnosis is usually based on your symptoms until the birth.
- Avoiding triggers may be sufficient.
- If symptoms are severe it may be necessary to take anti-inflammatory drugs or steroid hormones, usually by enema. This needs to be done by a doctor who is a gastroenterologist used to treating such bowel problems. Steroid enemas are reputed to be safe in low doses (p.389).
- Your obstetrician needs to monitor your baby's growth because it may be reduced (p.488) if your diarrhoea is severe and leads to mineral and vitamin deficiencies.
- Your nutrition will need to be monitored and blood tests will check for anaemia. You may need extra vitamins, minerals and iron.
- If you choose homeopathy, visit your homeopath for a remedy to fit your precise symptom picture.

DISPROPORTION IN LABOUR
See LABOUR, DISPROPORTION

DOWN'S SYNDROME & OTHER CHROMOSOMAL ABNORMALITIES
....
See also CONGENITAL ABNORMALITIES; Down's syndrome testing (p.84)

There are 23 pairs of chromosomes in every cell. The term trisomy describes the presence of three chromosomes. If a baby is born with three of the number 21 chromosomes she has trisomy 21, more commonly known as Down's syndrome. It is the most common trisomy disorder.

A Down's syndrome child may be floppy because of reduced muscle tone and has specific physical features, including low-set ears, a relatively large tongue, a small round face, a flattened back of the head, almond-shaped eyes that slant upwards and small hands with one palmar crease instead of two. Hearing and visual development may be delayed, affecting language development, and there may be associated HEART problems and congenital abnormalities of the digestive system. There is always significant reduction in mental development. Emotional development is specific: Down's syndrome children are vulnerable and often find it difficult to express their emotions and to read accurately the emotions of others. Nonetheless, a child with Down's syndrome is usually very loving and enthusiastic. Expected life span for a person with Down's syndrome is about 55 years although

susceptibility to leukaemia, thyroid disease and Alzheimers is increased.

What happens
Of babies with Down's syndrome, 95% have trisomy 21 – a triple set of chromosome 21 in every cell. Occasionally an extra chromosome 21 is attached to another chromosome; this is called translocation Down's syndrome (3–4% of cases). This is the only form that can sometimes be inherited from a parent, although a parent may show no signs of the defect. In 2%, mosaic Down's syndrome occurs when some cells have an extra chromosome 21 while others have the normal pair.

Action plan
Screening in pregnancy
Screening for Down's syndrome is now a standard part of antenatal testing, using the 12-week (nuchal) ultrasound scan and a triple blood test (p.84). If these screening tests suggest a risk of Down's syndrome that is greater than 1:250, you will be offered an AMNIOCENTESIS OR CVS, which enables your baby's chromosomes to be analysed. Some parents choose not to have these screening tests. The risk of Down's increases with a mother's age and in many hospitals women over 35 years are offered an amniocentesis or CVS. As the ultrasound and blood tests improve in accuracy, the need for amniocentesis and CVS decreases. If you go ahead and the result comes back positive, you will be faced with a difficult decision: you may consider terminating your pregnancy, or want to find out more about Down's syndrome and make choices for your future as a family. You may wish to contact your local Down's syndrome support group. Increasingly sophisticated antenatal tests detect most Down's babies during pregnancy.

Screening after birth
If your baby has not been diagnosed in pregnancy but shows signs of Down's syndrome at birth, your birth team will advise testing your baby's blood to study chromosome 21. Awaiting the results is an anxious time and you will most likely need support during this period.

Treatment and care
No specific treatment is available for Down's syndrome, but your baby will be thoroughly examined to ensure that she has no other physical problems. The degree of learning difficulty varies and early educational opportunities will help to maximise her potential.

Your baby will need regular medical follow-up and treatment, usually given by a paediatrician with a special interest in the condition. It is best to treat any hearing or visual problems before they hinder language development. The best treatment for your baby is receive love, attention and care and to be welcomed as part of your family.

Other chromosomal abnormalities
Trisomy with an extra chromosome may affect any chromosome pair. The extra chromosome is associated with a much higher chance of MISCARRIAGE or severe defects. The defects are often detected on ultrasound scans in pregnancy. Down's syndrome is the most common condition resulting

from a trisomy. Others include **Edward's syndrome**, with trisomy of chromosome 18, and **Patau's syndrome**, with trisomy 13. These rare disorders either lead to miscarriage or a combination of birth defects, including severe mental retardation, as well as health problems involving nearly every organ system in the body. Of babies born with trisomy 18 or 13, 90% die by age 1. The birth defects may mean that a baby does not come home from hospital after birth, and families need a great deal of support. There is no cure and, to date, no way to prevent any incidence of trisomy.

Turner syndrome (monosomy X) occurs in 1:2500 girls who are born with only one X sex chromosome, rather than the usual pair (XX). The missing sex chromosome usually comes from the sperm cell, and there is no link with maternal age nor is it inherited. The condition may be detected in pregnancy if ultrasound findings (swollen tissue in the neck) have prompted amniocentesis and chromosomal testing. Some babies with Turner syndrome have other health problems involving the heart or kidneys and have a webbed neck with low hairline or ears. Roughly one-third of affected girls show characteristic features at birth, and a blood sample can give an accurate diagnosis of the chromosomes. A third display signs in childhood and a third are diagnosed in their late teens, when there have been no signs of puberty. Affected girls are born with absent ovaries, do not grow to full adult height and cannot go through puberty. Hormone therapy can increase growth and promote menstruation. Infertility cannot be corrected, however. Intelligence is often normal but there is an increased incidence of learning disabilities.

There are a number of other less common chromosomal disorders. These include a disorder with 23 extra chromosomes (giving a total of 69 instead of the usual 46), which leads to miscarriage and does not tend to recur. Deletions of parts of the chromosome or absent chromosomes are usually associated with miscarriage. The abnormality is confirmed by placental culture. Sometimes there is a translocation where a part of one chromosome has moved on to another chromosome. If the translocation is balanced by a part of the other chromosome moving across, then it is compatible with normal life. If it is not balanced, miscarriage usually results. A culture of the parents' blood may show the translocation is inherited from one parent. With translocation there may be miscarriages but there is usually a pregnancy resulting in a healthy baby.

DRUGS, RECREATIONAL

See also ALCOHOL; SAFETY (p.388); SMOKING

The use of drugs in pregnancy presents health risks to a mother, may threaten pregnancy and can harm a baby, in some cases severely. Medications for illness need to be prescribed by your doctor with concern for the of your baby. Usually women who become pregnant are keen to avoid recreational drugs. But for some, stopping is not easy, not only because addictions are hard to kick, but because the underlying emotions that contribute to the need for relief can be difficult to address. Some 50% of people under 35 have experimented with

recreational drugs. One-third are regular users and 3% have an addiction problem. Women who consume drugs have HIGH-RISK PREGNANCIES.

Unfortunately, women with addictions may feel that many midwives and obstetricians have a flimsy grasp of the issues. Some mothers do not seek antenatal care, often because they feel guilty or worry that they will not receive sympathetic treatment but many who confide in a medical team receive support, which continues after birth.

Your feelings
When you become pregnant there may be an internal battle between your desire to continue the drug and the wish to do the best for your baby, and a fear of the feelings that may surface if you do stop. If it proves difficult to stop, you may feel guilty and angry. Guilt prevents many women from admitting their problem and seeking help. Acknowledging your feelings may be the first step towards seeking a way out.

What happens
The effect of drugs on a baby is directly proportional to the amount taken during pregnancy and will be combined with any adverse effects from poor diet, smoking or regular alcohol consumption, both of which commonly accompany drug use. When drug use involves sharing implements there is a higher risk of infection, particularly with needles that can spread diseases such as HEPATITIS B and C and HIV. The effect of usage before and during pregnancy has not been conclusively proven for all drugs, but guidelines do exist. Many babies exposed to drugs in the womb show withdrawal symptoms after birth (neonatal abstinence syndrome, opposite) and reduced performance at school age.

Street drugs taken in pregnancy
Amphetamine (speed): Causes a severe effect with constriction of the blood vessels and reduction in oxygen for the unborn baby. It also suppresses a mother's appetite, reducing nutrition for her baby, and increases the risk of PLACENTAL ABRUPTION, PREMATURE BIRTH, INTRAUTERINE GROWTH RESTRICTION (IUGR) and stillbirth (p.509).

Cannabis/marijuana: This is the most common recreational drug used by pregnant women. Usually it is mixed with nicotine before being smoked, and it is the nicotine that carries the greatest risk. Consumed alone, cannabis may be linked to IUGR and other effects on the baby. Cannabis is less hazardous than amphetamine, cocaine and heroin or alcohol.

Cocaine and crack: These constrict the blood vessels, reducing oxygen flow to the foetus, and have a major effect on foetal development and health. Cocaine suppresses the appetite so a mother may not provide adequate nutrition for her unborn baby. Regular use carries a high chance of congenital abnormality of the HEART, intestine, brain or limbs (35%) and of IUGR (30%). The effects may be worse than heroin. There is also risk of MISCARRIAGE, placental abruption and stillbirth, and of premature birth because cocaine stimulates uterine contractions. Where brain growth has been affected there may be slow mental development for life. It may also be connected with sudden infant death syndrome (p.510).

Heroin and methadone (opiates): These cross the placenta and increase the risk of death in-utero and premature birth. A baby's withdrawal symptoms can be severe, often coming on a few days after birth and lasting weeks (below).

Everyday drugs

The most significant drugs used as part of everyday life are alcohol and nicotine. Both can have implications if consumed in pregnancy. These are covered separately.

Caffeine intake has been linked with an increased risk of miscarriage and small babies (IUGR). In addition, when a mother consumes caffeine in tea, coffee, colas, energy drinks or chocolate, her baby feels the same effects as she does and after birth may experience withdrawal. During the second half of pregnancy caffeine is cleared very slowly from your body and this is the time to reduce the intake substantially.

Action plan

The best thing to do is to stop drug consumption. The less you consume, the smaller the potential effect on your baby, and the better your own health. When you are pregnant, you do not have the luxury of time to phase out consumption. Stopping may require effort and commitment. You may find it useful to take the steps outlined below and to approach the change with the use of the Wheel for Living (p.58). When drug use continues, it is best to let your medical team know so they can act in the best interests of safety for you and your baby.

Tips for quitting

Eat well: Vitamin and mineral deficiencies are common in women who smoke, drink or take drugs, perhaps because there is a reliance on 'fast' or packaged foods or a suppression of appetite. Attending to your nutrition will improve your health and is good for your baby (p.332).
Exercise and rest: Exercise taken on a regular basis kick-starts the body into health, improves circulation and metabolism and makes the body less reliant on substances that are not good for it. It may also help you let go of a psychological habit. Meditation, visualisation or yoga can be similarly powerful.
Lifestyle: If you regularly do activities that are linked with drug consumption, cut down on the activities. If your drug habit is linked to places you visit, or your pattern of relaxation at home, you may be able to get through usual consumption times more easily if you are occupied doing other things. A quitting or help group may make this easier.
Consider why you use drugs: If you want to give up, you'll need to look at how the drug affects your feelings. Many people find this difficult, particularly because taking a drug is often a way of skirting difficult emotions. You could keep a diary of your feelings before and after consumption. This will increase your awareness and help you look at practical ways to change. Hypnotherapy may be helpful to stay off medication.

Stopping

When you give up a drug you may experience physical symptoms of withdrawal and experience powerful urges to consume again. Strong feelings may also surface and you will not be able to take the drug to suppress these emotions. One of the key commitments for successfully giving up is to 'be in your feelings' and experience the discomfort of being upset or angry or afraid. In the short term this can be very difficult, and you will need lots of support. In the long run you may feel stronger and more in touch with yourself.

Medical care

Your doctor can advise you about the type of drug you are using and the safer alternatives for you and your baby. Nicotine replacement therapy doubles the quit rate for smoking but during pregnancy patches may be damaging for your baby, as are replacement drugs for opiates.

Homeopathy

If you visit your homeopath, you will be prescribed specific remedies. Broadly speaking, the following may be useful, but should be taken under guidance.

Use *Arsenicum* to deal with the effects of long-term alcohol abuse if you are usually chilly, pale and emaciated with extreme anxiety, restlessness and guilt; *Nux Vomica* as a detox remedy and to address the effects of withdrawal such as shaking, twitching, trembling and irritability; *Quercus* for diminishing alcoholic cravings – can be used daily in low potencies (6c) over a period of time; *Sulphur* also for detox, particularly when energy and moods fluctuate.

Support groups

Stopping drug use often requires medical support and emotional counselling or therapy. A quitting or support group may provide an environment where you are supported as you acknowledge and attempt to shake off your addiction.

Craving and slipping up

Try not to be upset when you feel a strong urge to smoke/drink/take your drug. Look to the deep-breathing techniques on p.346 and acknowledge the physical and emotional feelings. It may take weeks or months for your cravings to pass but they eventually do diminish.

Most people slip up from time to time. Try to accept your addiction, acknowledge you gave in to your urges, and re-commit to keeping away from the drug. To make things easier, try not to rationalise – 'I have given up for a while and a small dose will make no difference.' This is not true because addictive drugs work on a physical level and your body takes time to shake off physical dependency.

Pregnancy is an opportunity to give up drug use once and for all. Yet, although many women do give up, it is surprisingly common for them to take up the habit again after the birth. If you have given up during pregnancy, you may make a commitment to stop permanently.

Neonatal abstinence syndrome

Neonatal abstinence syndrome (NAS) is what a baby experiences when withdrawing from drugs. Foetal alcohol syndrome refers to withdrawal symptoms following alcohol use in pregnancy. Some drugs are more likely to cause NAS. Opiates like heroin and methadone cause withdrawal in over half of the babies exposed. This may occur with cocaine, too, but the main symptoms in the baby are due to the effects of the drug in the womb. Amphetamines, barbiturates, narcotics and benzodiazepines (e.g. Valium) can also cause withdrawal.

What happens

Addiction begins in the womb and dependence continues after birth. The drug is no longer available and the baby's central nervous system becomes over-stimulated. Symptoms of withdrawal vary depending on the drug, the quantity used and if a baby is premature. They may begin 24 hours after birth or not until 10 days later, and could last for months.

The most common symptoms of NAS are: tremors (trembling); irritability (excessive and high-pitched crying); SLEEP PROBLEMS; hyperactive reflexes; FITS or seizures; stuffy nose and sneezing; poor feeding and suck; vomiting and/or diarrhoea; sweating or unstable temperature. In addition to withdrawal symptoms, some babies may need special care for the effects of the drug. Babies suffering from withdrawal are often hard to soothe and swaddling (p.203) may help. Medical treatment will be directed by your paediatrician.

EAR, HEARING DIFFICULTIES

If your baby appears to have difficulty hearing, or hears nothing at all, it is useful to know there are three types of hearing loss, and deafness may be temporary. For most babies the problem is a conductive hearing loss, caused by wax blockage or glue ear (p.454). After investigation you can consider the best course of action, and get support if your baby does have permanent hearing loss. The sooner you do this, the greater his chance of developing language and communication skills at the same rate as hearing children. About 1:1000 babies born in the UK each year is deaf.

Signs of hearing difficulties
- In the first days and weeks your baby doesn't startle, blink or open his eyes in response to a sudden sound.
- At 1 month he doesn't stay still to listen if you make a sudden, continuous sound.
- At 3 months he doesn't calm down as your voice quietens.
- At 6 months he doesn't turn towards the sound of your voice when you are across the room or when you make a quiet noise to the side of his head.
- At 9 months he has not begun to babble, or does not look for a sound that is made by something he cannot see.
- At 12 months he does not respond when you call his name.
- As time goes on, you may notice your toddler is late learning to speak, shouts and is inattentive, especially at story time. He may not respond to music, give inappropriate answers to questions and have difficulty distinguishing between similar-sounding words, particularly when the words begin with f, sh or s. He may turn his head to favour one ear when listening.

What happens

Conductive hearing loss: Reflects a problem with the outer or middle ear. This includes temporary hearing loss caused by EAR INFECTIONS such as glue ear and colds and ALLERGIES. It is usually mild but can delay understanding and language development if the underlying cause is not treated.
Sensory hearing loss: Occurs when there is malfunction of the inner ear or damage to the auditory nerve. When the nerve is damaged, hearing loss is usually permanent. This can be genetic, or may be caused by a serious illness like MENINGITIS. It can also occur in the womb if the mother contracts RUBELLA or has LISTERIA infection. PREMATURE babies and those who have severe asphyxia (p.472) at birth may also suffer deafness.
Central hearing loss: Can be hereditary or caused by damage in the brain's auditory centre.

Action plan
Diagnostic tests
At present, babies routinely have their hearing tested when they are 7 or 8 months old (p.250). The test is only around 50% reliable, however, and if a difficulty is discovered this is late in terms of a baby's development. Some babies have hearing difficulties that remain undetected for 3 years. A new neonatal hearing test is therefore being introduced that will detect deafness and allow earlier communication training and parental awareness. Targeted neonatal hearing screening is already used in many hospitals for babies who are known to be at risk and in some areas testing is standard for all babies. The new test – universal neonatal hearing screening (UNHS) – will soon be offered to every baby.
- The test can be carried out within 2 days of birth and is not painful. It measures a reflex response to sound, called the oto-acoustic emission, or may involve the measurement of the brain's electric response to sounds.
- The person carrying out the test will insert a tiny probe just inside your baby's ear. This probe makes a small sound. If your baby can hear, his ear produces a kind of 'echo' that is picked up by the probe. If there is no echo it does not mean your baby is definitely deaf but he will be given more tests.

Treatment
- If deafness is caused by glue ear and the infection does not pass on its own (which it often does), a simple operation to fit a grommet can correct your child's hearing.
- If your baby's hearing difficulties may be helped by a hearing aid, you will need to visit a specialist centre. Conventional hearing aids work by amplifying sounds and can be used from as early as 6 weeks.
- If your child is given a hearing aid and this does not help, a cochlear implant may be considered. This is an electronic device that turns sounds into tiny electrical pulses, and, without needing to use the middle or inner ear structures that do not work properly, sends the signals directly to the hearing centres in the brain. Cochlear implants cannot yet restore hearing to normal. A cochlear implant has internal and external sections and needs to be fitted under surgery.

If your child is deaf
As soon as you knowif your child is deaf you can begin to communicate with him without using sounds. If you have no experience of deafness, this is a challenge but your baby needs his parents as supporters and your role is integral to his learning and development. It is best to know about deafness as early as possible and you may need EMOTIONAL ADVICE and training as you are taught to communicate by signing, and he learns to lip-read.

What happens once your child's difficulty has been diagnosed depends on the degree of hearing loss. You will be given extensive support from the medical team and your local education service will probably arrange for you to be in contact with a visiting teacher of the deaf. You may find national support groups for the deaf have valuable information and can put you in touch with other parents of deaf children. Many parents emphasise that communication without sound can never begin too early – your baby has an incredible capacity for communication (p.32).

EAR, INFECTION & PAIN: BABY

Ear pain, which may or may not be caused by ear infection, can make a baby very distressed. Ear infections are one of the most common reasons children see a doctor. Only rarely do they have serious consequences.

What happens
Ear pain may be part of an ear infection illness and your baby may have a high temperature, be restless, tug at or hit his ears, have a runny nose or a cough, shake his head and seem reluctant to suck. This group of symptoms may relate to other causes of discomfort, such as TEETHING or a common cold (p.438). If hearing (p.452) seems to be affected, he may have glue ear (overleaf). The only way to diagnose ear infection is to have your child's ear inspected by a doctor.

Pain in or around the ear could represent:
- An infection in the middle ear cavity (otitis media) when the middle ear is filled with mucus and pus. If tension builds up it may rupture the eardrum (above right) and the ear will ooze.
- A blockage of the pressure-equalizing Eustachian tube leading from the ear into the back of the nose. This causes a pressure build-up and pain behind the eardrum. It is similar to the pain that many people experience during a flight.
- Teething or a toothache or gum problem where pain travels to the ear.
- An infection in the external ear canal – otitis externa or 'swimmer's ear'.
- A scratched ear canal or pain from a foreign object in the ear (e.g. a bead, stone or insect). This is rare under 1 year of age.
- Extremely rarely, an underlying MENINGITIS infection may cause ear pain, also with FEVER and a rash that does not fade when a glass is pressed on to it, and a stiffened neck.

Ear wax
Ear wax keeps the ear canals clean. It is a sticky substance that coats the ear canal and traps any dirt or foreign objects. The wax accumulates and works its way out towards the outer ear. If wax gets wet, it expands and may gently touch the eardrum and hinder its movement. This is why water in the ear seems to affect hearing and balance. As the wax dries out under the influence of body heat, hearing returns to normal.

The only reason that wax may need to be removed from a baby's ear is so the eardrum can be looked at during a medical examination. It is not done to improve hearing. It is dangerous to poke around in your baby's ear, and cotton-wool buds are best used for cleaning the outside, never the inside of the ear. It is safest to put nothing smaller than your elbow in your child's ear.

Ruptured eardrum
If your baby has had symptoms of ear pain and a white or yellow pus-like fluid drains from the ear canal, he has probably suffered a ruptured eardrum resulting from a middle ear infection. This runny ear relieves pressure on the sensitive middle ear structures and the infection drains and resolves. The eardrum may heal in a few days with no trace of a scar and totally normal function. Occasionally the eardrum may scar and reduce hearing.

The ability of the eardrum to heal without complication led many doctors in the 'old days' to use a tiny knife to slit the eardrum to relieve pressure and pain. This cured the infection and the bacteria involved could be identified from a culture. The practice is being re-introduced increasingly in modern medicine because of concerns regarding antibiotic resistance of the bacteria that cause middle ear infections.

Action plan
It is not always easy to know whether your baby actually has ear pain. If he seems uncomfortable, soothe him, encourage him to drink and give him infant paracetamol to reduce pain and high temperature. Visit your GP if symptoms are severe or last longer than 3–4 days.

Medical care
- A small minority of doctors advocate treating all ear infections with antibiotics since there is a very small risk that an infection may worsen and infect bone surrounding the middle ear, or even the tissues surrounding the brain (MENINGITIS).
- Most doctors believe no treatment aside from pain control is required for the first 3 days because 85% of infections clear themselves and many are caused by viruses (which do not respond to antibiotics). Leaving them initially prevents the unnecessary use of antibiotics for most children. The risk of overuse of antibiotics, leading to resistance, may outweigh the small risk of complications.

Diet
The mucus-producing effect of cow's milk is so well known that many parents and paediatricians remove cow's milk from the diet of a child who is prone to chronic ear infections. About 30% of children with ear infections have an ALLERGY OR INTOLERANCE and in most cases the allergen is cow's milk. Reactions include nasal congestion and sore throats, and when the passages become blocked and irritated, ear infection often follows. A very high proportion of children with chronic ear pain improve when cow's milk is taken out of their diet. If you breastfeed your baby, he will be at a far smaller risk of developing ear problems. Your breast milk will have a protective effect when it comes to ear infections.

Complementary care
Many people feel alternatives to conventional medicine have

significantly helped their children, particularly when there have been several ear infections and no improvement despite medical treatment. These include homeopathy, herbal medicine, craniosacral osteopathy and acupuncture.

Homeopathy
Homeopathy can be an extremely effective treatment of acute ear infections and ongoing problems. Even if an ear infection is self-limiting, it can help relieve symptoms and boost recovery. When pain comes on suddenly or is acute, begin treatment quickly with the most indicated remedy (30c) hourly for 4 hours before reassessing. Symptoms may change from hour to hour, indicating a different remedy. Once the acute stage is passed, give the remedy 4 times a day for 2–3 days. If your baby has chronic or recurrent pain, ask for a constitutional remedy and, when pain is bad, treat the acute situation.

Use *Aconite* at the onset of earache with sudden symptoms, possibly around midnight when your baby screams in pain, is hot, frantic, anxious and restless and may have a dry cough and nasal congestion; *Belladonna* for a sudden onset, high fever, a flushed, hot face and head, perhaps dilated pupils and glazed eyes and the affected ear looks red – it is usually the right side – and is worse for light and movement; *Chamomilla* for earache that accompanies teething where the ears look red, one cheek is red and the other pale, your baby is irritable, alternating from temper tantrums to miserable weeping, wants something and then refuses it, hates being examined and feels better for being carried; *Hepar Sulph* at the established stage if there are few distinguishing characteristics or if your baby's ears are extremely sensitive and he is irritable, reluctant to be touched and feeling cold; *Merc Viv* for recurrent ear infections where ear pain tends to be accompanied by a sore throat, swollen glands and bad breath and profuse sweating at night, excess salivation and the ear may produce a gluey, pussy, yellow/green, smelly discharge; *Pulsatilla* for ear pain, perhaps worse on the left, with swollen glands and nasal congestion with thick yellowish mucus, your baby is clingy, weepy, whiny, feels worse in a warm stuffy environment and in the evenings – this is an excellent remedy for lingering problems.

Glue ear
See also EAR, INFECTION & PAIN: BABY

Glue ear is a condition in which thick sticky fluid collects in the middle ear, causing impaired hearing or temporary hearing loss. It affects up to 20% of children and is also known as chronic secretory otitis media, and can lead to ear pain and develop into acute otitis media. Glue ear usually occurs between the ages of 2 and 5 years, but can affect babies, particularly those who are prone to allergy, live with adults who smoke or have a CLEFT PALATE.

What happens
Hearing loss is the most common symptom of glue ear, because sound waves are not conducted properly through the fluid. Early detection and treatment could prevent a delay in acquiring speech. Normally each middle ear is ventilated by a Eustachian tube, a channel running from the middle ear to the back of the nose. If the tube is blocked or fails to function, fluid can accumulate. If your baby develops a viral infection with a cold, it may spread to the ear – the ear, nose and throat are closely related. Young children are more susceptible than adults because the Eustachian tubes block easily, and their adenoids (lymph tissue at the back of the nose where the Eustachian tubes open) are more likely to be enlarged.

Action plan
Diagnosis
Your doctor may conduct a number of tests.
- Audiometry: Measures hearing across a range of frequencies and there are techniques for babies.
- Otoscopy: This involves looking at the eardrum with a hand-held instrument to see bubbles of trapped fluid. It is also possible to check the pressure in the eardrum.
- Tympanometry: This is a measurement to assess how the eardrum moves in response to sound, but it does not directly measure hearing. It is a useful test even in babies under a year old.

Treatment: grommets
Glue ear does not always need treatment. Around 50% of cases get better on their own within 3 months, 75% within 6 months, and 90% within 12 months. If your child has frequent earache or may be at risk of developing speech problems, he may benefit from treatment. Some doctors advise a period of 3 months to watch for improvement before surgical treatment.

Surgical treatment for persistent glue ear is the insertion of grommets (in one or both ears). These are tiny tubes made of Teflon and placed into the eardrum to allow air to pass freely between the middle ear and the outside, and equalise the pressure. A small incision into the eardrum helps to remove most of the fluid and the grommet is then inserted. The operation is done under a general anaesthetic as a day-case, and afterwards most children have near-normal hearing. The change can be quite dramatic. Many children who need grommets have enlarged adenoids too, so they often benefit from adenoidectomy at the same time. Grommets usually stay in for 3–12 months, after which they fall out or are removed because if they are left in place for too long this could lead to permanent perforation of the eardrum. The eardrum usually heals quickly after grommets have been removed. If grommets fall out prematurely or glue ear recurs, your child may need to have them reinserted. It is fine to swim with grommets but diving, when he is older, is not advised because this may drive water into the middle ear under pressure.

Other treatments
- Some experts advocate a long course of antibiotics (2–4 weeks or more). This may treat infection but does not necessarily avoid the need for grommets, especially if both ears are involved. Steroids do not help.
- Some ear, nose and throat specialists recommend decongestant medicines containing pseudoephedrine. These are sometimes effective, although they can have side effects and the blockage can be increased when the effect wears off. Hearing aids can be used, but grommets are usually preferred.

EAR, SHAPES

It is quite common for a baby's ears to be pressed or bent slightly because of the way his head lay in the womb, and the ear usually reshapes itself naturally. Sometimes ears are naturally pointy. Because the cartilage of the external ear is soft and malleable, for the first few weeks it can be formed and allowed to 'set' to correct many common problems, either by taping the ear to the skull, or using a simple splint or spring. If your child has 'bat' ears that do not respond to simple treatments, you may consider plastic surgery when he is older.

EATING, CRAVINGS & PICA

Pregnancy commonly alters taste and smell and craving a particular food is extremely common. Yet many cravings have their basis in good nutrition – your body requires a balance of vitamins and minerals, and may call out for some foods to make up for something lacking in your diet or to quell NAUSEA. Cravings are not a problem if you can fulfil them without causing an imbalance in your diet. If you crave non-nutritional things that carry excessive calories, are very expensive or carry health risks in pregnancy (such as pâté, raw meat or fish or soft cheeses), it is best find an alternative.

Pica
When the craving is for a non-food, such as soil, coal, paper, starch or ice (and stranger things . . .) and you consume it, there may be risk to pregnancy. Craving for something with no nutritional value is known as pica. It is more common among women of African origin. Women who practise pica are often ashamed of the compulsion. The cause is unknown but it may be linked to iron-deficiency ANAEMIA.

What happens
The most common cravings are for sweets and dairy products, sour fruits and spicy or salty foods and junk foods. Cravings for salty foods such as pickles or crisps may indicate a need for minerals because blood volume and body fluid has increased in pregnancy. You may crave sugar because it is a quick energy source and helps reduce nausea. Recurrent cravings for sugar often reflect a poor diet containing too many fast-burning carbohydrates and a pattern of hypoglycaemia (p.336), or insufficient exercise: exercise releases hormones that trigger the release of glucose from the glycogen stores into the blood. Another cause may be anxiety, which is associated with adrenalin release and this stimulates the appetite for sugar. DRUG addiction, including SMOKING and caffeine consumption, can also increase cravings.

Action plan
- Aim for a nutritious diet with regular meals and a good balance of nutrients, focusing on slow-burning foods, and consider taking vitamin and mineral supplements (p.345).
- Try to include approximations of what you crave in your balanced diet, e.g. if you fancy orangeade, eat an orange; if

you want ice cream, try frozen yoghurt. Eating an apple or oat biscuit instead of chocolate does not give the same initial hit, but will satisfy your sugar requirement for longer.
- Sometimes thirst can be interpreted as hunger. Drink 6–8 glasses of water a day and try herbal teas.
- Try not to use pregnancy as an excuse to 'eat for two'.
- If you are bingeing or eating for comfort or have an eating disorder, you may need loving support while you look at the triggers.

Cravings usually fade as pregnancy progresses. Pica usually reduces but is not confined to pregnancy. A craving for sugar and chocolate may intensify after the birth when you feel the emotional effect of parenthood and have less time to cook and shop. If a craving becomes a problem, advice for EATING DIFFICULTIES & DISORDERS may help you.

EATING, DIFFICULTIES & DISORDERS

See also Eating and weight (p.332); EATING, CRAVINGS & PICA

If you have a less-than-happy relationship with food – perhaps you binge from time to time or are preoccupied with losing weight – you are not alone. Many women and a significant number of men feel uncomfortable about their weight and use eating as a way of venting difficult emotions. With pregnancy you may feel a new burst of health and responsibility and feel motivated to change, or you may feel confronted and your eating habits may intensify. For a small minority of women an eating disorder is present and it may be difficult to change.

Being over- or underweight means you are not as healthy as you have the potential to be, and may not enjoy your pregnancy, your baby or your partnership as you could. You may also compromise your baby's health in the womb. The most serious risks occur if you are underweight and poorly nourished prior to conception.

What lies behind an eating disorder?
Many factors contribute to eating disorders. Abnormal levels of brain chemicals may predispose some people to anxiety, perfectionism and obsessive–compulsive thoughts and behaviours that are then reflected in eating. Emotional issues such as depression (p.462) also play an important part. In spite of personal achievements, people with eating disorders commonly feel inadequate and tend to take the blame for troubles in their environment. Deeply ingrained feelings are hidden, often beneath starving or stuffing. There may often be a link with childhood eating patterns (e.g. using sweets to take the pain away), family attitudes to eating and weight, or perceptions of attractiveness formed in teenage years or later.

An eating disorder may also be associated with ALCOHOL or DRUG abuse. Sometimes the addiction may be to laxatives, enemas and appetite suppressants if weight loss is an issue. All of these carry risks in pregnancy.

Being overweight & obesity
Pregnancy is one of the most common times for a weight problem to begin. If you develop a habit of eating excessively

and if the weight gain continues after birth, or the excess is not lost, you may begin a long struggle with dieting.

Triggers for excessive weight
Being overweight and the extreme, obesity, carries considerable health risks. Obesity is defined as weighing more than 20% above expected weight for age, height and body build – that's an excess of approximately 15.9 kg (35 lb) or a body mass index (p.332) of 30–40. In the west, obesity is far more common than being underweight.

- Being overweight results from eating more calories than are burned by the body, and often this means eating lots of non-nutritious food (common culprits are calorie-laden fruit juice and colas, chocolates and sweets), eating when you are not hungry and not exercising sufficiently.
- There may be a gene that controls weight and metabolism and predisposes to excess weight.
- Dieting reduces the metabolism of the body to burn food. Any extra calories are then laid down as fat stores for reserve energy. This is why dieters are vulnerable (p.337): 98% of dieters regain all the weight they initially lose, plus roughly 4.5 kg (9 lb 15 oz) extra within 5 years.
- You may become overweight if you have been bulimic and are controlling your purges but not your food intake.
- Biological problems such as malfunctioning thyroid or pituitary glands can be a cause and it is worth visiting your doctor to be checked.

Implications for pregnancy
If you begin pregnancy overweight or gain excessively, the health risks rise in relation to the excess. A slight rise does not add a great health risk to your baby, particularly if you are well nourished and consume adequate vitamins and minerals. If your weight gain is significant, you are at greater risk of experiencing gestational DIABETES, high BLOOD PRESSURE, carrying a LARGE BABY and having difficulties in labour, and are susceptible to complications necessitating anaesthesia and a CAESAREAN SECTION. Your doctor may find it difficult to examine your abdomen and need more scans to monitor your baby. Extra fatty tissue can cause breathlessness, increase abdominal pressure with INDIGESTION & HEARTBURN, and stress the knee joints. Being overweight can contribute to depression also.

Compulsive overeating and bulimia nervosa
Compulsive overeating (binge eating) is an 'addiction' to food that often reflects a need to be loved. Binge eating may occur in fits and starts when you are faced with difficulties and you feel stressed or it may be your way of life. Some people who compulsively overeat control their weight gain by purging with self-induced vomiting or enemas or the use of diet pills, laxatives and diuretics. This is bulimia nervosa. In some countries one-fifth of young women display temporary bulimic symptoms.

Most women with bulimia have a normal pregnancy and birth, but there is an increased risk of MISCARRIAGE, PREMATURE BIRTH and depression. Excessive vomiting may cause dehydration and severe heartburn and abdominal pain, and nutritional deficiency. Laxatives and purgatives may be dangerous for a baby during pregnancy and when breastfeeding.

Being underweight
Being slightly underweight is rarely a health issue, particularly if your diet contains sufficient vitamins and minerals that allow you and your baby to thrive, but losing weight is not a good sign in pregnancy. You and your doctor or midwife will decide if your weight loss is of concern. If you have been very underweight you could find it hard to accept the weight gain of pregnancy. Some women react by eating small amounts so they grow with pregnancy but after birth they remain underweight. Dieting or depriving yourself of food will affect the nutrients your baby receives and may inhibit his growth, so seek help. Your nutrition, vitamin and mineral status and weight at conception are more important than worrying about weight gain because your baby is able to draw on your nutritional reserves.

Anorexia nervosa
Anorexia is defined as being below 85% of the expected weight for height and being afraid of gaining weight. Despite the low weight, most anorexic women feel fat (about 50% of people with anorexia subsequently develop bulimia). Anorexia is at its most threatening during pregnancy and to the baby in the womb. It reduces the chance of conception, so is an issue for only a small number of pregnant women. Many health-care specialists recommend delaying pregnancy until the illness is in remission. Most anorexic women who successfully treat their eating disorder regain their ability to conceive.

When anorexia and pregnancy coincide, the risks are considerable. Insufficient weight, sub-nutrition and vitamin and mineral deficiencies can lead to ANAEMIA, exhaustion and depression, miscarriage, CONGENITAL ABNORMALITIES, INTRAUTERINE GROWTH RESTRICTION (IUGR) and premature birth. The risks increase if laxatives and emetics are used and reduce with vitamin and mineral supplements. After birth, exhaustion and depression often continue.

Compulsive exercising (anorexia athletica)
Repeatedly training beyond the requirements for good health is often linked with an obsession about weight and diet. In pregnancy this may be a problem if it leads to overheating, dehydration or exhaustion or if the exercise carries a risk to your baby (e.g. excessive running or high impact sports). This may be a subtle form of abusive behaviour. With a good diet the risks to a baby are low but there is a higher chance of IUGR and premature birth. After birth, excessive exercise may lead to reduced breast milk flow.

Action plan for eating difficulties
Pregnancy brings an urgent need to attend to an eating problem and may be a catalyst for acknowledging some difficult emotions. It is very difficult, if not impossible, to step out of destructive eating patterns without help: almost all severe eating disorders need to be addressed through professional counselling, combined with loving support and encouragement from friends and/or family, before they are completely resolved.

Realistic steps to recovery are diverse and require considerable effort and perseverance. With support, you will be able to try, perhaps stumble, fall back into a pattern and emerge again, continuing to aim for the ultimate goal of eating well and maintaining a healthy body weight. On the way to this goal there is a chance to resolve emotional issues and re-examine some relationships that may be central to your life. The closer you are to a normal body weight, the safer it is for you and your baby.

Medical care

You are likely to receive the best medical care if you let your medical team know about any eating problem you have.

- Not all mild eating disorders need medical care. In pregnancy your nutrition and eating will be discussed and your midwife will alert you if your weight gain is too small or too large. Her advice and encouragement may help you to improve your diet.
- If your doctor believes you have a major eating problem, she may refer you for EMOTIONAL ADVICE AND SUPPORT.
- You may be helped at a support group.
- If you have been using enemas or laxatives ask your doctor for advice to gradually reduce use and to substitute natural foods such as linseeds to help your bowel movements. You can expect to be anxious if you don't pass a motion for a while but your body needs time to regulate itself and relearn how to respond to natural cues.
- Many alternative therapies can be helpful.

Diet and weight gain

Keeping an eye on weight gain is important for every woman in pregnancy (p.332). If you have a tendency to over- or under-eat, monitoring your weight is helpful. You or your midwife can weigh you regularly and keep records.

- Follow a plan for eating regularly and well that will keep your energy levels stable, reduce cravings and avoid sugar-laden, fast-burning foods.
- Try to avoid getting too hungry or feeling too full.
- If you recognise triggers for your eating habit, try to eliminate them.
- If you cannot give up vomiting or purging, try to delay it until nourishing foods have been digested.
- If you find you are likely to binge after eating a meal, try washing up immediately and throw away all leftovers. This will keep you busy for those difficult first minutes.
- You may find it helpful to tell someone about the warning signs to watch for so they can help you.
- If you are consuming alcohol or drugs that exacerbate your eating problem, seek help to quit.
- Go easy on yourself and allow time for your body and your mind to get used to becoming a mother and to a new approach to food and nutrition.

Exercise and lifestyle

Exercise can help keep weight in balance although it needs to be appropriate to pregnancy, leaving you with enough energy to nurture your baby and avoid exhaustion. If you are gaining weight excessively, exercise can help you to burn calories and could reduce your craving for food. Refer to the chapter on exercise (p.357) and seek advice so you know that the exercise you do is beneficial.

- Yoga and dance can boost body image and physical fitness.
- Do what you can to get enough sleep – being tired is sometimes an excuse for eating.
- You may find visualisation (p.370) helps to avoid vulnerable times or change your view of your body.

With your baby, after the birth

Like many mothers, you may find your eating disorder surfaces or spirals out of control after birth when physical and emotional demands pile up. It is important to continue with support and counselling: you need all the energy you can get through your nutrition so you don't become exhausted and can maintain a good milk supply. You will also find it easier to cope if you have practical help.

- Try to let yourself feel proud that you are a good parent, and take time to be with your baby and let yourself love and feel loved in return. You may find the information in Part IV helpful if you are facing difficult emotions.
- Many women with an eating difficulty who breastfeed enjoy nourishing their babies and find breastfeeding an important part of the recovery process.
- After birth you may need help to learn to recognise natural hunger signals from your baby. This may help you recognise signals in yourself and alter a set eating routine.
- If you are alone a lot, try to get company from your network of friends and family. This will help you to avoid loneliness (and perhaps depression) and may reduce tendencies to binge or purge.
- At night when you are up with your baby and it is quiet, you will need a lot of self-control if you feel an urge coming on, either to binge, purge or starve yourself.

If you slip back into a destructive pattern

Remember that a slip doesn't have to lead to a full-blown relapse, and a relapse doesn't have to lead to total collapse. If you do slip up, try to view the incident as a learning experience. Ask yourself what was happening that triggered your familiar coping device and then look back at the action plan for ways to avoid resorting to your old habits. Remind yourself that change is difficult and commit to trying once again. Don't forget the support network around you.

ECTOPIC PREGNANCY

In an ectopic pregnancy the fertilised egg implants in the fallopian tube instead of implanting in the uterus. As the embryo develops, the placenta burrows through the thin walls of the tube and there is bleeding into the pelvis and abdominal cavity. The bleeding may be intense and cause shock, as is a life-threatening emergency.

An ectopic occurs in 1% of pregnancies but the rate is rising with fertility treatment. In an ectopic pregnancy the baby cannot survive other than in exceptionally rare circumstances where the placenta implants outside the uterus in the pelvic cavity (in an extra-uterine pregnancy). Discovering that you have an ectopic pregnancy can be harrowing and involves the unavoidable loss of your pregnancy. You may need continuing support to absorb the news and choose the best course of action. All parents experiencing LOSS OF A BABY, regardless of the reasons, are likely to go through a period of grief, sadness and mourning. With an ectopic, this is mixed with a sense of relief that the condition was detected and treated.

Some ectopic pregnancies occur without an apparent reason. Certain conditions can increase the risk, although it is important to remember that ectopic is still unlikely.

- Previous infection with scarring of the fallopian tube usually caused by CHLAMYDIA.
- Previous surgery to the fallopian tube, including a previous ectopic because scar tissue distorts it.
- Becoming pregnant when an intrauterine contraceptive device (IUD) is in place, or while using the progesterone-only mini pill. These may affect the rate the ovum travels in the tube.
- With in-vitro fertilisation (IVF) and intrauterine insemination (IUI) the incidence of ectopic pregnancy is 4%.
- Women over 35 years of age are also at increased risk.

What happens

Almost every ectopic pregnancy is accompanied by pain. It usually begins on one side of the lower abdomen and is due to internal bleeding from the affected fallopian tube. It may last for hours and stop and start as the blood is released and reabsorbed. If the bleeding is profuse, pain spreads over the abdomen and becomes more intense. The loss of blood from your circulation into your abdomen may induce shock, with symptoms that may include weakness, light-headedness and shivering. If this happens, the situation is a life-threatening emergency requiring medical attention: call an ambulance.

Menstrual periods may stop when a pregnancy is ectopic but occasionally bleeding occurs at the expected time. The hormone levels from the ectopic fluctuate and as the levels rise and fall, the lining of the uterus sheds partially and bleeding occurs. The menstrual bleed may be heavier and more prolonged than usual because the lining of the uterus is thickened by the pregnancy hormones. The bleeding may be irregular and confused with spotting that occurs with a threatened MISCARRIAGE.

Symptoms may be minimal early on but if you have pain or spotting, a scan at Weeks 6–8 may reveal the ectopic before it ruptures with internal bleeding. If the ectopic receives too little blood in your fallopian tube, the pregnancy will be absorbed. Modern ultrasound scans show that many ectopic pregnancies occur without the mother having symptoms.

Diagnosis

If you are in pain or suspect an ectopic pregnancy because of irregular bleeding or a positive pregnancy test, you must tell your doctor as soon as possible. She can best visualise the pregnancy through an internal ultrasound scan using a probe in the vagina. An internal vaginal examination is less accurate.

In the first 14 days after the first missed period, the stretching of the fallopian tube may be minimal and the actual ectopic is small and may be difficult to see on a scan. The scan may need to be repeated the following week. If you are not pregnant and are ovulating normally, each month your ovary forms a corpus luteum after the egg is released and this might be difficult to distinguish from an ectopic on the scan. A pregnancy test detecting human chorionic gonadotrophin (HCG) levels (p.62) will also be done. If an ectopic is suspected, your GP or specialist can request an urgent blood HCG test. In a normal pregnancy, the HCG levels double every 3–4 days. A slower rise indicates pregnancy failure, either an ectopic or an impending miscarriage. If HCG is not detected an ectopic pregnancy is unlikely and your pain is from another cause.

Action plan

An ectopic is a serious and potentially life-threatening condition that is best treated by early diagnosis and either 'conservative' or operative care.

Conservative care

If the ectopic is seen to be small on a scan – detected before Week 8 – and the levels of HCG are low and rising slowly, the placenta may stop functioning. When this happens, the ectopic is absorbed by your body and there is no need for intervention. If your hospital has the facilities, it is safe to observe progress closely with follow-up scans and HCG blood tests every 2 or 3 days. Many women prefer to wait because the alternative is an operation. The scans show the pregnancy sac getting smaller but it may take 4–10 weeks to disappear and be reabsorbed.

When conservative treatment is an option, it is important to discuss the advantages – an increased chance of conceiving again and less likelihood of an ectopic occurring in the future – against the disadvantages of the uncertainty of waiting to see whether surgery is needed.

It is possible to speed up natural absorption of the ectopic by injecting a powerful drug (methotrexate, used for the treatment of cancer) that travels through your bloodstream and kills the foetal and placental cells. The drug is not used very often because it does have potential side effects.

Operative care

An ectopic with internal bleeding requires an operation to remove it. Modern techniques are minimally invasive, and the operation is done under general anaesthetic. A laparoscopy is performed: a tiny camera is inserted through your umbilicus into the abdomen to visualise the fallopian tubes and ovaries, and the ectopic. If the tube appears to be damaged it may be removed together with the ectopic, because it is likely to cause another ectopic pregnancy. If it appears unharmed it can be opened and the ectopic teased out, so the tube is preserved. There is an increased chance of another ectopic if the tube is left in place and some women choose to have the tube removed, even if it appears normal, as long as the other tube is normal. The laparoscopy operation usually leads to full recovery within a week.

If the ectopic is large because it has been detected after Weeks 8–10, a full laparotomy with an incision in the abdomen is required and the tube is removed. It takes longer to recover and is similar, in this respect, to a CAESAREAN SECTION. If you have lost a large amount of blood then either a BLOOD TRANSFUSION during surgery or using vitamins and iron afterwards will prevent ANAEMIA and aid a speedy recovery.

The next pregnancy

The fertility rates after ectopic are over 60%, with a higher rate of conception among women who had conservative treatment (without surgery). The chance of another ectopic occurring is 4–5% and it is highest in women who undergo IVF treatment or where the other tube is scarred. If the tube has been removed you may have to wait longer to conceive until you ovulate on the correct side. Vitamin and mineral supplements may aid conception. If you want to go on contraception, avoid an IUD or a progesterone-only mini pill. If you become pregnant again have an ultrasound scan as early as possible, using a vaginal probe to confirm where the baby is implanted.

EMOTIONS, ADVICE & SUPPORT

During pregnancy and after birth you may find you need more support than in the past as huge changes in your life present challenges and make you more emotionally volatile. The impact is similar for men and women but women are deeply affected by hormonal changes.

The foundation for effective support is acknowledging your feelings. Once you have admitted them to yourself and have shared them with someone else, you have begun the process of recovery. In some cases, the initial cause of emotional upset is indisputable – this applies if you have suffered a loss or received bad news. In other cases, the cause may seem elusive. Depending on your background it may be easier to talk about physical symptoms than it is to admit that you are depressed. For some people it is easier to admit to depression than to reveal the truth about abuse and everyone hides difficult emotional experiences in their unconscious mind.

In the first instance, you might find it helpful to turn to Part IV where common issues are explored, and review the way you are caring for yourself (p.51). If you address difficult feelings during pregnancy you may be able to avoid postnatal depression. Progress will depend on what you feel is wrong and the options available to you. During pregnancy and the postnatal period you may find it easier to access friends and family, support groups and professionals. People unite around a baby and your child's energy may boost your wellbeing.

Action plan

Depression is often the manifestation of underlying anxiety, anger, fear or sadness. Anxiety alone may be your main feeling. Finding your way through can take time and a number of different approaches. Committed changes to your lifestyle may make a real difference. Your health team may use a specially designed depression questionnaire to assess your wellbeing. Your GP, midwife, or another member of the medical team may suggest counselling or therapy and might put you in touch with someone who has had similar emotions. If you are depressed after birth, a postnatal support group could give valuable support and companionship.

Taking one day at a time

When you are in the midst of negative feelings it may not be possible to see light at the end of the tunnel, particularly if your baby is ill. Trusting that life moves on and things change is not easy, but it may be helpful. Remember not to expect too much: take one day at a time, set yourself small, achievable daily goals such as 'a walk', 'a bath', 'meet a friend', and reward yourself when you have done them. It is also helpful to accept there will still be bad days, even when you are feeling good about life. You could use the Wheel for Living (p.58) to make exercise, healthy eating, meditation and relaxation part of your daily life, and as a way to seek information. Even with difficult situations full information is preferable.

Counselling and therapy

Sometimes speaking to someone outside your family or network of close friends makes it easier to focus on difficult issues and feel heard without being judged. You can do this with a counsellor or as part of psychotherapy. Therapy does different things for different people. Sometimes three sessions can resolve a problem that has lingered for decades and sometimes three sessions a week may be needed for years before there is lasting benefit.

In psychotherapy, your relationship with the therapist may allow you to express and explore difficult emotions and experiences with the goal of feeling more balanced. Psychotherapy is available for individuals, couples, families or groups. It may help you live more positively and can be particularly helpful if you need to take medications, by offering insight into the underlying issues, promoting self esteem and reducing reliance on medication when setbacks and frustration occur. If, in therapy, something 'clicks' and you come to a realisation that had previously eluded you, it has been worth it. This can take a long time and is often progressive. Your choice of approach will depend on what is available in your area and the advice that you get from your medical and social group.

Psychoanalytic and psychodynamic psychotherapies: Based on Freudian theory and looking at early life events that were traumatic but are no longer consciously remembered, with the aim of resolving past issues and approaching conflicts without resorting to old patterns.

Analytical psychology: Considers the memories and emotions stored in the unconscious mind that can affect feelings, actions and relationship choices. It is linked to Jung's theories.

Behavioural and cognitive psychotherapy: Looks at the relationship between thoughts, feelings, behaviour and lifestyle, and family/social environment to focus on what is happening 'here and now' and alter behaviour patterns.

Experiential constructivist therapies: Aim to identify interpretations of experience(s), and look at the 'story' that may not be in proportion to the event itself but now influences actions and choices. This approach constructs a model for seeing things in a different light. Neurolinguistic programming (NLP) is one of the best-known approaches.

Family, couple, sexual and systemic therapies: Aim to look into patterns of belief and the roles and behaviours that become established in relationships, and then to establish new and more fulfilling patterns.

Humanistic and integrative psychotherapy: Includes different psychotherapies that consider a person in terms of his or her body, feelings, mind and spirit and uses the relationship between therapist and client as a vehicle for experience, growth and change that can lead towards a greater tolerance of life's experiences. These include humanistic, existential, transpersonal and integrative psychotherapy.

Hypno-psychotherapy: Uses hypnosis to bring about a state of relaxation that allows a shift in awareness. During hypnosis, the therapist can tap into a person's deeper levels of consciousness and draw attention to new possibilities and different patterns of behaviour and emotions.

Medication

If you have an emotional disorder that is extremely disruptive to your life, medication may bring immediate relief and help you approach the source of your upset. Medication can help with panic attacks, anxiety symptoms, depression, obsessive behaviour, violent and anti-social behaviours, and psychosis. Sometimes drugs alone can achieve good results, but it is usually preferable to combine medication with counselling, emotional therapy and practical support. If your doctor, psychiatrist or therapist believes medication may help, it is best to find the most suitable drug. You need to weigh up the pros and cons - depression can, for some women, carry a greater risk of harm to their baby and family life than the risk associated with anti-depressant drugs.

Depression: Antidepressants boost the level of neurotransmitters important in fighting depression. Each of the major classes of antidepressants – monoamine oxidase (MAO) inhibitors, tricyclics and selective serotonin re-uptake inhibitors (SSRI) – affects different neurotransmitter systems in a different way. MAO inhibitors are not safe to use during pregnancy. Tricyclic antidepressants are preferred, and are also used for severe obsessive–compulsive disorders. SSRIs such as Fluoxetine (Prozac), Sertraline (Zoloft) and Paroxetine (Aropax) may present a risk and are best reserved for severe depression and reduced or avoided after Week 25 and when breastfeeding. When there is a history of depression or severe pre-menstrual tension some doctors advise daily progesterone injections or vaginal pessaries immediately after birth to prevent a rapid withdrawal of the hormone as the placenta is born. It may help with postnatal mood swings.

Bipolar disorders: Commonly treated with lithium but it is advisable to stop lithium or carbamazepine before conception. An alternative is a high-potency antipsychotic agent. Sodium Valproate may be the safest mood stabiliser during pregnancy and when breastfeeding, although it is certainly not without risk. Lithium is secreted in breast milk, and the levels can be high. However, for a bipolar disorder it is usually recommended that lithium be restarted promptly after delivery as a precaution against postnatal depression.

Anxiety: Until recently benzodiazepines were standard treatments, but these are best avoided in pregnancy. Many of the drugs used for depression are also effective for severe anxiety, phobias and compulsive behaviour.

Alternative therapies

It is good to know that alternative therapies can be very powerful and have few side effects. They can help you stay calm and relatively balanced as you process an event in your life and begin to move forward once again. If you are suffering from depression the remedies for anxiety or anger given below may also suit you.

Homeopathy

Homeopathy is effective, and can be used for acute stages or with a constitutional approach for on-going problems. While you are waiting to see your homeopath and symptoms are intense you could try one of the following remedies in 200c potency, 3 times a day. After 3 days, reassess your choice and use 30c, morning and night. If you are treating depression, take your remedy (30c) 3 times a day for a week and then reassess.

Anxiety based on fear: Use *Aconite* if fear is so overwhelming that you are afraid you may die – it is good before a procedure such as amniocentesis or caesarean, or during labour; *Argentum Nitricum* if you have panic attacks or anticipatory anxiety, fear losing control and your adrenalin is pumping; *Arsenicum* suits raw fear and panic, particularly in the early hours of the morning, perhaps accompanied by vomiting and/or diarrhoea; *Gelsemium* if you fear losing control or worry about something that is about to happen (e.g. labour) to the extent that you become stiff or shaky, dizzy or apathetic.

Anxiety based on worry: Use *Aconite* if concern appears suddenly or is overwhelming, you feel terror and panic in a certain situation and cannot sleep; *Arsenicum* if you worry about everything and anything, need to control your life and project the worst scenario on to an ordinary event; *Arg Nit* for anticipatory anxiety that can result in panic attacks, you feel constantly rushed, forgetful and tormented by thoughts that something has gone wrong, sometimes with claustrophobia, and a craving for sweet and salty food; *Gelsemium* if you worry about how you appear to others or what could happen next and seize up mentally and physically, feel exhausted, weak, perhaps dizzy and shaky and unco-ordinated; *Lycopodium* for a sense of inadequacy (although you may be critical of others and appear haughty), and bloating or severe abdominal wind.

Depression: Use *Pulsatilla* in the early postnatal days if you feel weepy and sensitive, your moods change rapidly and you want attention and advice but become easily overwhelmed – you may feel worse in hot, stuffy rooms and seldom thirsty; *Ignatia* in the days after labour, particularly if you feel circumstances do not meet your hopes – you may reproach yourself and have wildly swinging moods, with lots of crying and sighing; *Sepia* (the 'hormonal balancer') after labour if you feel complete exhaustion, despondence, indifference and no bonding with your baby – you may cry yet shun consolation, and one thing that makes you feel better is vigorous exercise; *Staphysagria* after a 'high-tech' labour, perhaps with stitching, or an emergency caesarean and you feel violated or resentful but keep quiet, are very sensitive and go over events on your own, perhaps in the night; *Cimicifuga* if you feel low yet agitated, swinging from depression to excitement, and feel trapped by responsibility and paranoid that something terrible is going to happen; *Aurum Metallicum* if you feel overwhelmed by sadness and guilty because you could have done better in labour and could do better as a mother – it suits people who are characteristically driven but thrown by motherhood; *Natrum Mur* if you have suffered a bereavement during pregnancy and your feelings do not hit you until after the birth when you feel extremely sensitive, yet may appear defensive and find it difficult to cry – you feel better on your own but this isolation contributes to your sadness.

Anger: *Nux Vomica* if you are driven and domineering, have a quick temper but let go easily, become angry through frustration, from being contradicted or hindered and usually express this verbally but may occasionally throw or smash things; *Lycopodium* if you feel deeply insecure and not good enough, although outwardly you are domineering and sarcastic, you are prone to sudden explosions of shouting although may be charming away from home; *Arsenicum* if you are anxious about your future and your health and need to be fastidiously organised, but irritable when things don't go as you wish – you can present a cold, rather self-righteous face; *Sepia* if you can fly into a rage, sometimes being nasty or picking on someone when you are exhausted and drained and have not got the energy to deal with things calmly.

Aromatherapy and massage

These can be very relaxing and are particularly suitable for depression. Use the oils in appropriate doses (p.378) for massage, bathing or inhalation.

Anxiety: Neroli brings peace, jasmine inspires confidence and clary sage helps to put things in perspective (but does inspire vivid dreams so don't use it at night). Sandalwood sedates while patchouli helps bring you down to earth. After Week 24 you can use lavender, a traditional soother, and frankincense in low doses, which helps to overcome fear, cut links with past uncomfortable experiences and encourages calm breathing.

Depression: Bergamot can be particularly good (but brings sensitivity to sunlight). If you feel very low and tired, melissa and lemongrass are uplifting. You can also use lavender or camomile as a general soother and neroli to promote sleep – particularly good with an oil and a gentle facial massage.

Herbal remedies and acupuncture

Herbs can powerfully assist emotional healing, but while you are pregnant or breastfeeding it is important to consult a medical herbalist who is clear about what is and is not safe. European, Chinese, ayurvedic and Native American herbal remedies can have powerful effects on anxiety and depression and because the two co-exist, combinations are often useful.

Anxiety: Kava has a relaxing effect and helps reduce anxiety, tension and restlessness without withdrawal symptoms. Valerian root has a strong sedative effect promoting relaxation and deep, restful sleep; Passion flower has mildly sedative properties, often combined with camomile, and valerian; Camomile is helpful for insomnia.

Depression: St John's wort is a traditional remedy for anxiety and moderate depression, with a therapeutic effective similar to anti-depressant drugs but far fewer side effects. It is usually taken for between 2 and 10 weeks. It can be used with drugs of the SSRI class but not with monoamine oxidase inhibitor drugs (opposite).

Restoration: Herbs that renew vitality include Siberian ginseng, Ginkgo biloba extracts (particularly good for headaches, emotional tenderness and anxiety) and Dong quai, which has a calming effect.

Acupuncture, acupressure and reflexology may be calming and re-balance underlying tension patterns in your body.

EMOTIONS, ANXIETY

See also EMOTIONS, ADVICE & SUPPORT

Anxiety is a normal human emotion that is a protective response. It is part of the integral human 'fight or flight' reflex and can also provide motivation. Anxiety may cause a slight increase in heart rate and muscle tension and can stimulate a release of hormones, such as adrenalin and insulin, to give an instant burst of energy and determination.

It is normal, and acceptable, to be worried or anxious about the events that are part of becoming a parent. If you become extremely anxious, however, you may feel unwell, experience normal discomfort as extremely painful and enjoy your pregnancy, or your baby, less. If you are constantly anxious, even when a threatening situation has passed or may never come to pass, or you become anxious about something that most people find unthreatening, you may have an anxiety disorder. More than 1:5 people are affected by anxiety states that are actually medical disorders. Often, anxiety and depression coexist.

What happens

The symptoms of anxiety are in many ways similar to those of stress. The difference is that if you are stressed, your symptoms disappear once the situation has passed. If you are anxious, you may continue to feel tense, pressurised, worried and/or fearful and your stress feelings continue. If anxiety is severe, you may have unrealistic fears about birth or something happening to your baby. You may feel tense and restless, exhausted, have chronic headaches, sweaty palms, a sore abdomen, CONSTIPATION or DIARRHOEA, palpitations in your HEART or feel an uncontrollable urge to smoke or eat, or go off food altogether. Anxiety disorders are often missed because of a belief that all expectant and new mothers are excessively anxious.

What might cause anxiety?

The causes for anxiety are similar to those associated with depression. In pregnancy you may encounter more causes for anxiety in a short time than you have before. This may be your first experience of medical attention and hospital, or hospital treatment may be stressful if you have had a previous traumatic experience with medical care.

After birth all new parents are anxious to some degree – it is normal to worry about whether you are doing the right thing and whether your baby is all right. In the 1st year after birth, more visits are made to doctors or nurses than at any other time of life. You may also feel pressurised if you have financial, housing or career worries, or difficulties in family relationships. If you are concerned about your health or have continual low energy, illness or discomfort, these could reflect underlying anxiety.

Can anxiety affect your baby?

Most women become anxious at some time during pregnancy as well as after birth. In pregnancy it is extremely unlikely anxiety will harm your baby although he may receive stress hormones as part of the intimate communication between you.

He also has the capacity to produce stress hormones. For a very small number of women extreme anxiety may lead to reduced blood flow to the placenta, although this may be linked to inadequate nutrition or to SMOKING or DRUGS. Reduced flow can be detected on an ultrasound scan in mid-pregnancy and may lead to placental insufficiency and INTRAUTERINE GROWTH RESTRICTION. There is also an association between extreme antenatal anxiety and a small percentage increase in hyperactivity in children.

After birth your baby learns from the way you react to situations. Honesty is the best policy and even if you are very stressed you can tell your baby you are worried, it is not his fault and you love him. If you recognise your reaction may be excessive, you could seek support so that your anxiety does not impinge on your relationship with your baby.

Types of anxiety disorders

When normal anxiety gives way to excess, it is called an anxiety disorder. There are different types and some may coexist.

Generalised anxiety disorder: Brings a constant state of tension that may last for months. You may feel on edge, tired, unable to concentrate, irritable and unable to sleep, in discomfort or pain. Your friends may know you as a 'worrier' and you know that your anxious thoughts are not controllable.

Obsessive-compulsive disorder: Involves recurrent or persistent mental images or ideas, resulting in compulsive behaviours with repetitive and rigid routines. Obsessive thoughts and compulsive behaviours do not always coexist. It is quite common to hide obsessive thoughts and ritualistic behaviours (e.g. bulimia). A compulsive disorder is not a psychotic illness, and does not make you lose touch with reality. However, stress can be huge and some people are unable to control thoughts of not parenting well or harming their babies that bring self-reproach years or decades later.

Panic disorder: An extreme form of anxiety, usually accompanied by a fear of impending death. Panic attacks are terrifying, with sweating, palpitations, shortness of breath, chest pain, dizziness and fear of losing control or dying. The frequency can vary widely and each episode may last 15–30 minutes, although severe residual anxiety can persist. Panic attacks may occur out of the blue or in response to a particular situation. Avoiding situations may become a way of life that could be very restrictive and may lead to phobias.

Phobias: Overwhelming and irrational fears that something bad will happen. Phobias relating to parenthood include fear of needles and hospitals, of developmental problems in the baby, loss of pregnancy or death of a baby. A phobia typically meets four criteria: it is out of proportion to the situation (and you will recognise this); you cannot adequately or logically explain it away; it is beyond voluntary control, and it leads to an avoidance of the feared situation or stimulus.

If you are extremely anxious about something but can think of resources to deal with it, you do not have a phobia but could still benefit from techniques to reduce your anxiety. If you have a true phobia, for instance of hospitals, it is best resolved before labour. You will need professional help – the very nature of a phobia means you cannot help yourself to face the situation without panic.

Post-traumatic stress disorder: A reaction to one or more traumatic events. During or soon after the event you may feel emotionally numb and block out the reality (amnesia): symptoms may not occur for weeks, months or even years when you may have flashbacks, feel emotionally tender or withdrawn, hopeless, unable to sleep, experience panic attacks, guilt and difficulty concentrating. Being in a hospital environment or feeling scrutinised or invaded during antenatal or labour examinations may bring a buried memory to the surface and trigger a post-traumatic stress disorder.

Action plan

Except when it is severe, the key is not to eliminate anxiety, but to accept it and use the drive it gives you to make the most of your situation rather than let its power become overwhelming. The suggestions for EMOTIONS, ADVICE & SUPPORT may help you to do this and begin to live a life less burdened by stress.

Treating a phobia

How you approach a phobia depends largely on whether you want to overcome the phobia altogether, or simply deal with a specific circumstance when it arises. For example, for a needle or hospital phobia you may choose to begin with therapy and look into the background to your phobia. Your therapist might talk you through hospital admission or the use of needles to try to desensitise you. Usually three or four sessions are needed. You may be encouraged to have hypnotherapy, practise relaxation techniques with breathing exercises, visualisations and meditations and combine these with therapies such as homeopathy or Bach Flower Remedies. If you do not want to delve into the reasons behind your phobia, one option is to have injections under hypnosis. With good training, you may be able to use self-hypnosis. There is also the option of using anaesthetic cream before an injection.

EMOTIONS, DEPRESSION

See also EMOTIONS, ADVICE & SUPPORT

Strong feelings are an inherent part of being a parent, and depression, often with anxiety, is more common at this time. As a recognised condition, postnatal depression affects an estimated 1:7 women. Many affected women do not receive adequate support as they are not correctly diagnosed or do not seek help. Depression may not begin until after the birth, sometimes months later, but is often established in pregnancy, peaking around Week 32. Women are prone to mood swings because of hormonal changes and at least 1:10 men are also affected. The course of ante- and postnatal depression varies. Without treatment, an episode may last 6 months or more. With treatment, the majority of people recover much sooner.

Becoming a parent may involve a number of stressful events and birth may be a shock. Your baby can make a significant contribution to the strain of parenting and depression may be increased if your baby is difficult, unwell or demanding. Depression comes in different forms:

The 'blues' (p.303): These come for a while and then pass after a few days. They occur most commonly in the first few days after birth but may happen at any time, even in pregnancy, and can be a reaction to an event like illness or leaving work.

Depression: This is more intense than the 'blues' and lasts longer, may have an underlying emotional basis needing more help and support. This is the common type people refer to as feeling depressed. Many people show depression in the form of anxiety or physical discomfort.

Psychosis: The most intense and dangerous form of depression, with pschosis you become out of touch with reality. The psychosis may be mainly depressive and alternate with euphoria. This is a bipolar disorder, previously called manic depression, and is usually present before conception. Other psychoses, such as schizophrenia, may also flare up during or after pregnancy.

What happens

One of the most disabling symptoms of depression is the fact that it 'saps the will' and makes doing anything an enormous effort. Depression is an extremely unpleasant experience, and most people with this condition want to do whatever they can to get well. Taking the first step – seeking support – may require a great leap of courage if you feel your depression is your fault or could be prevented if you were a 'better' person. This applies particularly if your family does not believe in acknowledging depression or emotional support. You may be inspired by the possibility of change if you look at your depression as an illness that can be treated. Taking it out of your life will be liberating. When depression lingers, it can lead to personal dissatisfaction and low self-esteem, obstruct the developing relationship between you and your baby, and can cause family break-up, career disappointment or emotional and behavioural problems in your child. When severe, the effects of depression can be massive and even lead to addiction, abuse or suicide.

How you may feel if you are down

Every mother has some or many of these feelings. Whether they constitute depression depends on their degree and whether there are more bad days than good days.

- The 'blues' may leave you feeling highly sensitive, tired with poor concentration, suddenly overwhelmed by feelings of helplessness and unable to stop yourself from weeping. Some women, before or after birth, feel out of control and frightened by the responsibility of motherhood. Some describe the feeling as one close to madness.
- You may feel irritable and angry at the way life is not fair.
- Postnatal depression may bring symptoms such as anxiety, persistent sadness, tearfulness or avoiding other people. You may feel inadequate and/or guilty, cry a lot and feel you are the only mother who cannot cope. This could be particularly intense if your baby does not sleep well and is difficult to care for.
- Depression may show itself as anxiety. One of the signs is excessive concern that you or your baby is ill or has an undetected health problem. Anxiety symptoms occur in 80% of people with depression.
- You may have a lack of energy and enthusiasm that stops you from doing daily chores or trivial tasks like deciding what to wear. You may find it hard to be interested in your

baby. You may find it difficult to sleep, even when you are exhausted, or want to do nothing else but sleep.
- You may go off food and lose weight or eat in excess and put on weight. Alcohol, drug and food abuse can all be symptoms of depression. For some women physical symptoms, with endless aches, pains and illnesses, are the main outward sign of depression.
- If you have experienced a traumatic event, you may be at risk of post-traumatic stress disorder. This is an anxiety state (p.461) that also involves depression.

Causes of depression

There is no single cause of depression. Parenthood triggers many emotions (p.300) that may make you feel sad or melancholy. How you may be affected depends upon the combination of hormones and your underlying personality and life circumstances. What is happening at this time – your job, parents, relationship, house, finances – and what has happened in the past affect your tendency to anxiety or depression. Fathers are similarly affected and may feel rejected if the mother becomes engrossed in her baby, be anxious about the responsibility and financial burden involved in caring for a family and confused or sad at losing sexual desire. Many men do not talk about their problems and will not seek support if they feel depressed.

There are suggestions that there is a chemical basis in the brain that predisposes some people and some families to depression. Another theory proposes that anxiety or depression is a learnt response to fearful situations. If you were traumatised emotionally or physically as a child, or later, you may be in the habit of feeling anxious and emotionally low. You might be unaware of this in-built way of being because the traumatic memory is held in your subconscious mind and powerfully but subtly influences you. This view is the basis for a number of different psychotherapies (p.459).

Depression can affect anyone. Most people who develop the condition have previously led normal lives. The intensity of birth may mean this is the first time a tendency to feel low is recognised as important. There are, however, indications of increased risk:

- When there is, or has been, depression, breakdown or postnatal depression.
- If there is a family history of depression or mental illness.
- When there is persistent anxiety that things will go wrong or a need to be in control, with perfectionist tendencies.
- If there have been 'negative life events' such as bereavement, MISCARRIAGE, termination or LOSS OF A BABY, or an unhappy childhood, particularly if there was violence or abuse or loss of a parent.
- When post-traumatic stress disorder exists.
- If there is a previous or existing ALCOHOL or DRUG addiction or EATING DISORDER.
- When there is a lack of emotional support from other people, especially the father of the baby or family members.
- If a partnership is difficult or tense, particularly where abuse or violence is present or the pregnancy is unplanned and unsupported.
- When social circumstances are hard, perhaps with unemployment, poor housing or money problems.

- If there are medical complications, particularly for the baby, that lead to anxiety and sadness.

The Edinburgh depression scale could be a good tool if you wish to rate yourself. It focuses on depression rather than on anxiety disorders and phobias. Underline the answer that comes closest to how you have felt in the past 7 days, not just how you feel today. Response categories are scored 0, 1, 2 and 3 according to increased severity of the symptoms. Items marked with an asterisk are reverse scored (i.e. 3, 2, 1 and 0). A score of 12+ indicates the possibility of depression, but not its severity. A score over 20 indicates depression is likely.

1 *I have been able to laugh and see the funny side of things.* (As much as I always could, Not quite so much now, Definitely not so much now, Not at all)

2 *I have looked forward with enjoyment to things.* (As much as I ever did, Rather less than I used to, Definitely less than I used to, Hardly at all)

3 *I have been anxious or worried for no good reason.* (No not at all, Hardly ever, Yes sometimes, Yes very often)

4 * *I have blamed myself unnecessarily when things went wrong.* (Yes most of the time, Yes some of the time, Not very often, No never)

5 * *I have felt scared or panicky for not very good reason.* (Yes quite a lot, Yes sometimes, No not much, No not at all)

6 * *Things have been getting on top of me.* (Yes most of the time I haven't been able to cope at all, Yes sometimes I haven't been coping as well as usual, No most of the time I have coped quite well, No I have been coping as well as ever)

7 * *I have been so unhappy that I have had difficulty sleeping.* (Yes most of the time, Yes sometimes, Not very often, No not at all)

8 * *I have felt sad or miserable.* (Yes most of the time, Yes quite often, Not very often, No not at all)

9 * *I have been so unhappy that I have been crying.* (Yes most of the time, Yes quite often, Only occasionally, No never)

10 * *The thought of harming myself has occurred to me.* (Yes quite often, Sometimes, Hardly ever, Never)

Action plan
Ideally, it is best to begin treatment before the birth. After birth, early and effective treatment may transform a difficult and overwhelming experience of parenting into one of joy and hope. A bout of depression may pass within days or, if severe, and particularly if linked with previous traumatic experiences, it may persist for months. Ongoing support and therapy can be very helpful while the condition improves. You will find suggestions for treating depression in EMOTIONS, ADVICE & SUPPORT. Even simple steps can be very powerful.

Pregnancy and birth number two
If you became depressed in your first pregnancy or after your first baby was born and you now feel more comfortable and well supported, you may not experience the problem again. Having been through it once before, you may also be on your guard. If your circumstances are similar, it is worth trying to arrange support in advance of the birth. Consider talking to your GP, midwife or health visitor to arrange an assessment and treatment before your baby is born so you can reduce the intensity of your emotions. If it was severe in the first pregnancy, you may wish to try medication (p.460).

Puerperal psychosis
Puerperal psychosis is characterised by being out of touch with reality, feeling depressed or manic, or both, with psychotic symptoms of racing thoughts, rapid changes of intense feeling states, and frequent changes of topic when speaking. About 1:500 women suffer from puerperal psychosis. An affected woman may repeatedly pick up her baby, yet seem unaware of her baby's needs, and may have delusions and hallucinations and a general loss of insight, as if blanking out reality.

A puerperal psychosis may last only days but it usually takes weeks or months to resolve. It does not follow on from a general depression but begins as a psychosis. Psychosis usually needs hospital treatment, preferably in a ward where mother and baby can stay together, and involves medication. Most women make a full recovery in a few weeks. Others improve but continue having residual symptoms or find it hard to get back to normal activities for several months. For a minority an episode of postnatal psychosis can lead to an ongoing psychotic condition. Early treatment is extremely valuable during future pregnancies.

ENGORGEMENT
See BREAST, ENGORGEMENT

EPILEPSY
See FITS: BABY; FITS & EPILEPSY: MOTHER

EPISIOTOMY
See LABOUR, EPISIOTOMY & TEARS

EYE, INFECTION: BABY
....

If your baby has swollen, red or discharging eyes, he may have an infection. Blocked tear ducts predispose a baby to infection.

Blocked tear ducts
Usually, aided by blinking, tears flow across the front of the eye and drain into the tear duct, passing down the back of the nose and throat. About 5% of newborns have a blockage to the tear duct. This is usually noticeable within 2 months when one or both eyes water continuously ('weepy eye'), and when crying, the nostril on the affected side remains dry. Newborn babies often have partially closed ducts and have a tendency to recurrent conjunctivitis (opposite) for a few months.

Action plan
The best thing to do is to keep your baby's eyes clean.
- Gently clean the eyes using cotton wool soaked in fresh, cooled boiled water. Use a separate piece of cotton wool for each eye. Wipe up the bony part of the nose, over the inner corner of the eye, then out over the eyelids. This also massages the tear duct and may open the blockage.
- If you are breastfeeding, squeeze a couple of drops of breast milk into the affected eye.

- In general antibiotics are not needed, but occasionally may help for severe infection.
- Your baby's tear ducts are likely to be normal within 18 months, without treatment. There is a small chance (5%) that discharge may continue for longer and the ducts will need to be cleared and dilated under an anaesthetic.

Styes

A stye (hordeolum) is a bacterial infection of a gland or hair follicle on the edge of the eyelid. It starts as a red spot and enlarges over 3–4 days, slowly filling with pus. It then bursts, and heals over 5–7 days. If your baby rubs his eyes a lot, he may get a stye in his other eye. The infection may be cured naturally by his immune system, but antibiotic ointment can help. Rarely, infection spreads and causes cellulitis of the eyelid, which definitely requires antibiotic treatment. If the same gland gets infected repeatedly, your baby may need minor surgery to drain the gland.

Conjunctivitis

The conjunctiva is a transparent membrane that lines the inside of the eyelid and the front of the eye. Conjunctivitis, also known as '**sticky eye**', most commonly occurs because of blocked tear ducts and bacterial or viral infection, but may happen if your baby has got a chemical spray (e.g. perfume) in his eye. It usually affects both eyes. If just one eye is affected, check to see whether your baby has something lodged in his eye or has any sign of injury. Although rare in babies below 1 year of age, conjunctivitis may be a symptom of ALLERGY.

Uncommonly, conjunctivitis may be a symptom of GONORRHOEA infection, especially if sticky eye appears within 24 hours of birth or CHLAMYDIA in the first 2 weeks. Both infections need specialist treatment with antibiotics and eye ointments to prevent scarring of the cornea.

Bacterial conjunctivitis: This gives the symptom of yellow sticky pus and is contagious. It is best to take a swab to find the organism and it usually settles rapidly with antibiotic drops and ointment. If your baby wakes up with crusty eyelids, wipe his eyes with cotton wool soaked in warm, previously boiled water. While your baby is infected do not share towels.

Viral conjunctivitis: This often makes the affected eye feel gritty and there may be a slight discharge. Your baby may have other signs of a viral infection, such as a sore throat. Viral conjunctivitis will not respond to antibiotics and can take 2–3 weeks to settle on its own. If the eyes are very sore, lubricant drops may give relief. If conjunctivitis occurs as part of a generalised viral infection, e.g. MEASLES, RUBELLA or HERPES, your baby needs specialist treatment and antiviral drops.

Action plan

Arrange to see your GP if swelling seems redder or more puffy then usual, if regular cleaning isn't helping, if swelling persists for more than 3 days or if the eyelids are being stuck together, especially overnight. If the infection is bacterial, antibiotics may help.

Homeopathic treatment
Give a remedy (30c) 3 times a day for 3 days and then reassess. When you bathe your baby's eyes, use *Euphrasia Tincture*,

diluting 8 drops to 250 ml (½ pint) of boiled, cooled water.

Arg Nit is a specific remedy for newborn conjunctivitis where the eyes are red, the lids swollen and there is a pus discharge; use *Apis* if your baby has puffy eyelids, is irritable and fidgety, rubs his eyes and seems sensitive to light; *Pulsatilla* if the lids stick together with a bland, yellowish discharge (often the left eye is worse) and your baby is clingy or whiny and feels better in the open air.

EYE, VISION DIFFICULTIES: BABY

At birth your baby's eyes are well developed and will probably be blue or grey – they will reach their permanent colour by 9 months. Visual development is rapid, if the eyes are stimulated, and he may have 20/20 vision by the age of 2–3 years. Development and visual ability are explored on p.20.

At birth, you may see a blood-red spot in one or both of your baby's eyes. This is a result of pressure that has caused blood vessels on the white of the eye to break. The blood will be reabsorbed and the spot disappears within a few weeks.

Eye crossing & squinting

Eye crossing or misalignment is common in the first 12 or so weeks because the eyes do not work together. They become synchronised soon after this. If your baby's eyes cross beyond the 3rd month, or he seems to have a squint beyond the 6th month, you need to refer your baby to an ophthalmologist.

A squint may result from being long- or short-sighted. This leads to poor focusing and the brain does not merge the images received by each eye. Each eye then adopts its own position. Treatment with glasses to correct the impairment allows the eyes to realign and move together. If the squint is not treated, binocular vision, which is required to judge depth and distance, will not develop.

Some squints result from a weakness of one of the eye muscles. The muscle may be strengthened by exercises, wearing glasses, and finally by an operation. Operations are usually done for cosmetic reasons and a loss of depth perception is not always prevented despite early treatment.

Visual impairment & blindness

Fewer then 1:10,000 babies are blind. This usually becomes obvious around 3 months, although some parents notice it sooner. If your child does not fix on or follow your face, or his eyes wander randomly, ask your health visitor or doctor to check his vision. He will be referred to a specialist in children's eyes. If his impairment is due to delayed maturation of the brain, his vision is likely to improve as he gets older.

Retinopathy of prematurity (ROP): A common cause of blindness that has all but disappeared in the west. All PREMATURE and low-birth-weight babies (p.563) are monitored for ROP and given prompt treatment to prevent it. Low lighting in neonatal units may help prevent the condition. ROP is caused by excess oxygen causing an initial constriction of blood vessels in the retina followed by rapid growth. New vessels may then leak and cause scarring. These scars later shrink and pull on the retina, sometimes detaching it. Most children recover well from low grades of ROP.

Cataracts: These account for the largest proportion of partially sighted and blind-registered children in the UK. Some are genetic or caused by RUBELLA infection in pregnancy. They make the eye opaque so vision is unclear and the lens is not stimulated to develop normally. A mild cataract may lead to a 'lazy eye' and severe cataracts may lead to very poor vision or blindness. Some congenital cataracts need surgery and vision may eventually become near normal with the aid of glasses.

Rare diseases: Rare diseases, which cause blindness or partial sightedness, include cortical visual impairment, optic nerve dysfunction and retinal diseases.

Action plan

If your baby has had eye problems at birth, regular examinations throughout life are important, as he may be susceptible to further problems. If your baby is visually impaired, your family may need to adjust dramatically many aspects of your lifestyle, with increasing compensation for his lack of vision as he becomes mobile. He will rely on his other senses to make up for the absence of effective vision. You can encourage his development and enjoy rich communication with the help of specialised teachers and therapists. Your local educational and health authority can put you in touch, and RNIB provide information and support.

FAILURE TO THRIVE
See WEIGHT, LOW GAIN OR FAILURE TO THRIVE

FAINTNESS
See BLOOD PRESSURE, LOW

FEET & HANDS
....

See also LEGS & ARMS

Club foot

In newborns club foot (talipes equinus varus) occurs where the sole of the foot is turned in and the four smaller toes sweep towards the big toe. Overall about 1:300 babies are affected. Very few need surgical treatment. Club foot is not painful and does not affect labour. There are variable degrees of club foot. The mildest, 'positional talipes', is caused by a baby's position in the uterus and corrects itself after birth. More significant degrees are probably caused by muscle imbalances or an underlying nerve disorder, and often run in the family. It can be seen on ultrasound after 20 weeks. In very rare instances club foot is due to CEREBRAL PALSY and accompanies other abnormalities of posture and muscle tone.

If your baby has significant club foot, it will give problems when she begins to try standing or walking. She may walk on the sides of her feet or on the tips of her toes, which leads to abnormal patterns of muscle development and walking may be clumsy. With appropriate treatment most children who begin life with club foot lead a completely normal life with no limitation to participation in sports or other activities.

Action plan

- Physiotherapy, massage or just gentle stretching advised by a children's physiotherapist or masseur or osteopath can help speed up the natural correction process.
- If club foot is due to an underlying nerve or muscle imbalance and if gentle stretching does not correct it, you will need specialist care from a paediatric orthopaedic surgeon, preferably in the 1st week after birth.
- The non-surgical Ponseti method involves gentle massage and manipulation to stretch the contracted tissues to achieve nearer-normal alignment and a cast is applied to maintain the correction. After approximately 7 days, the muscles and ligaments stretch enough to make further correction possible: the cast is removed and massage and manipulation and reapplication of the cast are repeated at intervals for approximately 6 weeks. Most babies need to have their Achilles tendon released before the application of the last plaster cast. The tendon reattaches naturally within 2–3 weeks.
- If the club foot is more intense, surgical operations may be needed over months or years to achieve the best functional and cosmetic result.

Extra digits
See also CONGENITAL ABNORMALITIES

At the birth counting fingers and toes is part of the welcoming ritual. If accessory digits are present it is reassuring to know they are common and cause no problems. Usually they occur beside the little finger or smallest toe. The extra digit may only be attached by a narrow band of tissue and be very small with a nail. It will contain an artery and vein as well as a nerve but probably no bony tissue.

The best treatment is for a plastic surgeon to cut off the accessory tissue at the base. This is usually done at 3–6 months, under an anaesthetic. Once removed there is no problem with either walking or using the hand.

Much more rarely, an accessory digit occurs beside the thumb or at the site of the big toe. These can be associated with other defects, including heart abnormalities. The extra digits are often complete duplications of the thumb or big toe and require specialist treatment by a paediatric plastic surgeon.

Flat feet

A baby has flat feet when the arch to the sole of the foot is flattened. In young babies a flattened sole is normal – any 6-month-old baby's footprint shows the whole of the sole of the foot. If flatness persists beyond the age of 2–3 years, or there are other symptoms, such as pain or stiffness, consult your doctor.

FEVER
....

At some point your baby will almost certainly develop a high temperature. This is a natural mechanism that helps the body fight infections. The average baby has around seven viral illnesses a year, which results in seven episodes of fever. Fever is also called febrile illness. When the temperature rises rapidly, some babies are rendered susceptible to febrile seizures (overleaf) .

What happens

Your baby's 'normal' body temperature is individual to her. Take a measurement when she is well so you know what is normal. As a general guide, consider a temperature of 38°C (100.4°F) to be a fever. Accompanying symptoms, such as your baby seeming unwell or too warm, having sweaty skin or if she is being unusually out of sorts, are also important. If you are worried, follow your instinct. Feeling your baby's forehead is not an accurate measure of temperature – use a thermometer to be sure. Your paediatrician may refer to the following figures:

	Normal	Fever
In the mouth	37°C (98.6°F)	37.5°C (99.5°F)
In the armpit	36.4°C (97.6°F)	37°C (98.6°F)
Rectal	37.6°C (99.6°F)	38°C (100.4°F)

Action plan

Call your doctor or the emergency services immediately if there is:
- Any fever below 8 weeks of age or, when she is older, a temperature more than 0.5°C (0.9°F) above normal.
- FITS.
- Uncontrolled crying or restlessness.
- A sudden rash or bruising.
- If she has had a rash for more than 3 days and it is not fading.
- Difficulty breathing (p.417).
- Drowsiness or irritability.
- Fever related to heat/humidity exposure (heat stroke).
- A rash does not fade when a glass is pressed against it and she has a stiff neck. This could indicate MENINGITIS.
- EAR PAIN (or ear rubbing).
- She becomes limp and floppy. A very sick baby may not show a fever, but may get cold instead (p.486).
- If she has persistent DIARRHOEA and VOMITING.
- She looks or acts sick and refuses feeds.
- Her temperature does not fall in response to the usual techniques. Your baby may get one illness closely followed by another, giving the impression that the fever is long lasting but it is best to be safe.

The secret to curing a fever is uncovering the cause. This is often viral infection in the ears, nose or throat, the digestive system or in the urine. Viruses are usually the cause and disappear without treatment. Antibiotics have no effect on viral infections.

Stopping a further rise in temperature

The goal is to stop the temperature from becoming higher. This will make your baby more comfortable and reduce the small risk that a rapid rise in temperature will lead to a febrile convulsion. Use the 'take temperature, treat temperature, take temperature' approach to see if your treatment is working.
- Give loving care.
- Keep your baby's room cool but avoid cold drafts.

- Keep her lightly dressed in cotton for comfort or take all her clothes off.
- Do not bring your baby into your bed where your body heat may boost her temperature.
- Use infant paracetamol in the correct dosage to treat the fever and reduce pain. It cannot mask more serious symptoms. Paracetamol suppositories placed in the rectum are useful if your baby cannot take the oral preparation, or is vomiting. The rectal dose is 50% higher than by mouth. Always follow the instructions exactly. Giving extra will not bring a temperature down more quickly and is not safe.
- Give her her favourite nutritious foods and drinks. She may enjoy juice or pop-ices.
- Sponge your baby with lukewarm (never hot) water. If the water is too cold the blood flow to the skin will reduce and that may make her temperature increase. The proper temperature is the same as your skin. It often takes 20–30 minutes of this to reduce the fever significantly.
- Try to keep your child calm because exertion may raise the temperature.
- Do not put a baby with febrile seizures in a bath or use alcohol on her skin. Never give a cold-water enema to a child with fever.
- Aspirin-containing preparations must not be used in childhood. Aspirin intake during a viral infection has been associated with Reye's syndrome, a rare condition that causes brain and liver damage and death.

Fevers generally get better within 3–4 days. If your baby continues to have a high temperature or her rash does not settle, visit your doctor to exclude other illnesses including bacterial or urinary infections requiring antibiotics.

Because your child may be infectious, it is best to keep her away from other children for 24 hours after the fever has cleared.

Homeopathy

Homeopathic remedies can be an effective method of reducing temperatures. As you get to know which remedies work best for your baby, it becomes much easier to prescribe. When using a remedy, give the most appropriate (30c) hourly for the first 3 hours and then reassess. If she seems to improve, continue with the same remedy every 2 hours for a further 8 hours. If after 3 hours there is no change, look at giving a different remedy and consult your homeopath. If your baby's temperature is high you must seek urgent medical attention.

Use *Aconite* with a sudden onset of symptoms usually around midnight (sometimes after getting chilled) with a dry heat, great thirst, anxiety and restlessness; *Arsenicum* for symptoms that are worse between midnight and 2am, a high fever with sweating, thirst, laboured breathing and perhaps vomiting or diarrhoea; *Belladonna* for a sudden onset of symptoms – often around 3pm or 3am, a 'Belladonna look' with flushed face, red lips, dilated pupils, glassy eyes, your baby's skin is hot to touch but despite the heat on the rest of the body her feet are usually cold and your baby has a strong racing pulse; *Chamomilla* if your baby has a burning heat, usually with sweating, particularly around the face and head and perhaps heat alternating with chills or one part of the body hot while another is cool, one cheek may be red and the other pale and she is extremely irritable and demanding; *Ferrum Phos* for fevers where there are very few other guiding symptoms, without sudden onset or intensity, nor irritability or restlessness, but with fever worse in the late afternoon and at night and relief from cold compresses and lying down.

Febrile seizures

A febrile seizure is a convulsion brought on by a fever and appears to be related to a rapid rise in temperature, rather than the height of temperature. It usually has no serious or long-term effects but witnessing your child fitting can be one of the most terrifying things. These types of fits occur in around 3–5% of children between the age of 6 months and 5 years and do tend to run in families.

What happens

During a febrile seizure your child will lose consciousness, her eyes may roll back in her head and there is usually stiffening followed by rhythmic jerking of the arms and legs. This lasts no more than 10 minutes and stops without treatment. Your child will probably be sleepy after the seizure but get back to normal, except for feeling ill from whatever is causing the fever, within 60 minutes. If the fit continues for longer than 10 minutes, your baby needs help to stop the seizure because a long fit may lead to damage. Call for an ambulance.

After the fit your baby may continue to shake or shiver – this is called a **rigor**, and is her response to the high temperature. The rigors will stop as the temperature comes down. Many children thought to have had a febrile convulsion have in fact had a severe rigor. These carry no risk of epilepsy or any other complication.

Action plan

If your child has a febrile convulsion, attend to the fit, which will be short lasting. Then your priority is to help her temperature to fall as you would do if she had a fever. As soon as you can, or if someone is with you, call your doctor or the emergency services.

Although you may be frightened, it is most helpful to stay calm. This will help you to do the best for your child and to observe the fit so you can describe it to a doctor: note whether it affects the whole body or just certain parts. The fit may appear to last longer than it actually does. If there is a clock in the room, it is a useful guide – your doctor will ask about the duration of the fit.

- While your child is jerking, lie her on the floor on her side and check her throat is not obstructed: she may be dribbling or vomiting and should not be upright.
- Do not put anything in her mouth or restrain her.
- Soothe her with your voice and a gentle touch and watch her closely.
- When the fit has passed, unless you have already undressed your baby, remove her clothes as a first step to cooling her. Do not cuddle her as this will prevent her from losing heat.
- Sponge her with water that is cool (not cold), roughly the same as your body temperature. If you have flannels or cloths to hand, soak them and lay them over your baby's body for a short time. Do not leave them there because they will soon begin to trap heat.

- Turn off any radiators or move your baby to a cooler room or use a fan and await the arrival of your doctor or the ambulance crew.
- Stay with your baby and reassure her that everything is all right and you are there, but do not heat her by cuddling. She may take around 5 minutes to regain consciousness and register your presence and then go back to sleep.
- If you have not given infant paracetamol in the last 4 hours, give a dose as soon as she is able to take it.

Medical care

Not all paediatricians recommend admission following a febrile convulsion. Your doctor will advise you. If your baby is in hospital:

- If there has been vomiting or diarrhoea, she may be kept in isolation. Her temperature will be taken regularly and she will be kept calm and regularly given infant paracetamol.
- Your doctor may check to exclude bacterial infection or meningitis-related illness. A urine test will check for urinary infection.
- If the doctors are happy that your baby has fully recovered and have observed her for 6 hours, she will be allowed to go home. Her temperature, related to the initial cause, may remain high for 3–4 days. Further fever-related fits are unlikely.
- If your baby is still fitting when help comes, she will be given oxygen and anticonvulsant medication. After a prolonged fit she will be monitored, with full medical follow-up that may include tests for infection.

What are the implications?

- If your child has had no previous signs of neurological problems and the seizure is related to her fever, there is no increased risk of developmental problems.
- If she has had a rigor there is no risk of complications.
- Once your child has had a febrile seizure, the risk of having another is around 35%. Next time her temperature rises, take early steps to reduce it.
- A febrile convulsion cannot cause epileptic fits. If your child is predisposed to epilepsy, however, the first febrile convulsion may be a trigger.

FIBROIDS
....

A fibroid is a thickening of the muscle fibres in the uterine wall. Fibroids can vary from pea- to grapefruit-sized, or bigger, and may occur singly or in groups. Their cause is unknown. They are benign and usually reduce after pregnancy. They are more common in women of African origin and may run in families. Most women with fibroids are able to have a normal labour and birth, and although the most common symptom is pain, many women have fibroids without symptoms.

What happens

Fibroids can form on the outer surface of the wall of the uterus, in the wall itself or impinge into the internal cavity of the uterus – the last are more likely to be troublesome. During pregnancy the muscle fibres of your uterus and the fibroid enlarge and symptoms are more likely.

- If the fibroids are near the fallopian tubes, they rarely cause difficulty conceiving and an ECTOPIC PREGNANCY is slightly more likely.
- A fibroid in the internal cavity of your uterus may prevent conception because it acts like a foreign object. An early MISCARRIAGE is also slightly more likely if the placenta has implanted close to the fibroid. Larger fibroids very uncommonly cause a late miscarriage.
- Large fibroids may swell further by retaining fluid. This 'degeneration' may cause pain, usually after Week 12. Intense swelling may block the blood supply to the fibroid and after pregnancy it may shrink and even disappear.
- Very rarely, extremely large fibroids may lead to PREMATURE BIRTH.
- Fibroids low down in your uterus may prevent your baby's head from engaging. Your baby may breech, or her head may fail to engage for birth – either event means it is safest to deliver by CAESAREAN SECTION.
- Large fibroids may cause bleeding after birth because they can prevent the wall of the uterus from retracting to seal the blood vessels supplying the placenta. You may require an oxytocin hormone injection to speed up placenta delivery and minimise bleeding (p.138).

Action plan
If you have abdominal or uterine pain, with or without bleeding (p.578), it is important to contact your doctor or midwife immediately. An examination and ultrasound can detect whether this is due to fibroids. Treatment of fibroids during pregnancy depends on an accurate diagnosis of the number and the site of the swellings.

- Fibroids causing pain and discomfort are best treated by rest; you may have to cut down on work and intense physical activity. If pain is severe, analgesic medication may be needed.
- Homoeopathic remedies may help reduce pain and swelling and need to be prescribed on a case-by-case basis.
- After birth fibroids tend to shrink and soon may become even smaller than before conception. Unfortunately, new fibroids tend to form and recur even after surgery.
- Most small fibroids can be safely left. Surgery is not done during pregnancy because of the risk of bleeding. A number of new techniques have been developed to treat fibroids after pregnancy or to assist conception. If you have small fibroids and the cavity of your uterus was not opened during surgery, a normal labour is feasible in a subsequent pregnancy. If the cavity of your uterus was opened it may be safer to have a caesarean section because of the small risk of the uterine wall rupturing during labour.

FITS: BABY

A baby's developing brain is an incredibly complex collection of cells, connections and chemical reactions. When something causes this system to malfunction, the resulting change in brain activity may cause a fit, or convulsion, which is also known as a seizure. Repeated seizures are called epilepsy.

Most fits are less serious than they appear, and a baby becomes calm within 10 minutes. If there is no improvement within 10 minutes, you must call for immediate medical assistance. A prolonged fit can cause a fall in blood oxygen levels and damage to the brain. Many babies who are thought to be fitting are often not fitting at all. One cause may be reflux of feed and stomach acid (p.561) – retching may appear like a mild convulsion. Some babies have febrile convulsions in relation to fever, which are usually harmless. Others have much milder 'rigors' that are not fits.

What happens
In a small baby a fit may cause only excessive lip smacking or staring, with a slight shaking of the limbs, often down one side or other, and sometimes a colour change to bright red or pale white. There might not be a change in alertness and feeding may be unaffected.

When fit-like activity does not affect a baby's level of consciousness, it is called a partial seizure. When consciousness is lost, the fit is said to be generalised. Babies who have had a genuine fit tend to fall asleep or appear sleepy for 2–3 hours after. They then usually wake up and appear quite normal, unless the fit was due to an infection in the brain (MENINGITIS), when the level of consciousness may remain altered.

Jitteriness, mycolonic jerks and funny turns
Jitteriness: Looks like shivering, stops when you touch the shaking limb gently, and is not associated with any other unusual activity, such as strange eye movements, sleepiness or poor feeding. It is quite normal and can persist to the age of 4–6 months. These movements may be caused by an immature and active developing nervous system.

Myoclonus: Similar to jitteriness but is a larger more rhythmic movement, which occurs only during sleep and mimics a seizure. The condition can be alarming to witness, but does no harm. Sometimes only one limb may move and can be associated with grunting. To exclude the possibility of fits, brainwave monitoring can show there is no abnormal electrical activity during these events.

Funny turns: Brief episodes of blankness, blinking, shaking, head turning and nodding but no change in consciousness. Most of these are harmless and are merely habits and others are for enjoyment. Most stop as a baby grows older. In a small number of babies in the first 6 months an underlying problem such as reflux, tummy pain, earache or headache may cause a funny turn. Rarely, if the episode is linked with a colour change to blue or white (pallid attack) it may indicate a HEART rhythm disturbance.

Fits below 1 month of age
Fits at birth are rare. They may signify:
- Reduced oxygen flow to the brain before or during birth, leading to FOETAL DISTRESS & ASPHYXIA with HIE (p.474). 1:1000 babies are affected.
- BIRTH INJURY with bleeding in the brain, which usually occurs in premature babies and may resolve naturally.

- Meningitis infection, which needs intensive treatment.
- HYPOGLYCAEMIA (low blood glucose levels), which usually passes once feeding is established.
- Withdrawal from DRUGS taken in pregnancy or if a baby has needed surgery and morphine after birth.
- Injury to the head or being shaken can also cause fits.

Neonatal seizures, occurring in the first 28 days after birth in a full-term infant or up to 1 month after the due date in a premature baby, affect roughly 1:1000 babies, usually within a few days of birth. They can be difficult even for neonatal nurses and doctors to spot.

Some babies have a family tendency of neonatal fits, others may fit because there is a problem in the brain or nervous system and it is important to investigate a possible cause. If fits are due to asphyxia, the outlook is best if asphyxia was mild. If no cause is found, a family history of neonatal seizures may suggest a good outcome. Roughly half of babies who have neonatal seizures have underlying abnormalities that may lead to learning or developmental difficulties – the rest have no long-term problems.

Fits between 1 and 6 months of age

Seizures may occur in as many as 1% of children between the age of 1 month and 14 years. The period from 1 to 6 months is an unusual time to develop a seizure, and if your baby has not had fits in the 1st month then a fit between 1 and 6 months usually signifies illness. Idiopathic epilepsy (two or more seizures with no apparent cause – opposite) does not begin until the end of this time period andfebrile convulsions (p.468) are very rare under 6 months of age. Some fits are due to developmental abnormalities of the brain, which began soon after conception.

Below 6 months the likely cause is an infection of the nervous system, such as meningitis. Reactions to VACCINATIONS may be another cause of a seizure, but even though there may be a fever at this time, the fit is not considered to be a febrile convulsion. The cause is usually due to irritation of the brain or the lining membranes.

Many children who experience a first-time seizure in this period may never experience a second seizure. However, a seizure at this time may be the start of a serious medical condition and extensive tests may be needed.

Fits after 6 months of age

Over 6 months of age fits may be due to a number of causes:
- Infantile spasms occur between 4 and 8 months and consist of benign mycolonic spasms upon awakening.
- Febrile convulsions may arise in response to fever.
- A small number of fits after 6 months relate to causes that may have led to fitting after birth (e.g. foetal distress and asphyxia, infection, hypoglycaemia).
- Some babies have a habit of BREATH HOLDING that can give fit-like symptoms.
- Partial seizures, such as petit mal epilepsy (opposite), involve blanking off or staring in frequent short episodes, perhaps as many as 100 times a day. Non-accidental head injury, including being shaken, now accounts for about 15% of all new cases of epilepsy; another 15% are caused by infection and meningitis. The remainder may be linked to

syndromes that are genetically determined or to a family history of seizures, and often no cause is found. Many childhood epilepsies are associated with generalised disorders of the brain, and are part of more generalised disorders of development.

Action plan

Watching a child of any age have a convulsion is terrifying. You may feel certain that your child is going to die, and this often leads to confusion and panic. Despite this natural reaction, it is important you do all you can to remain calm and to help your child breathe. She is likely to be frightened and will need reassuring, either straight away or when she has come round from a brief spell of unconsciousness.

- Do not pick up your baby because, if she thrashes around, you may drop her. If she begins to have a fit while you are holding her, lie her down on the floor, on her side. Being upright only increases the chance of her vomiting and fainting.
- If your baby is unconscious, deal with the ABC (p.383).
- If your baby is hot with a febrile convulsion (p.468), cool her by removing clothing, opening a window or gently fanning. Do not put her in a cool bath – this may bring on a renewed fit and she may breathe in the water.
- Give a medicine designed to reduce FEVER, such as infant paracetamol suspension if she is able to swallow. Do this even if there is no apparent fever because often a convulsion precedes the fever.
- If recovery is complete, with return to normal behaviour, normal pupil size, and your baby is fully conscious within 30 minutes then arrange to see your GP within 24 hours.
- If recovery is not complete within 30 minutes, or the fit continues beyond 10 minutes call an ambulance or GP or NHS Direct. For a continuing fit your baby needs oxygen and anticonvulsant medication.
- Follow-up care after a prolonged fit may include a brain scan. An EEG reading can help doctors predict the likelihood of further fits occurring.

Homeopathy

If your baby has a fever with a fit while you are awaiting medical help, you can give *Aconite* (30c) in a soft tablet that can dissolve easily every minute for up to 3 doses. This is the no. 1 remedy for shock. For further treatment, consult your homeopath.

After a fit

Following a seizure your main concern may be whether your baby will be completely normal. If she was normal before the fit, the chances of any problem are low.
- If the cause of the fit (e.g. low blood sugar) is corrected, the risk of damage and further fits is considerably reduced.
- If the fit was caused by a febrile convulsion, the risk of damage is extremely low, and you can be reassured there will be no long-lasting effects.
- If the fit was prolonged and difficult to stop, taking 30–60 minutes to bring under control, the risk of a longer-lasting problem begins to rise. If the cause is a viral illness there is a risk that this has damaged the brain.

- For the large proportion of babies who have a fit, there is no significant effect. It may, however, take anything up to 5 years to ensure that there has been no subtle damage.

Epilepsy

Epilepsy is the name given to the condition of recurrent seizure activity, unrelated to fever, and there are several different types. Epilepsy in babies is rare – it more commonly affects older children. When it happens there may be repeated episodes of blanking out. If your baby shows this, or has had seizures, you will need a specialist opinion to diagnose the condition. Children known to have convulsions frequently are often provided with medicines called anticonvulsants, to help stop prolonged fits. If your child is epileptic it is essential that everyone who cares for her knows about the condition and what to do in the event of a seizure. The outlook is very good with modern drug therapy.

FITS & EPILEPSY: MOTHER

Fits (convulsions) are extremely rare. If you have a history of fitting because of epilepsy, it is important to receive specialist care while you are pregnant, and preferable to have counselling before conceiving. Specialist medical advice is constantly being updated and over 90% of epileptic women who become pregnant have completely normal pregnancies. In pregnancy a possible cause of fits is eclampsia, resulting from very high BLOOD PRESSURE.

Risk to your baby
If you are susceptible to fits, you need to take anticonvulsant medication. Some of these medications have been linked with an increased risk of congenital abnormality in babies: 7–10% compared to 5%. It is preferable to use single medications rather than a combination. If you have high blood pressure or pre-eclampsia that is kept under control, the risk of eclamptic fitting is very low. Eclamptic fits are more prolonged than epileptic fits and carry a higher risk.

Although your baby is protected, severe trauma from an intense seizure may cause PLACENTAL ABRUPTION or premature rupture of the membranes (p.501) and foetal asphyxia (p.472). There is a small risk you may injure yourself.

Action plan
If you have a fit in pregnancy
- Whoever is with you needs to call for medical help immediately. A fit is an emergency.
- You need to be protected from injuring yourself, without being tightly restrained. It is best for you to be laid on your side, and tight clothing loosened. The person with you will need to check you can breathe freely. A medical team can administer drugs to control your convulsion.
- If your fit is eclamptic, you will be given medications to control fits and your blood pressure. You may need artificial ventilation and intensive care. If pregnancy is sufficiently advanced, the team will deliver your baby by emergency CAESAREAN SECTION.

Preventing fits
- Good nutrition and emotional support to reduce stress are both helpful.
- Some doctors recommend combining medication with special diets as mineral deficiencies are often linked with epilepsy: your specific needs will be indicated by your medication and advice from a nutritionist may help.
- Some medications may increase the risk of CONGENITAL ABNORMALITIES of the baby and your doctor will advise you about the safest drugs. Vitamin K deficiency may be more likely in your baby with some drugs and a vitamin K injection at birth reduces the risk of neonatal bleeding (p.226).
- Eclamptic fits are usually prevented with measures to control high blood pressure.

During and after labour
- During labour it is important to have access to anticonvulsants in case they are needed. Your doctor will advise on the optimal drug to avoid depressing your baby's breathing reflex after birth.
- After birth the treatment you and your baby receive depends on the level of medication you have had during pregnancy. The higher the level, the more intense observation and treatment need to be.
- Your baby will be watched for bleeding and signs of withdrawal (p.451) from any anti-epileptic drug you have been taking, and may be given a vitamin K injection.
- If you are breastfeeding and taking anti-epileptic medications, your baby is unlikely to be affected. If she continually appears drowsy, inform your doctor.
- While you are caring for your baby, especially if you are breastfeeding, take care of yourself and get extra sleep whenever you can – lack of sleep may trigger seizures.
- Practical help and love and emotional support will help reduce stress and the likelihood of fitting. See the Wheel for Living (p.58) for some tips.
- It will help to use medical support – your health visitor, neurology nurse or occupational therapist may have good advice to suit your lifestyle.
- If you are prone to seizures, it is safer to feed and change your baby on the floor. If you are alone, give your baby a wash with a sponge rather than a full bath. Always use a safety harness in a pram or pushchair and take precautions against everyday hazards – a fire guard, stair gate, etc. will keep your baby safe if you have a seizure.

FLATULENCE: MOTHER

Excess wind is usually related to diet. In pregnancy feeling bloated and passing excessive wind is very common because of slower movement of food through the intestine combined with a change in diet. This is particularly the case if you are sensitive or ALLERGIC to certain food(s). Sometimes, more often in late pregnancy, flatulence is accompanied by a feeling of swelling and bloating and uncomfortable INDIGESTION & HEARTBURN.

What happens

Swallowed air is one cause of flatulence. You may swallow air quite unconsciously: as you talk, especially when upset, excited or nervous, when eating or drinking in a hurry, chewing gum or smoking, drinking carbonated beverages or swallowing excess saliva.

Another common cause is diet. Some foods are not digested in the stomach but pass into the colon where they are processed by intestinal bacteria, which produce gas. Common examples include foods rich in soluble fibre (fruits, beans, corn, peas and oat or wheat bran); foods containing the 'simple' sugar fructose (figs, dates, prunes, melons, pears and grapes and, in lesser quantity, onions, asparagus, broccoli, cauliflower, Brussels sprouts, artichokes), and wheat and artificially sweetened 'diet' drinks. Lactose, a sugar found in milk, may be difficult to digest if you are lactose intolerant (p.393).

Flatulence can also accompany NAUSEA or morning sickness, often because there is a change in diet to alleviate the nausea, and can accompany DIARRHOEA as a symptom of irritable bowel syndrome. After labour it may be caused by damage to the anal sphincter (p.557).

Action plan

An appropriate diet will help prevent excessive flatulence. If you are worried the distension is caused by an underlying problem with your baby, a clinical examination or an ultrasound scan will put your mind at rest.

Diet

- Eat and drink slowly and chew your food thoroughly before you swallow.
- For a few days, avoid the foods most likely to cause flatulence (above). Then gradually add them to your diet again, one by one, while keeping track of your symptoms. There are no general rules and if you are observant you will notice the foods that are a problem for you. If you have increased fibre rapidly, this may be a cause, so keep the increase gradual.
- Try peppermint, camomile or fennel tea after eating and cut down on gassy or carbonated drinks and alcohol. Aduki beans are thought to reduce wind, particularly if they are well cooked, and for some people cooking with garlic and ginger helps.
- You could eat live yoghurt and a variety of herbs that aid digestion: lemon balm, rosemary, sage, thyme, caraway and fennel seeds are all good.

Homeopathy

Take 1 tablet (30c), 4 times a day for 3–4 days, then reassess.

Use *Carbo Veg* if you have gas in the upper abdomen, acid reflux, your tummy rumbles, loud belching relieves, you feel heavy and full, sluggish, chilly and worse from wearing tight clothes and 30 minutes after food; *China* if there is lots of belching, distension, rumbles and gurgles, colicky pains, particularly in the afternoon, a good appetite but food tastes bitter, you crave sour fruits and feel better from pressure on your abdomen; *Lycopodium* if you feel bloated all the time, hungry but quickly feel full and worse after eating cold food or

beans, cabbage, onions or sweets, and much worse from 4–8pm; *Nux Moschata* when flatulence begins immediately after eating and there is a feeling of distension with cramping pressure in the abdomen, your mouth and throat remain dry yet you are not thirsty, you crave spicy foods and may feel a bit spaced out and chilly; *Nux Vomica* if you want to pass wind but can't, feel pressure in an upward motion, colicky spasms, lower back pain and nausea, worse about 2 hours after eating, crave spicy foods, feel uptight, irritable and stressed.

FOETAL DISTRESS & ASPHYXIA

Foetal distress is a term that implies a baby is receiving a reduced amount of oxygen. Reduced oxygen is called **hypoxia**. If it continues there may be changes in the physiology of the cells in the baby's body, particularly in the brain. This effect is called asphyxia. The terms asphyxia and foetal distress are used interchangeably but asphyxia may be the result of the distress and is the more accurate term.

You may hear these terms being used by midwives and doctors, particularly in relation to labour. This might worry you but in most cases the distress is minimal and asphyxia is absent. Attention for signs of asphyxia is one of the cornerstones of good midwifery and obstetric care: a medical team is ready to act quickly and effectively and can usually prevent a dangerous degree of asphyxia occurring.

What happens

If oxygen flow stops completely, an adult would have brain damage in about 5 minutes but babies can recover completely after 10 or more minutes. During this time a baby's cells are protected and function by drawing on energy reserves stored within the body. Fortunately, it is very rare for oxygen flow to stop completely. The most common time for oxygen flow to be interrupted is during the contractions of labour, but this is intermittent and it returns between contractions.

In a process called anaerobic respiration the energy reserves – sugar stored as glycogen in the liver and other organs – can provide glucose for your baby's organs, including the brain, to use when oxygen is low. During pregnancy the majority of babies are able to build up sufficient glycogen stores, most of which are laid down in the last 10 weeks. Babies who are PREMATURE, have undergone INTRAUTERINE GROWTH RESTRICTION (IUGR) or HIGH-RISK PREGNANCIES, and those few who have a developmental disorder or infection are more likely to have low reserves and are at a higher risk of asphyxia in a shorter time if the oxygen concentration drops.

If hypoxia occurs, the effect depends on the severity of the reduction in oxygen flow and the duration of the low flow. Foetal distress is mild if hypoxia is short-lived. If asphyxia is intense, levels of stress hormones rise, the 'feel good' endorphin hormones normally released during labour fall and a baby shows the pattern of what would be described as anxiety or panic in an older child or adult. After birth the baby may be shocked and take time to recover, and will benefit from resuscitation followed by loving contact and frequent feeding.

Severe asphyxia is rare, and occurs if hypoxia continues

and energy reserves have been used up. Then the body tissues release lactic acid and this leads to **acidosis**, changing the metabolism of the body cells and altering their ability to function normally. If the condition persists, the cells may be damaged permanently. The changes affect all the organs, including the heart, lungs, kidneys and liver, but the brain is the most sensitive. Because of these risks modern obstetric care is geared to checking babies during regular antenatal appointments, using ultrasound scans and heart beat monitoring and with close monitoring during labour. This monitoring is more intensive in high-risk pregnancies.

While labour is the most common time for asphyxia to occur, some babies are susceptible during pregnancy. When antenatal monitoring indicates this, early birth, often by elective CAESAREAN SECTION, is advised. On the other side of the spectrum a very small number of babies who develop asphyxia at birth do not show signs of foetal distress in pregnancy or during labour.

Asphyxia in pregnancy

Foetal distress and hypoxia in pregnancy are rare. Babies are more susceptible if pre- or postmature, when a mother has high BLOOD PRESSURE with pre-eclampsia or PLACENTAL ABRUPTION, or there is IUGR. If a baby has IUGR the diminished foetal nutrition must be very severe for the oxygen levels to fall before labour. Maternal DRUGS consumption and SMOKING increase the risk, as do CONGENITAL ABNORMALITIES and intrauterine infections. Signs of distress in pregnancy usually prompt urgent delivery to avoid complications.

Asphyxia in labour

In labour the flow of oxygen to your baby, from your blood via the placenta, usually decreases during a contraction and then returns to normal levels. A normal, well-grown baby can easily cope with this but if your baby's glycogen stores are low, it may lead to asphyxia. Asphyxia in labour is usually mild. Your medical team will be alert for signs:

Abnormal heart rate: Oxygen affects the sensitive heart muscle as well as the hormones and nerves that originate in the brain and control heart rate. Heartbeat monitoring is an integral aspect of modern obstetric care in preventing and diagnosing foetal distress. Although not 100% reliable, it is a good indicator and an abnormal variation prompts the medical team to observe your baby and your progress closely, and to monitor heart rhythm more intensely (p.125). Occasionally the heart rate may appear normal while a baby is distressed and a problem may not be detected earlyon . On the other hand an abnormal heart pattern may not indicate asphyxia because pressure on the head in labour can cause changes in heart rate anyway.

Meconium staining of amniotic fluid: Greenish meconium staining of the amniotic fluid is evident when your waters break, which indicates that your baby has passed her first bowel motion in the womb. The bowel movement can be normal (it happens in 30% of normal labours), and is more likely in older babies, particularly after Week 40, but may be stimulated by hypoxia. It does not indicate foetal distress unless the heart rate is abnormal or the meconium is very thick

and there is a reduced volume of AMNIOTIC FLUID. The greatest risk associated with passing meconium is meconium aspiration (overleaf).

Blood oxygen levels: If distress is indicated by your baby's heart rate during the 1st stage of labour, a doctor may take a blood sample from your baby's scalp. The oxygen and carbon dioxide content is assessed for acidosis within 10 minutes. The results help the doctor to decide whether it is safe for your baby to continue with labour. The practice of taking a blood sample in this way is becoming less common because there is a risk of scalp infection to the baby and transmission of HIV and HEPATITIS virus from the mother.

In addition to risk factors that identify babies who are more susceptible, asphyxia may occur in labour for other reasons:

- An excessive fall in blood flow to the placenta, which may affect the supply of oxygen to your baby. The flow may fall if the uterine muscle contracts excessively, sometimes following the use of oxytocin or prostaglandin to boost contractions. The flow may fall if you lie flat and your uterus presses on the blood vessels supplying the placenta.
- Epidural anaesthetic, particularly if you lie on your back.
- UMBILICAL CORD COMPRESSION from a reduced amniotic fluid volume or if the cord has become tight around your baby's neck or if the cord has prolapsed.
- Prolonged rupture of membranes or a slow prolonged labour particularly if there is intrauterine infection. Difficult forceps or ventouse delivery may cause distress.
- Placental abruption in labour.

Asphyxia after birth

If a baby has been deprived of oxygen during labour, she may be born asphyxiated and have difficulty breathing. This is called neonatal asphyxia or birth asphyxia. When mild it is easily corrected by administering oxygen.

In a minority of cases neonatal asphyxia is severe and there has been insufficient oxygen to the brain and other vital organs. A baby may show signs of brain injury with hypoxic ischaemic encephalopathy (HIE, overleaf). This is very rare and in its severe form affects 1:1000 babies. When breathing cannot be established, a baby is stillborn after labour; this tragic event occurs in 1:2000 deliveries in the UK.

Action plan
In pregnancy
Modern antenatal care aims to identify high-risk pregnancies and provide additional monitoring for mother and baby. This allows the medical team to detect any early signs of hypoxia and foetal distress prior to the natural onset of labour and be aware of a baby's susceptibility to asphyxia during labour. This is the main method of prevention, although a minority of high-risk pregnancies are not detected before labour.

If your baby is at a very high risk of asphyxia, an elective caesarean section may be suggested. You will need to give birth in a hospital with a SPECIAL CARE BABY UNIT (SCBU), particularly in the case of PREMATURE BIRTH. If the risk is lower, but still significant, an induction of labour (p.497) will be considered when your pregnancy is closer to term or if it is postmature. The early birth usually means that factors that could lead to asphyxia, such as postmaturity, are avoided.

Labour and birth

In the majority of cases where there are signs of distress and the birth team intervenes, a baby is born safely and has no long-term difficulties. Close monitoring during labour enables midwives and obstetricians to intervene at the appropriate time. Preventing birth asphyxia in labour is not always possible, however: even after an apparently healthy pregnancy, a baby may become distressed in labour.

Because of the risk of cerebral damage, if oxygen deprivation is prolonged your obstetrician may be keen to expedite the birth. The action chosen will depend upon the level of foetal distress, the stage of labour and your opinion.

- If significant foetal distress is apparent in the 1st stage, your birth team will treat the obvious causes. They may help you alter your position so that you are not lying on your back and are, preferably, upright (p.97), reduce an oxytocin infusion and/or adjust fluid replacement during epidural anaesthesia. If this is not successful, a caesarean section will be advised, particularly if your baby is at high risk.
- If the heartbeat is causing concern during the 2nd stage, when you are pushing, the birth team may recommend using an upright position to improve your pushing power or an assisted delivery with forceps or ventouse (p.496) or a caesarean section.
- If the foetal heart pattern at any time indicates there is a significant risk of neonatal asphyxia that could lead to HIE (right), your baby needs to be born within 10 minutes. When there is concern a paediatrician will be called to be present at the delivery to treat your baby at birth.

After birth

At birth the midwife or doctor will check your baby immediately. If there is asphyxia your baby may have difficulty establishing breathing, her heart rate may be slow and muscle tone floppy. This is assessed within 1 minute and the Apgar score (p.139) is assigned. If it is below '7' of a maximum of '10', your baby requires oxygen and resuscitation, and this is usually a simple and effective procedure. A score below '3' indicates severe asphyxia and the need for intense resuscitation. Most babies who receive help to begin breathing are fine within a few minutes.

- The first step is to remove liquid blocking your baby's airway. This is done gently, using a soft plastic suction catheter in the mouth or nose. Contact with the cooler air in the room normally stimulates breathing.
- If the onset of breathing is delayed, gentle stimulation will probably initiate breathing, and extra oxygen may be given by blowing it on her face.
- If after 1 minute your baby is not breathing regularly, artificial ventilation is started, initially using a face mask, but a plastic tube may be inserted into her airway. In mild asphyxia the initial gasp of oxygen is enough.
- For a tiny number of babies more treatment is needed and will be given by a paediatrician or midwife. The lungs may be ventilated. Usually this is sufficient to restart breathing and the tube can be safely removed after 5–10 minutes.
- If the asphyxia is severe, it may indicate HIE and so your baby would require ventilation and medication followed by transfer to a SCBU.

Your emotions

As parents, concern during pregnancy, labour and the anxious moments of silence after the birth as your baby is assisted may be very difficult. If the medical team is large enough, you may receive support and attention but most of the attention will be focused on your baby. This is an incredibly difficult time. Parents often feel helpless and can do nothing but wait and hope for the best. Even if your baby is fine within minutes, which is usually the case, coming to terms with what has happened may take time and involve talking over what happened with your medical team. Sometimes there are no clear reasons why a baby was in difficulty.

Meconium aspiration

Meconium aspiration into the lungs occurs if there is reduced amniotic fluid volume (the usual causes are postmaturity and IUGR) combined with the passing of meconium into the amniotic fluid and severe asphyxia that makes a baby gasp and inhale meconium before birth. Detecting reduced amniotic fluid volume and inducing labour often prevent meconium aspiration, as does reducing foetal distress in labour.

- If asphyxia occurs in labour, your baby may make gasping movements in the womb. Aspiration begins before birth.
- If there has been intense meconium staining, the midwife or doctor present at birth will apply suction to the back of your baby's mouth to remove meconium from the throat and larynx and prevent any more entering the lungs. Your baby is likely to respond well and may begin to breathe easily.
- In about 1:500 births the lungs contain thick meconium and oxygen cannot enter easily. These babies require the insertion of a tube into the trachea for suction and assistance with breathing. They are transferred to a SCBU for oxygen monitoring, ventilation and antibiotics to prevent a chest infection. The meconium clears in a few days but a baby may be ill during this time.

Hypoxic ischaemic encephalopathy (HIE)

Neonatal HIE is rare. It results from asphyxia with insufficient oxygen and reduced blood flow to the brain and other essential organs during the birth process and may cause brain injury. It may be temporary (Grade 1) or potentially permanent (Grade 2 or 3). It has serious consequences for about 1:1000 babies.

Neonatal HIE can only be diagnosed when there is evidence of severe foetal distress and asphyxia at birth with altered behaviour, such as needing intensive resuscitation and ventilation, excessive sleepiness, poor muscle tone and feeding, altered consciousness or FITS that are consistent with brain injury. Another indicator is an Apgar score below 3 at 10 minutes or later after birth.

What happens

With HIE there has been reduced oxygen to the brain and the nervous system becomes irritated or suppressed. The extent of symptoms, such as unconsciousness, reduced muscle tone and weak reflexes, reflects the degree. Grade 1 HIE is mild, usually passes within 48 hours and is rarely associated with long-term effects. Grade 2 is moderate and leads to fitting in 50% of cases and usually improves within 3–5 days, although some babies show long-term effects. Grade 3 is the most serious and may leave a baby unresponsive or unconscious and lead to fits. An affected baby may not survive, or may pull through with brain damage or developmental disability (CEREBRAL PALSY).

Action plan
If your baby has signs of HIE, the medical team will give breathing assistance at birth by ventilating the lungs. Intensive resuscitation with medication may be needed. This may include cardiac massage and intravenous fluids and adrenalin. This is often very frightening for parents – the medical staff can be extremely supportive, however. Intensive care in a SCBU is necessary. Treatment will be needed to correct HYPOGLYCAEMIA, breathing difficulties, fits and kidney failure. The long-term outlook is assessed by taking a number of factors into account, including the grade of HIE; how the baby responds in the first few days; the oxygen and acidosis levels in the cord blood at birth; the Apgar score at 10 minutes, and results from EEG as well as CT and MRI brain scans. Modern obstetric and paediatric care is geared to detecting hypoxia and reducing the long-term effects of asphyxia.

FORCEPS & VENTOUSE
See LABOUR, FORCEPS & VENTOUSE

GASTROENTERITIS
See DIARRHOEA: BABY

GENITALIA, AMBIGUOUS

See also CONGENITAL ABNORMALITIES

When a child's genitals do not appear clearly male or female, this is extremely distressing for the parents. Fortunately, it is very rare, affecting only around 1:25,000 babies per year in the UK. Most commonly, a female has severe virilising (overproduction of male hormones) and appears to have a small penis, or a male has an abnormally small penis that resembles a clitoris. Very few affected babies have genitals that are so ambiguous that a gender determination cannot be made at birth. True hermaphroditism, where a baby has both male and female internal genitals and the external genitals may be indistinct, is extremely rare. The ideal care is a team approach, including parents, neonatologists, geneticists, endocrinologists, surgeons, counsellors and ethicists.

What happens
In many cases the cause cannot be identified and the genetic disorder appears to occur by chance, but there are some known causes. **Congenital adrenal hyperplasia** (CAH), present in about 1:15,000 babies, is the most common cause of females to be masculinised. The condition is related to a gene that affects the over production of masculinising hormones from the adrenal glands and a deficiency of cortisone that leads to salt deficiency in the body's tissues. A paediatric endocrinologist may suggest medication to suppress the production of male hormones and replacement cortisone. In families with the

disease the diagnosis may be established by antenatal testing and steroid treatment may begin before birth for the mother.

Action plan
The discovery is usually unexpected: you will be offered counselling and put in touch with support groups. In most cases gender can be determined relatively soon and a baby's chromosome analysis will be done on a blood sample.

Treatment depends of the type of the disorder, but usually includes corrective surgery, hormone replacement and close follow-up. Some children born with ambiguous genitalia may have normal internal reproductive organs that do not interfere with fertility. At puberty treatment with oestrogen and progesterone may be used for girls with absent or non-functioning ovaries to bring on pubertal changes, of breast development, change in body proportions and body hair. In some girls the vaginal opening may need to be enlarged.

There is controversy concerning issues of gender because gender assignment by doctors and family may not correlate with gender preference by the patient in adulthood. The most important organ for gender assignment is the brain, which may undergo hormonal imprinting in the uterus. Intersex activists and some doctors have called for a moratorium on gender reassignment surgery until studies have been completed on the long-term effects. The best approach is to gather as much information as possible.

GERMAN MEASLES
See RUBELLA

GONORRHOEA

Gonorrhoea is rare and is usually easily treated. It is a highly contagious sexually transmitted bacterium that tends to infect the cervix. It may sometimes affect the urethra, the rectum or, less commonly, the throat. In men it infects the penis, urethra and prostate gland. If you have unprotected sex – oral, vaginal or rectal – with an infected person, you have a 90% chance of catching it. When gonorrhoea is present there is often an accompanying infection of CHLAMYDIA and TRICHOMONIASIS.

What happens
Around half of the women infected don't experience symptoms. Others have a vaginal discharge and may have vaginal pain and redness and perhaps pain when passing urine. Men have urinary or penis symptoms. If the infection is not treated, it may cause pelvic inflammatory disease, which may cause blockage of the fallopian tubes and increase the likelihood of ECTOPIC PREGNANCY and infertility. Rarely, it leads to severe pelvic inflammation after delivery. The baby is protected during pregnancy but bacteria present during birth may cause conjunctivitis (p.465). Gonorrhoea may also cause septicaemia in a baby, requiring intensive antibiotic treatment.

Action plan
A vaginal and urethral swab provides a sample that can be tested for gonorrhoea, chlamydia and trichomonas.

Medical care
The standard treatment during and after pregnancy is penicillin by injection, although there are alternative antibiotics if necessary. A vaginal swab after treatment ensures the bacteria have been eliminated. Your partner also needs to be treated and tested for other sexually transmitted infections. After birth your baby's eyes may be swabbed to test for infection and treated with antibiotic drops..

HAEMORRHOIDS
See PILES & ANAL FISSURE

HEAD & HEAD SHAPES

The average head circumference of a newborn is about 32 cm (13 in). Nature prepares your baby for the pressures of birth with skull bones that can easily slide over one another, and the head may mould into an alarming shape. The moulding will smooth out within a few days, but two areas known as fontanelles remain soft for longer. They are a part of the skull structure, enabling it to expand as the brain enlarges.

Fontanelles
Each of the two fontanelles consists of a sheet of tough fibrous material, which bridges the gap between the growing bones. This area is not more sensitive than any other area of the skull and is immensely strong. When your baby is quiet you may be able to see or feel her pulse here. The posterior (back) fontanelle cannot usually be felt beyond the 4th month, while the larger, anterior (front) fontanelle remains obvious until it closes around 18 months. Early or late closure of the anterior fontanelle is not usually a cause for concern. Very rarely, the posterior fontanelle may close before the 3rd month when the skull bones fuse early – this is usually linked with an unusually small head.

The fontanelles do rise and fall with normal breathing, and are of no concern. If they appear sunken, accompanied by a dry mouth and perhaps sunken eyes this may be a sign of dehydration (p.446). If they appear to bulge this may indicate MENINGITIS or hydrocephalus (right), when there is swelling within the brain. For sinking or swelling visit your doctor.

Large head: megancephaly
A larger-than-normal head (megancephaly) is usually noticed at the 6-week check. It is rarely a cause for concern, and often runs in families, so it is useful to check a parent's head circumference. It can prompt further investigation, however, due to confusion with hydrocephalus.

Small head: microcephaly
About 40% of babies whose heads are smaller for age and gender have no abnormalities related to development. However in 60% the head size relates to an abnormally small brain and there are associated learning difficulties, perhaps also a high-pitched cry, poor feeding, FITS, or spasticity (p.424).

A small brain is usually caused by early failure of brain growth in pregnancy due to chromosomal abnormalities,

infection, recreational DRUGS or excessive ALCOHOL abuse. After birth microcephaly may occur as a result of severe FOETAL DISTRESS & ASPHYXIA with brain injury, infection, or an underactive THYROID gland. Close follow-up is usual, but the extent of the problem is usually not evident for 7–9 years.

Microcephaly may be associated with fusion of the skull bones earlier than the usual 5th or 6th month after birth. Early fusion can restrict space for the brain to grow and may make the head look small or oddly shaped, depending on which skull bones fuse. Sometimes surgery may be needed to prevent damage to the developing brain.

Flattened head: plagiocephaly
If your baby's head appears flattened on one side behind the ear, this is most likely due to sleeping position as she habitually turns her head to one side. She may have a bald patch on the favoured side. You could alter your baby's head position from night to night to cure this. Otherwise, it will right itself when she begins to sit. Rarely, a flattened head may be a sign of WRY NECK, where there is tightness or tearing in one of the strap muscles. This can be treated with physiotherapy or osteopathy.

Hydrocephalus

The term hydrocephalus comes from two Greek words meaning 'water in the head'. It affects 1:6000 babies in the UK. The 'water' is cerebrospinal fluid (CSF) that does not drain away as usual. Because it is constantly produced but cannot get out, CSF accumulates, causes raised pressure, the brain tissue stretches and is squashed, and the head gets larger. The effects of hydrocephalus include pressure on the eyes, that may lead to a squint or impaired vision and symptoms related to raised intracranial pressure (e.g. VOMITING, drowsiness, FITS, failure to thrive, p.563). Later in childhood there may be effects on concentration, memory or co-ordination.

PREMATURE BIRTH is the most common cause because there is a higher risk of bleeding into the brain (p.407), which may block the absorption system. Before birth, a congenital abnormality such as SPINA BIFIDA or infection with TOXOPLASMOSIS may be a cause. MENINGITIS after birth may also cause inflammation that blocks the CSF pathways. Cysts and tumours are extremely unusual causes.

Action plan
Hydrocephalus may be diagnosed in pregnancy by ultrasound scan. After birth every baby has a head measurement to check for an unusually large head. Early diagnosis allows treatment to begin soon, and improve the outcome.
- Hydrocephalus is usually treated with an operation that allows the CSF to drain, via a shunt, into the bloodstream. Occasionally a shunt may be put in place using amniocentesis during pregnancy and will be replaced with a permanent shunt after birth. More recent techniques for making an opening in the skull instead of using a shunt are suitable for some types of hydrocephalus.
- Most children with hydrocephalus are educated in mainstream education – sometimes with extra help if they have learning difficulties. If the treatment is working

effectively, the prospects are good. The system of shunting has been used since the 1960s and many adults have grown up with their shunts without complications.

HEARING DIFFICULTIES
See EAR, HEARING DIFFICULTIES

HEART: BABY
....

See also CONGENITAL ABNORMALITIES

Heart rhythms and murmurs
Babies often have minor abnormalities of heart rhythm. The most common is a fast heart rate called supra ventricular tachycardia (SVT). This rarely causes serious problems, but can be picked up before birth, and it may lead to emergency delivery as the fast rate is interpreted as foetal distress. A slow heart rate may be caused by drugs or a congenital heart block of the impulse that governs the contractions. Babies with fast or slow heart rates may require medication after birth and sometimes a pacemaker is inserted to control the rate.

Heart murmurs are commonly heard in just under 10% of newborn babies. Most arise from the sound of blood flow through the heart and the blood vessels, and are completely innocent. If the murmur is found with other signs of possible heart problems, then further investigations are needed.

Heart defects
Around 8:1000 babies have a heart that has not formed correctly; the most common of the congenital abnormalities. For many the defect is not serious. Symptoms may not show until weeks or months after birth, and sometimes a defect may not become apparent until adulthood. The abnormality may sometimes cause breathing and circulation problems, which may begin early. Increasingly, an abnormality may be detected on ultrasound scan antenatally.

It is good to know that with increasingly sophisticated surgical skills many conditions can be addressed effectively. In some cases, the defect presents few problems or relatively simple surgery is required and the outlook is very good. For other babies a series of operations may be necessary. In up to 1:100 babies with a significant heart problem little can be done and the focus is on supporting the baby and parents.

If you receive the news that your baby has a heart problem, your initial response will soon be followed by the need to make practical plans. The specialists caring for your baby will be able to give you details of your baby's condition, the options for treatment and the long-term outlook.

What happens
In a normal heart the chambers, the ventricle and atrium on the left side, receive blood that has passed through the lungs and been oxygenated. The ventricle sends the blood to the aorta, the main artery, from where it is passed through the body. Blood then returns to the right side of the heart on to the lungs and back into the left side and around the body once more. Most defects of the heart reduce normal blood flow between the heart, lungs and body, or cause the blood to flow in an abnormal pattern. After birth a heart defect may cause one or more symptoms. These include breathlessness or rapid, shallow breathing; blue appearance; a heart murmur (some murmurs may not be a sign of an abnormal heart); poor feeding, listlessness, slow growth and failure to gain WEIGHT, and susceptibility to respiratory infections, e.g. pneumonia (p.441).

Diagnosing a heart defect
A defect may be suspected during pregnancy. After birth your baby will be referred to a paediatrician who specialises in cardiology. Your baby may be given a chest x-ray and an electrocardiogram (ECG), which monitors electrical activity of the heart and an ultrasound ECHO test that shows the anatomy of the heart and the direction of blood flow, and can indirectly measure the pressures in the heart.

Causes of heart abnormalities
A baby born with an abnormal heart is said to have a congenital heart defect. In most cases the cause is not known. Rarely, a viral infection in pregnancy, such as RUBELLA, may interfere with heart development. Some chromosomal abnormalities such as DOWN'S SYNDROME can involve the heart. If a mother consumes an excess of ALCOHOL, or recreational DRUGS such as crack cocaine, this may increase the risk of having a baby with a heart defect.

Action plan
The course of action and outlook for recovery and resumption of normal health depends on the problem, the extent of the abnormality and whether or not surgery is needed. You and your family need to be supported as you absorb the news, live with the difficulty and await the results of tests and operations, and look towards the future. Your medical team will be your first line of help and there are support groups.

With almost all cardiac defects there is a risk of a heart infection during any form of surgical treatment, including some dental work. To reduce this risk, it is important for your baby to take antibiotics after surgical procedures.

Types of congenital heart defect
Abnormalities that interfere with healthy heart function are numerous. Types of defect can be divided into the following categories. If your baby is diagnosed with any of these conditions, specialist care will depend on her exact condition.
Patent ductus arteriosus (PDA): An improper closing of a natural passageway in the heart that allows a baby to draw oxygen from blood flowing through the placenta during pregnancy and bypass the lungs; the passageway ordinarily closes after birth (p.35). It accounts for 10% of congenital heart diseases and is more common in premature babies. When it remains open some blood that should flow to the body returns to the lungs and the rest of the body does not receive enough oxygen. The persistent ductus may close by itself (60%), require a drug called indomethacin or surgery.
Stenosis: An obstruction of blood flow in the heart or the veins or arteries connected to it. Pulmonary stenosis involves the valve on the right side of the heart and this may give cyanosis

(blueness) because less blood reaches the lungs. Aortic stenosis is narrowing of the aortic valve leaving the left ventricle – it usually gives no symptoms and remains undetected until adulthood. The aorta itself may be narrowed (coarctation) and less blood flows to the lower part of the body. Symptoms can develop early or not until adulthood. Surgery may be needed if stenosis or coarctation is severe.

Septal defect, also known as 'hole in the heart': An opening or hole between the chambers of the heart. These account for 50% of congenital heart disease, allowing blood to flow between the heart's right and left chambers, which are ordinarily separated by a muscular wall. Oxygenated blood from the lungs mixes with deoxygenated blood. **Atrial septal defect** is an opening between atria, the two upper chambers, and may give few symptoms. **Ventricular septal defect** is an opening between the ventricles, the lower chambers: if small, it doesn't strain the heart but there is a loud murmur; if large, the heart has to over-work to pump extra blood and may enlarge. When this is combined with pulmonary high blood pressure and an abnormal aorta (in Eisenmenger's complex), the condition is very serious and may be fatal if untreated. Atrioventricular canal defect is a particularly large hole in the centre of the heart involving the atria and the ventricles. As a result of its size, it often inhibits normal growth and makes a baby look blue. Many babies with septal defects require surgery.

Cyanotic defects: An incomplete or incorrect formation of the heart that stops blood from being oxygenated sufficiently before being passed around the body. These conditions account for about 25% of congenital heart disease. The blood contains less oxygen than normal, causing blue discoloration of the skin (cyanosis). The term 'blue babies' is often applied to infants with cyanosis: they require expert surgical and medical care. The outlook depends on the severity of the defect.

Tetralogy of fallot involves a ventricular septal defect and a narrowing (stenosis) of the pulmonary valve and an abnormal aorta. If the condition is severe, an early operation is needed. **Transposition of the great arteries** is when the aorta is connected to the right side so most of the blood bypasses the lungs and the pulmonary artery is connected to the left ventricle, so most of the blood returning from the lungs goes back to the lungs again. Babies with this condition are very ill: the long-term outlook depends on the severity of the defects. **Tricuspid atresia** is a lack of a tricuspid valve, which means no blood can flow from the right atrium to the lungs for oxygenation unless there is also an abnormal opening in the internal heart walls (a septal defect) to allow the baby to survive. Surgical shunting procedure is needed to increase blood flow to the lungs. **Pulmonary atresia** is a lack of a pulmonary valve so blood can't flow on to the lungs. The only source of lung blood flow is the PDA (p.477). A surgeon can create a shunt between the aorta and the pulmonary artery to help increase blood flow to the lungs.

Hypoplastic left heart syndrome

This syndrome accounts for fewer than 10% of congenital heart defects. The left side of the heart is underdeveloped and to keep blood oxygenated the heart relies on the PDA. A baby may seem normal at birth, but when the ductus naturally closes, she will become ashen, have rapid and difficult breathing and also have difficulty feeding. This heart defect is often fatal.

HEART: MOTHER

Pregnancy hormones widen your blood vessels, increase blood volume and affect the way your heart responds to the increased load. Initially your heart copes by increasing the amount of blood ejected with every heartbeat but if this is not sufficient your heart rate may also rise. You will probably not notice the different beat unless you are exercising.

Palpitations & murmurs

Palpitations are fast or irregular heartbeats and are very common during pregnancy: your heart has to work up to 25% harder to keep the blood circulating around your body. Palpitations usually cease after birth. They are rarely linked with an underlying heart condition.

- Palpitations are more common with TWINS or if you have ANAEMIA or iron and vitamin deficiency. If you are very anxious, your heart may beat faster.
- Heart rate may increase if you get hungry or your blood sugar falls: this triggers a release of adrenalin to raise blood sugar, which also increases the heart rate.
- If your BLOOD PRESSURE falls when you sit still or stand suddenly, your heart may compensate by beating faster.
- During and after labour you may be aware of palpitations if you become dehydrated. The effect is intensified if you lose blood excessively during the birth. Your midwife will help to keep the bleeding to a minimum and provide you with fluids to prevent dehydration.
- Coronary artery disease or an abnormal electrical circuit that transfers the tiny electrical signal for every heart contraction at each beat may lead to palpitations and an irregular beat.

A murmur may be detected during a routine examination. The most common cause in pregnancy is the sound the increased blood flow makes as it passes the valves in your heart. This normal effect occurs in many women with a normal heart. Occasionally the increased flow during pregnancy brings an abnormality of one of the heart valves to light and the murmur is due to the blood flowing over the valve.

Action plan

If you are well nourished and look after yourself with a balance of exercise and rest, this will encourage good circulation. Be aware of your posture, avoiding slouching or lying down for long periods.

Medical care

If you have frequent palpitations, it is best to see your doctor and request a heart examination. This consists of listening to your heart to detect a murmur, and possibly an electrocardiogram (ECG) to check the regularity of your heart beat. Although heart disease is rare, your doctor may want to make investigations.

- Your blood may be tested for anaemia as a cause.

- If a murmur is detected, an ultrasound test will allow examination of the valves of your heart . If you do have an abnormal valve you will be offered antibiotics to prevent infection during the birth.
- If the beat is irregular and symptoms are intense, you may have to wear an ECG monitor for 24 hours.
- You may be advised to have further tests to monitor your heart after the birth.

Homeopathy
Use a remedy that suits your symptoms (30c) 4 times a day for 3 days and then reassess.

Use *Aconite* if palpitations occur suddenly, usually after a shock and are worse at night; *Arg Nit* when there is anxiety or a sense of being out of control or you're worried about your health; *Natrum Mur* when there's a feeling of heat – 'hot and bothered' – constriction in the chest and the heartbeats feel as if they are shaking your entire body.

Heart disease

Heart disease is uncommon in pregnancy. If you were aware of a problem, it is best to consult your cardiologist about the effect of the increased load on your heart in pregnancy. Unusually, a condition is discovered for the first time in pregnancy.

Medical care
- Your baby will be checked with ultrasound by a specialist ultrasonographer performing foetal echocardiography around Weeks 20. This will ensure her heart is developing normally and monitor her growth and development. This check is particularly important if you were born with a congenital heart problem.
- You will be advised to eat well and take supplements to prevent anaemia so the load on your heart is minimised. It has to deal with the largest load in the 12 hours after birth when the placental pool of blood is squeezed into your circulation before the fluid is excreted by your kidneys.
- Your doctor may advise rest and frequent visits to review your symptoms and alter drug treatment. If a very irregular heartbeat is compromising the function of your heart, you may be given beta-blocking drugs to regulate the heart rate.
- At delivery you will be asked not to bear down in order to keep the load on your heart to a minimum. Your contractions may provide enough downward force but there is an increased chance your baby will require assistance with forceps or ventouse (p.496). You can have an epidural, with care to prevent you being given too little or an excess of fluid, which would increase the volume in circulation and raise the load after birth.
- Birth of the placenta will be carefully controlled to ensure you do not lose excess blood because a sudden drop in blood volume may cause shock and compromise your cardiac function. Ergometrine (p.138) is not used to assist this stage as it can raise blood pressure and increase the strain on your heart.
- Women with cardiac problems are usually offered antibiotics to cover labour and birth to prevent an infection developing on one of the valves in the heart.

HEPATITIS

Hepatitis is an infection of the liver that may be caused by a number of different viruses. It is extremely rare for women to be infected for the first time in pregnancy. Hepatitis infection in children is uncommon except in areas where the viruses are endemic or when a child has been exposed to the infection in the womb. Not all people who contract hepatitis have symptoms, and this is particularly true among children. When symptoms appear they typically include abdominal pain, dark urine, fever, jaundice with yellowing skin and whites of the eyes, enlarged liver, malaise and tiredness, nausea and vomiting. Less common symptoms include joint pain, diarrhoea or light coloured stools and itchy skin.

Most cases of acute hepatitis lead to recovery within a few weeks. In some cases, however, more commonly when HIV infection or malnourishment also exists, hepatitis A, B, D and E can lead to severe illness and even liver failure. Hepatitis B and C can lead to a chronic liver disease. Fortunately, most people who have hepatitis infection recover fully. Pregnancy does not appear to induce deterioration of liver disease in women with hepatitis B or C, nor does the presence of hepatitis B or C increase the risk of obstetric complications. Hepatitis B is routinely screened for in pregnancy. You may request a blood test for other strains if you have been at risk of infection.

Hepatitis A & E
Hepatitis A is not significant in pregnancy but is the most common form of hepatitis in children, usually as a mild infection. Sometimes an infected baby has DIARRHOEA (gastroenteritis). Hepatitis A is present in the stools of infected individuals and also spreads in contaminated water and food and through close personal contact. The infection can pass and then relapse months later. VACCINATION for adults is available and effective, and is advisable if you are at risk. Attention to hygiene, particularly if you are changing nappies, is also an important preventative measure. Research is being conducted on the best method of vaccination for young children.

Hepatitis E virus is spread in the same way as hepatitis A and gives similar symptoms. There is no vaccine. After infection the illness usually passes and does not appear to develop into a chronic form.

Hepatitis B
Hepatitis B is potentially more serious than hepatitis A. Although most people make a full recovery, 10–15% succumb to chronic infection, which may lead to cirrhosis and, in a small number of cases, liver cancer. The risk of developing chronic infection is greatest in childhood. Hepatitis B is spread through contact with blood and body fluids (sexual contact or injections) and can be passed from a mother to her baby, most commonly during birth. There is no evidence to suggest that it can be passed through breast milk, but the virus may pass through blood if a mother's nipples are cracked and bleeding. There is no risk of transmission through kissing.

Hepatitis B virus has three parts that evoke antibodies. If you have a blood test and you are 'e' antigen or 'core' antigen positive, you are highly contagious. If you have 'core' or 'surface' antibodies present, you are immune and no longer susceptible. But if you are surface antigen positive, you are a carrier with a 10–20% chance of transmission to your baby.

Passive immunisation consists of injecting hepatitis B immunoglobulin within 12 hours of birth. This provides your baby with antibodies that will prevent infection while your baby develops her own antibodies. Active vaccination begins 12 hours after birth and stimulates your baby's immune system to develop its own antibodies and a repeat vaccination is needed at 2 months and 6 months. The vaccination is over 85% successful. In the very unlikely event that your baby does develop hepatitis B, she is likely to make a full recovery.

Hepatitis D
Hepatitis D cannot exist without hepatitis B. There is no treatment or vaccination for hepatitis D, so the best way to prevent it is to avoid infection with hepatitis B. A combination of hepatitis B and D seems to reduce the chance of infection reaching the chronic stage.

Hepatitis C
Hepatitis C infection is becoming an increasingly important health issue, with infection rates of 0.1–6% worldwide. Infection is most prevalent among intravenous DRUG users and can also be spread through sexual contact and exposure to semen, saliva and urine. Acute hepatitis C usually causes no symptoms or only mild fatigue. In 25% of cases it causes jaundice and it is estimated that 25% of infected people develop liver cirrhosis, with a smaller number developing liver cancer. The hepatitis C virus has at least 80 sub-types, all of which can be detected through laboratory blood tests, but because of this range there is not yet a hepatitis C vaccine.

If you test positive for hepatitis C, you may need therapy, although the standard drugs cannot be used in pregnancy. After pregnancy you may begin a course of interferon that leads to 10–50% viral clearance but may have side effects. You will need to decide whether to breastfeed – no studies have yet proved that transmission is possible, except when there are cracked and bleeding nipples.

If you have developed hepatitis C antibodies, these will be transferred to your baby and will remain in her blood for up to 15 months. She can be screened at 18 months – if she is infected she will have produced her own antibodies. Infection in babies is extremely rare and you will need to see a specialist for advice on treatment.

HERNIA: BABY
....

Abdominal hernias
An abdominal hernia occurs when a section of intestine protrudes through a weakness in the muscles of the abdominal wall – a soft bulge can be seen beneath the skin. The most common hernias are around the belly button (umbilical) or in the groin (inguinal). Umbilical hernias occur in around 10% of babies, with a higher incidence in Afro-Caribbean children; inguinal hernias occur in fewer than 3% of babies. PREMATURE babies are at a higher risk of developing a hernia, as are babies with CYSTIC FIBROSIS, or if there are problems with the TESTICLES when descent is delayed or if there is a family history of hernia.

Abdominal hernias are often reducible, which means they can be gently pushed back into the abdominal cavity. When a hernia is not reducible, the loop of intestine may become caught in the weakened area of abdominal muscle. This may lead to the blood supply being reduced and obstruction of the intestine. If the obstruction cuts off supply to the intestine completely, in a strangulated hernia, this is a surgical emergency. Surgery corrects the defect and saves the bowel.

Much more rarely, there may be a defect in the abdominal wall, allowing the abdominal contents to protrude into the diaphragm (congenital diaphragmatic hernia, opposite). Also rare, an exomphalos (opposite) occurs when a defect allows the abdominal contents to protrude in a sac near the belly button.

What happens
Hernias are usually apparent in a newborn, particularly when she is crying or straining, although they may not be noticeable until several weeks or months after birth. If you push gently on the bulge when your child is calm and lying down, it will usually get smaller or go back into the abdomen. If you cannot push it back, it requires urgent medical examination. Many hernias require surgery.

Umbilical hernia: There is a small opening in the abdominal muscles through which the umbilical cord passes that gradually closes after birth. Sometimes the muscles do not grow together and a hernia results. In most cases, an umbilical hernia is small and heals without the need for surgery.

Inguinal hernia: As a boy develops during pregnancy, his testicles descend from the abdomen through the inguinal canal into the scrotum. If the inguinal canal does not close off completely after birth, a loop of intestine can cause a hernia. Although girls do not have testicles, they do have an inguinal canal and can develop hernias here. The swelling is more common in the right groin, although it can occur on either side. In a boy similar symptoms may arise from hydrocoele fluid around the testicles, which is harmless, or from twisting of the testicles, which needs emergency treatment.

Epigastric hernia: This protrudes through a narrow hole in the ligament connecting the two rectus muscles that run down the front of the abdomen above the umbilicus. It is usually small and may occur between the umbilicus and the sternum bone in the chest. Sometimes fat or parts of the bowel get caught in the hernia and cause pain that mimics COLIC. Rarely, it can cause bowel obstruction and usually requires surgery.

Femoral hernia: Very rarely, the bowel pushes its way down the femoral canal, which is a channel running from the groin area in the abdomen to the thigh. Because this canal is small a femoral hernia is likely to cause bowel obstruction and needs surgical repair. The swelling appears in the inner part of the groin adjacent to the labia or the testicles.

Action plan
Your doctor will diagnose the hernia by feeling it. If the hernia cannot be pushed back, abdominal x-rays or ultrasound examinations may be used to visualise the intestine. If the intestine is obstructed, emergency surgery may be needed.

- Umbilical hernias usually close on their own without surgery. Most parents are advised to wait for this to happen. Surgery may be recommended if the hernia becomes bigger or is still present after the age of 3 years. Tape applied across the navel will not repair a hernia.
- An inguinal hernia needs to be surgically repaired soon to prevent obstruction to the intestine, under a general or local anaesthetic. After the operation most babies feel fine within a day or two and the incision is checked a few weeks later.
- An epigastric hernia is usually operated on after the age of 3, but if it causes pain early treatment may go ahead.

Congenital diaphragmatic hernia
See also CONGENITAL ABNORMALITIES

A diaphragmatic hernia is a rare congenital abnormality, affecting 1:3000 babies. It results from the improper formation of diaphragm muscle so the abdominal organs, such as the stomach, small intestine, spleen, part of the liver and the kidney, appear in the chest cavity. The lung tissue on the affected side has usually not developed fully, a condition called **hypoplastic lung**. BREATHING DIFFICULTIES usually develop shortly after birth because the diaphragm cannot move effectively and the lungs are unable to expand.

The cause is unknown and there is no prevention. It is usually an isolated abnormality, but can be associated with some HEART or chromosome conditions. Antenatal ultrasound may establish the diagnosis by Week 20 and a few specialist centres attempt in-utero surgery. At birth a baby needs immediate intensive care and ventilation, and an operation to replace the abdominal organs and repair the diaphragm. Multiple operations may be needed. The decision about whether to agree to surgery is extremely difficult for parents because babies who survive with a hypoplastic lung may have severe breathing problems and need long-term oxygen therapy. Life for them and their families can be very difficult.

Exomphalos
See also CONGENITAL ABNORMALITIES

Exomphalos (omphalocoele) is a defect in the wall of the abdomen allowing some of the internal organs to protrude in the vicinity of the umbilical cord, beneath a protective membrane. The opening occurs in 1:5000 babies. Many babies born with an exomphalos also have other serious genetic, chromosomal or organ abnormalities. It is often visible on a pregnancy scan and amniocentesis may be offered to diagnose chromosomal anomalies.

Since some or all of the abdominal organs are outside the body, infection is a concern after birth. There is also a risk that an organ may become pinched or twisted and lose its blood supply, then be damaged. If a baby with an exomphalos has another congenital abnormality, the outlook will also depend in part on that condition. If the exomphalos is small, and there is no other abnormality the outcome is usually excellent after an operation following birth. If it is very large, a series of operations may be needed, and a baby may need temporary ventilation assistance if the abdominal organs reduce space for the lungs to expand. If the abdominal cavity is too small to accommodate all the organs, this may lead to long-term problems with intestinal function and digestion.

HERNIA: MOTHER

Normally the muscles and ligaments of the abdominal wall protect the contents of the abdomen. A hernia occurs when there is a weakness in the wall of the abdomen (as described for hernias in a baby) and pressure of walking, coughing or moving causes the abdominal organs, usually the bowel, to protrude into the defect, causing a bulge beneath the skin. If you have a hernia during pregnancy, it is unlikely to cause problems. Rarely, a hernia becomes strangulated and causes pain, and does need urgent treatment. You may be more likely to get a hernia if you have had abdominal surgery, are overweight or have a family history.

What happens
Hernias in the groin: These are the most common. Less commonly, an inguinal hernia may occur above the crease with the thigh. A hernia in the femoral canal emerging from the groin to the outer side of the labia is rarer. Varicose veins in the groin may appear similar to a hernia.
Umbilical and epigastric hernias: Hernias may occur in the belly button (umbilical hernia) or above it (epigastric hernia).
Divarication of the rectus muscles: This occurs when the two strap muscles that run from the ribs to the pubic area move apart. The abdomen, mainly below the belly button, looks stretched and the uterus may protrude through the defect.
Diaphragmatic hernia: This may occur in the area of muscle where the oesophagus meets the stomach and weakens the valve that stops food from refluxing. This hernia is much smaller than diaphragmatic hernias in babies and is not visible. It may lead to painful reflux, INDIGESTION & HEARTBURN.

Action plan
- If you are aware of an umbilical, inguinal or femoral hernia before pregnancy, it is best to have it repaired before conception. Recurrence is uncommon.
- If you suspect a hernia during pregnancy, your doctor will ask you to cough as he feels for a bulge. If a new hernia appears, it is best to wait until after the birth for surgery. An abdominal support belt may help to reduce pressure.
- Only in the rare event that a hernia becomes strangulated will you need an operation that can be performed with very little risk to you or your baby.
- Divarication of the rectus muscles is usually not treated by surgery: a support belt is useful. After birth abdominal exercises encourage the muscles to move closer together.
- If you have a hernia it is possible to have an active birth. Pushing will not damage the tissues or cause strangulation. The skin on your abdomen will not burst.
- If you have a diaphragmatic hernia, you can reduce pressure by not gaining excessive weight and sitting and sleeping upright. Attention to diet and eating small meals may decrease discomfort from indigestion and heartburn, which can also be relieved with antacids.

HERPES

....

Herpes simplex virus (HSV) invades the nerves and then gives rise to skin blisters and ulcers that heal. There are two herpes simplex viruses: Type 1 and Type 2. Either can infect the mouth or genitals but, most commonly, HSV-1 occurs above the waist as oral herpes (cold sores or fever blisters), and HSV-2, below as genital herpes. Genital herpes occurs 2–20 days after contact with an infected person as white blisters in clusters, although a single spot may appear alone. The blisters burst and form painful open sores that may make urinating painful, and there is often a profuse vaginal discharge. Sometimes bacteria infect the sores and cause painful swelling in the lymph glands in the groin.

The first attack is the most painful. This stimulates the production of antibodies and any further attacks, coming on when the dormant virus in the nerves reactivates, are likely to be less intense. It is estimated that 1:10 women in the UK are affected, although attacks are less likely in pregnancy.

If you have had herpes but do not have an active attack when pregnant there is no risk to your baby. If you have genital herpes in labour it is safest to give birth by CAESAREAN SECTION because in a vaginal birth your baby may become infected. If you experience your first attack of herpes when you are pregnant, your baby is at risk of infection and you will need close medical care. If you have a depressed immune system (e.g. HIV) the herpes virus can be lethal.

What happens
During pregnancy your existing antibodies cross the placenta and provide protection to your baby. Herpes may be painful for you, but providing there is no genital infection at birth, your baby will be unaffected. If you have a long-standing herpes infection, your baby's immunity will be strong, and the chance of passing the virus to your baby, even if it is present in your vagina during delivery, is extremely small.

In the extremely unlikely event that you become infected for the first time in pregnancy, your baby is at risk of infection and this can lead to neonatal herpes. The risk is lowest if you are infected before conception or in the 1st trimester, and highest if you acquire the infection for the first time in the 3rd trimester, when there is less time for you to make sufficient antibodies to give your baby protection.

Infection in a baby
Around 1:44,000 babies are born with neonatal herpes. This may cause a severe illness involving the brain, eyes, skin and lungs if the herpes is not treated early. In most cases herpes is transmitted during birth. A small number of babies (5% of the total infected) are born with herpes acquired in the womb. After birth all babies are at risk of acquiring herpes, which can be passed on by being kissed by someone with oral herpes.

Action plan
Diet and lifestyle
- If you have sores, take care of the affected skin area. Keep the area dry and clean to help healing. Avoid physical contact with the area until all sores are healed.

- You can still breastfeed provided you wash your hands.
- Do not kiss your baby when you have oral herpes, and avoid sexual intercourse with your partner when either of you has genital herpes.
- With genital sores, wear cotton underwear and avoid tight clothes, as moisture and heat delay healing.
- A nutritious diet with appropriate vitamins and mineral and antioxidant supplements may increase your immunity and reduce the chance of recurrence. Lysine appears to be an effective agent. It is present in many foods, including fish, chicken, beef, lamb, milk, cheese, beans, brewer's yeast, mung bean sprouts and most fruits and vegetables.

Medical care
- A diagnostic test for the herpes virus can be made from a sample taken from the sores before they have healed. The symptoms of herpes may be confused with CYSTITIS (p.552) or SYPHILIS (open sores), which need different treatment.
- If you do not have herpes lesions at the time of delivery, you may safely continue with a vaginal birth as your baby is protected by your antibodies.
- For a first herpes infection in the last trimester, particularly between Weeks 36 and 40, many obstetricians recommend a caesarean delivery but some feel a vaginal delivery is acceptable if no lesions are present.
- In the rare event that you have an acute attack when you go into labour, a caesarean section may be recommended within 4 hours of spontaneous rupture of the membranes because the virus can travel into the uterus and infect your baby.
- If you have had genital herpes, your medical team may want to keep a close eye on your baby for the first 14 days in case sores develop.
- Antiviral drugs can be used to treat you after birth, and your baby if she is infected.
- The use of antiviral drugs for recurrent herpes is not recommended and has not been cleared for safety in pregnancy. The drugs may reduce the severity of attacks but do not reduce the likelihood of recurrence.

Homeopathy
Constitutional homeopathic treatment under the care of a qualified homeopath is by far the best way to deal with herpes. However, in an acute attack one of the following remedies may be useful (6c), 3–4 times a day. Reassess if there is no change after 2 days.

Natrum Mur for lesions that are often circular, hot, puffy and pearl coloured, with dry surrounding skin, and may appear when you feel vulnerable or after an emotional period of time; *Rhus Tox* for blisters that burn and itch, are red and swollen and then become crusty and you feel restless; *Hepar Sulph* for itching, inflamed sores that often converge, give stinging pain and can bleed and weep and you can feel extremely edgy and irritable; *Graphites* for burning, crusty eruptions that can ooze a honey-coloured sticky fluid and with very dry skin in the surrounding area. *Calendula* tincture is very useful as an adjunctive treatment – dilute 10 drops in 250 ml (½ pint) water and bathe the affected area 2–3 times a day to accelerate healing.

HIGH-RISK PREGNANCY

Pregnancy is not usually a high-risk condition, and most pregnancies have a healthy, happy outcome. Around 8:100 are identified as high risk. This does not mean that a problem will develop, but there is a higher chance, so antenatal monitoring is more intensive, as is attention during labour and provision of facilities for care after birth. High-risk pregnancies account for 70–80% of complications; there are also pregnancies where risks have not been identified that result in complications.

If you are told there is a cause for concern, you may become anxious (p.382). You may need considerable support and your medical team will give you the facts. Their highest priority is the health and safety of you and your baby. Often, extra care is a standard precaution and the outcome is fine.

What happens
Sometimes risk rises because of a mother's physiology, sometimes it relates to a baby's development, it may be caused by genetics or it may stem from environment and lifestyle during pregnancy. Usually a complication is out of the mother's control. Some conditions that may prompt the medical team to give close monitoring are listed here. There are details of the causes, care options and medical procedures and outlook for each within this health guide.

Mother
Age: Girls below 15 are more likely to develop high BLOOD PRESSURE with pre-eclampsia and deliver underweight babies – PREMATURE or INTRAUTERINE GROWTH RESTRICTION (IUGR). After 35 years of age there is an increased risk of high blood pressure, DIABETES, or FIBROIDS in the uterus and having a baby with a chromosomal abnormality such as DOWN'S SYNDROME.
Weight: Being underweight increases the likelihood of IUGR; being overweight raises the chance of DIABETES, high blood pressure and having a LARGE BABY.
Medical conditions: These may increase pregnancy risks – diabetes, chronic high blood pressure, kidney disease, HEART disease, epilepsy, sickle cell ANAEMIA, THYROID problems and BLOOD-CLOTTING problems.
Physiology: An abnormally shaped UTERUS may increase risks; so may an incompetent cervix (p.426) and fibroids.
Family history: If you or your partner have any hereditary disorders there may be a risk; this also applies to non-identical TWINS.

Previous pregnancies
Loss: If there have been three consecutive MISCARRIAGES there is a chance of another; if you have previously lost a baby through stillbirth or neonatal death (p.510) and the cause has been found it may indicate a risk in this pregnancy.
Premature birth: The cause of most premature births is unknown but the more pre-term deliveries a woman has had, the greater the subsequent risk.
IUGR: If you have previously had a growth-restricted baby it may happen again, depending on the cause.
Large babies: If you have previously had one or more large baby it may happen again (and could indicate diabetes).
More than five pregnancies: This increases the likelihood of weak contractions and rapid labour, and of bleeding after.
Rhesus incompatability: This is rare now that anti-Rh D immunoglobulin is routinely given to rhesus negative mothers (p.410).
Hypertension and pre-eclampsia: These are likely to recur, particularly if there is underlying high blood pressure.
Genetic disorders or birth defects: These may or may not recur – your obstetrician or geneticist can predict the risk.
Placental abruption: With antenatal bleeding this may recur.

Events in pregnancy
Something occurring in pregnancy may increase risk factors:
Exposure: To chemicals or radiation.
Infection: This may present a risk of infection in the womb or complicate delivery.
Medical condition related to pregnancy (e.g. CHOLESTASIS): This may require early delivery.
Drugs: Certain pharmaceutical or recreational DRUGS can harm the foetus and the mother.
Smoking: SMOKING can affect a baby's lungs and development and compromise the mother's health.
Excessive alcohol intake: ALCOHOL can affect mental and physical foetal development.
Bleeding: Caused by PLACENTA PRAEVIA or PLACENTAL ABRUPTION.
Amniotic fluid (p.397): Excessive or inadequate volume.
Premature rupture of the membranes (p.501) and premature labour.

Baby
Restricted growth (IUGR): Predisposes to problems such as FOETAL DISTRESS & ASPHYXIA.
Excessive growth (being large): May add to complications during vaginal delivery.
Twins or more babies: Are more likely to be born prematurely or receive inadequate nutrition in the womb.
Postmaturity (p.500): When a baby remains in the womb beyond Week 42 placental reserves may fall.
Congenital abnormality (p.433): May require special care.

In labour
The purpose of modern care in labour is to prevent foetal distress and asphyxia and BIRTH INJURIES. Babies with high-risk pregnancies are more susceptible to distress, particularly if they are fragile from prematurity or IUGR. Premature and very large babies are more likely to be injured during birth, as are babies who are not positioned optimally (p.498) or who are subjected to a prolonged labour.

Action plan
Before conception
If you are aware of any health problem or condition that may place you in a high-risk category, it is best to consult your doctor prior to conception.
• Many conditions can be treated before pregnancy to reduce risk, and if you need to take medications you can check the safety issues and take alternatives if necessary.

- If you take other drugs, drink ALCOHOL or SMOKE you may need support to give up.
- Nutrition (p.332) is very important and being optimally nourished improves your health and your baby's health.
- You may need to consult a genetic counsellor (p.434) if you have had a baby with a developmental problem, or have a family history of a condition. You may choose to consult before pregnancy even if you believe you are in good health.

In pregnancy
It is best to remain as healthy as possible with a balanced diet, regular appropriate exercise and a careful balance between rest and energetic activities (p.51). If your pregnancy holds risks, the medical team can take steps to ensure you and your baby are as safe as possible. Some conditions simply require extra observation, some can be managed easily and some need specialist attention. You will be able to discuss tests and options for care. If a problem is suspected with one test, further tests are often required for diagnosis. These may range from additional blood tests (e.g. for infection) to AMNIOCENTESIS OR CVS (e.g. if there is a risk of congenital abnormality).

If your baby is considered to be at high risk in the second half of pregnancy you will be checked frequently. The following tests may be suggested to help you and your doctor to decide on when and how your baby is born.

- You will need more frequent antenatal visits so your midwife can examine and record your baby's growth and the amniotic fluid volume and treat any medical disorder.
- You will be asked to observe your baby's movement. Normal movements indicate health. Movements may reduce when your baby sleeps, but if you are concerned that there are fewer than 10 movements a day, there is an indication to be examined and checked.
- You may be offered regular ultrasound scans with Doppler blood flows (p.81) with a frequency depending on the degree of risk associated with your pregnancy. The scans assess blood flow in your baby's vessels and indicate placental function and supply of nutrients to the brain and vital organs; the rate of growth; amniotic fluid volume, and foetal movements and muscle tone are also measured. In combination with a non-stress test (below), scan results give a 'biophysical profile' that assesses your baby's reserves and is the best indicator of when it is safest to be born.
- Foetal heart tracing (CTG non-stress test) is useful between scans and is done with a foetal heart monitor on your abdomen. As the predictive accuracy of health improves on scans, foetal heart tracing is used less frequently. If the pattern is normal, you can be reassured your baby will be fine for 24 hours; if there is an abnormality the test will be repeated and acted on if it is confirmed.
- A foetal heart trace (stress test) is similar to the CTG non-stress test but oxytocin is also injected to provoke uterine contractions and observe the reaction of a baby's heartbeat. Not all hospitals use it and improved ultrasound information has largely replaced the test in the birth timing. Your birth team will assess the results of the tests on an ongoing basis. The main indication for early birth is reduced Doppler blood flow, amniotic fluid volume or an abnormal CTG. If they consider the risk to your baby is high, an elective

CAESAREAN SECTION may be suggested and it is essential to give birth in a hospital with a SPECIAL CARE BABY UNIT. Your doctor will discuss the balance of risks. In rare instances being premature is less hazardous than remaining in the uterus. In a lower-risk situation an induction of labour will be considered when your baby is sufficiently mature. When the risk is not so significant, you can wait for labour to begin spontaneously and go ahead with a vaginal delivery.

In labour and birth
A high-risk baby will be closely monitored during labour and birth to detect and prevent foetal distress and asphyxia.

- In the highest-risk situation you will be advised to have a caesarean section.
- When the risk is lower you will be advised to be upright to maximise the blood flow to the placenta and choose a mobile epidural and adequate fluid replacement if you require these.
- If your baby is large, you will need careful help in the 2nd stage to reduce the chance of your baby's descent being obstructed (p.493).
- In the event of bleeding, premature birth or foetal distress, your doctor may request the help of a paediatrician to care for your baby and provide resuscitation if needed.
- After birth, all high-risk babies are monitored to prevent HYPOGLYCAEMIA (low blood sugar) and HYPOTHERMIA and to maintain breathing and oxygen flow.
- Early feeding helps prevent hypoglycaemia and aids weight gain. Premature babies or babies with specific problems have special requirements that are routinely checked.
- Often labour progresses normally and the baby is fine. It is always best to be prepared and the focus of care improves the outlook for mothers and babies.

HIPS, CONGENITAL DISLOCATION

During the standard neonatal paediatric check, the midwife or doctor will bend and flex each of your baby's hips in the Barlow and Ortolini's test. If there is a click (hence its commonly used name, '**clicky hip**'), it is probably due to the natural sliding of the ligaments. The test is repeated at 6 weeks. In roughly 1:300 babies a click indicates congenital dislocation of the hip (CDH) so every click is followed up with further investigation.

CDH affects girls more often than boys and is more likely to occur in the left hip. In about 25% of cases both hips dislocate. It can be caused by the way the legs are positioned in the womb, is more common in breech babies (p.492) and may run in families. It is more likely to occur in TWINS and may be associated with other congenital conditions such as SPINA BIFIDA or DOWN'S SYNDROME. There is no way to prevent the condition or to detect it in pregnancy.

What happens
With CDH the hip joint forms incorrectly so the head of the thighbone can be dislocated from the joint located in the pelvic bone. Usually the socket in the pelvis is shallow, allowing the

femur to slip out. The most common symptom is the 'click'. CDH may also lead to unusual skin folds on the upper legs and some babies have trouble spreading their legs for a nappy change. The condition does not give any pain, yet if it is not treated the joint may continue to develop poorly and there is an increased chance of arthritis and pain in adulthood. CDH does not delay walking, but could lead to a waddling gait.

Action plan
All babies with clicky hip, breech position or a family history of CDH are offered an ultrasound within 6 weeks of birth. The ultrasonographer can see how the head of the femur and the pelvis socket are formed. A baby with CDH will be referred immediately to a specialist orthopaedic surgeon – early treatment increases the chance of normal hip development.

- If there is a click but the bones appear to be functioning normally, the joint will be painlessly splinted by using two nappies instead of one for a few weeks.
- If there is dislocation or the hip socket is shallow, an orthopaedic brace or harness may be used for a few months. The harness has Velcro straps to hold the legs in a frog-leg position to put the hip ball into the socket. It is painless. The brace can be removed in seconds for nappy changes and does not interfere with feeding, bathing or sleeping. It needs to be worn until the hips are felt to be stable in the socket and then your baby is weaned off, usually by 6 months.
- If treatment is needed after 6 months, a plaster cast may be used. For a small number of babies surgery enlarges the socket: this is usually carried out before walking begins.

HIV (AIDS)

Human immunodeficiency virus (HIV) is responsible for acquired immune deficiency syndrome (AIDS). Becoming pregnant does not appear to endanger the health of an HIV-infected woman, but does carry implications for her baby. Yet treatment can dramatically improve a baby's outlook as well as a woman's health during and after pregnancy. Screening for HIV is routine in the UK although not everyone has the test. In some hospitals there are specifically trained HIV counsellors.

What happens
HIV is most commonly transmitted through sexual contact without a condom and through the use of contaminated needles, often in connection with DRUG use. A person who is 'HIV positive' does not necessarily have AIDS, but can transmit the virus to others. Antibodies may not show up in a screening test until 3 months after infection. It can take 10 or more years for an HIV-positive person to develop AIDS. A person with AIDS has a deficiency of the immune system and is more susceptible to infections, certain cancers and other problems that can be life threatening or fatal.

HIV and pregnancy
If you are HIV positive and become pregnant, the pregnancy is unlikely to affect your health. It is, however, sensible to care for yourself as well as possible, with a nutritious diet, vitamin and mineral supplements, and regular exercise and rest, and avoid people you know to be infected with contagious illnesses. It is best to avoid SMOKING and taking drugs that have not been prescribed for you. If your partner is HIV positive and you test negative, you refrain from unprotected sex and then test negative again after 3 months, you are clear of HIV and your baby will not be infected.

Transmitting HIV to your baby
The likelihood that you will transmit HIV to your baby in pregnancy ('perinatal transmission') directly correlates with viral load. If you have developed AIDS, you will have a greater number of viral particles in your circulation and transmission is more likely than if you are HIV positive without AIDS. Treatment in pregnancy can reduce the viral load, thus helping to prevent transmission.

When HIV testing first became available without treatment, transmission of HIV to a baby occurred in up to 27% of cases. The risk of transmission can be cut to just 2% if you take AZT (zidovudine) during the last 6 months of pregnancy, deliver your baby by CAESAREAN SECTION, bottle feed, and your baby receives drug therapy (AZT).

Action plan
Drug treatment in pregnancy
AZT is the usual medication given in pregnancy. It has not yet been linked with significant side effects. Some babies develop mild ANAEMIA that clears when the drug is stopped but continue to develop normally. Sometimes AZT is taken with other drugs, which has advantages as well as disadvantages. Drug therapy is continually evolving and it is best to discuss all your options with your specialist doctor.

Treatment after birth for a baby
Symptoms of HIV infection do not develop until some time after birth. All babies of HIV-positive mothers need to be treated with AZT for 6 weeks after birth, and need to avoid breast milk, which may carry the infection.

Testing a baby for HIV
During pregnancy your antibodies are passed to your baby, so an early blood sample will therefore test positive. This doesn't mean your baby is infected. She will keep your antibodies until she begins to make her own between 6 and 18 months of age. If your baby is infected with HIV, she will make antibodies, thus testing positive continually. New technologies are promising accurate testing 3 months or earlier after birth.

HIV-infected babies
HIV is a devastating infection for a baby. About 20% of HIV-infected babies develop AIDS in the 1st year and die before age 4. Most of the rest develop AIDS before the age of 6 years. Early diagnosis and treatment can help reduce susceptibility to infection. Yet because of immune system vulnerability, babies with AIDS may get MENINGITIS, which may lead to developmental delays, they often fail to gain WEIGHT or grow slower than expected, and frequently have DIARRHOEA.

If your baby is diagnosed with HIV, she may be treated with a combination of three HIV-fighting drugs, including

AZT. The combination therapy slows the progress of the disease but is not a cure, and may have side effects. It is very important that your baby receives VACCINATIONS, including yearly vaccination against INFLUENZA, starting at 7 months of age, and the pneumococcal vaccine at age 2, but avoids CHICKEN POX vaccine and the live polio vaccine. She will need the care of a paediatrician experienced in the treatment of AIDS because new technologies are constantly evolving.

Living with HIV

If you are diagnosed with HIV you will need to adapt to the changes in your body, as you would with any chronic illness, and the effects that drug therapy have on you and your family. If your baby is infected, coping with her physical symptoms may be extremely upsetting.

Perhaps the most difficult thing about living with HIV is uncertainty. In the past, HIV-positive people often faced death in the near future. Today, with daily medication, the prognosis is less grim. Although some drugs have unpleasant side effects, there is a chance that you could feel quite well and the effect on your life could be minimal for years. Living a normal life, enjoying your family, keeping a job and having the courage to fall in love with your children may not be easy when you are unsure about length and quality of life. Help from your family and friends, your medical team and HIV support groups could help enormously as you face this challenge. Other challenges include feeling stigmatised and worrying about your children being isolated because of your condition, and more so if they are infected. Your whole family, including your partner, will benefit from support.

HYPOGLYCAEMIA: BABY

Hypoglycaemia is a condition in which the amount of glucose (sugar) in the blood is lower than normal. It is reasonably common among newborns but if it becomes prolonged and severe it can cause brain damage because a baby's brain requires sugar to function. Fortunately, it is easily preventable with close blood glucose monitoring of babies who are at risk. Symptoms include sweating, jitteriness and jerky movements, rapid breathing, rapid heart rate, pallor or even apnoea (p.418). Approximately 1:500 newborns develop symptomatic hypoglycaemia.

What happens

During pregnancy, your baby receives glucose from your bloodstream. Some of the glucose is stored as glycogen in your baby's liver, heart and muscles. These stores are important for supplying her brain with glucose during labour and after she is born before feeding is established. If blood sugar levels are low, the body releases adrenalin, the hormone that stimulates the body to release stored glucose. Babies who are more likely to develop hypoglycaemia include:

- Babies whose mothers have DIABETES with high blood glucose in pregnancy, because the baby produces high levels of insulin to break down the glucose coming from the mother's blood. The insulin levels remain high after birth

and there is a rapid fall in blood sugar once the source of glucose is removed.
- Small or INTRAUTERINE GROWTH RESTRICTED babies may have low levels of stored glucose.
- PREMATURE babies, especially those with low birth WEIGHT, often have limited glycogen stores or immature liver function, because the glycogen stores are mainly laid down in late pregnancy.
- Babies who suffer from severe FOETAL DISTRESS & ASPHYXIA, where glycogen stores are used up during birth.

Action plan

A hypoglycaemic baby needs a rapid-acting source of glucose. Often the best source is breast milk or formula milk, although some babies need glucose given intravenously. For most babies the risks of hypoglycaemia pass after 48 hours, when regular feeding is established and blood glucose measuring can stop. In extremely rare cases where episodes recur for days or weeks, a specialist endocrinologist advises on treatment to stabilise blood sugar levels because some babies have an overactive pancreas and produce excessive insulin that leads to hypoglycaemia.

HYPOTHERMIA & COLD INJURY

In a newborn baby temperature regulation is not efficient and there is a greater risk of excessive cooling or overheating. It is important to keep your baby at a reasonable temperature (p.214). The main factors that may make your baby too cold are being exposed to cold draughts in a cold room or outside and being allowed to cool excessively when her skin is wet.

What happens

If your baby becomes too cold, her temperature will fall below 35°C (95°F). She is more susceptible to a reduction in temperature if her birth WEIGHT was low because she can more easily lose heat and is less able to produce it: she has a larger surface area of skin, less fat and low blood sugar levels (p.486).

Signs of being too cold include a cold head and body, apathy and poor feeding. A very cold baby will become apathetic and not feed, cry feebly and have depressed reflexes, a slow heart rate and reduced urine production. Deceptively, she may have ruddy cheeks and extremities, but will feel cold to the touch.

Hypothermia may make a baby have difficulty maintaining blood sugar levels, have BREATHING DIFFICULTIES and problems with BLOOD CLOTTING.

Cold injury refers to the rare event of severe hypothermia with a core body temperature of 32°C (89.6°F) or less. Risk factors include birth into a cold room or cold water, air conditioning blasting cold air on to a wet naked baby or exposure to a cold atmosphere when inadequately dressed. Severe cooling may make the body tissues become damaged and swell, giving a woody feel to the limbs. The death rate of cold injury is high because of severe hypoglycaemia, low blood oxygen levels and bleeding into the lungs and brain, and risks linked with re-warming.

Action plan
Prevention
At birth your baby will be at the optimal temperature if you hold her, naked, against your skin. Alternatively, she will be kept warm in a warm dry towel or in a warm cot.
- Premature babies below 1.8 kg (4 lb) are usually nursed in an incubator and the skin temperature kept at 36.5°C (97.7°F). Sometimes a plastic heat shield is used to lessen heat loss. Woolly bonnets are ideal for preventing heat loss through the head.
- If your baby becomes moderately cold, a cuddle, a hat and a feed will usually warm her. If you are worried that she is excessively cold, you need medical help.

Treatment
If your baby becomes too cold you need to contact the emergency services urgently.
- She will need re-warming in an incubator. Her temperature will be raised at around 1.5–2°C (2.7–3.6°F) per hour.
- She will be monitored for hypoglycaemia and treated if necessary with intravenous warmed dextrose water to prevent low sugar levels.
- The doctors will check whether an infection has caused the low temperature and give antibiotics as a precaution.
- She will be given oxygen while she is being re-warmed.
- When her temperature is back to normal she will be kept under observation to ensure that it remains normal at room temperature. It is best to continue to monitor temperature for a few days after recovery.

INCONTINENCE & VAGINAL PROLAPSE
See VAGINAL LAXITY, INCONTINENCE & PROLAPSE

INDIGESTION & HEARTBURN
....

Pregnancy hormones relax and soften the muscles in the valve between the oesophagus and stomach and the pressure of the uterus on the stomach may allow gastric acid to flow upwards into the oesophagus. When this irritates the sensitive lining it causes heartburn and pain. Indigestion may also accompany NAUSEA & VOMITING, excess FLATULENCE or CONSTIPATION.

What happens
Indigestion may cause distension and pain or discomfort in the upper abdomen. Heartburn causes a burning feeling extending up into the chest with belching when food and gastric juice refluxes into the oesophagus.

Heartburn often becomes more severe in late pregnancy and when lying down. It may be related to a change in diet and is more likely if you are overweight and have a LARGE BABY or TWINS. Very occasionally, pregnancy may bring to light a hiatus HERNIA where there is a weakness in the valve between the stomach and the oesophagus, giving heartburn. Stomach or duodenal ulcers cause indigestion but they are very uncommon during pregnancy.

Action plan
Diet and lifestyle
- It is best to eat a healthy, balanced diet with meals and small snacks every 3 hours. Relax before and after meals, don't rush, and sit straight to prevent acid reflux. Eat a light, slow-burning snack before sleep, perhaps a rice cake, oat biscuit or raw carrot. Avoid ALCOHOL, strong coffee, fizzy drinks, highly refined food, SMOKING and fatty or heavy meals.
- Alkaline antacid foods such as milk or yoghurt, which neutralise stomach acid, may ease heartburn but in some women the stomach reacts by producing more acid 30–90 minutes later. Light acids such as a dilute fruit juice can reduce acid production. The only way to find out what works for you is to experiment.
- Cut down on fluid during a meal to reduce the volume in your stomach – get your daily intake between meals. Try different water: some tap water is very acid. Mint tea is a good herbal remedy; camomile tea also helps.
- Iron supplements may cause heartburn but try organic iron preparations (p.345) taken 1 hour before a meal.
- Avoid slouching and adjust your sleeping position, perhaps by supporting your upper body with pillows or raising the head of your bed on two bricks.

Medical care
Heartburn usually settles after pregnancy unless there is an underlying hiatus hernia. If indigestion is severe, consult your doctor or midwife.
- There is a variety of antacids available that act like alkaline foods. Avoid preparations with a high sodium or particularly high aluminium content. H2 receptor antagonists and proton pump inhibitor drugs inhibit the production of gastric acid but they are not licensed for use in pregnancy. Check with your doctor which are the safest in pregnancy and reserve them for very severe indigestion where other treatments are not effective.

Homeopathy
Take 1 tablet (30c), 4 times a day for 3–4 days and reassess.

Use *Arsenicum* if heartburn is accompanied by nausea, you are chilly, restless and agitated, worse at night and better from sips of warm drinks, and crave company; *Lycopodium* to calm an acidic feeling with bloating and abdominal rumbling, burning from the stomach up to the throat, belching with acidic taste, indigestion that's worse from eating cabbage, beans, onions and cold food and drinks and comes with anxiety; *Nux Vomica* if you have a sour or metallic taste in the mouth, feel stressed, uncomfortable around 2 hours after eating, have a headache, constipation or nausea, feel full, are irritable, chilly or crave spices; *Pulsatilla* for heartburn and nausea after a meal of rich food, a dry mouth without thirst, weepiness and reduced symptoms after a good cry, and crave company and fresh air. Do not take *Pulsatilla* until after Week 12 of pregnancy.

Aromatherapy
Use lemon or ginger oil in the bath, in massage or as a compress. From Week 24 try lemongrass in low dosage and camomile.

INDUCTION OF LABOUR

See LABOUR, INDUCTION & AUGMENTATION

INFLUENZA

If you get influenza (flu) during pregnancy, you will feel unwell but there is little threat to your pregnancy. Rest as much as you can, and treat your symptoms as you would for a COUGH OR COLD. If your baby gets flu after birth he is likely to be unwell and then recover fully.

Flu is a highly infectious illness caused by the influenza virus. It tends to start suddenly with symptoms such as FEVER, chills, headache, aching muscles and feeling generally unwell, together with a cough or sore throat. Flu may lead to a bronchiolitis (p.440). VACCINATION is generally only recommended for babies who are at risk of complications, e.g. those with HIV, ASTHMA or HEART illnesses. The vaccine is developed from eggs, so if your baby is allergic to eggs or chicken, discuss this with your doctor.

Action plan

Most babies with flu require treatment for a fever as well as the symptoms usually associated with coughs and colds, plus rest and loving comfort for a few days, and then begin to recover. Give your child plenty to drink. If you also have flu, do what you can to get extra help. Arrange to be seen as soon as possible or call your doctor urgently if:

- Your child has an earache, ear drainage, or severe pain in his face or forehead; this could signal sinusitis or an EAR INFECTION.
- He has persistent chest pain and fever, or is wheezing and coughing up discoloured mucus; these might be signs of pneumonia (p.441).
- He is straining to breathe while lying quietly.
- He quickly bounces back from the flu but becomes sick again soon after.
- He has a high fever for more than 3–4 days.

INSOMNIA

See TIREDNESS, LOW ENERGY & INSOMNIA

INTRAUTERINE GROWTH RESTRICTION (IUGR)

If the exact date of conception is known, intrauterine growth restriction (IUGR) indicates the baby has a weight that would be attained by fewer than 5% of normal babies at that stage of pregnancy. Many but not all babies with IUGR have a low birth WEIGHT; this is usually defined as weighing less than 2.5 kg (5 lb 8 oz) after Week 37. Other terms for IUGR include small for gestational age, small for dates or foetal growth restriction. Some babies who weigh over 3 kg (6 lb 8 oz) were genetically meant to be big – possibly over 4 kg (8 lb 12 oz) – but do, in fact, have IUGR.

During antenatal checks if your midwife or doctor thinks your baby is small, she may refer you for an ultrasound scan.

Measurements are considered together with your baby's gestational age and sex and your ethnic origin, weight and height. Of every 100 babies who are thought to have IUGR, some are healthy at birth; about 70 are small and constitutionally healthy; around 10 need intensive monitoring and only one or two are severely affected.

Where IUGR is mild and birth goes ahead without complications and feeding begins soon, a baby thrives. Babies with severe IUGR are more susceptible to FOETAL DISTRESS because their energy reserves may be low. With increasingly sophisticated care it is possible to time the birth to minimise this risk. Where IUGR is severe, a baby may require more medical support after birth until feeding has been established and weight gain begins. If a baby is PREMATURE and has IUGR, there is a higher chance that special care will be needed.

What happens

The normal pattern of growth during pregnancy can be divided into two main phases. In the first 20 weeks there is rapid division of cells as the building blocks for body and brain are laid down. In the second 20 weeks the rate of cell division slows but the cells enlarge, and after Week 28 fat and muscle accumulate. Your baby gains over 90% of his weight during the last 20 weeks of pregnancy.

Growth inhibition during the first 20 weeks produces a smaller than usual baby who is said to have **symmetrical IUGR**, so called because the growth of the head and body are affected equally. If there are factors inhibiting growth after Week 20, a baby compensates by releasing nor-adrenalin and selectively diverting blood to the heart, brain and the head, where growth continues, while the other organs slow down, a phenomenon called the 'brain-sparing effect'. This leads to **asymmetrical IUGR** where the head is relatively larger than the abdomen. These babies have fewer fat stores and a smaller liver, with lower glycogen stores. Ultrasound measurements of the abdomen and head can distinguish between symmetrical and asymmetrical IUGR. Sometimes babies with IUGR are affected throughout pregnancy and there is a combination of symmetric and asymmetric growth restriction.

What may cause IUGR

Modern testing can detect babies with IUGR and can often determine the cause, so that complications may be reduced or avoided. However, not all IUGR babies are spotted in pregnancy and some may only be detected when they are weighed at birth. Medical care increases the chances of a baby reaching his full growth potential.

Maternal health

Your baby's environment for growth and nutrition in the womb partly depends on your health. Usually a baby is efficient at obtaining all the necessary nutrients, and minor illnesses, including morning sickness, do not have an adverse effect. Larger health problems may have an impact by reducing the efficiency of the placenta. IUGR is more likely with a HIGH-RISK PREGNANCY.

- If you have already had a baby with significant IUGR there is a higher risk of recurrence. IUGR may run in families.
- The importance of nutrition in foetal development is

undisputed. The current consensus is that low maternal weight before pregnancy, and a gain of less than 10 kg (22 lb) during pregnancy, is a risk factor. Many studies point to malnutrition or vitamin and mineral deficiency in early pregnancy as most significant.

- DRUGS may significantly affect development, and there is a correlation with the type of drug and the amounts consumed. SMOKING is probably the most significant cause of IUGR worldwide – perhaps causing as many as 40% of small babies – but alcohol, cocaine, amphetamines and heroin are powerful drugs that affect growth.
- An underlying medical condition may reduce the efficiency of the placenta. The most significant are: high BLOOD PRESSURE and severe pre-eclampsia, particularly if the elevated blood pressure was present before conception; BLOOD-CLOTTING DISORDERS with excess clotting; sickle cell and thalassaemia forms of ANAEMIA, and severe medical disorders requiring intensive medication.

Abnormality of the placenta and blood flow

IUGR may occur when there is a reduction in the function of the placenta, which means that blood flow to the baby, together with oxygen and nutrients, is reduced. This may be for one of several reasons:

- If placental cells do not embed deeply enough when they implant and do not invade the arteries in the wall of the mother's uterus, this may lead to a reduction in the volume of blood flowing to the placenta. This is most commonly beyond a mother's control but is more likely to happen if she has poor nutrition or a medical disorder (opposite).
- IUGR occurs in 15–25% of TWIN pregnancies and is particularly likely with identical twins where one baby receives less blood from the placenta.
- Placental function may become less efficient if there is significant BLEEDING DURING PREGNANCY that leads to PLACENTAL ABRUPTION. This is an uncommon but significant disorder.
- Occasionally the umbilical cordcontains a single artery in place of two (p.551): this may result in reduced cord blood flow.

Abnormality in the baby

Some developmental abnormalities reduce growth and lead to symmetrical IUGR, with the head and the body retaining the usual proportions.

- About 5% of IUGR babies have CONGENITAL ABNORMALITIES such as DOWN'S SYNDROME or heart or skeletal defects.
- Approximately 10% have restricted growth because of maternal infections in pregnancy, such as RUBELLA or CYTOMEGALOVIRUS. Some infections, such as SYPHILIS and TOXOPLASMOSIS, can be treated with antibiotics.

Action plan

Only a minority of IUGR babies are ill. In the majority of cases the screening tests confirm the baby is growing well. When measurements confirm there is IUGR, the course of action depends on the extent of growth restriction. The lower the weight the higher degree of risk. Often extra vigilance is needed not because of low weight, but to assess coexisting issues such as twins or high blood pressure.

Detecting and diagnosing IUGR

Antenatal examinations are geared to monitoring foetal growth. External estimations are not very accurate – about 70% of IUGR babies are detected this way. It is also common for the date of conception to be incorrect, so a midwife may expect the uterus to be larger than it is. Sometimes the examination will miss an IUGR baby, particularly if the mother is overweight.

IUGR can be best diagnosed with ultrasound scans where the date of conception is known. The earliest date that slow growth rate can be detected is around Week 12 but this is very unusual and applies to very severely affected babies. The rate of detection increases progressively beyond Week 20. The number and dates of scans vary across the country.

Scan 1: In the 1st trimester, preferably before Week 14; can accurately assess the date of conception. Markers of some congenital abnormalities can also be seen.

Scan 2: Between Weeks 18 and 22, checks growth and detects any further markers. After Week 20 a Doppler scan (p.81) can measure the rate of blood flow in the uterine artery: this may show there is a likelihood of IUGR developing. In most hospitals this is the last routine scan.

Scan 3: Between Weeks 30 and 34, can check foetal growth and monitor Doppler blood flow in the umbilical blood vessels to assess placental function. It can help distinguish between asymmetrical and symmetrical IUGR, and babies who are constitutionally small but healthy. A routine 3rd-trimester scan often detects unsuspected IUGR and is more accurate than an abdominal examination.

Scan 4 (or more): To monitor a baby who is thought to have IUGR. Measurements observe how well the baby is moving and analyse growth of the head and abdomen, the amniotic fluid volume and blood flow in the umbilical and cerebral arteries to check the flow of oxygen and nutrients.

While IUGR babies are often detected antenatally, allowing pregnancy to be monitored closely, some babies who are diagnosed with IUGR are born normal in size and perfectly healthy. Some so-called IUGR babies are genetically small but very healthy. At the same time some babies with true IUGR remain undetected. This includes babies who are born below their potential birth weight but appear normal. For instance, a baby who is genetically programmed to weigh 4 kg (8 lb 12 oz) at birth and is born weighing 3 kg (6 lb 8 oz) may not be considered small but will have IUGR. The distinction can be made after birth when signs include loose folds of skin and a nagging hunger.

Antenatal care

If your baby has IUGR you are likely to be examined more frequently. If your baby is small but growth is steady and there is no evidence of ill-health, then no extra care is needed, although your baby will continue to be monitored as a high-risk pregnancy. In a minority of severe IUGR cases detected early, an AMNIOCENTESIS may be necessary to check for CONGENITAL ABNORMALITIES. If the cause of slow growth is within control (e.g. high blood pressure or poor nutrition) you may be able to decrease the risk.

Extra care during labour and birth

Babies with severe IUGR are more likely to develop foetal distress and asphyxia with low Apgar scores (p.139). Severe IUGR may necessitate a CAESAREAN SECTION prior to labour. Babies with moderate IUGR may require induction of labour (p.497) , particularly in the amniotic fluid volume is reduced (p.397) In labour it is important to monitor foetal heart rate continuously or regularly in accordance with procedures for a high-risk pregnancy. The majority of babies with mild IUGR have a natural labour and birth although birth teams are more inclined to recommend a caesarean section at an early stage if there are signs of distress.

After birth

If vaginal or caesarean birth goes without complications and your baby begins feeding soon to boost his blood sugar levels, he is likely to thrive. Your birth team will be alert for problems specifically related to a low birth weight. A paediatrician will assess the IUGR, to exclude any underlying problem and provide extra care if necessary.

Potential difficulties after the birth

Hypothermia: Low fat reserves and a low capacity for producing heat increase the risk of low body temperature. It is important to keep your baby warm, preferably with skin-to-skin contact, and stay in a warm room.

Hypoglycaemia (p486): A smaller baby may have low sugar stores. If these are not boosted sufficiently after birth, there is a risk of reduced glucose and oxygen to the brain. This can usually be avoided with early feeding, and occasionally with medical support.

Polycythaemia: If an increased number of red blood cells formed because of a reduced concentration of oxygen before the birth, this may lead to JAUNDICE.

Prematurity: If your baby is born early and has IUGR, he may have additional problems if some body systems are immature – usually the lungs and breathing are affected. Assistance and treatment in a SPECIAL CARE BABY UNIT may be the best option. If the IUGR has been severe or prolonged, your baby may be more susceptible to BREATHING DIFFICULTIES.

Growth and development

With good feeding, catch-up growth with weight gain can be very rapid (within days), particularly if your baby is born in good condition with asymmetric IUGR. If your baby is genetically small, he will remain small. If the IUGR is severe and if there is an underlying cause, he may remain small. The only way of assessing growth is by monitoring it for years.

Except where IUGR is linked with a congenital abnormality or is very severe and began in early pregnancy, small babies tend to develop perfectly normally when given loving attention and good nutrition. Touch, loving contact and frequent feeding in the days and weeks after birth can have a very positive effect on development. Many of the care issues relating to premature babies (p.527) apply to IUGR babies.

The long-term effect depends on how long and how severely nutrition was reduced during crucial stages of brain development. In humans there is an intense brain growth spurt beginning in mid-pregnancy and continuing until the age of 2

years. If asymmetric IUGR occurs in the second half of pregnancy, with the 'brain sparing' effect, there may be no long-term effects on mental development. If there was an underlying cause such as an infection or chromosomal problem or severely reduced placental blood flow, it may affect future development. Conditions that begin early in pregnancy are likely to exert a greater effect. Yet even with severe IUGR most children develop normally.

Behaviour and relationships

A small number of babies whose growth has been severely restricted, where birth weight is below 2.27 kg (5 lb), may behave differently from babies with normal growth. With big differences from baby to baby, there is a general pattern of passivity, inconsolability when upset, more volatile emotions and a reduced ability to concentrate during the 1st year. Some people might say that IUGR babies 'speak a different language' and can be very challenging. If your baby acts like this, it may sometimes feel hard to engage his attention. Seeing him for the way he is rather than as a 'difficult' baby might make it easier for you to summon patience and put extra effort into your time together. You may need extra support, particularly if sleep is patchy. The rewards will be considerable and as your baby grows the challenge may get smaller. Vulnerable babies have a higher risk of emotional difficulties if they are not understood. It is important, for the whole family, to get as much practical and emotional support as possible (p.58).

IRRITABLE BOWEL SYNDROME
See DIARRHOEA: MOTHER

JAUNDICE

In the womb your developing foetus has more red blood cells than she will need after birth. The haemoglobin in these cells enables her to obtain sufficient oxygen from the transfer across the placenta. After birth, the extra red cells are broken down and eliminated. In the process, a yellow pigment called bilirubin is produced. This is then processed by the liver in preparation for excretion.

When bilirubin is produced more quickly than it can be excreted, the pigment is deposited in the skin, the whites of the eyes and the mucous membranes (e.g. the inside of the mouth). If this happens, your baby will look yellowish. This is extremely common: approximately 60% of the babies born each year develop neonatal jaundice and it is more common among PREMATURE babies. It rarely poses any problems.

What happens

Jaundice usually develops in the first few days following birth. This is because liver function is temporarily immature, and bilirubin is processed slowly. Yellowing becomes apparent 24 hours or more after birth and involves the entire skin, spreading from head to toe, peaking after 3–4 days. It usually passes within 7–10 days, with no complications, and does not recur. If your baby was premature, she may become jaundiced after birth, and it may not clear for up to 2 months. Some jaundice needs medical treatment and responds well.

Kernicterus

If jaundice is very intense, bilirubin pigment may be deposited in the brain and cause permanent changes that damage cerebral function. This is called kernicterus and is preventable provided bilirubin levels are kept below the danger line indicated on a chart that takes the baby's age and weight into account. In the early days after birth the baby's brain is more susceptible, particularly if birth was premature.

Breast milk jaundice

Around 5–10% of breastfed babies remain jaundiced for up to 10 weeks. It is unclear why breastfeeding and prolonged jaundice are related, although it may be that hormones in breast milk interfere with the breakdown of the bilirubin and slow the maturing of the liver. Jaundice is usually mild, giving a baby a healthy sun-tanned appearance, and does no harm. If you switch to bottle feeding, jaundice will reduce rapidly, but this is not necessary for a healthy, thriving baby.

If your baby appears to have breast milk jaundice but it is prolonged beyond 2 weeks, your midwife, doctor or health visitor may request blood tests to confirm your baby does not have abnormal liver or THYROID function. If the level of jaundice is not high enough to warrant treatment, nothing more needs to be done because as your baby feeds regularly and frequently the bilirubin levels in the blood will fall.

Insufficient feeding and jaundice

Some babies develop jaundice as a result of insufficient calorie and fluid intake, usually in the early days while feeding is being established. Because many mothers go home within 48 hours of birth, before the usual peak of jaundice, health visitors routinely monitor jaundice levels and weight. Excessive WEIGHT loss (more than 15%) may be associated with a high level of jaundice. A blood test assesses bilirubin levels.

Less common causes of jaundice

Many conditions and processes can contribute to the development of neonatal jaundice. In the most severe cases, several causes may be present.

Blood group incompatibility: If you and your baby have different blood group types, you may produce antibodies capable of destroying your baby's red blood cells. Rhesus (p.410) is very rare with modern prevention methods but ABO incompatability (p.410) is not preventable and may cause jaundice, needing treatment.

Premature birth: The liver may not be sufficiently mature to process bilirubin.

Breakdown of blood: Excessive amounts of blood are released into muscles from bruising during birth (p.404).

Polycythemia: The presence of excessive red blood cells in a baby is quite common and there are usually no symptoms. Polycythemia does not need treatment but the jaundice does.

G6PD deficiency: This is an inherited disorder of the enzyme G6PD and is more common in families of Mediterranean or Asian origin. The deficiency weakens the red cell and makes it break down more readily.

Late jaundice (after 1 month)

After 3 months a slight yellowy-orange tinge, particularly to the bridge of the nose and palms of the hands, is more often due to an excess of carrots than to jaundice: organic varieties seem to have a greater effect because they have a high volume of the naturally occurring food pigments carrotenoids. If you are concerned, however, do visit your doctor. Although extremely rare, apparent jaundice after the 1st month may indicate **biliary atresia**, where the normal connection between the liver and bowel needs to be surgically corrected, or neonatal HEPATITIS, which needs medical treatment.

Action plan

If your baby is jaundiced in the first 2–4 days after birth, ask your midwife to check weight and bilirubin levels. If jaundice is due to insufficient calorie or fluid intake, establishing comfortable and successful feeding is important – help with latching on and positioning (p.188) may steadily bring up your baby's weight. Most babies clear excess bilirubin without needing treatment. If your baby is unable to eliminate bilirubin sufficiently, simple treatment can help. The extent of jaundice is measured with a total serum bilirubin blood test, made on a drop of blood taken from your baby's heel.

Phototherapy

The most frequently used treatment is phototherapy. This involves exposing your baby's skin to ultraviolet light that has the effect of altering the bilirubin in the bloodstream as it circulates in the small capillaries under the skin. The altered bilirubin then passes into the urine and level drops rapidly. Phototherapy may be administered through a fibre-optic blanket connected to an ultraviolet light source or more intensively beneath overhead ultraviolet lights in a warm incubator. To protect her eyes she will either wear an eye pad or a tinted head box. A baby's skin appears blotchy under the phototherapy lights because it absorbs light at different rates.

While your baby is being treated, you do not need to be separated: you can feed and care for her as usual. Even if you feed every hour, your baby can be away from the lights while she feeds. You may be advised to feed her more frequently to increase bilirubin excretion. Bilirubin levels will be measured every 8–12 hours and when the level drops below the chart's phototherapy line, treatment can be discontinued. Intensive or prolonged phototherapy may be needed for prematurity, ABO incompatibility and extensive bruising during labour.

Exchange transfusion

Rarely, severe jaundice does not respond to phototherapy. An exchange transfusion can reduce the level of bilirubin and prevent the rare but serious complication of kernicterus and brain damage. This procedure removes small quantities of a baby's blood, replacing them with adult donor blood (not the mother's) that do not break down so easily.

Homeopathy

The main remedy for neonatal physiological jaundice is *Chelidonium*, an organ support remedy that helps the liver to function optimally. It may suit your baby if she is cold, has clammy yellow skin, marked yellowness on the nose and cheeks, and is lethargic. In the first 24 hours give *Chelidonium* (6c) every 2 hours for up to 6 doses, and then 3 times a day for up to 4 days. If there is no improvement, consult a homeopath.

LABOUR, ABNORMAL

See also CAESAREAN SECTION; Labour and birth (pp.118–41); When a helping hand is needed (p.164)

Many women prepare enthusiastically for a smooth unassisted labour, only to find that on the day they need help. This is common, and if you need a helping hand, it is best to remember that you and your baby both play important roles in the birth process and you are not able to be fully in control. Obstetric and midwifery care treats safety of mother and baby as the highest priority and assistance is available to ensure the best outcome. Most often, a problem is minimal and the action needed is simple and effective. With high-tech care, serious complications with long-term effects for mother or baby are rare. Statistics for complications and assistance in labour vary widely from hospital to hospital. The national average for total caesarean is: 20% (emergency 12%, elective 8%); induction: 20% ; episiotomy: 20%; ventouse: 7%, and forceps: 4%.

What happens
When there are signs that you or your baby needs assistance, in all but rare emergencies there is a chance to discuss your options. Usually monitoring is intensified and continuous as for a HIGH-RISK PREGNANCY and you will be informed and supported. Yet it is usual to feel worried, particularly when there is an emergency and decisions and procedures need to be made quickly or a paediatrician needs to be called. This is when the support of a birth partner can be especially helpful.

Whatever level of assistance you and your baby require, it is normal and acceptable to feel upset or disappointed or grateful and relieved or a combination. It is important for you to find space and time to talk through your feelings. EMOTIONS, ADVICE & SUPPORT may be helpful. Your baby may be resilient and recover well, but all babies react differently to the birth process (p.148) and all benefit from loving care and comfort in the days and weeks after birth.

LABOUR, BREECH BIRTH

Between Weeks 32 and 36 most babies settle into the optimum head-down position. In around 3% of pregnancies the buttocks are down in a breech position. There are various types of breech. In a frank breech, which is the most common, both hips are flexed, the knees are at the level of the baby's nipples and the feet are by the head. In a complete breech knees and feet are flexed and the feet tucked under the buttocks as if the baby is squatting on the inlet to the mother's pelvis. At birth the buttocks and feet emerge at the same time. In a footling breech one or two feet are lower than the buttocks as if the baby is standing at the pelvic inlet and one or both legs are born before the buttocks. In this situation there is a small risk of UMBILICAL CORD PROLAPSE alongside the leg when the membranes rupture.

What happens
In most cases there is no obvious reason for a baby being in a breech position; it may simply be that this position is more comfortable. A minority of babies may take the breech position for a specific reason, such as: being small through prematurity (p.526) or INTRAUTERINE GROWTH RESTRICTION (IUGR); being one of TWINS; if there is excess AMNIOTIC FLUID that allows the baby to move around; in PLACENTA PRAEVIA a low placenta prevents the head from engaging; an unusually shaped bicornuate UTERUS may make a baby's head more comfortable. CONGENITAL ABNORMALITY of the baby's limbs or spine are a rare cause and can be detected by a scan.

Action plan
If your baby is breech after Week 34, you will be given a clinical examination and an ultrasound scan may be suggested to exclude the above causes. Many babies, particularly in a second or third pregnancy or where there is plenty of amniotic fluid, will turn head down in the last 4 weeks before labour.

Exercises
There are exercises that can encourage a baby to turn and can do no harm. Kneel on the floor with your knees and legs wide apart and your buttocks in the air. Place your forearms on the floor with your hands on opposing elbows and rest your head on your forearms. Keep your buttocks in the air for 3–5 minutes with your pelvis higher than your head. This will encourage your baby's buttocks to disengage from your pelvis and the head may turn. Repeat the exercise 4 times a day.

Acupuncture
Acupuncture has been used with great effect for centuries. The treatment can begin from around Week 30. It involves moxibustion heat or a needle applied to an acupuncture point on the outer side of the little toe. The treatment is repeated on alternate days. The acupuncture point may also be stimulated with acupressure by massaging the outer part of the little toe 2 or 3 times a day for 1–2 minutes.

Homeopathy
Pulsatilla is used to turn breech babies. It is usually prescribed over a period of 4 days in ascending potencies, beginning around Week 34 or 35. It is not advisable to self-prescribe so consult a homeopath who may advise using the remedy in conjunction with acupuncture and exercise.

Medical care
Your obstetrician may attempt **external cephalic version** (ECV), which involves manipulation and massage of your abdomen. The procedure is usually done after Week 36 when the risks of prematurity have passed and the baby has had time to turn spontaneously. Where this technique is carried out it is successful in 60% of cases. First, an ultrasound scan assesses the size and condition of your baby and the amniotic fluid volume. If there is a reduction in amniotic fluid or any

sign of IUGR or the umbilical cord is around the baby's neck then an ECV is not recommended. The scan is often used during the turning and the obstetrician will be watching for changes in your baby's heart rate that may indicate tension on the umbilical cord or disturbance of the placenta that could lead to a PLACENTAL ABRUPTION. These risks are very low but if they occur, FOETAL DISTRESS may follow.

Once turned, most babies remain in a head-down position; returning to breech position may happen if there is an excess of amniotic fluid or it is not the first pregnancy and there is more room in the uterus. In some hospitals ECV is done in conjunction with using a drug to relax the wall of the uterus and it is usually performed on the labour ward. Your baby's heartbeat (CTG) will be monitored immediately after the procedure. If there are signs of foetal distress or placental abruption an immediate caesarean section is essential.

Breech birth

If your baby remains in a breech position at term, you may be able to have a vaginal delivery if hospital policy and your medical team support it. The safest route for your baby is caesarean section because there is a risk of birth asphyxia or injury (p.472) occurring in a vaginal birth. Some women elect to have a breech vaginal delivery in full knowledge of the risks. Statistically, 97% of breech babies born vaginally will not be seriously compromised. If you plan to have a caesarean section, a time will be set, usually after Week 38, to reduce the risks of prematurity and BREATHING DIFFICULTIES after birth.

What happens

If your obstetrician practises breech birth, she may agree to a vaginal birth if you have completed at least 36 weeks of pregnancy and you have not had a previous difficult birth. It is important your pelvic capacity is large and your baby weighs less than 3.8 kg (8 lb 5 oz), which can be assessed through ultrasound. There must be facilities for emergency caesarean delivery in case labour does not progress smoothly.

In a vaginal delivery when the body is born the umbilical cord may be compressed (p.550) between your baby's chest and your vagina and pelvic bones. When compression occurs a baby receives less oxygen from the placenta and the head must be born within 5–7 minutes after the umbilicus is visible. If the birth is delayed it may result in severe foetal distress and asphyxia that could have long-term effects on development.

Action plan

With a vaginal birth, close monitoring of your baby is absolutely essential. In the 1st stage of labour a vaginal examination will confirm that your baby's foot has not slipped into the cervix. Your baby's heartbeat is monitored to ensure there is no foetal distress. In the 2nd stage you must not bear down until your cervix is fully dilated because the cervix could delay the birth of the head. An upright supported squatting position (p.152) will help your pelvis to open maximally and allow you to push with optimal force when it is time. Alternatively you may use an epidural anaesthetic and be lying down but the mechanics of this position are less advantageous. If there is a delay or difficulty in delivering the head, forceps (p.496) may be used. An emergency caesarean

can be performed at any time until the birth of the buttocks and umbilical cord: when these have passed the vaginal entrance there is a commitment to a vaginal birth.

After birth the 3rd stage is normal. A breech baby will have different head moulding from a baby born head first, usually with the back of the head being prominent. The head shape normalises over months. Breech babies have a higher incidence of dislocated HIPS because of the leg position in the womb.

LABOUR, DISPROPORTION

See also LABOUR, MALPOSITION & MALPRESENTATION; LABOUR, SLOW PROGRESS; LARGE BABIES

During pregnancy the position your baby chooses will largely depend on him and to a lesser extent on the amount of amniotic fluid or the size and shape of your pelvis. Cephalopelvic disproportion occurs when the fit between a baby's head and the mother's pelvis is tight and it is difficult for the baby to advance through the birth canal. Disproportion cannot always be predicted in advance.

What happens

Cephalopelvic disproportion occurs if your baby is very LARGE or your pelvis is small or its shape is not optimal for birth. Your pelvis is fully grown by 17 years of age and the size will be optimal if you were well nourished as a child and teenager. If you are shorter than average height and your baby is big, this may lead to disproportion. In some women the pelvis is shaped with the pubic bones in front of the bladder forming a narrow triangular-shaped arch. This allows less space for the baby's head to fit and engage in the pelvis. In a few women an accident may have caused a fractured pelvis and an obstetrician will assess whether this might interfere with birth.

Action plan
Prevention

- It may be possible to prevent your baby from growing too LARGE by attending to your nutrition and treating DIABETES. His size is not entirely in your control and antenatal care detects most very large babies.
- Pelvic x-ray to determine the size of your pelvic bones is not recommended because of the radiation risks and the results would not help significantly in decisions about birth.

Pregnancy and birth

- Your midwife or obstetrician may anticipate disproportion if your baby appears large or has a non-engaged head in late pregnancy (p.499).
- With slow progress your midwife or doctor can assess the shape of your pelvis and your baby's position and extent of engagement through an internal vaginal examination. If there is a tight fit, your baby's head is more likely to be positioned awkwardly (occipito posterior) (p.499).
- If progress is slow and your birth team decide there is sufficient space for a safe birth, labour may be augmented by rupturing the membranes or administering an oxytocin infusion (p.496). Your baby may need help with the birth,

either by you being upright to maximise your power to push and open the pelvic cavity as much as possible, or with forceps or ventouse (p.496).

- If your birth team decide it would be safer for your baby, they may advise a CAESAREAN SECTION, either before labour begins or during the 1st or 2nd stage.

LABOUR, EPISIOTOMY & TEARS

See also Episiotomy (p.165); LABOUR, FORCEPS & VENTOUSE

Your vagina is designed to stretch at birth, but it may tear. This sounds worse than it is in reality – with the pressure and the force of birth, few women notice they have torn, and tears usually heal relatively quickly. Many tears do need to be stitched, however. An episiotomy is a cut that extends from the back wall of the vagina to the side of the anus along the perineum to enlarge the vaginal opening. It includes the vaginal and perineal skin and the underlying muscles. Tears and episiotomy are less common in subsequent vaginal births. Some women feel an episiotomy is an acceptable part of having a baby. Some are upset if an episiotomy is performed and would prefer to have torn or have had no tear. Others, who are afraid of tearing, elect to have an episiotomy.

Episiotomy is used frequently in some countries, with a variation in rates: from 8% in the Netherlands, to over 90% in the Eastern European countries. Research evidence suggests that a rate above 20% is not medically justified. Obstetricians tend to be more convinced than midwives that an episiotomy is an integral part of managing a first birth.

Arguments against routine use of episiotomy

Episiotomies became popularised by Dr Lee in the USA in the 1920s. They were thought to prevent perineal damage as well as vaginal and pelvic floor prolapse, and protect a baby from BIRTH INJURY or FOETAL DISTRESS by reducing the pressure of birth. These theoretical benefits have since been disproved and there is little justification for its routine use. But it is accepted that when episiotomy is used selectively it is an effective way to widen the vaginal entrance and allow a baby's head to emerge. This may be necessary when birth needs to be speeded up because there is evidence of foetal distress, the tissues are too tight to stretch, particularly if a baby is LARGE, or when an extra pulling force (forceps or ventouse) is needed.

- If a woman does not have an episiotomy, she may still have a small tear, but with rare exceptions the tear will be no worse than an episiotomy. Many women will not tear at all. An episiotomy does not prevent deep tears into the vagina or into the anal muscle.
- An episiotomy does not prevent birth injuries.
- It can increase the amount of maternal blood loss (p.406).
- Pain after birth is likely to be greater with episiotomy, as is persistent pain during intercourse.
- An episiotomy does not heal more quickly or more efficiently than a stitched tear, nor is it easier to repair.
- Tears of the anal sphincter muscle are more common with episiotomy and may lead to flatulence or anal incontinence (p.557). Yet an episiotomy does not reduce the chance of

urinary incontinence, nor reduce laxity of pelvic floor muscles, nor promise better sex after birth.

How you can help your vagina to stretch

During pregnancy perineal massage and pelvic floor exercises are helpful (p.98). During labour your input and your birth team's skill and assistance can help. This includes supporting you to be upright, facilitating slow delivery of the head while supporting the perineum, delivering the shoulders one at a time and assisting delivery in water. Some midwives gently massage the perineum to encourage stretching when birth is drawing near. Yet even with preparation and care during labour, you may tear or need an episiotomy.

What happens

Tears

If you tear you may not feel it, instead sensing only the pressure and power of birth. It may help to remember that the medical details can sound scary but the experience often is not. The most common place to tear is backwards along the perineum, between the vagina and the anus, but a tear may involve the front of the vagina and the labia and may go towards the clitoris. If you are on your back, tears tend to involve the back wall of the vagina whereas if you are upright or leaning forwards, the tear may be more superficial towards the front of the labia. Every woman is different and some have more elasticity in their vaginal tissues than others.

A superficial tear in the vaginal or labial skin is classed as 1st degree. If the underlying muscles are involved, which is less common, this is a 2nd-degree tear. On very rare occasions the tear is 3rd degree – that is, it extends into the anus. The likelihood of a 3rd-degree tear increases with episiotomy and forceps delivery, large babies – over 4 kg (8 lb 12 oz) – and prolonged 2nd stage of labour. Extremely rare 4th-degree tears involve complete disruption of the muscle of the anal sphincter and the lining of the anus.

Episiotomy

If you and your team decide to go ahead with an episiotomy, your vaginal area will be numbed with local anaesthetic delivered by injection, unless you already have an epidural in place. The injection will give a small, stinging sensation and the anaesthetic will become effective immediately. Your midwife or obstetrician will then perform the cut and you will not feel anything.

There are two types of episiotomies: midline (straight down toward the rectum) and mediolateral (down and off to one side). US and Canadian doctors may favour midline episiotomies while mediolateral cuts are preferred in Europe. Midline episiotomies are less painful, heal better, are less likely to cause pain with sex and cause less blood loss, but there is a risk that the incision may extend during the birth and the anus may tear. Mediolateral episiotomies are the opposite.

Action after episiotomy or tears

When the birth is over and your placenta has been born, your midwife or obstetrician will assess the need for stitches. Minor, 1st-degree tears heal spontaneously and often do not require stitching. 2nd-degree tears, if long or deep, are usually stitched. 3rd- and 4th-degree tears need to be stitched and a senior member of the obstetric medical team usually does this. An episiotomy is always stitched.

You will be asked to lie on your back and the head of the bed may be raised so you can hold your baby; you may breastfeed. The area is numbed and the stitching process usually takes 15–30 minutes. Depending on the area involved, the stitches are in three layers: the vaginal lining, the muscles and the external skin. Skin sutures dissolve in 4–6 days while muscle sutures take a few weeks.

Healing and recovery
Whether you have unstitched tears or a stitched tear or episiotomy, you may be uncomfortable. The degree of discomfort you feel and the rapidity of healing depend on the length and depth of your tear or cut, the skill of the obstetrician or midwife and the quality of suture material. While the area is healing you can care for your vagina and perineum and keep pain to a minimum. A tear or an episiotomy may contribute to blood loss after birth.

Pain
Pain may arise from a number of areas. The healing skin may be tender; pelvic muscles may be under tension from the stitches or because of spasm as a reaction to pain from the pelvic joints (p.519) or ligaments that may have stretched during the birth; or from PILES. You may notice discomfort for the 1st week – this can be relieved with painkillers. Pain from skin or muscle sutures usually passes in 10–14 days. Muscle spasm and ligament strain may continue for many weeks or even for months in some women who have needed stitches. Postnatal examination by your doctor will help to define the cause of the pain and if it is joint or ligament or muscle spasm then physiotherapy or osteopathy is useful. For around 5% of women discomfort takes months to settle because of muscle spasm and scar tissue forming in the deep tissues.

Posture and movement
You may find it helps to lie on your side instead of sitting, or to sit on a rubber ring. After the first few days it is good to walk and to do postnatal pelvic floor exercises and to begin gentle yoga stretches (p.346). The exercises may be uncomfortable or even painful but they will increase the blood flow to the muscles and help healing. Modern sutures are very strong and will not break if you contract your muscles.

Swelling and bruising
The vaginal tissues are able to expand and swelling may be caused by fluid passing into the tissues from the pressure of the birth. This usually settles in a few days but if the area is infected or there has been bruising, the swelling may increase. Your midwife can examine you for signs of infection or bruising. Bruises usually heal in 7–10 days, while infection may require antibiotic treatment.

Urination and opening your bowels
If there is stinging or burning, try pouring lukewarm water over your labia as you urinate. Initially you may find it easier to urinate in the bath or the shower. If your urine continues to burn after a few days, you may have cystitis (p.552), particularly after a long labour or if your midwife used a catheter to empty your bladder. Although it is rare, you may experience urinary incontinence or flatulence (p.557). This may be associated with prolapse and usually passes in a few days but it may sometimes persist.

Many women feel sore after birth. You may be afraid that the stitches will open but modern sutures last for weeks and will not break with a bowel action. Discomfort from stitches or piles may reduce your sensation and awareness of needing to open your bowels. During the first few days it is best to eat a high-roughage diet and drink lots of fluid to reduce CONSTIPATION, because passing a hard stool will increase your discomfort and anxiety. Some women need a suppository.

Scar tissue
The vaginal area usually heals well with little scar tissue. Sometimes parts of the internal lining of the vagina or the deeper tissues stick together and cause adhesions, which are bands of scar tissue. This may cause pain with sex and even narrowing of the vaginal opening. The usual site for this is on the back wall at the junction of the vagina and the perineum. Occasionally an operation is needed to remove the scars.

Homeopathy
After birth these remedies will speed up healing and ease discomfort, each taken in 200c, 4 times a day for 3 days then 3 times a day for 4 days.

Arnica reduces swelling, promotes healing of bruised tissue, reduces aching and soreness and assists in the effective reabsorption of blood; *Hypericum* works particularly on nerve pain and damage and is good for shooting or tearing pains; *Bellis Perennis* helps to heal deep tissue, relieves soreness and sensitivity and throbbing pains and is good in conjunction with *Arnica*; *Calendula* speeds up the healing process.

Calendula tincture can be applied externally in conjunction with the above. Add 10 drops to the bath or bidet or soak a sanitary towel or cotton wool in diluted tincture (10 drops in a bowl of water) and bathe the area. If it stings to urinate you can pour this diluted tincture over yourself as you sit on the toilet. *Staphysagria* is helpful when you feel emotionally bashed, almost cut and raw after an episiotomy or tearing badly. Take 3 x 200c tablets within 24 hours.

Aromatherapy
A few drops of comfrey, calendula or marigold or a decoction of the herbs themselves in a warm bath will soothe and help the healing process.

Making love again
Within 4 weeks the site of an episiotomy cut or tear will probably be completely healed and sexual intercourse is safe. The muscles may take time to regain normal strength, and the oestrogen output from your ovaries will be low, making the vaginal skin thinner and particularly sensitive. This effect lasts longer if you are breastfeeding and occurs even without stitches. When you resume penetrative sex, try gentle penetration (lying side to side or with you on top) and

lubricating the area with pure oil before intercourse. The back of the vagina near the perineum is the most sensitive, and lying on your back is not advantageous. Over the next weeks uncomfortable sensitivity is likely to disappear. If it does not, visit your doctor and ask for a check.

A minority of women feel violated and take time to get back in touch with their vagina as a sexual object. Men are often affected by what happened during birth and are concerned about contributing to more pain. Libido and sexuality may be altered for many months. Sometimes a difficult birth may lead to post-traumatic stress (p.462) that lowers self-esteem. Support may help you avoid depression and difficulties in your partnership. If there is an underlying physical problem that needs attention, it is best to have it investigated sooner rather than later.

LABOUR, FORCEPS & VENTOUSE

Forceps consist of two metal blades shaped like salad spoons that are put into the vagina and placed on either side of a baby's head. Their introduction in 1598 was a milestone in obstetric history, allowing intervention in difficult births when the lives of mother and baby might otherwise have been lost. The ventouse or vacuum extractor, invented in 1957, is an increasingly popular alternative. The ventouse is a plastic cup that is placed on a baby's scalp and connected to a vacuum pump. The cup is held on the baby's head by suction and the obstetrician pulls to give an extra downward force (traction) while the mother pushes. Modern cups are soft and pliable, mould well to a baby's head and cause minimal trauma. The ventouse is used more frequently because it occupies less space and there is less risk of tearing – an episiotomy is not always essential. A safety feature is that the cup will come off if too much pressure is applied during traction.

Forceps or ventouse are used in about 11% of births. Antenatal preparation and active upright birth positions may reduce the chances that your baby will need assistance, and second labours less commonly need to be assisted. The circumstances, however, cannot always be in your control. Your baby may need help for one of several reasons:

- The 2nd stage of labour may be prolonged (p.504) or you may lack energy to continue.
- Your baby's head might be large in relation to your pelvis (although a very LARGE BABY will need to be born by CAESAREAN SECTION).
- Your baby may be in an occipito posterior position (p.499). His head can be rotated with forceps or ventouse, after which delivery follows easily.
- Your baby may be breech (p.492) and the assistance helps his head to be born.
- If your baby has FOETAL DISTRESS, assistance helps speed up the birth and maximises safety.
- If you have had an epidural (p.159) this can reduce your pushing force (a mobile epidural is preferable to enable you to change position).
- You may have a medical condition that makes bearing down unsafe, e.g. high BLOOD PRESSURE.

Safety is the key issue and if the force needed is excessive, or the obstetrician feels the assistance may be too traumatic for your baby, an emergency caesarean section will be needed.

What happens
Forceps or ventouse can only be used when your baby's head has fully entered and engaged in your pelvis. Before the procedure priority will be given to effective pain relief. You may have the option of an epidural if an anaesthetist is present; alternatively you may be offered a pudendal block given by injection (both are discussed on pp.159–60). If you already have an epidural in place, it can be topped up.

You will be asked to lie on your back with your legs supported by stirrups. This position helps the obstetrician deliver your baby as safely and as quickly as possible. A catheter tube will be passed into your bladder to empty it and protect it from damage during delivery. Your partner will probably be welcome to stay, although some men do not feel comfortable. He may sit by your head during the procedure, and be there to hold your baby.

The forceps or ventouse are applied to your baby's head and pulled with carefully controlled pressure with each contraction. The pulling force will combine with your pushing force. Most women feel as if they are definitely doing most of the work. If your medical team believe that an episiotomy (p.494) is necessary (less common with ventouse) it will be done as you push. Birth usually occurs within three contractions after the application of the instrument.

Action plan for recovery
After birth you may feel sore and bruised in the front and back pelvic joints, which may open more than usual. The pelvic muscles may also have stretched, giving a sensation of bruising. Ventouse is less likely to cause muscle tears or excess stretching. You may feel uncomfortable if you have had an episiotomy and healing may take a few weeks.

Your baby after forceps or ventouse
Your baby feels the pulling force of forceps during two or three contractions, each lasting less than 1 minute. He may feel a strong tug and may feel pain. After birth there may be marks on his cheeks or jaw for a few days. If a ventouse has been used he will feel suction on his scalp for some minutes and this might be uncomfortable. His scalp may be swollen and red; this settles in a day or two. Some babies appear to have a headache. Frequent sucking at the breast or bottle is a good remedy, and is reassuring because of the warmth of a loving embrace. Cranial osteopathy (p.376) can be effective.

LABOUR, INDUCTION & AUGMENTATION

Induction is artificially starting the process of labour. The incidence in the UK overall is 10–20% but it varies from hospital to hospital. It is more common to induce a first baby. There are a number of complementary methods thought to bring on labour but medical methods using synthetic hormones are the most common.

Most women accept induction if they believe it is safer for their babies yet induction is a very emotional issue. Many women enjoy being certain that labour will not be prolonged beyond a set date. Some would prefer labour to be initiated by baby and mother. The decision to induce is not always an easy one, and you will probably want to talk through the pros and cons with your midwife, obstetrician and your partner.

Modern induction is usually successful and the failure rate is decreased by careful selection of technique by midwives and obstetricians. You may need patience to wait until your uterus responds to being stimulated and if the contractions are very painful you may also need pain relief. If induction fails, which only happens in a minority of cases, your baby will need to be born by CAESAREAN SECTION.

In some cases dilation of the cervix is slow or contractions become ineffective, whether labour has been induced or begun spontaneously. If this happens, labour can be supported with the same medical methods that are used for induction; this is called augmentation. Induction procedures are usually considered for one of the following reasons:

Postmaturity (p.500): Going beyond the due date is the most common reason.

Intrauterine growth restriction (IUGR) (p.488): If your baby is small it may be safer to be born than remain in the womb. The effects of IUGR are more marked in late pregnancy as placental function may naturally decline at this time.

Premature rupture of the membranes (p.501): This is particularly the case if it appears the amniotic fluid or your baby may be infected.

A medical condition: This may affect placental function (e.g. pre-eclampsia, p.410, or kidney disease). If you have DIABETES, labour may be induced if your baby is growing too LARGE or if your obstetrician is concerned about PLACENTAL FUNCTION.

Choice: If it suits the family to have the birth on a particular day. This is not an option in all hospitals. It is essential to be sure of the dating of pregnancy to prevent premature birth.

False labour (p.500): If you have been having runs of contractions that are not associated with dilation of your cervix for several hours or days you may become tired. If you are at or past full term, your birth team may consider augmentation.

Slow progress (p.502): If you are established in labour but your cervix is dilating slowly, your midwife will assess the cause and may augment your labour using oxytocin.

What happens

You might want to try some traditional methods of induction. If induction is more pressing and your doctor recommends it, you will probably go ahead directly with the medical process.

Traditional methods

Stimulating your nipples releases oxytocin, which in turn stimulates your uterus to contract. If your cervix is ripe, sexual intercourse may trigger labour because the semen contains prostaglandin to stimulate the uterus. These approaches only work if labour is about to happen within a few days. They cannot cause premature labour. If the waters have broken, sexual intercourse is not recommended.

Sweeping the membranes

Your midwife may be skilled in the centuries-old technique of 'stretching the cervix and sweeping the membranes' that may bring on contractions if the cervix is ripe. In outpatients she will insert her finger into your vagina and reach up to the cervix, then sweep the membranes gently away from the lower part of the uterus. This releases prostaglandin from the uterus and may lead to the onset of regular uterine contractions. The sweep may be repeated the following day. Most women find the procedure slightly uncomfortable but a minority do experience pain, and the midwife can stop. Sweeping may cause bleeding, similar to a show, from tiny blood vessels in the internal lining of the cervix. It is a safe procedure, but it is contraindicated if you have a PLACENTA PRAEVIA.

Complementary methods

A gentle massage or a soak in the bath with a soothing aromatherapy oil, such as lavender, may relieve any tension that is hindering the start of your impending labour and some essential oils help to stimulate contractions. The oils suggested on p.163 may be useful before labour begins – whether or not they influence your contractions, being relaxed and at ease may make a difference to your progress once labour does start. Acupuncture (p.377) may help and treatments may be needed over a few days.

You may have heard of castor oil as a remedy, which is most palatable if mixed with orange juice. The dose is 60 ml (2 fl oz) mixed with an equal volume of juice. It may, however, bring on diarrhoea and theoretically could cause your baby to pass a bowel movement in the womb: it is best to check with your midwife if you wish to take it. It is best avoided if the baby's AMNIOTIC FLUID volume is reduced.

Homeopathy

If there are no known complications, your baby is ready, and a well-indicated remedy is prescribed, it is rather like flicking a switch. While it may be difficult to be objective about yourself (and it is ultimately best to consult a qualified homeopath), you and your partner may choose something by looking at what may be preventing labour from establishing. If a remedy suits, take it in 200c and repeat 2 hours later. If there has been no change, reassess your symptoms and try another remedy.

Try *Aconite* if you have a raw fear and panic and feel tense with anxiety; *Gelsemium* if you have anticipatory anxiety and you think labour may be a huge ordeal; *Natrum Mur* if you are a self-conscious type, feel inhibited, or even subconsciously have set yourself high standards about your performance in labour; *Pulsatilla* if you have had runs of false labour; *Caullophylum* if you have weak labour pains and a rigid cervix.

Induction in hospital

Before induction your baby's gestational age is checked to prevent premature birth and because before term your uterus may be unresponsive there is a greater chance that you will need a caesarean section. Your baby's size and position and relation to your pelvic capacity will also be checked. Any contraindications, such as a malpresentation (p.498) or previous extensive uterine surgery will be discussed and your doctor will examine the ripeness of your cervix, because induction is more successful if it is ripe. If your cervix shows no signs of ripening and an ultrasound scan shows the placenta is still providing adequate nutrition, you may delay induction.

Prostaglandin

The majority of inductions are now undertaken using prostaglandin, which is a hormone produced by the lining of the uterus to stimulate muscle contractions and ripening of the cervix. It is in gel form and is inserted into the vagina with an applicator no thicker than a pencil. The dosage needs to be carefully controlled if you have high blood pressure or a HEART condition, have had ASTHMA, a previous caesarean section or more than four babies, are carrying TWINS or have an excessive volume of AMNIOTIC FLUID. Once the prostaglandin has been inserted it is best to rest in bed for an hour or two.

Your baby's heartbeat will be closely monitored electronically. Your uterus may respond rapidly and contractions could begin within an hour or two, giving a feeling of period-like cramps. If your cervix is not ripe the initial doses of prostaglandin are given to ripen the cervix and contractions may take longer to begin. Prostaglandin will be inserted every 6 hours and after your cervix is ripe, labour usually begins. Most women experience gentle contractions that gradually become stronger and more closely spaced, and normal labour occurs. If labour has not begun within 24 hours, which happens for a small number of women, it may be necessary to rupture the membranes and use oxytocin.

Possible side effects of prostaglandin include DIARRHOEA, NAUSEA and VOMITING, which affect 5% of women and usually disappear in a few hours. For a similar number of women the uterus may respond by contracting excessively, which may lead to intense discomfort requiring pain relief and sometimes to FOETAL DISTRESS. Close foetal heart monitoring is essential if your contractions are very frequent.

Artificial rupture of the membranes (ARM)

Some birth teams choose to break the waters manually to augment slow progress or to induce labour if the cervix is ripe and partly dilated, usually in second and subsequent pregnancies. When the membranes break, the lining of the uterus releases prostaglandin and labour usually begins. The waters are broken during a vaginal examination as the doctor or midwife inserts a thin plastic instrument into the cervix and punctures the membranes. It may be slightly uncomfortable.

Artificial rupture of membranes may not be the preferred choice if your baby is in an awkward position or the head is very high or you have a vaginal infection, particularly *Strep B*, because once the membranes have been ruptured they no longer protect against bacterial organisms in the vagina. Most hospitals are keen that birth follows no more than 24 hours later. If the contractions do not begin within a few hours, an oxytocin hormonal infusion is usually started to boost them.

Oxytocin

Oxytocin (also called Syntocinon) is a synthetic preparation with properties identical in action to the hormone oxytocin produced by your and your baby's pituitary glands. The hormone stimulates the muscle of your uterus to contract. Your pituitary releases oxytocin throughout pregnancy but towards term the muscle of the uterus becomes more sensitive and more responsive. If prostaglandin and rupturing the membranes are unsuccessful, oxytocin may complete the induction. It can also be used alone or with rupturing the membranes to augment a slow labour. The oxytocin is administered using an intravenous drip and your baby will be monitored closely for foetal distress. Your midwives will carefully regulate the dose if you have high BLOOD PRESSURE.

During an oxytocin infusion there is a small chance that the uterine muscle may contract excessively and this reduces the flow of oxygen to the placenta. This is particularly significant if you have had a previous caesarean section or have had more than three babies. The amount of oxytocin infused is gradually increased every 15–30 minutes but if hyperstimulation or foetal distress occurs, your midwife will reduce or stop the infusion. If you are given oxytocin to augment your labour, contractions will probably take 1–2 hours to reach maximum power. Sometimes delay in the 2nd stage of labour may be corrected by using oxytocin to boost contractions.

Induction of labour is usually successful and if your pregnancy is carefully assessed is likely to lead to a normal labour and birth. If there is a medical indication for induction, or there is slow progress, there is a higher chance that your baby may need assistance with forceps or ventouse (p.496), or perhaps delivery by caesarean. This depends on the cause (e.g. your baby may be large).

LABOUR, MALPOSITION & MALPRESENTATION

See also LABOUR, BREECH BIRTH; UMBILICAL CORD, COMPRESSED OR PROLAPSED

The way your baby is positioned in the womb has a great effect on the way labour progresses. Most babies prefer the occipito anterior position, but it is quite common for a baby to lie in a different way that may make the birth process more difficult. Sometimes there is a clear reason for this, but often it seems a baby simply prefers the position he has chosen. Your midwife will assess your baby's position. There are illustrations of positions on p.120.

Although a less usual position is not always a problem, it can contribute to complications in labour. You may choose to aim for 'Optimal foetal positioning' (p.95) with measures including attention to posture, avoiding slouching and toning your abdominal muscles through exercise. This cannot guarantee how your baby lies, but may help.

Occipito anterior position: normal

The majority of babies prefer the occipito anterior position when the crown of the head is down towards the cervix and the chin is tucked on to the chest. Your baby's spine faces the front of your abdominal wall on the left or right side. When his head enters your pelvis, his face turns towards your sacrum and the occiput (the bone at the back of the skull) faces anterior (toward your bladder at the front of your pelvis). This ensures the widest diameter of his head is in line with the widest diameter of your pelvic outlet. This is the most helpful position, and allows him to negotiate the birth canal in the most effective way.

Occipito posterior position: back to back

In an occipito posterior or 'back-to-back' position, your baby's spine is towards your spine and his limbs and front face your abdominal wall. The occiput (back of the head) points posteriorly back towards your sacrum and your baby's face looks towards your bladder. You may feel kicks at the front rather than on the side. This occurs in 20% of labours.

- Some babies find it is more comfortable to face the placenta if it is implanted on the front wall of the uterus. Labour is minimally affected and this applies to most occipito posterior babies.
- If the shape of your pelvis is more triangular than oval, with the widest space at the back, the angle between the pubic bones at the front allows less space for your baby's head. It is easier for your baby to be occipito posterior because the head's diameter is widest at the back and there is a better fit in the back part of the pelvis. If your pelvic capacity is large and your baby is normal in size, labour is not affected but when there is a tight fit labour may be prolonged.

There are a number of things you can do to help:

In the 1st stage: Labour may progress normally. However, your baby's chin may not tuck in so his head is deflexed and may press on your sacrum, giving you back pain. If you are active it may increase the contractions, birth may be easier; if your uterus contracts strongly, the power encourages the head to flex. Water and massage may help relax the muscles surrounding your pelvis and increase its capacity, while movements such as rotating your hips and kneeling (p.155), may encourage your baby to rotate during transition. If your pelvic muscles are tight an epidural may relax them and help your baby to turn.

In the 2nd stage: Staying upright in a supported squat maximises the opening of your pelvic bones and encourages your baby's head to flex and rotate. Occasionally assistance may be needed with forceps or ventouse (p.496) to rotate the head and help it to descend. If your baby's head remains high and your obstetrician judges it would be safer, a CAESAREAN SECTION may be the best option.

Breech position: bottom down

In breech position (p.492) your baby remains head-up with his buttocks nearest your pelvis. It occurs in 3–4% of pregnancies. This can make labour difficult and may indicate the need for a caesarean.

Brow & face position

Instead of flexing his head, your baby may extend his head back so his chin moves away from his chest. This occurs in about 1:500 births. If the head is half-way back, this is a 'brow' because the forehead comes first. This is an inefficient position because the head's widest diameter usually does not succeed in passing through the pelvis. A caesarean section is usually needed. In a 'face presentation', the head is thrown back and the diameter is smaller. This makes a vaginal birth possible

unless the fit is too tight. A baby born after this position often shows facial bruising that resolves in a few days.

Transverse lie

Very rarely (fewer than 1:500 births), a baby lies sideways (transverse) in the uterus, with a hand, shoulder or the umbilical cord presenting nearest the cervix. If diagnosed early, transverse lie may be changed by external cephalic version (p.492), but if the position cannot be altered and labour has started, a caesarean section is necessary.

If your baby is in a transverse lie and your waters break there may be a risk of UMBILICAL CORD PROLAPSE. This can be dangerous for your baby and you need an ambulance and immediate medical attention.

Many women whose babies are in a transverse lie do not need help because when labour contractions begin, the baby turns and the head will have made its way down into the pelvis. Your midwife will tell you your baby's presentation when she examines you – you need to contact her as soon as labour starts or when your waters break, whichever occurs first. If the lie is still transverse, a caesarean is undertaken.

LABOUR, NON-ENGAGED HEAD

Your baby's head will be engaged when the widest part (level with the ears) enters the pelvic brim. With your first baby this will probably happen some time after Week 36. In a second or subsequent pregnancy engagement often does not occur until labour begins. If your baby's head is not engaged before labour, there is probably no cause for concern but non-engagement signifies the need for extra surveillance.

What happens

When your midwife or doctor feels your abdomen, if she can feel more than three-fifths of your baby's head above your pelvic brim, it is not engaged. You may be aware of this if you feel your baby pushing up under your ribs. Your baby's head may not be engaged for a number of reasons:

- The most likely cause is that the ligaments supporting your uterus and cervix are attached high up to your pelvic bones and your baby's head will only be able to descend when your cervix has dilated fully. There is no lack of space for your baby to descend.
- Your baby may be encouraged to stay high if there is an excess of AMNIOTIC FLUID or PLACENTA PRAEVIA.
- If your baby is LARGE, or your pelvis is small, or both, the head cannot enter the pelvis (cephalo pelvic disproportion). In this instance 'five-fifths' of your baby's head may be felt when your abdomen is examined
- Your baby may be in an awkward position (p.498).

Action plan

- In most pregnancies the head will engage in labour and normal birth follows.
- If your ligaments hold the cervix high there is nothing to do but wait for full dilation. Contractions will probably encourage your baby's head to descend.

- Excessive amniotic fluid is not treatable but if the membranes rupture before labour begins you will need to be seen urgently, because these conditions increase the chance of UMBILICAL CORD PROLAPSE, which may cause FOETAL DISTRESS.
- If your baby is large or if your pelvis is very small, you cannot do much to remedy the situation. Depending on the extent of disproportion, you may be monitored closely and advised to have a CAESAREAN SECTION if labour is prolonged.
- If your baby is in an awkward position after Week 36, particularly occipito posterior, then attending to your posture and doing yoga may help optimal positioning (p.346). During labour the power of contractions may help your baby's head to rotate and negotiate the birth canal. If the malpresentation continues, the birth may need assistance with forceps or ventouse or a caesarean section.
- If you are having your second or subsequent baby, and none of the above conditions apply, the head engages.

LABOUR, POSTMATURITY

See also LABOUR, INDUCTION & AUGMENTATION

Most women deliver between Weeks 37 and 42, but a first pregnancy is more likely to go beyond the due date. A pregnancy that lasts more than 42 weeks is considered prolonged or postmature. One reason for going beyond your expected date of delivery (EDD) may be inaccurate calculation. If you have a long menstrual cycle, ovulation may be later and the due date needs to be adjusted (p.63). Using the last menstrual period as a starting point for calculations, 7.4% of babies are postmature; when using early ultrasound scans for dating, fewer than 3% of babies are postmature.

What happens
Most postmature babies born after an uncomplicated pregnancy are healthy. Despite knowing this, you may feel anxious about your baby and labour, and you may be uncomfortable and unable to sleep well. This can be a vulnerable time. If you are desperate for labour to start, you might be able to request induction; if you are keen for labour to begin spontaneously, you may resist induction.

Generally, being late is not dangerous. It is estimated that out of 500 babies born after induction because a pregnancy has passed the due date, only a few avoid risks associated with a late delivery. The small risks increase as pregnancy continues, particularly after Week 42. If your pregnancy is prolonged, your baby is likely to be LARGE and his size may contribute to a longer labour and possibly the need for a CAESAREAN SECTION. Though your placenta will probably continue to function well, its efficiency may fall after Week 40. This will be of particular concern if there have been signs of slow growth (p.488) in the 3rd trimester. Placental function can be assessed using ultrasound. The well being of your baby and the AMNIOTIC FLUID volume can be similarly assessed: fluid volume naturally decreases at the end of pregnancy but if the decrease is significant there may be an increased risk of

UMBILICAL CORD COMPRESSION during labour, which may contribute to FOETAL DISTRESS. The rate of stillbirth (p.519), although still very rare, rises after 42 weeks.

Action plan
If your pregnancy is prolonged the main priority will be to prevent complications for you and your baby. Policies regarding postmaturity and the need to induce labour vary from hospital to hospital. You could choose from a number of complementary therapies to encourage LABOUR INDUCTION and for relaxation while you wait you might use massage (p.365), aromatherapy (p.378), meditation or visualisation (p.370).

Medical care
Once your pregnancy goes 7–10 days beyond the due date, you and your baby will be monitored more closely with ultrasound scans and foetal heart monitoring, as for a HIGH-RISK PREGNANCY. The intensity of monitoring depends on your pregnancy. If monitoring shows that it would be safer, you may be encouraged to induce labour.
- After Week 42 CTG heartbeat monitoring every 1 or 2 days is advisable in addition to ultrasound scans To check amniotic fluid volume and blood flow in the baby's cord and brain.
- Postmature babies are more likely to have a bowel movement before birth with meconium staining of the amniotic fluid. If amniotic fluid volume is reduced and there is also foetal distress there may be meconium aspiration (p.474), causing BREATHING DIFFICULTIES after birth.
- During labour your baby will be closely monitored and the team will be aware that postmaturity is associated with potential difficulties particularly if the amniotic fluid volume is low. If your doctor is concerned that foetal distress has occurred or that your baby is too large to navigate your pelvis, a caesarean may be recommended.

LABOUR, PRE- & FALSE LABOUR

For some women, 'practice' or Braxton-Hicks contractions seem very strong, perhaps from as early on as Week 25. If you are sensitive to the activity of your uterus, you may have the feeling that labour is beginning, although there is no dilation of the cervix. It happens more often in second or subsequent pregnancies. This is known as pre- or false labour. Usually the contractions are irregular or when they are regular they come in clusters that may last many minutes and then disappear.

Other organs in your abdomen may also contract and mimic the uterus. This applies to your bowel if you have CONSTIPATION or irritable bowel syndrome (p.448), either of which may be brought on if you are anxious. It may apply to your bladder from pressure or if you have cystitis, or to the muscles in your abdominal wall. The way to distinguish uterine contractions is to sit quietly and place your hand flat on your abdomen over your belly button. With a contraction you will feel your uterus hardening when you feel discomfort.

The term false labour is also used to describe apparent

labour where the cervix remains below 3-cm dilation; this can be called the latent phase of the 1st stage and many women would class this as true labour because there can be considerable pain. It can last for days. True labour begins when dilation progresses beyond 3 cm (p.121).

Action plan
If you are concerned, contact your birth team, particularly if you have been told that you are at increased risk of premature labour, perhaps because you have previously had a premature birth or you have CERVICAL INCOMPETENCE.

Medical care
- A midwife will monitor your baby's heartbeat and your contractions.
- An internal examination will show the state of your cervix. If you are in labour it will be shortened and softened and at least 3 cm dilated.

What you can do
- If you are a long way off your due date it is worth taking it easy, doing what you can to reduce anxiety. Homeopathy or acupuncture may be helpful.
- If you are close to the due date and are having runs of painful Braxton-Hicks contractions it is best to maintain your energy for when true labour begins by caring for yourself (p.123).
- There may be a gentle gradation between pre-labour and the 1st stage of true labour, so keep in touch with the birth team. If you are at term but becoming tired and unable to sleep, they may suggest induction or augmentation (p.497).

LABOUR, PREMATURE RUPTURE OF THE MEMBRANES
....

See also PREMATURE BIRTH

Spontaneous rupture occurs when the chorion and amniotic membranes surrounding your baby leak, releasing amniotic fluid into the vagina. When this happens before Week 37, it is referred to as premature rupture of the membranes (PROM) and after Week 37 as pre-labour rupture or spontaneous rupture of the membranes. Premature rupture affects 3–5% of all pregnancies and is the most common cause of PREMATURE BIRTH. The membranes confine the amniotic fluid and protect your baby and the umbilical cord and provide a barrier against infection. The earlier in gestation rupture of the membranes occurs, the greater the likelihood that normal development may be adversely affected.

Although in most instances the cause of PROM is unknown, it may be connected to triggers for premature labour (p.527). There may be an increased risk if there is a vaginal infection, VAGINOSIS or CHLAMYDIA. The organisms may reduce the strength of the membranes and stimulate the release of prostaglandin hormones that encourage uterine contractions. The incidence rises if there is increased intrauterine pressure due to excessive AMNIOTIC FLUID or if you are carrying TWINS or more babies. The risk increases for women who work with industrial machines in late pregnancy. It is true that good maternal nutrition and health can reduce the risk of prematurity.

What happens
If your membranes rupture, a large volume of amniotic fluid may gush out of your vagina. There may be a little bit of blood mixed in it. Sometimes it is not so obvious because if the rupture occurs behind your baby near the top of the uterus in a 'hind water leak', a small volume of fluid may trickle out and you may mistake it for a heavy VAGINAL DISCHARGE or urinary leakage. Amniotic fluid is the colour of light urine and watery (unlike discharge) and has a sweet smell, unlike urine.

The most significant risk to your baby is prematurity. The complications relate to his age and become less common after Week 34. The other risk is of infection entering into the uterus, in which case you are more likely to need a caesarean section. Less common complications include UMBILICAL CORD COMPRESSION OR PROLAPSE, or PLACENTAL ABRUPTION.

In a minority of cases the leak may seal and the flow ceases. Amniotic fluid is constantly being formed, mainly by your baby swallowing and urinating. If there is a slow leak the fluid can be replaced and the volume remains normal. If the leak begins before Week 28, the amniotic fluid volume may drop (p.397), putting your baby at risk of premature birth and INTRAUTERINE GROWTH RESTRICTION, and your baby's body may become compressed, particularly before Week 26. Significant fall in fluid volume usually leads to the onset of labour.

Action plan
If you think your membranes have ruptured, at whatever stage of pregnancy, call your doctor or midwife.
- A diagnosis can be made using a speculum to visualise the fluid emerging from your cervix.
- The fluid can be tested with Nitrazine, a dye that changes colour in amniotic fluid, but it is only 90% reliable: seeing the fluid is optimal.
- Your baby's wellbeing will be assessed on an ongoing basis by foetal heart monitoring and by ultrasound scan to check growth, amniotic fluid volume and placental blood flow.

PROM after Week 37
- A swab from the vagina detects infection and can be repeated often until birth. If an infection is detected in the amniotic fluid antibiotic therapy can begin immediately. Prophylactic antibiotics are used in some hospitals but this is less necessary than for PROM earlier in pregnancy.
- Labour may begin spontaneously. It is safe to wait provided there is no sign of infection, your baby is well and amniotic fluid volume remains normal.
- If there is a sign of infection or concern about your baby's health, or you state a preference, labour may be induced using prostaglandin gel or oxytocin (p.497).
- If there is concern about your baby's wellbeing a caesarean section may be the best option.

PROM before Week 37
The medical approach to rupture of the membranes has

changed considerably since techniques to delay labour were introduced. The aim is to avoid infection and premature birth.

- You will be given frequent examinations to check for infection, your baby's heart rate will be monitored and his wellbeing and growth and amniotic fluid volume assessed through ultrasound scan. After the initial assessment it is best to reduce internal vaginal examinations, which may increase the chance of infection.
- Before Week 32 monitoring and treatment may be in hospital and you may need to stay in.
- You may be given antibiotics that help to delay birth and reduce infections. The antibiotics used cover the most common infections STREP B and vaginosis. Further treatment depends on test results. If there are any signs of infection in your uterus, you will be offered intensive antibiotic therapy and advised to deliver your baby early.
- Prolonged rupture may stimulate your baby's lungs to mature and release surfactant, thus reducing BREATHING DIFFICULTIES after birth. Before Week 34 you may be given corticosteroids, to further help your baby's lungs to mature. This is standard procedure prior to premature birth. If your baby is premature, he may need special care after birth (p.536).

LABOUR, SHOULDER DYSTOCIA

See also BIRTH INJURIES; LARGE BABIES

Shoulder dystocia is the failure of the shoulders to pass spontaneously through the pelvis in the 2nd stage of labour. Following birth of the head, the shoulders become wedged at the inlet to the pelvis and the baby is stuck. This happens in 1:200 vaginal births, and is more likely to occur in large babies. Although half of all shoulder dystocia affects babies weighing less than 4 kg (8 lb 12 oz) at birth, the incidence rises as the birth weight increases: at least 1:10 babies weighing more than 4.5 kg (9 lb 15 oz) are affected. Large babies due to maternal DIABETES are at even higher risk, because they have significantly greater shoulder–head ratios.

The risk of shoulder dystocia also relates to maternal size. If you are short or have a small pelvic capacity, the risk is higher. If you have had a previous baby with shoulder dystocia, you are a little more likely to have another. During labour, if the 2nd stage is prolonged or difficult, or your team needs to assist your baby's descent with forceps or ventouse (p.496), this may sometimes indicate that your pelvis is a tight fit for your baby and there is a risk of shoulder dystocia.

What happens
With shoulder dystocia, as your baby descends through the birth canal the front or anterior shoulder remains hooked behind your pubic bone close to your bladder. This stops the shoulders from descending, so once your baby's head has been born, his chin will be pressed against your perineum. This is an emergency requiring specialist midwifery and obstetric skills. After the head has been born, the UMBILICAL CORD may be compressed between your baby's chest and the side of your vagina. This can rapidly lead to FOETAL DISTRESS &

ASPHYXIA. Your birth team needs to act quickly to ensure your baby's body is born because if asphyxia persists for longer than 10 minutes there is a risk of brain damage.

Action plan
If clinical and ultrasound measurements suggest that your baby is over 4.5 kg (9 lb 15 oz), you may plan a CAESAREAN delivery. If shoulder dystocia arises in labour, your team is trained to act quickly. Most instances can be managed without excessive trauma to mother or baby. There are a number of manoeuvres that can reduce the risk of asphyxia and action needs to be swift and careful: inappropriate force to deliver the shoulders may cause birth injuries, such as a broken clavicle or damage to the nerves in the neck.

The midwives may flex your thighs and apply pressure over your lower abdomen to nudge your baby's shoulder through the pelvic brim. This may be sufficient, although during the birth you may get significant vaginal tears. If this is insufficient your obstetrician may advise an episiotomy and she may need to turn your baby's back shoulder by placing her hand into your vagina to ease it around. You will be asked to help by pushing and bearing down. If your knees are flexed, you will be able to summon maximal strength. Forceps or ventouse may have been used earlier for the birth of the head.

After the birth your baby may need resuscitation and will then be examined and observed during the first 24 hours to ensure there are no signs of clavicle or nerve palsy injury (p.405) or asphyxia. Most babies who have had shoulder dystocia recover well with no long-term effects. Cranial osteopathy (p.376) and massage (p.365) may be very useful.

You may find the birth very stressful. Being with your baby will be the beginning of the healing process, although the emotional impact of the experience may not hit home for some time and you may experience post-traumatic stress (p.462).

LABOUR, SLOW PROGRESS

See also Birth: a natural process (p.127)

Every labour is different and there is a wide variation in the overall time between the first sign to the birth of the placenta: it is difficult to build a simple definition of 'normal' labour. Slow progress (**dystocia**), is upsetting for women and for their birth attendants. It may lead to tiredness and a range of emotions. Although most mothers and babies are healthy and well after a long labour, slow progress can indicate things are not going well and prompts midwives and doctors to monitor mother and baby closely, keeping safety as the top priority. Sometimes a helping hand is needed to assist progress.

Labour can be divided into pre-labour and the 3 stages. These are the estimated times for each stage (refering to a first labour): 1st stage: 2–20 hours; 2nd stage: 5 minutes–2 hours; 3rd stage: 5 minutes–1 hour. When labour has begun, progress is slow if you exceed the upper limit of the timings. Second and subsequent labours are usually – but not always – faster.

Your doctor or midwife will probably use a partogram to chart the dilation of your cervix and the descent of your baby's head: progress is defined according to the slope of the line.

Some hospitals intervene if the cervix does not dilate at a defined rate within 4 hours. Others acknowledge that there is a huge difference in each woman's energy and pain threshold and take their lead from the mother, providing the baby is safe. Many women prefer the individual approach.

With foetal heart monitoring your baby's wellbeing can be assessed, and your midwife will observe your strength and energy, your emotional state and the strength of your contractions. If there is any indication that labour needs to be speeded up because it is safer for you or for your baby, your midwife will suggest augmentation (p.497).

Slow progress in the 1st stage

If the 1st stage appears slow, your birth team will assess whether labour is established because the diagnosis of slow progress can only be made during true labour. The medical definition of true labour is regular contractions with a minimum of 3-cm dilation of the cervix. Women who experience a long pre-labour may feel that labour has begun as the cervix is dilating to 3 cm. The latent phase (0–3 cm) usually takes the most time. The more intense active phase rarely takes longer than 6–8 hours. At the end of the active stage you will be in transition before you have the urge to bear down and give birth. Transition may take anything from 5 minutes to 2 hours, it is longer with an epidural anaesthetic.

What happens

There are a number of factors that may prolong the 1st stage. They reflect an intricate mix of emotions and physical changes and the close partnership between you and your baby. Dystocia is more common with elective induction of labour, particularly before term, which is why induction is best done as late as possible. Possible causes include:

You may be tired: This may occur if you have had a long pre-labour (latent phase), poor sleep and have not eaten and your contractions may be less powerful.

You may be anxious and become tense: This could hinder the release of oxytocin and endorphin hormones – your uterine muscle works best when you feel relaxed.

The birth environment: The right environment can encourage your body to release labour hormones and help you relax.

Mobility and water: These may each reduce your pain and assist progress. The birth pool is best used after 6-cm dilation because immersion earlier may slow contractions. Upright positions (p.97) have many advantages including improving the action of the uterus and reducing pain.

Slow activity of the uterus (hypotonic labour): This involves infrequent contractions accompanied by progressive dilation of the cervix. This is also called low-intensity labour and there is time to rest between contractions. With patience this is relatively easy to handle because you can keep yourself nourished and energised. If labour has been progressing well and uterine activity slows in the active phase (known as secondary arrest), it may indicate that your baby's position or size does not fit your pelvis optimally.

Unco-ordinated uterine activity: This involves strong and painful contractions but slow dilation as there is not good co-ordination between the upper half of the uterus, pulling upwards, and the lower half, stretching as the cervix dilates. It

may be due to your baby's size or position, or may occur if your cervix is not ripe when contractions begin or after induction.

The position and size of your baby: These may make birth difficult, either because of malpresentation (p.498) or a poor fit between his size and your pelvis (p.493). In both cases, contractions may become unco-ordinated or hypotonic.

Action plan

Some women choose to augment labour because they feel too tired to let the 1st stage continue; others are able to rest and sleep intermittently and keep up their energy. When the 1st stage is very long, the risk of FOETAL DISTRESS rises.

Medical assessment

Your midwife will do a full abdominal and vaginal assessment to establish whether your cervix has dilated and with ongoing examinations will know whether dilation is progressing. She will also check the position, size and descent of your baby, the quality and tone of your contractions and the size of your pelvis and note whether the membranes have ruptured. Your birth team will discuss what might be causing the slow progress and you will be involved in the plan of action.

If your midwife decides you are having a long latent phase and false labour – contractions without progressive dilation of the cervix – you may be encouraged to go and rest in the comfort of your home until you enter the active phase of labour. If you have been having days of discomfort you and the team may decide that induction is a good option.

Self-help

The advice for keeping yourself energised in labour (p.156) may help if the 1st stage is prolonged. Steps include eating nutritious snacks and drinking well, making your environment comfortable, using movement and breathing. Your partner or another supporter can help you. If you have moved from your home to the hospital, or from the ward to the labour suite, your contractions may pick up again once you feel settled.

Pain relief

You may want stronger pain relief (p.158) and, if this helps, your energy may rise and assist labour progress. An epidural anaesthetic might also relax your pelvic floor muscles and aid the descent of your baby. A low-dose epidural is preferable as a dense block can delay progress and increase the need for oxytocin and operative intervention. The epidural may wear off so you can summon power to push in the 2nd stage.

Homeopathy

In combination with movement and breathing techniques, and with medical augmentation if this has been recommended, homeopathy can be very powerful in labour. The remedies on pp.162–3 may encourage good progress.

Medical augmentation of labour

If labour has started but is progressing slowly, your midwife may suggest augmentation (p.497) through artificial rupture of the membranes, which is often useful if contractions are slow and hypotonic or unco-ordinated. Your baby's heart rate will be monitored for decelerations after the amniotic fluid is released. Sometimes rupturing the membranes gives labour a sufficient boost. Your doctor may also suggest administering oxytocin (Syntocinon) through intravenous drip. Oxytocin is often effective for hypotonic labour and may also help to co-ordinate uterine contractions, although in a small number of women the uterus is overly sensitive and co-ordination does not improve. If your baby is in a slightly awkward position oxytocin may boost your contractions enough to help him negotiate the birth canal in readiness for the birth. It may also encourage a baby in an occipito posterior position (p.499) to turn and move down. With a drip in place you may receive intravenous fluids if you are dehydrated to improve your energy levels.

In most hospitals oxytocin is begun slowly and the rate is gradually increased using a pump while the baby's heartbeat and uterine contractions are continuously monitored. A possible complication is hyperstimulation of the uterus, giving excessive contractions that may reduce the flow of blood in the placenta and lead to foetal distress. The rate of oxytocin flow can be safely controlled or stopped if necessary, and oxytocin will not be given if there are any signs of foetal distress. It is used cautiously after a previous caesarean.

Caesarean section
If, in spite of using oxytocin, the rate of dilation of your cervix does not improve, or if your baby appears to be distressed, a CAESAREAN SECTION may be the best option. One of the most common indications for caesarean is failure to progress in the 1st stage of labour. If your birth team believes that malpresentation or disproportion makes it unlikely that your baby will be born safely this is also an indication for a caesarean section.

Slow progress in the 2nd stage
The 2nd stage of labour runs from full dilation until your baby is born. Although this stage can last as little as 5 minutes, many hospitals regard 120 minutes as acceptable for a 1st birth and up to 90 minutes for subsequent births. Your medical team will revise their expectations if you or your baby become distressed. If you have had an epidural, the 2nd stage might be longer.

What happens
Some women enjoy this stage and have a boost of confidence and are pleased to be active and bear down to give birth. Others feel afraid and exhausted, or nervous about opening their bowels in public (midwives and obstetricians welcome this as a sign that the baby is about to be born). Factors that may contribute to slow progress in this stage are similar to those affecting the 1st stage.

Pain relief and weak pushing reflex: If you have had a large dose of pain-relieving opiates or a dense epidural anaesthetic, you may find that the reflex to push is not strong. Many women feel more capable of pushing once the effects have worn off. It is safe to wait for this provided your baby's heartbeat is normal.

Slow uterine activity: If you are having a hypotonic, low-intensity labour, the contractions may be infrequent and lack

power. This may be compounded if your baby has a malpresentation or there is disproportion and a tight fit through your pelvis.

Low energy: If the early stages have been very long and you are tired and dehydrated, the 2nd stage may be prolonged.

Action plan
Your midwife will continue to monitor progress of labour and your baby's condition. If there is no cause for concern, with encouragement and support you may find the energy and stamina to continue and to take a few practical steps to help this stage progress.

What you can do
- If your baby is healthy it is best to delay pushing until the head descends and presses on your pelvic floor and you have the urge to bear down.
- If you can get into an upright position, either on the bed or in a supported squat, this may help considerably. If you are in pain it may be hard to change position and you will need to rely on your supporters, who can also guide your breathing. Draw on your antenatal preparations and try to relax your pelvic floor while bearing down.
- Being in water may prolong the 2nd stage and it may be best to be upright on land for maximum pushing power.
- The people with you may be able to help by gently massaging you or putting slightly firmer pressure on your lower back – they will follow your directions. If you are nervous or upset, their support might help enormously.
- Homeopathic remedies (p.162) can help shift your mood, reduce your fears and help increase your urge to push.
- In the 2nd stage the force of birth and the accompanying adrenalin may trigger the urge to moan or scream. Being expressive may help you to go with the flow of your labour. Some women find it is better to be quieter and direct their energy downwards: your midwife will guide you.

Medical assistance
Some mothers feel absolutely exhausted and certain that they cannot go on. If your labour has been very prolonged, you may need an intravenous drip to provide fluids and minerals to boost your energy.

Pain relief: It is often best to let an epidural wear off because this inhibits pushing power.

Augmentation: If your contractions lack power an oxytocin infusion may help, but this will not be an option if your midwife believes your baby is too LARGE to pass through your pelvis.

Assistance with forceps, ventouse and caesarean: If your baby's head is deeply engaged in your pelvis but there is no advance after you have been pushing and you are very tired your obstetrician may decide your baby needs help from forceps or ventouse (p.496). Once the instrument is in place your baby will be born with two or three contractions. If your baby's head is not deeply engaged in the pelvis, your obstetrician may advise caesarean section. The decision may also be taken if there are signs of foetal distress or of disproportion or malpresentation, which could put your baby under too much pressure.

Slow progress in the 3rd stage

The 3rd stage of labour begins after the birth of your baby and ends when the placenta is born. In the majority of births this is a joyous time when the baby is welcomed, and the placenta is born without complications, usually within 5–30 minutes. It is prolonged if it lasts longer than 60 minutes.

In many hospitals women are routinely given an injection of oxytocin (Syntocinon) on its own or combined with ergometrine (Syntometrine) very soon after the baby is born, and this speeds up the separation of the placenta. This 'active management of the 3rd stage' is considered to reduce the risk of excessive bleeding (p.406) as the placenta separates and does speed up the 3rd stage. If left to follow its natural progress, the 3rd stage may take up to 1 hour. Your contractions may be encouraged if you breastfeed, because this stimulates oxytocin release. Resting in a supported sitting position will also help because gravity will be in your favour. Some midwives gently massage the uterus to encourage separation.

If Syntocinon or Syntometrine is injected, your midwife will be under time pressure to deliver the placenta within 5–15 minutes before the muscle of the uterus clamps down and traps it. She will apply a gentle pulling force on the umbilical cord to help the placenta to separate. This carries a slight risk that fragments of the placenta will not separate from the uterine wall and need to be surgically removed (p.407).

Action plan

If the 3rd stage is left to progress naturally but continues for more than 1 hour, it is likely you will be given an injection of Syntocinon or Syntometrine to stimulate uterine contractions and the placenta will be born within roughly 10 minutes. If you have been given an oxytocin injection but there is delay and if the umbilical cord tears while the midwife applies gentle traction, you then have a retained placenta. If this happens, the obstetrician will have to perform a manual removal under an epidural or general anaesthetic. This is covered in the section on medical care on p.407. The main risk associated with a prolonged 3rd stage of labour is excessive bleeding.

Most labours are not prolonged and with modern care the long ones are dealt with safely. Most women are pleased to be helped if they feel there has been sufficient time given for the labour to progress and the intervention was for safety.

LARGE BABIES

Your baby's birth weight can never be known accurately before birth, but during antenatal tests your midwife, obstetrician or ultrasonographer may suspect that he is larger than usual for the stage of pregnancy. A large baby (macrocosmic) generally weighs more than 4 kg (8 lb 12 oz) at birth. Some 10% of babies fall within this weight range and 2% weigh more than 4.5 kg (9 lb 15 oz).

Not all large babies have difficulty during birth but there is an increased risk of difficulty passing through the pelvic cavity (p.493); BIRTH INJURIES and shoulder dystocia (p.502), where there is difficulty delivering the shoulders. A mother is also at

risk of 3rd- and 4th-degree vaginal tears (p.494). If you know your baby is very large a vaginal birth will be closely monitored, or a CAESAREAN SECTION may be recommended.

What happens

Birth weight often relates to a mother's size and body build, and her own weight at birth. Size also relates to ethnicity. While one-third of large babies are born to mothers with no apparent risk factors, there are some factors that may contribute to a large birth weight. These include: maternal DIABETES; a previous pregnancy with a large baby; high weight before pregnancy; excessive weight gain in pregnancy; and pregnancy lasting more than 42 weeks (p.500).

Action plan

During antenatal checks your baby's size will be assessed by the feel of your abdomen and with ultrasound scans, both of which allow size, as well as amniotic fluid volume, to be calculated. Neither, however, is very accurate: feeling the abdomen gives an average error of around 330 g (11½ oz) and is more difficult if you are overweight or tall; ultrasound scans carry a similar margin of error, although accuracy is increasing with more sophisticated measuring techniques.

Controlling your diabetes, and blood sugar and keeping to a nutritious diet (p.332) is a sensible preventative measure to avoid excess weight gain. Avoiding fast-burning foods is important, as regular consumption of these has the same effect on a baby's growth as diabetes.

Birth

In general suspected high birth weight alone is not sufficient to prompt an elective caesarean section. If your baby's weight is estimated to be above 4 kg (8 lb 12 oz) but below 5 kg (11 lb), you may be encouraged to give birth vaginally, depending on hospital policy. If your baby might weigh more than 5 kg (11 lb) a caesarean is probably the safest option. The decision will also rest on your experience in any previous births, and your own stature – if you are small the risks of complications during birth increase. After Week 37 a baby's weight gain usually slows but inducing labour before or near term has not been shown to prevent the complications associated with large babies, or reduce the caesarean section rate. If you go ahead with a vaginal delivery you will be monitored closely. It is worth familiarising yourself with upright positions (p.152) because these will assist your baby's descent.

- If the 1st stage is prolonged and you are given oxytocin, this needs to be controlled. If your baby appears to be having difficulty descending through your pelvis, a caesarean section is safer than a difficult forceps or ventouse delivery.
- If you have previously had a caesarean section and this labour is prolonged, another caesarean may be advised.
- If you have already given birth vaginally but the birth was complicated by shoulder dystocia (p.502), your team will consider whether your current baby appears to be smaller: if so, the problem is unlikely to recur. But if your baby is as big or labour is prolonged, a caesarean may be the safest option.

Large babies who have had an uncomplicated birth are usually robust and adapt well to being born and usually feed well and gain weight normally. Some may behave like diabetic babies and need to be checked for HYPOGLYCAEMIA and BREATHING DIFFICULTIES. The size and weight of your baby in adulthood depends more on his genetic mix than on the birth weight.

LEGS & ARMS

See also FEET & HANDS

Bow legs

A baby is said to be bow-legged if the knees do not touch when the ankles are pressed together. This is quite normal for the first 2 years – almost all children have bow legs when they first learn to walk and gradually lose the tendency. If you are concerned the gap between your baby's knees is pronounced, or the 'bow' effect only appears in one leg, check with your doctor or health visitor. If your baby's legs are bowed once he has started walking, massage (p.368) and cranial osteopathy (p.376) can speed up the straightening process and he may be given special boots or splints to wear at night.

Knees or elbows that click

If you feel your baby's knees or elbows clicking, don't worry – this is very common and is due to the loose ligaments sliding over the bones. Over the next 6 months his ligaments will firm up and the tendency to click will pass. Sometimes a click persists but is of no consequence and can be safely ignored.

Knock knees & in-toeing

When your baby starts to stand or walk, his knees may meet and knock together and his ankles may seem far apart. Knock knees (femoral anteversion) is outgrown except in very rare cases when they simply become part of a child's life.

In-toeing is commonly caused by a twist in the shinbones (tibial torsion), which corrects itself as walking helps the bones straighten along the line of stress bearing. In-toeing may also be caused by a twist in the thighbone or femur (femoral torsion). The feet bones remain straight, but the softer ligaments mould more easily and cause the feet to curve inwards. This is usually nothing to worry about – if the feet straighten when you gently hold them in a forward-facing position, you can be confident they will straighten up over time. If they feel stiff or you are concerned, physiotherapy and foot-stretching exercises may help to loosen them and assist the natural process of straightening. One in 3000 babies need specialist orthopaedic care to speed up the straightening.

LISTERIA

Listeria is a food-borne bacteria that uncommonly causes infection, which is usually fought off by the body's natural defence system without symptoms. If it does cause illness, symptoms include TIREDNESS, DIARRHOEA, NAUSEA & VOMITING, FEVER and flu-like feelings. Very rarely, the illness may be more serious, with septicaemia, MENINGITIS or pneumonia. During pregnancy women have a lower resistance to the bacteria. Infection in pregnancy is very rare but carries a small risk to your baby and may lead to late MISCARRIAGE or stillbirth (p.519). An infected baby may remain perfectly well but could show effects ranging from conjunctivitis to neonatal pneumonia.

Action plan
Prevention
Listeria monocytogenes is found in soil and water and may travel into your digestive system if you eat unwashed vegetables, raw or undercooked meats or unpasteurised dairy products. All pregnant women are advised to avoid soft cheeses such as feta, Brie, Camembert and blue-veined cheese, undercooked eggs or pâté and not to eat leftover or ready-to-eat foods without thoroughly reheating them. Hard, processed, cream and cottage cheeses or yoghurt made from pasteurised milk need not be avoided. Discard any uneaten food that has been left out of a refrigerator for 2 hours or more.

Treatment
- Listeria is not routinely tested for in pregnancy and the infection is difficult to diagnose.
- If you contract listeria, you will need antibiotics in high dosage, usually a combination including ampicillin or penicillin. If treatment begins soon enough, it can prevent your unborn baby from becoming infected.
- You can safely breastfeed without passing on the infection.
- If your baby is infected after birth he can also be given antibiotics.

LOSS OF A BABY

Losing a baby, at any stage of pregnancy, at or after birth, is one of the most devastating and traumatic experiences in any person's life. During pregnancy both parents expect new life and are eager to welcome their child. The same happens during labour – the expectation is that at the end of all the hard work there will be a beautiful baby to greet. When things do not go as planned, this hope of new life is taken away.

Fortunately, it is the minority of pregnancies that do not result in the birth of a live baby, and death during or soon after birth is rare, affecting 3–6:1000. MISCARRIAGE is the most common cause of loss in pregnancy and it is most likely to happen early but may occur up to Week 20. If a baby dies in the womb between Week 20 and birth, this is defined as a stillbirth (p.519) – the baby will not be born alive. Death within 4 weeks of birth is a neonatal death (p.510); later than that it is an infant death. Sudden infant death syndrome (p.510) was previously referred to as a cot death and affects 1:1600 babies.

What happens
The reaction to losing a baby is individual. You will have your own feelings and act these out in your own unique way. You and your partner may be surprised that you respond very differently to your loss. One of you may cry more than the other, one may be quiet and feel cut off, some days one of you may be angry, and there may be a difference in how intimate you wish to be with one another. You are both deeply hurting

and are each overwhelmed by your own feelings and questions. It is important to recognise that what you are going through is a period of grieving. You may feel shock, anger, disbelief, despair, guilt, confusion and a need to lay blame. These powerful and traumatic feelings can linger for a long time and fluctuate in intensity.

The loss of a baby can sometimes be anticipated if a problem has been diagnosed. Knowing that you may lose your baby does not reduce the impact of your actual loss, but gives some time and space to begin to gather a team of loving support. If your baby was unwell at birth, you may have spent time in a SPECIAL CARE BABY UNIT. You may have felt helpless, angry and frightened, and will need a lot of support as you move on to the next stage and begin to grieve for your lost baby and a lost future. Accepting the reality and grieving are often made more difficult if a cause for death cannot be found or the death is sudden, or if there has been a miscarriage and the baby felt part of you but you may not have seen him.

In many ways, living with loss follows a pattern similar to that related to receiving bad news, as you feel shocked by what has happened, react to the reality, adapt your life accordingly and begin to find ways to orientate yourself. Facing the true loss of a baby is shocking and many parents feel completely numb.

Fortunately, most hospitals offer support and counselling to help parents begin a process of grieving and acceptance, but the need for support continues, perhaps for years. Less fortunately, some women and men do not feel they received sympathetic care and are deeply scarred not only by their grief, but also by the physical procedures. This may be the case during examinations at a miscarriage, if a baby has died in the womb and birth is induced, or if a baby is extremely unwell at birth and is taken away quickly before the mother and father have had a chance to greet him.

Grieving
While everybody is different, grief brings on a number of common symptoms: crying, feelings of intense loneliness and isolation, the need to talk about it, anger, guilt, an urge to allocate blame, anxiety, insomnia, a lost appetite or compulsive overeating or taking DRUGS or ALCOHOL. You may find it hard to concentrate or to remember events and facts and lose sight of your goals and all hope or enthusiasm for the future. Physically, you may feel tense, achy or breathless and there may be secondary symptoms, such as digestive problems.

Grieving, mourning and healing are each long processes and you will have ups and downs. It is common to have thoughts that are painful and may not have answers, such as: 'Why did this happen to my baby?', 'Why did it happen to us? To me? To our family?', 'Why didn't I do something better to stop this from happening?', 'Could I have acted sooner?', 'Why didn't the medical team stop it from happening?' 'If only . . .'

Whatever circumstances have led to the loss, you will need to be supported as you take the reality on board and tend to practical details. You may find support among your family and friends, your medical team, other parents who have had similar experiences, and/or local or national help groups. It may be some time before you find the right person to talk to about your experience. Don't forget the team who cared for

you. Talking may enable you to voice your experience and come to terms with the fact that it is real. Some people find writing things down helps. Over time when troubling thoughts quieten you may find it easier to move on.

What you may do
Most parents have a powerful need to say goodbye. Some choose to be with their baby for a couple of hours or days, and hospitals often have a space where this is possible. The contact and quiet time together can be a crucial part of the grieving process. Although it is very painful to see your baby, this short time is precious and can provide a chance for you and your partner to welcome your baby, bid him farewell, and share your feelings with each other. You may also take this opportunity to name your baby and you might take away comforting memories of seeing, holding, loving and caring for him. Many parents choose to have a photograph or keep a footprint or a lock of hair. Some people find these keepsakes too emotive and choose instead to keep some blankets or a nursery toy, hospital records, sympathy cards and perhaps scan pictures or photographs taken during pregnancy.

Practicalities
If your baby's death was unexpected, your doctors may ask you to consider allowing a post-mortem examination to be carried out on your baby. They cannot do this without your permission except with a sudden infant death. The tests cannot be guaranteed to identify a cause. You may want to talk to your midwife, obstetrician or a genetic counsellor about the pros and cons of testing. If you are considering another pregnancy, it might be helpful to know whether any future babies may be at risk. You may find it easier to make up your mind if you can talk to a number of people in the medical team as well as your family or friends.

Parents who have lost a baby after Week 20 are given a medical certificate of stillbirth or death. This needs to be taken to a registrar before a certificate of burial or cremation can be issued. Some hospitals undertake burial or cremation on parents' behalf. Alternatively, you may make your own arrangements. Some parents find that organising the ceremony helps them feel more involved in their baby's short life, while others prefer not to face this. In the event of a late miscarriage, having a funeral or cremation may be an important way of saying goodbye. Some people find actions and ritual help the mourning, while others put all their energy into the practicalities and only feel the intensity of their grief when things are quieter. Some delay a memorial service until later.

Other aspects of life
After the shock and sadness of losing a baby, many parents feel desolate and, even with love and support, are prone to depression (p.462). Consider asking your friends and family to care for you in a practical way, to ensure you eat well and rest in the early days and get out of the house, perhaps exercising, regularly. Remember that you will need to take care of yourself as your body adapts and heals after pregnancy and birth. You may need to put major plans, such as moving house or changing jobs, on hold, and your network of friends and supporters can help with the practicalities.

Often people are unsure about what to say or how to act. You might come across a number of 'stock' phrases that may seem like platitudes but are, probably, uttered because those who love you are trying to say something that might lessen your pain. For instance: 'Don't worry, you will have more children', 'You were lucky that it was so early in pregnancy', 'It is a good thing you never brought your baby home from hospital', 'At least you are fit and well.' Let those who are close to you know how important your baby was and is to you. Sometimes it may help to ask them simply to listen. It may be up to you to keep in contact. This is often worthwhile – with your encouragement others may soon feel more comfortable listening to you and feel better about sharing their own grief, and about sharing joy and laughter as well. Letting them know just what they can do to help you and being honest about the way you feel may reduce their feelings of helplessness.

As the days and weeks pass – some more easily than others – you will continue to benefit from support. You may meet other parents who have been similarly affected through your hospital or a support group. They may make good listeners and could become close friends; they may also help you to believe that your pain will soften over time.

Depression and anxiety

Feeling depressed and anxious is very common after losing a baby and is a natural part of bereavement, and may be severe if you are already prone. As time passes you will notice the feelings lift but this may take many months. Consider reading the advice in EMOTIONS, ADVICE & SUPPORT. It deals with practical issues and complementary, medical and lifestyle advice.

Your partnership

It is common for couples to come together in a time of loss and crisis, but it is also fairly common for anger and frustration to affect the partnership and some underlying relationship problems to surface at this time of vulnerability. Sometimes mothers and fathers blame one another for the event, or for everything else that seems wrong. It is common for the mother to be blamed as if it was her fault and she let the baby down. It can be helpful to know that people may react in this way.

If your relationship is feeling the shock waves, try to acknowledge the difficulties and, with appropriate support, listen to one another and work through areas of conflict. This may help to save your partnership. The advice on p.290 aims to support you. Taking it step by step may be useful while you are both physically, mentally and emotionally exhausted. What you communicate verbally presents just a small part of what you truly feel, and taking space and time to acknowledge each other's moods and unspoken concerns can be an important aspect of your healing and the strength of your partnership. Intimacy can also create conflict, as one partner needs closeness, or reassurance that some of life remains the same, while another cannot think about sex in the light of what has happened. Sex can be a particularly difficult subject (p.285).

There is no set timetable for recovery, no goals that you 'should' reach, either together or separately. You cannot change what has happened, yet you can move forwards without belittling your feelings or the life that you lost. Your relationship may be uncomfortable for some time – this does not mean that it will always be uncomfortable.

Breastfeeding and lactation

If you have lost your baby in late pregnancy or after birth, your breasts may produce or continue to produce milk. This might be extremely upsetting and it is best to take practical steps to reduce and stop the flow (p.189) and ease discomfort from a build-up of milk.

Surviving siblings

If you have other children they will feel the impact of the loss, even if there has been an early miscarriage. When you are with your other child(ren) give them space to express their feelings, and bear in mind that they may do this more through actions than words. Even so, the words of young children can be powerfully direct and honest, and even a 2- or 3-year-old can express himself. If your child talks about the death, let him continue and give your full attention to him while he does. If he does not express his reaction through words, you may decide to encourage him to tell you. Many bereavement organisations have support groups and reading material especially for children and there are groups for children who have experienced the death of a brother or sister.

Anniversaries

You may find your feelings come back with force on anniversaries of the loss, of conception or of your baby's birth or due date. These dates may remain embedded in your mind. You may like to do something special on the given day and acknowledge how you feel now and how you felt at the time. Even 5 minutes of quiet time can be useful.

Looking ahead to another baby

The decision to have or not have another baby belongs to you and your partner. There is no 'appropriate' waiting period. No matter what decision you make regarding a subsequent pregnancy or adoption, it will probably not change the length of your grief for your baby who died, and conceiving again is not a quick-fix way to fill the gap in your life.

Although most parents who lose a baby are unlikely to lose another, you may want to talk to a genetic counsellor about the possible causes. In another pregnancy it is also important to remember that you may be more emotionally stressed. Grieving takes a lot of energy and enjoying pregnancy while you are still mourning may be challenging. Your support network will be extremely important: this begins with your partner and includes the medical team. You will be helping yourself if you ask as many questions as you need to regarding the safety of your pregnancy and the wellbeing of your baby and request extra antenatal testing. Hearing your baby's heartbeat or seeing the ultrasound scan will be reassuring and if you are informed you may be likely to act appropriately if there are signs that could be a cause for concern.

You may choose to involve people who can help you balance your life and work towards optimum health with exercise, a good diet and enjoyable activities, which could help you to be positive as well as realistic about your pregnancy. There are also organisations (e.g. the Stillbirth and Neonatal

Death Society: SANDS) that offer support for women who are expecting a baby after a loss. Success stories are often encouraging. Other women who have made it through a subsequent pregnancy are living proof that it is possible to give birth to a healthy baby after a traumatic loss.

Homeopathy for loss/grief

Any mourning process can be complex, confusing and full of many possible emotions. The list is unique to each individual. The remedies suggested below can in no way suppress or eradicate grief, but they can support you and allow your grief process to unfold so you can deal with your loss in a manner that is appropriate for you.

In the early stages: Take a high potency (200c), 3 times a day. *Aconite* is useful in the first instance when the loss is unexpected and you are deeply shocked or afraid; *Ignatia* is good in the early days when your emotions are all over the place and often contradictory (laughing/crying, shaking/still) yet you are often on the verge of tears; *Arsenicum* helps if you are acutely agitated and hyped up, which may lead to insomnia, and you are frightened by loss of control – DIARRHOEA is common with this remedy picture; *Pulsatilla* suits grief with long bouts of weepiness and a need to be consoled and supported with loving company.

After 4–5 days: Use 200c twice a day for a week, and then reassess. *Natrum Mur* helps if your grief is stopping you from moving on, you feel hurt to the core yet bottle up your feelings and do not want to break down in public and may develop physical complaints and become deeply depressed; *Aurum Metallicum* is helpful for grief with a deep, black despair, a sense of hopelessness, self-blame and a feeling you have failed, leading to severe depression; *Staphysagria* is often needed in the established phase of grief where emotion has been suppressed or after a succession of losses that have never been dealt with and you feel anger and resentment towards the person who has died and towards yourself for being in some way to blame; *Sepia* suits grief characterised by emotional apathy, withdrawal and indifference even to your closest friends, with strong mood changes, irritability and extreme fatigue, often leading to depression.

LOSS OF A BABY, STILLBIRTH

See also LOSS OF A BABY; MISCARRIAGE

Stillbirth is a devastating loss, yet it is rare. In the UK approximately 6:1000 babies die before birth. A stillbirth follows the death of a baby in the womb after Week 20. Sometimes loss can be anticipated but 50% of stillbirths happen without warning. Most occur before labour. The minority (14%) become apparent in labour. The loss can be extremely difficult to accept, and the process of coming to terms with the reality may be long. Over the past 20 years stillbirths have declined by nearly 50%. This is largely due to better attention to nutrition, monitoring in pregnancy and improved diagnosis and treatment of maternal conditions including high BLOOD PRESSURE, DIABETES, CHOLESTASIS, rhesus disease (p.410), and DRUG avoidance.

The cause of stillbirth is not always known. Where a cause is found it is most commonly due to developmental problems linked with CONGENITAL ABNORMALITIES, and these are often detected by a 2nd trimester ultrasound scan. Sometimes a stillbirth follows late elective termination when a diagnosis of a debilitating condition is made after Week 20. The chance of a stillbirth is increased in HIGH-RISK PREGNANCIES, particularly when there is severe INTRAUTERINE GROWTH RESTRICTION. Occasionally the death of a baby in pregnancy may be caused by a PLACENTAL ABRUPTION. With modern monitors, stillbirth in labour is increasingly unlikely (about 1:1000).

What happens

The first sign of death is usually an absence of foetal movements. A healthy baby can be expected to move at least 10 times a day either as a single run of ten kicks or spaced out. During labour the absence of the baby's heartbeat is the diagnostic sign.

Action plan

If you notice a change in your baby's kicking pattern and have felt fewer than ten movements in 24 hours, contact your midwife or doctor. You will be assessed with an electronic monitor to listen to your baby's heartbeat, which can be confirmed using an ultrasound scan. In most instances decreased movement turns out to be insignificant but it can be an indication of a problem. In rare cases heartbeat is absent and the baby is no longer alive. If you are told this tragic news, your emotions may range from total shock and numbness to extreme anger or tearful hysteria. Your midwife will be there with you and a doctor will confirm the diagnosis.

Most hospitals now have counselling facilities so you may be offered help and support as you face giving birth to your baby who is no longer alive. You and your partner will need to decide whether you wish labour to be induced or come on spontaneously. As long as your health is not in danger, you can take a day or two to come to terms with the enormity of what has happened before you make your decision.

Most couples choose to have labour induced in hospital. Some opt for immediate induction and a minority prefer labour to begin spontaneously. If labour has not begun after 7 days, induction is recommended because there is a small risk of bleeding from a clotting abnormality that can develop after this time. You may wish to have your baby by CAESAREAN SECTION but because the recovery process is longer and there are more risks involved, you will probably be advised to give birth vaginally.

Labour

Talk to the midwife or another member of the medical team about your hospital's protocol. You may meet the doctor(s) who will care for you. Induction of labour is often handled with careful sensitivity and it is helpful to know in advance what level of support you are likely to receive and what pain relief is available. Another couple who have had a similar experience in your hospital may be able to give you valuable advice. You may choose to have a close friend or family member with you so you receive emotional and physical support.

Early induction of labour may be a slow process because your cervix may not be ripe. Some couples find the waiting period gives the first real chance to begin grieving. Induction (p.497) begins by inserting into your vagina a gel containing prostaglandin that helps to ripen the cervix. This may be followed by an intravenous oxytocin infusion. Labour then follows the usual progress at full term and may be very long and very painful. With the knowledge that your baby will not be alive, your energy may be low and you will need lots of support from your medical team and birth partner. Some women choose to avoid pain relief altogether, which can be a useful part of the grieving process. Others choose to have an epidural.

Stillbirth in labour
If FOETAL DISTRESS & ASPHYXIA occurs in labour, in most instances a baby is delivered safely. If intense asphyxia leads to a stillbirth, it comes as a great shock. You will not be forewarned and you and your partner will have to greet and say goodbye to your baby at a time when your hormones and hopes are geared to welcoming. This is a confusing nightmare for both of you.

After the birth
Most hospitals have bereavement rooms where the parents can remain with their baby after the birth. This time together is an excruciatingly painful yet constructive part of the grieving and healing process. If your doctor advises that tests or a post-mortem be carried out on your baby and you agree, it may be some time before you can lay your baby to rest. The long-term process of healing and recovery, plus the practicalities involved when a baby is lost, are covered from p.506.

LOSS OF A BABY, SUDDEN INFANT DEATH SYNDROME (SIDS) & NEONATAL DEATH

See also LOSS OF A BABY

SIDS is the term given to unexpected death after the 4th week. The UK rate is around 1:1600. This is three times less common than ten years ago, partly due to education and awareness of reducing the risks by attention to health in pregnancy and with care after birth. If you are worried you may lose your baby, you might be reassured by these figures. You share your fear with almost all parents.

There is no single cause for unexpected infant death, although after investigation a cause can be found for around 2:3 cases. SIDS is more common among PREMATURE babies (affecting 10:1000), among TWINS AND HIGHER MULTIPLES, babies who had severely restricted growth in the womb (p.488), and among boys. Not all deaths happen at night or in bed, which is one reason why the term 'cot death' has been replaced.

Preventative measures begin in pregnancy by looking after yourself and avoiding SMOKING, and continue in the way you care for your baby, with particular attention to his temperature and 'feet-to-foot' sleeping position (p.203). You may also be

less anxious if you learn the basics of resuscitation (p.383). Your GP or health visitor can direct you to a class.

Action plan
In the unlikely and traumatic event of unexpected death you will find your baby not breathing and lifeless. You and your partner will need a great deal of loving support from your friends and family. Your hospital may wish to conduct x-rays and post-mortem tests. Permission is not required by the coroner. A coroner's officer looks into unexpected deaths and you may be visited by a police officer. Although officers aim to be sensitive, you may feel under suspicion. These practical arrangements may seem like an invasion and an insult at a time of such sadness. Your GP, midwife or health visitor might be an important member of your supportive team.

Neonatal death
Neonatal death is the term given to death within 4 weeks of birth. During this 4-week period, 3–4:1000 babies die, most commonly within the 1st week. Around 25% of neonatal deaths occur because babies have severe genetic or chromosomal abnormalities (p.433) or developmental problems, most commonly affecting the heart. Usually when this is the case pregnancy ends in an early MISCARRIAGE, but some pregnancies continue to full term. Sometimes a problem is detected antenatally and parents can prepare in some ways for the short time they will have with their babies. Often, however, parents anticipate the birth of a healthy baby and are shocked when their baby is born very ill and is not expected to survive. Early death is also associated with very early premature birth. Rarely, death follows infection in pregnancy or FOETAL DISTRESS & ASPHYXIA during labour.

If your baby is born very prematurely or is very sick, he may be rushed into intensive care or the SPECIAL CARE BABY UNIT. If he needs to be transferred to another hospital it may be extremely traumatic for you and your partner to be separated from him. Soon after the initial shock, you may find yourself watching your baby fight for life in an unfamiliar setting that may feel intimidating. It is common to feel helpless, frightened, angry and emotionally overwhelmed and you will need a great deal of support from your family, friends and medical team. Even if your baby survives for only a short time, being with him and being involved in his care in whatever way is possible may make you feel you have helped, and provide you with memories for the difficult times ahead.

Your consent must be obtained for further examination or investigation to discover the cause of death, unless the death has been reported to a coroner. If the doctors looking after your baby cannot give a cause of death the case will be referred to the coroner. It is likely that you will be offered follow-up support and told about the investigation results. Some parents find it easier to say goodbye if a cause has been discovered. Knowing a possible cause and discussing any chance of recurrence with a genetic counsellor is helpful if planning future pregnancies.

LOW MILK FLOW
See BREAST, LOW MILK FLOW

MALPRESENTATION
See LABOUR, MALPOSITION & MALPRESENTATION

MASTITIS
See BREAST, BLOCKED DUCTS, MASTITIS & ABSCESSES

MEASLES

Measles is very unusual under 1 year of age, due to the presence of maternal antibodies in 95% of babies, and not common after this age due to VACCINATION. A child with measles is usually unwell for 8–14 days, often with a COUGH OR COLD, FEVER and EYE INFECTION. A dull red and slightly raised rash starts behind the ears. It is usually associated with EAR INFECTION and lasts 5–7 days before clearing up. There may also be a rash inside the cheeks. The illness is infectious from 2 days before the rash appears until 4 days after it has appeared. Measles infection is often confused with RUBELLA, the pink rash ROSEOLA INFANTUM OR PARVOVIRUS.

Measles infection can have serious complications, including pneumonia (p.441), deafness and encephalitis if the brain becomes inflamed. Extremely rarely, there may be progressive loss of brain function, years after the initial infection.

Action plan
If you require confirmation, your baby can be tested for antibodies using a sample of saliva or blood.
- Treat the fever with infant paracetamol or ibuprofen in appropriate doses. If the fever does not fall, or rises again after falling, call your doctor.
- Keep her comfortable and encourage her to drink plenty of fluid. She may be soothed by soaks in a warm bath.
- If a chest infection ensues, your doctor may prescribe antibiotics.
- Your homeopath may prescribe a suitable remedy.

MENINGITIS

Meningitis is infection of the meninges, the membranes that line the brain. It is a very rare disease in babies under 9 months, although for the small number affected, there may be complications. Usually meningitis is viral and is not serious. But because the illness can develop suddenly and there is a small risk of a serious infection, it is helpful to be aware of the symptoms that denote an emergency.

What happens
When the meninges are infected, the virus or bacteria cause inflammation with swelling of the membranes and an increase in the volume of cerebrospinal fluid that surrounds and protects the brain. These effects give classic symptoms of FEVER and headache and neck stiffness.
Viral meningitis: May be caused by one of many different viruses. It can be a mild illness, where your baby has a high fever, is off feeds and has a headache. There are no long-term

problems for the vast majority of infected babies. A very small number, however, have a severe illness with long-term effects.
Bacterial meningitis: More rare. In the newborn baby, Group B streptococcal meningitis (p.511) is the usual bacterium involved. Premature babies are at greatest risk and the infection may occur in labour if the mother is a carrier of Strep B.

In babies older than 3 months the three most common bacteria that cause meningitis are: haemophilus influenzae Type B (Hib), which has nearly been wiped out in the UK since the Hib vaccine was introduced in 1992; pneumococcus, for which a vaccine is to be introduced soon; and meningococcus Groups A, B and C. Meningococcus Group B is the most common, but Group C is more severe and can be fatal. About 1500 cases of Group C meningitis are reported in the UK each year. Unfortunately, there is no safe and effective vaccine against Group B, but Group C VACCINATION is effective and is offered to all babies in the first 3 months.

The majority of children with viral illnesses recover from meningitis easily without long-term effects. In some children, particularly with bacterial infection, meningitis may lead to FITS and damage to the brain. This may result in mild to severe learning difficulties, with deafness being the most common complication. As a result of widespread vaccination, the once-common bacterial meningitis is now very rare indeed.

Symptoms
Meningitis can develop very quickly. A baby can seem perfectly well then, just a few hours later, be extremely ill. The symptoms of meningitis are very difficult to detect. Unfortunately they are similar to symptoms connected with many other common childhood illnesses. The Meningitis Trust produces an excellent leaflet about diagnosing meningococcal diseases. Things to look out for include the following. They may not all occur, or occur at the same time:
- Altered level of consciousness.
- VOMITING and/or refusing feeds.
- Fever and a blank, staring expression.
- Fretfulness and a high cry, particularly when picked up.
- Pale skin and cool limbs with toes and fingers that are cold and appear blue despite high temperature.
- Doziness and reluctance to wake.
- Tense or bulging fontanelles.
- The neck may be arched backwards.

Call your doctor immediately if:
- Your baby has a fever: temperature of or above 38°C (100.4°F).
- She has a rash that does not fade when a glass is pressed against it (overleaf).
- She develops a sudden rash or bruising beneath the skin.
- She has a stiff neck with fever.
- She is having difficulty breathing.
- She appears to be having a convulsion, with stiffened body followed by shaking.
Meningococcal rash: Some bacteria that cause meningitis can also cause infection of the blood (septicaemia). Meningococcal septicaemia causes a rash to appear under the skin that starts as a cluster of tiny spots of blood, like pin-pricks. Without

treatment these grow larger and look like bruises, with bleeding under the skin. The rash can appear anywhere on the body and is difficult to see in the case of dark skin.

The classic way to test for this is to use the glass test. If a glass tumbler is pressed firmly against a septicaemic rash, the spots/bruises do not turn white and will show through the glass – the glass test is positive. Call your doctor immediately – although most children with indicative rashes do not have meningococcal disease, it is best to begin medical investigation.

Action plan

If your doctor suspects meningitis infection, a lumbar puncture test can be done so the cerebrospinal fluid can be analysed. If there are more than the normal number of white cells, which fight infection, this indicates infection. Hospital admission is usually necessary for the first 24 or 48 hours while the bacterial test results come back.

- Your baby may be given antibiotics even though these do not fight a viral infection, because it is safer to begin at once in case of bacterial infection – bacterial culture tests take 48 hours to give a result.
- If no bacteria are found, the infection will be viral and your baby is likely to recover within 3–5 days.
- If a bacterial meningitis is confirmed, intravenous antibiotics can be given at home by a specialist nurse or by daily visits to hospital. The course will be completed in 7–10 days, depending on the nature of the bacteria.
- After treatment has been completed, some doctors repeat the test on the cerebrospinal fluid by doing a second lumbar puncture to make sure all bacteria have been killed.
- A hearing test is usually done after about 4 weeks, as deafness is the most common complication of bacterial meningitis.
- If your baby has meningitis it may take months to get completely back to normal sleeping and behaviour. By about 3 months after the infection it is usually possible to check for evidence of damage to the brain. Sometimes, however, minor degrees affecting learning skills do not become apparent until the age of 5–7 years.

MISCARRIAGE

See also BLEEDING, DURING PREGNANCY; LOSS OF A BABY

A pregnancy that ends spontaneously before Week 20 is called a miscarriage or a spontaneous abortion. Many embryos are lost before they implant in the uterus and a woman may never be aware of the pregnancy. Of the pregnancies that are recognised, 15–25% end in miscarriage, most often between Weeks 6 and 12 and miscarriage is less common after this time. After Week 20 the loss is called a stillbirth (p.509). At any time in pregnancy the loss may be devastating and many women and men take a great deal of time to come to terms with what has happened. This is explored from p.506, together with advice on dealing with practical issues.

The first 12 weeks of pregnancy are the most vulnerable period for a baby. With each week that passes, the risks

decrease rapidly but there is usually no way to predict a miscarriage. The most common reason for early loss is because the embryo has not developed normally; there are other, less common, reasons that may be related to recurrent miscarriage, although the likelihood of this is low. Among women in their 20s the rate of clinically evident miscarriages is 10%; in the 30s this rises to 15% then to 33% in the early 40s and over 50% in the late 40s. This is related to the age of an egg and to lower progesterone levels after conception.

What happens

The earliest sign of miscarriage is bleeding, although it is helpful to remember that not all BLEEDING DURING PREGNANCY signifies miscarriage. The greater the volume of blood loss, the higher the chance the pregnancy will miscarry, particularly if there is pain and blood clots are being passed. If there is light bleeding with no pain, you may be having a **threatened miscarriage**; the chances are high that your baby is alive and your pregnancy will continue.

A missed abortion

A missed abortion occurs when an embryo dies early in pregnancy but the placenta continues to grow. It is also known as a **blighted ovum**. A pregnancy may continue for as long as 14 weeks with placental hormones keeping the pregnancy tests positive even though there is no baby. An ultrasound scan will reveal a missed abortion; miscarriage occurs eventually but many women prefer to have the placenta removed by dilation and curettage (D&C, p.407) instead of waiting.

Action plan

If you have bleeding, an obstetrician or midwife may perform a gentle vaginal examination and if your cervix is dilating, a miscarriage is inevitable. The definitive diagnosis is made on ultrasound scan where the amniotic sac can be visualised and the foetal heartbeat observed.

If you have had a 'threatened miscarriage' with bleeding but loss is unlikely, you will probably be advised to take it easy, avoid strenuous exercise and cut down on work. You must also avoid sexual intercourse until bleeding has stopped. This is an anxious time so support and tranquil surroundings will help you to relax as much as possible. Over 70% of all mothers diagnosed as having a threatened miscarriage in the first 12 weeks carry their pregnancies to term. Early bleeding is often your blood, related to the placenta implanting, and is not an indication of a developmental problem with the baby.

Medical care

- If you have a true miscarriage early in pregnancy, you may pass blood and clots before you get to hospital. It is best to keep the clots to be inspected by your doctor or nurse.
- If you begin bleeding and an ultrasound scan confirms the embryo is not viable before Week 8, you will miscarry with blood loss similar to a very heavy menstrual period. This usually happens within a week of the initial bleeding. If it has not occurred in this time you may need to go to hospital for a D&C. After you miscarry it is wise to have an ultrasound to confirm the uterus is empty of placenta.
- If pregnancy has progressed beyond Week 8, you will

probably be admitted to hospital so that surgical dilatation of the cervix and curettage of the uterus can be performed under general anaesthetic. This is to ensure your uterus is clear of all placental and membrane fragments, to avoid infection. The decision to do a D&C is based on the size of the uterus and the ultrasound scan findings.

- You will be given a BLOOD GROUP test: if you are rhesus negative you will be given an anti-Rh D injection to protect future pregnancies.
- The placental tissue may be sent for microscopic examination but the cause of miscarriage is not usually identified. You may choose to have the chromosomes from the placenta cultured to discover the gender and chromosome count of the foetus.
- If you have a miscarriage after Week 12 it is like labour and there may be a lot of pain and bleeding. Sometimes the placenta has to be removed surgically if it does not separate.

Emotional recovery
Many women feel that the baby was part of them and feel bereft because they have not had the 9 months of pregnancy to separate as two individuals. Early miscarriage may be like losing part of yourself and you may be surprised by intense emotions. In early miscarriage you will not see the baby but after a loss you may choose to begin the grieving process by spending time together, or you may wish to arrange a ceremony or funeral. You may need emotional support because as well as grief you may feel confused or guilty. It may be helpful to remember that miscarriage is usually a chance occurrence and is not a mother's fault. Women are often blamed.

Physical recovery
After a miscarriage it will take time for your body to return to normal – the process is longer the later in pregnancy you miscarry. Periods usually return within 4–6 weeks, but could take longer. Some women wish to conceive again as soon as possible, but it is best (although not essential) to wait for at least three menstrual cycles – waiting reduces the statistical risk of miscarrying again. Taking vitamin and mineral supplements for both partners (p.345) before conceiving, particularly folic acid and zinc, may also lower the risk.

Recurrent miscarriage
It is natural that any woman who has miscarried is anxious about doing so again. Yet in most cases miscarriage is a chance occurrence. Only 1% of all women experience three or more miscarriages and of these up to 75% go on to have a successful pregnancy without the need for special treatment. Recurrent miscarriage is diagnosed after the third successive miscarriage because having two miscarriages may be unlucky chance.

If you have recurrent miscarriage you and your partner will be offered blood tests and you may be given an ultrasound scan to examine your pelvic area and assess the condition of your ovaries, uterus and cervix. Your medical team may look into the following potential causes, some of which may be considered after a single miscarriage.

Genetic factors: 60% of miscarriages before Week 12 are caused by abnormal embryonic development. Many conceptions pass unnoticed or lead to a late period. Although foetal chromosomal abnormalities (p.433) are the most common cause of sporadic miscarriage, they are less commonly the cause of recurrent miscarriage. Some 3–5% of expectant parents who experience recurrent pregnancy loss carry a chromosomal abnormality, often a translocation of one part of one chromosome on to another chromosome (p.449).

Ovulation abnormalities: Recurrent miscarriage may be caused by defects in the ovulation cycle. Appropriate treatment gives a promising outlook for future pregnancies.

Low progesterone levels: Some early miscarriages are a result of insufficient levels of progesterone, which is usually produced by the ovaries for the first 10–12 weeks before the placenta takes over production. Low levels are more common among women over 38 years old or those with polycystic ovaries. It is possible to supplement progesterone levels using injections, vaginal pessaries or tablets.

Blood-clotting disorders (p.409): These may lead to miscarriage if untreated. Around 15% of women with recurrent miscarriage test positive for thrombophilia where the blood clots excessively and placental blood flow and foetal nutrition is reduced. The causes of thrombophilia include antiphospholipid antibodies and treatment that begins in early pregnancy using aspirin or heparin to thin the blood is usually effective (p.408).

Drugs: Intensive medications prescribed for malignancy and diseases of the immune system can increase the risk of miscarriage. Other drugs, including ALCOHOL and recreational *drugs*, may cause miscarriage if used in high dosage for a long period of time.

Infections and illnesses: A tiny fraction of miscarriages are caused by unusual infections such as RUBELLA and LISTERIA, but recurrent miscarriage is not.

The uterus: CERVICAL INCOMPETENCE can cause miscarriage in the 2nd trimester. A stitch can strengthen the cervix in future pregnancies.

Psychological factors: Some people believe anxiety can affect the hormonal system. However, many women across the world have borne children in extremely stressful situations. Believing that stress can influence miscarriage may incline a mother to blame herself for an event that was not within her control. Some women also blame themselves for exercising too much or even for flying in an aeroplane, but there is no evidence that any of these increases risk.

Poor nutrition: It is difficult to predict when poor nutrition may threaten pregnancy but it is true that vitamins and minerals taken by both partners before conception and avoidance of alcohol, drugs and SMOKING may reduce the overall incidence of miscarriage.

Occupational exposure: Little reliable evidence exists for exposure to things like herbicide spraying, electromagnetic fields, chemical inhalation, anaesthetic gases or VDU usage as causes of recurrent miscarriage.

Recurrent miscarriage leaves parents upset and perhaps struggling with the conflict between hope and despair. With increasingly good medical care and ever-advancing technology, however, the underlying causes are more frequently diagnosed and recurrent miscarriage can often be prevented.

MORNING SICKNESS
See NAUSEA & VOMITING

MUMPS
....

Mumps is very rare in babies under 1 year of age as they are usually protected by their mothers' antibodies and thereafter VACCINATION is effective, available for children as part of the MMR vaccination (measles, mumps, RUBELLA). Actually having the disease confers life-long immunity and the vaccine has a similar effect.

What happens
Mumps is a viral infection that typically causes enlargement of the two salivary glands in the cheeks. This gives a look akin to a hamster with food in its cheeks. It gives symptoms of a dry mouth and FEVER with headache and difficulty swallowing that generally improve over 4 days and do not usually cause lasting effects. Yet mumps can have serious side effects. Around 1:25 people have deafness following infection, which gets partly or completely better. Infection after puberty may cause swollen, inflamed testicles (in 1:5 males) and can lead to sub-fertility. It may also cause inflammation of the pancreas and, rarely, inflammation of the central nervous system causing MENINGITIS. Infection can lead to MISCARRIAGE. Vaccination is important to protect people of all ages. Mumps is transmitted mainly by infected saliva although the urine also contains virus particles. The saliva is infectious for about 6 days prior to the onset of swelling and for up to 2 weeks after.

Action plan
Your doctor will probably make a diagnosis based on the swelling of the cheek salivary glands. Laboratory tests are available but usually unnecessary. If your baby has mumps:
* Help to bring down the FEVER and relieve pain with infant paracetamol.
* Rinse her mouth regularly and encourage her to drink lots.
* Let your doctor know what is happening.
If an adult develops mumps:
* Consult your doctor, especially if a male is infected and has swollen, painful testicles or if there is infection in pregnancy.
* Treat fever, drink plenty and rest.
* Avoid contact with young or unimmunised babies.

NAPPY RASH
See SKIN, NAPPY RASH

NAUSEA & VOMITING
....

Nausea with vomiting occurs in 70% of pregnancies, typically starting by Week 4 or 6, peaking by Weeks 8 or 12 and resolving spontaneously by Week 16. It can occur at any time of day or night, although may be more intense in the morning, hence the term 'morning sickness'. Some women feel queasy at intervals during the day and some vomit once or more daily for weeks. Around 20% experience sickness in late pregnancy. Nausea and vomiting are usually not a cause for concern. More severe vomiting that leads to weight loss and dehydration is called hyperemesis (opposite). Nausea tends to be worse in a first pregnancy and in women who have a poor diet, and for women carrying TWINS.

What happens
The exact connection between vomiting and pregnancy is not well understood. The centre for nausea is in the brain and it is unclear how hormonal changes affect this. It is interesting that nausea usually diminishes around Week 10–12, a time when the hormones (human chorionic gonadotrophin and relaxin) released by the placenta are reaching a peak, but their levels are maintained after the nausea decreases.

Nausea can be brought on by muscle tension, particularly in the diaphragm or upper abdomen, that is often aggravated by poor posture (p.346). A vicious circle begins with nausea giving rise to fatigue, and fatigue bringing increased muscle tension, a tendency to flop rather than sit upright, and increased nausea. If you have an underlying tendency to nausea, for instance travel sickness, you may be more susceptible. Nausea may reflect anxiety about your personal and family circumstances or ambivalence at becoming a mother. Later in pregnancy nausea may return as your enlarging uterus presses on your stomach.

Implications for you and your baby
The majority of women function fine in spite of nausea, even though it can be tiring and upsetting. Physically, there are no long-term health problems related to nausea, although if you eat an excess of sugary foods to reduce nausea you may gain excessive WEIGHT. Occasionally an underlying emotional or stressful issue is brought to light and persistent and severe vomiting may put a strain on family relationships or lead to depression (p.462). Some women feel so upset they consider terminating the pregnancy. The passing of sickness is usually accompanied by a joyful high.

Your developing baby obtains adequate nutrients from your reserves of vitamins, minerals, proteins and fatty acids that have been stored before conception. Even if you have intense vomiting in early pregnancy that settles on treatment, your baby is likely to continue to grow normally. Babies born after severe vomiting and hyperemesis treatment may weigh on average 200 g (7 oz) less than average but their development is normal provided twins have been ruled out on antenatal testing (multiple pregnancy may cause excessive vomiting).

Action plan
If you are well nourished before you become pregnant, you are less likely to suffer from nausea and if it does occur your energy levels will be higher. To cure sickness, try homeopathy or acupuncture first – these are safest. To alleviate nausea, your best resource is a balanced diet.

Diet and lifestyle
* Where you can, avoid the sight and smell of things that

make you nauseous. If your home or workplace smell is a problem, try burning an aromatic essential oil.

- Try to eat small quantities of slow-burning food (p.332) every 3–4 hours to avoid sugar lows (p.336) and keep your stomach acids neutralised. If you eat lots of refined sugary food and drinks because they make you feel better, take care because these are potent causes of excess weight gain, although the weight gain may be less important for a few weeks than keeping yourself going. Nuts and seeds are usually well tolerated.
- Give yourself 15–20 minutes to relax and have a snack before getting up in the morning. Also have a snack before sleep or if you wake at night. A complex carbohydrate is best, something like a wholewheat or oat biscuit or a rice cake. Carry snacks around with you so you don't find yourself without food in the late afternoon, often a queasy, low-energy time.
- Even if you cannot tolerate food it is important to keep drinking – dehydration will make you exhausted and weak and, if severe, may lead to hyperemesis (right). Drink small amounts every hour or two to avoid distending your stomach and focus on water and a variety of herbal teas: ginger, mild mint or hot water with a slice of lemon. Fruit or vegetable juices or soups contain essential electrolytes and minerals as well as liquid. For vitamin and mineral supplements you may prefer a tonic to a tablet or could crush pills and put the powder on your food.
- Rinse your mouth with a gentle fluoride rinse each time you vomit so that you feel fresh and also protect your teeth from the acid of the stomach contents. Use a very soft toothbrush twice a day – not after each vomit because stomach acids may soften enamel and excessive brushing could cause erosion.
- Reducing stress may reduce nausea. If you are feeling isolated or anxious try to find ways of improving your circumstances (p.459). If you have been feeling nervous about your baby, seeing him on an ultrasound scan may help to allay your anxiety. Visualisations or meditations (p.370) may decrease stress. Slow, restful yoga postures and breathing techniques (p.346) may help to release muscle tension.

Homeopathy

Match your symptoms to a remedy picture below and take a tablet in the 30c potency, 4 times a day for 3–4 days, then reassess the situation.

Use *Arsenicum* for persistent nausea and vomiting leading to exhaustion, faintness, restlessness, anxiety and chilliness, with relief from sips of hot drinks, but cold foods and drinks exacerbate symptoms; *Ipecac* if you are pale and prostrate with nausea, salivation and empty retching, no thirst, no relief from vomiting or eating and worse from any motion; *Nux Vomica* for nausea with difficult but relieving vomiting, CONSTIPATION and irritability, gagging and retching, a feeling of stress from doing too much and relief from sleep, lying down and quiet; *Sepia* for constant nausea, empty feeling in the stomach, a desire to eat but the thought or smell makes things worse, you're better for eating little and often, very tired, irritable and upset, worse first thing in the morning and 3–5pm.

Aromatherapy

Massage with essential oils can be powerful in breaking a cycle of vomiting and replacing tension with calm. You could also add a few drops of essential oil to a warm bath and have a good soak. Ginger is good; try lavender after Week 24.

Acupuncture

Acupuncture can be very effective. The point Pericardium 6 is the usual focus, and in full treatment this would be combined with other acupuncture points according to your needs. Pericardium 6 is where you wear a watchstrap, two finger-widths above where your wrist and your palm meet, in line with your middle finger. You can buy acupressure travel sickness wristbands from chemists, with instructions for locating the acupuncture point – you can press the buttons to increase stimulation. You could massage this point with your thumb in an anti-clockwise direction, with moderate pressure, for 2 minutes on each wrist, 2 or 3 times a day.

Medical care

- If you are vomiting and have INDIGESTION OR HEARTBURN you may be prescribed medication to reduce acid production.
- Anti-nausea medication may be essential if the vomiting is causing you to feel weak or dehydrated or shows the characteristics of hyperemesis. The medication acts on your brain to reduce vomiting. None of the anti-nausea medications are licensed for use in pregnancy because of the possible side effect on a developing foetus, but if vomiting is severe your doctor may consider treatment essential. Dopamine antagonist drugs (e.g metoclopramide and prochlorperazine) have been used for decades and to date there is no association with any harmful effects for developing babies, although some women do feel drowsy. Your doctor will tailor medication to your needs and suppositaries are useful if you vomit excessively.
- On very rare occasions an inner ear infection may cause vomiting and can be treated, but this is usually associated with dizziness.

Hyperemesis

Hyperemesis is a condition characterised by excessive vomiting, dehydration and the loss of more than 5% of original body weight. Fortunately it is very uncommon (3:1000 pregnancies) and usually responds to hospital treatment involving intravenous fluid therapy, to replace water, electrolytes and sugar, and anti-nausea medication. A tiny proportion of women require prolonged treatment and support, particularly those carrying twins. Excessive vomiting may lead to inflammation of the oesophagus and even bleeding from the inflamed area. It may be necessary to treat the acidity with antacids or drugs to reduce acid production and replace vitamins and minerals as part of the treatment programme.

NEONATAL DEATH

See LOSS OF A BABY, SUDDEN INFANT DEATH SYNDROME (SIDS) & NEONATAL DEATH

NIPPLES

See BREAST, NIPPLES, CRACKED; BREAST, NIPPLES, INVERTED & FLAT

OBESITY: BABY

See WEIGHT, OBESITY: BABY

OBESITY: MOTHER

See EATING DIFFICULTIES & DISORDERS

OEDEMA

See SWELLING (OEDEMA)

OLDER MOTHERS & FATHERS

The concept of an 'older parent' is not the same now as it was a few decades ago. In the 1960s most women had babies in their early 20s and 'middle age' began at 40. Today the average age for a first baby is almost 30 and the 40s are in the upper range of youth. Many doctors and midwives would not consider you to be 'old' for a first baby – 'elderly prima gravida' – until the age of around 37 years.

There are pros and cons of a later pregnancy. Some risks increase but there are additional benefits and most women who have a baby after the age of 40 thrive, as do older fathers. Few of these 'older' parents feel old.

What happens

Whether planned or not, on the road to parenthood you will face the same issues that are faced by parents in their 20s. Later in life, though, you may have the advantage of being financially stable and have an established network of support. You may also feel better about giving up less healthy aspects of your lifestyle, such as SMOKING, late nights and parties, to focus on your baby and your family's wellbeing. This could reduce anxiety or depression that can arise if you feel conflict between responsibility and independence (p.300). Another advantage is that you may feel emotionally more prepared – research suggests that older mothers tend to be more patient and relaxed. A number of older parents also feel fulfilled in their careers, perhaps ready to cut down or stop work, or very well established and able to negotiate suitable timetables. Waiting for pregnancy later in life may be the best thing for some people who had a difficult childhood and needed time to live comfortably with past experiences.

The slightly increased risk of complications in pregnancy is often overstated, but is worth acknowledging. Some are less significant than they were a few decades ago because of advances in medical technology and because more women are physically active, fit and healthy. After an uncomplicated pregnancy and delivery your baby is as likely to thrive as a baby of a younger mother.

- Some women conceive quickly, others wait for up to 2 years. Fertility reduces progressively after 35 years of age.

- There is a higher risk of MISCARRIAGE if you're 40 or over. This is partly because of the age of your eggs and partly because your ovaries may produce less progesterone (treatment with additional progesterone may prevent miscarriage).
- The risk of your baby having DOWN'S SYNDROME rises progressively to 1:100 after age 40.
- You are more likely to conceive two or more babies (p.548).
- You have a higher likelihood of developing medical conditions such as DIABETES, FIBROIDS and high BLOOD PRESSURE with pre-eclampsia, but seen in context the majority of women over 40 do not have these problems.
- Many women have perfectly normal and natural births over 40 but a higher proportion have a CAESAREAN SECTION, sometimes through choice, sometimes because of complications such as high blood pressure and sometimes because an attending obstetrician is more wary of potential complications. Sometimes an older uterus may be less efficient but the majority function normally.
- You may find the physical and emotional demands of parenting harder than you might have earlier. This depends on many things, including your baby's health and character, your fitness, your relationship, your support network and time management. Some women find it easier because they are more relaxed.

Being an 'older' father

Many men are even keener than their partners to begin a family later in life, or to extend an existing family. This is often the case in a second or third marriage when a child can cement a relationship. Some feel ambivalent and can become distanced – often when a pregnancy comes as a surprise. This is no different from the range of reactions among fathers of any age (p.292), although an older man may be more 'set in his ways' and could take longer to adjust to the idea of a baby.

You may feel less pressurised about financial issues and be able to afford more help. If you are retired you might have plenty of time and energy and enjoy this new beginning. As an older man you will probably have a wide network of male friends who can offer advice and encouraging stories based on their experiences of bringing up children. In fact, this is more likely than if you were younger and most of your friends were still without children.

Action plan

If you take care of yourself with a balanced nutritious diet and regular exercise balanced with rest, you are doing the best for yourself and your baby, whether you are 18 or 45 years old. It helps to think about the balance between time for your baby, time for you and time for your partnership, and time at work if you stay on. Organisation (p.54) can reduce TIREDNESS AND LOW ENERGY and improve your relationships.

- Obstetricians and midwives sometimes treat older women differently but the prejudice is quickly disappearing. Different treatment reflects the concern for a good outcome, particularly in a first pregnancy after fertility treatment. You will be monitored as usual and the team will bear in mind any risk factors; they may be less keen for pregnancy to become postmature (p.500) if labour is delayed.

- After birth there is no difference between an older woman and a younger woman – both benefit from practical help and loving support.
- Breastfeeding is usually successful in older mothers. If you have other children who are also young, you will need a lot of energy to keep on top of things. If you have children who are grown, you may have extra help from them.
- You may take longer to get your figure back after birth – this depends on keeping fit and exercising regularly, and eating well. Some older mothers need to focus hard on pelvic floor exercises (p.357), especially if they have had children before.

Emotions and feelings

Although pregnancy in later life is becoming more commonplace, many men and women feel distanced from friends their own age who have grown-up children or have declared themselves child-free. It may be difficult to feel at ease at antenatal and postnatal groups where most other women are younger than you. If you already have grown-up children, you may feel sad that you had regained your independence and will be putting this on hold while you bring up your baby.

It's more common for older parents to have ageing mothers and fathers who may need care. Some have lost their own parents. If this is true for you, you may be upset that the generation link will not be there for your baby, and miss the wisdom your mother or father might have passed to you. At the same time you may feel more decisive, and happy with your role as the head of your new family.

If you give birth at or after 40 you might be anxious that you will be pushing 60 when your children are in their teens, and wonder what implications this will have. Remember that if you feel happy at 40 you may be happy at 60. Your age may improve your ability to love and care for your children, and to bring them up feeling wanted and adored.

OSTEOPOROSIS

Bone is constantly breaking down and rebuilding. Osteoporosis occurs when bone breaks down faster than new bone is formed, so there is a decrease in bone density. Although severe pregnancy-associated osteoporosis is rare, it is worth being aware of how to protect your bones, particularly if there is a family history, because lesser degrees of low bone density may precede osteoporosis in later life. Osteoporosis may not give any symptoms, but could lead to back or hip pain, weight loss and vertebral or hip fractures.

What happens

Bone loss does not occur during pregnancy. Your body actually increases absorption of calcium from foods and responds to your baby's calcium demands by increasing vitamin D levels. High oestrogen levels also give protection, and the load-bearing exercise of carrying your baby encourages bone strengthening. Bone density increases with an increased number of pregnancies and births. This may be partly related to high oestrogen levels in highly fertile women.

Bone loss can occur during breastfeeding. The increased calcium demand depends on the amount of milk produced and on how long you continue. While you are feeding, prolactin levels rise and this reduces oestrogen levels. The loss of bone tends to be temporary, with full recovery of density 6 months after stopping feeding. Susceptibility to osteoporosis increases if you have a family history, are not adequately nourished or have an EATING DISORDER, do not exercise regularly, have THYROID problems, are on cortisone or heparin medications, SMOKE or drink ALCOHOL heavily.

Preventative measures are important. Eat well, with a regular, balanced intake of minerals including calcium, magnesium, zinc and boron, and avoid excess phosphate, found in fizzy drinks. Carry your baby in a sling or papoose – the weight bearing is good for your bones. Weight causes your bones to deposit calcium and increases density. Exercise regularly, including weight-bearing exercises. If you are on cortisone, heparin or thyroid medication, ask for regular bone density monitoring.

PAIN, ADVICE & SUPPORT

Pain is a symptom of something happening in the body and there is a huge range in individual pain thresholds. Those who experience pain acutely may visit the doctor frequently, whereas stoical people usually make fewer visits. There is no 'right' way of responding to pain. If you are a frequent patient, the downside is that you may be very anxious and the advantage is that you will receive early attention if there is a problem. If you are less affected or more stoical, you may hardly ever visit the doctor, although you may overlook the importance of symptoms that indicate something is wrong.

During and after pregnancy your body undergoes an amazing number of changes. Some of these may be accompanied by aches and pains, most commonly in the later stages when the uterus is large and the baby heavy. Most do not point to any significant problem but it is vital to remember that pain may be a symptom of an abnormality and that if it is severe or continues for a long time it is essential to be examined. Even when there is no significant medical problem, there may be several ways of reducing pain and alleviating the stress that persistent discomfort can bring to daily life.

The emotional aspect of pain

After you have investigated physiological causes, it is helpful to consider the emotional issues (p.459) that may underlie, cause or exacerbate pain. Often women who have a tendency to anxiety feel pain more acutely, and being in pain brings anxiety. Pain may drain energy, reduce optimism and add to depression (p.462). It may be helpful to know it is 'normal' to feel low if you have ongoing pain, and also there are a number of things you can do to alleviate anxiety. In some families it is acceptable to be in pain but it is not to feel depressed.

Where the pain is

The body is interconnected. The spine runs from the pelvis to the top of the skull and a problem in one area may result in discomfort in another. For instance, there may be imbalance in the pelvis that brings on a headache, or a pain in the lower back that results from poor posture. Pregnant women are usually most concerned by pain in the abdomen and pelvic region. Most times pain in these areas indicates muscle or ligament strain and does not signal a serious problem.

Factors contributing to aches and pains

Posture: The physical and hormonal changes of pregnancy alter the normal curve of the spine, your abdomen becomes heavier and your abdominal muscles are stretched, so there is more strain on your back. In pregnancy the lower spine curves forwards while the upper spine (in your chest area) curves back. Your workstation may accentuate strains.

Ligament and joint laxity: As pregnancy progresses, there is increased production of the hormone relaxin, which allows your pelvic joints to expand. Your joints may feel more lax in second and subsequent pregnancies.

Birth: During birth the pelvic joints open and the ligaments in the pelvic area and in the lumbar spine may be stretched.

Daily babycare: After the birth feeding and carrying your baby may impose additional tension on your back.

Fatigue: Tiredness is exaggerated by poor posture.

Previous back problem, or pain with a previous pregnancy: Old areas of discomfort (perhaps caused by a past injury, an intervertebral disc abnormality or a habitual sitting posture) may be resolved and a new balance established. In some cases the changes may aggravate an underlying tension pattern or give rise to a new area of discomfort.

Take your pain seriously and seek medical advice if:
- There is pain in the area of the uterus, especially if you have bleeding and the pain increases in intensity, spreads or is severe to begin with.
- If you feel ill.

For less serious pain resulting from muscle tensions, you may try a combination of rebalancing and calming techniques (below). Although most tensions disappear after birth, attend to any discomfort to prevent a long-term strain pattern.

Action plan

The majority of pregnancy and postnatal pain relates to the changes described above. It may also arise from the normal physiological changes in the bowel, bladder and other internal organs. Seeking medical or midwifery advice improves safety for you and your baby. If you have had pain in a previous pregnancy, or are carrying more than one baby, you are more likely to have discomfort.
- Exercise (p.357) is very good for toning muscles and improving flexibility. You will need to take advice from a professional if you have pain. Some exercises will help and some need to be avoided. Always warm up and cool down and stretch before and after exercise.
- Yoga (p.346) is excellent for balancing the body, gently strengthening it and calming the mind. Some postures may not be suitable: for example, if you have pelvic pain, avoid postures that involve opening the legs wide.
- Meditation, relaxation and visualisations (p.370) help to calm the mind and this often reduces discomfort and pain.

- Osteopathy is a safe and effective way of resolving tension patterns (p.376). Postnatal pelvic discomfort is best treated early before the ligaments harden.
- Massage and/or aromatherapy oils can be effective (p.378).
- A good diet will give your body the nutrients it needs and spacing meals every 3–4 hours avoids sugar lows that make you feel tired and tense.
- Homeopathy can be very effective: the remedy depends upon the type of pain.
- Medical analgesics can be useful, providing they are safe for pregnancy and breastfeeding. Medication for depression and anxiety may reduce pain.
- Posture has a profound effect on energy levels and moods. Good posture helps your body stay in balance and avoids strain, and is particularly important during and after pregnancy (p.348).
- Emotional support may help you deal with your feelings and reduce symptoms of pain. Pain is a way that many people have of showing what is happening emotionally.
- Time is a great healer. Minor aches and pains associated with the stretching and softening of muscles and ligaments settles down after the birth, but your body takes time to revert to its non-pregnant state. Resting, through sleep, relaxation postures and moments of calm, perhaps with visualisations is a great help. Remember that ligament and joint changes may take 6 months to return to normal.

PAIN, IN THE ABDOMEN

See also PAIN, ADVICE & SUPPORT

You may feel abdominal or pelvic discomfort to varying degrees throughout pregnancy. As your growing uterus reaches your rib cage, the muscles that support your abdomen stretch and the ligaments that support your spine and pelvis and the surrounding muscles soften and expand. The ligaments supporting your uterus also stretch and your bladder is pushed forwards and up and your bowel is pushed up. It is hardly surprising that many women experience aches and pains. Discomfort may also arise from internal organs (uterus, bladder, kidneys, stomach, colon) or from the muscles and ligaments or the joints in your back, abdomen or pelvis.

Pain in the uterus & ovaries
Common pain

In early pregnancy: Pain often arises from the ovary as the corpus luteum enlarges. Discomfort is usually felt on one side of the pelvis and may radiate into the lower part of the abdomen on that side. This is relatively common and can be diagnosed on ultrasound scan. It may be quite intense but diminishes by Week 10.

Round ligament pain: The round ligaments that run from the top of the uterus to the inguinal area in the groin lengthen a lot during pregnancy. Sometimes there is tension on these ligaments giving discomfort on the upper part of the uterus, often on one side. The pain may also radiate into the groin.

Contractions in pregnancy: The muscle wall of your uterus contracts throughout pregnancy in Braxton-Hicks or 'practice'

A B C D E F G H I J K L M

contractions. You may feel your uterus becoming hard and if you touch the outside of your abdomen it will feel tight. As pregnancy advances the power increases and these contractions are a common feature in late pregnancy. The pain perception associated with them varies enormously. Usually the contractions are felt as runs of discomfort. They may last for minutes or hours. Awareness of them does not indicate you are more likely to have a premature labour.

Labour contractions: As labour approaches, contractions are more likely to cause pain. When labour begins, contractions become strong and the intensity of pain increases, reaching its peak at the end of the 2nd stage (p.132).

After the birth: Your uterus reverts to the non-pregnant size by contracting, a process that gives rise to 'afterpains' for a week or two. Breastfeeding stimulates contractions. Afterpains are often more intense with subsequent births and some women describe them as worse than labour contractions. You may be able to ride through them by focusing on your breathing, as you did in labour, or you may require painkillers.

Homeopathic remedies for afterpains (in 200c potency, every 2 hours for 6 hours) include *Arnica*, particularly after a long, arduous labour; *Sepia* for pains with a strong bearing down sensation, often after a second or subsequent birth; *Cimicifuga* for violent spasms low in the pelvis moving to the abdomen and groin; *Pulsatilla* for protracted and changeable pains worse during breastfeeding if you feel weepy, clingy and not thirsty; *Chamomilla* for unbearable pains making you irritable and very difficult to please.

Less common pain

In the vast majority of pregnancies pain arising from the uterus and ovaries does not indicate a serious problem. Occasionally, pain may signal the need for medical attention.

Severe pelvic pain: At the front of the abdomen, often low down on one side and perhaps intense and knife-sharp, may indicate an ECTOPIC PREGNANCY. This is a rare occurrence but may be life threatening because there is internal bleeding.

Strong uterine contractions: In early pregnancy that are in the centre of your pelvis and come and go may indicate a threatened MISCARRIAGE if the pain is accompanied by bleeding. Contractions usually last about 30 seconds and then recur every 3–5 minutes. In PREMATURE labour, the symptoms may be similar.

Later in pregnancy: A very rare but potentially serious cause is internal bleeding related to PLACENTAL ABRUPTION. The bleeding is between the placenta and the wall of the uterus and the pain over the front wall of the uterus is usually constant, unlike contractions that come and go. If you experience pain that is spreading and severe, urgent, medical advice is essential particularly if you feel shocked and are bleeding.

Fibroids (p.468): In some women parts of the uterine muscle thicken and condense to form fibroids. Often these cause no symptoms, but there may be pain over the area of the fibroid that tends to last for days or weeks and then gradually fades.

Infection: If an infection occurs in the uterus after the birth, particularly if there are fragments of placenta in the cavity (p.407), you will feel tenderness in the lower abdomen and pelvis. There is always an associated vaginal discharge or bleeding and you may have a FEVER.

Bladder & kidney pain

The ureters are tubes that transfer urine from your kidneys to your bladder. During pregnancy they are distended due to the combined effect of hormonal changes and an increase in pressure from the uterus. This may sometimes cause discomfort and very occasionally pain on one side, often on the right. It may radiate from the groin up towards the kidney area at the back of the abdomen under the lower ribs.

- Around 5% of women are susceptible to URINARY TRACT or kidney infections during pregnancy. If there is a bladder infection, the main symptoms are a need to pass urine frequently and burning as the urine emerges. Pain in the ligaments and joints of the pubic symphysis (overleaf) in front of the bladder may mimic CYSTITIS but the pubic joint is tender to the touch and this distinguishes the two.
- If the infection extends up to the kidneys, which is rare, you may feel tenderness extending into the back of your abdomen. A severe kidney infection (pyelonephritis, p.552) may cause pain and a fever.

Stomach & bowel pain

Although stomach and bowel pain may be caused by digestive problems, such as nausea or INDIGESTION, some women feel discomfort in the upper abdomen from spasm of the muscle in the wall of the stomach or the oesophagus.

- Severe pre-eclampsia (p.410) may cause upper abdominal pain in late pregnancy and needs urgent attention.
- Pains in the lower abdomen may arise from spasm in the wall of the colon or the rectum. In a small number of cases this may occur as part of an underlying bowel disorder, for example an irritable bowel syndrome (p.448), but it may also be associated with CONSTIPATION or DIARRHOEA. Contractions of the lower colon bowel wall can feel like uterine pain and give rise to fear of premature labour.
- Sometimes pain in the anal area is associated with PILES.

PAIN, IN THE BACK & PELVIS

See also PAIN, ADVICE & SUPPORT

About half of all pregnant women get low-back pain. It can usually be addressed and relieved with simple attention to posture, exercise and relaxation (p.518). Some women suffer severe pain that may continue for months or years after the birth. If you have had back pain before, you are more likely to have discomfort in pregnancy.

What happens
Lumbar pain
Lumbar pain involves the lumbar vertebrae behind the lower part of the abdomen and can occur with or without radiation to the legs. It often stems from the joints between the vertebrae, the surrounding muscles or ligaments or the nerves that run from the lumbar spine into the lower abdomen and legs.

Sometimes tension arises from deep muscles on the front of the vertebrae and may cause symptoms that mimic uterine or bowel pain. The nerves adjacent to the muscles may be affected and the pain interpreted by your brain as arising from an abdominal organ rather than the tense muscle. Occasionally, low back pain may be attributable to a herniated vertebral disc.

Pelvic pain

The pelvic girdle is made up of three large bones, the sacrum (base of the spine) and two pelvic bones that form a joint at the front, the pubic symphysis, and join with the sacrum at the back, at the sacroiliac joints. The coccyx or tailbone is attached to the sacrum. It is thought that 20–30% of pregnant women experience both lumbar and sacroiliac pain. In pregnancy the symphysis pubis and the sacroiliac joints soften.

The symphysis pubis widens throughout pregnancy from its normal width of 5 mm (¼ in) to a maximum of approximately 12 mm (½ in). As it widens, the pubic and sacroiliac joints move excessively and can cause discomfort when pain-sensitive ligaments are stretched.

Sacroiliac joint pain: Felt in the buttock, usually on one side, and may radiate down the back and outer side of one thigh, usually to the level of the knee and, rarely, to the calf. It is four times more common than lumbar pain. Symptoms of sacroiliac joint pain often continue several months after delivery.

Symphysis pubis dysfunction (SPD): Also called diastasis symphysis pubis (DSP), may give pain low down over the joint, in the vagina, groin and lower abdomen, over the bladder. If the sacroiliac joint is involved it can radiate down to the thighs. It is usually worse when walking, rolling over in bed, parting the legs (e.g. getting into a car) or putting weight on one leg (e.g. using stairs). Sometimes a clicking can be heard or felt. SPD occurs if softening of ligaments allows excessive movement and an abnormally wide gap in the pubic joints. This puts tension on the surrounding ligaments. Following delivery, the space decreases within days but the supporting ligaments take 3–5 months to return fully to their normal state and the pain may continue. SPD pain is increased if one or both sacroiliac joints are unstable and this leads to extra stress on the symphysis.

Sciatica: Involves the sciatic nerve. It is rare and accounts for a small percentage of low-back pain in early pregnancy. It can cause discomfort in the low back and in the sacroiliac joint in the buttock region or deep in the vagina. You may feel it more on one side and the pain might radiate down one thigh. In late pregnancy sciatica may bring on sharp pain, cramp, pressure or aching in the hips or buttocks. As babies tend to lie more heavily to one side, the discomfort can be stronger in one hip.

Nocturnal pain: Occurs in the low back only at night in bed and may follow daytime SPD and sacroiliac pain. There are many theories about night pain that include muscle fatigue after exercise in the day, stress from imbalanced posture and changes in circulation.

Postnatal backache: It is very common as joints and ligaments take months to return to normal after birth. Sacroiliac strain can increase if you have a forceps- or ventouse-assisted delivery (p.496). Your abdominal muscles may take up to a year to regain pre-pregnancy tone, and meanwhile do not provide maximum support for your back. The way you carry and hold and feed your baby may compound the problem. If you have intense symptoms it is best to treat them before attempting to become pregnant again.

Action plan
Medical care
- It is best to discuss your pain with your midwife or doctor, particularly if it is severe or there are other concerning symptoms. For instance, if the pain is associated with loss of sensation or tingling in the thighs or feet or muscle weakness, a prolapsed intervertebral disc may be considered.
- You may be advised to use a TENS machine (p.158) or take paracetamol in safe doses.
- You might be referred to a physiotherapist who can give you specific exercises and postural advice. Some recommend the use of support straps, corsets or belts.
- Osteopathic treatment can be a very powerful aid.

What you can do
Be aware of your posture and look over the general principles for approaching pain on p.517. You can also try:
- A warm bath or a hot-water bottle for lower backache and/or a massage.
- Lying on your back with your feet propped approximately 60 cm (2 ft) above your hips on a cushion or low chair for about 20 minutes, 4 times a day.
- Exercise (p.357) and yoga (p.346), but with SPD don't open your legs.
- Try not to get downhearted. If you have back pain in pregnancy this won't necessarily make labour harder, and if your pelvic joints have opened wide this could mean that labour is in fact easier. If you are feeling low, your emotions may affect the way your body feels, and could also make you slouch, exacerbating any areas of imbalance. You may benefit from EMOTIONAL ADVICE AND SUPPORT.

Homeopathy
In addition to attention to your posture and lifestyle, a homeopathic remedy may be useful. *Kali Carb* is good if your back feels weak, stiff or bruised with dragging pains in the lumbar region and the coccyx, you wake regularly at 3am and sweat at night, feel worse sitting for any length of time or walking and better lying on a hard surface or with pressure on the back; *Rhus Tox* if you have stiffness in the lower back, feel as if the muscles seize up when you rest and get better for movement and warmth; *Arnica* is generally used to alleviate bruising and may help pain in the back if you have no clear symptoms. Take one of the above in 30c, 3–4 times a day for 1 week and reassess. If back problems persist, take *Calc Phos* and *Calc Fluor* 6x in a combination remedy am and pm for up to 4 weeks, but only after Week 12 of pregnancy.

PAIN, IN THE HAND

See also PAIN, ADVICE & SUPPORT

During pregnancy body fluid increases significantly (p.38) and it is quite common to get slightly puffy fingers. If your fingers feel numb, your tissues may be retaining fluid (p.539) and your finger joints may ache. This happens to roughly 5% of women. When fluid is retained in the **carpal tunnel syndrome**, which is made up of bone and ligaments in the wrist, this puts pressure on the median nerve, often leading to numbness, pins and needles and pain in the thumb, index and middle fingers. Sometimes pain radiates up the arm. When there is general swelling, all the fingers may hurt. There may be a combination of the two. Because fluid collects throughout the day, the symptoms are often worse at night.

Action plan

- If your sleep is disturbed, your doctor may suggest wearing a wrist splint to relieve pressure on the nerve. Try sleeping with your hands raised on a pillow.
- You could try massaging your wrists, concentrating on the front of the joint near the hand.
- You can gently stretch your ligament to encourage fluid to dissipate: kneel with the palms of your hands on the floor and your fingers pointing towards your knees (wrists facing away from you) and keep your elbows straight. Slowly move your knees back until you can feel a stretch in the wrists. Repeat 3–4 times a day, including last thing at night.
- The section on SWELLING describes a variety of tips to reduce fluid retention.
- When the syndrome is bad, you may be offered mild painkillers in the form of non-steroidal anti-inflammatory drugs: these are usually only necessary in late pregnancy.
- This condition normally resolves after delivery but very occasionally simple surgery is needed to release the ligament on the front of the carpal tunnel.

Homeopathy

Take the remedy that suits in a 6c potency, 3 times a day for 1 week and then reassess the situation.

Ruta is the no. 1 remedy for an aching pain when the area feels bruised, worse on first moving and better with warmth and by rubbing the area; *Calc Carb* if you have tingling and numbness in the fingers, swelling in the wrist and pain from the elbow to the wrist, usually on the right side; *Rhus Tox* if you have a tearing pain, stiffness and your hand and wrist feel hot and better from continual gentle motion, worse in damp weather; *Causticum* is good when the fingertips, first finger and thumb are affected with a ra w pain with tingling, numbness and stiffness, better from warmth and damp weather.

PAIN, IN THE HEAD

See also PAIN, ADVICE & SUPPORT

Headaches are common during and after pregnancy. The most likely cause is tension due to changes in muscles and ligaments. A headache may also be linked to pain or imbalance in the back (p.519) or to TIREDNESS or anxiety (p.461). There are other less common but potentially serious reasons for headaches. Call your doctor if you have a sudden or extremely intense headache. A slowly progressive headache that is due to muscle tension needs less urgent attention.

- Tension headaches are due to changes in muscles and ligaments and usually involve the brow, often worse on one side, sometimes radiating to one eye. Tension headaches are more common in women who are working and after the birth. They often stem from poor posture.
- Conditions unrelated to pregnancy may cause the problem. Tooth pain and sinusitis are examples that can be treated.
- Migraine is more likely if you have had it before, although it may occur for the first time. Migraine may be associated with other symptoms including visual disturbances and vomiting, which may also signal pre-eclampsia (p.410) so it is important to check your blood pressure. Migraines are often reduced by avoiding triggers such as stress, hypoglycaemia (p.336) and allergenic substances (p.391).
- An intense headache may indicate high BLOOD PRESSURE and severe pre-eclampsia, particularly if it is associated with visual changes, swelling in your legs and upper abdominal discomfort. It is worth reporting to your midwife because, in rare instances, pre-eclampsia can lead to extremely dangerous eclamptic fits and treatment is preventive.
- After birth if you have had a spinal or epidural anaesthetic this can lead to an alteration in the cerebrospinal fluid pressure, called a dural tap, and cause a headache that usually disappears within 5 days. It is most effectively treated by resting flat in bed.
- Very rare but acute problems involving bleeding or blood clots in the brain can cause headache: sudden onset of severe pain associated with vomiting or muscle weakness warrants a full neurological examination.
- Postnatal headaches in the early weeks and months are often due to tiredness or stress, and to the way you hold your baby. They may reflect dehydration too if you are forgetting to drink enough.

Action plan

If a headache is new or severe, a full examination is needed to exclude pre-eclampsia and rare causes. For a moderate headache remember that tension may be linked with backache. You can begin to treat a headache with many of the principles outlined on p.517. Pregnancy and the few weeks following the birth are an excellent time to focus on releasing tension in your muscles and improving your strength and posture. It may be possible to alter an underlying tension pattern through rest, yoga postures (p.346) or osteopathy (p.376).

- A balanced diet that avoids sugar highs and lows and drinking plenty of water may help.
- You could make simple changes to your posture.
- If your headache is related to another medical condition, from high blood pressure to a common cold (p.442), treating that cause will often relieve the headache.
- Persistent headache may be related to ALLERGY and is often linked to SMOKING.
- Paracetamol painkillers in a safe doses may help.
- You may also need to tend to anxieties, perhaps on an ongoing basis: feeling emotionally at peace is a great step towards reducing headaches.

Homeopathy

For acute headaches one of the following may suit you. This is by no means a comprehensive list and you may want to consult your homeopath if your symptoms are not met here; headaches are sometimes difficult to self-prescribe for. Take the most suitable remedy in 30c, 3–4 times a day and then reassess. For chronic ongoing headaches, migraines or cluster headaches, consult a homeopath.

Bryonia for a bursting, crushing, severe headache that often settles above one eye, worse for any movement whatsoever, particularly when stooping, a desire to apply firm pressure to the pain and to keep as still as possible – a very useful remedy for a sinus headache; *Gelsemium* for a congestion-type headache that gives the sensation of having a tight band around the head or over the eyes and pain tends to move from the back of the head forwards, you feel heavy-lidded, often dizzy and exhausted and may have flu-type symptoms; *Sepia* for heavy-headed shooting pains that often settle over one eye (usually the left), can come on because you skip meals, you feel exhausted and worn out, may be accompanied by nausea and dizziness or backache and improves for fresh air or some form of exercise; *Nat Mur* when your head is being hammered with pain settling on the top of your head or over your eyes, worse from coughing, moving your eyes or direct sunlight, better when you are alone, quiet and in the fresh air; *Nux Vomica* for headaches that follow over-indulgence of food or drink or a period of loss of sleep and stress, that give a dull pressure, often with nausea and make you extremely irritable and sensitive to noise and light.

PAIN, IN THE LEG

See also PAIN, ADVICE & SUPPORT

Leg cramps are due to tightness and spasm in the calf muscles and are more common in the second half of pregnancy. If you are getting cramps you can prevent and treat them. If you get a severe pain in your calf that does not go away, consult your doctor to exclude the very small chance that you have a blood clot (thrombosis) in a deep VEIN in your calf.

What happens
Tight muscles arise if you frequently wear high-heeled shoes and do not stretch your Achilles tendons and calves, so that over time the muscle fibres shorten. Short muscles are more liable to go into spasm. Doing aerobic exercise without stretching increases the likelihood of cramp. Another cause is inadequate nutrition: reduced intake of calcium may lead to the muscle being more irritable and contracting.

Action plan
In addition to the guidelines for pain in general (p.517), the following techniques may reduce the occurrence of cramp and/or relieve it when it occurs.

Exercise and rest
- Yoga stretches the muscles of the lower back and thighs, calves and feet and cures cramps. To focus on your calves, stand facing the wall, 60 cm (2 ft) away, and rest your elbows, forearms and wrists on the wall. Now leave one foot stationary and move the other away from the wall with the knee straight until there is a feeling of tightness in the calf muscle. Maintain the stretch for 1–3 minutes and then

change legs. Try to repeat the exercise 4 times a day.
- Stretch all your main muscle groups before walking or exercise and when you finish (p.364).
- Resting with your leg up is helpful.

Diet and lifestyle
- Eat calcium-rich foods – there are many sources besides cow's milk (p.339).
- Reduce phosphorus by avoiding fizzy drinks and pre-prepared instant soups because phosphorus competes with calcium and renders the muscle more sensitive.
- Vitamin and mineral supplements with additional magnesium help to provide the background nutrients for the muscles to contract.
- Wear comfortable shoes with a flat heel; trainers or walking shoes are preferable.

Massage
- Lightly rubbing or massaging the cramped area can help. To break the spasm, straighten your leg and flex your toes towards your knee.
- In massage, in the bath or as a compress, try a base oil mixed with the essential oils tangerine, orange or lemon and from Week 24, lavender or geranium.

Homeopathy
A suitable remedy you can take is *Mag Phos* 6x (an anti-spasmodic) morning and night for 2–3 weeks alongside one of the following remedies (30c), 3–4 times a day for 1 week and then reassess.

Sepia helps to improve circulation and relieves cramp in the calves, toes and soles of the feet, is worse at night and while walking and leaves you irritable, snappy and worn out; *Nux Vomica* for cramp felt in toes, calves, soles of feet, numbness or pins and needles in arms and hands with pains that can radiate over the whole body and you are hypersensitive, irritable, nervy and quarrelsome, feel chilly and better from rest and warmth; *Ledum* is useful if your legs and feet feel cold and numb and yet are relieved by cold applications; *Cuprum Met* helps for severe cramps in the feet and legs that begin with twitching in the muscles.

PALPITATIONS
See HEART: MOTHER

PARVOVIRUS B19

Parvovirus B19 is a virus that lives within the red blood cells. It is also sometimes called '**slapped-cheek disease**' or '**fifth disease**'. It most commonly infects children, giving a facial rash, pale lips and a generalised rash on the trunk. In adults symptoms usually involve joint pains and stiffness in the hands, wrists and knees. Symptoms begin 4–14 days after infection and commonly pass within a couple of weeks, although some people have symptoms and rash for months. Around 20% of infected adults have no symptoms at all. The rash is similar to RUBELLA rash. If you have been infected in childhood, you will be immune. There is no vaccine.

If you are not immune and have contact with an infected person, you have a 30% chance of catching the virus. If you become infected before Week 20 there is a higher than normal risk of MISCARRIAGE. Most babies of infected pregnant mothers do not become infected, but there is a small risk that your baby, if infected in the womb, may develop ANAEMIA. In a tiny minority of cases, infection can lead to stillbirth (p.509).

Action plan

- If you develop parvovirus in pregnancy, you cannot be treated. A sample of your blood will be tested for antibodies to confirm the diagnosis. Your medical team will monitor your health and your baby's wellbeing.
- Scans can detect whether your baby has developed anaemia by looking for excess fluid in the abdomen, an enlarged liver and SWELLING (oedema) of the limbs. Treatment depends on the degree of anaemia and the stage of pregnancy. If foetal anaemia is severe, an intrauterine blood transfusion may be recommended.
- If your baby has foetal anaemia your medical team will monitor birth closely, because the low haemoglobin level increases the risk of FOETAL DISTRESS & ASPHYXIA.
- At birth your baby's blood will be checked for anaemia and transfusion given as necessary.

PENIS, HYPOSPADIAS & CHORDEE

Hypospadias is a birth defect that occurs in roughly 1:350 boys and affects the position of the urethra, the opening through which urine passes. The defect may occur anywhere along the underside of the penis down to the scrotum, but most commonly it is close to the normal opening site. The foreskin may appear split or hooded. Males with hypospadias usually have normal testes and can father children. Chordee is a downward curve of the penis associated with hypospadias. Boys with uncorrected chordee often have to sit to urinate and it can make intercourse impossible. Fortunately, treatment for both conditions is usually successful.

What happens

Around Week 10 of pregnancy the urethra begins to fold and close and the penis grows. If the folding is incomplete, hypospadias occurs. The cause is unknown but it is more common when the mother is over 35 years old. If two people in a family have hypospadias, the chance of recurrence is 20%.

Action plan

Hypospadias and chordee are suspected during normal checks at birth and your baby then needs to be inspected by a specialist surgeon. CIRCUMCISION must not take place, as some of the foreskin may be needed to reconstruct the opening. An ultrasound scan is often done to check the anatomy of the genital organs and the kidneys.

The best age for corrective surgery depends on the size of the penis and degree of the defect. It is usually done at 6–12

months on an outpatient basis. Some 90% of corrections are completed in one operation that corrects the chordee and extends the urethra to the tip of the penis. More extensive operations may involve creating a tube from the foreskin or using skin grafts. Surgery usually results in a penis that looks and functions as normal.

PHENYL KETONURIA (PKU)

This rare disease occurring in about 1:125,000 newborns is caused by a defective gene that regulates metabolism of the amino acid phenyl alanine. As a result of the defect, harmful phenyl ketones build up in the bloodstream; in high levels they are toxic to the developing brain. Treatment beginning in the first few weeks of life can prevent the build-up of toxins, and standard testing (through the heel prick test, p.226) identifies all cases. Without early treatment, a child would suffer irreversible brain damage and develop learning disability.

Treatment involves a special diet low in phenyl alanine, including special milk. To maintain normal growth and intellectual development a child needs to keep to the diet for the rest of his life. For girls with PKU not on the diet there is a risk of damage to babies in pregnancy through high phenyl alanine levels, which can affect brain development.

PILES & ANAL FISSURE

Piles (haemorrhoids) are small, blood-filled swellings caused by dilated veins. Initially, they are located just inside the anus (internal haemorrhoids) but can sometimes protrude (external haemorrhoids). Haemorrhoids are not dangerous. During pregnancy increased blood flow to the pelvic area may cause the veins to swell and this effect is increased with hard stools and CONSTIPATION. The pressure in the veins increases as pregnancy advances and is at its height during birth. Piles often coexist with varicose veins (p.559). Small piles affect many pregnant women and usually resolve soon after birth. Large piles may very occasionally prolapse out of the anus.

What happens

Small piles – pea size – can exist without giving any symptoms. If they reach the size of a grape, or larger, the anal muscle may go into spasm. This causes burning on passing a stool, particularly if the stool is hard. There may be mucus discharge and irritation from inflammation of the lining of the anus or bright red bleeding during a bowel movement. Large piles may protrude. Small piles may only be visible on anal examination using a proctoscope, a small instrument that enables a doctor to visualise the lining of the anus. Your doctor may also perform a gentle examination with her finger.

Piles are biggest after the pushing force of birth and may enlarge if the pelvic muscles go into spasm following a vaginal tear with stitches, because the blood may not drain freely from the veins. After the birth piles get better over a 6–12 week period. Even large ones may disappear completely.

Action plan

If you have piles, your discomfort will depend upon their size and the degree of irritation of the anus.

Diet and lifestyle

• Follow the advice for avoiding constipation to prevent straining. This stops piles from getting worse.
• To reduce pressure on the rectal veins avoid standing for long periods of time. When large piles are present and cause pain, you could sit on an inflatable ring or lie on your side, particularly after the birth.

Exercise and aromatherapy

• Try regular pelvic floor exercises (p.98), beginning by tightening the anus. These help the blood flow to the piles and may reduce the symptoms.
• Apply cypress or lemon oil in a cold compress to the piles for 20 minutes, 3 times a day, but not longer because the anal skin may crack and cause a fissure if the compress is left on too long. Alternatively apply 1–2 drops to the piles every 8 hours. Keep cypress oil away from stitches.

Medical care

Lubricating the anus with glycerine suppositories or a pure vegetable oil (such as almond or grapeseed) after each bowel movement or using a suppository containing a local anaesthetic and a mild steroid (cortisone) may prevent irritation and muscle spasm pain.

It is best for your doctor to check your piles after birth. Usually no further treatment is needed but occasionally an operation may be required to remove the varicosities. Piles tend to recur in subsequent pregnancies and if you are constipated and strain on passing a stool. Extremely rarely, where anal bleeding does not stop, there may be a rectal polyp or cancer and further examinations will be needed.

Homeopathy

Take a suitable remedy (6c) 3–4 times a day for 5–7 days and then reassess. External creams are available.

Use *Aesculus* to relieve prolapsed, purple, bleeding piles that give a constricted feeling in the anus with burning and sharp splinter-like pains, large, hard and dry stools, with discomfort lingering for a long time after passing a stool, worse in the morning, from standing, walking and in cold weather, better for bathing with cool water; *Collinsonia* for chronic internal or protruding piles, itching and burning in the anus, intermittent bleeding, splinter-like pain, alternating DIARRHOEA and constipation with hard, dry stools, worse at night and better in the mornings; *Hamamelis* if the piles protrude, are bluish in colour, bleed profusely, give pulsating pain, pricking and stinging accompanied by pains in the back; *Nux Vomica* for sensitive, inflamed piles that bleed easily with stitching pains that can be felt up the spine, constipation with ineffectual straining, the rectum feels constricted and the piles feel large and inflamed, worse at night and when stressed, better later in the day and from resting; *Sepia* when there is a strong bearing-down sensation, large, hard and protruding piles that can bleed, the feeling of a ball in the rectum and you generally feel run down and miserable, with mood swings.

Anal fissure

A fissure or crack in the anal skin may mimic piles by causing bleeding and pain. It is most common after the birth. It is usually caused by constipation and heals when stools are softer. On rare occasions it may signal an underlying inflammatory bowel problem (p.448). Most fissures heal with the use of a cream or suppository, measures to soften the stool and the use of sitz baths (soaking the anal area in plain warm water for 20 minutes, several times a day). The small numbers that do not heal rapidly may need an operation.

Prolapsed piles

If the rectal muscles go into intense spasm, pressure in already swollen veins increases, and the piles may swell further and protrude in a painful condition known as prolapsed piles. It usually occurs after birth and is treated with rest in bed, painkillers and application of a local anaesthetic cream a few times a day. Ice packs, cold compresses or cabbage leaves kept in the fridge and applied to the area for 20 minutes every 3–4 hours bring relief and can reduce swelling. The piles usually recede within a few days and the process is speeded up if they are gently pushed back into the anus. Surgery is very rarely needed before or soon after the birth and even large piles may not be visible 6 months later.

PLACENTA ACCRETA

See also BLEEDING, DURING PREGNANCY

In placenta accreta the placenta does not embed in the decidual lining of the uterus as usual, but grows through the decidual layer into the muscle wall of the uterus and becomes firmly attached. The condition is very rare and is more likely to occur in women who have had surgery to the uterus or a prior CAESAREAN SECTION. It may accompany PLACENTA PRAEVIA (low-lying placenta).

During the 3rd stage of labour a placenta accreta does not separate. This stops the uterus from contracting and retracting, and there is a risk of heavy bleeding. In the majority of cases the placenta requires surgical removal in the operating theatre under epidural or general anaesthesia by an obstetrician who inserts her hand into the vagina to reach the uterus and define a plane of separation from the wall. This is similar to a curettage (p.407) but a sharp instrument is not used. If the placenta is removed completely there is a normal amount of postnatal bleeding but there is a slightly higher risk of the problem recurring in the next pregnancy. On exceptionally rare occasions the placenta penetrates the wall of the uterus completely and a hysterectomy is needed.

PLACENTA PRAEVIA

See also BLEEDING, DURING PREGNANCY

When the placenta implants in the lower half of the uterus (the lower segment) and it extends to cover partially or completely the internal opening of the cervix, it is called a low-lying placenta or placenta praevia. In early pregnancy the placenta covers most of the cavity of the uterus and a placenta praevia is a very common finding. As pregnancy progresses, the placenta becomes confined to one portion of the uterus, usually clear of the cervix. By mid-pregnancy, fewer scans show a low placenta and by Week 32 less than 1% are praevia.

When the placenta partially covers the internal opening of the cervix, it is a 'minor' placenta praevia; when the cervix is completely covered there is a 'major' placenta praevia and there is likely to be bleeding in pregnancy. Modern ultrasound scans are usually reliable in detecting a placenta praevia, provided the scan is performed with an empty bladder and can therefore define the exact situation of the placenta. If ultrasound is not available, a diagnosis can be made during a vaginal examination to investigate the cause of bleeding but this is not recommended as it may provoke dangerous further bleeding and is not as accurate as a scan.

What happens
The main symptom of a placenta praevia is painless bleeding. This may occur at any time but is more common after Week 30. The bleeding is usually bright red, can be light or heavy, may occur with no obvious reason or might follow intercourse or straining. The first bleeds are usually light but later on the blood flow may increase and become heavier; bleeding usually stops and starts again. Some women with a placenta praevia don't experience any bleeding in pregnancy and it only occurs as the cervix dilates in labour. Major placenta praevia tends to cause bleeding earlier and may even begin before Week 20, when it is defined as a threatened MISCARRIAGE.

Bleeding occurs because the lower part of the uterus normally stretches during pregnancy as the cervix effaces and ripens before labour but the placenta cannot stretch; instead a small area of placenta separates and bleeding occurs from exposed blood vessels in the uterus. Bleeding from the placenta does not usually interfere with function.

The majority of cases of low-lying placenta occur without any obvious cause. The risk is slightly increased when previous pregnancies have been followed by gynaecological curettage operations (p.407), there have been a previous CAESAREAN SECTION or uterine surgery. The chance of placenta praevia rises with TWINS because the placenta is larger.

Action plan
Your placenta will probably function normally even though it is praevia and your baby is likely to develop and grow normally. His growth and wellbeing will be checked regularly with ultrasound and clinical examination of your abdomen. If the praevia has kept your baby's head high, he may be in a breech or awkward position (p.498), and a caesarean will be recommended. The main health risk is to you, from heavy bleeding or haemorrhage. If a placenta praevia has bled, you will be admitted to hospital so that you and your baby can be assessed. Having a placenta praevia is very taxing emotionally when there is a threat of haemorrhage, and anxiety is natural. It is common to have a false alarm before your baby needs to be born and it is very useful to have support from friends, family and your medical team.

Lifestyle
If bleeding is light or stops completely, you may be allowed home yet advised to take it easy. You must avoid sexual intercourse and heavy exercise. It is essential to have access to hospital within 15 minutes and to have an adult available 24 hours a day who can contact the services and admit you to hospital if bleeding recurs. You need to be booked into a hospital with facilities to perform emergency caesarean sections and to administer an urgent BLOOD TRANSFUSION.

Medical care
- If bleeding is significant you will have to remain in hospital until your baby is mature enough to be delivered. Depending on the blood loss and your haemoglobin level you will need iron and vitamin supplements or, rarely, a blood transfusion. The aim of your medical team will be to keep pregnancy going until your baby is not PREMATURE.
- If bleeding becomes life threatening at any time your baby will be born immediately by caesarean section and you may need a blood transfusion. The obstetrician needs to deliver the placenta carefully because it may be embedded in the wall of the uterus (PLACENTA ACCRETA, opposite). The main concern is your blood loss during and after the operation – you need to be attended by an experienced obstetrician and anaesthetist, especially if you have a higher risk of complications because of previous uterine scars or associated placenta accreta.
- If you have not bled and have a major placenta praevia, your baby will need to be born by caesarean before labour starts because the risk of bleeding as the cervix dilates makes labour dangerous.
- Intense nursing care is essential after birth to ensure your uterus is well contracted and to prevent or treat excessive bleeding from the placental site.
- If your baby is premature he will need to be cared for in a SPECIAL CARE BABY UNIT.

PLACENTAL ABRUPTION

See also BLEEDING, DURING PREGNANCY; PLACENTA PRAEVIA

This condition occurs in fewer than 1% of pregnancies when a normally positioned placenta separates from the wall of the uterus. It may be 'revealed' when blood escapes from the uterus into the vagina or 'concealed' when blood loss becomes trapped between the wall of the uterus and the placenta. Usually some blood flows into the vagina and some is retained. The most common symptoms of abruption are bleeding and pain.

Minor degrees of concealed abruption may not cause symptoms and have no effect on your baby. If the abruption is more evident it may affect placental function and your baby's growth, leading to INTRAUTERINE GROWTH RESTRICTION. Severe abruption may cause a medical emergency.

Most often, abruption occurs without an obvious cause. There are a number of conditions where the risk increases. These are: severe high maternal BLOOD PRESSURE (pre-eclampsia); increased maternal blood clotting from thrombophilia (p.408); a diet deficient in vitamins, minerals, antioxidants and essential fatty acids, particularly before conception (these deficiencies may cause inadequate placental implantation); SMOKING or taking DRUGS, particularly cocaine and crack; carrying TWINS, or an accident involving an intense blow to the abdomen. Very rarely, women have placental abruption in more than one pregnancy: it may be associated with an underlying problem such as high blood pressure, kidney disease or excessive blood clotting. In such cases, close antenatal care is essential, along with rest and good nutrition for the mother.

What happens

Placental abruption usually becomes obvious in the second half of pregnancy. If separation occurs in a small area there may be minimal symptoms. A large degree of separation causes intense bleeding and severe abdominal pain, with a tender uterus that feels hard. Blood is usually dark in colour, with or without clots. Internal bleeding may bring on contractions and labour.

If a large part of the placenta separates, oxygen exchange is reduced and your baby may suffer from severe FOETAL DISTRESS & ASPHYXIA. Heavy blood loss may be accompanied by shock and you may feel faint, cold, clammy and ill. If heavy bleeding continues, natural blood-clotting factors may be used up and bleeding can increase further. This can become a life-threatening emergency and urgent action is essential.

Action plan

Modern emergency maternity care has dramatically reduced the risks associated with placental abruption. With prompt expert intervention, almost all mothers with severe placental abruption and more than 90% of babies survive; foetal distress and PREMATURE BIRTH present the greatest risk to babies. Long delays and heavy bleeds are the most dangerous, so contact your hospital in the event of sudden pain in your abdomen or vaginal bleeding in the second half of pregnancy.

Treatment depends on how much of the placenta has separated, the amount of blood lost, your baby's wellbeing and the stage of pregnancy. Any other difficulties you are having (e.g. high blood pressure) will also be taken into account. Placental abruption is potentially life threatening and needs to be treated as an emergency, early and intensively.

- If the abruption is minor, your baby is not in distress and your own condition is stable, you may be able to go home after observation in hospital and you will be advised to rest. You will be offered frequent visits and close monitoring and ultrasound scans for the remainder of your HIGH-RISK PREGNANCY. If there are signs of reduced placental blood flow and function, your doctor may advise you that it is safest to deliver your baby early.
- If the abruption is major you will be treated in hospital as an emergency. If there is a major degree of separation, the diagnosis is usually obvious. Your doctor will give you an intravenous drip and take blood tests to ensure your blood is able to clot properly and your baby's heart beat will be monitored on CTG and ultrasound scan.
- If separation is major but your baby shows no signs of foetal distress and you are stable, your doctor may advise

induction of labour (p.497) and a vaginal delivery if you have passed Week 36. Your obstetrician will insure that your uterus contracts properly after delivery because you are at increased risk of BLEEDING AFTER BIRTH. You may require oxytocin medication to stimulate contractions.

- If your baby is showing foetal distress, your doctor will recommend immediate delivery by CAESAREAN SECTION and if birth is premature your baby may need care in a SPECIAL CARE BABY UNIT.
- If you lose a lot of blood you may need a BLOOD TRANSFUSION and require treatment for shock. If your blood is not clotting normally the clotting factors will be replaced during the transfusion. This will reduce the risk of bleeding during and after delivery as the clotting factors are made in your liver and they return to normal in a day or two.

PNEUMONIA
See COUGH & COLD: BABY

POSTMATURITY
See LABOUR, POSTMATURITY

POSTNATAL & ANTENATAL DEPRESSION
See EMOTIONS, DEPRESSION

PRE-ECLAMPSIA
See BLOOD PRESSURE, HIGH

PREMATURE BIRTH

See also EMOTIONS, ADVICE & SUPPORT; SPECIAL CARE BABY UNIT (SCBU)

Premature birth is when your baby is born before the 37th week of pregnancy (up to and including day 259 of pregnancy). In the UK, 5–10% of babies are born early. Like many parents you may be surprised if labour begins early. Even if you have time to prepare for the birth, coping with prematurity is still a challenge.

During the important last weeks of pregnancy your baby's organs mature. If birth is early, he will need to mature fully without the protection of the womb. The earlier birth occurs, the greater this challenge becomes for your baby and for the medical team, and the risks to health also increase if some of his body systems are not working optimally.

It is good to know that babies born after Week 32 usually do very well . With earlier birth the risk of complications rises, although advanced neonatal care has greatly improved the outcome. Babies born between Weeks 26 and 28 have an 80% chance of survival, with 70% of survivors having no long-term physical problems, and many babies born as early as Week 25 benefit from excellent neonatal nursing, although a larger proportion may have developmental difficulties.

Premature birth, expected or not, commonly makes parents anxious and can be frightening and upsetting. This is an entirely normal reaction that is the beginning of what may be a lengthy process of acceptance and adaptation by all the family. Being informed about what may lie ahead may help you prepare or you may prefer to take each day at a time. Part of dealing with an early birth is gathering a support network and finding which members of the medical staff understand you best. When your baby is born it may take courage to let yourself fall in love with him, particularly if he is not well and you are afraid you may lose him.

Depending on how early your baby is born, it may take days, weeks or months of care by the neonatal team to ensure he develops and reaches his full potential. Babies who have severe INTRAUTERINE GROWTH RESTRICTION (IUGR) may be born early and then need intensive care to recover from the combined effects of IUGR and prematurity.

What may cause premature birth?

The majority of premature births are not predictable, and for many the cause cannot be identified. There are, however, some pointers that may increase the possibility of prematurity. For more information on each of the following, turn to the appropriate entry.

- CERVICAL INCOMPETENCE of the valve of the cervix.
- A previous premature birth.
- A pregnancy with TWINS OR HIGHER MULTIPLES.
- Poor maternal nutrition (p.455) causing a deficiency in minerals and vitamins.
- Infection in the vagina and cervix, particularly VAGINOSIS, which can cause premature rupture of the membranes (p.501) , the most common trigger for premature labour.
- SMOKING and the use of DRUGS inappropriate for pregnancy.
- Complicated pregnancies that may warrant early delivery: PLACENTA PRAEVIA, DIABETES, high BLOOD PRESSURE and severe IUGR.

What happens: premature labour

If you believe you may be in premature labour, whatever the time of day or night, call your doctor or midwife. If you are in labour a vaginal examination will confirm your cervix has begun to dilate. You will probably have painful and regular contractions. Depending on your stage of pregnancy and your baby's wellbeing, your medical team may want to delay birth. If you need to give birth to your baby early for medical reasons, your doctor will arrange the necessary medical care.

After Week 34

If you go into labour after Week 34, your medical team will want to ensure there is no risk of FOETAL DISTRESS & ASPHYXIA and then you will be able to go ahead with an active vaginal birth. Babies born around Weeks 35–37 rarely have major problems, although establishing feeding and maintaining temperature may mean a longer hospital stay.

Before Week 34

If you go into labour before Week 34, your medical team may want to delay labour to allow time for you to be given cortisone (dexamethazone) injections to stimulate the development of your baby's lungs, thus reducing the risk of respiratory distress and BREATHING DIFFICULTIES at birth. To reduce your contractions you may be given intravenous tocolytic medication and you and your baby will be closely monitored. The medication usually delays labour for 24–48 hours, sometimes longer.

In labour

In labour, your baby's heartbeat will be monitored frequently because he is more susceptible to foetal distress, particularly if he also has IUGR. You may be anxious by unexpectedly being in labour and you will benefit from the support and some calming techniques you practised in pregnancy, such as breathing (p.346), visualisation (p.370) and massage (p.365).

Your medical team may avoid a number of procedures. Because a premature baby's skull is prone to excess moulding or bruising, it is best not to break the waters to speed up slow progress (p.502), as they protect against excess pressure. You may also be advised to avoid pethidine for pain relief (p.161) because a small baby may be very sensitive and the drug may depress breathing at birth. An epidural anaesthetic is better. Your birth team may advise delivery by CAESAREAN SECTION if your baby has a malpresentation (p.498) or shows signs of foetal distress or asphyxia because your less mature baby is less able to cope with stress caused by low oxygen supply.

Premature babies

How your premature baby copes after birth depends on how early birth is, the cause of prematurity and his weight. If your baby is born between Weeks 33 and 37 and has no underlying abnormalities, there is an excellent chance he will adapt quickly to life outside the womb and, after a short spell in a SPECIAL CARE BABY UNIT (SCBU), will be fit and feeding confidently and can come home. If he is born earlier he will need more intensive care. Smaller premature babies may be very ill and need intensive support but with advances in care, neonatal death (p.510) is increasingly rare. It is usually related to very premature babies or those who are very sick at birth.

Time together

However young or small your baby, he will benefit from your presence and loving touch. You may be able to stay with him and hold him, or your time together may be limited to a few hours a day and touching him through the sides of the incubator. It is preferable to spend as much time with your baby as your circumstances allow.

If he is very tiny in the early days you may rarely touch him but will be able to watch him. The memory of looking into your baby's eyes will stay with you when you are separated. You may want to have a photograph so you can see him when you are apart. As time passes, you will be able to lay your hands on him, gently massage his limbs and stroke his face.

When you can take him out of the incubator, you can hold him close and massage him all over and you may be able to carry him, preferably with skin-to-skin contact. This kangaroo care (p.537) has been proven to give positive results relating to a baby's recovery. It provides emotional contact between you and your baby and gives him the feeling of warmth and the sound of your breathing and heartbeat that are familiar from the womb. If you carry your baby like this, frequent feeding is easy. The neonatal team can help you and your partner. Both of you may need to take extra time off work in the first few months. This early time together is very important and it is best if it is not rushed.

Feeding and nourishing your baby

Premature babies have special nutritional needs and the younger they are, the more intense their need. A premature baby requires adequate calories, proteins, minerals, a wide range of vitamins and fluids. Breast milk is the best fluid, containing antibodies as well as all the constituents for body and brain development, and during the feed your skin provides the perfect temperature for your baby. Many babies need feeds designed for premature infants in addition to, or instead of, breast milk.

If your baby is relatively large – over 1.5 kg (3 lb 5 oz) – he may be able to breastfeed successfully. If he is smaller he may be too small to suck and will need to be fed via a nasogastric tube that is passed down his nose and into his stomach until he can breastfeed – he can be fed your milk in this way. The sucking reflex is usually present after Week 29. If he is very young and his digestive tract is still immature, he will need an intravenous drip to provide glucose and essential amino and fatty acids, which are crucial to the normal development of the brain. The exact constituents of your baby's feed will depend on his individual requirements.

Breastfeeding tips

Emotionally, many mothers feel better if they can breastfeed their babies, and they and their babies benefit from long periods of close body contact. If your baby is not able to suck from birth, you may need a high degree of motivation to keep your breast milk flowing through expressing (p.195). Many hospitals supply breast pumps and provide a private place for expressing or breastfeeding.

- Colostrum is the early milk and it is highly nutritious and it may be very useful for your baby in the early days.
- Your milk will flow more if you are able to express every 3 hours, even at night. You can freeze milk for later use but an excess is unlikely in the first weeks.
- When your baby is able to suck, your milk flow will adapt to his needs. If your baby has been taking a bottle, it may be possible to encourage him back on to your breast.
- Because your baby is small you may need to help him more as he learns to feed and latch on. If you have been expressing your milk, it may take a few days for your baby to stimulate the let-down reflex to provide the nourishing hind milk. There is no hurry and the neonatal staff will help.
- If your baby needs to be monitored, you may still be able to breastfeed while the nurses take measurements.
- In the early months your baby will be weighed frequently to check he is getting adequate nourishment. Weight gain will be charted and your neonatologist will let you know whether he needs more frequent breastfeeds and/or supplementary milk.

Special care

Babies born before Week 35 are generally cared for in a neonatal intensive care unit (p.536). If your baby is older and he is well, he may be cared for in a SCBU.

Risks for premature babies

Premature babies are at greater risk of health problems and difficulties after birth, and for any parent a list of possibilities is daunting. The risk rises for a baby born before Week 32. Some babies seem to be strong-spirited and get through very difficult stages with relative ease; others find it upsetting and hard and take longer to become independent. Below is a list of potential complications, each covered in full in this guide:

Hypoglycaemia (p.486): A drop in blood sugar, which is guarded against with appropriate feeding.

Hypothermia (p.486): A fall in temperature, which is usually prevented with the constant temperature of an incubator or through kangaroo care.

Breathing difficulties (p.417): The lungs may be immature. Ventilation assistance may be needed and a cortisone injection to boost the lungs prior to birth is often helpful.

Internal bleeding (p.407): Into the brain.

Heart abnormalities (p.477): May occur in a tiny minority and exacerbate breathing difficulties.

Infection: A risk because of an immature immune system and the need for special care treatment.

Eye & vision problems (p.465): Rarely impaired vision and retinopathy may occur.

Jaundice (p.490): Caused by an immature liver and bruising at birth.

Taking your baby home

Like most parents you may feel a mixture of excitement and anxiety when it is time to take your baby home. The SCBU will have discharge guidelines and specific details relating to your baby. Before leaving, he may be given immunisations (p.554), screening tests (e.g. vision and hearing) and you will be given guidance for any special care he still requires.

Your baby will probably be ready to come home when he is gaining weight, has a stable temperature in an open cot, can feed from a bottle or the breast without difficulty and has a mature and stable heart and is breathing well. There may be a room for you to stay with your baby before discharge.

At home it may take time for all of you to adjust and for your baby to adopt a day–night routine after the brightly lit ward. The transition is often smoother if both parents have time to be at home and with kangaroo care – this helps your baby feel secure. Equally importantly, it may help you to relax with your baby, and get used to having your baby at home.

Long-term outlook

Requiring ventilation support after birth rarely leads to long-term breathing difficulties, although ASTHMA is a little more common. Babies who have been born early do, however, tend to have more than their fair share of COUGHS AND COLDS, some no doubt due to increased susceptibility to infection.

Your baby's age is calculated from the date of birth but this does not take into account that he may have missed up to 3 months of developmental time. This is very important during the 1st year but by the 3rd or 4th year the differences disappear. Paediatricians correct for the effects of prematurity until the age of 3 years, when they conduct routine development tests. It is preferable for you to take things as they come and interact according to what your baby can do.

Premature babies thrive on close contact and mental and physical stimulation to achieve their full potential. Massage, swimming and exercise are all useful when your baby is strong enough to do them. In the SCBU your baby will have spent a lot of time lying on his back so being carried and placed on his abdomen while you're with him can be very beneficial.

Into childhood

You may be concerned about how he will catch up in terms of growth and development. It is helpful to remember there are several factors other than the timing of birth that determine weight at birth. One is inheritance – if you and your partner are tall, for instance, your baby is likely to be tall, and if you are both smaller than average, he is also likely to be small. Another factor contributing to size in the womb is IUGR.

If your baby was born weighing more than 1.5 kg (3 lb 5 oz) he is likely to catch up with other children as he grows. However, if he weighs less at the time of birth than expected and there has been IUGR, he may remain small.

Slow growth

If your baby is tiny and finds it hard to feed in the early days, he may lose weight and take up to 2–3 weeks to regain his birth weight. There is also an increased risk that he could be unwell – a sick baby may not tolerate intravenous nutrition and it may take longer to catch up. Babies in the uterus grow very rapidly during the last trimester and it is very hard for a premature baby to keep up with this pace if he is sick.

If a premature baby does not grow, or grows more slowly than usual, he will start to fall off the growth chart. Luckily, the phase of slow growth usually rights itself and soon the baby is able to put on weight as fast as a baby in the uterus.

Faster growth

When the faster growing phase begins, brain growth is given priority, next your baby will put on weight and lastly his length will increase. His body proportions differ from those of a full-term baby and this fast growth phase helps to reverse any nutritional defects as long as adequate minerals and vitamins are included in the diet. There are special milks and additives for meeting the increased nutritional needs of premature babies.

Catch-up growth

For your child to become the same size as his full-term peers, growth needs to be faster than usual. This is called catch-up growth. Some 85% of premature infants have catch-up growth and then follow a normal growth chart by 2 years of age. Catch-up growth can continue until a child reaches normal size at adolescence. Most premature babies are not below average size in adulthood. Some common reasons a child may not catch up fully by 2 years of age include:
- Starting out very far below the growth chart with a long, long way to catch up.
- Ongoing problems that increase nutritional requirements or make it hard to obtain calories if metabolic rate is increased.
- Illness and a consequential reduction in feeding.
- A tendency to have a low appetite and need ongoing encouragement to feed.

Development in childhood

Your baby will be given follow-up assessments by a paediatric team to check for problems that occur more commonly among premature babies. These include developmental delays, growth problems and vision and hearing difficulties and rare but major handicapping conditions such as CEREBRAL PALSY, mental retardation, blindness and deafness (more common among babies born before Week 25). The earlier any condition is detected, the sooner treatment can begin, and this greatly improves the outlook.

As a group, babies born prematurely are known to have poorer concentration and many need extra support when they begin school but individual children may function normally. You will probably be keen for your child to attend all the usual health checks or have extra tests. For instance, if hearing is impaired, this could delay language development. Most premature babies are referred to a 'developmental follow-up' clinic, where tests are geared to detect problems associated with prematurity. Reassessment occurs over the first 5 years as many developmental difficulties emerge slowly over time. The clinic may also be a valuable source of support for you and a place where you can meet other parents of premature babies.

RASH

See SKIN, RASHES, IRRITATION & SPOTS: BABY; SKIN, RASHES & IRRITATION: MOTHER

REFLUX

See VOMITING: BABY

RESPIRATORY DISTRESS SYNDROME

See BREATHING DIFFICULTIES: BABY

RETAINED PLACENTA

See BLEEDING, IN LABOUR & AFTER BIRTH

RHESUS FACTOR

See BLOOD GROUP, RHESUS FACTOR

RICKETS

Rickets, a decrease in bone density, is very rare in the UK where the population is generally well nourished. It is based on a deficiency either of vitamin D, or of the basic building blocks of the bones, calcium and phosphorus. It occurs rarely in PREMATURE babies, resulting in fractures and impaired growth, and respiratory distress. Vitamin D-deficiency rickets may appear in children unable to absorb the vitamin because of disorders of the bowel or the liver. Almost all babies are cured after treatment with vitamin D and calcium. Only in severe cases may there be some deformity of the leg bones with bow LEGS and knock knees.

ROSEOLA INFANTUM

Roseola infantum is a viral illness caused by herpes virus Type 6 and Type 7 that most commonly affects children aged 7–13 months. It brings on a cold or respiratory illness that may be followed by a high FEVER lasting 2–5 days. Your child may have a sore throat with swollen glands in the neck. As the fever ends, a pink, raised rash appears on the trunk. The pink-red spots turn white when you touch them, and individual spots may have a lighter area or 'halo' around them. The rash usually spreads to the neck, face, arms and legs, and fades after 1–3 days, and they can appear when a baby otherwise seems well.

Action plan
If your child becomes infected with roseola, treat her fever and keep her cool, encouraging her to drink well and rest. She will be infectious for 5–15 days following initial exposure, although the disease is not extremely contagious. Adults rarely become infected as they will have acquired immunity in childhood.

RUBELLA

Rubella is usually a mild, self-limiting disease. Most adults in the developed world have been infected or vaccinated as children and are now immune. Routine VACCINATION is available for children as part of the MMR (measles, MUMPS, RUBELLA). For the very small number of women who are infected in pregnancy, rubella carries serious implications because it may lead to foetal infection and developmental damage. This is known as congenital rubella syndrome.

Rubella infection brings on a rash of pink flat spots on the face and ears that spreads to the trunk. It is similar to the PARVOVIRUS rash, and may be accompanied by pain and swelling of the small joints of the hands, feet and knees, a slight fever and swollen lymph glands. Symptoms begin 2–3 weeks after exposure and pass in a few days. An infected person may infect others for around 1 week before symptoms begin, and for a few days after they have passed. Rubella is spread by breathing in infected particles shed into the air.

Action plan
All pregnant women are tested for rubella immunity: over 90% are immune. If your test is negative, you are 'rubella susceptible' and need to take care not to be in contact with any infected person. You may have been immunised and your antibody levels have dropped but you will still be partially immune. You will be offered vaccination after birth but not while you are pregnant. However, if you receive the vaccine while you are unaware of your pregnancy this does not imply that your baby is at risk: there have been no cases of CONGENITAL ABNORMALITIES associated with the vaccine.

- If you develop a rash, with or without other symptoms, visit your doctor. Rubella infection can be confirmed through a blood test. If your initial test is negative it can be repeated 2 weeks later to see whether antibodies develop.

- If rubella is confirmed before Week 12, your baby is highly likely to be infected. Congenital rubella brings an 80% chance of congenital abnormalities that may range from cataracts and deafness to HEART defects and learning difficulties. You will need a great deal of support as you plan for the future. Termination may be an option.
- If you become infected between Weeks 13 and 17, your baby is at risk only of deafness; infection after Week 17 carries no risk to your baby.
- If your baby is born with congenital rubella, she may have a low birth WEIGHT, a rash due to low platelets and an enlarged liver and spleen with *jaundice* and may remain contagious for months.

Rubella in a baby
In the very unlikely event that your baby gets rubella from contact with the infection after birth, reduce her FEVER with appropriate doses of infant paracetamol. Your homeopath may also prescribe remedies. Keep your baby away from any pregnant women or women planning to get pregnant. As adult infection is more common in men, it is a good precaution to warn all adults with whom you will be in contact. Recovery is usually complete, although there is a minimal risk of deafness.

RUPTURED MEMBRANES
See LABOUR, PREMATURE RUPTURE OF MEMBRANES

SHOULDER DYSTOCIA
See LABOUR, SHOULDER DYSTOCIA

SICKLE CELL DISEASE
See ANAEMIA: BABY; ANAEMIA: MOTHER

SKIN, ECZEMA: BABY

Dermatitis and eczema are often considered synonymous. Eczema is an inflammation of the skin with swelling, redness, itching or a burning sensation. Sometimes the inflammation is felt, rather than seen, as it is just beneath the skin's surface. Reddened spots, scales, crusts or blisters may be present, either alone or in combination. It usually affects the trunk and limbs.

If your baby has eczema, he will be uncomfortable when it flares up. It may also be difficult for you because eczema can be unsightly and feels scaly and strange. With treatment, eczema may be helped. Few cases persist beyond childhood, and the eczema rash does not scar. Eczema is not contagious. Up to one-fifth of school-age children have eczema and 70% are virtually clear by the time they reach their mid-teens.

What happens
Atopic eczema
Atopic or allergic eczema is thought to be hereditary. It is the most common form of eczema and is closely linked with the allergic reactions ASTHMA and hay fever. Affected people are

sensitive to allergens in the environment (p.395): the immune reaction leads to inflamed, irritated and sore skin. The most common symptom is itchiness, which can be almost unbearable, and there is often dryness. Constant scratching can cause the skin to split, leaving it prone to infection. In infected eczema the skin may crack and weep. Treatments include emollients to maintain skin hydration and steroids to reduce inflammation, plus avoidance of allergens where possible.

Allergic contact dermatitis develops when the body's immune system reacts against a substance in contact with the skin. The allergic reaction often develops over a period of time through repeated contact with the substance and is not common in infants. It may be caused by contact with detergents and chemicals or washing powders and soaps.

Cradle cap

Cradle cap (seborrhoeic dermatitis or napkin psoriasis) is a flaky rash of dry, scaly and brownish-red skin. It is a type of eczema often found on the head, but it can also affect the nappy area and the torso. Although it looks unpleasant, it is not sore or itchy and does not cause your baby to feel uncomfortable or unwell. The cause is unknown and it usually clears in a few months.

Cradle cap on the head usually responds quickly to a special shampoo, available over the counter. Other remedies include rubbing a pure oil, such as almond, olive or grapeseed oil, into the scalp. You can mix the oil – 60 ml (2 fl oz) – with 1 drop of tea tree essential oil and 1 drop of lavender.

Try a suitable homeopathic remedy – 6c, 3–4 times a day for 3 days – and then reassess. Use *Graphites* when the scalp is encrusted and weepy, the hair matted and smelly; *Lycopodium* if the rash is dry and scaly, but not infected, moves to the eyebrows and has cracks behind the ears; *Sulphur* if the scalp is dry and itchy, your baby is irritated, hot and bothered.

Action plan

To make an accurate diagnosis of a severe rash it is best to have the help of a specialist, a nutritionist or a paediatrician. There is currently no cure for eczema but there are many ways to minimise discomfort – the foundation is effective skin care. Many people find complementary therapies helpful.

Emollients

- Emollients reduce water loss from the skin. This provides a barrier and the skin becomes less dry and itchy.
- Emollients are safe to use as often as is necessary and are available in various forms including ointments for very dry skin and creams and lotions for mild to moderate or 'wet' eczema. Some are applied directly to the skin, while others are used as soap substitutes or can be added to the bath. Avoid standard soaps.
- Test a small amount on the skin first, as emollients contain substances to which some people are sensitive. You may need to try several different types before you find one that suits your baby.

Medical care

- When eczema is under control, only emollients need to be used. However, when the skin becomes inflamed, a steroid

cream often reduces inflammation. It is very rare that steroids are needed in young babies because the other forms of treatment usually work. Steroids may have side effects if used in high potency for a long time. Oral steroids taken by mouth are never prescribed under 9 months of age.
- If the skin becomes infected, an antiseptic cream may be needed, and perhaps antibiotics. Liberal use of antihistamines to discourage itching is often effective.
- In the early months, your doctor may discuss wet-wrap bandaging to soothe dry, itchy skin.

Helping your baby to be comfortable

The itchiness of eczema can be very distressing and there are some things you could try as you make your baby more comfortable and reduce his urge to scratch.
- Cotton clothing and bedding keep the skin cool and allow it to breathe.
- Using a non-biological washing powder and avoiding fabric softeners can help.
- Keep your baby's nails short and use scratch mitts if itching is very bad.
- When bathing your baby avoid soap, because it produces an alkaline reaction in the skin and removes its natural acid protection, tending to aggravate eczema. Bacteria are more likely to grow, and cause infection, in an alkaline medium.
- A few drops of natural oil (almond, wheat germ, olive or grapeseed) in the bath may nourish the skin. You could also use this for a soothing massage (p.368). Touching your baby lovingly is also very positive – many people shy away from touching the dry skin of eczema and this can undermine self-esteem.

Avoiding allergens

If you suspect or identify an allergen, you will help your baby by avoiding it or minimising exposure (p.394). When you wean your baby, do so slowly and watch for skin reactions. This is a large and complex problem.

Complementary therapies

Many people explore complementary therapies in addition to conventional treatments. It is essential to let your doctor know if you are starting another course of treatment, since interactions can occur between certain medications; it is equally important not to stop conventional treatment suddenly or without consultation. Homeopathy views eczema as a complaint of the whole system that manifests through the skin. *Calendula* cream, *Aveeno* cream and bath sachets, and *M-folia* cream and ointment can be very helpful. For specific remedies, you need to consult a homeopath. Acupuncture works to release the body's toxins.

SKIN, NAPPY RASH

Almost every baby has a rash in the nappy area at some point. Contrary to popular belief, this is not exclusively caused by the contact of urine and faeces with the skin, or by the nappy itself. A rash may also occur as a result of something your baby has eaten or it may be due to a fungal infection or an ALLERGY. The term 'nappy rash' actually covers a variety of rashes, each of which looks different. Some rashes do not seem to irritate, others itch or sting, and may become inflamed or raw. Once identified, a nappy rash can almost always be treated quickly and simply. A rash may begin or be exacerbated:

- If your baby becomes dehydrated, either in hot weather or if the house is overheated.
- If your baby is TEETHING or has a COUGH OR COLD, or another mild illness or if your baby cries a lot and becomes hot.
- If your baby is red-headed, he may be more susceptible due to an altered skin pH.
- If you are using washable nappies in which the plastic liner traps heat and moisture.
- If any nappy you use is too tight or has abrasive sections that rub his skin or you do not change it often enough.

Most rashes have a characteristic appearance, and while the prevention and treatment (right) applies to all, if you can identify the type and target the treatment, a rash is likely to clear up very soon. Complementary therapies combined with chemical or over-the-counter treatments are powerful healers.

Ammoniacal dermatitis

Faeces contain bacteria that may act on urine, breaking it down to release ammonia. This burns your baby's soft skin, producing a moist rash of angry-looking red patches around the genitals, although it seldom affects the skin creases. The skin thickens and wrinkles and then peels and becomes raw. The burn may be aggravated by cow's milk, acid water mixed with formula milk, or plastic pants. The most common cause is leaving wet and soiled nappies on for too long.

Change your baby's nappy frequently, wipe the skin with water and often expose it to air. Don't keep a wet nappy on for longer than half an hour during the day, and change a soiled nappy straight away. Apply barrier cream over the rash.

Candida albicans

The fungal infection thrush is a frequent cause of nappy rash that does not clear easily in newborn babies, causing white patches surrounded by a reddened skin starting around the anus and spreading across the buttocks. It may also affect the mouth, and often mother and baby are affected at the same time. Treatment is discussed on p.423.

Eczema

If your baby's nappy rash begins as a red area, which then becomes raised and itchy, and perhaps dry, it may be ECZEMA, which is a symptom in the skin of an allergic response (p.530).

Action plan
Preventing rashes

It is not possible to prevent your baby from ever getting a rash, but extra care will help. Keep him clean and dry around the nappy area and the rest of his skin, and be observant.

- Change his nappy regularly, roughly every 3 hours, and straight away if he has passed a stool. At night you needn't change his nappy if he has no rash and it means waking him; but when he has a nappy rash, one or two changes will help him feel more comfortable.

- Your baby's skin is delicate and might be very sensitive to detergents and soaps. Wherever possible, use mild soaps and laundry detergent – the detergent is significant if you are using washable nappies.
- Use just water to clean your baby's bottom, saving baby wipes for changes away from home. Moisturise the nappy area with a light, pure oil (grapeseed or almond), which allows the skin to breathe and improves resilience.
- Every day give your baby time without a nappy on.
- Don't give your baby cow's milk to drink before he is 1 year old. If you are breastfeeding, reduce spicy or acidic foods if these seem to irritate your baby.
- Try to avoid antibiotics if you are breastfeeding, or giving them to your baby when another approach may treat an illness. This reduces susceptibility to candida (below left).

Treating rashes

When your baby gets a rash, the priority is comfort – often simply by leaving the nappy off whenever you can – and to treat the cause. There are general steps to take for any rash.

- Clean your baby's bottom gently with just water, and let it dry well – drying in air is best.
- To soothe the area, you can use a conventional cream, such as Sudocrem, Morhulin, Vaseline, zinc and castor oil or Metanium. These are usually very effective, but only use a small amount because if you use too much, the cream will trap moisture on the skin and worsen the rash. When the rash has settled, return to pure oils (almond or grapeseed).
- Gentler creams include calendula-based creams. *Calendula* tincture is also effective – 10 drops per 250 ml (½ pint) of water for a light wash with a sponge, or 10 drops in a bath.
- Acupuncture or acupressure applied to the legs correctly can get rid of accumulated toxins.

Homeopathy

Choose a remedy according to your baby's symptoms and give it in the 6c potency, 3–4 times a day for up to 3 days and then reassess. You may also want to refer to remedies for cradle cap (p.531), which can give similar symptoms in scalp and nappy area, or ask your homeopath for a tincture.

Use *Apis* for a rash that is shiny, sore and bright red, makes your baby very restless and fidgety; *Cantharis* for severe inflammation with a burning heat, worse when your baby urinates and makes him very distressed and unable to sleep; *Mercury* when the area is moist and sweaty and your baby is salivating a lot; *Rhus Tox* for a spotty, itchy rash, worse from exposure to heat; *Sulphur* for a red rash that is markedly worse after any form of heat and is obviously itchy.

SKIN, RASHES, IRRITATION & SPOTS: BABY

Your newborn baby may have red skin in parts of, or all over, his body. This is normal and is due to a high number of red blood cells. As these are broken down there may be a slight yellowing (p.490), which usually passes by the end of the 1st week. You may also notice spots or rashes: 70% of babies have a neonatal spotty rash (erythema toxicum , below) and usually becomes soft-skinned cherubs within a few weeks.

Throughout the 1st year your baby may get a number of rashes. Sometimes their cause is not obvious and they fade almost as suddenly as they appear. Occasionally, a rash may be uncomfortable or indicate a medical condition, such as an infection, that requires treatment.

When to seek medical help
Call a doctor immediately if there is a temperature of 38°C (100.4°F) or higher; your baby has a rash and FEVER after exposure to heat (heat stroke); if a rash appears suddenly and does not fade or turn white when pressed beneath a glass – this may indicate MENINGITIS. Visit your doctor if your baby has a rash that does not disappear after 3–4 days or appears to be getting worse, or you suspect the rash is related to an infection such as CHICKEN POX, MEASLES or PARVOVIRUS.

Acne
Around 1:5 babies are born with neonatal acne (milia), often spread across the nose and cheeks. The spots may be red or have a small yellow head on them. Milia is harmless and passes within weeks with normal skin care. It does not indicate a predisposition to develop acne as a teenager.

Blue skin
Blue skin (acrocyanosis) involves a change in flow of blood with a bluish tinge to the skin, particularly in the hands, feet and around the face. There is no swelling. It is harmless and resolves when the skin is warmed. It may occur with DOWN'S SYNDROME and disappears by 1 month of age. **Cyanosis** is another condition causing blue colour to the lips and tongue due to low oxygen in the blood. This remains when a baby is warm and may indicate a HEART or lung abnormality.

Candidiasis
Candidiasis is a fungal infection that often begins as a nappy rash, causing a red area, usually flat with sharper borders and, sometimes, small pustules, usually in skin creases where there is warmth and moisture. The rash on the skin is often associated with oral thrush, with white spots in the mouth, or genital thrush. If your baby is affected you may be too. Treatment is suggested for you both on p.423.

Erythema toxicum
Erythema toxicum is a harmless newborn rash consisting of multiple red blotches with pale or yellowish bumps at the centre, which give the rash a hive-like appearance. It occurs in 70% of full-term infants. This rash usually blossoms a day or two after birth and goes within a week. It differs from acne because with acne the skin is pale and the bumps are separate from one another. Blisters containing clear fluid may suggest a *herpes* infection that will be diagnosed by a paediatrician.

Heat rash
Heat rash (prickly heat), as its name implies, is a rash that appears when your baby is too hot and sweat clogs the skin pores. Some babies develop this simply from being over-dressed or overheated in an already warm atmosphere. It

appears as clusters of little red spots and can occur anywhere on the body, often in skin folds and where clothing fits snugly – on the neck, under the arms or near the edges of the nappy. First remove unnecessary clothes. Keep your baby in a cool room and if he still appears hot, use a fan or sponge him gently with a flannel or cloth soaked in cool, but not cold, water. The rash will disappear within an hour unless your baby is still too hot. If it persists it is best to check your baby's temperature and begin to treat any fever. The rash will disappear as his temperature falls. Some viral illnesses give a fever and a rash.

Meningoccocal rash
The rash associated with meningitis is one that parents hope to be able to recognise. It consists of red spots larger than 2 mm (⅛ in) diameter, which spread rapidly and do not disappear when a clear glass is pressed to the skin. The rash almost always coincides with other symptoms, such as signs of illness.

Mongolian blue spots
Mongolian blue spots, more common among babies of black, oriental or Asian families and appearing over the lower back and buttocks, are often mistaken for bruises. In fact they are areas where the skin's pigment is blue or blue grey. They are harmless and tend to fade with age.

Naevi (birth marks)
A naevus is a mark apparent at birth or appearing within a few weeks of birth.
Vascular naevus: The most common birthmark, this is a salmon patch or 'birth stork mark' over the nape of the neck or over the eyelids. It forms because of dilated blood vessels and tends to disappear within the 1st year. The mark is not related to the birth process.
Port wine stain: A flat, red mark that is present at birth (2:1000 newborns). A stain tends to persist, unchanged, during childhood and may be associated with dilated and malformed blood vessels, under the skin. If your baby has a large, easily visible port wine stain, laser treatment may be effective.
Haemangioma (strawberry mark): Consists of dilated blood vessels that are rarely present at birth but appear within 4 weeks in 10% of babies. They tend to be more common in pre-term babies. A haemangioma begins as a barely visible small red mark that grows over weeks to form a bright red compressible area of dilated small capillary blood vessels. Growth usually stops by 12 months and the mark usually shrinks and disappears without treatment by 2 years.

Scaly rashes
In rare circumstances the skin of a newborn feels scaly, which may be caused by an inherited developmental anomaly called icthyosis, literally 'fish scales'. Your doctor may require a series of tests to establish a diagnosis. Mildly scaly skin usually responds well to an emollient cream that prevents dryness and a cream to reduce the formation of keratin, which causes the scaly appearance. Cradle cap (p.531) may appear scaly.

Urticaria (nettle rash, hives)
A red rash can commonly occur on the forehead, thighs and abdomen. It is not eczema and may wax and wane. It usually

disappears by 3 months and has raised areas. It is caused by an ALLERGY to food or to substances touching the skin. The treatment is similar to that for the allergic type of eczema (p.530).

The main homeopathic remedies used for urticaria are (6c, 3 times a day for 3 days before reassessing): *Apis* when the skin is inflamed, hot, red, itchy and looks shiny, worse from heat of any kind and much better for cold applications; *Natrum Mur* for recurrent or ongoing urticaria, usually at the joints, particularly the hands or ankles, white in appearance and perhaps linked with emotional stress; *Rhus Tox* when the rash is very itchy, can form blisters, is concentrated on forearms or hands and makes your baby restless; *Urtica Urens* should your baby get the rash from stinging nettles or another plant, bringing on white weals with a red centre. The tincture of *Urtica* is good for bathing – 10 drops in a bath or a sponge wash with water and tincture (10 drops to 250 ml/½ pint).

SKIN, RASHES & IRRITATION: MOTHER

During pregnancy your skin undergoes many changes. It stretches and the moisturising sebaceous glands that produce natural oils and the sweat glands that control heat loss become more active. It also darkens. A number of women experience uncomfortable changes, ranging from dryness or excessive oiliness, to acne and rashes. In most cases, these conditions settle after birth. Some improve greatly with attention to nutrition. Many women find skin condition improves through massage and with the use of appropriate essential oils. Common changes are covered on p.43. Other changes include:

Acne: This may arise because the sebaceous glands swell and become blocked by oily secretions due to an increase in testosterone in pregnancy. It can also reflect diet. Acne retinoid medications are contraindicated in pregnancy. The best treatment is to keep your skin clean with water and a mild, natural cleanser, and attend to your diet (overleaf).

Dry skin: The best treatment is to drink plenty of water and use a natural moisturiser (vitamin E cream is good).

Itching and irritation: This is common – up to 1:5 pregnant women complain of a generalised itch, commonly beginning over the front of the abdomen. It may begin early but it is usually most intense in the last 10 weeks. Usually itching without rash is of no concern. It can, however, be a symptom of the rare condition CHOLESTASIS, and is worth investigating.

Skin tags: These are tiny polyps that sometimes occur where skin rubs together or rubs on clothing; under the arms, beneath the bra or on the neck, for instance. They are caused by excessive growth of the superficial layer of skin, and disappear after pregnancy.

Stretchmarks: These are due to a loss of elastin fibres and an increase in collagen. They occur in the last 3 months as red marks that fade slowly months after birth. You are more likely to have them if they occur in your family, if you have a dry skin and rapid weight gain. Natural oils and creams can help skin retain moisture, and massaging stimulates the skin. This combination could minimise stretchmarks.

Skin rashes in pregnancy
If you are prone to dermatitis, acne, allergic reactions or another skin condition, it may flare up in pregnancy. Eczema may often improve. Some women develop ALLERGIES in pregnancy, and these usually clear after birth. There are also a number of pregnancy-specific skin conditions that may have an autoimmune or allergic cause. These include:

Pruritic urticarial papules of pregnancy (PUPP): The most common rash related to pregnancy, and can be severe and really itchy. It may begin on the abdomen and spread to the thighs, arms and buttocks, with angry raised spots or bumps, but does not spread to the face. The cause is not known, it presents no risks to baby or mother, may last for months and clears within weeks of birth. Sleep can be disrupted and may lead to such exhaustion that induction is considered.

Prurigo of pregnancy: More common in women who have a family predisposition to allergic dermatitis. The skin appears red, is very itchy and may form small red dots and nodules that weep. It usually begins in the second half of pregnancy, particularly in the last few weeks, on the limbs and abdomen, usually on stretchmarks. It may become worse after birth but clears in 1–3 months. It does not present any risk to the baby.

Papular dermatitis of pregnancy: An extremely itchy rash of red, raised spots that look like insect bites and are spread out all over the body. Some spots may scab over. The spots continue to appear until childbirth when they clear rapidly.

Herpes gestationis: A rare disease that is not related to the viral infection HERPES simplex. It causes pustules that may resemble the blisters of herpes or CHICKEN POX. In severe cases, it may lead to FEVER and need hospital treatment. It usually resolves in late pregnancy but may flare up after birth. Babies can be born with this rash, but it usually clears up within a few weeks without treatment.

Infections causing rashes
A number of infections may cause rashes in pregnancy and it is worth asking for a medical examination. Infections that cause rashes and may affect your baby in pregnancy include RUBELLA, TOXOPLASMOSIS, PARVOVIRUS and CYTOMEGALOVIRUS (rash on the body); herpes or another sexually transmitted infection. After birth a rash on your nipples may indicate CANDIDA, a fungal infection that can be passed to your baby, causing nappy rash (p.531) or discomfort in the mouth.

Action plan
Medical care
Ask your doctor to assess you in case the cause of the rash has implications for you or your baby. Itching without a rash, particularly of the palms and soles, needs to be investigated to exclude cholestasis, which can affect your baby.
- Your doctor may prescribe emollients to maintain skin hydration. They work in the same way as for a baby (p.531).
- If a rash is severe and does not respond to nutritional changes and gentle remedies, it may respond to cortisone that is sometimes added to skin creams. There is some absorption into the bloodstream but your baby is unlikely to be affected if a mild cream is used. For an extreme rash, steroid tablets may very occasionally be prescribed.

Diet and lifestyle

- Focusing on nutrition may improve acne, skin quality and the connective tissue. The essential main elements are antioxidants, essential fatty acids, vitamins and minerals. Ensure you are drinking enough water – 6–8 glasses a day. Avoid fried and fatty food and dairy products and eat whole grains and vegetables to provide roughage.
- Try calamine lotion or aloe vera to soothe your skin. You can moisturise it with a pure oil (lanolin-free vitamin E or grapeseed, for instance) in a light massage or in the bath. Use no unscented soaps and bathe once a day.
- Use cotton bed linen and try a different washing powder. Wear loose, cotton clothing and ensure you do not overheat.
- Avoid overheating and drying the air in your house through air-conditioning and central heating: humidifiers often help, as does additional ventilation.

Aromatherapy and acupuncture

- Use neroli, tangerine or orange oil in a bath or add to a carrier oil (almond or grapeseed) for a light massage. If you have stretchmarks, apply the oil 3 times a day. After Week 24 use lavender, frankincense and geranium in low dosage.
- Calendula cream may be soothing.
- Acupuncture can help reduce itching or dryness.

Homeopathy

For chronic skin conditions such as eczema it is best to consult a homeopath as constitutional treatment will be needed.
For stretchmarks: Use *Calc Fluor* 6x as it helps promote elasticity of the skin.
For irritating itching and rashes: The following remedies may bring some relief in 6c potency, morning and night for a week. Use *Arsenicum* for a ticklish, crawling itch that burns after scratching, dry, rough skin that may bleed from excessive scratching, usually worse after midnight and better from warmth, and makes you feel restless, anxious and chilly; *Dolichos* for itching in pregnancy without visible eruptions when the more you scratch the worse the itch, worse at night and exacerbated by warmth; *Sulphur* when the skin feels red, hot and dry and burns after scratching, your whole body feels hot, worse after contact with water, in bed and after exertion. **External applications:** *Calendula* is soothing, used in tincture form (10 drops in a bath) or in a prepared cream applied twice a day; *Graphites* cream is good when skin becomes excessively dry or cracks; *Urtica Urens* cream helps where the itching burns after scratching. It is possible to have combination creams made up by the homeopathic pharmacies.

SLEEP DIFFICULTIES: BABY

In sleep, your baby, like you, rests and gains energy for a new day and his unconscious mind processes events. He also grows while he sleeps and may become irritable and difficult if he does not get enough or has a very disrupted sleeping pattern. How he sleeps influences the entire family's life and wellbeing.

The variation in normal sleeping patterns from birth to 9 months is vast. It is covered in Part III on p.202 (0–12 weeks),

p.238 (4–6 months) and p.260 (7–9 months), with suggestions on encouraging a pattern that suits your baby. It is helpful to remember that sleep may be influenced by the spacing of meals during the day, what a baby eats, how much he stretches and exercises, his comfort, and by illness. It may also reflect his emotional state (which may mirror your own), as well as his personality – some babies sleep lightly, some dream more vividly than others, and some sleep long and deeply on all but a few occasions. If you worry about your baby's sleep, talk to your doctor in case there is an underlying illness, such as EAR or URINARY TRACT INFECTION. She may put you in touch with a sleep clinic or a support group for families who are having difficulties.

Homeopathy

If your baby is unable to fall asleep easily, give a remedy (30c) in the evening and again on first waking. Try this for 3–4 nights and then reassess. If he goes to sleep easily but wakes from around midnight, give the most appropriate remedy at the first waking time and again if he wakes subsequently. Try this for 3–4 days and then reassess. If disturbed sleep becomes an ongoing problem or if none of the suggested remedies fit the symptom picture for your baby, visit your homeopath.

Use *Aconite* if your baby seems to be woken by fear or anxiety and can be restless and jumpy even in sleep (often good for a newborn after a difficult labour); *Chamomilla* if your baby wakes frequently between midnight and 2am, seems oversensitive and is difficult to please, wails pitifully, seems desperately tired but cannot sleep, is fine while you carry him but wakes when you try to put him down; *Coffea* if he seems hyped up and excited and if you are breastfeeding and drink a lot of coffee (in which case it's best to cut down and see if your baby sleeps better); *Phosphorus* if your baby is easy-going during the day but out of sorts during the evening, tired but cannot fall asleep or wakes soon, troubled, and likes to be stroked back to sleep (these babies often develop strong imaginations as they grow older and have vivid dreams and nightmares at night; they are very scared of the dark); *Pulsatilla* if he is frightened of separation – when he wakes he may hate the dark and want soothing and contact rather than a feed; *Stramonium* for twitchy babies who have had a difficult labour, wake frequently in a panic and are jumpy and unsettled.

SMOKING

See also DRUGS, RECREATIONAL

One in 4 adults in the UK smoke cigarettes, receiving the highly addictive drug nicotine and endangering their health. Given the widespread and well-known side effects of smoking, this figure is surprising and also an indication of how extremely addictive nicotine is. Maternal smoking remains the largest cause of PREMATURE BIRTH, INTRAUTERINE GROWTH RESTRICTION, disability and death. The odds of developing ASTHMA are twice as high among children whose mothers smoke more than 10 cigarettes a day, and babies exposed to smoke (passive smokers) more frequently get coughs and colds and ear infections. Nicotine consumption during pregnancy can affect mental development in later life and predispose a child to take up smoking. For a mother, smoking increases the likelihood of developing chest and respiratory infections, heart disease, lung disease, cancer and dying prematurely.

What happens

Nicotine causes spasm of the arteries, affecting circulation, and may reduce blood flow to the placenta. Smokers inhale nicotine and carbon monoxide, which reach the baby through the placenta and block the flow of nutrients and oxygen. This may have intense effects because oxygen is needed for the normal growth of body and brain. Smoking in pregnancy interferes with a baby's growth and is linked with a high-risk of MISCARRIAGE and complications that include vaginal bleeding (p.406), early PLACENTAL ABRUPTION, premature birth and premature rupture of the membranes (p.501). Passive smoking also adds a risk to pregnancy.

Stopping smoking during pregnancy, particularly early on, reduces the effects on a baby. If you smoked before pregnancy but stop at conception there is still a slight risk of miscarriage but there is little risk to your developing foetus. After birth, smoking around a baby makes the baby a passive smoker, with all the health risks associated with active smoking. Babies have very small lungs and airways that get even smaller when they breathe smoke-filled air. It can cause COUGHS from bronchitis and pneumonia that could need hospital treatment. If you smoke, your baby ingests nicotine in the breast milk.

Action plan

You may find that becoming pregnant is sufficient to make you want to stop. If not, these 10 steps may help. There is additional advice for cutting out addictive drugs on p.451. You may need considerable support as you go through withdrawal symptoms and at first you may feel unsettled. No matter how long you have been smoking, quitting will benefit your health.
1 Set the quit date and stick to it.
2 Get help and advice.
3 If you've tried before without success, consider using low-dose nicotine replacement therapy with advice from your doctor.
4 Don't have even one puff.
5 If your partner smokes, ask him to stop with you.
6 Get rid of all cigarettes and ashtrays and never hold or light cigarettes for anybody else.
7 Avoid the people, times and places where you used to smoke.
8 Do something active when the urge hits.
9 Things will get easier as time goes by.
10 Resolve to stay a non-smoker after your baby is born.

SPECIAL CARE BABY UNIT (SCBU) & NEONATAL INTENSIVE CARE UNIT (NICU)

See also EMOTIONS, ADVICE & SUPPORT

Each year, about 10% of all babies are admitted to a special care baby unit (SCBU). The majority are born at term and have minor problems. A small number are ill, often PREMATURE, and require intensive care. Most babies admitted to the neonatal intensive care unit (NICU) are born before Week 35, have low birth WEIGHT – less than 2.5 kg (5 lb 8 oz) – or a condition that requires special care. There may be a need for continued care for babies who are not severely unwell but require specialised nursing. Larger hospitals usually have a NICU.

Very immature babies, usually under 26-weeks gestation, may require tertiary care with the most sophisticated facilities and highly trained specialists. If your baby needs to be transferred, he will travel in a portable incubator accompanied by one of the staff.

What happens

A NICU is usually brightly lit and filled with equipment. There is usually a lot of activity, with babies, doctors, nurses and parents in the same room. The babies are usually naked, except for a nappy, or they wear caps to prevent heat loss from their heads.

Your baby may have a variety of high-tech attachments that can be off-putting at first but you may soon get used to them. They may include ventilation, tubes for feeding, suction to clear the lungs and lines to monitor heartrate, breathing, oxygen tension and temperature. A 'long' intravenous line may be inserted to allow intravenous nutrition and blood sampling. Phototherapy lights help in the treatment of JAUNDICE.

The medical team

Your baby may be subjected to tests, procedures, noises and lights very different from the warm, dark, comfort of the womb and the team will do what they can to provide comfort. The role of the team is to provide the best possible environment for your baby to thrive. There have been many advances in the care of sick and premature babies, not just in technology and medicine, but also in meeting both their emotional and developmental needs. Today's high-tech treatment is designed to provide your baby with oxygen, nutrition and all the factors needed to continue his development outside the womb.

Developmental care also involves helping babies feel secure and develop normal sleep patterns, decreasing stimulation from noise, lights or procedures, and following a baby's rhythms and signals so care can be given when the baby is awake and least stressed. Change based on research into developmental care is bringing all manner of benefits for premature babies, including shorter hospital stays, fewer complications, improved weight gain, better feeding and enhanced bonding.

The neonatal team are likely to be very encouraging if you wish to be involved. They will help you to change nappies, wash and feed your baby, while they gently act as supervisors, and encourage you to breastfeed and express milk (p.195). They know that it will take you time to get used to SCBU jargon and understand that you may need to ask many questions. As your baby's medical needs diminish and you become more confident, your mothering role will increase.

If you are not happy about some aspect of care, it may be difficult to question or criticise those on whom your baby's life depends, but if you express your concern tactfully you will fulfil your obligation to yourself and your baby. The unit may offer an independent counsellor or parent representative who can help you present your views to the staff. Most parents get on well with many of the staff and keep in contact for months or years after discharge.

Your feelings

While you may feel relieved that the intensive care is available for your baby, you may also be frightened and upset. Some parents feel angry if something went wrong, some feel ashamed their baby is so small and fragile. You may feel guilty and resort to a string of 'If onlys'. This is a common reaction. You and your partner will need support and advice about whether your feelings are reality-based as you go through an emotional period.

It may be difficult to allow yourself to fall in love with a tiny baby who requires intensive medical help and who may not survive. In the short term you may find it easier to remain objective and rational. Once outside the high-tech environment of the SCBU, it may be easier to go into your range of feelings. Research suggests that emotional expression helps parents to accept the reality of the situation and move forward and bond with their babies. If you feel supported, then you will have more emotional strength and reserves for your baby.

There is no doubt that it is better to bond with and love your baby even if he does not survive. If your baby is in care for several weeks, support may diminish as family and friends become more involved in their own lives. But you will still need to care for yourselves to keep your energy going, and you may need to rely more heavily on the medical team and counsellors.

You and your baby

Parenting a premature or sick baby is a very stressful experience. You may be worried about long-term effects on his physical and mental development. You may also be worried about bonding if you do not have close contact in the first few hours and days. Yet relationships and love develop over time. One of the characteristics of the human brain is plasticity and the ability to adapt to circumstances and you will have opportunities to make up for a period of separation. Young babies are very sensitive to being touched and you will be shown how to hold, stroke and massage your tiny baby. Being with him, offering love and encouragement, gentle touch and eye contact, are powerful ways to cement your relationship in hospital. If you are separated because the hospital is far from your home, you might find that a photograph of him is comforting while you are away.

Fathers

Fathers are very important after a premature or traumatic birth. As a father you offer support to the mother and to your baby. In the early days you may spend extra time visiting your baby, particularly if your partner is unwell. Your strong feelings may or may not be similar to hers, and could include anger at lack of action or a medical mistake that might have led to the need for special care. You also need support and gentle encouragement to acknowledge and process your feelings.

A father often sees his role as the technical supporter and is keen to know the practical issues of care. It may take time to accept that some aspects of care are based on opinion rather than hard scientific facts: if you need explanations it may be best to arrange to meet the senior member of staff, particularly if you usually visit when they have gone home. Another aspect of your managerial role may be to create a schedule that allows you and your partner to visit your baby, together and separately, and to relax and find time to spend with one another. Parenting a sick baby can put strain on a partnership and time together may be the first and most important step towards maintaining closeness.

Siblings

Your older children may feel very confused. They were expecting a baby and were probably not expecting you to be away for any length of time. Even if your children are very young, spend time telling them what happened. They may not understand the details but will sense from the tone of your voice how you feel. Explain that you love and adore them and your new baby needs your attention, and a special room and nurses to help her. The NICU may agree to siblings visiting; you or the nurses can explain about all the wires and tubes and it may be possible for your older children to touch your baby. You may have a present waiting for your older child when she comes to visit and you might like to give her something to give the new baby.

A long hospital stay

Hospitals differ in their policy about when babies are able to go home. A baby who is very healthy but small will be discharged at a lower birth weight than a baby who is unwell. Usually babies who have been born prematurely need to weigh over 2 kg (4 lb 7 oz) before they go home, unless the system of 'kangaroo' is in operation.

Kangaroo care originated in Columbia in the late 1970s and has been adopted world wide because of the advantages for premature babies. Kangaroo care means holding a baby skin-to-skin (against your chest) for varying lengths of time. Premature and sick babies that 'kangaroo' appear to relax and become content. Numerous studies have shown that it has many health benefits that include higher blood oxygen levels and improved sleep, breastfeeding and weight gain. Kangaroo care also helps parents feel close to their baby, and gives them confidence in their ability to meet their baby's needs. Mothers who 'kangaroo' also show improved breast milk production.

Coming home

Most pre-term infants, even those with very complicated problems, go home. The transition may lead to a withdrawal state for you and your baby. If there has been a lack of day–night rhythm because the lights are on for 24 hours in the SCBU, your baby's sleep pattern will reflect this and it will take time to change. You may feel nervous without the back-up of nurses. You and your baby will begin a new stage as you have more contact, and get to know one another more deeply. You will mirror one another: your baby will reflect your mood in his behaviour, feeding, crying and overall development, and you will be affected by his mood, and rhythms.

Different babies vary in their response to the treatment they received. Some take the difficulties in their stride while others show signs of strain by being irritable and crying a lot. Massage and cranial osteopathy combined with lots of contact are a great help. It may take a few weeks to settle at home and it is important for your baby to be held and carried in a sling with warmth and body contact to make up for the isolation of the incubator. Sharing a bed can also be a lovely way to get to know your baby and for him to feel comfortable.

SPINA BIFIDA & NEURAL-TUBE DEFECTS

See also CONGENITAL ABNORMALITIES

Neural-tube defects are serious congenital abnormalities that involve incomplete development of the brain and spinal cord. If the embryo's neural tube (which develops into the brain, spinal cord, and vertebral column) fails to form properly during the first 4 weeks of development, this results in varying degrees of permanent damage. The reason for incorrect formation is not clear. Spina bifida is the most common of the neural-tube defects and it is the most frequent disabling birth defect, although folic acid supplements reduce the incidence. The other two neural-tube defects are anencephaly and encephalocoele. Around 1:1000 babies are affected.

What happens

In spina bifida the spinal cord is not protected in the bony spinal column. **Spina bifida occulta** is the mildest form where one or more vertebrae are malformed but they are covered in skin. It affects roughly 5% of people, and most are unaware of it and it causes no problems. The membranes around the spinal cord or even the cord are exposed in more severe forms. This is a **meningocoele**. **Anencephaly** results in an incomplete skull and underdeveloped brain, and a baby will not survive after birth. **Encephalocoele** is a hole in the skull through which brain tissue protrudes; most babies with this do not live.

With spina bifida and a meningocoele there may be nerve damage with either loss of motor power (paralysis) or sensation (numbness). The effect is related to the number of vertebrae involved and the level of the spinal defect and may include bladder and bowel dysfunction, muscle paralysis and orthopaedic problems including spinal curvatures, hip dislocation or club feet (p.466). Some children born with spina bifida walk without assistance; others need braces and some require a wheelchair. About 80% with severe defects develop hydrocephalus, where the cerebral spinal fluid builds up, causing pressure within the brain and an enlarged HEAD, and may also have learning difficulties. A small number have difficulty feeding and swallowing.

Action plan

Prevention
Taking folic acid before and during early pregnancy reduces the risk of neural-tube defects. It is best to take 400 mcg of folic acid every day before becoming pregnant. Nutritionists believe other vitamins and minerals are also important for normal

development and a well-formulated multivitamin and mineral supplement is preferable to folic acid alone. In future, bread may be fortified with folic acid. If you have a previous pregnancy with a neural-tube defect or have spina bifida yourself, you need a higher dose of folic acid. It is best to consult your doctor before becoming pregnant. Do not take the extra by taking more multivitamins because too much of some of the other vitamins could be harmful (p.343).

Prenatal diagnosis and care
Antenatal ultrasound scanning is increasingly accurate in detecting neural-tube defects. Severe defects may show at the 12-week scan; smaller defects are visible on later scans. AMNIOCENTESIS & CVS are not used to diagnose neural-tube defects. If your baby shows signs of a neural-tube defect, you will need the advice of your obstetrician, paediatrician or genetic counsellor, and considerable support. The medical team will discuss the potential effect on your baby's future and options for surgical treatment. You may elect a termination of pregnancy. Foetal surgery at around Week 25 is being tried but the long-term results are not known and there are risks, including PREMATURE BIRTH.

After birth
Babies with spina bifida require extensive health evaluations and treatment after birth. The treatments range from surgery to ongoing care in a stimulating and loving environment. Babies with open spina bifida usually have surgery within 24–48 hours of birth to repair the spinal cord, skin defect and treatment for hydrocephalus if needed. This reduces the damage, although it frequently cannot prevent some permanent disability. A baby may require multiple operations. Most children born with spina bifida live well into adulthood as a result of sophisticated medical techniques and are able to join in normal life, displaying a sense of fun and love. If massive hydrocephalus is not present at birth, intelligence is often normal but some children with spina bifida do experience learning problems.

STILLBIRTH
See LOSS OF BABY: STILLBIRTH

STREP B OR GROUP B STREPTOCOCCUS

Strep B (Group B streptococcus) infection is borne by one of many bacteria that live naturally in the human gut. Approximately 25% of women carry it in their vagina. The risk of a baby developing a Strep B infection decreases with age – it is maximal in PREMATURE newborns, less common in full-term babies, rare after 1 month of age.

What happens

Few Strep B carriers are aware of it; occasionally it causes a VAGINAL DISCHARGE or a URINARY TRACT INFECTION. It may also cause a postnatal pelvic infection. The vast majority of babies whose mothers have the infection do not become infected. The small number who do acquire Strep B (less than 1% of those at risk) do so during birth by inhaling or swallowing vaginal secretions, and show symptoms within 2 days. Strep B is the most common severe neonatal bacterial infection, affecting 1:1000 babies. Premature babies where the membranes ruptured for many hours before birth (p.501) are at increased risk. The typical signs of infection include grunting, poor feeding, lethargy or irritability and abnormally high or low temperature, rapid heart rates or breathing rates.

The infection presents the greatest risk to the small number of babies who develop signs more than 2 days after birth when it may lead to septicaemia or MENINGITIS. Of these babies, roughly 33% have long-term effects. The warning signs of late-onset Strep B infection may include FEVER, poor feeding and/or VOMITING, change of consciousness, a shrill cry or whimpering, dislike of being handled, a tense or bulging fontanelle, jerking movements or floppiness, altered breathing patterns, and pale or blotchy skin.

Routine testing for Strep B in pregnancy is not current in all UK hospitals, and is not 100% accurate. Your baby is three times more likely to be exposed to Strep B and, if susceptible, to develop the infection if: Strep B has been discovered in your urine or vagina at any time during or before pregnancy; you have the organism and your baby is born prematurely; you have the organism and premature rupture of the membranes (before Week 37); you have the organism and the membranes rupture more than 18 hours before the onset of labour; you have a raised temperature that is 37.8°C (100°F) or higher during labour.

Action plan
Pregnancy and birth
If you test positive for Strep B or have been positive in the past, antibiotic treatment in pregnancy is unlikely to be effective. Once the bacterium has colonised your intestines, antibiotics do not eradicate it. You will be advised to receive intravenous antibiotics from the onset of labour, or if the membranes rupture and your waters have broken, until birth. A minimum of 4 hours is recommended from the initial injection. This is effective in preventing most Strep B infections in babies and is also advised if you have previously had a baby with Strep B. The usual antibiotic is penicillin or amoxicillin but there are alternatives for allergic people.

After birth
- The Strep B bacteria can be passed through touch, so it is very important that all adults make sure their hands are clean before handling your newborn baby.
- If you have tested positive in pregnancy, your newborn baby will be checked by a paediatrician. He will not require treatment unless there are clear indications of infection. If you have not been able to receive antibiotics for at least 4 hours prior to delivery and the membranes have been ruptured for a significant time, he may be offered antibiotics until the doctors are certain that he is not infected. Opinions vary and many paediatricians do not recommend routine antibiotic treatment in these circumstances.
- More than 2 days after birth if your baby shows signs

consistent with late onset Strep B infection or meningitis (left) call your doctor immediately. Early intensive treatment could prevent potentially serious consequences.

SUDDEN INFANT DEATH SYNDROME (SIDS)
See LOSS OF A BABY, SUDDEN INFANT DEATH SYNDROME (SIDS) & NEONATAL DEATH

SWELLING (OEDEMA)

During pregnancy the amount of water in your body increases. Oedema occurs when extra fluid seeps out of the cells into the tissues and causes them to swell. It can be a common but completely harmless side effect of pregnancy but may indicate pre-eclampsia (p.410) so it is important to investigate it. If you swell, press the skin over your shinbone. If there is a white, pitted mark that lasts for over 30 seconds, it is oedema. If you feel bloated this may be connected to FLATULENCE from poor digestion.

What happens
Oedema is more common with TWINS, if you are overweight (p.455) or if your family has a tendency to retain fluid. Swelling in pregnancy often settles after birth. It can be worse in hot weather and after standing for a long time, and increases towards term, reducing when you rest in bed at night. After birth, as excess body fluid is excreted, your legs may swell excessively for 2–3 days.

Sometimes oedema relates to a cause that needs treatment. It may be a symptom of pre-eclampsia, also indicated by a puffy face, high BLOOD PRESSURE, protein in the urine, headaches or abdominal pain. A rare cause of oedema is kidney disease: regular urine tests assess this. Oedema can be associated with varicose veins (p.559). Swelling of one calf, with pain, may indicate deep vein thrombosis (p.560).

Action plan
Visit your doctor if you have a sudden increase in swelling, pain or facial puffiness.

Exercise, yoga and diet
- Exercising improves circulation and redistributes retained fluids – walking is very effective. Swelling is often most marked in the legs, feet, hands and abdomen, so you may choose yoga postures and exercises that encourage circulation in these areas.
- As part of a good diet (p.332), exclude excess salt and include 6–8 glasses of water a day (not tea, coffee or fruit juice) to help your kidneys eliminate excess fluid.
- Herbs and vegetables that assist kidney function include celery, dandelion, nettles and cleavers. Fennel is good for reducing bloating and can be added to most dishes, but should not be taken in concentrated form in pregnancy.
- Essential fatty acids and fish oils may help oedema associated with pre-eclampsia.

Posture

- When you rest, lie on your side as often as possible: this enhances kidney function. Try to do this several times a day for 20–30 minutes each time, and at night.
- If your legs are bloated, don't cross them and rest with them raised when you can. This reduces pressure on the veins draining the extremities. You might find support tights comfortable, particularly if you have varicose veins.

Homeopathy

For oedema in your ankles, feet, hands and fingers: use *Apis* when you cannot tolerate heat in any form, your fingers and toes may swell quite severely and you feel stinging or burning in the affected area, worse from 3 to 5pm and better with cool applications, cool bathing, cool air; *Natrum Mur* if there is a feeling of heaviness with swelling that may also be in the legs, you feel restless and want to keep moving the swollen area, worse from heat and after eating, better from rubbing the area and after perspiring. Take the remedy that suits your symptoms in 6c, 4 times a day for 4–5 days, then reassess.

If you have swelling of the vulva: Use *Ferum Met* if you feel swelling and pulsation, are over sensitive and better from moving slowly; *Sepia* if you have a strong bearing-down sensation as if everything were about to fall out from the vagina, a sensation of congestion and feel better from exercise. Take either in 6c, 3 times a day for 3–4 days and then reassess.

Aromatherapy

Try sandalwood, patchouli and from Week 24 lavender and geranium (geranium needs to be in low dosage) in a bath or diluted with a carrier oil and used for massage.

SYPHILIS

Syphilis is an uncommon sexually transmitted disease (STD) caused by the bacterium *Treponema pallidum*. Fortunately syphilis can be treated during pregnancy. The primary stage of syphilis is usually marked by sores (called chancres) appearing, which are similar to HERPES but less painful and last 3–6 weeks. If antibiotics are not administered, the infection progresses to the secondary stage in months, marked by a non-itchy rash, FEVER, swollen lymph glands, weight loss and tiredness. Without treatment, the infection progresses in years to the tertiary stage with damage to organs, including the brain and the nerves. There is around a 40% chance that your baby may die, leading to a stillbirth (p.509). There is a similar risk of congenital syphilis with FITS, developmental delay, skin and mouth sores, infected bones, ANAEMIA, JAUNDICE, or a small HEAD (microcephaly). These can be prevented with treatment.

Action plan

Standard blood analyses of pregnant women in the UK test for syphilis. If your test appears positive, you may be offered a second test to verify the result. A single dose of penicillin is enough to treat an infection less than 1 year old but for long-term infection you will need a course of antibiotic injections. If you are allergic to penicillin, other antibiotics can be used. A low level of antibodies will stay in your blood for years after treatment. There are no over-the-counter treatments. It is sensible to be tested for other infections including CHLAMYDIA, GONORRHOEA and HIV. At birth, a sample of your baby's cord blood may be sent to confirm there is no infection and he may be given follow-up blood tests at 1 and 6 months. If infected, he can be successfully treated with antibiotics.

TAY-SACHS DISEASE

Tay-Sachs disease is a fatal genetic disorder in which harmful quantities of a fatty substance called ganglioside GM2 accumulate in the nerve cells in the brain. The condition is caused by insufficient activity of an enzyme called hexosaminidase A. It is more common in Ashkenazi Jewish families and can be detected through a blood test taken before or during pregnancy. Babies with the disease appear to develop normally for the first few months after birth. Then, as nerve cells become distended with fatty material, a relentless deterioration of mental and physical abilities occurs. The child becomes blind, deaf and unable to swallow.

Patients and carriers of Tay-Sachs disease can be identified by a simple blood test that measures hexosaminidase A activity. Both parents must be carriers in order to have an affected child. When both parents are found to carry a genetic mutation in hexosaminidase A, there is a 25% chance with each pregnancy that the child will be affected and an AMNIOCENTESIS is advised. If your baby is diagnosed with Tay-Sachs, you will be offered counselling as you consider the implications for the future. Presently there is no treatment. Children with Tay-Sachs disease usually die by age 5.

TEETH & GUMS: MOTHER

It is a myth that a woman loses a tooth for each child she bears in today's society with a combination of improved nutrition and lifelong dental care. Even so, many women experience oral and dental problems during and after pregnancy. The most common is gum inflammation, or gingivitis. Vomiting may encourage erosion and loss of enamel but holes occur as a result of poor dental hygiene, not as a result of pregnancy. Mouth ulcers tend to become less common in pregnancy.

Pregnancy gingivitis

Gingivitis causes very red gums that are often swollen, shiny and tender and bleed when brushed or hard foods are chewed, together with bad breath or a bad taste in your mouth. Symptoms often begin in the 2nd trimester, reaching a peak by the 8th month. Hormones and increased blood flow can cause swelling but the main cause of gum disease is the bacteria in dental plaque that settle where the teeth meet the gums. Bacteria are likely to build up if you snack on or drink high-sugar foods and neglect oral hygiene. If your gums are soft because of gingivitis, you may also notice your teeth moving slightly. This usually returns to normal in the postnatal period.

Action plan

There is nothing about being pregnant that unavoidably jeopardises the health of teeth and gums and it is as important as ever to look after your dental health with attention to oralhygiene and what you eat.

Diet

Sugars are easily fermented and can combine with harmful bacteria in the mouth and the sticky layer of plaque on the teeth. The combination results in the production of acid, which can dissolve the minerals in the enamel and dentine of teeth.

- If you eat a sugary snack between meals, rinse your mouth with water or brush your teeth. If you need to eat between meals, nibble on raw vegetables or fruits that encourage saliva flow, which helps to balance acid levels in the mouth.
- Avoid sugary drinks, particularly carbonated colas, as well as sweets (including minty 'breath fresheners').
- Avoid SMOKING, which can cause gum disease.

Dental care

- Continue to care for your teeth with brushing and flossing morning and night. Your dentist can advise on toothbrushes and flossing techniques.
- If you vomit, use a soft toothbrush and don't brush every time because too much brushing can erode enamel and dentine. Rinsing with a dilute neutral fluoride solution is refreshing and helps to re-mineralise softened tooth tissue.
- See a dentist twice in pregnancy and regularly after birth so early signs of gingivitis can be spotted. Your dentist (perhaps with a dental hygienist) may remove plaque to guard against cavities and gum disease.
- If you have cavities, it is safe to have them treated while you are pregnant. The care is generally free to women in the UK during pregnancy. Avoid x-rays if possible, although they can be done if necessary while you are screened with a lead apron to protect your baby. It is safe to have a local anaesthetic – the amounts that enter your bloodstream will not affect your baby. Filling material presents no risks to you or your baby.
- If you have pain or infection, ensure that medications are safe for pregnancy.
- In the 3rd trimester turn slightly on your side in the dentists's chair so the pressure of your uterus is directed away from the big blood vessels that run along the back of your abdomen.
- If you have not visited your dentist in pregnancy and discover after the birth that you have gingivitis, a programme of 3-monthly cleaning and plaque removal combined with a healthy diet and good brushing and flossing can help your gums return to normal.

TEETHING

Very few babies are born with any teeth. Most wait for 2–3 months or longer before feeling the first pangs of teething. Although some babies are unaffected most have symptoms commonly including general grumpiness and crying, sore ears, reluctance to eat, dribbling, red cheeks and red gums, waking in the night and fussiness over feeding, and some can seem frantic with pain. Often, teething is accompanied by nappy rash (p.531), a COUGH or even a FEVER – whether these are coincidental or related to teething cannot be certain. Some doctors say that teething simply produces teeth, and that all other symptoms just happen to occur at the same time. Whatever your view, don't forget that your baby may co-incidentally develop a common illness. If you are concerned, visit your doctor.

What happens

The first teeth to appear are usually the lower or upper front teeth, some time after 6 months, but perhaps earlier or considerably later. Variation is normal and a baby may get 3–4 bottom teeth before the top teeth come through. The other teeth appear progressively, with a full set by the age of 3 years. As a tooth emerges, the gum may appear red and swollen. Sometimes your baby may show all the signs of teething and then calm down hours or days later without a new tooth. Often the first teeth cause the greatest irritation, and molars may erupt (from 13 months onwards) with considerable pain. All baby teeth are replaced by adult teeth from 6–7 years of age.

Action plan

Every baby is different when it comes to teething, and some remedies may work some, but not all, of the time.
- Cooled or frozen rubber teething rings can give relief.
- Try rubbing ice on sore gums.
- Teething (anaesthetic) gel available in chemists may help.
- If your baby is eating finger foods, chewing on a piece of apple, dried fruit or a crust of toast may give her relief.

Homeopathy

For acute teething use 30c potency, 2-hourly for the first 8 hours and then repeat 3–4 times a day for 3 days. Then reassess – if there is no improvement, consult a qualified homeopath. While teething, your baby could benefit enormously from constitutional treatment. Her inherited immunity from you starts to wane around 6 months, so if her system is stressed by teething she may be more susceptible to other ailments.

Chamomilla is the no. 1 remedy, good if the gums are inflamed and your baby is clearly in pain, is sensitive, irritable, wants something then refuses it, cannot be pacified, has one flushed cheek and one pale, may be colicky and have watery, greenish stools and is better for being carried and having something in her mouth. Use *Arnica* for gum inflammation and pain (may be given in addition to another remedy); *Belladonna* for teething accompanied by a fever and distress with symptoms that occur suddenly and intensely, a flushed face, red gums, hot mouth, perhaps ear pain (usually on the right), a hot head and cold feet, worse for sudden movement and bright light; *Pulsatilla* if teething is accompanied by ear problems, congestion and yellowish mucus with snuffling, crying, clinginess and improvement after fresh air. If teeth are appearing late, and there may be digestive problems, particularly with wind or DIARRHOEA *Calc Phos* can be given with another teething remedy, in low 6x potency morning and night for up to 2 weeks.

Caring for your baby's teeth

Primary tooth development begins between the 2nd and 3rd month of pregnancy, and permanent teeth begin to form several months before birth. It is important for you to eat a well-balanced diet with enough protein, calcium, phosphorus and vitamins (especially A, C and D). After birth even before your baby's teeth push through her gums, and certainly once they appear, they are vulnerable to decay (evident if there are white, yellow or brown spots that won't brush off or if a tooth seems sensitive to hot or cold liquids).

Limit or avoid sweets and sweet drinks. Remember that a bottle of juice or milk in bed allows liquid to pool in the mouth, providing an environment for bacteria to grow. If your baby enjoys drinking from a cup, encourage her to let go of the bottle by around 12 months because sucking on it is more likely to encourage tooth decay. Not all parents or health professionals agree with this approach, however, as some babies benefit enormously from the soothing effect of sucking.

Once your baby's first teeth appear, clean them with a wet cloth, a moistened cotton-wool bud or very soft baby toothbrush. Do not use toothpaste at first – the early days are to get your baby used to a dental-care routine with a 'brush' morning and night (with the evening clean most important). Introduce baby toothpaste gradually, in small amounts. Cleaning is essential because however careful you are about what and when your baby eats and drinks, bacterial plaque will continually form and needs to be removed.

Fluoride supplementation is recommended from 6 months onwards in areas where there is not enough fluoride in the water. You can check levels with your water board – too much fluoride can be more harmful than too little.

TESTICLES, SWOLLEN

A **hydrocoele** is a collection of fluid around the testicle in the scrotum that affects about 20% of all newborn males. The swelling is painless. In pregnancy fluid from the abdomen passes through the neck of a balloon-like structure that runs along the spermatic cord and around the testicle. If it fails to close as usual, fluid continues to seep through and causes swelling. This usually settles in a few months. Hydrocoeles require repair if swelling is still present after 2 years, which is the case for 1:1000 boys affected at birth. If it has a big enough opening, a HERNIA can occur. To check, your doctor will hold a torch behind the scrotum – if the light does not shine through, a hernia is present.

TESTICLES, UNDESCENDED & RETRACTILE

During foetal development a boy's testicles form inside the abdomen and around Week 36 they descend into the scrotum through the inguinal canal. One testis is normally higher than the other. When a testicle does not move, it is undescended and sometimes it only moves partly down. This happens in

1:125 boys. In 15% of cases both testicles are involved. In boys with undescended testicles, 50% descend by 6 weeks, 66% by 3 months and 75% by 9 months, all without intervention. After 9 months, referral to a paediatric surgeon is recommended. If a testicle remains within the abdomen, the higher body temperature may inhibit normal sperm production and future fertility. An undescended testicle is also frequently associated with inguinal HERNIA, and is more vulnerable to injury.

Retractile testicles

This occurs when a testicle has moved into the scrotum but then moves into the groin because it is pulled up by the cremaster muscle. The testicle(s) will reappear when the outside temperature is warmer, perhaps when your baby is in a warm bath. This condition requires no treatment as retraction is a normal reflex pattern in response to a cold temperature.

Action plan

If an undescended testicle is suspected, your doctor checks for a retractile testicle. If one or both remain undescended, an ultrasound scan can check the location. The testis may be in the inguinal canal on the way to the scrotum (85%) or remain in the abdomen (15%). You may be advised to wait to see if the testes descend of their own accord. Be observant for swelling in the groin, which may indicate an inguinal HERNIA: this needs prompt treatment. If there is no descent by the end of the 1st year, surgery can bring the testis into the scrotum. The procedure causes little discomfort. When your child gets older, let him know that he needs to examine his testicles periodically – there is a tiny increased risk of testicular cancer with undescended testicles, which is reduced by surgery in infancy.

Very rarely (1%), a testis may be absent. This may be because of torsion (twisting) in pregnancy that cuts off the blood supply, or an indication of a sex chromosome disorder or ambiguous GENITALIA: a specialist paediatric urologist needs to look into this. **Testicular torsion** is caused by an abnormality of the covering that allows it to twist within its sac. It is mainly a problem in boys over 7 years old but can happen in babies on rare occasions. Twisting can cut off the blood supply, bringing pain and swelling of the scrotum and endangering the testis, and is a surgical emergency.

THALASSAEMIA
See ANAEMIA: BABY; ANAEMIA: MOTHER

THRUSH
See CANDIDA

THYROID: BABY

See also CONGENITAL ABNORMALITIES

When your baby has a heel prick test (p.226) in the 1st week after birth (day 5–7) one of the conditions she will be tested for is **congenital hypothyroidism**. The disorder results in an underactive thyroid gland so levels of thyroxin hormone are low. Thyroxin is essential for development. Screening is vital because early treatment of the disorder is important.

Around 1:4000 Caucasian babies and 1:30,000 non-Caucasian babies are affected in North America and Europe. Among these, some babies have temporary congenital hypothyroidism, which gives similar symptoms. The treatment for both is the same. After the age of 2 or 3 years medication can be reduced to ascertain whether the condition is permanent and, if it is, replacement of the thyroid hormone is then needed for life. Rarely, the thyroid gland is absent.

What happens

In most cases there is no specific reason why the thyroid gland did not develop normally, although occasionally the disorder may be inherited. Babies with congenital hypothyroidism often appear normal at birth, usually because they have a small amount of functioning thyroid to get them going in the first few weeks or thyroxin comes across the placenta. Some have symptoms: reluctance to feed, JAUNDICE that does not clear, a puffy face with a flattened bridge of the nose and occasionally a swollen tongue, low muscle tone, persistent CONSTIPATION, umbilical HERNIA and failure to gain WEIGHT. The long-term effects include reduced mental and physical development.

If the standard heel prick tests shows normal thyroid function, you will probably not be informed. With a positive test result another confirmatory blood test is usually done, and your baby may be given an ultrasound scan that examines the state of the thyroid gland.

Action plan

Treatment involves replacement of the missing thyroid hormone in pill form. It is extremely important that these pills be taken because thyroxin is essential for all the body functions and for intellectual development. Your paediatrician will prescribe a dosage that suits your baby's weight and current thyroid function. The pill can be crushed, then administered in a small amount of water or formula or breast milk. Thyroxine should not be mixed with soy formula as this product interferes with its absorption. With early replacement of adequate thyroid hormone and proper follow-up and care, the outlook for most children is excellent.

Graves disease

In Graves disease the antibodies that stimulate the mother's thyroid may pass into the foetal circulation and rarely neonatal thyrotoxicosis occurs. It usually does not begin until 7–10 days after birth if the mother is on medication. The condition may be severe and cause failure to thrive, jaundice and a variety of other symptoms. The diagnosis depends on the doctor making a link with the mother's thyroid problem, and an affected baby needs intensive medication to prevent a severe illness. Thyroid antibodies can be measured in the mother's blood during pregnancy to predict neonatal thyroid overactivity.

THYROID: MOTHER

The thyroid gland in the neck produces thyroid hormones that act as a metabolic thermostat. Thyroid hormones cross the placenta and are important in early foetal development, and it is important they are kept at normal levels. When a thyroid gland does not function optimally, it may be over or under active. Thyroid hormones contain iodine and if there is a deficiency in the diet, which is rare in Europe because the food manufacturers add iodine to salt, the gland may enlarge. This is called a goitre. Thyroid function is easy to measure with a simple blood test. Rarely, a thyroid disorder in a mother may result in abnormal thyroid function in a baby.

Thyroid overactivity

Approximately 2:1000 pregnant women have an overactive thyroid (thyrotoxicosis/hyperthyroidism). It is most commonly caused by an autoimmune disorder called Graves disease where the immune system produces antibodies that stimulate thyroid hormone production. A diagnosis is usually made before pregnancy where there is swelling in the neck that may be accompanied by swollen bulging eyes, insomnia, palpitations, feeling anxious and weight loss.

Action plan
Medical care

- It is preferable to begin treatment before conception with tablets that decrease the excess thyroid output. This improves fertility and reduces the risk of MISCARRIAGE. Sometimes the excessive activity is reduced by the injection of radioactive iodine, which is taken up by the thyroid and the radiation destroys the cells. Although a very effective treatment, it should never be given during pregnancy because the baby's thyroid gland could be damaged and it is only used if drug treatment is not successful.
- In pregnant women, propylthiouracil is the safest drug. Because it can also affect the baby's thyroid gland, it is very important to be monitored closely with blood tests so the dose can be adjusted.
- Some of the symptoms caused by too much thyroid hormone, such as tremor or palpitations, can be improved by beta-blockers. These are useful to control symptoms rapidly and to enable the dose of propylthiouracil to be reduced.

Thyroid underactivity

About 3:1000 women of childbearing age develop thyroid underactivity (**hypothyroidism**). However, it often remains undetected because there may be no obvious physical signs or symptoms. The underactivity is usually caused by the development of antibodies against the thyroid gland in a condition called autoimmune thyroiditis (**Hashimoto's disease**). An overactive thyroid gland may, over time or with surgical or radioactive thyroid treatment, become underactive. An underactive thyroid can cause weight gain, tiredness and depression and may cause infertility and recurrent miscarriage if untreated. Children born to mothers with untreated hypothyroidism during pregnancy score lower on IQ than those on thyroid replacement.

If you have been treated for hypothyroidism, the medication dose may be increased during pregnancy according to your needs, determined with tests every 2–3 months. There are no side effects as long as the proper dose is used. After birth, the levels needs to return to pre-pregnancy dose and thyroid function tests will be reviewed after 2 months. It is safe and essential to continue taking the medication if breastfeeding.

Thyroid problems after pregnancy

Within a few months of birth, 1:20 women develop thyroid inflammation, a condition called **postpartum thyroiditis**. It is painless and causes little gland enlargement. Thyroid hormone output may rise causing overactivity that lasts for several weeks, followed by a fall in levels, and underactivity. The symptoms are sometimes missed and mistakenly attributed to lack of sleep, nervousness or postnatal depression. Beta-blockers may help if there is overactivity with symptoms such as tremor or palpitations. Thyroxin can be used to treat underactivity for up to 6 months. The condition passes within 4 months but may recur after subsequent pregnancies. Some women develop a permanently underactive thyroid gland.

TIREDNESS, LOW ENERGY & INSOMNIA

One of the most commonly held beliefs is that women bloom throughout pregnancy, shine with health and feel better than they ever have before. This does happen sometimes but most women experience a combination of high and low energy. After birth most women are tired and it may take weeks for normal energy to return, and many women (and men) do not get a full night of unbroken sleep for weeks or even months.

It is important to do what you can to care for yourself (p.51). This will help you maintain and replenish your energy as much as possible and enjoy your pregnancy, your labour and the early months with your new baby. If tiredness persists or becomes extreme, you may feel low and depressed.

What happens
Physical and medical causes
- Hormones alter the metabolism of your body and it changes from being designed to perform intensive aerobic tasks to longer, slower, repetitive activity. Physically carrying your baby before and after birth, together with natural changes to your circulation may drain energy.
- Medical issues such as NAUSEA & VOMITING or heartburn (p.487), HEART or chest problems and back or pelvic pain (p.519) may sap strength. After birth, and maybe before, ANAEMIA and thyroid underactivity may reduce energy.
- Insomnia is common in late pregnancy. When your uterus is large, you may have to pass urine frequently, it may be harder to get comfortable in bed and it is extremely common to sleep in short patches. Sleep deprivation is also common in early motherhood.
- If labour has been long, tiring and/or traumatic it may take days or weeks to feel you have your strength back.
- Some medics believe that chronic health conditions can contribute to lethargy. There are many names for such conditions, including candidiasis (p.524), chronic allergy, ME and chronic fatigue syndrome.

Emotional demands
- The emotional demands of the transition into parenthood may be considerable (p.285) and take up a lot of energy, particularly if there is conflict in any of your relationships.
- If you are low this will contribute to a general feeling of listlessness and fatigue. Antenatal and postnatal depression are common and troubling emotions may add to insomnia.
- Anxiety and vivid dreams may also make sleep less restful.
- You may have more time to reflect on troubling emotions and feel tired as a result.

Daily life
- If you are unfit, you may feel exhausted by the physical demands of being pregnant and caring for your baby.
- A diet deficient in vitamins and minerals can contribute to low energy, particularly if you eat lots of sugary foods that give initial highs followed by energy lows. Sugar lows can contribute to nightmares.
- After the birth your baby may interrupt your sleep.

Action plan
Improving and balancing energy will improve your enjoyment of pregnancy and birth and help you to welcome and enjoy your new baby. There are many possibilities for change that you can try and apply if they suit you. If you were physically fit and emotionally healthy before pregnancy, it is highly likely that you will return to that state afterwards. It does take commitment to look after yourself before and after the birth if you are going to maintain optimum energy levels.

Sleep
Many people expect to sleep 8–9 hours but neurological research suggests that 5–6 hours of restful sleep is all that is required each day. Although there is variation in how much sleep individuals need, it might help to assess the adequacy of your sleep not by the number of hours but by how you feel. Many adults are unconsciously concerned about not getting enough sleep and underlying anxiety or a feeling of being deprived can contribute to insomnia. To improve your quality of sleep, consider the following:
- Do what you can to make yourself comfortable. Use cushions in bed to support your bump or prop yourself up if you have INDIGESTION & HEARTBURN. Keep the room ventilated and avoid getting too hot.
- Check your mattress – if it is too soft your body may not relax as efficiently as it could on a more supportive surface.
- If you have insomnia, try to lie down and rest, even if you don't sleep, for 7–8 hours a day. Try not to sleep for long periods in the day. You may find short cat naps energising.
- A visualisation (p.370) may help you unwind or you may find a massage, yoga stretch or breathing (p.346) restful before retiring at night. Exercise (p.357) in the day may help you to sleep peacefully.
- After birth you may find it easy to rest when your baby sleeps: being in rhythm with one another helps you to pace yourself through each 24-hour period.
- If your baby's breathing keeps you awake, try using ear plugs or turn down the baby monitor if you are in separate rooms. You will wake in any case when she cries.

Medical care

You may want to be examined by your doctor to exclude a medical problem. If you have a medical condition, once treatment begins you may notice a considerable improvement. A common cause of tiredness after birth is anaemia, which can usually be relieved by taking supplements. An underactive THYROID also causes fatigue. Your doctor may also help you attend to any persistent pain that reduces your energy and affects sleep.

For a chronic condition (e.g. ME), treatment usually requires major changes at home, for instance by removing allergens. You may be advised to make changes to your diet, perhaps by restricting some foods. Some changes are simple, like a candida-inhibiting diet designed to reduce fungal growth, but the process of identifying an allergen may take months and is difficult in pregnancy. The restrictions can be stressful, and anxiety contributes to tiredness. Make changes under the supervision of a nutritionist who is fully aware of the other demands in your life, including pregnancy.

Emotions

Hormonal changes may contribute to your moods but the issues in your life – from becoming a parent to coping with your relationships – will continue regardless of your hormones and will also affect your partner. Living with challenging emotions and moving forward can be a rewarding part of parenting. If you are constantly worn down by your feelings, you may be able to improve your outlook and energy, by confiding in a friend or family member. It may be helpful to take steps to make time for you and your partner to be together, to feel supported by one another (p.290).

If uncomfortable emotions do not lessen, you may have depression or anxiety and EMOTIONAL ADVICE AND SUPPORT may be useful. Therapy can help relieve depression. In severe cases, medication is a useful support.

Complementary therapies

Massage, particularly with the essential oils lemon, grapefruit and jasmine, can be wonderfully relaxing and energising. The oils can also be used in a bath. Lemongrass and melissa are good for an energy lift after birth. To relax before sleep, try lavender (after Week 24) or some tangerine oil, perhaps in a warm bath or for a gentle face massage. Osteopathy (p.376) and acupuncture and reflexology (p.377) may all be very helpful. Yoga (p.346) and visualisation (p.370) may be very powerful for you.

Homeopathy

Aconite is the no. 1 remedy for sleeplessness, particularly when you are restless, anxious or have vivid dreams and wake up in a panic. In the 3rd trimester *Kali Carb* is helpful, particularly if you have backache and night sweats. *Coffea* may help if you are over excited and just can't close your eyes, and *Nux Vomica* is good if you sleep lightly, wake easily and can't get to sleep again, and have exhausting dreams. Take any of these in the 30c potency before bed and then again on waking during the night. Another good remedy for the 3rd trimester is *Avena Sativa*, *Passiflora* and *Valeriana* combined in a 6x potency.

For an energy pick-up, select from *Kali Phos* if you feel overloaded and stressed, perhaps with backache; *Phosphoric Acid* if you feel absolutely exhausted, want to be alone and crave refreshing drinks and fruit; and *Gelsemium* when you feel physically and emotionally weak and drowsy. Take the remedy in 30c, 3 times a day for a week, and then reassess.

TOXOPLASMOSIS

Toxoplasmosis is an infection caused by a microscopic parasitic organism. Many people are immune following an infection that did not cause symptoms. In some people it causes flu-like symptoms including sore throat and muscles, swollen glands and tiredness. Infection in pregnancy is rare, affecting fewer than 2:1000 women in the UK. The infection may lead to serious health complications for a baby, however.

What happens

Although the parasite *Toxoplasma gondii* is found in many animals, it is only in the cat that the infective forms are passed on through the faeces. Kittens are most likely to carry the parasites. If you have lived with cats before becoming pregnant, there is a chance you have contracted toxoplasmosis and are immune. Infection can also be acquired through eating raw or undercooked meat but not from raw fish.

If you become infected in the first 3 months of pregnancy there is a risk of around 45% that your baby will be infected. The infection is likely to be mild but there is a small (9%) chance of MISCARRIAGE or stillbirth (p.509), and a higher chance (around 30%) of damage to her eyes and/or brain. If you are infected in the last 3 months, your baby is much less likely to contract the disease. Signs of the disease may not be present at birth, but may appear later. Some affected children eventually suffer eye damage but the proportion is uncertain.

Action plan
Prevention

Most importantly, avoid the risk of contracting toxoplasmosis.
- If you have a cat, dispose of soiled litter daily, wear gloves to do so and wash your hands afterwards. Wear gloves if you are gardening as cat faeces are a hazard.
- If you have a sandpit, use a secure lid to prevent cats from using it as a litter tray.
- Thoroughly cook all meat and wash salads, fruit and vegetables.

Diagnosis and treatment

In the UK, pregnant women are not routinely tested for toxoplasmosis. A specific blood test can detect antibodies, and if they are present a repeat sample taken 2–4 weeks later checks whether the antibodies are of the IgG or IgM type and this enables accurate dating of the initial infection. If there are mainly IgM and the IgG has a low avidity (ability to stick to the toxoplasma organism) then the infection is recent. Infection more than 3 months before conception gives rise to protective antibodies and your baby is unlikely to be affected. If your doctor predicts a high likelihood that your baby is affected, you may be referred to a specialist centre for ultrasound scanning and possibly foetal blood sampling. If your baby is diagnosed with the infection you will also be offered counselling as you consider the options for treatment and future implications. Drug treatments in pregnancy may reduce the effects of the disease but they are not completely effective in treating an unborn infected baby, and do have side effects.

TRAVEL IN PREGNANCY

Many women travel in pregnancy and thoroughly enjoy it. While you are pregnant the main things to consider are: your comfort, your baby's health and the stage of pregnancy. Against this you'll also need to consider any particular health care you require. If you are on holiday the time off may be so relaxing that many unpleasant symptoms disappear. Remember your energy is needed to nurture your body and your growing baby, so don't overdo it.

When to call a doctor
If you are away from home and you experience concerning symptoms, consult a doctor immediately. These include bleeding, abdominal cramps, contractions, ruptured membranes, excessive leg swelling or headaches.

When is the best time to travel?
1st trimester: Travelling, whether by car, train or aeroplane, may bring difficulties such as NAUSEA, perhaps with vomiting, and fatigue. Travel wristbands based on acupuncture can alleviate nausea, and plenty of rest and relaxation is the first step to take if you have TIREDNESS AND LOW ENERGY.
2nd trimester: You will probably begin to feel more lively. This is the best time to make a long journey, and there is least risk of needing medical care: the risk of MISCARRIAGE greatly reduces after Week 12 and the risk of PREMATURE labour remains low unless you have a past history.
3rd trimester: You may choose to stay at home or within easy reach of your surgery or hospital. From Week 32 your antenatal appointments will become more closely spaced. You may not be able to fly from Week 32 and insurance companies may not provide cover in any case.

When travel is not recommended
It is always best to consult your doctor if you are travelling far from medical facilities. Your doctor will be able to assess the risks, recommend precautions and advise you of any reasons to avoid travel. You may be advised against travel if you:
- Have a history of recurrent miscarriage (this risk reduces after Week 12).
- Have CERVICAL INCOMPETENCE (no travel until the stitch is safely in).
- Have a history of premature labour or premature rupture of membranes (p.501) (travel inadvisable after Week 27).
- Have a baby with INTRAUTERINE GROWTH RESTRICTION or a PLACENTA PRAEVIA.
- Are carrying TWINS or more babies.
- Have pre-eclampsia (p.410) or DIABETES, unless it is well controlled, or another health condition that requires

frequent medication or observation.
- Have severe ANAEMIA, because when you fly your baby may receive less oxygen than she needs.

Where it's not advisable to go
- High altitudes – above 2000 m (6500 ft).
- Areas with ongoing outbreaks of life-threatening food- or insect-borne infections or chloroquine-resistant *Plasmodium falciparum* malaria is endemic.
- Areas where live-virus vaccines are recommended.
- Areas that are excessively hot unless you are able to acclimatise gradually and you increase your fluid and salt intake accordingly.

What to take with you
- Your medical notes.
- Your doctor's phone number.
- Plenty of healthy snacks and fresh water to drink, to keep up your energy levels on the journey.
- An extra cushion for comfort, particularly after Week 20.
- Light loose-fitting clothes – you may feel warmer than usual – and comfortable shoes that allow your feet to expand if you are flying or stay seated for long periods.
- Support stockings if you have any swelling or prominent veins in your legs. They prevent deep vein thrombosis (p.560) and swelling during flying or long car journeys.

Your medical kit
Some additions to your everyday First Aid kit might include:
- Pregnancy multivitamins and minerals, and folic acid tablets in the 1st trimester.
- Oral rehydration powder in case of DIARRHOEA.
- Anti-fungal cream and pessaries to treat vaginal candida.
- Insect repellent that is preferably free of DEET (diethyltoluamide) or containing a low percentage (10–35%) because the chemical is absorbed by your skin and may, in theory, affect your baby. You can spray it on clothing rather than directly on your skin. There are a number of herbal repellents available, but these too need to be cleared for safe use in pregnancy. A mosquito net is useful at night.
- Sunscreen with a high sun-protection factor.
- In the 3rd trimester you may want to take urine dipsticks so you can check for protein to rule out pre-eclampsia.
- A homeopathy travel kit advised by your homeopath.

Travelling by car
When you travel by car, always wear a seatbelt. As your abdomen grows, fix the lap section of the belt beneath – not over – your abdomen, across your pelvis, with the other strap passing over one shoulder, between your breasts and around the side of your bump. You may prefer to sit in the back, where it is safer. If there are air bags fitted, move your seat back as far as is comfortable. In the event of an accident, be examined urgently. Use support stockings for long trips.

Travelling by plane
Commercial air travel poses no special risks to a healthy pregnant woman or her baby. Each airline has its own policy, so it is best to check when booking. You may need to carry

documentation stating your expected date of delivery. Domestic travel may be permitted until Week 36, while international travel is commonly disallowed beyond Weeks 32–34. Flying does not bring on labour but there are practical difficulties involved if a woman goes into labour on a plane.

Air pressure and oxygen: It is not safe in pregnancy to fly in an unpressurised cabin, but on commercial planes the cabin pressures are safe. The amount of oxygen in the atmosphere is lower than on land but your baby experiences an even smaller drop. The effect is insignificant unless you have anaemia.

Metal detectors and radiation: Security checks, which may involve a magnetic field, do not present any risk. Cosmic radiation is known to increase at altitude and the effect is related to the time in the air. Exposure is unlikely to pose any risk to your developing baby if you fly just once or twice.

Keeping hydrated: The main risk associated with air travel is dehydration, because of low humidity. Drink plenty of water at regular intervals – at least 1 litre (2 pints) for every 2–3 hours flying – and eat healthy snacks to maintain your energy levels.

Movement: Walking around, up and down the aisle, every 2 hours or so will help keep your circulation moving, reduce swelling, stiffness and cramp, and reduce the risk of deep vein thrombosis. If there's room, stretch your arms and tense and relax the muscles in your legs for a few minutes.

Where to sit: You may be able to book a seat with more leg room.

Preventing deep vein thrombosis: You are advised to wear support tights for any flight longer than 4 hours, drink water and avoid alcohol, move around the cabin every 2–3 hours. A 75 mg aspirin before the flight is safe to thin the blood.

Vaccinations for international destinations

If you plan to travel to an area where immunisation is advised, you will need to consult your doctor, perhaps in conjunction with a travel health clinic or centre for tropical diseases. Some vaccines use a live (attenuated) virus and there is a theoretical risk that a mother could become infected and pass the infection to her baby, and this could carry a risk of developmental damage. Thus live vaccines are best avoided, especially during the 1st trimester while your baby's organs are developing. It is also best to avoid them in the 3 months prior to conception.

While you are away

• Find out the address and contact numbers for local doctors.

• Do not drink water unless you know it is safe; either filtered, boiled or bottled. In pregnancy, using an iodine purification system is not recommended. Avoid ice and ice-based drinks.

• While enjoying food, take precautions. Eat food that has been well cooked; avoid cold or lukewarm food that has been exposed to air; avoid salads if local water quality is dubious. Avoid unpasteurised milk.

• If you suffer from diarrhoea, guard against dehydration by drinking adequate clean water and medically prepared rehydration solution. Rice milk is an effective substitute to rehydrate. You can take a stool sample to a health clinic or hospital for analysis.

• If you travel to a country where malaria is a risk, it is important to take precautions, remembering that a number

of other insect-borne diseases may be prevalent. Try not to go out of doors between dusk and dawn, especially if you are near a river or swamp. When you do go out, wear long sleeves, trousers and socks and a hat. Sleep with a mosquito net and use measures such as insect repellent and mosquito coils. Discuss malarial prophylactics with your doctor.

TRAVEL WITH A BABY

Babies are great travelling companions. They usually travel for free, offer good company and amusement to others and need little maintenance. As a newborn, your baby will sleep most of the day, so in theory you will be relatively free to organise your time as you wish. When older, particularly when she's mobile, you may have less chance to rest during the day but your nights could be less disturbed. When travelling, your priorities need to be your baby's safety and comfort, combined with your own comfort, rest and enjoyment.

Within sensible limits most travel is possible with a young baby, from car trips and train journeys to transatlantic flights and some adventure holidays. There are a number of specialist holiday companies for families who want extra help. It is inadvisable to take your baby on a plane before she is 2 weeks old if she was born at term, or 2 weeks after her due date if she was PREMATURE. Insurance is important. Check the policy closely, paying close attention to medical cover.

If you are going to an area where prophylactics and vaccinations are needed, appropriate advice must be sought prior to departure. If you are breastfeeding your own medication will not pass to your baby in the milk: she needs her own protection.

When to call a doctor

Some babies adjust to travelling easily. Some find it unsettling. While you may take this into account if your baby doesn't appear her normal self, it's also worth getting medical attention soon if you are at all concerned. This applies particularly if you are in a country where there are contagious diseases and you are not familiar with the symptoms.

Your medical kit

A medical kit is an essential piece of travelling equipment. In addition to general First Aid remedies (p.387), you may want to pack the following:

• Barrier cream: your baby may become hot or slightly dehydrated, both of which may lead to nappy rash.

• High-protection sun block formulated for babies.

• Insect repellent specially formulated for babies. Mosquito netting impregnated with permethrine is ideal.

• Rehydration powders for if you and your baby get DIARRHOEA.

• Homeopathic remedies recommended by your homeopath.

On the move

• Always use an approved car seat for your baby, but never put it in a seat where there is an air bag. Make sure the straps fit snugly so that neither your baby nor the seat can move more than two finger widths. When she is very small if she slips down in the seat, place a rolled up cloth between her nappy and the strap that passes through her legs.

- If you are flying, dress your baby in loose, comfortable clothing. Reduced air pressure in the cabin makes air in the bowel expand and can cause abdominal, colicky pain.
- Feed her during take off and landing. Sucking and swallowing helps equalise ear pressure and reduces ear pain. If she is not hungry, offer a bottle of water or diluted juice. Let her breastfeed or drink from a bottle whenever she wants. Babies become dehydrated in the dry cabin air more quickly than adults.
- Many companies provide cribs and can fix them securely.
- After a flight, watch for signs of ear pain. If your baby is uncomfortable she may cry or scream within half an hour of landing, become restless and irritable, particularly if she is lying down, or be unable to sleep. Some babies shake their heads. Pain usually passes by the following morning.
- While you are away, take similar precautions about hygiene as you would in pregnancy and find out about medical facilities nearby.

TRICHOMONIASIS

Trichomoniasis is the infection caused by a single-celled organism, trichomonas vaginalis. It is transmitted through sexual contact and inhabits the vagina, urethra and urinary tract. It is often present without symptoms, but can cause a thin, frothy and yellow-green discharge, with an unpleasant fishy smell. The discharge makes the skin around the vagina sore and inflamed and there may be itching and pain on passing urine. Trichomonas can spread to cause cystitis (p.552).

A very small number of women are infected in pregnancy, often with other sexually transmitted infections (commonly GONORRHOEA and CHLAMYDIA). Rarely, trichomoniasis may be responsible for pneumonia in the newborn (p.441). A cervical smear or vaginal swab test can diagnose infection. Both sexual partners need treatment with metronizadole, although this is not suitable in early pregnancy. It is safe in late pregnancy and during breastfeeding. Once treated, trichomoniasis will not recur unless there is reinfection from another person.

TWINS & HIGHER MULTIPLES

Today, with routine scans, it is extremely rare for twins to be missed. Discovering twins can be a shock, even after fertility treatment. Anxiety about how you will give birth and cope as a parent may be intense, but you can look forward to double rewards as well as an increased workload. There are support groups for parents of twins and you could make contact during pregnancy and perhaps spend time with a family who has twins: this might help you to prepare for what is to come. If you have triplets or more, you may receive extra help from local social services.

There is no doubt that twins, particularly if they are identical, have a deep bond and a close understanding. They grow together in the womb and communicate with one another non-verbally on a level that few people can access: sometimes twins are late in using verbal language because of this, and they often rely heavily on one another for emotional support. Ultrasound scans show twins from 6 months in the womb touching through the membranes that divide them.

What happens

Identical twins: These develop from a single fertilised egg that divides into separate embryos. The babies are the same sex, the same genetic make-up and very similar physically. Identical twins occur randomly and do not run in families. These **monozygotic twins** occur in 3–5:1000 pregnancies and share a single placenta, although each has an amniotic membrane and sac and umbilical cord. Two-thirds of identical twins share a chorion, the second and the outer membrane (monochorionic), and the other third of identical twins each have their own chorion. Monochorionic twins need to be monitored particularly closely during pregnancy as they are at a higher risk of developing complications because one of the twins may have a lower blood flow and grow less well.

Non-identical or dizygotic twins: These result from the fertilisation of two eggs, each by a separate sperm, and are no more alike than other siblings. They have completely separate membranes, placenta and umbilical cord. Non-identical twins occur in 5–7:1000 pregnancies. The tendency to release two eggs at ovulation is inherited, rises with fertility treatment and is more common over the age of 35 years.

Siamese or conjoined twins: These are very rare with only 12 cases in the UK in the last 50 years.

Complications associated with multiple pregnancies

Symptoms of pregnancy, such as NAUSEA & VOMITING, are often more severe with twins, and your uterus will be 'large for dates'. You will feel heavier in the later stages than if you were carrying only one baby. Throughout pregnancy you will be more closely monitored. Half of all twin pregnancies result in healthy full-term babies, usually at about Week 37, with no complications. The other 50% of twin births are premature (before Week 37), and these babies usually require a period of time in a SPECIAL CARE BABY UNIT.

- The most significant potential complication is PREMATURE BIRTH, often due to excess AMNIOTIC FLUID, particularly with monochorionic twins. After birth, premature twins are more prone to the problems of immaturity than a premature singleton.
- INTRAUTERINE GROWTH RESTRICTION (IUGR) is common. It is usually mild but there may be a dramatic difference in size and one baby may be up to 1 kg (2 lb 3 oz) smaller than the other. Severe IUGR may necessitate an early birth.
- Twin-to-twin transfusion only occurs in some monozygotic (identical) twins. This means that while the babies share a placenta, part of the blood flow is diverted from one twin to the other. This results in the twin who receives less blood being under nourished and showing IUGR and even ANAEMIA during pregnancy. Early birth may be needed to rescue the smaller twin but new techniques are evolving to

reduce the cross-over of blood. The diagnosis is made on ultrasound scans to check growth and blood flow.

- There is an increased risk of PLACENTA PRAEVIA, where the placenta is low and may cover the cervix, necessitating delivery by CAESAREAN SECTION.
- The incidence of foetal loss is higher in twin pregnancies, particularly with identical twins. An early ultrasound scan under 6 weeks may reveal two amniotic sacs but one of the embryos has been absorbed. An obvious MISCARRIAGE may occur. In a tiny minority, the baby may stop growing after 12 weeks and the foetus that would have miscarried will shrink and will be born after the living twin. Very rarely, particularly with identical twins, one foetus does not receive sufficient placental blood flow and may be STILLBORN (p.509). The impact from the LOSS OF A BABY is significant and difficult because there is joy that one baby is normal and sadness for the other.
- Pre-eclampsia (p.410) is more common, particularly with identical twins. You may be uncomfortable from pressure on your back and internal organs: you may have PAIN IN THE BACK OR PELVIS, or SWELLING (oedema) in your legs, INDIGESTION & HEARTBURN, and BREATHLESSNESS. The incidence of iron-deficiency ANAEMIA, URINARY TRACT INFECTIONS, PILES and varicose veins (p.559) is higher than with a single baby.

Action plan

Antenatal care is important for you as well as for your babies, and you will probably be offered more frequent check-ups with your midwife and obstetrician or a foetal medicine specialist. Caring for yourself is important, too (p.51), because there are even higher demands on your body than with a singleton pregnancy and twins are at an increased risk of complications. Close care will reduce complications.

Medical care in pregnancy

Close monitoring ensures your blood pressure, digestion and back and pelvis are not causing concern and checks your babies. You may be offered ultrasound scans at 4-week intervals or more frequently if your doctor is concerned about one of your babies.

Later in pregnancy their foetal heart patterns (CTG) may also be monitored. If there is any suggestion of IUGR, monitoring will intensify and you may be advised to stop working relatively early in pregnancy.

Nutrition and exercise

A balanced diet (p.332) is very important. It is not necessary to eat twice as much, however, nor is it safe to take double the dose of vitamin and mineral supplements recommended for pregnancy. You can expect to gain more weight than in a singleton pregnancy – 15.9–20.5 kg (35–45 lb) is the average weight gain (p.332) – so watch your diet and avoid calories that will add to this gain. You may need to eat smaller amounts more frequently, as your stomach will be under pressure from your growing uterus. With the extra weight and the energy required to nourish your babies, you'll need to rest regularly and choose gentle yet effective exercise – walking, swimming and yoga.

Planning ahead

It's a good idea to look into the financial and practical implications of paid help if you won't be getting assistance from your family: parents of twins do need help. And because twins are more commonly born early, prepare from Week 28: you'll need two of everything.

Labour and birth

Some twins are born vaginally, yet because of an increased risk of complications during labour most twins in the UK are born by caesarean section. The method of delivery will be your choice, but if your doctor anticipates any problems or if you go into labour before Week 37, a caesarean may be the safest option. Sometimes the first twin may be delivered vaginally but because of awkward positioning the second may need to be delivered by caesarean. It is usual to give birth in a high-dependency unit rather than a cottage hospital so extra medical help is at hand.

In an active birth the cervix usually dilates more rapidly and labour is a little shorter. If you are comfortable being upright, the flow of blood to the placenta will be maximised. The birth team will monitor the wellbeing of your babies with extra vigilance. It is common practice to ensure there is an anaesthetist and a paediatrician available.

The main difficulty with twin births is the delivery of the second twin. The most common presentation is for both twins to be head down but often the second is breech (p.492). Your doctor will check your babies' positions with ultrasound before or during labour, and after the first twin is born, your second baby's position is re-checked. If the head is down, the membranes around the amniotic sac may be ruptured to encourage birth and if contractions do not begin within 10 minutes, you may be given oxytocin to stimulate your uterus. If the second twin changes position and is breech or lying transversely (p.498), a caesarean section will be advised. Triplets are usually delivered by caesarean.

During a vaginal birth the delivery of the placenta is usually managed actively, which means you will be given an injection of oxytocin to encourage delivery, and your midwife will apply a light pulling force to the umbilical cords (p.138). This is to reduce excessive bleeding, which is more likely because of the large surface area of the placentas.

After the birth

After the birth you will quickly focus on caring for your babies. There is a long-established belief that only women who cope well with babies have twins, so rest assured you will probably be fine. If everything goes well with the birth, you will have both babies with you soon afterwards and you can establish breastfeeding as soon as possible.

- Because newborns eat often, you may be feeding almost constantly, and provided your nipples do not become painful, this is good because the more your babies feed, the more milk you will produce. When you are used to it, both babies can feed at the same time provided you are comfortable and they are well supported on pillows.
- If one or either of your breasts is red or lumpy, change your feeding position and alternate your babies: one may suck more strongly.

- You will need to maintain a high fluid intake and nourish yourself adequately. This will be easier if there is someone who can cook and clean for you, at least in the early days. If you are planning to bottle feed your babies then you will need to be very well organised and have a 24-hour supply of bottled milk made up in advance every day, ready to be warmed.
- It is hard to hold and feed two babies at once: most parents cradle one baby and rest the other on a pillow, and then swap for the next feed.
- Some mothers find that alternating bottle feeding and breastfeeding for each baby helps avoid exhaustion and anxiety. If one or both of your babies are taking a bottle, you can share the feeding times with your partner or another adult.

However you feed, it helps to feed both babies at the same time or you will be feeding virtually non-stop. When one wakes for a feed, wake the other – during the night and the day. With luck you will all fall into a reasonably predictable pattern, although you may be unlucky and find they have wildly different sleeping rhythms.

Feeding takes up a lot of time and, as with every other aspect of babycare, you need to be very well organised and have adaptable babies if you are going to get sufficient rest in the first few months after birth. Use the help that you've arranged during pregnancy and rest as often as you possibly can. If your mind is buzzing and you find it hard to relax, try visualisation (p.370) or yoga-based breathing exercises (p.346) to help you switch off.

How you may feel
Parents say that having twins is double the trouble but also double the joy. There may be knock-on effects to your relationship so it helps to have undisturbed time with your partner as soon, and as often, as you are able. You will need lots of extra support to make this a reality (use the Wheel for Living, p.58). You have twice the work and perhaps twice the stress faced by parents of single babies, and you'll benefit from space to yourself twice as much.

From the beginning your twins will learn to accept that you cannot be in two places at one time and you will learn how to switch off and ignore some of the crying. If you are very sensitive, ear plugs are helpful for a few hours a day to help you get some rest. As the weeks pass your babies will be focused on and amuse one another and you will have more time for other things. This aspect of life with twins is one that many mothers of single babies envy, and it gets better as twins grow and play together.

You may feel confused or guilty if your feelings for your babies are not the same for them both, particularly if one is in special care and the other is not. Whatever happens, each baby has a unique personality: one may be dominant, one placid, one big and hungry, the other slight and quiet. There are years ahead to get to know one another and interact as a family where differences as well as similarities find a place. Make use of special groups for twins where you can contact other parents and health professionals who can offer support and advice over the weeks, months and years.

UMBILICAL CORD BLOOD & STEM CELLS

Cord blood is a richer source of stem cells, the building blocks of blood and the immune system, than bone marrow. Banking is the process of collecting blood from the umbilical cord immediately after delivery and freezing it for long-term cryogenic storage. Stem cells collected and stored at birth can be stored with a commercial service, and saved for your baby's future use, or in a state-run bank, where they are available for unrelated patients. They may be used in transplant medicine to regenerate a patient's blood and immune system or after chemotherapy or radiation, to treat malignancies including leukaemia, sickle cell and thalassaemia ANAEMIA and inborn genetic errors. Future possibilities rely on advances in molecular biology.

UMBILICAL CORD, COMPRESSED OR PROLAPSED

Oxygen and other nutrients are passed from you through the placenta and the umbilical cord to your baby. The umbilical cord is naturally protected: it has two arteries wrapped around a vein and protected in a substance called Wharton's jelly. The cord skin allows it to slide and prevents it being trapped between the baby's head and your pelvis, and the amniotic fluid protects it as well. If there is a cord accident and the blood flow is reduced, it may lead to FOETAL DISTRESS & ASPHYXIA with low oxygen flow to your baby.

Umbilical cord compression very rarely happens in late pregnancy and occurs in roughly 1:10 deliveries. It is usually mild and intermittent during a contraction and there is sufficient time for a baby to recover by using sugar stores for energy until the oxygen supply returns between contractions. The birth team is alert for signs of distress, and if there is prolonged cord compression, the treatment is urgent delivery.

Babies frequently have the cord around the neck, but if it is not pulled tight it is insignificant. The cord is usually long enough to prevent the vessels being narrowed, but as the baby descends in the 2nd stage the cord may tighten, particularly if it is short. Cord compression is more likely to cause foetal distress and asphyxia for a baby who is already at risk. Compression is more likely if the amniotic fluid volume is low (p.397), particularly with INTRAUTERINE GROWTH RESTRICTION (IUGR) or postmaturity (p.500), and the risk rises after the membranes rupture and particularly in labour. If the umbilical cord has prolapsed (opposite), there is a greater chance of compression.

What happens
When the umbilical cord is compressed there may be a reduction in blood flow to your baby and this could cause foetal distress and asphyxia. The midwife can detect this from an altered heartbeat (p.125). The effect of compression depends on the energy reserves your baby has and the duration and intensity of compression. A stoppage of blood flow for longer

than 10 minutes, or less time for a baby with severe IUGR, may have long-term effects and cause asphyxia.

Action plan
Medical care antenatally and particularly in labour is geared towards detecting signs of compression or of the cord tightening around the neck and foetal heart CTG monitoring is intensified for HIGH-RISK PREGNANCIES. If there are signs of compression from your baby's heart rate:
- Your midwife may gently press on your abdomen, where your baby's back is and encourage him to shift off the cord. Not all midwives practise this.
- If you are in the 2nd stage of labour she may encourage you to be upright and push or recommend forceps or ventouse (p.496) to speed progress.
- A CAESAREAN SECTION may be needed if labour has not begun or birth is still a long way off.

Your baby
If cord compression has not been prolonged, your baby is likely to be fine. If it has been severe he may need resuscitation (p.383). Most babies recover from this easily. Rarely, if cord compression leads to severe asphyxia there may be long-term effects from oxygen deprivation. Fortunately, with modern obstetric care this is increasingly rare. Some babies who are born with a tight cord around the neck can be red-faced at birth, but this usually resolves over a few days.

Umbilical cord prolapse
A rare complication of labour involves a prolapsed umbilical cord, occurring when a loop of the umbilical cord is presenting between the baby's body and the cervix before the head engages. It is more common if a baby is PREMATURE, breech or a transverse lie (p.498) or if there is excess AMNIOTIC FLUID. If the umbilical cord is presenting below your baby and the membranes rupture before the head has engaged, the cord can slip or prolapse through the cervix. The main risk after prolapse is cord compression if your baby's head descends and pushes the cord against your pelvic bones.

Action plan
If your waters break you need to contact your midwife immediately, particularly if your baby's head is high, he is in a breech position or you have an excess of amniotic fluid. Any of these situations increase the risk of prolapse.
If the cord does prolapse and it can be felt in your vagina this is an emergency.
- You need an ambulance to get you to hospital.
- Remain on all fours with your head lower and your bottom higher to slow your baby's descent and reduce the pressure of his head on your cervix. Your midwife may hold your baby's head up by inserting her fingers into your vagina until a caesarean section can be performed.
- If the cord protrudes from your vagina, it is dangerous because exposure to air can cause spasm of the blood vessels and reduced blood flow to your baby. If the cord is exposed your midwife will replace it into your vagina – you will need to do this if it becomes exposed before medical help arrives.

UMBILICAL CORD, INFECTION

Occasionally a cord stump becomes inflamed and infected (**omphalitis**), making the skin around it red, perhaps with pus or discharge and a foul smell, and a FEVER. It is important to tell your midwife or doctor because although this can clear up quickly, infection may spread to deeper structures.

Action plan
Luckily, the best way to prevent infection is to leave the area well alone and expose it to air whenever possible – the bacteria on the skin allow the cord to soften and separate. If antibiotic powders are used as a preventative measure, the process takes longer. It is safe to clean the area in a bath or with cotton wool dipped in cooled, boiled water.

Medical care
Your doctor or midwife may advise you to use a special alcohol solution or an antibiotic powder or ointment to clear the infection. Very, very rarely, the cord continues to ooze a clear fluid, representing a persistent connection between the bladder and umbilicus, called a patent urachus. This can be closed through simple surgery.

Homeopathy
Add 10 drops of *Hypercal* to your baby's bath and give 1 dose of *Hypericum* (30c) in the morning and 1 at night, as well as *Hepar Sulph* (30c) mid-morning, lunchtime and mid-afternoon. Do this for 2 days and reassess. If there has been no improvement, consult your doctor. As a preventative measure, add 10 drops of *Hypercal* tincture to the bath from immediately after delivery.

UMBILICAL GRANULOMAS

Umbilical granulomas occur within 6 months of birth in roughly 1:20 babies. The granuloma is a small piece of pink, fleshy tissue that has not been covered by skin after the umbilical cord has separated. It contains no nerves and your baby will not feel anything if it is touched. It may produce discharge and can bleed. Most umbilical granulomas disappear in a few months. Some need to be cauterised in a simple painless process involving application of a silver nitrate stick.

UMBILICUS, SINGLE ARTERY

Ordinarily, the umbilical cord contains three vessels: two arteries and one vein. Around 5% of babies, however, have just one artery, occasionally detected on antenatal ultrasound scans. The condition is more common among TWINS. Since a foetus can function with only one umbilical artery, this poses no problem. Yet in 15% of affected babies this abnormality is linked with other CONGENITAL ABNORMALITIES and it will prompt a full examination and possibly further investigation.

URINARY TRACT INFECTION: BABY

A urinary tract (kidney and bladder) infection is not always easy to detect. Infections are more common in baby girls, affecting 5%, because their urethra is shorter than boys'.

What happens

If your baby is unwell, with FEVER, irritability or DIARRHOEA, is refusing feeds or has poor WEIGHT gain and his urine smells strong, this may indicate a urinary tract infection. Normal urine is sterile and is free of bacteria, viruses and fungi. An infection occurs when micro-organisms, usually bacteria from the colon, cling to the opening of the urethra, the tube that carries urine from the bladder to the outside of the body, and travel into the bladder where they begin to multiply.

Action plan

For most babies simple remedies such as adequate fluid intake help to prevent infections. Always wipe your baby girl from front to back to reduce the chance of bacteria travelling from the bowel to the bladder. A urine test can detect infection.

- A urinary infection may be treated with antibiotics, possibly for a long period if the infection recurs. Your baby may also need infant paracetamol to relieve pain.
- Your baby needs increased fluids to help flush the kidneys.
- When a urine infection is confirmed, a specialist will investigate the underlying cause. The tests mainly look for obstruction and reflux (below) and your baby may require further testing to visualise the urinary tract.

Urinary obstruction & reflux

A very small number of babies have an obstruction to the flow of urine or reflux of urine back from the bladder to the kidneys that increases the tendency to infection. This may lead to long-term kidney damage that treatment may prevent, so all babies with urinary infections are referred for specialist assessment.

What happens

If the urine flow along the ureter, the tube between the kidney and the bladder, is obstructed or refluxes, it leads to a condition called **hydronephrosis**: the ureters and the kidney become dilated and distended with urine. This may be visible on an ultrasound scan during pregnancy (in about 2% of babies) or after birth, or the problem may become apparent with a urine infection in the first few months.

Hydronephrosis may be caused by urinary reflux, where the valve between the ureter and the bladder is not working and urine flows in the reverse direction from the bladder towards the kidney when the bladder contracts. Ureter obstruction is common in boys and results from a developmental problem with narrowing of the ureter. The majority of babies found to have dilated ureters have normal kidneys.

Very rarely, in boys, the ureter or the bladder outlet is blocked, giving severe hydronephrosis that damages developing kidneys. With complete blockage the distension is often visible on an antenatal ultrasound scan by Week 20.

Action plan

Some foetal medicine specialists place a catheter to drain the urine by amniocentesis during pregnancy and relieve the effects of pressure. This may not, however, prevent damage to the kidneys. If hydronephrosis is suspected, after birth your baby may be given a low dose of antibiotics to prevent infection while tests are being done. In many babies the condition seen in pregnancy resolves spontaneously and treatment is stopped.

- After birth the tests include ultrasound scan to check for two normal kidneys.
- In some centres a micturating cystourethrogram is done by passing a catheter tube into the bladder via the urethra, injecting a dye and taking x-ray pictures to see if the urine refluxes. It involves a number of x-rays and the more up-to-date equivalent using ultrasound imaging.
- Other tests involve injecting radio-isotopes into a vein and using a gamma camera to see the function of the kidneys and observe reflux or narrowing of the ureter.
- Babies found to have obstruction or reflux are usually started on a preventative, low dose of antibiotics. This is to reduce the risk of infections damaging the kidneys through scarring. Urinary obstruction and reflux generally improves by the age of 1–3 years after which antibiotics are stopped because the risk of new scarring is minimal. Your baby will be followed up and surgery may occasionally be needed.
- After the birth of one baby with hydronephrosis there is around a 30% chance that a subsequent baby may be affected. Even if scans are normal before birth, it is advisable for a baby to have an ultrasound scan after birth.

URINARY TRACT INFECTION: MOTHER

See also TRICHOMONIASIS; VAGINA, DISCHARGE & INFECTION

The urinary tract consists of the kidneys, the ureters (tubes connecting the kidneys to the bladder) and the bladder. Urinary infections affect up to 10% of women. Infection usually begins in the bladder, where it is called **cystitis** and causes increased urinary frequency as well as burning as the bladder empties. Infection may extend to the kidneys in a very small number of women, where it is called **pyelonephritis** and gives symptoms of FEVER and loin pain, usually in addition to bladder symptoms. Occasionally urine may contain bacteria without causing cystitis; this is **bacteruria** and may not cause symptoms, but women with this condition are predisposed to cystitis. Bacteruria is also associated with vaginal infections (p.556) and slightly increases the risk of PREMATURE BIRTH.

What happens

Urinary infection is more frequent during pregnancy because the tone in the muscle of the bladder wall and the ureter relaxes and slows the flow of urine so bacteria have longer to multiply. It also increases the chance that bacteria from the bowel or vagina may enter the bladder. Flow may slow further as the pressure of the uterus on the bladder increases. After birth, cystitis may occur after bruising following an operative delivery or when a catheter has been used. If there has been VAGINAL PROLAPSE, this predisposes to an infection.

An irritable bladder, also known as **chronic cystitis**, may cause symptoms similar to a urinary infection but the urine does not contain organisms. There is usually a history of the condition prior to pregnancy but the urine must be cultured to exclude an infection. **Kidney stones** may also cause urinary blockage with resultant kidney infection.

Action plan
Medical care
- If you have bladder or kidney pain, you need to visit a doctor – there is more urgency if you have a fever.
- Your doctor will ask you to take a mid-stream urine sample: do this by holding the labia apart and catching a small amount as the urine flows.
- Infection needs to be treated with antibiotics. After treatment you will be offered another urine analysis to check all the bacteria have been eliminated. Women with recurrent urinary infections may require long-term antibiotics.
- You may be offered an ultrasound scan if you have loin pain to check whether the ureter is excessively dilated, which usually indicates a pregnancy effect or, rarely, a stone. Most stones pass into the bladder and operations to remove them are usually deferred until after birth.
- Infection caused by vaginal prolapse diminishes when the condition is treated.

Diet and lifestyle
- After passing urine, wipe the labia from front to back to reduce the chance of transferring organisms from the anus or vagina to the urethra and bladder.
- Drink more water to flush the bladder and the ureter, preferably before 6pm to help your sleep.
- Onions, garlic and chives help to prevent the growth of harmful bacteria. Barley water (without sugar) is famously good for soothing urinary infections.
- For cystitis, unsweetened cranberry juice, drunk 3 or 4 times a day, reduces the adherence of organisms to the bladder wall so they are more easily flushed out. Don't drink the sugared variety, which may increase your susceptibility to CANDIDA (thrush), and be a potent cause of weight gain.
- If you are prone to calcium stones, eat less dairy products. Reducing consumption of spinach, chocolate, rhubarb and nuts can prevent oxalate stones forming.

Homeopathy
If you have a fever, severe kidney pain or blood in the urine, you will need a medical examination and opinion. For recurrent bouts of cystitis it is advisable to consult a qualified homeopath, who may recommend *Berberis*, a bladder-support remedy, in low potency.

For an isolated attack of cystitis take a suitable remedy in 30c, 2-hourly for 12 hours and then reassess. If there is no improvement, consult a qualified homeopath or see your GP.

Use *Apis* for fluid retention and extreme sensitivity to heat, irritability and restlessness, a constant desire to urinate, a scalding sensation when urinating and improvement with cool air and cold compresses; *Arsenicum* for cystitis accompanied by anxiety, restlessness and chilliness and a feeling that the bladder is not emptying well, with nausea and DIARRHOEA and better for warmth; *Cantharis* if the burning pain is severe, worst after urination, you constantly want to urinate and it feels your bladder can't empty and only small amounts of urine are passed, you have lower back pain and feel irritable and worse for movement; *Merc Cor* for an intense and constant urge to go despite urinating that is passed drop by drop with pain, and there is anxiety, thirst, chilliness and possibly faintness; *Staphysagria* after catheterisation, intervention during labour, or after sexual intercourse, pain after urinating and urine is passed drop by drop, you are easily angered or offended, better from warmth and resting.

Aromatherapy and acupuncture
Sandalwood and patchouli, used in the bath or on a compress, can soothe. After Week 24 you can try lavender and camomile. Acupuncture can bring relief.

URINE FREQUENCY & INCONTINENCE
See VAGINAL LAXITY, PROLAPSE & INCONTINENCE

UTERUS, ABNORMAL SHAPE – BICORNUATE
....

The uterus consists of two halves that fuse together and a cavity forms. A normal uterus is pear-shaped and contains a regular cavity that connects the cervix below to the fallopian tubes above. A wide range of abnormalities is possible that range from a minor indentation at the top of the uterus to a more overtly heart-shaped uterus (bicornuate), or, very rarely, to a complete double system with a double uterus and cervix.

What happens
The most common abnormality is an indentation (a septum) in the cavity at the top of the uterus. This is a septate uterus and usually causes no symptoms or complications. The next in frequency is a bicornuate uterus where there is one cervix but the septum is more pronounced and the cavity is heart shaped. These uterine variants are quite common and 3:100 women are affected, with no genetic tendency. If only one side of the uterus forms, it may be associated with abnormal development of the kidney on the absent side.

Most women with uterine variations do not have problems. Difficulties are more likely if the uterus is heart-shaped and are related to the degree of abnormality. If the heart shape is severe there is an increased risk of CERVICAL INCOMPETENCE and MISCARRIAGE; breech presentation (p.499); PREMATURE BIRTH; INTRAUTERINE GROWTH RESTRICTION (IUGR), and the need for CAESAREAN SECTION. After the birth there is more likelihood the placenta may be retained (p.407).

Action plan
If you are aware of a bicornuate uterus before conception, tell your doctor, particularly if you have had previous miscarriages, a breech baby or a retained placenta.

Investigation may include ultrasound scans with 3-D imaging, x-rays and laparoscopy. Treatment before pregnancy may include division of the septum by minimally invasive vaginal surgery, although only a minority of women need this if there has been infertility or recurrent miscarriages.

During pregnancy

During pregnancy your doctor will see you frequently. You may be offered ultrasound scans to check the cervix for incompetence by measuring the canal diameter, to check for IUGR and breech presentation and see where the placenta has implanted. If the canal of the cervix is dilated, a cervical cerclage suture (p.426) is performed (Weeks 12–15) to prevent a miscarriage and reduce the chance of premature birth.

- Early birth may be considered if there is severe IUGR.
- Labour may be very painful or progress slowly because the two sides of the uterus may not synchronise well.
- After a vaginal birth you may be offered oxytocin to speed up the birth of the placenta and prevent excessive bleeding.

VACCINATIONS

Like a number of parents you may struggle with the decision about whether or not to vaccinate your child – you want to do the best for her. Like countless others, you will be aware that widespread vaccination has all but eradicated many potentially harmful or fatal diseases from the UK that were once common. You will also be aware of ongoing controversies regarding the safety and appropriateness of vaccine administration. Volatile debates are fuelled by a mixture of personal experiences, medical opinion and research, media intervention and scare mongering. Some people fully support vaccination campaigns. Some are keen to support it but want very clear explanations of the risks and benefits involved. Some feel that research is not yet sufficient and are concerned that vaccination may put – and has already put – some children at risk of damage from side effects.

If you are unsure what steps to take, read as much literature as possible and consider the views of both sides. There is no alternative way to immunise your child against disease. Homeopathy cannot offer vaccination but does offer remedies that can strengthen the immune system or increase resistance to disease and remedies that can be used with standard vaccinations to reduce side effects. If your choice is not to immunise, you have a right to exert your responsibility, even if that means putting your child at risk of contracting the infection against which the vaccine is offered. On the whole, however, vaccinations have had a very positive effect on children's health.

What happens

The standard immunisation programme recommended by the Department of Health is constantly being updated and you will need to take the advice of your GP or paediatrician. The programme may begin when your baby is 8 weeks old. If your child is ill or on medication of any kind you must ensure your GP is aware of this before immunisation.

Some vaccines are given together. This is because they may enhance the way each one works or because it is easier to ensure that some vaccines are not omitted if they are given individually. If you spread out vaccinations your baby may develop a needle phobia. The recommendation to vaccinate a baby at 2, 3 and 4 months is made because there are fewer reported side effects at these times.

Action plan

Standard programme for babies and children

Diphtheria, tetanus, pertussis (DTP) and haemophilus meningitis (Hib) + meningitis C: Four vaccines in a single injection given in the upper forearm or thigh, a single injection of the **meningitic C** vaccine together with **oral polio** at 2, 3 and 4 months of age.

Hepatitis B: May be given at birth and repeated at 1 month and 6 months only where a baby is at risk (p.479).

Measles, mumps, rubella (MMR): Primary dose can be given at any age over 12 months. If there is a local outbreak of measles, it can be given from 6 months.

Booster DTP and oral polio: Given pre-school.

MMR: 2nd dose is given 3 years after completion of primary course, usually pre-school. It is not a booster, but is given to increase the numbers of children who successfully respond to the vaccine from about 75% to 89%. All children are given the 2nd dose because this is more practical than testing all children to see who has not responded to the first dose.

Tuberculosis (BCG): May be an option in the first 8 weeks, depending on where you live and travel.

Influenza: The INFLUENZA vaccine is only recommended for 'at risk' babies, e.g. those who have HEART disease or another major illness, and can be given from 3 months of age.

The diseases that standard vaccines protect against

Diphtheria: This is now very rare in the UK, but can damage the heart and nervous system and can be fatal.

Haemophilus influenzae Type B (Hib): This is an infection that may cause illnesses, including haemophilus MENINGITIS, pneumonia (p.441), septicaemia and EAR INFECTION.

Meningitis C: Meningococcus Type C is a bacterium that is the cause of one type of meningitis, meningococcal meningitis. If the bacteria are in the blood, not confined to the meninges and brain, it is meningococcal septicaemia, which is a severe and life-threatening illness, usually associated with a red purpuric rash. Meningococcus also exists as Types A and B. The Type B causes a similar disease and is generally less common. There is no effective vaccine against Type B at present. Type A may cause epidemics of meningitis and there is an effective vaccine.

Polio: This virus attacks the nervous system and can cause paralysis in the limbs or affect the chest muscles and can be life threatening. Because of vaccination it is unheard of in Europe. The vaccine is given as an (altered) virus in drop form into your baby's mouth. In some areas mothers are offered polio at the same time as their babies. The virus may be present in faeces for up to 4 weeks following immunisation and cross infection can occur, so always wash your hands after nappy changing and wash or cover changing mats used by other babies who may have received polio immunisation. With good hygiene, the risk of cross infection is minimal. If a baby is accidentally infected with the polio virus from another recently vaccinated baby, then the child may develop a high FEVER and be quite unwell, but will recover fully.

Tetanus: Also known as 'lock jaw', this is a rare disease in developed countries that affects the muscles, can cause breathing difficulties and can be fatal if not treated. It is a common problem in undeveloped rural communities. It can be caught from cutting or burning the skin, leaving it open to infection from tetanus bacteria, which are usually found in soil and especially in gardens treated with horse or cow manure.

Whooping cough (pertussis) (p.441): A very tiring and potentially serious illness for a child, especially under the age of 1 year. In the UK, nine babies die from this illness every year – 90% of them are too young to have been immunised and many have caught the illness from unimmunised children. Currently the Department of Health recommends pertussis vaccination at 2, 3 and 4 months because of the real risk of babies catching pertussis from older bothers and sisters. A second (acellular) pertussis vaccination has now been added at pre-school age to boost immunity and reduce the number of older children and adults carrying the pertussis. The acellular vaccine is not as effective in the younger babies, yet in older children causes fewer side effects than the whole cell vaccine.

Indications for avoiding vaccination

- Don't vaccinate your child if she has a fever on the day that the vaccine is due to be given. If she has a cold, runny nose or cough but no fever you can still go ahead.
- The only other medical reason to avoid vaccination is if your baby has a severe medical problem, particularly if an accurate diagnosis of the problem has not yet been made. Your paediatrician will advise you.

Inform your doctor

- Let your doctor or nurse know if your baby has a high fever, has had a bad reaction to any other immunisation, has had or is having treatment for cancer, has a BLEEDING PROBLEM, has had FITS in the past or has had any severe allergic reactions.
- Let your doctor or nurse know if your child or any member of the family has an illness or is having treatment depressing the immune system. There is a risk posed by the live virus immunisations – polio, MEASLES, MUMPS and RUBELLA – to people whose immune system is not functioning well.

Some parents are anxious about the safety of vaccination for other reasons. You are advised to go ahead even if:

- Your child has had the illness that the vaccine is designed to prevent. Prior infection may not give full protection and the diagnosis of a previous infection may often be wrong. Many infections cause a similar looking rash.
- Your child has had a mild reaction to a previous dose of the vaccine.
- Your child has an egg allergy. This is not necessarily a contraindication (see MMR, p.556) but may be a consideration if your child needs the influenza vaccination.

Your baby's reaction

Although most children have no reaction, all children are different.

- Sometimes redness and swelling may develop within 6–8

hours where the injection was given. If this happens, don't worry – it will slowly disappear. Sometimes a small lump develops where the injection was given. This lump can last for several weeks.

- It is quite normal for a baby to be miserable within 48 hours of immunisation. Some babies become irritable and show signs of a headache, sometimes with a fever. Doziness, crying, irritability or a raised temperature can last for up to 24 hours and there may be mild DIARRHOEA following oral polio immunisation.
- A dose of infant paracetamol as directed by your health visitor or doctor will help reduce discomfort for your baby and bring down her temperature if it rises.
- If you are concerned about your child because she has a high fever or shows other signs of distress, contact your GP.
- Homeopathy (prescribed) can help to boost the immune system before immunisation and reduce reactions.

Less common and delayed reactions

- Very rarely, children can have allergic reactions straight after immunisation. As a caution, you will be asked to stay in the health clinic for 10–15 minutes. If your child does react and is treated quickly, usually with an injection of adrenalin (epinephrine) and antihistamine medicine, recovery will be complete. People giving immunisations are trained to deal with these allergic reactions.
- Convulsions due to vaccination are very rare, and usually the baby will make a complete recovery. It may be a febrile convulsion (p.468) caused by a rise in your baby's temperature. While most parents are wary of continuing with further vaccines, many will persevere and complete the course with no further problems. Often in this situation the vaccines are split up, with the whooping cough vaccine being given separately. Immunisation for DTP-Hib later than 4 months increases the chances of fits.
- A mild rash, perhaps with a mild fever and swollen glands, may occur within 5–12 days of measles immunisation.
- The BCG vaccination is a small amount of the bacteria injected under the skin. This causes a local reaction at the site of the injection with a small pus-filled blister. This then bursts and needs to be kept clean until it heals, a process that takes 3–12 weeks.

Thiomersal in vaccines

There has been recent media-provided information giving rise to anxiety about the safety of a mercury-based preservative used in some vaccines to prevent or kill bacteria growing in the vaccine and its connection with autism and autistic spectrum disorders (p.403). At the moment there is no evidence linking an apparent rise in the occurrence of autistic spectrum to exposure to Thiomersal. It has been in use for over 60 years and plays an important part in making vaccines safe.

The vaccines in the UK that contain Thiomersal are diphtheria, tetanus and pertussis. It is not used in any of the MMR, BCG, Hib, Meningitis C or oral polio vaccines. Children in the USA receive many more routine vaccinations than in Britain. As a result, American children are exposed to twice the amount of Thiomersal but there is no difference in the numbers of children affected by autistic spectrum disorders.

However, it has been recommended that manufacturers of vaccines phase out their use of Thiomersal wherever possible.

MMR: measles, mumps, rubella

This single injection protects against three diseases that are becoming less common due to immunisation programmes. Each may have long-term effects and can present serious health risks. Measles, which causes a high fever and a rash, can lead to chest infections, fits and even brain damage in a small number of infected children. Rubella, or 'German Measles', is mild in children but can severely damage babies of infected pregnant women. Mumps can lead to deafness and fertility complications and was once a very common cause of viral meningitis in young children. Measles and mumps are both rare conditions under the age of 1 year. This is one of the reasons for not immunising until a child is 12 months old.

Currently, many parents have safety concerns about the MMR vaccine. You may want to research the facts long before your child's first birthday. Although extensive independent research from around the world has not confirmed any evidence of a relationship between MMR vaccine and either childhood autism or Crohn's disease of the bowel, there is still a need for further detailed research to improve the understanding of the causes of autistic spectrum disorders.

In the US, MMR has been given for more than 25 years and around 200 million doses have been used. Autism and Crohn's disease have not been linked with MMR there. In Finland, where children have been given 2 doses of MMR since 1982, reactions reported after MMR were followed up. There were no reports of permanent damage due to the vaccine. A special study in Finland also showed no link between MMR and autism and Crohn's disease. Some parents worry that giving all three live viruses in MMR together challenges the immune system. Most doctors are confident that the immune system of a healthy baby is constantly subject to a barrage of potential infecting viruses and is easily able to cope. Giving the vaccines separately may be possible by private arrangement but may not be safer in terms of complications and it prolongs the period of time during which your baby is susceptible to the diseases mumps, measles and rubella. It also reduces the number of babies who are immunised because the parents forget to keep to the schedule.

The MMR vaccine is prepared using chick cells to grow the virus. There is no egg protein in the vaccine and therefore no need to be concerned if your baby has an existing egg allergy. The usual signs of a serious allergic reaction are a rash that covers the face and body, a swollen mouth and throat, breathing difficulties and shock. This type of reaction is actually triggered by the child being sensitive to the small amount of antibiotic present in the vaccine to prevent infection in the vaccine during storage, not to egg or any egg protein.

VAGINA, DISCHARGE & INFECTION

A thin and milky, mild-smelling vaginal discharge is normal because microbes live in the healthy vagina. In pregnancy the cervix excretes an increased amount of mucus and discharge may increase. If you feel discomfort or itchiness, or develop a discharge that is yellowish, greenish or foul smelling, you may have an infection. In addition to discomfort, some infections carry a risk of harming the foetus so it is important to inform you doctor or midwife. In pregnancy vaginal infections often recur and may not resolve completely until after the birth.

What happens

Bacterial infections: Include VAGINOSIS, CHLAMYDIA, GONORRHEA and SYPHILIS and can be treated and cured in pregnancy to clear symptoms and protect an unborn baby. STREP B may not give symptoms but does carry risks to your baby so you may wish to be treated in labour

Fungal infections: Those such as CANDIDA can be treated.

Viral infection: With HERPES or HIV these cannot be cured, but there are treatments that can ease symptoms and greatly reduce the risks to a baby.

Occasionally a discharge of clear urine coloured fluid signifies rupture of the membranes and it is amniotic fluid leaking. Sometimes irritation and itching may be a SKIN rash, often related to an ALLERGY.

Action plan

If you have symptoms, arrange to be examined and have a vaginal swab sent for culture. Different swabs are needed to test for bacterial, viral and chlamydia infections and your doctor will recommend the most appropriate. Strep B may only be detected on a rectal swab. Routine testing for vaginal infection differs from hospital to hospital.

Sometimes a test is negative but there is an infection and if symptoms continue it is worth being tested again. If you test positive for a vaginal infection that may be sexually transmitted, it is sensible to ask to be tested for other sexually transmitted diseases and for HEPATITIS B and C and HIV. Testing involves a vaginal swab or a blood test. You may want your partner to be tested. If your discharge is heavy:

- If you have a proven infection, consult your doctor for treatment.
- Try wearing a panty liner. Change it regularly to keep the area fresh and clean. Do not use tampons, which could introduce bacteria and lead to infection.
- You may feel better if you wear loose-fitting clothes and cotton underwear.
- It could help to avoid perfumed toiletries as they can cause irritation and make matters worse.
- Do not douche during pregnancy; there is a danger of altering the normal vaginal bacteria and making an infection more likely.

Homeopathy

Following your specific symptoms, use one of the following in 30c, 4 times a day for 4 days. If there is no change in 2 days, try another remedy; if there is improvement, continue until you are symptom-free. When you bathe, 10–15 drops of *Calendula* tincture in the bath may ease itching and burning.

Kreosotum for an excoriating, profuse, foul-smelling discharge (can smell like rye bread) that stings and burns, is milky or yellow in colour, itches and irritates and can be accompanied by pains in the lower back and general weakness; *Nitric Acid* for a pinkish or greenish stringy, smelly discharge that itches, irritates and burns, comes with splinter-like pains and feels worse in the evenings (often indicated for chronic vaginitis); *Pulsatilla* for thick milky or creamy-yellow bland discharge, accompanied by itching but not as much irritation and excoriation compared to the other remedies and you may feel weepy and want consolation; *Mercurius* for thick, lumpy, excoriating discharge, foul-smelling, itchy and burning and you feel chilly and sweaty; *Sepia* for watery, stringy or lumpy discharge in the day, white or yellow with an offensive odour, and you have dragging pains or a heaviness, itchiness, irritation or dryness, mood changes and you don't want sex.

VAGINAL LAXITY, PROLAPSE & INCONTINENCE

Carrying a baby through pregnancy and, more significantly, giving birth vaginally, puts pressure on your pelvic floor area and the muscles and ligaments around your vagina. Your body is designed to cope, and will be better equipped if you are committed to performing pelvic floor exercises (p.98) that strengthen the pelvic floor and the valves of the bladder and the anus. For some women, damage to the pelvic floor leads to problems. Usually these are short term and there are effective methods of treatment, but they may continue for longer.

There is not a clear relationship between the number of vaginal deliveries and the risk of pelvic floor disorders. The first delivery may carry the highest risk for some types of pelvic floor damage, such as anal sphincter disruption; there may be a cumulative risk of damage with subsequent births that contribute to the eventual development of a clinical pelvic floor disorder. Factors that may contribute include prolonged 2nd stage, use of forceps or ventouse (p.496), being overweight, or coming from a family where there is low resilience in the connective tissue and ligaments that support the vagina and the uterus. Routine use of episiotomy does not prevent prolapse; a midline episiotomy (p.494), however, may increase the risk of anal sphincter damage.

Giving birth by elective CAESAREAN SECTION does reduce the likelihood of prolapse. The reduction is less evident if the operation is done late in labour. However, many mothers and medical professionals believe the other risks associated with caesarean outweigh this potential benefit. Caesarean birth does not reduce the laxity of muscles resulting from weight bearing and hormonal changes in pregnancy.

Stress incontinence of urine
This is a 'storage' problem in which the strength of the bladder sphincter (valve) reduces, and is not able to prevent urine flow against increased pressure from the abdomen. Small leakages of urine are common in pregnancy, usually brought on by a cough, sneeze or laugh, or a sudden movement like running or jumping, particularly in the later stages. Up to 20% of women experience it for a short time after birth but many find that with regular pelvic floor exercises incontinence does not persist for more than a few weeks. Roughly 10% experience

occasional incontinence 9 months after birth. It is more likely to affect women who have given birth vaginally. A heavy VAGINAL DISCHARGE or rupture of the membranes with the passage of amniotic fluid may be mistaken for incontinence.

Vaginal prolapse
Vaginal prolapse occurs when the vaginal walls drop below their normal limits because the supporting ligaments and muscles have been stretched by the birth. Prolapse occurs in about 10% of women after birth but it is usually mild and does not need to be repaired. A minority of women who have delivered vaginally do not develop prolapse and it may be associated with urinary incontinence. Prolapse symptoms may not become apparent until years after childbirth.

Anal incontinence
A disruption of the anal sphincter muscle allows for involuntary passage of gas or faeces. This is more likely during instrumental delivery with forceps or ventouse and affects roughly 4% of mothers. Women who already have one pelvic floor disorder, such as prolapse or urinary incontinence, are more likely to suffer from anal incontinence as well.

What happens
During birth the pelvic organs and structures may be injured. If the ligaments that attach to the side wall of the pelvis to support the vagina are stretched or torn, the vaginal walls may become lax and descend (prolapse). The muscles of the pelvic floor may also tear, and these include the valve-like sphincters that control outflow from the bladder and the bowel. If these sphincters are disrupted incontinence may, but will not always, follow. Another cause of damage is bruising or injury of the nerves along the side walls as your baby's head descends through your pelvis. If the pelvic nerves do not function normally, pelvic muscle tone may be reduced and add to the prolapse and the incontinence. After a few months the vagina recovers, the tissues regain their tone and symptoms are less frequent. Not all women recover fully, however.

Moderate or severe pelvic floor injury will give discomfort or pain and may lead to a variety of symptoms.

- There may be an ache in your lower back or pelvis from tension on the ligaments that support the vagina. If you had stitches or if the joints and ligaments in your pelvis were stretched, the discomfort may increase after birth.
- If the bladder sphincter is disrupted, urine may leak on coughing or straining (stress incontinence).
- The bowel may be unaffected or it may be difficult to empty completely. If the muscle that protects the sphincter at the anal opening is stretched or torn there may be faecal incontinence or FLATULENCE.
- If it feels as if something is coming down in the front or back of your vagina there may be prolapse. The front is affected if the bladder descends (a **cystocoele**). When the back is affected and the rectum descends, it is called a **rectocoele**.
- If there is a cystocoele you may pass urine more frequently, occasionally there may even be difficulty emptying the bladder, and a URINARY TRACT INFECTION is more likely.
- Prolapse may sometimes give a sensation of a wide vagina and reduced sensitivity during intercourse.

Action plan

If you have symptoms of prolapse or urinary or anal incontinence, visit your doctor. At your 6-week postnatal visit the tone of your pelvic floor muscles and ligaments will be checked but your doctor will examine you in more detail if you are concerned. Few women find it easy to admit to faecal incontinence, but treatment can be very effective.

What you can do

- Pelvic floor exercises in pregnancy help strengthen the muscles around the vagina, anus and pelvis and are good preparation for the pressure of birth. After birth begin the exercises as soon as possible and build up gradually. You can concentrate on tightening your anus as well as your vaginal area. Try contracting and releasing your pelvic floor 30 times every time you feed your baby.
- When you urinate, tighten your muscles mid-flow so the flow stops and then release and let it recommence. It may take a week or two before your pelvic floor responds. You may also hold your urine for a progressively longer time, up to 5 minutes, to strengthen the muscles. Sex is a great way to strengthen all the muscles in the vagina.
- There are no certain ways to prevent prolapse but using upright postures in birth (p.152) may reduce the time spent bearing down, when pressure is maximal, and reduce the likelihood that you will need assistance. If your baby does need help, it is preferable to use ventouse instead of forceps. The ventouse takes less room, and provided it is only applied when your cervix is fully dilated, it is less disruptive on your tissues than forceps.
- Being well nourished and eating optimal amounts of vitamins, minerals and antioxidants improves the tone of your connective tissues and reduces the severity of prolapse if it occurs. Eating well also allows your body to recover more easily.

Medical care

- An ultrasound scan can identify pelvic floor damage and tears to the anal sphincter. MRI, x-ray and bladder-pressure studies that can be done if the symptoms persist for months.
- If the ligaments are very stretched or if the pudendal nerves in your pelvis are bruised, you may find it difficult to contract your pelvic floor selectively. A physiotherapist may recommend exercises and the use of cones to improve the muscle strength and control. They are very easy to use and within 4–6 weeks, you are likely to notice an improvement.
- Biofeedback is another simple method that can assist with exercises and cones. Electrodes are placed on your abdomen and along the anal area. A monitor shows which muscles are contracting and which are at rest and you can use this to identify the correct muscles for performing pelvic floor exercises. Of the people who used biofeedback, about 75% report improved symptoms.
- Electrical stimulation therapy uses low-voltage electric current to stimulate and contract the correct group of muscles. This may be done in a clinic or at home if you prefer. The current is delivered using a battery-operated probe in the anus or vagina. Treatment sessions usually last 20 minutes and may be performed every day for months

Stimulation is effective if the pelvic nerves are not functioning.

- If you have prolapse you may have an increase in urinary or anal incontinence in the next pregnancy but it usually settles after the birth. The next birth is likely to be straightforward because the vaginal tissues stretch easily and an episiotomy will probably not be needed.
- It is rare, but if prolapse is severe your doctor may insert a ring to hold your vagina in place postnatally. The ring can be removed when your vaginal ligament tone improves.
- A surgical operation may be required to treat severe prolapse, particularly if it is associated with incontinence and/or anal sphincter damage. It is preferable to postpone the operation until your childbearing is completed. After a prolapse operation, birth is usually by caesarean section to avoid damaging the repair.

Homeopathy

These homeopathic remedies may help stress incontinence. Take in 30c, 3 times a day for up to 1 week and then reassess.

Use *Causticum* if involuntary urination is worse during the first part of the night and if you feel chilly; *Pulsatilla* if leakage occurs particularly at night or while lying down and you feel thirstless, weepy and your moods are changeable; *Sepia* if leakage is accompanied by a bearing-down sensation, is worse from walking, you are irritable and feel chilly.

Urinary urgency incontinence

If your bladder is irritated by infection (e.g. chronic cystitis, p.553), inflammation or bruising, it may be more liable to contract so small volumes of urine give a feeling of fullness and urgency, and there may be leakage when you need to pass urine but it flows before you are ready. It is also known as **irritable bladder**. Strengthening through pelvic floor exercises and physiotherapy techniques (left) usually helps. If a narrowing of the urethra causes the irritability, it may need to be dilated under surgery. Inflammation may not be infectious but caused by an ALLERGY.

Once you have been checked for infection and diagnosed with irritable bladder, try one of these homeopathic remedies if it suits your symptoms in 6c, 4 times a day for up to a week, and then reassess.

Use *Equisetum* with a constant desire to urinate, often urgently, a sensation of fullness in the bladder, general tenderness and aching, a cutting or pricking pain in the urethra while you pass large quantities of light-coloured urine, worse at the end or after urination; *Staphysagria* if you used a catheter and/or have a frequent urge with a sensation of pressure but difficulty urinating, burning during urination (drop by drop) with a continued urge and pain afterwards.

Urinary retention & overflow incontinence

Pressure during birth may lead to swelling of the tissues of the urethra in the bladder outlet and cause retention of urine so the bladder fills excessively and then overflows. Inserting a catheter tube to drain the urine until the swelling reduces treats retention. The bladder usually recovers spontaneously within 24–48 hours.

The following homeopathic remedies may be useful in 30c, every hour for 4 hours. *Staphysagria* particularly if forceps were used; *Aconite* if labour was emotionally shocking and delivery was very fast, there is a frequent urge to pass urine with pressing pains accompanied by anxiety; *Opium* if retention follows shock and the sphincter of the bladder is in spasm, you are confused and feel spaced-out.

VAGINOSIS

Bacterial vaginosis, previously known as gardnerella vaginitis, is one of the most common causes of vaginal discharge. It is called non-specific vaginitis and can be present without symptoms. It may be transmitted through sexual contact but this is not an exclusive route, and although men also carry the bacteria they do not show symptoms. The infection cannot be spread by sharing eating utensils or clothes or in swimming pools. Nor can it be spread from a pregnant woman to her unborn baby, but it has been linked to premature rupture of the membranes (p.501) and PREMATURE BIRTH, so early treatment is worthwhile.

What happens
Vaginosis bacteria often live in the vagina in small numbers without presenting any problems. The bacteria favour conditions that are not too acid and increase if the environment is more alkaline, as in pregnancy, perhaps giving a vaginal discharge with an unpleasant fishy odour. The smell may be strongest after sex but there is unlikely to be any itching.

Action plan
- A vaginal swab can be tested for organisms. Treatment is with antibiotics in tablets or as an antiseptic vaginal gel. The usual choice is metronidazole for use once the 1st trimester has passed. If treatment eradicates the infection, it may reduce the risks of premature birth.
- If you have had premature birth in a previous pregnancy, you may consider asking for a test.
- Pro-biotic yoghurt or pills may help to replace the lactobacilli in your bowel and vagina, thus preventing the gardnerella bacteria from thriving (for details of how to take this, see CANDIDA).
- Nutrition can build up your immunity to this and other common infections.

VEINS: MOTHER

The veins in your body undergo many changes during pregnancy. Blood volume increases; pregnancy hormones relax and dilate the vein walls; and the veins expand, particularly in the pelvis, labia and thighs and legs. In some women, problems range from harmless visible veins to a rare but potentially life-threatening condition, thrombosis (overleaf).

Spider veins
Sometimes blood vessels become visible as red spots that are

spider shaped and may be up to 3 mm (⅛ in) in diameter. These consist of capillary blood vessels dilated by the hormones and will disappear if you touch them lightly, then reappear when you release the pressure. They will become invisible when pregnancy is over.

Prominent & varicose veins
When veins swell because of increased blood flow, they become prominent, visible as blue lines beneath the skin and perhaps slightly raised. They are most common on the abdomen and breasts. Sometimes as a vein expands, the valves in the wall stretch and lose their competence to stop the backflow of blood and the vein becomes varicose. They are most common in the legs and labia and also appear on the thighs and around the anus. Probably 30% of women get them. Varicose veins often run in families (due to thin connective tissue), are more common with TWINS, in overweight women or women whose occupations involve standing for long periods.

Varicose veins often throb, particularly at the end of the day and may be associated with slight swelling, often in the legs. The varicosities present no risk to a baby. After pregnancy, varicosities usually improve. Labial veins always disappear completely after birth but varicose leg veins may not resolve completely if the extent of stretching means that the valves are no longer strong enough to prevent the build-up of pressure. You might find that varicosities increase in subsequent pregnancies.

Action plan
Medical care
- If you have pain in the veins that does not disappear when you rest or if they are red and sore, further investigation is needed to exclude **phlebitis** (inflammation) or deep vein thrombosis (p.560).
- Surgical removal is not recommended during pregnancy because of the high blood flow in the veins at this time. It is best to wait for 3–6 months after birth, and in this time the veins may shrink. You may prefer to wait until you've completed your family because each pregnancy puts additional strain on your venous system.

Lifestyle, diet and exercise
- Good-quality elastic support tights are essential to minimise pressure on the veins. If the veins are severely affected, use the tights whenever you are out of bed. Support is very important after delivery (a high-risk time), particularly during and after CAESAREAN SECTION, to prevent a deep vein thrombosis, and will help veins return to their normal state.
- Avoid clothing that restricts blood flow. This includes tight trousers and socks with elastic tops.
- Reducing the pressure on your legs may prevent or decrease the extent of varicose veins. Try to put your legs up above the level of your uterus for an hour or two during the day and raise the foot of your bed by about 15 cm (6 in) at night.
- If you are taking a long flight, use support tights, drink water and walk around regularly and take a single dose of aspirin (75 mg) before the flight.
- Avoid gaining too much WEIGHT. A diet rich in vitamins and

minerals and antioxidants reduces the risk of thrombosis.

- Exercise by walking or swimming often to maintain circulation and prevent thrombosis.

Aromatherapy and massage

A cold compress can offer relief, as can a gentle massage: massage in gentle upward strokes and never massage directly over a varicose vein. Try lemon essential oil mixed into a carrier and after Week 24 you can use geranium in a low dose.

Homeopathy

Take a remedy in 6c, 4 times a day for up to 2 weeks and then reassess. If there is no change see a homeopathic practitioner. If pain is severe and persists seek medical advice.

The no. 1 remedy for varicose veins is *Hamamelis*, for soreness, congestion, heaviness of legs and thighs, a constricted, stinging feeling in the veins, worse from pressure and movement and better at night, perhaps with a history of poor circulation. *Sepia* helps for purple varicosities on the vulva and legs with a feeling of heaviness, when the whole system feels sluggish (perhaps with CONSTIPATION or PILES) but better for fast movement and warmth; *Pulsatilla* for poor circulation with cold hands and feet, bluish, swollen veins, changeable symptoms, turbulent emotions, better for gentle exercise, fresh air and pressure on the affected area; *Fluoric acid* for chronic varicose veins in women who have had many children, knotted and sensitive with a burning sensation, better for fast motion and from bathing in cool water; *Carbo Veg* if you feel chilly, particularly your hands and feet, yet veins are burning and itching and your skin appears mottled, pain reduces in fresh air; *Lachesis* for hard, ropy, purple, distended veins, usually on the left leg, with pulsating pains exacerbated by heat and worse after sleep.

Phlebitis, deep vein thrombosis & pulmonary embolism

From conception, the blood-clotting system is very active and is at its most coagulable in the first week after the birth. This prevents excessive bleeding but it also increases the risk of developing a blood clot, venous thrombosis, a rare but potentially serious problem that usually occurs in the pelvic or leg veins. Phlebitis is inflammation of the vein wall, usually associated with varicose veins.

The risk associated with thrombosis is that if the clot is dislodged it may travel to the heart and block the pulmonary veins in the lungs, causing a pulmonary embolus. This rare event can be life threatening as it reduces the amount of oxygen the blood receives. Early diagnosis and treatment prevents serious complications.

What happens

When a leg vein becomes inflamed (phlebitis) it feels hot, red and tender and the leg may swell, usually only around the swollen vein. With care this will not necessarily progress to thrombosis. In the more dangerous deep vein thrombosis the usual symptoms are pain and swelling of the calf or the thigh but in 50% of thromboses there is neither swelling nor pain, particularly if the clot is in one of the pelvic veins. The 'silent' thromboses are more dangerous because they are not treated

early. The pain of a deep vein thrombosis is not relieved by bed rest or elevating the leg. If the clot travels to the lungs to give a pulmonary embolus, symptoms may vary from minimal BREATHLESSNESS to severe chest pain, shock and collapse. A number of factors increase susceptibility: prolonged bed rest before or after the birth; a previous episode of deep vein thrombosis or embolus formation; existing large varicose veins or inflammation in the veins; being overweight; SMOKING; following operative surgery, including caesarean section; a family history of pulmonary embolism or deep vein thrombosis. If you have thrombophilia (p.408) the risk is significantly increased.

Action plan

Call your doctor immediately if:

- You have a swollen vein or leg with pain that does not improve with bed rest.
- You have even mild symptoms associated with pulmonary embolus, such as breathlessness. Severe chest pain or shock needs urgent medical attention.

Preventative measures

- If you have a caesarean section you can reduce the risk of thrombosis by using elastic stockings and being mobile within hours of surgery.
- If you have had a previous thrombosis or embolus or thrombophilia, using blood-thinning anticoagulants (aspirin or heparin) is a standard precaution.
- Superficial phlebitis (inflammation) carries minimal risk of an embolus provided there is no underlying deep vein thrombosis and the swelling is treated with anti-inflammatory tablets and cream. The legs must be supported with tights and it is important to remain mobile to reduce the risk of the clot extending into the deep veins. Anticoagulants may be needed.

Treatment for thromboses

- A deep vein thrombosis is confirmed by ultrasound scan and can be treated with anticoagulants. Heparin is the drug of first choice because it does not cross the placenta. It is administered by injection under the abdominal skin once or twice a day. However, if heparin is used for more than a few months, it may cause OSTEOPOROSIS. After pregnancy it can be gradually replaced with warfarin to keep the blood thin. The doses must be carefully monitored to prevent over-thinning and internal bleeding. Depending on clot size, the treatment may continue for a few months. Aspirin may be used in conjunction with heparin in pregnancy.
- A pulmonary embolus is an emergency treated with heparin to thin the blood and prevent further clot formation. If the embolus is large, additional intravenous medication may be administered to break down the clot and improve blood flow to the lungs. During pregnancy a pulmonary embolus cannot be confirmed with the usual ventilation and perfusion scan because of the radiation risk to the baby. This test can be performed after birth.
- You are at greatest risk in the 1st week after birth and this is the time to ensure you are mobile and receiving anticoagulants if these are needed.

VOMITING: BABY

All babies bring up a small amount of milk (around 2–3 tsp) after some, most or all of their feeds for the first few months, often without any force. This is possetting, and is completely normal and rarely causes distress. **Reflux** is where the valve between the stomach and the oesophagus is weak and the milk comes back up. Providing your baby is gaining weight, it is not a cause for concern. Vomiting involves bringing up a large amount of stomach contents through the mouth and sometimes the nose. All babies vomit some time in the early months.

Vomiting under 12 weeks
By far the most common reason for babies to vomit is if they have been fed too much. The milk returns much the same as it went down, although it may be curdled if it has spent more than a few minutes in the stomach acid. Effortless reflux and possetting is equally common, and the milk just trickles out the mouth, or can be burped a few inches. Occasionally, early vomiting before 12 weeks may indicate gastroenteritis infection (p.446). Very rarely, often when vomiting is projectile, it may be a sign of a obstruction to the digestive system such as pyloric stenosis (p.563).

Vomiting after 12 weeks
If your baby begins vomiting when she is older, it may indicate an infection of the digestive tract, often accompanied by DIARRHOEA and FEVER, or a URINARY TRACT INFECTION. If she has had an injury to the head, it may be a symptom of concussion.

When vomiting is not a cause for concern
Although it may upset your baby, and alarm you, occasional vomiting is seldom linked to a serious health concern. A single vomit may simply be a sign that your baby is a little unwell or overfilled with milk, and is usually self-limiting.

When vomiting may be serious
If your baby doesn't usually vomit and has repeated vomiting of sudden onset, particularly if it is linked with diarrhoea or a fever, it may be a sign of infection. In a small number of cases, ongoing vomiting (particularly if projectile) is a sign of a obstruction in the digestive tract. Usually the main concern with repeated vomiting is that it may cause dehydration – where your baby does not have enough fluid or salt in her system. Dehydration (p.446) can lead to fluid and mineral imbalance and weight loss and when severe it needs hospital treatment to prevent long-term effects.

What happens
When a baby vomits, contractions of the stomach force food contents up the oesophagus and out of the mouth and nose. The milk or food is often partially digested and may have a curdled appearance, and because it contains stomach acid it may make also your baby uncomfortable with heartburn. If your baby inhales while she is vomiting or while vomit remains in her mouth, she may cough and gag, become breathless and panic until the vomiting has stopped and the airway is clear.

Vomiting itself is seldom dangerous – it is the resulting dehydration that presents a problem. A normal healthy baby will not choke on vomit unless she is unconscious for another reason. Even when she is asleep your baby has well-developed reflexes that prevent anything from being aspirated into the lungs.

Reflux
At the level of the stomach the oesophagus is closed off by the lower oesophageal sphincter (valve), which relaxes to let food into the stomach and closes to prevent food mixed with stomach acid from refluxing back up into the mouth. If food does come back, even part of the way, this is called reflux or gastro-oesophageal reflux.

All babies reflux: this is part of the process that lies behind possetting. If the reflux causes pain as acid comes back up the oesophagus (giving heartburn), your baby may appear unsettled after feeding or be reluctant to feed; the reflux may also appear as vomit. The reflux is likely to pass as your baby grows older, either when she begins to eat solid food, or when she learns to stand and walk and spends more time upright.

There are many simple treatments that make a baby more comfortable and could resolve the problem.
- Prop up your baby during and after a feed. Give her less milk at each feed, feed more often and ensure she is winded.
- If she is over 4 months and eating solids, increasing the solids in her diet may be effective. Do not add any cereal or other thickener to formula milk, or use more formula powder than instructed – this could increase the sodium content to dangerous levels and cause dehydration.
- A very few babies with reflux fail to gain WEIGHT, and this is probably the only group for whom medical treatment with antacid or anti-reflux drugs, or, rarely, surgery is needed. There are also thickened milk feeds, such as Enfamil. Your paediatrician may prescribe drugs that improve the movement of food through the bowel or to reduce stomach acid. Reflux can be a symptom of milk ALLERGY OR INTOLERANCE. You will oten need an alternative formula milk.

Disorders of the digestive system
Early vomiting rarely occurs because of a disorder of the digestive system. If your newborn baby vomits forcefully after each feed and brings up bright yellow or green vomit, there may be an **obstruction** to the passage of food and fluid through the bowel. This needs to be checked urgently by your paediatrician who may order an x-ray or ultrasound scan. The obstruction may be due to intestinal atresia (p.563) or her bowel may be slightly twisted (intestinal malrotation). These rare conditions also lead to CONSTIPATION. Pyloric stenosis (p.563) is a rare condition that leads to projectile vomiting beginning in the 3rd–12th week after birth.

Infection
About 90% of vomiting after the 12th week is caused by viruses, predominantly **rotavirus**. Occasionally there may be infection earlier but your baby is protected by your antibodies,

particularly if you are breastfeeding. You may suspect bacterial infection if your baby has abdominal pain and bloody stools, has been in contact with known cases or travelled abroad. When accompanied by diarrhoea, vomiting is often a sign of a bowel infection such as gastroenteritis or food poisoning.

Vomiting is also commonly linked with almost any viral infection such as a COUGH OR COLD. Excess mucus on the chest leads to coughing and that can cause your baby to vomit. It is more likely to happen while your baby is not upright and mucus is more difficult to expel. Vomiting may be symptom of a throat or EAR INFECTION. It may also be a sign of a urinary tract infection. More serious infections that may lead to vomiting include MENINGITIS. When an infection has passed, perhaps after treatment, the vomiting clears up on its own.

Vomiting with blood
If your baby vomits and you can see blood in the regurgitated stomach contents, this is not necessarily a cause for concern. If you are breastfeeding and have cracked nipples (p.416) your baby will be taking in blood. It is safe to continue feeding and the blood will do no harm.

Blood in vomit may, however, be a symptom of a BLEEDING PROBLEM and you need to consult your doctor urgently who will check blood clotting. Bloody diarrhoea with vomiting may on rare occasionas indicate **haemolytic uraemic syndrome**, a disease usually triggered by a bacterium called E. coli that is commonly spread in partly cooked meat. Treatment requires hospital admission and specialist care and although recovery is usually complete, kidney damage may result.

Injury
Vomiting may result from an injury to the head and could be a symptom of concussion. If your baby has had an injury and also appears sleepy or listless, consult your doctor urgently.

Action plan
Calling your doctor
You need to visit your doctor if your baby:
- Has signs of dehydration (p.446) (dry lips but wet inside the mouth), is troubled but not overly fretful and tires easily.
- Is under 6 months and has been vomiting for more than 12 hours.
- Is over 6 months and has been vomiting for more than 24 hours.
- Has other symptoms that are of concern; e.g. ear pain, diarrhoea, fever, listlessness.

You need to call your doctor urgently and you may need to take immediate First Aid measures (p.383) if:
- There is blood in the vomit, unless you have cracked nipples.
- The vomit is bright yellow or bright green – this bilious vomiting could indicate a bowel obstruction.
- Your baby's abdomen appears to be more swollen or the veins have become more prominent then usual.
- Your baby seems to have abdominal pain for more than 2 hours, lasting longer than a usual attack of COLIC.
- Your baby has signs of dehydration – mottled or pale skin, listlessness, dry lips and mouth, absence of urine. Your baby

cannot keep down any fluid.
- Your baby has a high fever above 38.5°C (101.3°F), particularly with a rash.
- Your baby has had an abdominal injury or a head knock.
- Your baby is having a FIT (convulsion).
- Your baby is on medicines for seizures or a heart condition and cannot keep these down.
- Your baby may have ingested a poison (plant, medicine, chemical).
- Your baby appears to be choking.

Medical care at home
The key to treating vomiting is to do what you can to avoid dehydration, i.e. give your baby fluids. When there is vomiting it is important to introduce the fluids gradually, and in small amounts. If you are breastfeeding, let your baby suck for a short time every 5 minutes. If not, offer your baby water or a rehydration solution an hour after the last vomiting attack because episodes of vomiting usually settle quickly. Begin with a sip or teaspoonful every 15 minutes.
- When your child is vomiting often, stop any medicines, unless critical (e.g. anticonvulsant or for a heart condition when, if more than 1 dose is missed, call your doctor).
- You can use infant paracetamol to bring down fever, if she has one. If she cannot keep this down, your doctor may prescribe paracetamol suppositories.
- Do not give your child anti-nausea medication or medicines to stop vomiting, which are only necessary if the vomiting is severe and then your child may be cared for in hospital.
- There is no correct lying position to prevent inhalation unless your baby is unconscious. If so, turn her on her side, and allow secretions to drain from the mouth.

Homeopathy
When not severe, vomiting can be treated with the diarrhoea homeopathic remedies listed on p.447.

Treatment of vomiting in hospital
If you take your baby to hospital, the doctors will note how frequently she is vomiting, when it began, whether it contains blood, if urine is being passed. Your baby's temperature will be taken and you will be asked about her recent feeding patterns and any contact she might have had with infection. Your baby will then be examined and tested for dehydration and other infections, including coughs and of the chest, meningitis, urinary infections, haemolytic uraemic syndrome (above left), and intestinal obstruction.

Most babies are then offered a feed of clear fluid of about 30–90 ml (1–3 fl oz). If this is tolerated and not vomited within 30–60 minutes, it is repeated. If your baby keeps down the fluid and appears well, she may be allowed home. The medical team will ensure you are confident and understand the situation. Continue with feeds as usual and supplement with extra oral fluids. Use oral rehydration solution or Dioralyte 4–8 hourly.

If your baby does not keep down the initial feed, fluid may be given through a vein, or through a tube into the stomach. Often this is sufficient to stop vomiting, and fluids by mouth can be restarted. If this is tolerated your baby will be observed for a few hours, and she may be discharged. Most babies recover within 48 hours on this treatment but others need longer. Occasionally antibiotics are used for bacterial infections.

Pyloric stenosis & other rare causes of vomiting

Pyloric stenosis affects about 2:1000 babies. It brings on progressively severe vomiting, usually starting by the 3rd week after birth and seldom later than the 12th week. It is more common in boys and is caused by an excessive thickening of the muscle, the pylorus, which obstructs the stomach at the exit to the small bowel and stops it from emptying. Projectile vomiting during or straight after feeding flies across the room and may travel as far as 1.5 m (5 ft), and your baby will look hungry afterwards. Weight loss can occur quickly. The cause is not known.

Occasional projectile vomiting is not a sure sign of pyloric stenosis. Many babies initially thought to have this condition are in reality being overfed, and stop vomiting when their feed is reduced. Before the onset of projectile vomiting, pyloric stenosis may produce symptoms that mimic other causes of vomiting.

Pyloric stenosis can be detected by feeling the hard pylorus muscle on examining the abdomen and can be confirmed with an ultrasound. If there is any doubt, your baby may be given a barium swallow x-ray. The treatment involves a relatively simple operation under general anaesthetic where the muscle is split. The need for an operation may make you anxious, but once the operation is complete feeding generally returns to normal and your baby's growth resumes. These babies quickly catch up in weight with their contemporaries. Rarely, the intestine may be blocked and this may cause vomiting and constipation.

Oesophageal atresia & tracheo-oesophageal fistula

Oesophageal atresia affects around 1:1800 babies and leads to vomiting and often excessive dribbling. Oesophageal atresia refers to malformations that block the oesophagus, the muscular tube that connects the mouth to the stomach. Sometimes the oesophagus ends in a closed sac or may be narrowed (stenosis). Most affected babies have a connection between the trachea (windpipe) and the oesophagus, a tracheo-oesophageal fistula. This is a serious defect and in one-third of cases accompanies other CONGENITAL ABNORMALITIES. With a fistula, swallowed food can get into the lungs, causing coughing and choking, pneumonia (p.441) and a blue tinge to the skin due to lack of oxygen.

Oesophageal atresia requires immediate surgery and possibly multiple operations. Your baby may have to be tube fed for much of the 1st year in a SPECIAL CARE BABY UNIT and may need medical and nutritional support for years. This is very demanding and you will need ongoing emotional and practical help.

WHEEZING: BABY

See ASTHMA: BABY

WEIGHT, LOW GAIN OR FAILURE TO THRIVE: BABY

In the first 2 years after birth most children gain relatively more weight and grow much more rapidly than they ever will in a similar period of time later on. Rapid growth is very noticeable in the first few months, but this is also a common time for parents to worry about inadequate growth. If you regularly plot growth in your baby's record book, you will notice an upward trend on the chart. At times your baby's weight gain may plateau or he may go through growth spurts and occasionally he may lose a little weight. This fluctuation is normal.

If your baby fails to gain weight as expected for 2 consecutive months, or drops down 2 or more percentile curves on the chart over a short period, your doctor will probably want to investigate his failure to thrive and work with you to promote weight gain. Only around 2% of babies truly fail to gain weight adequately, although 4% are referred for investigation when the charted line falls a single centile.

What happens

'Failure to thrive' is a general diagnosis of a condition rather than a specific disease, with many possible causes. Children who fail to thrive don't receive or are unable to take in or retain adequate nutrition. The condition is more common in premature babies, when it is often linked to medical problems associated with an early birth.

The first month

A full-term baby loses up to 10% of his birth weight in the first week after birth. This is because fat and glycogen stores in the body are used for energy while feeding is established. After this, normal weight gain is progressive. A PREMATURE baby or one who has INTRAUTERINE GROWTH RESTRICTION may not lose as much weight initially, and many small babies gain weight rapidly to catch up their 'normal' weight. Breastfed babies often gain weight more slowly than bottle-fed babies in the first 2 weeks, due to low milk flow. This is usually due to feeding difficulties (p.412) because it can take time and guidance to establish breastfeeding. For guidance , expect your baby to have a milk feed 8-12 times in every 24-hour period.

Babies who gain weight slowly are often referred to hospital, and are occasionally found to be mildly dehydrated, slightly JAUNDICED and have lost between 11 and 15% of birth weight. The main medical concern is to ensure there is no underlying cause such as an undiagnosed URINARY TRACT INFECTION or perhaps even a HEART condition. Most often feeding, with attention to latching on and position (p.188), type of formula milk or the introduction of supplementary feeds for a few days is enough to increase calorie intake and weight gain. A mother may need time, support and rest if she feels anxious, because anxiety may affect milk supply.

Up to 6 months, and beyond

By the 2nd or 3rd month, it is usual for a baby to have 6-8 milk feeds a day, although each milk feed will be larger now. Milk continues to provide essential calories when solid food is introduced, usually at or after 4 months. The average baby born at full term doubles his birth weight by 6 months and triples it at 1 year. A premature baby attains his birth weight from about 10 days after birth, and then his weight increases as normal, providing he is able to tolerate his feeds.

In general babies who fail to thrive simply because they have feeding difficulties are rarely miserable, except at feeding times. Although thin and wide eyed, they are often happy. If poor nutrition persists and a baby continues to grow more slowly than expected, he may become apathetic and irritable, and may not reach milestones like sitting up and experimenting with language at the usual age. And because a baby's brain grows so much in the 1st year, very poor nutrition may have permanent effects on mental development. This only occurs in the most severe cases, and is usually also associated with emotional deprivation.

What causes failure to thrive?

The causes of failure to thrive may be broadly sorted into 3 categories: a baby is eating but not being given enough milk and/or food; he has a medical problem that interferes with proper digestion; or his requirements are higher due to some illness or infection. Sometimes paediatricians cannot pinpoint a specific cause. A baby's personality also plays an important role. The distinction between medical causes and causes linked to care or environment is not always easy to make. This is because a medical cause could make a baby fractious at mealtimes, and a parent may also become tense and spend less time feeding.

Possible causes

- Difficulty sucking in the early weeks is a common cause, more usual among premature babies or babies with a CLEFT LIP OR PALATE. Some full-term babies take time to get used to feeding from a breast or bottle.
- Poor feeding position, incorrect latching on or not feeding for long enough may mean a breastfed baby does not get enough milk. A mother may have low milk flow (p.415).
- When a baby begins to eat solids there may be a temporary plateau or slowing of weight gain as the body adjusts to new food types. Occasionally an ALLERGY OR INTOLERANCE affects gain, and for a small number of babies milk intolerance affects gain before solids are introduced.
- Digestive difficulties resulting from conditions such as chronic DIARRHOEA or reflux (p.561), which makes eating painful and may lead to VOMITING, can slow weight gain or lead to weight loss.
- CONGENITAL ABNORMALITIES such as CYSTIC FIBROSIS, liver disease, metabolic disorders and coeliac disease (p.393) that limit the body's ability to absorb nutrients may affect growth, even if a baby seems to eat enough.
- Infections, especially urine infections if left untreated, place great demands on the body and force it to use nutrients rapidly, sometimes bringing about short- or long-term failure to thrive.
- A host of other medical causes - including neurological, cardiac, endocrine and respiratory conditions - can be suspects as well. Babies with IUGR or autistic spectrum disorders may be very difficult to feed.

- Parents' attitudes or behaviours may be a cause. Some parents restrict the amount of calories they give their babies, perhaps due to a fear of excess gain or a mistaken belief that a low-fat adult diet is suitable for babies. A small number of children fail to thrive as a result of neglect: they are simply not fed enough.

Action plan

Diagnosing the cause

When your baby's growth is slower than expected, your doctor will begin to investigate possible causes. A blood count, urine analysis and various blood chemical and electrolyte tests can give useful information. If the paediatrician suspects a particular disease or disorder, she may perform tests to identify that condition. Perhaps with the help of a dietician or breastfeeding counsellor, she will also ask you what your baby eats and how he behaves when he eats, and may recommend you keep a food diary, which can be used to calculate your baby's calorie intake. You may be asked about your own diet and lifestyle if you are breastfeeding.

Treatment

The duration of treatment varies. Weight gain takes time, so several months may pass before your baby is back in the normal range. Sometimes gain increases within a week and behaviour becomes more settled.

Breastfeeding

If you are breastfeeding, a midwife, health visitor or breastfeeding counsellor may help you address problems. Most commonly, difficulty latching on, poor positioning or not having time are at the root of slow feeding or low milk flow.

Nutrition and extra feeding

Most cases of failure to thrive are due to inadequate intake. These can be tackled through a change in diet. Often moving from breast milk to formula milk, or supplementing breast with bottles, leads to weight increase. If this does not work, your doctor may prescribe a high-density milk formula or recommend high-calorie foods if your baby is weaned. If your baby shows an allergy or intolerance, different formulae may be tried before his weight stabilises and he begins to gain.

If the feeding difficulty has not been solved or helped by the more general approach of reassurance and monitoring of weight, you and your baby may be supported by a nutritionist and perhaps also by an occupational or speech therapist who can address any problems with sucking and swallowing that your baby may have, and look at the interaction between you both at feeding times.

If your baby has a more persistent case of failure to thrive, he may need to be admitted to hospital, often as a day case for investigation. Infrequently, he may need to be tube fed, particularly if he is ill, or weight gain has been poor over a period of observation. This can sometimes be done at home. Usually a liquid milk or supplemented liquid milk is given. With supplementary feeding at night the tube does not interfere with activities during the day and he may continue to eat normally in the day. About half his calorie requirements can be delivered at night through a continuous drip into the

Growth charts provide a useful tool for parents and health professionals who need to assess whether a baby is thriving. In the UK health checks are spaced at increasingly wide intervals, and a child's weight and height plotted in the parent-held record book. If a doctor is concerned about a child's health, any abnormal growth patterns can be easily spotted this way. Very rarely, a failure to gain weight may first be noted with the use of these charts.

There are separate charts for boys and girls, because their average birth weight and rate of growth differs. On both charts, however, the principle is the same. To record your baby's height and weight, find his age in weeks along the bottom (horizontal) axis and the weight or length on the side (vertical) axis. Draw a line from each: where they meet, mark a dot. Over time each chart will show a line of dots, and joining them gives your baby's growth curve.

The lines already marked on the chart are called centiles or percentiles. The central line is the 50th centile – 50% of children fall below this line, 50% above. The top and bottom centiles represent the extremes of height and weight – 0.5% of normal babies fall beyond these. Your baby's growth curve is likely to run parallel to the 50th centile. Small deviations from this line are not a cause for concern, and every baby fluctuates from his or her average with growth spurts and minor illnesses.

Downward-sloping lines: If your baby's measurements join to form a downward-sloping curve, this suggests he is not growing optimally (the term used is 'failure to thrive'). In most cases this is not significant and the downward trend is temporary, yet it is best for a health visitor or doctor to check your baby's wellbeing.

Upward-sloping lines: These cross upwards across the percentiles and usually indicate catch-up growth. If your baby's weight for height or length is 50% more then expected you will need to take care that you are not overfeeding him. Early weight gain may be an indicator for obesity (right) in early childhood.

Premature babies: A premature baby's birth weight is plotted at the week of birth rather than at '0'. Over the next weeks the extent of prematurity is subtracted from the real age. For instance, if your baby is born at Week 36, birth is plotted at 36; when your baby is 4 weeks old the measurement will be plotted above '0' in the chart; and when he is 10 weeks old, above '6'. This assesses your baby according to his expected delivery date and accounts for the shortfall in growth. The subtraction usually continues to the end of the 12th month after birth, although some authorities continue to the end of the 24th month.

Postmature babies (p.500): These are usually plotted from Week 40 as a correction for 2 weeks makes no difference.

tube. Once he has gained weight, he will feel better and the tube can be removed.

Treatment in hospital

If your baby continues to fail to thrive and seems to be losing weight despite food supplementation, he may need to be admitted to hospital where he can be fed and continuously monitored. The hospital team will attempt to identify any underlying medical causes. They can also help if you are experiencing breastfeeding difficulties and may offer advice and support if there appear to be any problems in his relationship with you or other carers.

Your baby will probably stay in hospital until weight gain is adequate. Very occasionally it can be many weeks until symptoms of severe malnutrition are no longer present. There are some units where mother and baby can remain together during tests and receive advice about operating as a team to maximise weight gain. If a chronic illness or disorder such as cystic fibrosis, has caused failure to thrive your baby may have to be monitored periodically and perhaps treated for a lifetime.

Extra care

Depending on the cause, a paediatric nutritional specialist may be part of your baby's care team. If the reason for slow growth is thought to be related to your baby's personality or environment rather than a medical condition, a social worker or psychologist may provide support. Sometimes the cause of the failure to thrive, and associated feeding behaviour problem, is due to a mother's emotional problems. In these cases the mother and baby may be admitted to a mother and baby unit. Skilled psychiatric and paediatric input usually results in improvement in the mother's emotional state and the baby's nutritional state.

Your baby plays an important role in what and how he eats. If he does not eat readily or becomes upset at mealtimes, you may become frustrated. It is common to feel you may be somehow at fault, even though the cause is often completely out of your control. Both you and your baby need love and support. Some days may be easier than others and it might help to remember that some babies are very fussy about food. Eating habits in your new family may soon fall into a pattern, and this might resemble habits from your own childhood. It might help to redraw your boundaries, keep them dynamic and take things day by day. Most babies respond to fun and love better than pressure to eat at mealtimes, and when this makes adults more relaxed, the family atmosphere may be less stressed. These behaviour problems are one of the biggest challenges to parents and childcare professionals. Working as an encouraging team that responds to your baby as an individual is usually the best route to having a thriving child.

WEIGHT, OBESITY: BABY

Only around 2% of babies show weight readings in the upper, coloured zone of the weight chart (see box, left), indicating obesity. Obesity in childhood (after age 5) is recognised as a global epidemic and does present risks to health, and research suggests that a baby can become prone to obesity during pregnancy. In the UK around 10% of children are obese by the age of 6. Obese children are twice as likely as normal-weight children to become obese adults, and face a number of physical and emotional challenges. Being overweight can lead to teasing, low confidence and poor achievement. Health risks relate to premature heart disease and high BLOOD PRESSURE, DIABETES, early-onset arthritis and aggravation of ASTHMA.

In pregnancy and in the 1st year after birth you can reduce

your child's tendency to become overweight in later life. Although childhood obesity is usually associated with parental obesity, this is a mainly reflection of habitual eating patterns and lifestyle: only a very small number of children become obese because of inherited genes.

What happens

There appear to be two types of obesity: endogenous obesity is caused by a specific chemical or disease and relates to a tiny fraction of obese children; exogenous obesity is caused by excessive calorie intake and family traits that influence the way the body burns calories. This is most common.

Everybody has fat cells, and these increase in number when calorie intake increases. This process begins in the womb and continues through adolescence. If a baby develops a high number of fat cells that he will be prone to becoming overweight. Inadequate exercise, an increasing phenomenon in western societies, can contribute to excessive weight gain.

Action plan

Prevention is possible and a powerful aid. Helping your baby build a good foundation may help him avoid obesity for life. Some families believe chubbiness denotes good health, for a baby and for a mother-to-be. Others believe that any sign of excess body fat is unhealthy. It might be useful for you and your partner to look at your values and see how this affects your approach to food and weight.

In pregnancy

Weight gain (p.563) is part of antenatal monitoring and is essential. If you are gaining excessively, your midwife may suggest ways to slow the gain.

- Eat well with regularly spaced, nutritious meals.
- Some researchers believe that what a mother eats in pregnancy affects a baby's taste sensitivity. Whether true or not, if you have sweet food or drink, you and your baby will experience a sugar high followed by an energy slump. This pattern of feeding may become habitual for him. Try to substitute slow-burning foods for sweets, and avoid colas and juices. A balanced diet supplemented by appropriate vitamins and minerals could help you avoid sweet snacks.
- If you are diabetic, you need to monitor your blood sugar levels closely because uncontrolled diabetes can be associated with above-average foetal growth.
- If you are concerned about your weight or have an EATING DISORDER, talk to your midwife, GP or a counsellor. You may benefit from EMOTIONAL ADVICE & SUPPORT. Eating disorders can influence an entire family's eating pattern.

After birth

- Breastfed babies very rarely eat more than they need. Overfeeding is more common among bottle-fed babies, but if you monitor the spacing and size of your baby's feeds, this is avoidable (p.198).
- If you think your baby seems overweight, first ask your health visitor or doctor to weigh him and check his height. He may appear chubby yet still be an acceptable weight. Your doctor will tell you if there is cause for concern.
- Try not to compare your baby to others, and follow the

advice of your health visitor. Every baby is an individual.
- If you are breastfeeding, continue to eat nutritious, well-spaced meals so your baby gets a healthy balance of nutrients and calories without regular high-sugar feeds.
- Listen to your baby's signals. He will indicate how much and how often he likes to eat. If you find it difficult to tell, or think your own view of eating and weight may be clouding your judgement, ask your health visitor for advice.
- When you wean your baby, go at his pace and begin with easily digested foods (p.243). Avoid giving sweet things that do not contain goodness. Some babies have a voracious appetite from the start and others take months to become keen eaters. Ask your health visitor if you are concerned that your baby eats too much or always seems hungry.
- Even when your baby is not mobile, encourage him to kick and play regularly. He needs this for normal development and for an efficient burning-up of calories.
- Remember that snacks between meals, particularly if they are sweet, are a potent cause of excess calorie intake, as is fruit juice. Keep these to a minimum.

WEIGHT, OBESITY: MOTHER

See Eating and weight (p.333); EATING, DIFFICULTIES & DISORDERS

WHOOPING COUGH

See COUGH & COLD: BABY

WRY NECK

Wry neck (**torticollis**) affects roughly 2% of babies, giving a small lump in the neck and causing a baby to hold his head towards the affected side. It involves tightness in one of the strap muscles that connect the breastbone, head and neck. The cause is unknown, though it may be due to position in the uterus with the head tilted to the side, cutting off blood supply to the neck muscle, or, less likely, to injury at birth.

Wry neck is not painful. The muscle can be lengthened and strengthened with gentle massage and physiotherapy and encouragement to turn away from the injured side. Osteopathy (p.376) is also effective. The swelling disappears in 4–6 weeks and normal neck movement can be established by 6 months. Because the head lies to one side, HEAD shape may be temporarily affected, but rights itself once a baby is sitting up confidently, which allows full motion.

XIPHISTERNUM

A xiphisternum is a part of the sternum, or breastbone. It is seen, or felt, as a soft piece of cartilage that protrudes in the midline just below the level of the nipples at the lower end of the rib cage. This may be mistaken for a swelling but it is quite normal and gradually becomes less obvious as the ribs and the cartilage around the ribs becomes firmer.

Index

Acknowledgements

The vision of one man, Dr Yehudi Gordon, has given us *Birth and Beyond*. Drawing on many years of experience as a practising obstetrician and father Yehudi has created this guide to pregnancy, birth and family life during the miraculous primal period. Yehudi has practised integrated health care since 1979 when he first supported the use of yoga, acupuncture, massage and osteopathy to enhance the care of families, using the safety net of conventional medical care. He is also one of the pioneers of active and water birth in England. Yehudi has celebrated the birth of many babies and he enjoys an ongoing relationship with many parents, midwifery, medical and complementary health professionals who form the basis for this book.

This book began life some years ago as a pamphlet given to parents-to-be at the Birth Unit at the Hospital of St John and Elizabeth in London. The midwives, obstetricians and paediatricians on the Birth Unit have practised integrated health care for many years. In partnership with Harriet Sharkey, Dr Andy Raffles, the Birth Unit midwives, and many other contributors, the small pamphlet matured into a booklet. Two years later, *Birth and Beyond* was born.

Birth and Beyond has resulted from inspired and committed teamwork, involving many people. At the heart of the core team with Yehudi Gordon are Harriet Sharkey, a writer and mother, who has worked in partnership with Yehudi to write and edit many parts of the book, and sculpted it into one comprehensive whole; Dr Andy Raffles, consultant paediatrician and father, who brings a wealth of practical and clinical experience and has contributed to the clear, no-nonsense tone that gives parents the answers to the everyday questions surrounding baby care; Felicity Fine, mother and practising homeopath, whose insight and indispensable advice is based on her considerable experience of working with families; and Genna Naccache, mother and photographer, whose wonderful images and loving touch give this book a unique quality.

Birth and Beyond was 'born' in the 70s in Nimbin, a small town in Australia, where midwives Mira and Tansen Stannard-Elliott set up a healing centre and a home birth movement with midwifery care, yoga, a library and a community support system for the whole family. They called the movement Birth and Beyond. Tansen used acupuncture, homoeopathy and naturopathy while Mira gave emotional support and the confidence needed to give birth naturally: 'All women have to do is get the mind out of the way. Know that you know is my best advice.' Birth and Beyond had a profound impact on birth in Australia and in the 80s Mira and Tansen came to London where they met Yehudi Gordon. This remarkable and inspiring meeting of hearts and minds continues to this day. The Birth and Beyond movement continues in Australia, India and Bali and provided the inspiration for this book.

The philosophy outlined in these pages is practised by the midwives and consultants on the Birth Unit of the Hospital of St John and St Elizabeth, London. The Birth Unit is well known for active and water birth and the midwives and consultants all practise integrated family support combining conventional and complementary care in pregnancy, birth and beyond. Many of the midwives have additional complementary skills and training and made an invaluable contribution to the book.

The incredible range of the book's contents is due to the input of many professionals who worked with the core team.

The Birth Unit team

The midwives' support has been considerable. Ann Herreb0udt ensured that this book remained true to reality. She shared her insight and wisdom as a psychologist, midwife and therapist, contributed to many parts of the book, particularly Part 3, talked us through difficult areas, and reviewed the text many times. Ann helped us appreciate things from a baby's point of view, understand the dynamics of family life, and address issues faced by so many mums and dads. Anita O'Neill acted as midwifery and aromatherapy consultant; Pat Scott was consulted on risk and safety; Catriona Muir contributed to the A–Z; Melissa Good gave advice for support in labour; Karen Robb advised on breastfeeding; Lynda Leach and Karen Taylor on massage, and Karen Arkle and Indira Carter provided insight into emotional support. Talha Shawaf, consultant obstetrician, gave unwavering support, and we also thank all the midwives and paediatric and obstetric consultants on the Birth Unit.

Integrated health and complementary therapies, in order of appearance in the book:

Kitty Hagenbach, transpersonal psychotherapist, has given insight into the emotional life of babies, adults and families.

Wendy Gordon contributed her wisdom on families and women's motivations in the 21st century.

Caron Barruw and Jonty Hurwitz gave tips on what it's like to be a father.

The nutrition chapter was founded on the expertise and advice of Dr Marilyn Glenville, nutritional therapist.

Yoga by Jill Benjoyer Miller, a mother, active birth and yoga teacher, who appears in the yoga photographs, with baby Jonah.

Exercise by Shirel Stemmons, mother and fitness and exercise consultant who also appears in many photographs with her family.

The massage chapter was created by massage therapists Tanya Gordon and Lynda Leach.

The meditation concept and guided visualisations by Mira and Tansen Elliott Stannard, and Dr Gowri Motha, obstetrician and visualisation guide.

Homeopathy by Felicity Fine.
Osteopathy by Lynn Haller, cranial osteopath.
Acupuncture by Meredith and Wainwright Churchill, traditional Chinese acupuncturists. The aromatherapy chapter was put together by Anita O'Neill.
Herbal medicine by Delphine Sayre and Helen Stapleton, medical herbalists. Delphine also contributed to single parenting.

The families and photographers
We would like to thank all the families who built up strong and trusting relationships with Genna Naccache so that we could share some of their most intimate and beautiful moments: Gabi and Paul Brogan and their baby Max; Andrea and Bertie De Rougement and their children Elyssia and Seraphina (who appears on the front cover); Oskarina and Tandile Gubevu, their son Welela and baby daughter Mihlali; Hisako and Shizaki Okajima, and their children Shoko, Nobuko and baby Masataka; Jacqueline (Jac) and Stephen Palmer, their daughter Chili and baby girl Olive; Shirel and Robert Stemmons and baby Jake, who joined brother and sister Robbie and Sophie; Christiana and Rory Webster, and their daughter Sasha and baby son Finn. Other photographs were from Tanya Gordon and Max Glicksman. Bill Smith graciously provided pictures and information on ultrasound scanning. Thanks also to Stephen Male, Oliver Chanarin and Adam Broomberg whose vision helped the book evolve.

Other support
Thank you to Lucy Bragz for research and writing original material, particularly in parts 1 and 2; to Peter Walker for inspiration on baby massage and to Paul Robinson and the Landmark Forum who inspired some of the practical lifestyle advice. For the insight into a baby's neurological development we would like to thank Professor Hugh Johnson and Eileen Mansfield at the Babylab at Birkbeck College, London; Professor Annette Karmiloff-Smith; Giep Franzen and Margot Bouwman and Dr Gill Harris.

In the production of this book we would like to thank all those who have been involved at Random House, particularly Fiona MacIntyre, who helped us all dive in at the deep end and come out smiling; Denise Bates for her patience and organisational skill; Emma Callery for diligence and astute and sensitive editing; Helen Lewis for exemplary design; Kate Parker for her proofreading skills; Tony Howard for his index; Amanda Williams for her clear illusrations, and Helen Brocklehurst for always being there. The team at Viveka Health helped and supported us.

The essential foundation
Behind the scenes we have had tremendous support from partners and families, particularly Wendy Gordon, Dee Sharkey, Jo Raffles and Barry Fine. Some of their words, ideas and concepts appear in this book and it would not have reached its full potential without their love and patience. Of course, none of this would have been possible without our children and grandchildren, particularly Rosa and Max who travelled through their own primal periods before our eyes as the book developed. We are deeply indebted to all the babies and families whose experiences have helped us ensure that the book is a real reflection of life during the primal period.

London, February 2002

Ebury Press
Random House, 20 Vauxhall Bridge Road, London SW1V 2SA

Random House Australia (Pty) Limited
20 Alfred Street, Milsons Point, Sydney, New South Wales 2061, Australia

Random House New Zealand Limited
18 Poland Road, Glenfield, Auckland 10, New Zealand

Random House (Pty) Limited
Endulini, 5a Jubilee Road, Parktown 2193, South Africa

The Random House Group Limited Reg. No. 954009
www.randomhouse.co.uk

Papers used by Ebury Press are natural, recyclable products made from wood grown in sustainable forests.

A CIP catalogue record for this book is available from the British Library

ISBN 0 09 185694 9

Editor: Emma Callery
Designer: Helen Lewis
Illustrations: Amanda Williams
Index: Tony Howard
Photographs: all photographs supplied by Genna Naccache except: pp.11, 64: Petit Format/Nestle/Science Photo Library; p.19: Neil Bromhall/Science Photo Library; p.28 picture courtesy of Centre for Brain and Cognitive Development, Birkbeck College, University of London.
The extract on p.280 is from *Life and How to Survive It* by John Cleese and Robin Skynner published by Arrow. Used by permission of The Random House Group Limited.

Printed and bound by Graphicom, Italy